Introduction to
Vascular
Ultrasonography

6th
Edition

Introduction to
Vascular
Ultrasonography

John S. Pellerito, MD, FACR, FSRU, FAIUM

Associate Professor of Radiology
Hofstra North Shore-LIJ School of Medicine;
Associate Chairman
Department of Radiology
Chief, Division of Ultrasound, CT, and MRI
Director, Peripheral Vascular Laboratory
North Shore University Hospital
Manhasset, New York

Joseph F. Polak, MD, MPH

Professor of Radiology
Tufts University School of Medicine;
Vice Chair of Business Development
Tufts Medical Center
Boston, Massachusetts;
Chief of Radiology
Lemuel Shattuck Hospital
Jamaica Plain, Massachusetts

ELSEVIER
SAUNDERS

1600 John F. Kennedy Blvd.
Ste 1800
Philadelphia, PA 19103-2899

INTRODUCTION TO VASCULAR ULTRASONOGRAPHY   ISBN: 978-1-4377-1417-3

Library of Congress Cataloging-in-Publication Data

Introduction to vascular ultrasonography -- 6th ed. / [edited by] John S. Pellerito, Joseph F. Polak.
    p. ; cm.
Includes bibliographical references and index.
ISBN 978-1-4377-1417-3 (hardcover : alk. paper)
I. Pellerito, John S. II. Polak, Joseph F.
[DNLM: 1. Vascular Diseases--ultrasonography. 2. Blood Vessels--ultrasonography. WG 500]
LC classification not assigned
616.1'307543--dc23   2012006759

Content Strategist: Pamela Hetherington
Content Development Specialist: Joanie Milnes
Publishing Services Manager: Anne Altepeter
Senior Project Manager: Cheryl A. Abbott
Design Direction: Ellen Zanolle

Printed in China

Last digit is the print number: 9 8 7 6 5 4 3 2 1

To Elizabeth, John, Alana, and Daniel for your support and encouragement. To Marie and Peter for being there for me from day one. And to my colleagues and sonographers for making work fun.
J.S.P.

To Jo-Anne and Alexandra.
J.F. P.

ACKNOWLEDGMENTS

I gratefully acknowledge the following individuals who have contributed to this sixth edition.

My co-editor, Joseph Polak, for his insights, expertise, and humor throughout the writing and editorial process.

All the authors who contributed their time, energy, and outstanding chapters.

My administrative assistant, Barbara Stanco, for her patience and support.

My co-workers in the Peripheral Vascular Laboratory, James Naidich, MD; Catherine D'Agostino, MD; Brian Burke, MD; Danielle Berne, RN; Bindu Rameshan, RVT; Jane Joo Ah Kim, RVT; John Torres, RVT; Glenn Prucha; Daniel Hernandez, RVT; and Christine Antoldi.

My chief technologists, Amalia Pose and Saiedeh "Nanaz" Maghool and all of the sonographers at North Shore for their commitment to excellence.

Joanie Milnes, Pamela Hetherington, Cheryl Abbott, Rebecca Gaertner, and all at Elsevier for their help and expertise.

Irwin Kuperberg and everyone at IAME for their dedication to medical education and their support of vascular ultrasound.

And always, my family, Elizabeth, John, Alana, Daniel, Peter, Mom, and Dad, for their continuing support and understanding.

John S. Pellerito, MD, FACR, FSRU, FAIUM

I gratefully acknowledge all of the individuals who have contributed to this sixth edition.

My greatest thanks go to my co-editor, John Pellerito, for sharing his knowledge and optimism throughout the writing and editorial process. I especially thank him for taking me on as his co-editor for this truly unique textbook of vascular ultrasound.

I would like to recognize the efforts of all of the chapter authors and co-authors who have spent so much of their precious time preparing their chapters, especially colleagues who have shared their knowledge when participating at various continuing medical education venues, primarily the long running Current Practice in Vascular Ultrasound (www.IAME.com), the AIUM (www.AIUM.org), the RSNA (www.RSNA.org), and the ACR (www.ACR.org).

I give my special thanks and gratitude to the sonographers who have contributed materials to this book: Jean M. Alessi-Chinetti, Gregory Y. Curto, and Richard J. Porter.

I thank all of the staff of Elsevier who had to put up with my sometimes finicky requests in order to prepare an improved edition of this book.

I especially thank my wife, Jo-Anne, and daughter, Alexandra, for putting up with my work habits and for my takeover of our living room to accommodate my workstation and its' 30-inch screen.

Joseph F. Polak, MD, MPH

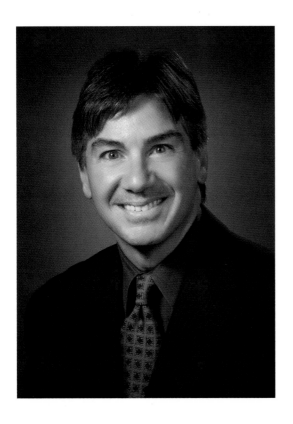

John S. Pellerito, MD, FACR, FSRU, FAIUM, is Associate Professor of Radiology at Hofstra North Shore-LIJ School of Medicine. He is Associate Chairman of Strategic Planning and Technology at North Shore University Hospital in Manhasset, New York. He is also Chief of the Division of Ultrasound, CT, and MRI; the Director of the Peripheral Vascular Laboratory at North Shore University Hospital; the Director of the Body Imaging Fellowship Program; and the author of multiple original articles, book chapters, web lectures, and DVD programs. His practice focuses on cardiovascular and gynecologic diseases. His current interests include new imaging technologies and approaches to the diagnosis of vascular and oncologic diseases. He is an acclaimed national and international speaker and contributes to multiple CME programs. Dr. Pellerito holds multiple editorial appointments and is a board examiner for the American Board of Radiology. He has served on the board of the Intersocietal Accreditation Commission for the accreditation of vascular laboratories and American Institute of Ultrasound in Medicine. He is a fellow of the American College of Radiology, Society of Radiologists in Ultrasound, and American Institute of Ultrasound in Medicine. He and his wife, Elizabeth, have three children: John, Alana, and Daniel.

Joseph F. Polak, MD, MPH, is Professor of Radiology at Tufts University School of Medicine, Director of the Ultrasound Reading Center at Tufts Medical Center, as well as Chief of Radiology at the Lemuel Shattuck Hospital in Boston, Massachusetts. A graduate of McGill University Medical School, he holds a master's degree in public health from the Harvard School of Public Health. He has co-authored more than 250 peer-reviewed articles and more than 80 non–peer-reviewed articles and chapters. He has served on the editorial board of *Radiology,* the *Journal of Neuroimaging,* the *Journal of Vascular Ultrasound,* and the *Journal of Ultrasound in Medicine.* He is a prior president of the Intersocietal Accreditation Commission for the accreditation of vascular laboratories. His research interests include interventional radiology, non-invasive vascular imaging, and the development of biomarkers for the detection and monitoring of early atherosclerosis. He has been principal investigator on two RO-1 grants studying the progression of atherosclerosis with carotid artery intima-media thickness and co-investigator on multiple other NIH grants.

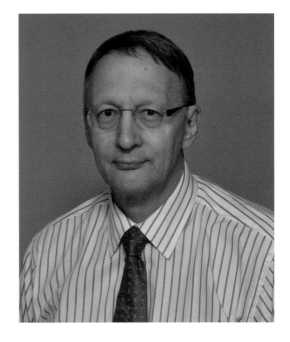

PREFACE

The sixth edition of *Introduction to Vascular Ultrasonography* is a major update to our previous editions. First, I would like to welcome my new co-editor, Joseph F. Polak, to this edition. Jo and I have collaborated for many years on multiple projects and at numerous meetings, most notably our Current Practice of Vascular Ultrasound program, which is approaching its twentieth anniversary. Having produced separate vascular publications, we decided to collaborate on this edition, hoping to create the definitive vascular ultrasound textbook. We are very pleased to find that this partnership produced an inclusive tome that surpassed our expectations. We added several new chapters that focus on growing areas of vascular ultrasound and updated previous chapters with the assistance of leading experts in our field. We believe the most popular text on vascular ultrasound is now significantly improved.

As an interventional radiologist and vascular specialist, Dr. Polak brings extraordinary experience in medical imaging and vascular medicine to this edition. Jo Polak is one of the true leaders in vascular ultrasound. His curriculum vitae includes many original papers utilizing duplex ultrasound in diagnosis of carotid and venous disease. His expertise extends to 10 chapters in this edition. New topics include evaluation of the abdominal aorta, screening for vascular disease, and correlative imaging with CT and MR angiography.

There are 29 authors involved in this edition. All the authors have contributed to the field of vascular ultrasound, and we are proud to include their material. Each has made a substantial contribution with expanded and new chapters. Significant additions to this edition include enhanced versions of the role of ultrasound contrast in vascular imaging, the role of ultrasound in management of cerebrovascular disease, and evaluation of the hepatic vasculature. New topics include assessment of carotid interventions, evaluation of organ transplants, and accreditation and the vascular laboratory.

John S. Pellerito, MD, FACR, FSRU, FAIUM

Andrei V. Alexandrov, MD
Professor and Director
Comprehensive Stroke Center
University of Alabama Hospital
Birmingham, Alabama

Clotilde Balucani, MD
Department of Neurology
University of Perugia
Perugia, Italy;
Research Fellow
Comprehensive Stroke Center
University of Alabama Hospital
Birmingham, Alabama

Dennis F. Bandyk, MD
Professor of Surgery
University of South Florida
College of Medicine
Tampa, Florida

Phillip J. Bendick, PhD
Director
Peripheral Vascular Diagnostic Center
William Beaumont Hospital
Royal Oak, Michigan

Carol B. Benson, MD
Professor of Radiology
Harvard Medical School;
Director of Ultrasound
Co-Director of High Risk Obstetrical Ultrasound
Brigham and Women's Hospital
Boston, Massachusetts

George L. Berdejo, BA, RVT
Director, Vascular Ultrasound Imaging Services
Moses, North, and Weiler-Einstein Divisions
Division of Vascular Surgery
Department of Cardiovascular and Thoracic
  Surgery
Montefiore
Bronx, New York

Edward I. Bluth, MD, FACR
Professor
Ochsner Clinical School
University of Queensland School of Medicine;
Chairman Emeritus Radiology
Ochsner Health System
New Orleans, Louisiana

Brian J. Burke, MD, RVT
Attending Radiologist
Department of Radiology
North Shore University Hospital;
Assistant Professor
Department of Radiology
Hofstra North Shore-LIJ School of Medicine
Manhasset, New York

Stefan A. Carter, MD, MSC, FRCP(C)
Professor of Physiology and Medicine
University of Manitoba
Winnipeg, Manitoba, Canada

John J. Cronan, MD
Professor and Chairman
Brown Alpert Medical School;
Department of Diagnostic Imaging
Radiologist-in-Chief
Rhode Island Hospital
Providence, Rhode Island

Joshua Cruz, RVT
Technical Director and Manager
Yale Vascular Laboratory
Yale University School of Medicine
New Haven, Connecticut

Daniel T. Ginat, MD, MS
Radiology Resident
University of Rochester Medical Center
Rochester, New York

Edward G. Grant, MD
Chairman and Professor
Department of Radiology
University of Southern California
University Hospital
Los Angeles, California

Ulrike M. Hamper, MD, MBA
Professor of Radiology, Urology, and Pathology;
Director, Division of Ultrasound
Russell H. Morgan Department of Radiology
  and Radiological Science
The Johns Hopkins University
School of Medicine
Baltimore, Maryland

Kelly Hodgkiss-Harlow, MD
Division of Vascular and Endovascular Surgery
University of South Florida College of Medicine
Tampa, Florida

Sandra Katanick, RN, RVT, FSVU, CAE
Chief Executive Officer
Intersocietal Accreditation Commission
Ellicott City, Maryland

Gregory M. Keck, MD
Interventional Radiologist
Southwest Medical Imaging Associates;
Department of Radiology
Midland Memorial Hospital
Midland, Texas

Evan C. Lipsitz, MD
Associate Professor of Surgery
Albert Einstein College of Medicine;
Medical Director, Vascular Diagnostic
    Laboratory Services
Chief, Division of Vascular Surgery
Department of Cardiovascular and Thoracic
    Surgery
Montefiore
Bronx, New York

Mark E. Lockhart, MD, MPH
Professor of Radiology
Chief, Body Imaging Section
Chief, GU Radiology
University of Alabama at Birmingham
Birmingham, Alabama

Mahan Mathur, MD
Department of Diagnostic Radiology
Yale University School of Medicine
New Haven, Connecticut

Michelle Melany, MD
Clinical Professor of Radiology
University of California Los Angeles David
    Geffen School of Medicine;
Vice Chair of Radiology
Greater Los Angeles VA Medical Center;
Chief of Women's Imaging
Cedars Sinai Imaging Medical Group
Los Angeles, California

Daniel A. Merton, BS, RDMS, FSDMS, FAIUM
Clinical Instructor and Technical Coordinator
    of Research
Jefferson Ultrasound Research and Education
    Institute
Department of Radiology
Jefferson Medical College
Thomas Jefferson University
Philadelphia, Pennsylvania

William D. Middleton, MD, FACR
Professor of Radiology
Mallinckrodt Institute of Radiology
Washington University in St. Louis
St. Louis, Missouri

Darius G. Nabavi, MD
Professor
Department of Neurology
Klinikum Neukölln
Berlin, Germany

Laurence Needleman, MD
Medical Director, Noninvasive Vascular
    Laboratory
Thomas Jefferson University Hospitals;
Associate Professor of Radiology
Jefferson Medical College
Thomas Jefferson University
Philadelphia, Pennsylvania

Marsha M. Neumyer, BS, RVT, FSDMS, FSVU, FAIUM
International Director
Vascular Diagnostic Educational Services
Harrisburg, Pennsylvania

Shirley M. Otis, MD
Director
The Brain Research and Treatment Center
Scripps Clinic
La Jolla, California

John S. Pellerito, MD, FACR, FSRU, FAIUM
Associate Professor of Radiology
Hofstra North Shore-LIJ School of Medicine;
Associate Chairman
Department of Radiology
Chief, Division of Ultrasound, CT, and MRI
Director, Peripheral Vascular Laboratory
North Shore University Hospital
Manhasset, New York

Joseph F. Polak, MD, MPH
Professor of Radiology
Tufts University School of Medicine;
Vice Chair of Business Development
Tufts Medical Center
Boston, Massachusetts;
Chief of Radiology
Lemuel Shattuck Hospital
Jamaica Plain, Massachusetts

Margarita V. Revzin, MS, MD
Assistant Professor of Radiology
Yale University School of Medicine
New Haven, Connecticut

E. Bernd Ringelstein, MD
Professor of Neurology
Department of Neurology
University Hospital Münster
Münster, Germany

Martin A. Ritter, MD
Consultant Neurologist
Head of the Stroke Unit
Department of Neurology
University Hospital Münster
Münster, Germany

Michelle L. Robbin, MD, MS
Professor of Radiology and Biomedical
    Engineering
Chief of Ultrasound
University of Alabama at Birmingham
Birmingham, Alabama

Kathryn A. Robinson, MD
Mallinckrodt Institute of Radiology
Washington University in St. Louis
St. Louis, Missouri

Deborah Rubens, MD
Professor of Imaging Sciences, Oncology, and
    Biomedical Engineering
Associate Chair, Imaging Sciences
Associate Director for the Center for Biomedical
    Ultrasound
University of Rochester Medical Center
Rochester, New York

Leslie M. Scoutt, MD
Professor of Diagnostic Radiology and Surgery
Yale University School of Medicine;
Chief, Ultrasound Service
Medical Director, Non-Invasive Vascular
    Laboratory
Yale-New Haven Hospital
New Haven, Connecticut

Steven R. Talbot, RVT, FSVU
Research Associate
Division of Vascular Surgery
Technical Director, Vascular Laboratory
Cardiovascular Services
University of Utah Medical Center
Salt Lake City, Utah

James A. Zagzebski, PhD
Professor and Chairman
Department of Medical Physics
University of Wisconsin
Madison, Wisconsin

R. Eugene Zierler, MD
Professor of Surgery
University of Washington School of Medicine;
Medical Director, D.E. Strandness, Jr., Vascular
    Laboratory
University of Washington Medical Center and
    Harborview Medical Center
Seattle, Washington

CONTENTS

Basics

HEMODYNAMIC CONSIDERATIONS IN PERIPHERAL VASCULAR AND CEREBROVASCULAR DISEASE

JOSEPH F. POLAK, MD, MPH; STEFAN A. CARTER, MD, MSC, FRCP(C);
and JOHN S. PELLERITO, MD, FACR, FSRU, FAIUM

The circulatory system is extremely complex in both structure and function. Blood flow is influenced by many factors, including cardiac function; elasticity of the vessel walls (compliance); the tone of vascular smooth muscle; and the various patterns, dimensions, and interconnections of millions of small branching vessels. Some of these factors can be measured and described in reasonably simple terms, but many others cannot be described succinctly because they are difficult to quantify and generally are not well understood.

With these limitations in mind, this chapter presents the basic principles of the dynamics of blood circulation, some of the many factors that influence blood flow, and the hemodynamic consequences of occlusive disease. These considerations are helpful in understanding the normal physiology of blood circulation and the abnormalities that can occur in the presence of vascular obstruction.

PHYSIOLOGIC FACTORS GOVERNING BLOOD FLOW AND ITS CHARACTERISTICS

ENERGY AND PRESSURE

For blood flow to occur between any two points in the circulatory system, there must be a difference in the energy level between these two points. Usually, the difference in energy level is reflected by a difference in blood pressure, and the circulatory system generally consists of a high-pressure, high-energy arterial reservoir and a venous pool of low pressure and energy. These reservoirs are connected by a system of distributing vessels (smaller arteries) and by the resistance vessels of the microcirculation, which consist of arterioles and to a lesser extent the capillaries (Figure 1-1).

During blood flow, energy is continuously lost because of the friction between the layers of flowing blood. Both pressure and energy levels therefore decrease from the arterial to the venous ends. The energy necessary for blood flow is continuously restored by the pumping action of the heart during systole, stored in the elastic wall of the aorta and large arteries, and released during diastole. The generated arterial pressure forces blood to move from the arterial system into the venous system and maintains the arterial pressure and the energy difference needed for flow to occur.

The high arterial energy level is a result of the large volume of blood in the arterial reservoir. The function of the heart and blood vessels is normally regulated to maintain volume and pressure in the arteries within the limits required for smooth function. This is achieved by maintaining a balance between the amounts of blood that enter and leave the arterial reservoir. The amount that enters the arteries during a cardiac cycle is the stroke volume. The amount that leaves depends on the arterial pressure and on the total peripheral resistance, which is controlled in turn by the amount of vasoconstriction in the microcirculation.

Under normal conditions, blood flow to all the body tissues is adjusted according to the tissues' particular needs at a given time. This adjustment is accomplished by local alterations in the level of vasoconstriction of the arterioles within the organs supplied. Maintenance of normal volume and pressure in the arteries thus allows for both adjustment of blood flow to all parts of the body and regulation of cardiac output (which equals the sum of blood flow to all the vascular beds).

FORMS OF ENERGY IN THE BLOOD AND ITS DISSIPATION DURING FLOW

This section considers the forms in which energy exists in the circulation and the important factors that govern the dissipation of energy during flow, including friction, resistance, and the influence of laminar and turbulent flow. In addition to reviewing Bernoulli's equation and Poiseuille's

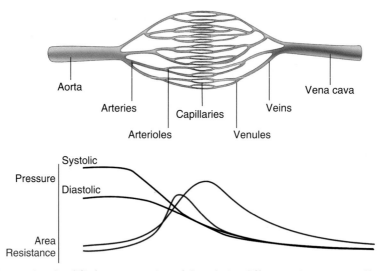

FIGURE 1-1 This diagram is a simplified representation of the relative differences in pressure, effective resistance, and overall vessel cross-luminal area at the different levels of the circulation.

law, an equation that summarizes the basic relationships between flow, pressure, and resistance, this chapter also reviews the effects of connecting vascular resistances in parallel and in series.

Forms of Energy

Potential and Kinetic Energy. The main form of energy present in flowing blood is the pressure distending the vessels (a form of potential energy), which is created by the pumping action of the heart. However, some of the energy of the blood is kinetic; namely, the ability of flowing blood to do work as a result of its velocity. Usually, the kinetic energy component is small compared with the pressure energy, and under normal resting conditions, it is equivalent to only a few millimeters of mercury or less. The kinetic energy of blood is proportional to its density (which is stable in normal circumstances) and to the square of its velocity. In essence, over relatively straight arterial segments, this balance of kinetic (blood flow) and potential (blood pressure) energy is maintained. The equation that summarizes this relationship is Bernoulli's equation (Figure 1-2). If the artery lumen increases, kinetic energy is converted back into pressure (potential energy) when velocity is decreased. Conversely, if the artery lumen narrows, the potential energy is converted into kinetic energy. Therefore, within certain limits, important increases in kinetic energy occur in the systemic circulation when blood flow is high (e.g., during exercise) and in mildly stenotic lesions where luminal narrowing leads to increases in blood flow velocities.

The effects of gravity due to differences in height of the blood vessel are normally neglected over short arterial segments.

Energy Differences Related to Differences in the Levels of Body Parts. There is also variation in the energy of the blood associated with differences in the levels of body parts. For example, the pressure in the vessels in the dependent parts of the body, such as the lower portions of the legs, increases by an amount that depends on the weight of the column of blood resting on the blood in the legs. This hydrostatic pressure increases the transmural pressure and the distention of the vessels. Gravitational potential energy (potential for doing work related to the effect of gravity on a free-falling body), however, is reduced in the dependent parts of the body by the same amount as the increase resulting from hydrostatic pressure. Therefore, differences in the level of the body parts usually do not lead to changes in the driving pressure along the vascular tree unless the column of blood is interrupted, as may be the case when the venous valves close. Changes in energy and pressure associated with differences in level are important under certain conditions, such as with changes in posture or when the venous pump is activated because of muscular action during walking.

Dissipation of Energy

During Laminar Flow. In most vessels, blood moves in concentric layers, or laminae; hence the flow is said to be laminar. Each infinitesimal layer

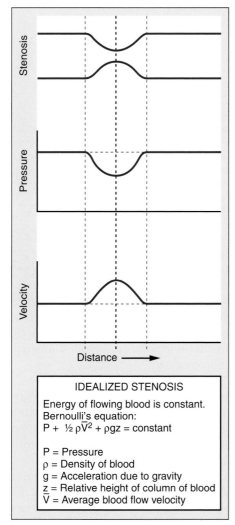

FIGURE 1-2 This diagram represents the complementary changes in potential and kinetic energy taking place at an idealized stenosis. Bernoulli's equation indicates that as velocity increases, the potential energy (pressure) of blood decreases. This idealized representation is not to scale and neglects viscous and inertial forces.

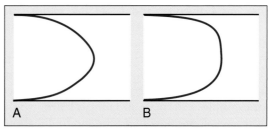

FIGURE 1-3 Blood flow velocity profiles across a normal arterial lumen. **A,** Parabolic profile of laminar flow. **B,** Flattened profile with a central core of relatively uniform velocity encountered in the proximal portion (inlet length) of arterial branches or with turbulent flow.

flows with a different velocity. In theory, a thin layer of blood is held stationary next to the vessel wall at zero velocity because of an adhesive force between the blood and the inner surface of the vessel. The next layer flows with a certain velocity, but its movement is delayed by the stationary layer because of friction between the layers, generated by the viscous properties of the fluid. The second layer, in turn, delays the next layer, which flows at a greater velocity. The layers in the middle of the vessel flow with the highest velocity, and the basic physics underlying this effect are such that the *mean velocity averaged across the vessel is half of the maximal velocity measured in the*

center. Because the rate of change of velocity is greatest near the walls and decreases toward the center of the vessel, a velocity profile in the shape of a parabola exists along the vessel diameter, and this type of blood flow is typically referred to as laminar flow (Figure 1-3).

Loss of energy during blood flow occurs because of friction, and the amount of friction and energy loss is determined in large part by the dimensions of the vessels. In a small-diameter vessel, especially in the microcirculation, even the layers in the middle of the lumen are relatively close to the wall and are thus delayed considerably, resulting in a significant opposition or resistance to flow in that vessel segment. In large vessels, by contrast, a large central core of blood is far from the walls, and the frictional energy losses are less important. As indicated later, friction and energy losses increase if laminar flow is disturbed.

Poiseuille's Law and Equation. In a cylindric-tube model, the mean linear velocity of laminar flow is directly proportional to the energy difference between the ends of the tube and the square of the radius and is inversely proportional to the length of the tube and the viscosity of the fluid. In the circulatory system, however, volume flow is of more interest than velocity. Volume flow is proportional to the fourth power of the vessel radius, because it is equal to the product of the mean linear velocity and the cross-sectional area of the tube. These important considerations are helpful in understanding Poiseuille's law, as expressed in Poiseuille's equation:

$$Q = \frac{\pi(P_1 - P_2)r^4}{8L\eta} \qquad (1\text{-}1)$$

where Q is the volume flow; P_1 and P_2 are the pressures at the proximal and distal ends of the tube, respectively; r and L are the radius and length of the tube, respectively; and η is the viscosity of the fluid.

Because volume flow is proportional to the fourth power of the radius, even small changes in radius can result in large changes in volume flow. For example, a decrease in radius of 10% would decrease volume flow in a tube model by about 35%, and a decrease of 50% would lead to a 95% decrease in volume flow. *Because the length of the vessels and the viscosity of blood do not change much in the cardiovascular system, alterations in volume blood flow occur mainly as a result of changes in the radius of the vessels and in the difference in the pressure energy level available for flow.*

Poiseuille's equation can be rewritten, therefore, as follows:

$$\frac{8L\eta}{\pi r^4} = \frac{P_1 - P_2}{Q} \qquad (1\text{-}2)$$

$$R = \frac{8L\eta}{\pi r^4} \qquad (1\text{-}3)$$

$$R = \frac{P_1 - P_2}{Q} \qquad (1\text{-}4)$$

The resistance term *(R)* depends on the viscous properties of the blood and on the dimensions of the vessels. Although these parameters cannot be measured in a complex system, the pressure difference $(P_1 - P_2)$ and the volume flow *(Q)* can be measured, and the resistance can thus be calculated. Because resistance is equal to the pressure difference divided by the volume flow (the pressure difference per unit flow), it can be thought of as the pressure difference needed to produce one unit of flow and, therefore, can be considered as an index of the difficulty in forcing blood through the vessels.

Vessel Interconnection and Energy Dissipation. Poiseuille's law applies with precision only to constant laminar flow of a simple fluid (such as water) in a rigid tube of a uniform bore. In the blood circulation, these conditions are not met. Instead, the resistance is influenced by the presence of numerous interconnected vessels with a combined effect similar to that observed in electrical resistances. In the case of vessels in series, the overall resistance is equal to the sum of the resistances of the individual vessels, whereas in the case of parallel vessels, the reciprocal of the total resistance equals the sum of the reciprocals of the individual vessel resistances. Thus, *the contribution of any single vessel to the total*

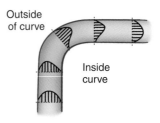

Outside of curve

Inside curve

FIGURE 1-4 Alteration in the velocity distribution of red cells in a curving arterial segment. The velocity distribution becomes asymmetric as red cells enter a curve. A laminar pattern is reestablished downstream over a distance that is mostly dependent on the velocity of blood and the diameter of the artery.

resistance of a vascular bed, or the effect of a change in the dimension of a vessel, depends on the presence and relative size of the other vessels linked in series or in parallel.

Deviations from the conditions to which Poiseuille's law applies also occur in relation to changes in blood viscosity, which is affected by hematocrit, temperature, vessel diameter, and rate of blood flow.

During Nonlaminar Flow. Various degrees of deviation from orderly laminar flow occur in the circulation under both normal and abnormal conditions. Minor factors responsible for these deviations include changes in blood flow velocity during the cardiac cycle as a result of acceleration during systole and deceleration in diastole and alterations of the lines of flow due to small changes in the diameter of the vessel. Alterations in the blood flow profiles occur at curves (Figure 1-4), at bifurcations, in branches that take off at various angles, and at stenotic lesions. Once altered, the laminar (parabolic) velocity profile is often not reestablished for a considerable distance. Instead, the velocity distributions can remain skewed after curves and branches or flattened within and just distal to stenotic lesions (plug flow) (see Figure 1-3, *B*).

In certain circumstance, laminar flow can evolve into a blood flow pattern that is mixed: a flow profile that has both forward and backward flow velocity components across the diameter of the artery. The transition zone where the lamina reach zero velocity is then referred to as the site of boundary layer separation. This phenomenon can occur at branch points and is classically described at the carotid artery bifurcation (Figure 1-5). Another situation is distal to stenotic lesions.

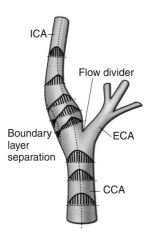

FIGURE 1-5 This representation of the carotid artery bifurcation displays the principal alterations that take place in a normal bifurcation. The flow profile in the distal common carotid artery (CCA) starts to deviate from a laminar pattern to one favoring the internal carotid artery (ICA). As the red cells enter the carotid sinus, a zone of boundary layer separation (where the effective velocity is zero) forms. To one side, blood flow is reversed, whereas blood continues forward on the other side. Blood flow reestablishes itself toward a laminar one more distally in the ICA. For purposes of illustration, the actual effects of the external carotid artery (ECA) on blood flow are neglected.

At the carotid bifurcation, the blood flow profile in the distal common carotid artery tends to diverge toward the internal carotid artery and then to evolve a zone of boundary layer separation in the proximal internal carotid artery (see Figure 1-5).

Laminar flow may be altered or become disturbed or fully turbulent, even in a uniform tube. The factors that affect the development of turbulence are expressed by the dimensionless Reynolds number (Re):

$$\mathrm{Re} = \frac{v\rho 2r}{\eta} \qquad (1\text{-}5)$$

where v is the velocity, ρ is the density of the fluid, r is the radius of the tube, and η is the viscosity of the fluid. Because the density (ρ) and viscosity (η) of the blood are relatively constant at 1.04 to 1.05 g/cm³ and 0.03 to 0.05 poise (g/[cm sec]), respectively, *the development of turbulence depends mainly on the size of the vessel and on the velocity of blood flow.* In a tube model, laminar flow tends to be present if the Reynolds number is less than 2000, is considered in transition between 2000 and 4000, and is absent as turbulence is established at values above 4000. However, in the circulatory system, disturbances and various degrees of turbulence are likely to occur at lower values because of body movements, the pulsatile nature of blood flow, changes in vessel dimensions, roughness of the endothelial surface, and other factors. Turbulence develops more readily in large vessels under conditions of high flow and can be detected clinically by the finding of bruits or thrills. This would typically be seen in dialysis access fistulas. Bruits may sometimes be heard over the ascending aorta during systolic acceleration in normal individuals at rest and are frequently heard in states of high cardiac output and blood flow, even in more distal arteries, such as the femoral artery.[1] Distortion of laminar flow velocity profiles can be assessed using Doppler ultrasound, and such assessments can be applied for diagnostic purposes. For example, in arteries with severe stenosis, *pronounced turbulence is a diagnostic feature observed in the poststenotic zone.* This is typically associated with soft tissue vibrations in the range of 100 to 300 Hz.[2]

Turbulence occurs because a jet of blood with high velocity and high kinetic energy suddenly encounters a normal-diameter lumen or a lumen of increased diameter (because of poststenotic dilatation), where both the velocity and energy level are lower than in the stenotic region. During turbulent flow, the loss of pressure energy between two points in a vessel is greater than that which would be expected from the factors in Poiseuille's equation and Bernoulli's equation (see Figure 1-2), and the parabolic velocity profile is flattened (see Figure 1-3, *B*).

PULSATILE PRESSURE AND FLOW CHANGES IN THE ARTERIAL SYSTEM

With each heartbeat, a stroke volume of blood is ejected into the arterial system, resulting in a pressure wave that travels throughout the arterial tree. The speed of propagation, amplitude (strength), and shape of the pressure wave change as it traverses the arterial system. The velocity of the pulse wave is strongly influenced by the varying characteristics of the vessel wall it traverses, and the shape is affected by reflected waves. The velocity and, in some parts of the circulation, the direction of flow, also vary with each heartbeat.

Correct interpretation of noninvasive tests based on recordings of arterial pressure and velocity, as well as pressure and velocity waveforms, requires knowledge of the factors that influence these variables. This section considers these factors as they occur in various portions of the circulatory system.

Pressure Changes From Cardiac Activity

As indicated previously, the pumping action of the heart maintains a high volume of blood in the arterial end of the circulation and thus provides the high pressure difference between the arterial and venous ends necessary to maintain blood flow. Because of the intermittent pumping action of the heart, pressure and flow vary in a pulsatile manner. During the rapid phase of ventricular ejection, the volume of blood at the arterial end increases, raising the pressure to a systolic peak. During the latter part of systole, when cardiac ejection decreases, the outflow through the peripheral resistance vessels exceeds the volume being ejected by the heart, and the pressure begins to decline. This decline continues throughout diastole as blood continues to flow from the arteries into the microcirculation. Part of the work of the heart leads directly to forward flow, but a large portion of the energy of each cardiac contraction results in distention of the arteries that serve as reservoirs for storing the blood volume and the energy supplied to the system (Figure 1-6). This storage of energy and blood volume helps maintain blood flow to the tissues during diastole.

Arterial Pressure Wave

The pulsatile variations in blood volume and energy occurring with each cardiac cycle are manifested as a pressure wave that can be detected throughout the arterial system. The amplitude and shape of the arterial pressure wave depend on a complex interplay of factors, which include the stroke volume and time course of ventricular ejection, the peripheral resistance, and the stiffness of the arterial walls.

In general, an increase in any of these factors results in an increase in the pulse amplitude (i.e., pulse pressure, difference between systolic and diastolic pressures) and frequently in a concomitant increase in systolic pressure. For example, increased stiffness of the arteries with age tends to increase both the systolic and pulse pressures through an increase in the magnitude of reflected pressure waves from natural branch points in the arterial system.

The arterial pressure wave is propagated from the heart distally along the arterial tree. The speed of propagation, or pulse wave velocity, increases with stiffness of the arterial walls (the elastic modulus of the material of which the walls are composed) and with the ratio of the wall thickness to diameter. In the mammalian circulation, arteries become progressively stiffer from the aorta toward the periphery. Therefore, the speed of propagation of the wave increases as it moves peripherally. Also, the gradual increase

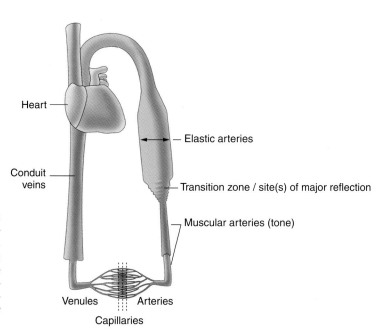

Heart

Elastic arteries

Conduit veins

Transition zone / site(s) of major reflection

Muscular arteries (tone)

Venules   Arteries

Capillaries

FIGURE 1-6 This simple representation of the circulatory system shows the principal elements of the circulatory system. Wave reflection can take place within the muscular arteries as well as in the larger elastic artery. The effective location of the principal reflection sites varies with age, migrating more centrally with aging.

in stiffness tends to increase wave reflection (discussed later) and in young people has a protective effect by decreasing central aortic pressures. With aging, the degree of stiffening increases to such a degree that the reflected waves return earlier and have a detrimental effect by increasing the pulse and systolic pressures in the aorta.[3-5] The pressure against which the heart ejects the stroke volume and the associated cardiac work are accordingly decreased at younger ages but increased with age.

Pressure Changes Throughout the Circulation

Figure 1-1 illustrates changes in pressure in the systemic circulation from large arteries through the resistance vessels to the veins. Because there is little loss of pressure energy from friction in large and distributing arteries, they offer relatively little resistance to flow, and the mean pressure decreases only slightly between the aorta and the small arteries of the limbs, such as the radial or the dorsalis pedis.[6] The diastolic pressure also shows only minor changes. The amplitude of the pressure wave and the systolic pressure actually increase, however, as the wave travels distally (*systolic amplification*), because of the increased stiffness of the peripheral artery branches, the preferential forward transmission of high-frequency components of the pressure wave, and the presence of reflected waves.[3] These waves arise where the vessels change diameter and stiffness, divide, or branch and are superadded to the oncoming primary pulse wave.[6] The reflected waves, at least in the extremities, are strongly enhanced by increased peripheral resistance.[6] Direct measurements of pressure in small arteries in experimental animals and humans, and indirect measurements of systolic pressure in human

digits, have shown that the pulse amplitude and systolic pressure decrease in smaller vessels, such as the digital vessels of the human extremities.[7-9] However, some pulsatile changes in pressure and flow may remain evident even in minute arteries and capillaries, at least under conditions of peripheral vasodilatation, and can be recorded by various methods, including plethysmography. The effect of peripheral vasoconstriction on pulsatility in the microcirculation is opposite to that seen in the proximal small or medium arteries of the extremities. *Pulsatile changes in minute arteries, arterioles, and capillaries are reduced by vasoconstriction and enhanced by vasodilatation. In small and medium arteries of the limbs, however, pulsatile changes are increased by vasoconstriction, as a result of enhanced wave reflection, and are decreased by vasodilatation.* Figure 1-7 shows arterial pressure pulses recorded directly from the femoral and dorsalis pedis arteries during peripheral vasoconstriction and vasodilatation induced, respectively, by body cooling and heating.

There is almost a complete disappearance of amplification in the dorsalis pedis artery in response to vasodilatation induced by body heating.[10] Similar changes in the distal pressure waves result from other factors that alter peripheral resistance; for example, reactive hyperemia and exercise. Exercise, by decreasing resistance in the working muscle, would be expected to decrease reflection in the exercising extremity. Because of vasoconstriction in other parts of the body during exercise (the result of cardiovascular reflexes that regulate blood pressure and circulation), however, the reflection may be increased and lead to a high degree of amplification. For example, it has been shown that during walking, the pulse pressure in the radial arteries can exceed that in the aorta by perhaps 100%.[11]

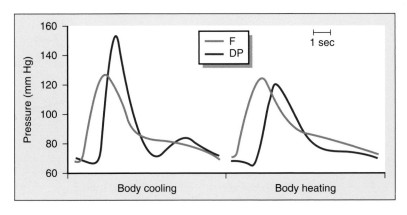

FIGURE 1-7 Pressure waves from the femoral (F) and dorsalis pedis (DP) arteries during heating and cooling. Note that the pulse pressure of the dorsalis pedis artery is greater with vasoconstriction (body cooling) and falls dramatically with vasodilatation (body heating). (*From Carter SA: Effect of age, cardiovascular disease, and vasomotor changes on transmission of arterial pressure waves through the lower extremities,* Angiology *29:601–616, 1978.*)

Differences between peripheral amplification of the pulse pressure and central augmentation of blood pressure due to reflected waves likely explain some of the physiologic differences seen between young and older individuals and those with atherosclerosis.[12,13]

These considerations are important for correct interpretation of pressure measurements in peripheral arterial obstruction. For example, brachial systolic pressure corresponds well to aortic or femoral systolic pressure and is used as a standard against which ankle pressure can be compared. The systolic pressure at the ankle usually exceeds brachial pressure in normal subjects; therefore, the finding of ankle systolic pressure that is even slightly lower than brachial systolic pressure indicates the increased likelihood of a proximal stenotic lesion. However, systolic pressure in human digits is usually lower than systolic pressure proximal to the wrist or the ankle. This observation has to be taken into account when measurements of digital systolic pressures are used as an index of distal arterial obstruction. In such cases, the appropriate norms for the differences between the proximal and digital systolic pressures have to be applied, for example by adopting a toe-brachial cut-off of 0.75 for the presence of obstructive arterial disease compared with 0.9 for the ankle-brachial index.[14,15]

Pulsatile Flow Patterns

Pulsatile changes in pressure are associated with corresponding acceleration of blood flow with systole and deceleration in diastole. Although the energy stored in the arterial walls maintains a positive pressure gradient and overall forward blood flow in the large arteries and microcirculation during diastole, temporary cessation of forward flow or even diastolic reversal occurs frequently in portions of the human arterial system.

How these phenomena occur may be clarified by considering pulsatile pressure changes at two points along the arterial tree. Figure 1-7 shows arterial pressure pulses in the femoral and dorsalis pedis arteries. The corresponding pressure gradient between the two arteries (Figure 1-8) varies during the cardiac cycle, not only because of differences in the shape and magnitude of the original pressure waves but also, more importantly, because the wave arrives later at the dorsalis pedis. The pressure gradient is greatest during the first half of systole, at which time the peak of the wave arrives at the femoral site. Thereafter, the gradient decreases, and by the time the peak arrives at the dorsalis pedis, the femoral pressure has fallen and a negative pressure gradient appears. Such negative gradients, related to different arrival times of the pressure wave at various sites in the arterial system, are commonly observed along human arteries and are conducive to the reversal of blood flow. Despite the reversal of the pressure gradient, however, the direction of flow may not be reversed if there is a large forward mean flow component.

The presence of reversed flow during diastole can also be understood if one imagines a major arterial segment, with a certain diastolic pressure, that has several branch vessels leading to areas with different levels of resistance. If one of the proximal branches leads to an area with low peripheral resistance, flow during diastole in the main vessel will occur toward this branch, and flow will reverse in the distal portion of the main vessel if distal branches supply areas with higher peripheral resistance. Such situations of transient flow reversal may exist in the limb during cooling (see Figure 1-8), but during

FIGURE 1-8 Pressure differences between the femoral and dorsalis pedis arteries obtained from the waves shown in Figure 1-7. Note the effect of vasodilatation (body heating) on the negative (reverse flow) component.

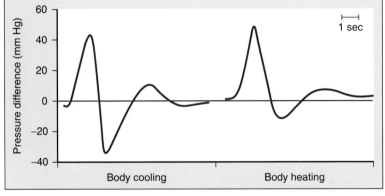

body heating, when peripheral resistance in the distal cutaneous circulation is reduced to a low level, reversed blood flow is decreased or may be abolished. Diastolic flow reversal is generally present in vessels that supply vascular beds with high peripheral resistance. It tends to be absent in low-resistance vascular beds or when peripheral resistance is reduced by peripheral dilatation, such as that which occurs in the skin with body heating, or in the working muscle during exercise or reactive hyperemia. These principles are important in assessing blood flow in arteries that supply various regions, including the cranial circulation. For example, flow reversal can be observed in the external carotid because extracranial resistance is relatively high, but it is absent in the internal carotid because the cerebrovascular resistance is low.

Another way of explaining these changes is to decompose the pressure and velocity waves into forward and backward components.[3,16,17] Pressure and blood flow waveforms can be viewed as the sum of the forward pressure waveform generated by the heart and of the reverse or backward component due to reflection at the site of distal resistance (impedance). Although the reflected blood pressure wave is additive to the overall pressure wave (Figure 1-9), the reflected blood flow waveform is subtractive (Figure 1-10). The combination of these forward and backward blood flow waves can lead to negative velocities. With heating, the backward wave decreases and the forward wave maintains blood flow during diastole. With cooling, the reflected wave is more significant and reversal of blood flow increases. Low-resistance beds do not generate prominent backward waves.

EFFECTS OF ARTERIAL OBSTRUCTION

Arterial obstruction can result in reduced pressure and flow distal to the site of blockage, but the effects on pressure and blood flow are greatly influenced by a number of factors proximal and especially distal to the lesion. One must be familiar with these factors when interpreting noninvasive studies, because they affect the pressure and velocity waveforms observed both proximal and distal to the obstructive lesion. In this section of the chapter, the concept of the critical stenosis is considered, as well as the pressure, velocity, and blood flow manifestations of arterial obstructive disease.

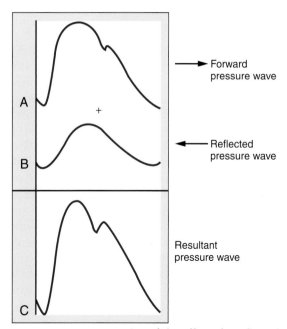

FIGURE 1-9 Representation of the effect of a reflected pressure wave on the final pulse pressure wave. The forward component of the pressure wave **(A)** is added to the reflected pressure wave **(B)** to form the final pressure wave **(C)**. The final shape depends on the location of the artery and the effective distance to the major reflecting point.

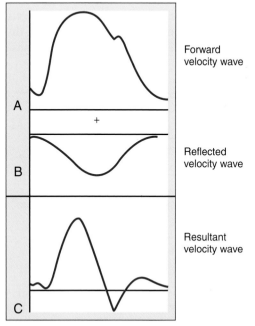

FIGURE 1-10 Representation of the effect of a reflected velocity wave on the final velocity wave. The reflected velocity wave **(B)** is reversed when added to the forward velocity wave **(A)** to form the final velocity wave **(C)**. The final shape depends on the location of the artery and the effective distance to the major reflecting point.

ARTERIAL NARROWING

Blood flow through a narrowed segment of the arterial or venous system is governed by the principle of conversation of mass: what goes in must come out. Therefore, the product of the average blood flow velocity and the cross-sectional area of the artery should be constant (Figure 1-11). While this global effect holds for the overall flow through a vessel without branches, it does not take into consideration the loss of blood flow velocity or kinetic energy that can take place at the level of a narrowing.

As discussed earlier, the energy of flowing blood is a combination of the potential energy of blood (gravity and blood pressure) and the kinetic energy of blood. This is normally described as Bernoulli's equation (see Figure 1-2). Under ideal conditions, and neglecting losses due to friction (viscous forces) or to acceleration/deceleration changes (inertial forces), conservation of energy will translate potential energy (blood pressure) against kinetic energy (square of the blood flow velocity).

However, this ideal scenario is not seen in real life. As indicated by Poiseuille's equation, friction (due to viscosity of blood) causes a progressive loss of energy of the column of flowing blood. These changes are exacerbated at more severe stenotic lesions. In addition, instability in the blood flow profiles due to turbulence can cause

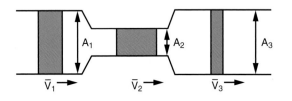

CONSERVATION OF MASS

Volume of blood flowing through a vessel without branches is constant.

Average velocity × Area = Constant

$$\bar{V}_1 \times A_1^2 = \bar{V}_2 \times A_2^2 = \bar{V}_3 \times A_3^2$$

FIGURE 1-11 This diagram is an idealized representation of the principle of conservation of mass as applied to a straight arterial conduit. Basically, the amount of flowing blood remains constant. Based on this principle, and assuming the same driving blood pressure, a very tight stenosis that decreases blood flow at the stenosis will decrease blood flow through the whole conduit. What is not shown here are the collaterals that normally divert blood flow when a segment becomes very stenotic.

additional energy losses distal to the stenosis (Figure 1-12).

CRITICAL STENOSIS

Encroachment on the lumen of an artery by an arteriosclerotic plaque can result in diminished pressure and flow distal to the lesion, but this encroachment on the lumen has to be relatively extensive before hemodynamic changes are manifested because large arteries offer relatively little resistance to flow compared with the more distal resistance vessels with which they are in series.

Studies in humans and animals have indicated that about 90% of the cross-sectional area (approximately 70% diameter narrowing) of the aorta must be encroached upon before there is a change in the distal pressure and blood flow, whereas in smaller vessels, such as the iliac, carotid, renal, and femoral arteries, the critical stenosis level varies from 70% to 90% reduction in cross-sectional area (approximately 45% to 69% diameter narrowing).[18,19]

It is important to differentiate between percentage decrease in cross-sectional area and diameter. For example, a decrease in diameter of 50% corresponds to a 75% decrease in cross-sectional area, and a diameter narrowing of 70% is equivalent to about a 90% reduction in area.

Whether a hemodynamic abnormality results from a stenosis and how severe it may be depend on several factors, including (1) the length and diameter of the narrowed segment; (2) the roughness of the endothelial surface; (3) the degree of irregularity of the narrowing and its shape (i.e., whether the narrowing is abrupt or gradual); (4) the ratio of the cross-sectional area of the narrowed segment to that of the normal vessel; (5) the rate of flow; (6) the arteriovenous pressure gradient; and (7) the peripheral resistance beyond the stenosis.

The concept of critical stenosis (i.e., a stenosis that causes a reduction in flow and pressure) has been treated extensively in the literature.[19-21] This concept has been accepted because there is generally little or no change in hemodynamics when an artery is first narrowed by disease, but a relatively rapid decrease in pressure and blood flow occurs with greater degrees of narrowing.[19] The critical stenosis concept is of practical significance, because lesser degrees of narrowing of human arteries often do not produce significant changes in hemodynamics or clinical manifestations. It must be recognized, however, that

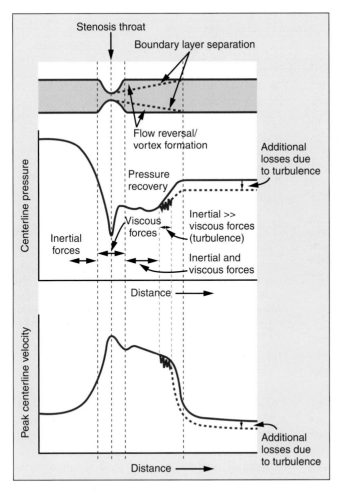

FIGURE 1-12 The effects of a stenosis that has generated a velocity jet are summarized in this diagram. The transition from large diameter to small diameter and the reverse transition are dominated by inertial forces. Viscous forces cause resistance in the stenosis proper. The post-stenotic region is a complex interplay of all of these forces. The velocity jet expands and the associated boundary separation decreases with distance from the stenosis. The development of turbulence occurs when the area of increased velocity delineated by the boundary zone becomes large enough to become unstable. This occurs over a short distance since viscous forces are also acting to decrease blood flow velocity with distance. Turbulence results in a nonrecoverable loss of energy as do the viscous forces at the stenosis proper.

the concept of critical stenosis is a gross simplification of a very complex interplay of numerous circulatory factors. In particular, changes in peripheral resistance, such as those occurring with exercise, may profoundly alter the effect of a given stenotic lesion.[22,23] These considerations dictate that the hemodynamic and clinical significance of stenotic lesions be assessed, whenever possible, by physiologic measurements; otherwise, erroneous conclusions may be reached.

In evaluating the hemodynamic effect of stenotic lesions, it is also important to recognize that two or more stenotic lesions that occur in series have a more pronounced effect on distal pressure and blood flow than does a single lesion of equal total length.[24] This difference is a result of large losses of energy at the entrance, and particularly at the exit, of the lesion resulting from grossly disturbed flow patterns, including jet effects, turbulence, and eddy formation. Thus, the energy losses in tandem lesions can exceed those that result from frictional resistance in a solitary stenosis, as represented in Poiseuille's equation.

PRESSURE CHANGES

Experiments with graded stenoses in animals have indicated that, whereas the diastolic pressure does not fall until the stenosis is quite severe, a decrease in systolic pressure is a sensitive index of reduction in both the mean pressure and the amplitude of the pressure wave distal to a relatively minor stenosis (Figure 1-13).[25] Also, damping of the pressure waveform, increased time to peak, and greater width of the pressure wave at half-amplitude can be detected distal to an arterial stenosis or occlusion.[26]

These abnormal features of the pulse wave correlate well with the results of measurement of systolic pressure and can be demonstrated by noninvasive techniques employing pulse waveforms recorded using various types of plethysmography (Figure 1-14). In the case of very mild

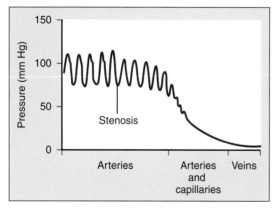

FIGURE 1-13 Decrease in pulse amplitude and systolic and mean pressures distal to a stenosis. In minimal stenosis, alterations in pulse pressure such as this may be evident only during high-volume flow induced by exercise or hyperemia. *(From Carter SA: Peripheral artery disease: pressure measurements ease evaluation,* Consultant *19[9]:102–115, 1979.)*

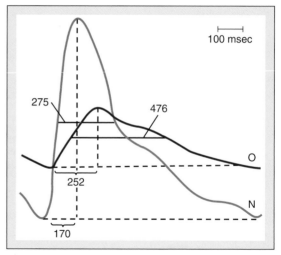

FIGURE 1-14 Dorsalis pedis pulse waves from a normal limb (N) and a limb with a proximal occlusion (O). The wave from the limb with occlusion shows a prolonged time to peak (252 msec) and increased width at half of the amplitude (476 msec). *(From Carter SA: Investigation and treatment of arterial occlusive disease of the extremities,* Clin Med *79[5]:13–24, 1972 [Part I];* Clin Med *79[6]:15–22, 1972 [Part II].)*

stenotic lesions, however, little or no pressure or pulse abnormality may be evident distal to the lesion when the patient is at rest. The presence of such lesions may be demonstrated if blood flow is increased with exercise or through the induction of hyperemia. Enhanced blood flow through the stenosis results in increased loss of energy since energy loss due to frictional (viscous) forces is proportional to velocity and accentuates the detectable decrease in pressure distal to the lesion.[23]

BLOOD FLOW CHANGES

At rest, the total blood flow to an extremity may be normal in the presence of a severe stenosis or even a complete obstruction of the main artery because of the development of collateral circulation, as well as a compensatory decrease in the peripheral resistance. In such circumstances, measurement of systolic pressure, as discussed earlier, is a better method of assessing the presence and severity of the occlusive or stenotic process than measurement of blood flow.[23] Resting blood flow is reduced only when the occlusion is acute and the collateral circulation has not had a chance to develop or, in the case of a chronic arterial obstruction, when the occlusive process is extensive and consists of two or more lesions in series. Although single lesions might not be associated with symptoms or significant changes in blood flow at rest, such lesions can significantly affect the blood supply when need is increased during exercise. In such cases, the sum of the resistances of the obstructions (stenosis,

collateral resistance, or both) and of the peripheral resistance may prevent a normal increase in flow, and symptoms of intermittent claudication may develop.

Arterial obstruction can lead to changes in the distribution of the available blood flow to neighboring regions or vascular beds, depending on the relative resistance and anatomic arrangement of these areas. For example, blood flow during exercise can increase in the skeletal muscle of the extremity distal to an arterial obstruction, but because the distal pressure is reduced during exercise, the muscle "steals" blood from the skin and the blood supply to the skin of the foot is diminished. Such reduction in flow to the skin may be manifested clinically by numbness of the foot, a common symptom in patients with claudication. In lower extremities with extensive large vessel occlusion and additional obstruction in small distal branches, vasodilator drugs or sympathectomy may divert flow from the critically ischemic distal areas by decreasing resistance in less ischemic regions.[27] Obstruction of the subclavian artery is known to cause cerebral symptoms in some patients because of reversal of flow in the vertebral arteries (the subclavian steal syndrome); similarly, obstructive lesions of the internal carotid artery may lead to reversal of flow in the ophthalmic vessels, which communicate with external carotid branches on the face and scalp.

BLOOD FLOW VELOCITY CHANGES

In normal arteries, blood flow velocity increases rapidly to a peak during early systole and decreases during early diastole, when flow reversal can occur. The shape of the resulting pulse velocity wave resembles the pressure gradient shown in Figure 1-8. The character of this velocity profile can be subjectively observed on the Doppler spectral waveform or quantified from Doppler waveform recordings by calculating various indices of pulsatility and damping.[28] Over normal peripheral arteries, double or triple sounds are heard; the second sound represents the diastolic flow reversal *(biphasic)*, and the third sound represents the second forward component *(triphasic)*. Whether the Doppler waveforms are *biphasic or triphasic* is probably not of practical clinical significance and may be related to a complex interplay of several factors. These factors include the basal heart rate and the shape of the pressure and blood flow waves. As discussed earlier, the latter factors depend on the degree of peripheral vasoconstriction and elastic properties of the arteries.

Distal to an arterial stenosis the pressure wave is more damped than normal and is similar in pattern to the pressure wave seen in Figure 1-14. Also, flow reversal disappears distal to an arterial stenosis. The calculated wave indices are thus altered, and the Doppler waveforms have a single component *(monophasic)* rather than the double or triple components usually heard.[11] The disappearance of reversed flow distal to a stenosis probably results from a combination of several factors, including (1) the maintenance of a relatively high level of forward flow throughout the cardiac cycle (because of the pressure gradient across the stenosis); (2) resistance to reverse flow created by the stenotic lesion; (3) a decrease in peripheral resistance as a result of relative ischemia; and (4) damping of the pressure wave by the lesion and a decrease in mean pressure, resulting in attenuated pressure pulses, which are less subject to the reflections and amplification that normally contribute to diastolic flow reversal. The latter would explain the presence of monophasic signals that extend only during systole (high resistance) rather than throughout the cardiac cycle (low resistance).

Assessment of blood flow velocities at and distal to arterial obstructions is useful in evaluating the significance of the occlusive processes. Doppler spectrum analysis allows the accurate detection and quantification of blood flow abnormalities resulting from stenotic lesions. This subject is considered in further detail in Chapters 2 and 3, but it is of interest to comment on the physiologic principles illustrated by the Doppler frequency spectra in normal and abnormal vessels. As noted previously, the velocity pattern across a stenotic vessel is flattened and has a more constant velocity distribution across the diameter of the artery (plug flow) (see Figure 1-3, *B*). As a result, the particles in the central core of normal arteries flow with relatively uniform and high velocities during systole. This can be demonstrated by Doppler spectral waveforms, which reveal a narrow band of velocities near the maximum velocity.[29] Stenotic lesions result in marked disturbance of flow with the occurrence of abnormally high velocities at the site of narrowing, jet effects extending from the stenosis, irregular travel of particles in various directions and at different velocities, and eddy formation (see Figure 1-12). The change in the direction of particle movement with respect to the axis of the vessel alters the observed Doppler shifts and also contributes to the occurrence of a large range of blood flow velocities registered with Doppler spectral analysis. These effects of arterial stenosis are manifest as widening or dispersal of the band of systolic velocity (spectral broadening), complete filling in of the spectral tracing, and reversal of blood flow due to eddies, as discussed in Chapter 3.

VENOUS HEMODYNAMICS

As shown in Figure 1-1, the pressure remaining in the veins after the blood has traversed the arterioles and capillaries is low for a subject in the supine position. Because of their relatively large diameters, medium and large veins offer little resistance to flow, and blood moves readily from the small veins to the right atrium, where the pressure is close to atmospheric pressure. Although the effects of arterial pressure and flow waves are rarely transmitted to the systemic veins, phasic changes in venous pressure and blood flow reflect changes in right atrial pressures in response to cardiac activity and because of alterations of intrathoracic pressure with respiration.

Knowledge of these changes is necessary for correct assessment of peripheral veins by noninvasive laboratory studies.

The final section of this chapter discusses changes in pressure and blood flow in various portions of the venous system that are associated with cardiac and respiratory cycles. Also considered are alterations in venous hemodynamics that occur with changes in posture, the important consequences of competence or incompetence of venous valves, and the effects of venous obstruction.

FLOW AND PRESSURE CHANGES DURING THE CARDIAC CYCLE

Figure 1-15 shows changes in pressure and flow in large veins such as the venae cavae that occur during phases of the cardiac cycle. Such oscillations in pressure and flow may, at times, be transmitted to more peripheral vessels. Characteristically, three positive pressure waves (a, c, v) can be distinguished in central venous pressure and reflect corresponding changes in pressure in the atria. The *a wave* is caused by atrial contraction and relaxation. The upstroke of the *c wave* is related to the increase in pressure when the atrioventricular valves are closed and bulge during isovolumetric ventricular contraction. The subsequent downstroke results from the fall in pressure caused by pulling the atrioventricular valve rings toward the apex of the heart during ventricular contraction, thus tending to increase the atrial volume. The upstroke of the *v wave* results from a passive rise in atrial pressure during ventricular systole when the atrioventricular valves are closed and the atria fill with blood from the peripheral veins. The *v* wave downstroke is caused by the fall in pressure that occurs when the blood leaves the atria rapidly and fills the ventricles, soon after the opening of the atrioventricular valves, early in ventricular diastole.

The venous pressure waves are associated with changes in blood flow. There are two periods of increased venous flow during each cardiac cycle. The first occurs during ventricular systole, when shortening of the ventricular muscle pulls the atrioventricular valve rings toward the apex of the heart. This movement of the valve ring tends to increase atrial volume and decrease atrial pressure, thus increasing flow from the extracardiac veins into the atria. The second phase of increased venous flow occurs after the atrioventricular valves open and blood rushes into the

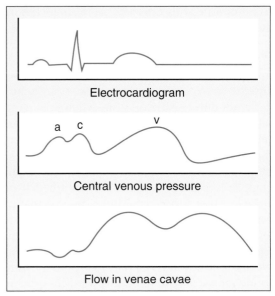

FIGURE 1-15 Schematic representation of normal changes in pressure and flow in the central veins associated with the cardiac cycle. a, a wave; c, c wave; v, v wave.

ventricles from the atria. Venous flow is reduced in the intervening periods of the cardiac cycle as the atrial pressure rises during and soon after atrial contraction and in the later part of the ventricular systole. Because there are no valves at the junction of the right atrium and venae cavae, some backward flow may actually occur in the large thoracic veins during atrial contraction as blood moves in the reverse direction from the atrium into the venae cavae.

The changes in pressure and blood flow in the large central veins that are associated with the events of the cardiac cycle are not usually evident in the peripheral veins of the extremities. This is probably the result of damping related to the high distensibility (compliance) of the veins, as well as compression of the veins by intra-abdominal pressure and mechanical compression in the thoracic inlet. Because the effects of right-sided heart contractions are more readily transmitted to the large veins of the arms, the pulsatile changes in venous blood flow velocity associated with the events of the cardiac cycle tend to be more obvious in the upper extremities than in the veins of the legs.

In abnormal conditions, such as congestive heart failure or tricuspid insufficiency, venous pressure is increased. This elevation of venous pressure may lead to increased transmission of cardiac phasic changes in pressure and blood flow to the peripheral veins of the upper and lower limbs. Such phasic changes may occasionally be found in healthy, well-hydrated individuals, probably because a large blood volume distends the venous system.

VENOUS EFFECTS OF RESPIRATION

Respiration has profound effects on venous pressure and blood flow. During inspiration, the volume in the veins of the thorax increases and the pressure decreases in response to reduced intrathoracic pressure. Expiration leads to the opposite effect, with decreased venous volume and increased pressure. The venous response to respiration is reversed in the abdomen, where the pressure increases during inspiration because of the descent of the diaphragm and decreases during expiration as the diaphragm ascends. Increased abdominal pressure during inspiration decreases pressure gradients between peripheral veins in the lower extremities and the abdomen, thus reducing blood flow in the peripheral vessels. During expiration, when intra-abdominal pressure is reduced, the pressure gradient from the lower limbs to the abdomen is increased and blood flow in the peripheral veins rises correspondingly.

In the veins of the upper limbs, the changes in blood flow with respiration are opposite to those in the lower extremities. Because of reduced intrathoracic pressure during inspiration, the pressure gradient from the veins of the upper limbs to the right atrium increases and blood flow increases. During expiration, blood flow decreases because of the resulting increase in intrathoracic pressure and the corresponding rise of the right atrial pressure. The respiratory changes in blood flow in the upper limbs may be influenced by changes in posture. With the upper parts of the body elevated, venous flow tends to stop at the height of inspiration and resumes with expiration, probably because of the compression of the subclavian vein at the level of the first rib during contraction of the accessory muscles of respiration.

The respiratory effects are usually associated with clear phasic changes in venous blood flow in the extremities; these can be detected by various instruments, including plethysmographs and Doppler flow detectors. The respiratory changes in venous velocity may be exaggerated by respiratory maneuvers such as the Valsalva maneuver, which increases intrathoracic and abdominal pressures and decreases, abolishes, or even reverses flow in some peripheral veins.

Also, the respiratory effects on venous flow may be diminished in the lower limbs in individuals who are chest or shallow breathers and whose diaphragm may not descend sufficiently to elevate intra-abdominal pressure. Venous flow then tends to be more continuous.

VENOUS BLOOD FLOW AND PERIPHERAL RESISTANCE

Blood flow and blood flow velocity in the peripheral veins, particularly in the extremities, are profoundly influenced by local blood flow, which is in turn largely determined by the peripheral resistance or the state of vasoconstriction or vasodilatation. When limb blood flow is markedly increased as a result of peripheral vasodilatation (e.g., secondary to infection or inflammation), the flow tends to be more continuous, and the respiratory changes in flow are less evident. When there is increased vasoconstriction in the extremities (e.g., when there is a need to conserve body heat and blood flow through the skin is decreased), venous flow is also markedly decreased and there may decreased Doppler flow signals over a peripheral vein, such as the posterior tibial vein. Also, severe arterial obstruction may decrease overall blood flow and velocity in the vessels of the extremities and lead to decreased velocity signals over the venous channels.

EFFECT OF POSTURE

In the upright position, the hydrostatic pressure is greatly increased in the dependent part of the body, particularly in the lower portions of the lower extremities. This increase in hydrostatic pressure, as indicated earlier, is associated with high transmural pressures in the blood vessels and, in turn, leads to greater vascular distention. In the veins, which have low pressure to start with and are distensible, considerable pooling of the blood occurs in the lower parts of the legs. The resulting decrease in venous return to the right atrium is associated with diminished cardiac output. When the normal compensatory reflexes that increase peripheral resistance are impaired, decreased cardiac output can lead to hypotension and fainting.

The movement of the skeletal muscles of the legs, such as that which occurs during walking, leads to decreased venous pressure because of the presence of one-way valves in the peripheral veins. Contraction of the voluntary muscle squeezes the veins and propels the blood toward the heart. Muscular contraction not only increases venous return and cardiac output but also interrupts the hydrostatic column of venous blood from the heart and thus temporarily decreases pressure in the peripheral veins (e.g., in the veins at the ankle). Activity of the skeletal muscles of the legs in the presence of competent venous valves therefore results in the lowering of pressure in the veins of the extremity, leading to decreased venous pooling, decreased capillary pressure, reduced filtration of fluid into the extracellular space than would otherwise occur, and increased blood flow because of increased arteriovenous pressure difference.

EFFECT OF EXTERNAL COMPRESSION

Sudden pressure on the veins of the extremities, whether caused by an active muscular contraction or external manual compression of the limb, increases venous blood flow and velocity toward the heart and stops blood flow distal to the site of the compression in the presence of competent venous valves. The responses to sudden pressure changes are affected by venous obstruction and damage to the venous valves. The detection of such changes is important when assessing patients for the presence of venous disease. (This is discussed further in Chapters 21 and 22.)

VENOUS OBSTRUCTION

Venous obstruction can be acute or chronic. Acute venous thrombosis may lead to potentially fatal pulmonary embolism due to embolization of thrombi in the leg veins and resulting obstruction of the pulmonary arteries. The clinical diagnosis of acute deep venous thrombosis is unreliable, and noninvasive venous ultrasound has become the primary means of making this diagnosis (see Chapter 22). In the case of severe chronic obstruction, edema may occur due to poor exchange of oxygenated blood in the peripheral soft tissues. Also, the nutrition of the skin in the affected region may be impaired, and characteristic trophic changes in the skin and venous stasis ulcers may result.

An audible Doppler signal should be present over peripheral veins; it can be easily distinguished from an arterial flow signal because of the absence of pulsatility synchronous with the heart. As indicated earlier, a signal may be absent in low-flow states, especially when the limb is cold and auscultation is carried out over small peripheral veins. Squeezing of the limb distal

to the site of examination should temporarily increase blood flow (augmentation) and cause an audible signal if the vein is patent. Spontaneous venous blood flow signals normally possess clear respiratory phases. However, if there is an obstruction between the heart and the examination site, the respiratory changes in venous blood flow velocity are absent or attenuated. Over larger, more proximal veins, such as the popliteal and more proximal veins, the absence of audible signals after an adequate search is indicative of an obstructed venous segment.

The presence or absence of obstruction is also gauged by increasing blood flow toward the examination site by squeezing the limb distally or by activating the *distal* muscle groups and thus increasing venous blood flow toward the flow-detecting probe (augmentation). Absence of increased blood flow signals or attenuation of the expected increase in blood flow signals is associated with obstruction between the probe location and the site from which the enhancement of venous flow is attempted.

Increase in blood flow is also elicited when manual compression of the limb proximal to the flow-detecting probe is released, because of filling of the proximal veins that have been emptied by the compression maneuver. If the proximal veins at or near the point of compression are occluded, the augmentation of blood flow after release of the compression is attenuated.

VENOUS VALVULAR INCOMPETENCE

When the valves are competent, blood flow in the peripheral veins is toward the heart. However, blood flow may be temporarily diminished or stopped soon after assumption of the upright posture, at the height of inspiration, or during the Valsalva maneuver. The peripheral veins normally fill from the capillaries, and the rate at which they fill depends on the peripheral resistance and arterial blood flow, as determined by the degree of peripheral vasoconstriction. When there are incompetent veins proximally, there may be retrograde filling of the peripheral veins, such as those in the ankle region, from the more proximal veins, in addition to normal filling from the capillary beds. This retrograde filling may have serious consequences because of a resulting chronic exposure to persistent levels of elevated hydrostatic pressure and filtration of fluid into the extravascular spaces in the upright position.

The presence or absence of the retrograde blood flow may be detected by examining the Doppler spectral waveforms obtained after the limb is squeezed distally. Various plethysmographic methods can detect the rate of venous filling by measuring changes in venous volume after the blood volumes have been decreased during muscular action such as flexion-extension of the ankle in the upright position. After such exercise, the venous volume and pressure increase more rapidly when the valves are incompetent, because the peripheral veins fill as a result of retrograde blood flow from the more proximal parts of the limbs. The application of a tourniquet or cuff with appropriate pressure compresses the superficial veins and allows localization of incompetent veins, not only to the various segments of the limbs, but also to the superficial veins as opposed to the perforating or deep veins.

SUMMARY

Doppler ultrasound measurements reflect key elements of arterial and venous hemodynamics. An understanding of the basic physiologic principles plays a critical role in the evaluation of arterial and venous disease.

REFERENCES

1. Carter SA: Arterial auscultation in peripheral vascular disease, *JAMA* 246:1682–1686, 1981.
2. Miller A, et al: Effects of surrounding tissue on the sound spectrum of arterial bruits in vivo, *Stroke* 11:394–398, 1980.
3. Latham RD, et al: Regional wave travel and reflections along the human aorta: a study with six simultaneous micromanometric pressures, *Circulation* 72:1257–1269, 1985.
4. Munir S, et al: Peripheral augmentation index defines the relationship between central and peripheral pulse pressure, *Hypertension* 51:112–118, 2008.
5. Murgo JP, et al: Effects of exercise on aortic input impedance and pressure wave forms in normal humans, *Circ Res* 48:334–343, 1981.
6. Carter SA: Effect of age, cardiovascular disease, and vasomotor changes on transmission of arterial pressure waves through the lower extremities, *Angiology* 29:601–606, 1978.
7. Gaskell P, Krisman AM: The brachial to digital blood pressure gradient in normal subjects and in patients with high blood pressure, *Can J Biochem Physiol* 36:889–893, 1958.
8. Lezack JD, Carter SA: Systolic pressures in the extremities of man with special reference to the toes, *Can J Biochem Physiol* 48:469–474, 1970.

9. Nielsen PE, Barras JP, Holstein P: Systolic pressure amplification in the arteries of normal subjects, *Scand J Clin Lab Invest* 33:371–377, 1974.
10. Carter SA, Tate RB: The effect of body heating and cooling on the ankle and toe systolic pressures in arterial disease, *J Vasc Surg* 16:148–153, 1992.
11. Rowell LB, et al: Disparities between aortic and peripheral pulse pressures induced by upright exercise and vasomotor changes in man, *Circulation* 37:954–964, 1968.
12. Sharman JE, et al: Pulse pressure amplification during exercise is significantly reduced with age and hypercholesterolemia, *J Hypertens* 25:1249–1254, 2007.
13. Nijdam M-E, et al: Pulse pressure amplification and risk of cardiovascular disease, *Am J Hypertens* 21:388–392, 2008.
14. Allen J, et al: Photoplethysmography detection of lower limb peripheral arterial occlusive disease: A comparison of pulse timing, amplitude and shape characteristics, *Physiol Meas* 26:811–821, 2005.
15. Williams DT, Harding KG, Price P: An evaluation of the efficacy of methods used in screening for lower-limb arterial disease in diabetes, *Diabetes Care* 28:2206–2210, 2005.
16. Westerhof BE, et al: Quantification of wave reflection in the human aorta from pressure alone: a proof of principle, *Hypertension* 48:595–601, 2006.
17. Westerhof N, et al: Forward and backward waves in the arterial system, *Cardiovasc Res* 6:648–656, 1972.
18. Schultz RD, Hokanson DE, Strandness DE Jr: Pressure-flow and stress-strain measurements of normal and diseased aortoiliac segments, *Surg Gynecol Obstet* 124:1267–1276, 1967.
19. Berguer R, Hwang NH: Critical arterial stenosis: a theoretical and experimental solution, *Ann Surg* 180:39–50, 1974.
20. Kreuzer W, Schenk WG Jr: Hemodynamic effects of vasodilatation in "critical" arterial stenosis, *Arch Surg* 103:277–282, 1971.
21. May AG, et al: Critical arterial stenosis, *Surgery* 54:250–259, 1963.
22. Young DF, Cholvin NR, Kirkeeide RL: Hemodynamics of arterial stenoses at elevated flow rates, *Circ Res* 41:99–107, 1977.
23. Carter SA: Response of ankle systolic pressure to leg exercise in mild or questionable arterial disease, *N Engl J Med* 287:578–582, 1972.
24. Li Z-Y, et al: The hemodynamic effects of in-tandem carotid artery stenosis: implications for carotid endarterectomy, *J Stroke Cerebrovasc Dis* 19:138–145, 2010.
25. Widmer LK, Staub H: Blood pressure in stenosed arteries, *Z Kreislaufforsch* 51:975–979, 1962.
26. Carter SA: Indirect systolic pressures and pulse waves in arterial occlusive diseases of the lower extremities, *Circulation* 37:624–637, 1968.
27. Uhrenholdt A, et al: Paradoxical effect on peripheral blood flow after sympathetic blockades in patients with gangrene due to arteriosclerosis obliterans, *Vasc Surg* 5:154–163, 1971.
28. Johnston KW, Taraschuk I: Validation of the role of pulsatility index in quantitation of the severity of peripheral arterial occlusive disease, *Am J Surg* 131:295–297, 1976.
29. Reneman RS, Hoeks A, Spencer MP: Doppler ultrasound in the evaluation of the peripheral arterial circulation, *Angiology* 30:526–538, 1979.

PHYSICS AND INSTRUMENTATION IN DOPPLER AND B-MODE ULTRASONOGRAPHY

JAMES A. ZAGZEBSKI, PhD

This chapter presents an overview of the physical and technical aspects of vascular sonography, including the following: (1) a brief review of relevant ultrasound–soft-tissue interactions, (2) pulse-echo principles and display techniques, (3) harmonic and chirp imaging, (4) the Doppler effect as it applies to vascular sonography, (5) continuous-wave (CW) and pulsed Doppler instrumentation, (6) the common techniques used for displaying Doppler signal spectral information, and (7) extended field-of-view and three-dimensional (3D) techniques.

SOUND PROPAGATION IN TISSUE

Sound waves are produced by vibrating sources, which cause particles in the medium to oscillate, setting up the wave. As sound energy propagates, it is attenuated, scattered, and reflected, producing echoes from various interfaces. In medical ultrasonography, *piezoelectric elements* inside an ultrasound transducer serve as the source and detector of sound waves. The design of the transducer is such that the waves travel in a beam with a well-defined direction. The reception of reflected and scattered echo signals by the transducer makes possible the production of ultrasound images and allows detection of motion using the Doppler effect. This section inspects factors that are important in the transmission and reflection of ultrasound in tissue.

SPEED OF SOUND

Most ultrasound applications involve transmitting short bursts, or pulses, of sound into the body and receiving echoes from tissue interfaces. The time between transmitting a pulse and receiving an echo is used to determine the depth of the interface. The speed of sound in tissue must be known to apply pulse-echo methods.

Sound propagation speeds depend on the properties of the transmitting medium and not

significantly on frequency or wave amplitude. As a general rule, gases, including air, exhibit the lowest sound speed; liquids have an intermediate speed; and firm solids such as glass have very high speeds of sound. Speeds of sound in common media and tissues are listed in Table 2-1. For soft tissues, the average speed of sound has been found to be 1540 m/sec.[1] Most diagnostic ultrasound instruments are calibrated with the assumption that the sound beam propagates at this average speed. Slight variations exist in the speed of sound from one tissue to another, but as Table 2-1 indicates, speeds of sound in specific soft tissues deviate only slightly from the assumed average. Adipose tissues have sound speeds that are lower than the average, whereas muscle tissue exhibits a speed of sound that is slightly greater than 1540 m/sec.

FREQUENCY AND WAVELENGTH

The number of oscillations per second of the piezoelectric element in the transducer establishes the frequency of the ultrasound wave. Frequency is expressed in cycles per second, or hertz (Hz). Audible sounds are in the range of 30 Hz to 20 kHz. *Ultrasound* refers to any sound whose frequency is above the audible range (i.e., above

TABLE 2-1 Speed of Sound for Biologic Tissue

Tissue	Speed of Sound (m/sec)	Change from 1540 m/sec (%)
Fat	1450	−5.8
Vitreous humor	1520	−1.3
Liver	1550	+0.6
Blood	1570	+1.9
Muscle	1580	+2.6
Lens of eye	1620	+5.2

From Wells PNT: Propagation of ultrasonic waves through tissues. In Fullerton G, Zagzebski J, editors: *Medical physics of CT and ultrasound,* New York, 1980, American Institute of Physics, p 381.

20

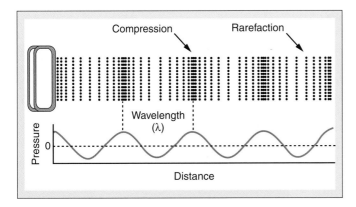

FIGURE 2-1 Sound waves produced by an ultrasound transducer. Vibrations of the transducer are coupled into the medium, producing local fluctuations in pressure. The fluctuations propagate through the medium in waves. The pressure amplitude is the maximum pressure swing, positive or negative. The diagram schematically illustrates compressions and rarefactions at an instant of time. The symbol λ is the acoustic wavelength.

20 kHz). Diagnostic ultrasound applications use frequencies in the 1-MHz to 30-MHz (1 million to 30 million Hz) frequency range. Manufacturers of ultrasound equipment and clinical users strive to use as high a frequency as practical that still allows adequate visualization depth into tissue (see section on attenuation). Higher frequencies are associated with improved spatial detail, or better resolution.

Figure 2-1 shows what might be called a snapshot of a sound wave, captured at an instant of time. It illustrates accompanying compressions and rarefactions in the medium that result from the particle oscillations. The wavelength λ is the distance over which a property of a wave repeats itself. It is defined by the equation

$$\lambda = \frac{c}{f} \qquad (2\text{-}1)$$

where c is the speed of sound and f is the frequency. Table 2-2 presents values for the wavelength in soft tissue, where the speed of sound is taken to be 1540 m/sec, for several frequencies. A good rule of thumb for tissues is the wavelength $\lambda_t = 1.5$ mm/F, where F is the frequency expressed in MHz. For example, if the frequency is 5 MHz, the wavelength in soft tissue is approximately 0.3 mm. Higher frequencies have shorter wavelengths and vice versa.

Wavelength has relevance when describing dimensions of objects, such as reflectors and scatterers in the body. The size of an object is most meaningfully expressed if given relative to the ultrasonic wavelength for the frequency of the sound beam. Similarly, the width of the ultrasound beam from a transducer depends in part on the wavelength. Higher-frequency beams have shorter wavelengths and are narrower than lower-frequency beams.

TABLE 2-2 Wavelengths for Various Ultrasound Frequencies

Frequency (MHz)	Wavelength* (mm)
1	1.54
2.25	0.68
5	0.31
10	0.15
15	0.103

*Assuming a speed of sound of 1540 m/sec.

AMPLITUDE, INTENSITY, AND POWER

A sound wave is accompanied by pressure fluctuations in the medium. The pressure profile that could occur for the wave in Figure 2-1 might appear as in the graph in the lower part of this figure. The pressure *amplitude* is the maximal increase (or decrease) in the pressure caused by the sound wave. The unit for pressure is the pascal (Pa). Pulsed ultrasound scanners can produce peak pressure amplitudes of several million pascals in water when power controls on the machine are adjusted for maximal levels. As a benchmark for comparison, atmospheric pressure is approximately 0.1 MPa, so it is clear that ultrasound fields from medical devices significantly exceed this mark. The high-pressure amplitudes of an ultrasound pulse can easily burst contrast agent bubbles (see later) that are sometimes injected into the bloodstream to enhance echo signals. Diagnostic levels, however, are not believed to create biologic effects in tissues if such gas bodies are not present.

The intensity (I) of a sound wave at a point in the medium is estimated by squaring the pressure amplitude (P) and using $I = P^2/2\rho c$, where ρ is the density and c is the speed of sound. Units for ultrasound intensity are watts per meter squared

(W/m^2) or multiples thereof, such as mW/cm^2. In water, a 2-MPa amplitude during the pulse corresponds to a pulse average intensity of $133\ W/cm^2$! This is a high intensity, but, fortunately, it is not sustained by a diagnostic ultrasound device because the duty factor (i.e., the fraction of time the transducer actually emits ultrasound) typically is less than 0.005. Therefore, the time-averaged acoustic intensity from an ultrasound machine, found by averaging over a time that includes transmit pulses as well as the time between pulses, is much lower than the intensity during the pulse. Typical time-averaged intensities at the location in the ultrasound beam where the maximal values are found are on the order of 10 to 20 mW/cm^2 for B-mode imaging. Doppler and color flow imaging modes have higher duty factors. Moreover, these modes tend to concentrate the acoustic energy into smaller areas. Time-averaged intensities for Doppler modes may be a few hundred mW/cm^2 for color flow imaging and as high as 1000 to 2000 mW/cm^2 for pulsed Doppler![2,3]

The acoustic *power* produced by a scanner is the rate at which energy is emitted by the transducer. Average acoustic power levels in diagnostic ultrasonography are low because of the small duty factors used in most equipment. Typical power levels are on the order of 10 to 20 mW for black-and-white imaging, but may be three to four times this value for color flow modes of operation.

ACOUSTIC OUTPUT LABELS ON MACHINES

The transmit level, or the output power, on most scanners may be adjusted by the operator. Increasing the power applies a more energetic signal to the transducer, thereby increasing the pressure amplitude and increasing the power and the intensity of the waves produced. Higher power levels are advantageous because they enable detection of echoes from more weakly reflecting interfaces in the body. The disadvantage of high power levels is that they expose the tissue to greater amounts of acoustic energy, increasing the potential for biologic effects. Although there are no confirmed effects of ultrasound on patients during diagnostic ultrasound exposures, most operators attempt to follow the ALARA (As Low As Reasonably Achievable) principle when adjusting the power level and other instrument controls that affect output levels.

It would be difficult to follow ALARA without labels on the machine to inform the operator

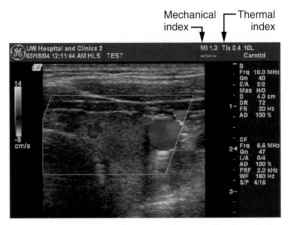

FIGURE 2-2 Ultrasound image showing display of the mechanical index (MI) and thermal index (TI).

"how much" ultrasound energy is being applied. Although some ultrasound machines display relative output indications, such as a transmit level percentage, a relative level in decibels, or simply the setting of a power control knob, such labels do not provide users sufficient information to help them understand the likelihood that the sound levels produced might be in an undesirable zone.

To help operators implement the ALARA principle, output labels are used that are related to the biologic effects of ultrasound.[4] One of the potential effects is "cavitation," which describes activity of small gas bodies under the action of an ultrasound field. When gas bodies are present, such as when there are contrast agents in the ultrasound field, cavitation increases the local stresses on tissue that are associated with the ultrasound waves. If the wave amplitude is high enough, collapse of the gas body occurs, and this is accompanied by localized energy depositions that significantly exceed depositions that might occur without cavitation. Cavitation is believed to be most closely associated with the peak negative pressure in the ultrasound wave. Scientists have developed a "mechanical index" (MI) that is derived from the peak negative pressure in the medium. For most ultrasound machines, the current maximum MI in the field is displayed in a prominent position on the display (Figure 2-2).

Another way that ultrasound energy may affect tissue is by heating through absorption of the waves. Absorption is one of the mechanisms that result in attenuation of a sound beam as it propagates through tissue. A corresponding index, the "thermal index" (TI) is displayed to indicate the likelihood of heating (see Figure 2-2). This is estimated using the time-averaged acoustic power or the time-averaged intensity, along with detailed mathematical models for the sound beam pattern and assumptions on the ultrasonic and thermal properties of the tissue. Depending on the application, a machine will exhibit either a soft tissue thermal index value (TI_s) or a thermal index for the case in which absorbing bone is at the beam focus (TI_b). TI_c is a thermal index that is used for Transcranial Doppler studies because heating is likely to occur in the cranial bones.

The acoustic output labeling standard calls for a clear display of MI and TI.[4] The standard is followed by most ultrasound equipment manufacturers, and it provides ultrasound system operators values of acoustic output quantities that are relevant to the possibility of biologic effects from the ultrasound exposures.

DECIBEL NOTATION

Decibels are used frequently to indicate relative power, intensity, and amplitude levels. Their use is a way to express the ratio of two signal amplitudes or two intensities. Suppose one wishes to express how much greater (or smaller) one intensity (I_1) is relative to another (I_2). Their relative value in decibels is given by

$$dB = 10 \log \frac{I_1}{I_2} \qquad (2\text{-}2)$$

Thus, the decibel relation between two intensities is just the log of their ratio multiplied by 10. The same equation holds for expressing the ratio of two power levels. The difference in decibels between two powers is found by taking the log of their ratio and multiplying by 10.

Sometimes amplitudes rather than the intensities of two signals are used to express decibels. For a given decibel level, one must account for the fact that the intensity is proportional to the square of the amplitude. Substituting the corresponding amplitudes (A_1 and A_2) into Equation 2-2, squaring them, and taking into account that $\log (x^2)$ is $2(\log x)$, we have the relationship

$$dB = 20 \log \frac{A_1}{A_2} \qquad (2\text{-}3)$$

Notice, the multiplicative factor is 20 rather than 10 when converting amplitude ratios to decibels.

TABLE 2-3 Decibel Differences Corresponding to Various Intensity and Amplitude Ratios*

Amplitude Ratio (A_1/A_2)	Intensity Ratio (I_1/I_2)	Decibel Difference (dB)
1	1	0
1.41	2	+3
2	4	+6
2.828	8	+9
3.16	10	+10
4.47	20	+13
10	100	+20
100	10,000	+40
1	1	0
0.707	0.5	−3
0.5	0.25	−6

*For example, if I_1 is 10 times I_2, it is 10 dB greater than I_2. A 20-dB difference between two signals corresponds to both a ratio of 10 for their amplitude or a ratio of 100 for their intensities, and so forth.

Table 2-3 lists decibel values for various intensity and amplitude ratios. Notice that a 3-dB increase in the intensity is the same as doubling the quantity. A 10-dB increase corresponds to a 10-fold increase, and a 20-dB increase means that the intensity is multiplied by 100. The lower half of the table shows decibel changes corresponding to reductions of the intensity. A 3-dB decrease is the same as halving the intensity, and so forth.

Frequently, decibels are used to describe the loudness of audible sounds. Here, the level of one sound often is expressed with no explicit comparison to another, such as "the sound intensity of the jet at takeoff was 110 dB." However, with airborne sounds, a reference intensity is implied when not stated explicitly. This reference is $I_2 = 10^{-12}$ W/m², the accepted threshold for human hearing.

ATTENUATION

As a sound beam propagates through tissue, its intensity decreases with increasing distance. This decrease with path length is called *attenuation*. Attenuation of medical ultrasound beams is caused by reflection and scatter of the waves at boundaries between media having different densities or speeds of sound and absorption of ultrasonic energy by tissues. As mentioned previously, absorption may lead to heating if beam power levels are sufficiently high.

The rate of attenuation in relation to distance is called the *attenuation coefficient*, expressed in decibels per centimeter. The attenuation coefficient

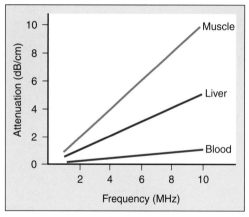

FIGURE 2-3 Variation of attenuation with tissue type and frequency.

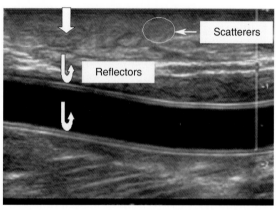

FIGURE 2-4 B-mode image of an arterial graft. Such images are constructed from echoes detected from large interfaces (arrows) and from small scatterers (smooth echo region). Bright dots on ultrasound B-mode images indicate high-amplitude echoes, and dim dots indicate low amplitudes. Notice how the echoes from the vessel wall vary as the orientation changes slightly, characteristic of a specular reflector. The highest-amplitude echoes occur when the interface is perpendicular to the ultrasound beam. The interior of the vessel appears anechoic because blood has a lower backscatter level (lower echogenicity) than surrounding tissues. Scattering from small interfaces produces the vast majority of echoes visualized throughout the image.

depends on both the medium and the ultrasound frequency. Figure 2-3 illustrates attenuation coefficients for a few tissues, plotted versus the frequency. Attenuation is quite high for muscle and skin, has an intermediate value for large organs such as the liver, and is very low for fluid-filled structures. For the liver, it is approximately 0.5 dB/cm at 1 MHz, whereas for blood, it is about 0.17 dB/cm at 1 MHz. An important characteristic of attenuation is its frequency dependence. For most soft tissues, the attenuation coefficient is nearly proportional to the frequency.[1] The attenuation expressed in decibels would roughly double if the frequency were doubled. Thus, higher-frequency sound waves are more severely attenuated than lower-frequency waves, and the high-frequency beams cannot penetrate as far as low-frequency beams. Diagnostic studies with higher-frequency sound beams (7 MHz and above) are usually limited to superficial regions of the body. Lower frequencies (5 MHz and below) must be used for imaging large organs, such as the liver.

REFLECTION

Figure 2-4 shows an ultrasound image of the carotid artery of a normal adult. The walls of the vessel can be seen because of reflection of sound waves. Echoes from muscle and other tissues are also produced by reflections and by ultrasonic scatter. Both reflection and scatter contribute to the detail seen on clinical ultrasound scans.

Partial reflection of ultrasound waves occurs when they are incident on interfaces separating tissues having different acoustic properties. The fraction of the incident energy that is reflected

depends on the acoustic impedances of the tissues forming the interface. The acoustic impedance (Z) is the speed of sound (c) multiplied by the density (ϱ) of a tissue. The amplitude or strength of the reflected wave is proportional to the difference between the acoustic impedances of tissues forming the interface.

The *reflection coefficient* quantifies the relative amplitude of a wave reflected at an interface. It is the ratio of the reflected amplitude to the incident amplitude. For perpendicular incidence of the ultrasound beam on a large, flat interface (Figure 2-5), reflection coefficient (R) is given by

$$R = \frac{Z_2 - Z_1}{Z_2 + Z_1} \qquad (2\text{-}4)$$

where the impedances Z_1 and Z_2 are identified in Figure 2-5.

Equation 2-4 shows that the larger the difference between impedances Z_2 and Z_1, the greater will be the amplitude of the echo from an interface, and hence, the less will be the transmitted signal. Large impedance differences are found at tissue-to-air and tissue-to-bone interfaces. In fact, such interfaces are nearly impenetrable to an ultrasound beam. In contrast, significantly weaker echoes originate at interfaces formed by

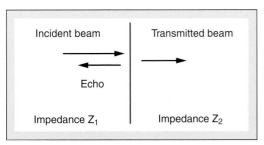

FIGURE 2-5 Reflection at a specular interface. The echo amplitude depends on the difference between the acoustic impedances Z_1 and Z_2 of the materials forming the interface.

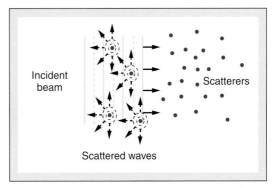

FIGURE 2-6 Scattering of ultrasound by small inhomogeneities.

two soft tissues because, generally, there is not a large difference in impedance between soft tissues.[5]

Large, smooth interfaces, such as those indicated in Figure 2-5, are called *specular reflectors*. The direction in which the reflected wave travels after striking a specular reflector is highly dependent on the orientation of the interface with respect to the sound beam. The wave is reflected back toward the source only when the incident beam is perpendicular or nearly perpendicular to the reflector. The amplitude of an echo detected from a specular reflector thus also depends on the orientation of the reflector with respect to the sound beam direction. The ultrasound image in Figure 2-4 was obtained using a linear array probe, which sends individual ultrasound beams into the scanned region in a vertical direction as viewed on the image. Sections of the vessel wall that are nearly horizontal yield the highest amplitude echoes and hence appear brightest because they were closest to being perpendicular to the ultrasound beams during imaging. Sections where the vessel is slightly inclined are seen as less bright.

Some soft tissue interfaces are better classified as *diffuse reflectors*. The reflected waves from a diffuse reflector propagate in various directions with respect to the incident beam. Therefore, the amplitude of an echo from a diffuse interface is less dependent on the orientation of the interface with respect to the sound beam than the amplitude detected from a specular reflector.

SCATTERING

For interfaces whose dimensions are small, reflections are classified as "scattering." Much of the background information viewed in Figure 2-4 results from scattered echoes, where no one interface can be identified but usually echoes

from many small interfaces are picked up simultaneously. The scattered waves spread in all directions, as suggested in Figure 2-6. Consequently, there is little angular dependence on the strength of echoes detected from scatterers. Unlike the vessel wall, which is best visualized when the ultrasound beam is perpendicular to it, the scatterers are detected with relatively uniform average amplitude from all directions. Echoes resulting from scattering within organ parenchyma are clinically important because they provide much of the diagnostic detail seen on ultrasound scans.

In Doppler ultrasound, blood flow is detected by processing signals resulting from scattering by red blood cells. At diagnostic ultrasound frequencies, the size of a red blood cell is very small compared with the ultrasonic wavelength. Scatterers of this size range are called *Rayleigh scatterers*. The scattered intensity from a distribution of Rayleigh scatterers depends on several factors: (1) the dimensions of the scatterer, with a sharply increasing scattered intensity as the size increases; (2) the number of scatterers present in the beam (e.g., Shung has demonstrated that when the hematocrit is low, scattering from blood is proportional to the hematocrit[6]); (3) the extent to which the density or elastic properties of the scatterer differ from those of the surrounding material; and (4) the ultrasonic frequency. (For Rayleigh scatterers, the scattered intensity is proportional to the frequency to the fourth power.)

NONLINEAR PROPAGATION

A sound wave traveling through tissue will also undergo gradual distortion with distance if the amplitude is high enough. This is a manifestation of *nonlinear* sound propagation, and it leads to creation of harmonic waves, or waves that have frequencies that are multiples of that of the

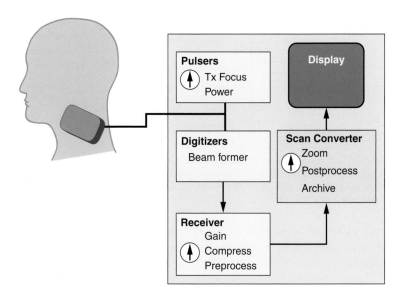

FIGURE 2-7 Simple block diagram of a pulse-echo ultrasound instrument.

original transmitted wave. When partial reflection of the distorted beam occurs at an interface, the reflected echo consists of both the original, "fundamental frequency signals" and harmonic components. A 3-MHz fundamental echo is accompanied by a 6-MHz second harmonic echo and so on. Higher-order harmonics are possible, but attenuation in tissue usually limits the ability to detect them. Although the second harmonic echoes themselves are of lower amplitude than the fundamental, it is possible to distinguish them from the fundamental in the processor of an ultrasound machine and to use them to construct an image, called a tissue harmonic image.[7]

A noteworthy character of tissue harmonic images is that they appear less noisy and have fewer reverberation artifacts than images made with the fundamental. This is believed to be related to the way the harmonic component of the beam forms (i.e., the harmonics gradually grow in amplitude with increasing depth). The harmonic is not present at the skin surface but gradually develops as the beam propagates deeper and deeper into tissue. The second harmonic reaches a peak at some intermediate depth in the patient, then reduces with further increases in depth. Any reverberations or other sources of acoustic noise generated when the transmitted pulse is near the skin surface preferentially contain fundamental frequencies because the harmonics have not built up to any appreciable level at that point. Examples of harmonic images are presented later in this chapter.

B-MODE IMAGING

RANGE EQUATION

Ultrasound imaging is done using pulse-echo techniques. An ultrasonic transducer is placed in contact with the skin (Figure 2-7). The transducer repeatedly emits brief pulses of sound at a fixed rate, called the pulse repetition frequency, or PRF. After transmitting each pulse, the transducer waits for echoes from interfaces along the sound beam path. Echo signals picked up by the transducer are amplified and processed into a format suitable for display.

The distance to a reflector is determined from the arrival time of its echo. Thus,

$$d = \frac{cT}{2} \qquad (2\text{-}5)$$

where d is the depth of the interface, T is the echo arrival time, and c is the speed of sound in the tissue. The factor 2 accounts for the round-trip journey of the sound pulse and echo. Equation 2-5 is called the *range equation* in ultrasound imaging.[8] A speed of sound of 1540 m/sec is assumed in most scanners when calculating and displaying reflector depths from echo arrival times. The corresponding echo arrival time is 13 μs/cm of the distance from the transducer to the reflector.

SIGNAL PROCESSING

To create images, pulses of sound are transmitted along various beam lines, each followed by reception and processing of resultant echo

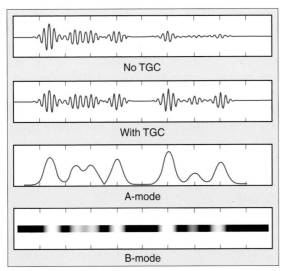

FIGURE 2-8 Signal processing for imaging. *From top to bottom*, the diagram illustrates the radio frequency signal versus depth for a single beam line; the same signal after application of time gain compensation (TGC); the demodulated, or A-mode waveform; and the B-mode display of the echoes for this line.

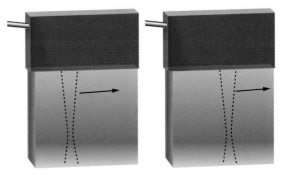

FIGURE 2-9 Ultrasound B-mode scanning using a linear array. Each sketch shows the position of an ultrasound beam line interrogating the scanned field. The resultant B-mode echo display trace changes with the position of the beam line.

signals. Imaging is done with transducer arrays, where echo signals are acquired by individual elements and are combined within a beam former into a single signal for each beam line. The role of the beam former will be discussed in more detail later. Following the beam former, echo signal processing for imaging consists of amplifying the signals; applying time gain compensation to offset effects of beam attenuation; applying nonlinear, logarithmic amplification to compress the wide range of echo signal amplitudes (called the displayed echo dynamic range) into a range that can be displayed effectively on a monitor; demodulation, which forms a single spike-like signal for each echo; and brightness-mode (B-mode) processing. The B-mode display is used in imaging. Signal processing steps are shown in Figure 2-8.

FORMING THE IMAGE

Two well-known echo display techniques are also illustrated in the lower two panels of Figure 2-8. The amplitude-mode (A-mode) display is a presentation of the echo signal amplitude versus the echo return time, or the reflector depth. This is a one-dimensional display portraying echo signals and their amplitudes along a single beam line (i.e., along one direction). In contrast, the more versatile B-mode display is used for gray-scale imaging. The display is formed by

converting echo signals to dots on a monitor, with the brightness indicating echo amplitudes.

In B-mode scanning, sound beams are swept over a region (Figure 2-9), and echo signals are registered on a two-dimensional (2D) matrix in a position that corresponds to their anatomic origin. Registration is done by placing the B-mode dots along a line that corresponds to the axis of the ultrasound beam as it sweeps across the scanned field; the proper depth of each echo is determined from the arrival time. In Figure 2-9, the sound beam is swept by electronic switching between groups of elements in a linear array transducer. The B-mode display on the monitor follows the axis of the ultrasound beam as it is swept across the imaged region. Usually, 100 to 200 or more separate ultrasound beam lines are used to construct each image. Most ultrasound systems have controls that allow the operator to vary the beam line density, either directly or indirectly when some other image-processing control is manipulated.

IMAGE MEMORY

An image memory, or *scan converter*, temporarily retains images for review and photography and converts the image format into one that can be viewed on a video monitor or that can be recorded on videotape. The scan converter is a digital device and may be thought of as a matrix of pixels (image elements); typically, 500 or more pixels are arranged vertically, and about 500 horizontally. The more pixels horizontally and vertically, the better the detail that is represented in the memory, which is particularly important if a postprocessing digital zoom is applied.

Image attributes such as the echo amplitude at each pixel location are represented using a sequence of 1s and 0s, as is the practice for digital devices. The fundamental unit of storage in a digital device is a singular entity called a bit. A single bit can take on a value of either 1 or 0, but by grouping bits into multibit storage cells, each multibit word can represent a large range of values because of the different combinations of 1 and 0 that can be accommodated. For example, "8-bit" memories divide the echo signal into 255 (2^8) different amplitude levels and store an appropriate level at each pixel location. Twelve-bit memories represent the echo amplitudes using 4096 (2^{12}) levels, and so forth. The more bits (amplitude levels), the more different shades of gray are possible from the stored image, especially during postprocessing (see later). Modern scanners also allow storage of cine loops, using a memory that can retain many separate images.

A variety of types of storage media are used in ultrasound. Some laboratories continue their use of hard copy, such as film or other print media. For studies where flow or other dynamic information must be viewed, video tape recorders can store significant quantities of information and facilitate archiving.

Today's ultrasound machines are equipped with digital storage devices, including fixed computer disks, removable magnetic media such as ZIP disks, and CD-ROMs, and these devices are used to archive study results. Software on the machine can be invoked to recall specific studies and display the image or cine loop sequence. In addition, the majority of installations now utilize computer networks for transferring images, making it possible to view study results on workstations and archive information in centrally organized digital collections. Picture archiving and communication system (PACS) software is available to do these tasks, either on the ultrasound machine itself or off-line. A standard file organization system, the Digital Imaging and Communications in Medicine (DICOM) standard, was created by the National Electrical Manufacturers Association and other standards bodies to aid in the distribution and viewing of ultrasound and other medical images created by equipment from different manufacturers. Each DICOM file contains a "header section" that has information including the patient's name, the type of scan, image dimensions, and more, as well as the image data itself. Some scanners require a converter box to accept the image data from the scanner, convert it to a DICOM file, and then transfer the file to the PACS network. More commonly, scanning machines themselves have software to convert files to DICOM format and communicate with the external PACS network. When files are in DICOM format, users with access either to the archived data on the scanning machine or from the network itself can employ DICOM readers available for workstations and personal computers to view, archive externally, print, and manipulate the image data.

FRAME RATE

In most applications, B-mode imaging is performed with "real-time" scanning machines. These machines automatically sweep ultrasound beams over the imaged region at a rapid rate, say 30 sweeps per second or higher. The *image frame rate* is the number of complete scans per second carried out by the system. Fundamentally, image frame rates are limited by the sound propagation speed in tissue. An image is produced in the machine by sending ultrasound pulses along 100 to 200 different beam directions (beam lines) into the body. For each beam line, the scanner transmits a pulse and waits for echoes along that beam line, all the way down to the maximum depth setting. Then it transmits a pulse along a new beam direction and repeats the process. Beam lines are addressed serially, meaning the scanner does not transmit a pulse along a new beam line until echoes have been picked up from the maximum depth in the previous line. The speed with which the pulse propagates through tissue, the depth setting of the scanner, the number of transmit focal zones, and the number of beam lines used to form a single image frame all intermix to establish the maximal possible image frame rate.

Using the range equation, if the maximum depth setting is D, it takes a time $(T = 2D/c)$ to receive echoes from the entire beam line. The amount of time for a complete image frame constructed with data from N beam lines is simply $N \times T$, or $2 ND/c$. If the maximum frame rate is FR_{max}, FR_{max} will be equal to the inverse of the time needed for a complete image. This may be written as

$$FR_{max} = \frac{1}{NT} = \frac{c}{2ND} \qquad (2\text{-}6)$$

For soft tissue in which the speed of sound is about 1540 m/sec, or 154,000 cm/sec, if the depth setting *(D)* is expressed in centimeters, Equation 2-6 also works out to

$$FR_{\max} = \frac{77,000}{ND(\text{cm})} \text{ Hz} \qquad (2\text{-}7)$$

For example, with $N = 200$ beam lines and an image depth of 15.4 cm, $FR_{\max}$ is 25 Hz.

Operators can easily verify that reducing the depth setting on the machine will increase the frame rate, and vice versa. Often, the machine is programmed to provide as high a frame rate as is practical for the operator settings. Some machines allow the operator to change N, the number of beam lines used to form the image, for example, by increasing the angular separation between beam lines. This, in turn, also affects the frame rate, as does changing the horizontal size of the image and changing the number of transmit focal zones.

TRANSDUCER PROPERTIES

An ultrasound transducer provides the communicating link between the imaging system and the patient. Medical ultrasound transducers use piezoelectric ceramic elements to generate and detect sound waves. Piezoelectric materials convert electric signals into mechanical vibrations and pressure waves into electric signals. The elements, therefore, serve a dual role of pulse transmission and echo detection.

Internal components of an array transducer are shown in Figure 2-10. In the figure, the elements are seen from the side, and the ultrasound waves would be projected upward. The thickness of the piezoelectric element governs the resonance frequency of the transducer. Quarter-wave matching layers between the piezoelectric elements and a protective outer faceplate are used on most transducers. Analogous to special optical coatings on lenses and on picture frame glass, the matching layers improve sound transmission between the transducer and the patient. This improves the transducer's sensitivity to weak echoes. Backing material is often used in pulse-echo applications to dampen the element vibrations after the transducer is excited with an electric impulse. Dampening shortens the duration of the transmitted pulse, improving the axial (or range) resolution. With optimized designs of the matching and backing layers, transducers can be made to operate over a range of frequencies. Hence, ultrasound machines provide a frequency control switch that

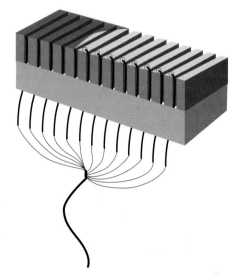

FIGURE 2-10 Drawing of an array transducer. A number of rectangular-shaped piezoelectric elements are mounted side by side within the array housing.

the operator manipulates to select the frequency from a menu of choices available for each probe. Some transducers have sufficient frequency range that harmonic imaging can be done, where a low-frequency transmit pulse is sent out, and echoes whose frequency is twice that transmitted are detected and used in imaging.

TYPES OF TRANSDUCERS

The operation of three principal types of array transducers is presented in Figure 2-11. The most important transducer for peripheral vascular applications is the "linear array." "Curvilinear arrays" and "phased arrays" also are used in the clinic but mainly for imaging deeper structures in the body. Their use in imaging superficial vessels is rather limited.

Linear (Sequential) Array Scanner

An array of perhaps 200 separate rectangularly shaped transducer elements is arranged side by side in the transducer housing. Conceptually, groups of perhaps 15 to 20 elements are activated simultaneously to produce each ultrasound beam. The beam line would be centered over the central element in the group, except when beam lines are near the lateral margins of the image and an asymmetric element arrangement would be used. An image frame is initiated by a group of elements on one end of the array. The group transmits a pulsed beam and collects the echo signals for this beam line. The active element group

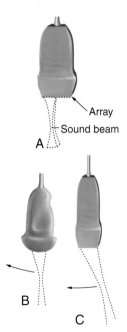

A
Array
Sound beam

B
C

FIGURE 2-11 Transducer types. **A,** Linear array transducer. **B,** Curvilinear array scanner. **C,** Phased array scanner.

is shifted (translated) by one element, forming a new element group, and the pulse-echo process is repeated along a second, parallel beam line. The active element group progresses from one end of the array to the other by switching among the elements. Beam lines are parallel to one another, and the resultant image format is rectangular.

The linear array image format may be expanded by applying "beam steering" that directs additional ultrasound beams at angles lateral to the transducer footprint. This approach borrows from phased-array transducer scanning methods, described later. It broadens the imaged field, particularly at depths away from the source, and improves overall visualization of mid-depth to deep structures.

Curvilinear Array Scanner

These arrays are similar to the linear array, only the elements are arranged along a convex scanning surface. The method for image formation is identical to that of the linear array, in which the active element group is switched progressively from one side of the array to the next. The fan-like arrangement of the element supports results in a sector shape for the imaged field. Compared with the linear array, the curved array provides a wider image at large depths from a narrow scanning window on the patient surface.

Phased-Array Scanner

Phased-array scanners consist of an array of 120 or so very narrow rectangular elements arranged side by side. In contrast to the operation of the linear and curvilinear arrays, all elements in the phased array are used for each beam line. The ultrasound beam is "steered" by introducing small time delays between the transmit pulses applied to individual elements. Time delays are also applied among echo signals picked up from individual elements during reception, steering the received directionality as well. An image is formed using perhaps 100 beams steered in different directions. The advantage of the phased array is that it provides a very broad imaged field at large depths, and this is done with a narrow transducer footprint. The transducer readily fits between the ribs or underneath the rib cage for cardiac scanning. It also makes easy the search for scanning windows in the abdomen, where wound dressings or gas bodies may be present to impede ultrasound beam transmission.

AXIAL RESOLUTION, LATERAL RESOLUTION, AND SLICE THICKNESS

Spatial resolution describes the minimum spacing between two reflectors for which they can be distinguished on the display. Important factors are the axial resolution, the lateral resolution, and the slice thickness. These define a "resolution cell," as illustrated in Figure 2-12. Like the size of a paintbrush affecting the detail on a painting, the dimensions of the resolution cell ultimately limit the tissue detail that can be resolved on an ultrasound image.

Axial resolution is the ability to resolve reflectors that are closely spaced along a sound beam axis. It is determined by the pulse duration, the length of time the transducer oscillates for each transmit pulse. Short-duration pulses enable the axial resolution to be 1 mm or less in imaging applications. Damping material attached to the back of the elements helps reduce the pulse duration and improve axial resolution. Axial resolution is considerably better at higher frequencies (Figure 2-13) because pulse durations can be made much shorter than at low frequencies. A measurement of the intima-media thickness of a blood vessel requires excellent axial resolution to visualize the interfaces and enable the operator to position the distance measuring cursors for an accurate result (Figure 2-14).

Lateral resolution refers to the closest possible reflector spacing perpendicular to the beam that

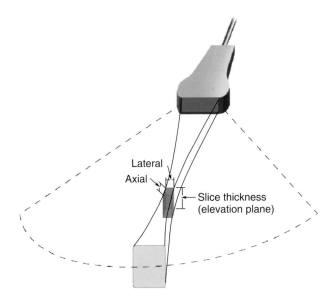

FIGURE 2-12 Typical pulse dimensions emerging from an ultrasound transducer along a single beam line. The pulse duration affects the axial resolution. The width of the beam in the scanning plane determines lateral resolution, whereas the dimensions of the beam perpendicular to the scanning plane determine the slice thickness.

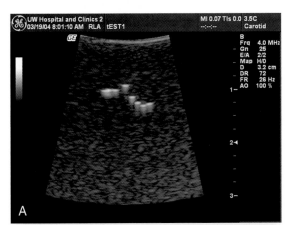

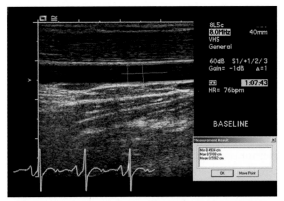

FIGURE 2-14 Intima-media thickness measurements in a brachial artery. Axial resolution is important in being able to make these measurements with high precision.

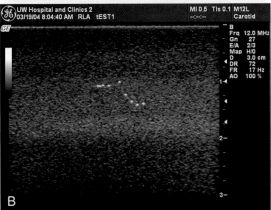

FIGURE 2-13 Images of a test object for determining resolution. The reflectors are spaced axially by 2 mm, 1 mm, 0.5 mm, and 0.2 mm. The horizontal row also has reflectors spaced at 2 mm, 1 mm, 0.5 mm, and 0.2 mm. **A,** Image obtained using a transducer running at 4 MHz. **B,** Image obtained using an 11-MHz setting on a different probe.

allows them to be distinguished. It is determined by the width of the ultrasound beam at the location of the reflectors. Beam forming with array imaging systems is a two-step process, first involving shaping a transmitted field and then focusing the sensitivity pattern during echo reception.[5]

The transmitted field from an individual element would spread quickly with distance if it were driven in isolation because the element is narrow. However, when a group of elements is excited, a directional beam can be formed. This beam can be focused by applying infinitesimal time delays to the transmit pulses applied to individual elements, exciting the outer elements of the group a little earlier than the neighboring inner ones, and so on, as in Figure 2-15. When the operator adjusts the "focus" of a machine, he or she is changing the focal distance of the transmitted beam. The machine responds by adjusting the precise arrangement of the time delays applied to the individual elements producing the beam. Focusing narrows the ultrasound beam at the focal depth. Multiple transmit focal depths are also possible. Usually, this is done by sending several different transmit pulses along each beam line, each transmit pulse focused at a slightly different depth. Because the system must wait for echoes from the focal zone of the previous transmit pulse before a subsequent transmit can be initiated, image frame rate suffers when multiple transmit foci are applied.

Focusing is also done on the received echoes. After a transmit pulse, echoes are picked up by each element of the active aperture. These are digitized and sent to the digital "beam former." The beam former combines the digital signals from each of the array elements and adds them together, forming one extended signal for each transmit pulse. However, the echo from any reflector will need to travel slightly different distances to be picked up by the different array elements. This will create phase differences between the signals from the individual elements. This is corrected by "receive focusing," where precisely programmed focusing time delays are applied to the individual signals before summation. The required delay pattern for focusing must change as echoes arrive from progressively greater depths following the transmit pulse. Therefore, the receive beam former is designed to adjust the time delays in real time. So-called "dynamic receive focusing" enables the

receive focus of the array to track the depth of the reflector as echoes arrive from deeper and deeper structures. Dynamic receive focusing is not affected directly by the transmit focus adjustment done by the operator, but rather it is internal to the machine. Some machines even run parallel beam formers during reception, creating several dynamically focused received echo beam lines for each transmit pulse.

Focusing reduces the beam width and improves the lateral resolution over a volume called the *focal region*. The beam width *(W)* in the focal region is approximated by

$$W = \frac{1.2\lambda F}{A} \qquad (2\text{-}8)$$

where F is the focal distance, A is the aperture (i.e., the length of the active part of the transducer when signals are picked up), and λ is the wavelength. Higher-frequency transducers, for which the wavelength is smaller, provide narrower sound beams and better lateral resolution than lower-frequency transducers. For a given focal depth, the larger the aperture, the narrower is the beam. Often, a system will employ a dynamically changing aperture, increasing A as the echoes arrive from progressively deeper structures, which maintains approximately the same pulse-echo beam width at all depths. In Figure 2-13, the images at both frequencies also include a horizontal row of reflectors, where the separation is from 2 mm to 0.25 mm. As is clearly seen, the detail is much better in the image obtained at a higher ultrasound frequency.

The *slice thickness* is the thickness of the scanned section of tissue that contributes to the image. It depends on the width of the ultrasound beam perpendicular to the image plane (see Figure 2-12), often called the elevational beam width. Many phased, linear, and curvilinear array transducers still use a one-dimensional array (Figure 2-16) along with a mechanical lens to provide focusing in this direction. While the in-plane beam width and, hence, the lateral resolution are exquisitely controlled by electronic focusing, the slice thickness for these units is not. The elevational focusing mechanical lens provides good detail near the focal zone but poor detail at depths proximal and distal to this zone (see Figure 2-16, *B*). Not surprisingly, therefore, slice thickness is the worst aspect of the resolution of array transducers.

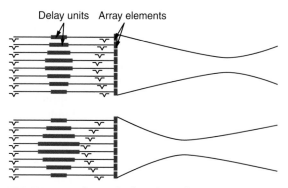

Delay units   Array elements

FIGURE 2-15 Electronic focusing of an array during pulse transmission. By exciting the outer elements of an array group slightly before the inner elements in the sequence shown, the waves from individual elements converge, forming a focused beam. The transmit focal distance is user selectable.

Manufacturers are rapidly developing "multi-D," such as "one-and-a-half–dimensional" arrays that will enable electronic focusing in the slice thickness as well as in the lateral direction (Figure 2-17). These arrays, though more complex and expensive, significantly improve the resolution of small spherical objects, as illustrated in Figure 2-17, *B*.

Transducers that are used with stand-alone CW Doppler units are not intended for imaging and therefore are much simpler. Most employ two elements, one for continuously transmitting and the other for receiving echoes. To detect echo signals from scatterers, the beams from the transmitter and the receiver are caused to overlap. This is done by inclining the transducer elements or by using focusing lenses. The area of beam overlap defines the most sensitive region of the CW transducer.

PRINCIPAL SCANNER CONTROLS

Ultrasound machine operators must be familiar with many instrument controls to produce optimal images with their equipment. Details and examples of different control settings can be found in standard textbooks.[5,8] The major controls found on scanners include the following:

- Transducer select, to activate one of two to four probes physically attached to transducer ports on the machine.
- Transducer frequency select, to select the center frequency of ultrasound pulses emitted by the transducer. Modern transducers can produce ultrasound beams covering a range of frequencies. This control is used to determine which frequencies are used in the image.
- Depth setting, to select the size of the imaged field.
- Transmit focus, to enable users to set the number and depth of transmit beam focal zones.
- Output power control, to vary the scanner sensitivity. Increasing the transmit power allows the operator to view weaker echo signals from the body. (Higher transmit power levels also increase the acoustic exposure to the patient.)
- Overall receiver gain, also to vary the scanner sensitivity. Gain describes the amount of amplification of echoes in the receiver.

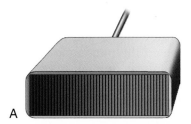

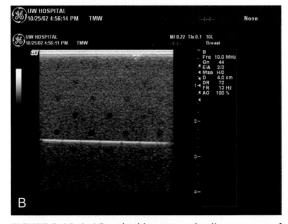

FIGURE 2-16 **A,** View looking toward a linear array of typical element cuts. **B,** Image of a test phantom containing 2.4-mm diameter spherical targets. Only targets in the mid-range for this transducer are visualized.

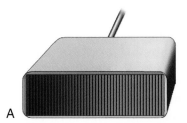

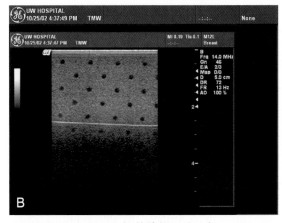

FIGURE 2-17 **A,** One-and-a-half dimensional array. **B,** Image of the same test phantom as in Figure 2-16, using a one-and-a-half-dimensional array.

Higher gains apply more amplification than lower gains; overall gain adjusts the gain throughout the imaged field.

- Time gain compensation, to compensate for attenuation of the ultrasound beam in tissue. With time gain compensation, the receiver amplification increases automatically with the depth of origin of the echoes, so echo signals from deep structures, which have undergone significant attenuation, are amplified more than signals from shallow structures that have undergone less attenuation. Time gain compensation is controlled in most machines using a set of six to eight gain knobs, each adjusting the receiver gain at a different depth.
- Compression, to vary the amplitude range (dynamic range) of echoes displayed as shades of gray on the image. Most machines apply logarithmic compression to the echo signals emerging from the receiver; the amount of compression is under user control.
- Other preprocessing, to alter the echo signals before they are sent to the scan converter. Some machines, for example, apply edge-enhancing filters to the signals. Others allow the operator to vary the "beam line density," packing more beam lines into the image in hopes of improving image quality but trading off image frame rate.
- Postprocessing, to change the appearance of echo signals, already stored in memory, on the image. Various postprocessing curves are available, each emphasizing different portions of the echo amplitudes stored in the image memory.
- Persistence, to include the images from several successive sweeps of the transducer with the current image. High persistence has the effect of smoothing out the image but at the expense of losing some temporal detail.

SPECIAL PROCESSING TECHNIQUES

COMPOUND IMAGING

B-mode images produced using conventional linear or curvilinear arrays appear "granular" or noisy, and this can contribute to uncertainties when interpreting scan results. The granular pattern originates from two sources. First, ultrasound images are subject to a process called speckle, which leads to the random arrangement of B-mode dots on images of organs. The speckle pattern originates from the presence of many unresolvable scatterers that contribute to the echo signal at each location in the image. Once the number of scatterers gets so dense that the imaging machine cannot resolve them, a distribution of dots occurs, whose origin is the underlying, random arrangement of scatterers. The second reason images appear noisy is that small surface reflectors, such as tissue boundaries, muscle fascia, and vessel walls, often are at an unfavorable angle to the incident ultrasound beam. Echoes are difficult to pick up, or are even lost, when the surface is at a steep angle (not perpendicular) to the ultrasound beam.

Compound imaging[5,9] addresses both of these issues by sweeping ultrasound beams that are oriented at different angles across the imaged region (Figure 2-18). The speckle pattern from any location will vary with the direction of the incident beam, because the positions of the individual scatterers relative to the ultrasound beam axis will differ. Therefore, by averaging the angled image data at each location, a smoother pattern can be produced. This improvement in image quality results in greater ability to visualize regions that exhibit subtle changes in echogenicity compared with the background tissue. Additionally, with interrogating beams incident at various angles, surfaces that may not be favorably inclined to the ultrasound beam for one beam direction may turn out to be so for other angles in the compound acquisition. Thus, there usually is more complete outlining of structural boundaries.

Figure 2-18 shows only three acquisition angles, but as many as 9 to 10 are available in some imaging systems. In these systems, operators can choose between different levels of compounding

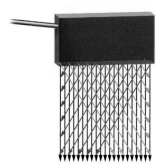

FIGURE 2-18 Compound scanning with a linear array transducer. Echo data resulting from scans done at several beam angles are superimposed on the same image.

when scanning. A greater degree of compounding requires longer scanning times and, hence, lower image frame rates.

HARMONIC IMAGING

We mentioned earlier that sound pulses undergo nonlinear distortion as they propagate through tissue (Figure 2-19). The distortion is accompanied by the production of harmonic frequencies (i.e., added components to the pulse that are integral multiples of the fundamental transmitted pulse frequency). A 2-MHz incident pulse has harmonic components of 4-MHz, 6-MHz, and so on, and echoes will contain mixtures of fundamental and harmonic components. These components, while not present in the transmit pulse emitted by the transducer, build gradually as the pulse makes its way deeper into the tissue. Because this is a nonlinear phenomenon, higher-amplitude pulses undergo much more distortion than lower-amplitude pulses, and the central portion of the ultrasound beam, where the beam intensity is highest, undergoes greater harmonic conversion than the weak edges of the beam.

Although the existence of harmonic distortion in ultrasound has been known for some time, the means to exploit this phenomenon has been only recently incorporated into ultrasound instruments. "Tissue harmonic imaging" is done by filtering out the low-frequency, fundamental components of the ultrasound echoes and using the second harmonic components to form B-mode images. Two signal processing approaches are common.[7] The first applies

frequency filtering to isolate the second harmonic frequency component of echo signals from the fundamental. The second method applies "pulse inversion" techniques, explained later.

The frequency filtering methods require special pulse shaping applied to the transmit pulse to ensure that there is no overlap between echoes within the fundamental frequency band and those in the harmonic spectrum. A short-duration pulse, optimized for achieving high axial resolution by its nature, contains a spectrum of frequencies; the shorter the pulse, the wider the range of frequencies. The filtering method sometimes is referred to as "narrow-band harmonics" because of the need to restrict the frequencies in the transmit pulse to be sure the higher-frequency components in the much stronger fundamental frequency echoes do not overlap with the low-frequency components of the harmonic echoes. Harmonics tend to be of much lower amplitude than the fundamental, so a significant overlap would offset the benefits to be gained in employing the harmonic mode.

The pulse inversion approach requires two transmit pulses along the same beam line (Figure 2-20). The first is a conventional imaging pulse of short duration and wide-frequency bandwidth. After echoes are collected for this transmit pulse, a second pulse is launched that is 180 degrees out of phase (i.e., the exact negative of the first pulse). The resultant echo signals from the two pulse-echo sequences are then added. For linear propagation, the two echoes should cancel each other, and no signal would be displayed along that beam line. However, when significant nonlinear propagation occurs, the echo signals from the different-shaped transmit pulses will not cancel, because the nonlinear distortion occurs more for the positive-going, compressional half cycles of the wave than for the negative, rarefactional half cycles. The noncanceling part is the harmonic signal (see Figure 2-20, *B*). The apparent advantage of pulse or phase inversion over narrow-band harmonics is the use of shorter-duration pulses with their inherently better axial resolution. A disadvantage of pulse inversion is the need to employ two transmit pulse-echo sequences for each beam line, decreasing the image frame rate.

Either method is supposed to help reduce reverberation noise in images and thus improve image quality. An example is presented in Figure 2-21. The echoes within this cystic mass in the breast are caused by reverberation of parts of the

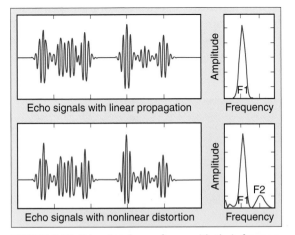

FIGURE 2-19 Echo signal waveforms with their frequency spectra for linear propagation *(top)* and nonlinear propagation *(bottom)* through tissues, with generation of harmonic signals.

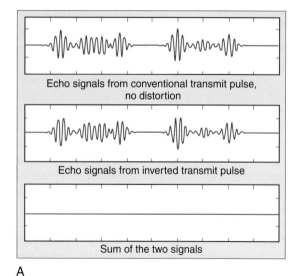

A

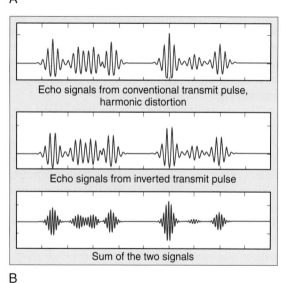

B

FIGURE 2-20 Pulse-inversion technique for extracting harmonic signals. Echoes from two successive pulse transmissions, one with a conventional pulse, the other with a pulse that is the exact negative of the first, are added. Linear parts of the echoes cancel **(A)**, whereas the harmonics combine **(B)**.

incident pulse as it progresses through the tissue layers proximal to the mass. Harmonic echoes are not as strongly affected by the reverberations taking place in the overlying tissues, because the harmonic components have not yet built up to an appreciable degree when the incident pulse is near the skin surface.

IMAGING WITH CONTRAST AGENTS

It is possible to enhance the echo signals from a region if small gas bubbles are present. This is exactly how contrast agents may be used to enhance the echo signals from blood. Ultrasound contrast agents consist of tiny gas bubbles, either air or a heavy molecular weight gas, stabilized with a type of shell. One of the earliest contrast agents available was Albunex (Mallinckrodt Medical, St. Louis, MO), manufactured by sonicating human serum albumin in the presence of air. A number of similar agents have evolved and are available commercially, each having a particular shell material or gas. The bubble sizes commonly are in the 1- to 5-μm range. Even though bubbles are small, they can produce large-amplitude echoes and so are used to intensify echoes from small blood vessels and sometimes from the chambers of the heart.

Special properties of gas bubbles can be exploited to help distinguish between echoes from contrast agents and echoes from tissues that have no agent present.[10] The first property is the ease with which the bubbles reflect nonlinearly, producing echoes not only of the frequency transmitted by the transducer but also at harmonics of the transmitted frequency. For example, when 3-MHz waves are reflected by contrast agent bubbles, fundamental (3-MHz), second harmonic (6-MHz), and higher, as well as subharmonic (1.5-MHz) echoes result. Tuning the scanner to pick out the harmonic frequencies helps isolate

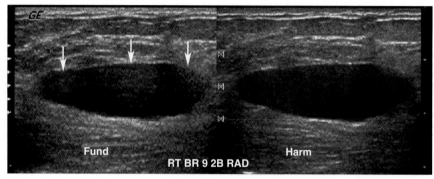

FIGURE 2-21 Image of a breast cyst with conventional processing *(left)* and with harmonic processing *(right)*.

the echo signals from the contrast agent. Ultrasound machines set up for contrast agent imaging sometimes apply complex pulse-echo sequences, where the resultant echoes can be combined in a way that draws out the echoes resulting from nonlinear reflections from the bubbles and cancels the echoes from other reflectors.

Another property that can be exploited in their detection is that contrast agent bubbles are easily destroyed by high-amplitude ultrasound pulses. Thus, bubbles are detected by transmitting a high-amplitude destructive pulse, collecting the echoes, then transmitting a second pulse and comparing the echoes from the two. Echoes from the contrast agent bubbles would be present for the first pulse but absent for the second because of the destructive effects of the first pulse. Manipulation of the echo signals is done to isolate signals from the agent only, which is sometimes useful to detect flow in small vessels. Ultrasound machines with contrast agent imaging modes may thus implement special pulse sequences to draw out the echo signal from the agent itself.

CODES AND CHIRPS

To achieve the best spatial resolution, equipment operators attempt to use as high an ultrasound frequency as possible when scanning. Unfortunately, high ultrasound frequencies are severely attenuated, so the need for adequate beam penetration usually limits the frequency that can be effectively used. If it were possible to increase the transmit power, sending more energetic pulses into the tissues, this might improve penetration of these high frequencies somewhat. The transmit power can be increased by increasing the amplitude of the ultrasound pulse emitted by the transducer. This works only up to a point, however, because nonlinear distortion, equipment limitations, and regulations on ultrasound equipment for safety purposes result in limitations on the amplitude of the transmitted pulses from the transducer. Related to the question of potential biologic effects, current practice by the U.S. Food and Drug Administration requires manufacturers of ultrasound equipment to limit the amplitude of the transmitted pulse to levels that have MI values of 1.9 or less.

Another way to provide a more energetic transmit pulse without exceeding the amplitude limits or equipment capabilities is to make the pulse duration longer. However, it is first necessary to encode the pulse in a special way that would enable recovery of a short-duration pulse with its accompanying good axial resolution after echoes are received. Use of "coded excitation" is one means of achieving this.

Coded excitation applies a unique signature to the transmitted ultrasound pulse. The pulse itself has a very long duration compared with conventional pulses applied in ultrasound. However, it is modulated by a specific pattern of 1s and 0s before being applied to the transducer. An example of a waveform detected from one manufacturer's coded transmit by a detector in water is presented in Figure 2-22. This long-duration transmit pulse undergoes reflections at interfaces, and echoes are detected once again by the transducer. After amplification and beam forming, the echo signals are sent to a special decoding process, often referred to as a matched filter, to recover signals exhibiting short-duration pulse properties. Certain codes require two pulse-echo sequences, each transmit pulse having slightly different timing features but the two together having complementary properties. When echo signals are combined, the process eliminates artifacts known as range side-lobes that sometimes

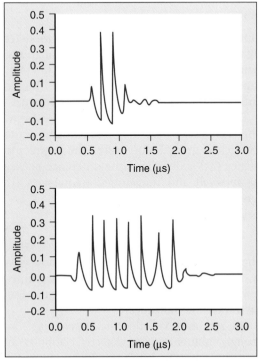

FIGURE 2-22 Comparison of transmitted waveforms using conventional pulsing *(top)* and coded excitation *(bottom)*. The short-duration nature of the system response is recovered following coded excitation by applying special decoding, or matched filter schemes.

are present when codes are used. Nevertheless, with coded excitation methods, it is possible to recover both the effects of having a short-duration pulse and a pulse of much higher amplitude.

Another type of code is a "chirp pulse."[11] A chirp is a brief transmit burst, or pulse, whose frequency varies over the pulse duration. Again, special decoding schemes allow the original short pulse duration to be recovered while providing much better beam penetration than would be provided with conventional, short-duration pulse transmission.

DOPPLER ULTRASOUND

The Doppler effect is a change in the frequency of a detected wave when the source or the detector is moving. In medical ultrasonography, a Doppler shift occurs when reflectors move relative to the transducer. The frequency of echo signals from moving reflectors is higher or lower than the frequency transmitted by the transducer, depending on whether the motion is toward or away from the transducer. The Doppler shift frequency, or simply the Doppler frequency, is the difference between the received and transmitted frequencies.

DOPPLER EQUATION

Ultrasonic Doppler equipment is used for detecting and evaluating blood flow. A typical arrangement is illustrated in Figure 2-23. An ultrasonic transducer is placed in contact with the skin surface; it transmits a beam whose frequency is f_o. The received frequency f_R will differ from f_o when echoes are picked up from moving scatterers, such as the red blood cells. The Doppler frequency (f_D) is defined as the difference between the received and transmitted frequencies. The f_D is calculated by the following:

$$f_D = f_R - f_o = \frac{2f_o V \cos\theta}{c} \qquad (2\text{-}9)$$

where c is the speed of sound, V is the flow velocity, and θ is the angle between the direction of flow and the axis of the ultrasound beam, looking toward the transducer.

The symbol θ is called the *Doppler angle* and strongly influences the detected Doppler frequency for a given reflector velocity. When flow is directly toward the transducer, θ is 0 degrees and $\cos\theta$ is 1. The Doppler frequency detected for this orientation would be the maximum one could obtain for the flow conditions. More

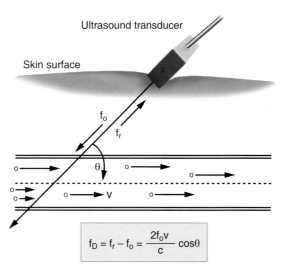

$$f_D = f_r - f_o = \frac{2f_o v}{c} \cos\theta$$

FIGURE 2-23 Arrangement for detecting Doppler signals from blood. The angle θ is the Doppler angle, which is the angle between the direction of motion and the beam axis, looking toward the transducer.

typically, the ultrasound beam will be incident at an angle other than 0 degrees, and the detected Doppler frequency will be reduced according to the $\cos\theta$ term. For example, at 30 degrees, the Doppler frequency would be 0.87 multiplied by what it is at 0 degrees; at 60 degrees, it would be 0.5 multiplied by its 0-degree value. Finally, when the flow is perpendicular to the ultrasound beam direction, θ is 90 degrees and $\cos\theta$ is 0; there is no detected Doppler shift! In practice, the transducer beam is usually oriented to make a 30- to 60-degree angle with the arterial lumen to receive a reliable Doppler signal.

CONTINUOUS-WAVE DOPPLER EQUIPMENT

CW Doppler is done in a variety of instruments, ranging from simple, inexpensive handheld Doppler units, to "high-end" duplex scanners in which CW Doppler is one of several operating modes. A simplified block diagram of the necessary components of a CW Doppler unit is presented in Figure 2-24. The transmitter continuously excites a transmit section of the ultrasonic transducer, sending a continuous beam whose frequency is f_o. Echoes returning to the transducer have frequency f_R. These signals are amplified in the receiver and then sent to a demodulator to extract the Doppler signal. Here, the signals are multiplied by a reference signal from the transmitter, producing a mixture of signals, part having a frequency equal to $(f_R + f_o)$ and part having

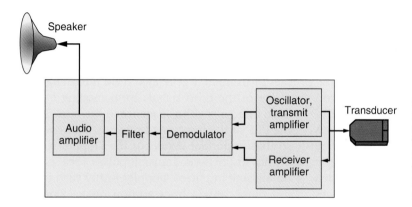

FIGURE 2-24 A continuous-wave Doppler instrument. The Doppler signal is obtained by demodulating the amplified echo signals and then applying a low-pass filter. Because the signals are generally in the audible range, a loudspeaker may be used to display the Doppler signals.

a frequency $(f_R - f_o)$. The sum frequency $(f_R + f_o)$ is very high—about twice the ultrasound frequency—and is easily removed by electronic filtering. This leaves signals with frequency $(f_R - f_o)$ at the output, which is the Doppler signal!

What are typical Doppler frequencies for blood flow? Suppose V = 20 cm/sec; the ultrasound frequency (f_o) is 5 MHz (5×10^6 cycles/sec); and the speed of sound (c) is 1540 m/sec. Let θ equal 0 degrees, so that cos θ is 1. Using Equation 2-9, we find

$$f_D = \frac{2 \times (5 \times 10^6 \text{ cycles/sec}) \times 0.2 \text{ m/sec}}{1540 \text{ m/sec}}$$
$$= 1299 \text{ cycles/sec}$$

(2-10)

or about 1.3 kHz, which is within the audible frequency range. The filtered output Doppler signal can be applied to a loudspeaker or headphones for interpretation by the operator. The signals can also be recorded on audiotape or applied to any of several spectral analysis systems (see later).

It is possible to eliminate signals of certain frequency ranges from the output. This is done in instruments that have additional electronic filters in their circuitry. For example, when studying blood flow, relatively low-frequency Doppler signals originating from movement of vessel walls may be eliminated from the output by applying a high-pass filter. The lower cutoff frequency of such "wall filters" is usually operator selectable.

CONTINUOUS-WAVE DOPPLER CONTROLS

Basic CW Doppler units usually have only a few controls, but operators should be familiar with those on their own equipment. Examples include the following:
- Transmit power, to vary the amplitude of the signal from the transmitter to the

transducer, thus changing the sensitivity to weak echoes. Some simple units omit this control, keeping the transmit level constant.
- Gain, to vary the sensitivity of the unit.
- Audio gain, to vary the loudness of Doppler signals applied to loudspeakers.
- Wall filter, to vary the low-frequency cutoff frequency of the wall filter.

DIRECTIONAL DOPPLER

A basic CW Doppler instrument allows detection of the magnitude of the Doppler frequency, but it provides no indication of whether flow is toward or away from the transducer (i.e., whether the Doppler shift is positive or negative). A common technique for determining flow direction is to use quadrature detection in the Doppler device. After the received echo signals are amplified, they are split into two identical channels for demodulation. The channels differ only in that the reference signals from the transmitter sent to the two demodulators are 90 degrees out of phase. Two separate Doppler signals are produced. They are identical except for a small phase difference between them, and this phase difference can be used to determine whether the Doppler shift is positive or negative.[12] Various schemes are used that combine the two quadrature signals to enable presentation of positive and negative flow in stereo speakers.[13]

PULSED DOPPLER

With CW Doppler instruments, reflectors and scatterers anywhere within the beam of the transducer can contribute to the instantaneous Doppler signal. A pulsed Doppler instrument provides for discrimination of Doppler signals from different depths, allowing for the detection of moving interfaces and scatterers only from within a well-defined sample volume (Figure 2-25). The sample volume can be positioned anywhere along the axis of the ultrasound beam.

The principal components of a pulsed Doppler instrument are shown in Figure 2-26. The ultrasonic transducer is excited with a short-duration burst, rather than continuously as in the CW instrument. Scattered and reflected echo signals are detected by the same transducer, amplified in the receiver, and applied to the demodulator. The output of the demodulator is then applied to a sample-and-hold circuit, which integrates (or averages) a portion of the signal, selected by a range gate. The gate position and duration are controlled by the operator. The gated signal, taken over a series of pulse-echo sequences, forms the Doppler signal heard over the loudspeaker of

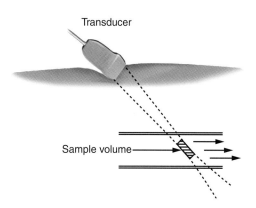

FIGURE 2-25 Sample volume in pulsed Doppler. Echo signals from a fixed depth are selected by a range gate. The size of the sample volume depends on the beam width, the duration of the gate, and the pulse duration from the transducer.

the device. In Figure 2-26, quadrature detectors are used to form two output channels, enabling the flow direction to be determined.

The Doppler signal produced by a pulsed Doppler instrument is generated from the changes in phase of the echo signals from moving targets from one pulse-echo sequence to the next. Thus, the PRF of the instrument must be high enough so that important details of the Doppler signal are not lost between transmit pulses. (See section on aliasing in pulsed Doppler.) After each transmit pulse, only a brief portion of the Doppler signal is available within the demodulated echo signals selected by the gated region. Multiple pulse-echo sequences are required to construct the Doppler signal heard over the loudspeakers. By filtering the sample-and-hold output from one pulse-echo sequence to the next, a smooth Doppler signal is formed.

DUPLEX INSTRUMENTS

A real-time B-mode imager and a Doppler instrument provide complementary information because the scanner can best outline anatomic structures, whereas a Doppler instrument yields information regarding flow and movement patterns. *Duplex ultrasound instruments* are real-time B-mode scanners with built-in Doppler capabilities. In typical applications, the pulse-echo B-mode image obtained with a duplex scanner is used to localize areas where flow is to be examined using Doppler.

The region of interest for Doppler studies may be selected on the B-mode image by placement of a sample volume indicator, or cursor (Figure 2-27). Most duplex instruments allow

Pulsed Doppler

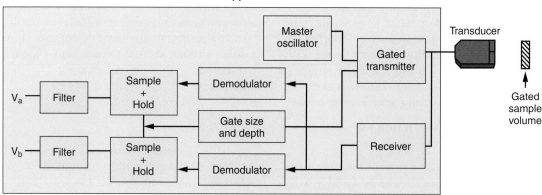

FIGURE 2-26 Principal components of a pulsed Doppler instrument. The transducer is excited by a brief pulse; echo signals are amplified in the receiver and sent to the quadrature demodulators. A portion of the demodulated waveform is held in the sample-and-hold unit, which forms the Doppler signal by using several pulse-echo sequences. V_a and V_b are quadrature signals that can be processed to indicate flow toward and away from the transducer.

the operator to indicate the Doppler angle or the direction of blood flow with respect to the ultrasound beam. The Doppler angle must be known to estimate flow velocity from the Doppler signal.

CHOICE OF ULTRASOUND FREQUENCY

Competing physical interactions govern the choice of the operating frequency employed in an ultrasound instrument. For Doppler work, the choice is usually dictated by the need to obtain adequate signal strength for reliable interpretation of Doppler signals. It was mentioned previously that the intensity of ultrasonic waves scattered from small scatterers such as red blood cells increases rapidly with increasing frequency, being proportional to the frequency raised to the fourth power. It thus would seem reasonable to use a high ultrasonic frequency to increase the intensity of scattered signals from blood. As the frequency increases, however, the rate of beam attenuation also increases (see Figure 2-3). In selecting the optimal frequency for detecting blood flow, these competing processes must be balanced, and the choice of operating frequency is often determined by the tissue depth of the vessel of interest. For small, superficial vessels, in which attenuation from overlying tissues is not significant, B-mode and Doppler probes operating at 7 to 10 MHz are commonly used. Doppler applications in the carotid artery usually employ somewhat lower frequencies to avoid significant attenuation losses, and frequencies of 4 to 5 MHz are typical. Frequencies as low as 2 MHz are used for detecting flow in deeper arteries and veins.

DOPPLER SPECTRAL ANALYSIS

For many structures of interest, the Doppler signal is in the audible frequency range. For some applications, adequate clinical interpretations can be made simply by listening to the signals. The listener then characterizes the flow according to the qualities of the audible signal.

In the case of blood flow, the Doppler signal is fairly complex because of the complicated blood velocity patterns found in most vessels. In a large blood vessel, the blood velocity is not the same at all points but follows some type of flow profile. If the ultrasound beam and the sample volume are large compared with the lumen diameter, scattered ultrasound signals are received simultaneously from blood that is moving at different velocities. The resultant Doppler signal, therefore, is complex.

A complex signal such as that shown in Figure 2-28, *A*, may be shown to be composed of many single-frequency signals (see Figure 2-28, *B*). Each of these has a particular amplitude and phase so that, when added together,

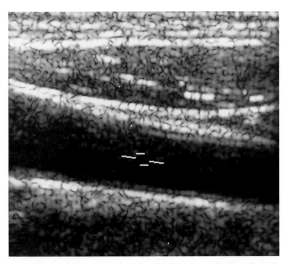

FIGURE 2-27 Image of a carotid artery obtained with a duplex ultrasound machine. A sample volume cursor is positioned to detect Doppler signals from within the artery, and a Doppler angle cursor is oriented to "angle correct" the Doppler signals for displaying the velocity.

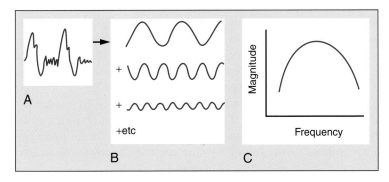

FIGURE 2-28 A complex signal waveform **(A)** can be generated by a combination of single-frequency signals **(B)**. **C,** Spectral analysis involves the separation of the complex signal into its frequency components and the display of the magnitude of each frequency component that contributes to the signal.

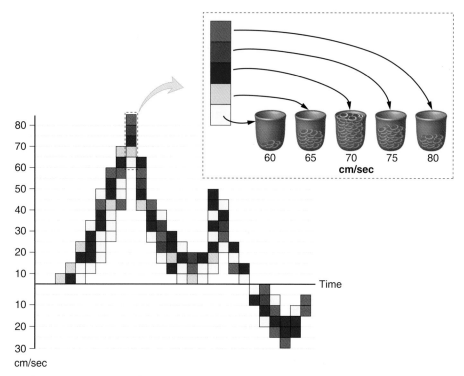

FIGURE 2-29 Information on a spectral Doppler display. Doppler frequency (or reflector velocity) is plotted vertically and time, horizontally. For each time segment, the amount of signal within specific frequency bins is indicated by a shade of gray. The amount of signal corresponds to the amount of blood flowing at the corresponding velocity.

they form the original signal. *Spectral analysis* is a way to separate a complicated signal into its individual frequency components so that the relative contribution of each frequency component to the original signal can be determined (see Figure 2-28, *C*). Often, the relative contribution is denoted by the signal power in a given frequency interval, and the spectrum is referred to as the *power spectrum.*

Most instruments use a Fast Fourier Transform to do spectral analysis of Doppler signals. The Doppler signal is fed into the spectral analyzer in small time segments (e.g., 5 msec). The power spectrum is computed and is displayed along a vertical line, where the height represents a frequency bin and the brightness represents the signal power or intensity for that bin (Figure 2-29). The relative intensity of Doppler signals depends on the amount of blood generating that signal, so the brightness of each frequency bin indicates the amount of flow at the velocity corresponding to that Doppler frequency. As the spectral signals from one segment are being displayed, a subsequent segment is being analyzed, producing a continuous display.

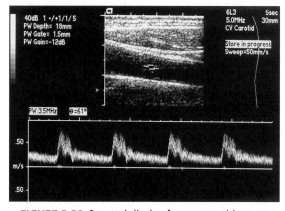

FIGURE 2-30 Spectral display from a carotid artery.

Duplex instruments display a B-mode image along with a Doppler spectral display. An example is presented in Figure 2-30. The vertical scale on the spectral display can be either Doppler frequency (in hertz) or velocity (in centimeters per second or meters per second). To display the velocity, the analyzer solves the Doppler equation to derive the velocity from the Doppler signal frequency. The spectral display is considered in detail in Chapter 3.

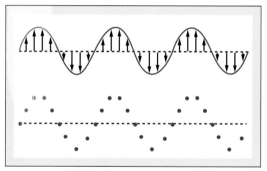

FIGURE 2-31 Sampling a Doppler signal. The *solid line* on top is a sine wave, and *arrows* represent the times when discrete samples of the signal are taken. The *dotted line* on the bottom is the sampled signal.

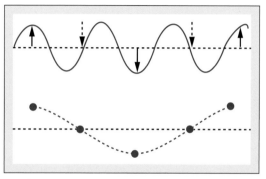

FIGURE 2-32 Production of aliasing when the sampling rate is less than two times the frequency of the signal. The upper curve is the signal, which is being sampled at the discrete times indicated by *arrows*. The lower curve is a lower frequency alias of the signal resulting from inadequate sampling.

ALIASING IN PULSED DOPPLER

With a pulsed Doppler instrument, a limitation exists on the maximum Doppler frequency that can be detected from a given depth and on the set of operating conditions. The limitation referred to is *aliasing* and, if present, can lead to anomalies on Doppler signal spectral waveforms.

Consider the situation illustrated in Figure 2-31. As mentioned earlier, a pulsed Doppler instrument forms the Doppler signal using multiple pulse-echo sequences. The Doppler signal is said to be sampled, and the sampling frequency is the PRF of the instrument. In Figure 2-31, the Doppler signal is represented by the *solid line*, and the *arrows* represent successive samples of this signal. The *lower waveform* depicts the sampled signal. In this case, the sampled signal is an excellent representation of the original signal because sampling occurred multiple times for each cycle of the original waveform.

Unfortunately, with pulsed Doppler, it is not always possible to have the PRF significantly higher than the frequency of the Doppler signal. As discussed in the next section, we must limit the PRF, so sufficient time is available to collect all signals from one pulsing of the transducer before a subsequent pulsing. This restriction on the PRF depends on the depth of the sample volume. The greater the distance to the sample volume, the longer it takes to pick up echoes from that region and the lower the PRF must be.

At a minimum, the PRF must be at least twice the frequency of the Doppler signal to construct the signal successfully. When the PRF equals twice the F_D, this is known as the *Nyquist sampling rate*. The Nyquist rate is the minimum sampling rate that can be used for a signal of a given frequency. If the sampling rate is lower than the Nyquist rate, aliasing occurs. Aliasing is a production of artifactual, lower-frequency signals when the sampling rate (the PRF) is less than twice the Doppler signal frequency.

Aliasing is illustrated schematically in Figure 2-32. The actual Doppler signal *(top)* is sampled *(arrows)* at a rate less than twice each cycle of the signal. The resulting sampled waveform (see *lower part* of Figure 2-32) is one whose frequency is less than that of the actual signal.

A common way that aliasing is manifested on a Doppler spectral display is illustrated in Figure 2-33. The Doppler spectrum wraps around the display, with high velocities being converted to reversed flow immediately at the point of aliasing and still higher velocities in the flow signal appearing as progressively lower velocities.

Several methods are used to eliminate aliasing. It can often be eliminated by increasing the velocity/frequency scale limits of the spectral display (see Figure 2-33, *B*). When the scale is increased, the Doppler instrument increases the PRF, keeping it at the Nyquist limit for the maximum Doppler frequency shown on the spectral scale. The operator can also adjust the spectral baseline, the line representing 0 velocity, assigning the entire spectral display to flow moving in just one direction (see Figure 2-33, *C*). This is successful when flow is in one direction only. Yet another way to eliminate aliasing may be to use a lower-frequency transducer. The Doppler frequency is proportional to both the reflector velocity and the ultrasound frequency (f_o), so a lower ultrasound frequency results in a lower-frequency Doppler signal for a given velocity.

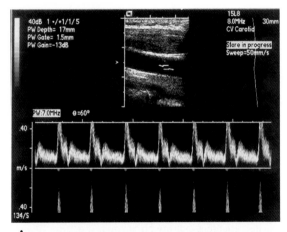

A

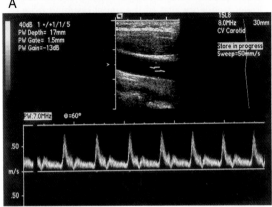

B

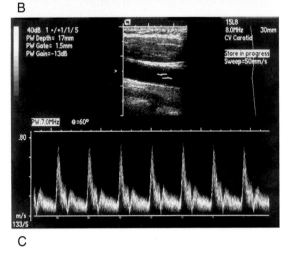

C

FIGURE 2-33 Manifestation of aliasing on a spectral display. **A,** The spectrum warps around. **B,** Correction of aliasing by increasing the velocity scale on the machine. **C,** Elimination of aliasing by adjusting the baseline.

MAXIMUM VELOCITY DETECTABLE WITH PULSED DOPPLER

As mentioned earlier, to detect a Doppler signal without aliasing, the PRF of the instrument must be at least twice the Doppler frequency. An

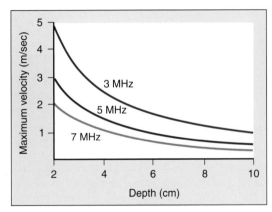

FIGURE 2-34 Maximum velocity detectable with pulsed Doppler versus sample volume depth for three different ultrasound frequencies.

upper limit on the PRF is established, however, by the time interval required for ultrasound pulses to propagate to the range of interest and return. If the time between pulses is insufficient, "range ambiguities" arise because of overlap of echoes from successive pulses. With the sample volume set at depth d, the minimum time needed between pulses (T_d) is $2d/c$ (from the range equation). The maximum PRF possible, PRF_{max}, is just the inverse of T_d. Thus,

$$PRF_{max} = 1/T_d = c/2d \qquad (2\text{-}11)$$

What is the highest flow velocity that can be detected, given the limitation expressed in Equation 2-9? The maximum Doppler frequency we can detect without aliasing will now be $PRF_{max}/2 = c/4d$. Using the Doppler equation and substituting for f_D, we get

$$\frac{2f_o V_{max}}{c} = \frac{c}{4d} \qquad (2\text{-}12)$$

where V_{max} is the maximum velocity detectable without aliasing. Solving for V_{max},

$$V_{max} = \frac{c^2}{8f_o d} \qquad (2\text{-}13)$$

Assuming a speed of sound of 1540 m/sec, the plots in Figure 2-34 were generated using Equation 2-10, relating the maximum reflector velocity that can be detected to reflector depth for three different ultrasound frequencies. As the sample volume depth increases, the maximum detectable Doppler signal frequency, and hence the maximum reflector velocity that can be detected, decreases. At any depth, lower ultrasound frequencies permit detection of greater velocities than higher frequencies.

In some instruments, higher velocities than those shown in Figure 2-34 can be obtained using a "high PRF" selection. In this mode, the PRF of the instrument is allowed to be increased beyond the limit set by Equation 2-9. Now, range ambiguity is present because the echo data from successive transmit pulses overlap. This is indicated on the display by the presence of multiple sample volumes displayed on the image. In general, however, the range ambiguities are not a problem, because the operator already has the area of flow sampling isolated before activating high PRF, and the exact origin of the Doppler signals is still known.

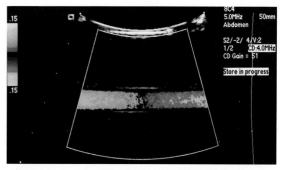

FIGURE 2-35 Color flow image of a horizontal vessel in a flow phantom. Flow is from left to right on the image, so for the sector transducer, it is directed toward the transducer on the left-hand side of the image and away from the transducer on the right-hand side.

COLOR FLOW IMAGING

FORMING COLOR IMAGES

Color flow imaging (or color velocity imaging) is done by estimating and displaying the mean velocity relative to the ultrasound beam direction of scatterers and reflectors in a scanned region. Echo signals from moving reflectors are generally displayed so that the color hue, saturation, or brightness indicates the relative velocity. Color flow image data are superimposed on B-mode data from stationary structures to obtain a composite image.

Several methods for processing echo signals to produce color flow images have been described. Some of these operate on the signals produced after Doppler signal processing,[5,14,15] whereas a few process echo signals directly.[16] (Specific mathematical details of the methods are given in the references, especially references 14 and 16.) For each method, a series of pulse-echo sequences are produced along a single-beam axis. Echo signals from each succeeding transmit pulse are compared with signals from those of the previous pulse, and phase shifts in the succeeding signals are then estimated. Once this is done for all pulse-echo sequences along the beam line, a mean Doppler frequency shift and, hence, a mean velocity are calculated. This process is carried out at all locations along the beam line, and the estimated velocity is displayed using a color. Then, another beam line is interrogated, and so on.

With most instruments, 10 or more transmit-receive sequences might be used to produce an estimate of mean reflector velocities along each beam line. The term *pulse packets* has been adopted to designate the transmit-receive pulse-echo sequences, with *packet size* designating the number of such sequences along each beam line.[17] Some instruments allow the operator to vary the packet size directly; most vary the packet size when the operator changes other control settings, such as color preprocessing.

Because data for each acoustic line that forms a color velocity image are acquired using multiple pulse-echo sequences, frame rates in color flow imaging tend to be lower than frame rates in standard B-mode imaging. In color flow imaging, noticeable tradeoffs are evident among factors affecting color-image quality and scanning speed or frame rate. Most instruments provide signal processing controls that allow the user to optimize imaging parameters for specific applications. Higher frame rates are often accompanied by reduced image quality, because fewer acoustic lines are used to form the image. In contrast, very detailed color images, sensitive to low-flow states, are frequently obtained at the expense of lower frame rates.

The direction of blood flow is indicated by the display color; for example, red might encode flow toward the transducer, and blue, away from the transducer. It should be kept in mind that the color processor displays motion relative to the ultrasound beam direction for each beam line forming the flow image. Different parts of a vessel are often interrogated from different beam directions, either because of the orientation of the vessel or as a result of the transducer scan format. The latter problem is illustrated in Figure 2-35, in which continuous flow through a horizontal vessel appears both blue (away) and red (toward) because of the different beam angles that interrogate the vessel when a sector scanner is used.

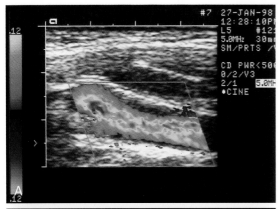

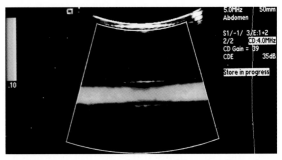

FIGURE 2-37 Power-mode image of the same flow phantom as in Figure 2-35. The energy mode image is almost insensitive to the Doppler angle.

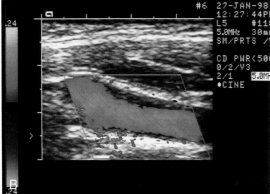

FIGURE 2-36 Aliasing in color flow imaging. **A,** Color flow image of a carotid artery, with aliasing. **B,** Same as in **A,** only the velocity scale has been adjusted to eliminate aliasing.

ALIASING ON COLOR DISPLAYS

The color velocity image is produced with pulsed Doppler techniques; therefore, the image is subject to aliasing, as discussed previously. A common manifestation of aliasing is a wraparound of the display, resulting in an apparent reversal of the flow direction (Figure 2-36, A). For example, aliased flow toward the probe is interpreted as flow moving away. Increasing the color flow velocity scale essentially increases the PRF of the processor and eliminates the aliasing problem if flow velocities remain within the allowable range of velocities on the instrument (see Figure 2-36, B). Also, changing the color baseline (the zero-flow position on the spectral display) can shift the allowable Doppler frequency range; this method is effective when flow signals are only in one direction.

ENERGY MODE IMAGING

Color flow imaging displays scatterer velocities relative to the interrogating ultrasound beam direction at positions throughout the scanned field. An alternative processing method ignores the velocity and simply estimates the strength (or power or energy) of the Doppler signal detected from each location. So-called power or energy mode imaging[18] has both advantages and limitations.

An energy mode image of the horizontal vessel in the flow phantom depicted in Figure 2-35 is presented in Figure 2-37. The energy mode image is continuous rather than divided into segments because of the different beam directions. In other words, the energy image is not sensitive to relative flow direction, as is the color velocity image. Another advantage of the energy mode image is that it is not affected by aliasing. The energy mode image does not depict velocities but only a value related to the strength of the Doppler signal, so the effects of aliasing are not manifested.

The advantages of this modality over color velocity imaging are, therefore, as follows:
1. Energy mode seems to be more sensitive to low- and weak-flow states than color velocity.
2. Angle effects on the Doppler frequency are ignored, unless the angle becomes so close to perpendicular that the Doppler signals are below the flow detectability threshold of the color processor.
3. Aliasing does not affect the energy mode display. Thus, a more continuous display of flow, especially in difficult-to-scan regions, is provided.

Disadvantages of energy mode imaging are also clear:
1. Information on reflector velocity and flow direction relative to the transducer is not displayed. Sometimes these features are important to a diagnosis.

2. Image build-up tends to be slower, and image frame rates lower, because of the use of more signal averaging in energy mode than in velocity mode. Consequently, problems with flash artifact caused by Doppler signals from slowly moving soft tissues are more severe in energy mode than in velocity mode.

BEYOND TWO-DIMENSIONAL IMAGING

EXTENDED FIELD OF VIEW IMAGING

Sometimes it is desirable to display a larger imaged region than that provided simply by the format of the ultrasound transducer. To some extent, this has already been addressed in technology that widens the image format of linear array transducers. It might be possible to produce images whose view is much larger than that provided by the transducer alone if the probe were attached to a mechanical translation system and the transducer were moved in a direction parallel to the image plane as image data are acquired. However, the idea of mechanically linking the transducer for the purpose of providing an image that has a wider format might not appeal to operators, who need extensive freedom to manipulate the probe to desired image planes. An alternative and effective method for extending the image field is one in which the operator freely translates the probe parallel to the image plane, and probe motion is tracked by changes in the image itself. As the transducer is translated manually, image-processing software identifies the amount of lateral motion from one frame to the next. This enables the software to register new image information in a location that correctly corresponds to its anatomic position with respect to structures appearing in the original image.

An image of the arm arteries shown in Figure 2-38 illustrates one result of this process. Although the original image from the linear array transducer used in creating the image would be only about 4 cm wide, careful translation of the probe along with the image registration software provides an extended view of the brachial and radial arteries.

THREE-DIMENSIONAL ULTRASOUND

The real-time nature of ultrasound imaging and the need to view structures through scanning windows that sometimes provide poor acoustic access

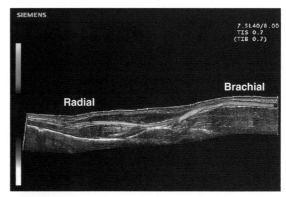

FIGURE 2-38 Extended field of view imaging. This image of the brachial and the radial arteries of the arm extends over 20 cm. It is constructed by tracking motion of the transducer during the scan using correlation processing applied to the B-mode image data. *(Courtesy of Siemens Medical.)*

has limited the use of 3D volume acquisition and display techniques. However, transducers that are comparable in size to conventional probes but with 3D capabilities are leading to a renewed interest in 3D imaging in ultrasound. Some applications appear to benefit greatly from using 3D, especially imaging the fetus and certain vascular structures (Figure 2-39). Three-dimensional scanning acquires ultrasound B-mode or color images over an entire volume. Besides the more extensive data set that is obtained using large numbers of 2D images, a 3D set enables new views that sometimes can save time during interpretation and analysis. Moreover, 3D images often are more intuitive than sets of conventional, 2D images for those who are not specialists in medical imaging, making communication with patients and referring physicians easier.

Typically, to acquire 3D data, the ultrasound transducer is translated perpendicular to the plane of the acquired image (Figure 2-40), and images are stored at predetermined spatial intervals. The stack of images so acquired may be thought of as a volume scan. We think of "acquired image planes" (i.e., images generated by the real-time beam sweeping methods discussed earlier) and "reconstructed planes," or new images generated using the entire 3D image data set. The shorter the distance between acquired planes, the better will be the resolution, particularly of reconstructed planes from the set, but the greater will also be the storage and image-handling requirements. "Freehand" scanning, mechanical movement within a specialized 3D probe housing, and 2D transducer arrays have all been implemented

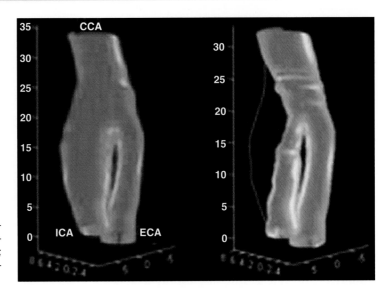

FIGURE 2-39 Surface-rendered three-dimensional image of the carotid bifurcation. CCA, common carotid artery; ECA, external carotid artery; ICA, internal carotid artery.

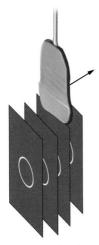

FIGURE 2-40 Arrangement for acquiring three-dimensional images by freehand translation of a transducer. Probe tracking methods vary from no tracking, where the assumption is made that the translation is at a uniform speed, to detecting changes in the image texture pattern when the changes can be associated with scan plane translation, to attaching sensors to the transducer so that the position and orientation of each recorded image plane are known precisely.

to translate the acquisition plane across the volume.

In the simplest freehand scanning method, the operator translates the probe over the scanned volume, and a loop of image data is stored during a preset time interval. Three-dimensional image reconstruction is then done by assuming that all image planes are equidistant from one another, with the interval between planes essentially being controlled subjectively by the operator.

Rough 3D data sets are thus acquired and can be displayed with this method, but the distance between image planes is not known precisely. The spatial relationship between any two structures that are not in one of the acquired image planes can be erroneous because it depends on the operator providing perfectly spaced scans, which is unlikely for this type of system.

More accurate tracking of the transducer position can be done by systems that process the image data to sense changes in the image texture patterns from one frame to the next while the operator does a freehand sweep. The texture changes are measured as reductions in the degree of information correlation within a region from one acquired image to the next. Once the rate of reduction with translation distance is calibrated, the system can use the image data to estimate distances between successive image planes and reconstruct 3D data sets.

A third freehand tracking scheme uses sensors attached to the transducer or otherwise placed in the scanning room and measures the position and orientation of the probe directly.[19] For example, one method uses video cameras to record the positions of small reflectors affixed to the transducer, whereas a more common tracking system uses an electromagnetic coil attached to the probe with transmitters distributed around the scanning room. These methods place each acquired image in a properly registered location and orientation in the 3D ultrasound data set. Reconstruction and display methods then can be used quite reliably for producing 3D images.

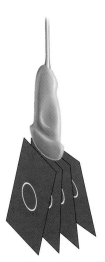

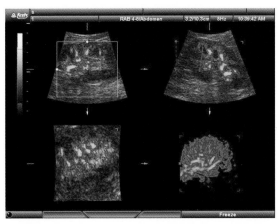

FIGURE 2-41 Commonly used three-dimensional trans-ducer assembly. In this arrangement, the image plane is translated by mechanical movement, within the trans-ducer housing, of a curvilinear array probe.

FIGURE 2-42 Display of three-dimensional ultrasound information from a kidney. *Top left*, One of multiple acquisition planes. *Top right*, Constructed plane orthog-onal to the acquisition planes. *Lower left*, Reconstructed c-plane (constant depth) representing a coronal view. *Lower right*, Volume-rendered image depicting the blood vessels derived using color flow imaging. *(Courtesy of General Electric.)*

More precise acquisitions of volumetric data are done using mechanically translated trans-ducer arrays within special-purpose 3D probes. Mechanical systems for 3D vascular imaging have been pioneered by Fenster and colleagues.[20] Com-mercial versions of the mechanically scanned arrays operate with special array transducers that are slightly larger than conventional one-dimensional arrays. With these, the image plane is manipulated by an internal motor system, such as the pivoting system shown in Figure 2-41, that translates the acquired image plane. Thus, a series of 2D images is acquired at volumetric scanning rates that are high enough to track slow move-ments, such as fetal limbs. However, blood flow in vascular studies usually requires electrocardio-gram gating, particularly when precise measure-ments of vessel sizes are being made.

Progress is being made gradually in the devel-opment of full 2D ultrasound transducer arrays.[21] These enable acquisition of volumetric data sets without the need for mechanical manipulations inside the transducer housing or translations of the probe by the operator. One such system is rapid enough to provide live images of the adult heart. Two-dimensional arrays require large channel counts to enable individual elements to be driven. For example, a typical high-quality one-dimensional array operates with a channel count of 128 or more elements. If one were to repeat the same channel density in two dimen-sions, it would require more than 10,000 chan-nels, which currently is prohibitive, given the status of miniaturization of circuits and other factors. Thus, the usual strategy is to get by on fewer elements. The Duke system, for example, uses randomly positioned elements.

There are various ways to display the volu-metric data during acquisition and for analysis. The preferred methods depend on the nature of the data and their potential uses. For example, in echocardiology, a simultaneous display of two orthogonal image planes that represent tradi-tional ultrasound acquisition planes, along with one or more reconstructed "C-planes" (constant-depth planes) depicting structures in a plane at a selected distance from the transducer, has been found extremely useful.[21]

Volumetric acquisition and display techniques often support multiview displays, as shown in Figure 2-42. The *image in the lower right* repre-sents the entire color data volume acquired from a kidney. The gray-scale echo data have been suppressed in this view. The other three images depict single image planes. The *top left* is the nor-mal acquisition plane, representing one of the planes used as input to the data set volume. An orthogonal, reconstructed plane is presented in the *top right image*. Although this image could have been generated simply by rotating the orig-inal scanning plane 90 degrees, here it is com-puted from the 3D data set. The *lower left image* is another reconstructed plane, this one at a fixed depth from the transducer. One of the very useful

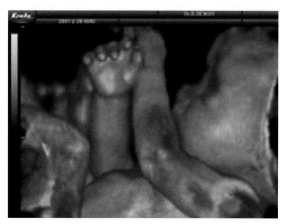

FIGURE 2-43 Surface-rendered image of a fetus, clearly depicting facial features and other anatomic details. *(Courtesy of General Electric.)*

aspects of this type of 3D scanning is the ability to generate new image planes, such as that shown here, which are not accessible with conventional, 2D imaging.

Besides multiview displays, various volume-rendering and surface-rendering techniques have been found useful for 3D ultrasound data. The fetal image in Figure 2-43 is one that uses thresholding and surface rendering to portray a view similar to a visual image of the structures. This method works in cases where the image contrast is sufficiently high that the surface can be detected by automated methods. Contrast with color flow imaging is also very good, so surface rendered images of major vessels (see Figure 2-39) can portray information on the lumen shape and diameter, the course of the vessel, and the relationship between flow features in adjacent vessels. Volume-rendered images, such as the kidney in Figure 2-42 can also be useful, particularly when the image includes vascular information displayed in color. The complex relationship among vessels of different diameters and locations can be readily appreciated with such methods.

As computational and image-processing techniques become more powerful and processor speeds intensify, we can anticipate that there will be increasing uses of 3D ultrasound. The tremendous data overhead that is required for these techniques used to be a burden, even for powerful workstations, but this is no longer the case. Furthermore, it is likely that the data-handling capabilities of tomorrow's processors will hardly be challenged by present-day approaches to acquisition, image processing, and display. Hopefully,

diagnostic capabilities of ultrasound machines will also continue to increase, benefiting greater numbers of patients.

EQUIPMENT SAFETY

In an ultrasound examination, acoustic energy must be transmitted into the tissue. The possibility that the energy could produce a detrimental biologic effect has been considered extensively by bioacoustics researchers; it continues to be studied to this day. At this time, most workers conclude that diagnostic ultrasound equipment is safe and that it is unlikely that bioeffects could result from prudent use of this modality, at least with current scanners. The American Institute of Ultrasound in Medicine's official statement on the clinical safety of diagnostic ultrasound instrumentation reads as follows:

> There are no confirmed biological effects on patients or instrument operators caused by exposures from present diagnostic ultrasound instruments. Although the possibility exists that such biological effects may be identified in the future, current data indicate that the benefits to patients of the prudent use of diagnostic ultrasound outweigh the risks, if any, that may be present.[22]

Readers should consult more detailed reports[23] on postulated mechanisms for bioeffects; acoustic exposure parameters of concern; reports of the nature of biologic effects, especially high-power and intensity levels; and acoustic output data from current scanners.[4]

The responsibility for safety of medical diagnostic ultrasound equipment falls on everyone involved in manufacturing, regulating, and using this equipment.[24] Until recently, manufacturers in the United States were required to adhere to "application specific limits" on the intensity, peak pressure levels, and acoustic power levels of scanners. When a new scanner or a new transducer was planned for marketing, the U.S. Food and Drug Administration considered acoustic output data submitted by the manufacturer of the device. If the intensities were lower than these limits, the product was considered satisfactory as far as acoustic output was concerned.

Most equipment manufacturers in the United States and Canada now follow the acoustic output labeling standard described earlier in this chapter (see Figure 2-2).[4] It requires manufacturers to provide output indicators on their scanners to inform users of levels as they relate to potential biologic effects. These quantities enable users to implement the ALARA principle. Although regulators continue to impose a 720-mW/cm^2 limit on the time-averaged intensity and a limit of 1.9 on the MI value, it is feasible that such upper limits could be relaxed at some future date. Presumably, this would open up the potential of still further diagnostic capabilities with medical ultrasonography. It would, of course, also place greater responsibility for clinical safety on the operator and physician responsible for the ultrasound examination.

Some individuals are concerned that the removal of application-specific intensity limits will not be recognized by ultrasound equipment users and they may operate a scanner at an unnecessarily high output setting. As the new labels become more familiar to ultrasonographers, the likelihood of this occurring will diminish.

REFERENCES

1. Wells PT: *Biomedical ultrasonics*, New York, 1977, Academic Press, pp 120–123.
2. *1993 Acoustical data for diagnostic ultrasound equipment*, Laurel, MD, 1993, American Institute of Ultrasound in Medicine.
3. Duck FA: Output data from European studies, *Ultrasound Med Biol* 15(Suppl 1):61–64, 1989.
4. *Standard for real-time display of thermal and mechanical acoustic output indices on diagnostic ultrasound equipment*, Laurel, MD, 1991, American Institute of Ultrasound in Medicine.
5. Zagzebski JA: *Essentials of ultrasound physics*, St. Louis, 1996, CV Mosby.
6. Shung KK: In vitro experimental results on ultrasonic scattering in biological tissues. In Shung KK, Thieme GA, editors: *Ultrasonic scattering in biological tissues*, Boca Raton, FL, 1993, CRC Press, pp 219–312.
7. Desser T, Jaffrey B: Tissue harmonic imaging techniques: physical principles and clinical applications, *Semin Ultrasound CT MR* 22:1–10, 2001.
8. Kremkau F: *Diagnostic ultrasound principles, instrumentation and exercises*, ed 5, Orlando, FL, 1993, Grune & Stratton.
9. Entrekin R, et al: Real-time spatial compound imaging: application to breast, vascular, and musculoskeletal ultrasound, *Semin Ultrasound CT MR* 22:50–64, 2001.
10. Burns P: Instrumentation for contrast echocardiography, *Echocardiography* 19:241–259, 2002.
11. Pedersen MH, Misaridis TX, Jensen JA: Clinical evaluation of chirp-coded excitation in medical ultrasound, *Ultrasound Med Biol* 29(6):895–905, 2003.
12. Taylor KJW, Wells PNT, Burns PN: *Clinical applications of Doppler ultrasound*, New York, 1995, Raven Press.
13. Beach K, Philips D: Doppler instrumentation for the evaluation of arterial and venous disease. In Jaffe C, editor: *Vascular and Doppler ultrasound. Clinics in diagnostic ultrasound series*, New York, 1984, Churchill Livingstone.
14. Omoto R, Kasai C: Basic principles of Doppler color flow imaging, *Echocardiography* 3:463, 1986.
15. Evans D: *Doppler ultrasound physics instrumentation and clinical applications*, New York, 1989, John Wiley & Sons.
16. Embree P, O'Brien W: Volumetric blood flow via time-domain correlation: experimental verification, *IEEE Trans Ultrason Ferroelec Freq Control* 37:176–185, 1990.
17. Kisslo J, Adams AB, Belkin RN: *Doppler color flow imaging*, New York, 1988, Churchill Livingstone.
18. Rubin JM, et al: Power Doppler US: a potentially useful alternative to mean frequency-based color Doppler US, *Radiology* 190:853–856, 1994.
19. Nelson TR, Pretorius DH: Three-dimensional ultrasound imaging, *Ultrasound Med Biol* 24:1243–1270, 1998.
20. Fenster A, Downey DB, Cardinal HN: Three-dimensional ultrasound imaging, *Phys Med Biol* 46(5):R67–99, 2001.
21. Kisslo J, et al: Real-time volumetric echocardiography: the technology and the possibilities, *Echocardiography* 17(8): 773–779, 2000.
22. *1997 Statement on clinical ultrasound safety*, Laurel, MD, 1997, American Institute of Ultrasound in Medicine.
23. *Exposure criteria for medical diagnostic ultrasound: II. Criteria based on all known mechanisms*, NCRP Report 140 Bethesda MD, 2002, National Council on Radiation Protection and Measurements.
24. *Medical ultrasound safety: bioeffects and biophysics; prudent use; implementing ALARA*, Laurel, MD, 1994, American Institute of Ultrasound in Medicine.

BASIC CONCEPTS OF DOPPLER FREQUENCY SPECTRUM ANALYSIS AND ULTRASOUND BLOOD FLOW IMAGING

3

JOHN S. PELLERITO, MD, FACR, FSRU, FAIUM, and JOSEPH F. POLAK, MD, MPH

SPECTRUM ANALYSIS

If blood flow were continuous rather than pulsatile, if blood vessels followed straight lines and were uniform in caliber, if blood flowed at the same velocity at the periphery and in the center of the lumen, and if vessels were disease-free, then each blood vessel would produce a single Doppler ultrasound frequency. However, blood flow *is* pulsatile, vessels are not always straight or uniform in size, flow is slower at the periphery than in the center of the vessel, and the vessel lumen may be distorted by atherosclerosis and other pathology. For these reasons, blood flow produces a mixture of Doppler frequency shifts that changes from moment to moment and from place to place within the vessel lumen. Spectrum analysis is needed to sort out the jumble of Doppler frequencies generated by blood flow and to provide quantitative information that is critical for diagnosis of vascular pathology.

THE DOPPLER SPECTRUM

The word *spectrum*, as derived from Latin, means *image*. You may think of the Doppler spectrum as an image of the Doppler frequencies generated by moving blood.[1-8] In fact, this image is a graph showing the mixture of Doppler frequencies present in a specified sample of a vessel over a short period of time.[1-3] The key elements of the Doppler spectrum are *time, frequency, velocity,* and Doppler signal *power*. These elements are best described in pictorial form; therefore, this information is provided in Figure 3-1, rather than in the text. Please review this figure now, directing particular attention to the four key elements cited previously.

THE POWER SPECTRUM

The Doppler frequency spectrum that you have just reviewed in Figure 3-1 is sometimes called a *power spectrum*,[1-3] because the power, or strength, of each frequency is shown by the *brightness* of the pixels. The power of a given frequency shift, in turn, is proportionate to the *number* of red blood cells producing that frequency shift. If a large number of blood cells are moving at a certain velocity, the corresponding Doppler frequency shift is powerful, and the pixels assigned to that frequency are bright. Conversely, if only a small number of cells are causing a certain frequency shift, the pixels assigned to that frequency are dim. The power spectrum concept is important for understanding power Doppler flow imaging, which is discussed later in this chapter. The concept of the power Doppler spectrum is nicely illustrated in Figure 2-29.

FREQUENCY VERSUS VELOCITY

The echoes that are reflected back to the transducer from moving cells in a sampled blood vessel contain only Doppler frequency shift information; yet the Doppler spectrum often displays both velocity (cm/sec or m/sec) and frequency (kHz) information. How does the instrument convert the Doppler frequency shift to velocity? This conversion occurs when the sonographer "informs" the duplex instrument of the Doppler angle,[1,2,9] which is shown in Figure 3-2. If the instrument "knows" the Doppler angle, it can then compute the blood flow velocity via the Doppler formula (see Chapter 2). You may note in this formula that the frequency shift is proportional to the cosine of the Doppler angle, theta. When the operator informs the ultrasound machine of this angle, the frequency shift is proportional to blood flow velocity. Voila! The frequency spectrum becomes a velocity spectrum. A Doppler angle of *60 degrees or less* is required to derive accurate frequency and velocity measurements. If the angle is greater than 60°, velocity measurements are unreliable. Although there is greater error in measurements obtained at higher angles, some applications (e.g., carotid examinations) are more easily performed at angles closer to 60°. It is generally recommended that the

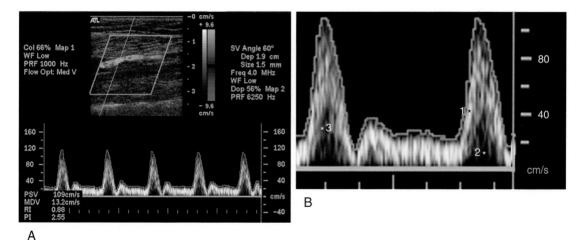

FIGURE 3-1 The Doppler spectrum display. The following information is presented on the display screen (**A,** Entire display; **B,** Magnified Doppler spectrum). *Color flow image*: The vessel, the sample volume, and the Doppler line of sight are shown in the color flow image at the top of the display screen. *Color flow information*: The "color bar" to the right of the image shows the relationship between the direction of blood flow and the colors in the flow image. By convention, the upper half of the bar shows flow *toward* the transducer. This is logical, as this part of the bar is nearest to the transducer in the image. The lower half represents flow *away* from the transducer. In this case, red/orange colors correspond to flow toward the transducers, and blue/green colors indicate flow in the opposite direction. A shift in color from red to orange or from blue to green represents increasing flow velocity. *Doppler angle*: The Doppler angle for the spectral Doppler appears at the upper right of the display screen, in this case 60°. *Time*: The time is represented on the horizontal *(x)* axis of the Doppler spectrum, at the base of the display. The lines represent divisions of a second, but typically a scale is not provided. *Velocity*: Blood flow velocity (cm/sec) is shown on the vertical *(y)* axis of the spectrum. In this case, velocity is shown on both vertical axes. On some instruments, the velocity is shown on one vertical axis and the Doppler-shifted frequency (KHz) on the other. *The distribution of velocities* within the sample volume is illustrated by the brightness of the spectral display (the *z*-axis). To better understand the *z*-axis concept, examine the magnified spectrum shown in *B* and imagine that the spectral display is made of tiny squares called *pixels* (for picture elements). You cannot see the pixels in this image because they are purposely blurred to smooth the picture. The pixels are there, however, and each corresponds to a specific moment in time and a specific frequency shift or velocity. *The brightness of a pixel (its z-axis) is proportionate to the number of blood cells causing that frequency shift at that specific point in time*. In this example, the pixels at *asterisk 1* are bright white, meaning that a large number of blood cells have the corresponding velocity (about 41 cm/sec) at that moment in time. The pixels at *asterisk 2* are black, meaning that no (or very few) blood cells have the corresponding velocity (about 12 cm/sec) at that moment. The pixels at *asterisk 3* are gray, meaning that a moderate number of blood cells have the corresponding velocity (about 35 cm/sec) at that moment. Got it? If not, read this again and remember that the brightness of each pixel is proportionate to the *relative* number of blood cells with a specific velocity at a specific moment in time. Since the brightness of the pixels also shows the distribution of flow energy, or power, at each moment in time, the spectrum display is also called a *power spectrum*. *Flow direction*: The direction of flow is shown in relation to the spectrum baseline. In this case, flow toward the transducer is shown above the baseline, and flow away from the transducer is shown below the baseline. Note that the number 40 in the lower right corner is preceded by a minus sign. This is because the area below the baseline corresponds to flow away from the transducer, which would generate a negative Doppler shift. The relationship between the flow direction and the Doppler baseline may be reversed by the operator, but flow toward the transducer will always be represented by positive velocity or frequency values. *Peak velocity envelope*: The peak velocity throughout the cardiac cycle is shown by the *blue line* outlining the Doppler spectrum. Based on this envelope, a numeric output is provided at the bottom left, showing the peak systolic velocity (PSV) and the minimum diastolic velocity (MDV). In this case, the MDV also corresponds to the end-diastolic velocity, but this is not necessarily the case. The instrument also automatically calculates the resistivity index (RI) and the pulsatility index (PI), as shown below the velocity values. *Pulse repetition frequency*: A noteworthy number shown on the display is the pulse repetition frequency (PRF). The PRF for the color flow image is shown at the left of the image (1000 Hz, or cycles, or pulses per second). The PRF for the spectral Doppler is much higher (6250 Hz), as shown to the right of the color flow image. This difference illustrates the fact that the color flow image is based on the average Doppler frequency shift or velocity, while the spectral Doppler values are shown as absolutes, without averaging. A higher PRF is needed for the spectral Doppler to ensure that systolic velocities are shown accurately, without aliasing.

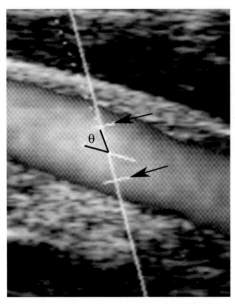

FIGURE 3-2 The Doppler angle and sample volume. The *nearly vertical line* is the Doppler line of sight. The *line in the center of the blood vessel* indicates the axis of blood flow. The angle formed by these two lines is the Doppler angle (θ). The parallel lines *(arrows)* indicate the length of the Doppler sample volume.

Doppler angle should be less than or equal to, but not greater than 60° for greatest accuracy.

In spite of potential measurement inaccuracy described in the previous paragraphs, it is desirable to operate the duplex instrument in the velocity mode rather than the frequency mode for two reasons.[1,2,9] First, velocity measurements compensate for variations in vessel alignment relative to the skin surface. For instance, the Doppler frequency shift observed in a tortuous internal carotid artery might be radically different from one point to another, but angle-corrected velocity measurements will be similar throughout the vessel, in spite of dramatic changes in vessel orientation relative to the skin. Second, the Doppler frequency shift is inherently linked to the output frequency of the transducer, but velocity measurement is independent of the transducer frequency. For instance, if the output frequency goes from 5 to 10 MHz, the frequency shift is doubled. Imagine the clinical consequences of such frequency changes. If transducers with different frequencies were used to determine stenosis severity, different diagnostic parameters would be needed for each ultrasound transducer (e.g., 3.5, 5, or 7.5 MHz). This problem is eliminated when the instrument converts the "raw" frequency information to velocity data.

AUDITORY SPECTRUM ANALYSIS

The human ear was the spectrum analysis instrument used initially for Doppler blood flow studies. The ear is a highly capable spectrum analysis instrument, which is evident in its ability to distinguish one person's voice from another. Even though duplex ultrasound instruments are equipped with electronic spectrum analysis devices, an audible Doppler output is provided as well, to take advantage of the human ear's capabilities. Certain features of the Doppler flow signal can be appreciated aurally that are difficult or impossible to display electronically, and as a result, the audible Doppler signal remains important in ultrasound vascular diagnosis. For instance, in very high grade carotid stenoses, a distinctive whining or whistling sound is heard. In spite of its abilities, however, the human ear has three major drawbacks. First, the ear is a purely qualitative device; second, it is not equipped with a hard copy output for permanent storage; and third, some ears work better than others—some cannot hear very high frequencies. Electronic spectrum analysis overcomes these obstacles.

THE SAMPLE VOLUME

The frequency spectrum shows blood flow information from a specific location called the *Doppler sample volume*, which is illustrated in Figure 3-2. You should be familiar with the following three characteristics of the Doppler sample volume: First, it is, in fact, a volume (three dimensions), even though only two of its dimensions are shown on the duplex image. The "thickness" of the sample volume cannot be shown on the two-dimensional spectrum display, and this can sometimes lead to errors of localization. Doppler signals may be obtained from vessels that are marginally within the sample volume but are not shown on the two-dimensional display. For instance, the ultrasound image may show the internal carotid artery, but you may actually be receiving flow signals from an adjacent external carotid branch. Second, the actual shape and size of the sample volume may be somewhat different from the linear representation shown on the duplex image. Third, and most important, the Doppler spectrum displays flow information only within the sample volume and does not provide information about flow in other portions of the blood vessel that are visible on the ultrasound image. Therefore, if the sample volume is positioned incorrectly, key diagnostic information may be overlooked.

FLOW DIRECTION

The frequency spectrum shows blood flow *relative to the transducer*. Flow in one direction, toward the transducer, is displayed above the spectrum baseline, and flow in the opposite direction is shown below the baseline. One must always remember that the flow direction is *relative* to the transducer and is not absolute. The apparent direction of flow can be reversed by turning the transducer around or by pressing a button on the instrument that inverts the spectrum! The arbitrary nature of this arrangement can lead to significant diagnostic error. Clues to the correct direction of flow can be found by comparing the color (e.g., red or blue) in the vessel to the color bar or color velocity scale and by checking whether the velocity information on the spectrum is positive (toward the transducer) or negative (away from the transducer). Another method to check direction of flow is comparison with a reference vessel in which the flow direction is known (e.g., when working in the abdomen, the aorta is a handy reference vessel).

WAVEFORMS AND PULSATILITY

In arteries, each cycle of cardiac activity produces a distinct "wave" on the Doppler frequency spectrum that begins with systole and terminates at the end of diastole. The term *waveform* refers to the shape of each of these waves, and this shape, in turn, defines a very important flow property called *pulsatility*.[1,2,10-28] In general terms, Doppler waveforms have low, moderate, or high pulsatility features, as illustrated in Figure 3-3. Please review this figure before proceeding to the material that follows.

Low-pulsatility Doppler waveforms have broad systolic peaks and forward flow throughout diastole (see Figure 3-3, *A*). The carotid, vertebral, renal, and celiac arteries all have low-pulsatility waveforms in normal individuals because these vessels feed circulatory systems with low resistance to flow (low peripheral resistance). Low-pulsatility waveforms are also *monophasic*, meaning that flow is always forward, and the entire waveform is either above or below the Doppler spectrum baseline (depending on the orientation of the ultrasound transducer).

Moderate-pulsatility Doppler waveforms have an appearance somewhere between the low- and

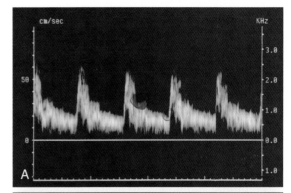

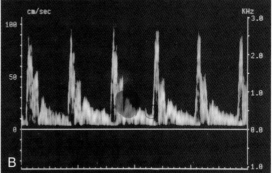

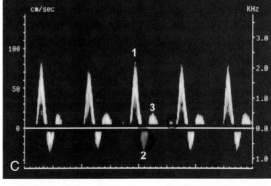

FIGURE 3-3 Pulsatility. **A,** Low pulsatility is indicated by broad systolic peaks and persistent forward flow throughout diastole (e.g., the internal carotid artery). **B,** Moderate pulsatility is indicated by tall, sharp, and narrow systolic peaks and relatively little diastolic flow (e.g., the external carotid artery). **C,** High pulsatility is characterized by narrow systolic peaks, flow reversal early in diastole, and absence of flow late in diastole. In this classic triphasic example, the first phase *(1)* is systole, the second phase *(2)* is brief diastolic flow reversal, and the third phase *(3)* is diastolic forward flow. Triphasic flow is seen in normal extremity arteries at rest.

high-resistance patterns (see Figure 3-3, *B*). With moderate flow resistance, the systolic peak is tall and sharp, but *forward flow is present throughout diastole* (perhaps interrupted by early-diastolic flow reversal). Examples of moderate pulsatility are found in the external carotid artery and the superior mesenteric artery (during fasting).

High-pulsatility Doppler waveforms have tall, narrow, sharp systolic peaks and reversed or absent diastolic flow. The classic example of high pulsatility is the triphasic flow pattern seen in an extremity artery of a resting individual (see Figure 3-3, *C*). A sharp systolic peak (first phase) is followed by brief flow reversal (second phase) and then by brief forward flow (third phase). High-pulsatility waveforms are a feature of circulatory systems with high resistance to blood flow (high peripheral resistance).

Pulsatility and flow resistance may be gauged qualitatively, either by visual inspection of the Doppler spectrum waveforms or by listening to the auditory output of a Doppler instrument. Qualitative assessment of pulsatility is often sufficient for clinical vascular diagnosis, but in some situations (e.g., assessment of renal transplant rejection), quantitative assessment is desirable. A variety of mathematical formulae can be used for this purpose, but the most popular measurements are the pulsatility index (of Gosling), the resistivity index (of Pourcelot), and the systolic/diastolic ratio,[24,26,28,29] all of which are illustrated in Figure 3-4.

Normal values for pulsatility measurements vary from one location in the body to another. Furthermore, both physiology and pathology may alter arterial pulsatility. For example, the normal high-pulsatility pattern seen in extremity arteries during rest converts to a low-resistance, monophasic pattern after vigorous exercise (because the capillary beds open and flow resistance decreases). Although this monophasic pattern is *normal* after exercise, it is distinctly *abnormal* in a resting patient and, in that circumstance, indicates arterial insufficiency resulting from obstruction of more proximal arteries. The point to be made here is that proper interpretation of pulsatility requires knowledge of the normal waveform characteristics of a given vessel *and* the physiologic status of the circulation at the time of examination. The status of cardiac function is also important; slowed ventricular emptying, valvular reflux, valvular stenosis, and other factors may significantly affect arterial pulsatility.

ACCELERATION

Acceleration is another important flow feature evident in Doppler spectral waveforms.[24,25] In most normal situations, flow velocity in an artery accelerates very rapidly in systole, and the peak velocity is reached within a few hundredths of a

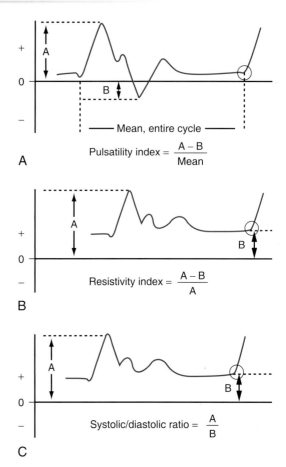

FIGURE 3-4 Pulsatility measurements. **A,** The pulsatility index (Gosling). **B,** The resistivity index (Pourcelot). **C,** The systolic/diastolic ratio.

second after ventricular contraction begins. Rapid flow acceleration produces an almost vertical deflection of the Doppler waveform at the start of systole (Figure 3-5, *A*). If, however, severe arterial obstruction is present proximal (upstream) to the point of Doppler examination, systolic flow acceleration may be slowed substantially, as shown in Figure 3-5, *B* and *C*. Quantitative measurement of acceleration is achieved by measuring the acceleration time and the acceleration rate (index), as illustrated in Figure 3-6. These measurements are used, for example, in evaluating renal artery stenosis.

VESSEL IDENTITY

As you may have already surmised, vessels can be identified by their waveform pulsatility features.[1,2,14,21-23,26] For example, Doppler waveforms readily differentiate between lower extremity arteries, which are distinctly pulsatile, and veins, which have gently undulant flow features. Doppler waveforms are particularly helpful in distinguishing the

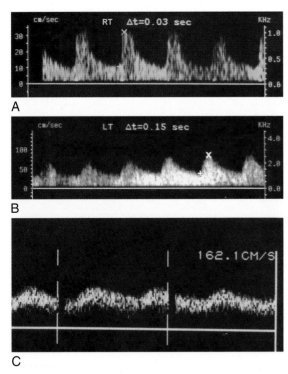

A

B

C

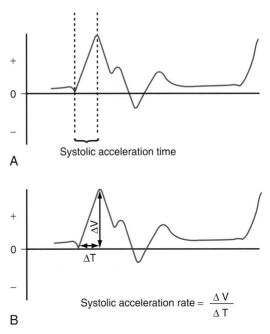

A

Systolic acceleration time

B

$$\text{Systolic acceleration rate} = \frac{\Delta V}{\Delta T}$$

FIGURE 3-6 Acceleration measurements: acceleration time **(A)** and acceleration rate **(B)**.

FIGURE 3-5 Acceleration and damping. **A,** The acceleration time (0.03 sec) is normal in the right kidney. **B,** The acceleration time is prolonged (0.15 sec) in the left kidney due to severe proximal renal artery stenosis. (**A** and **B** are from the same patient.) **C,** Severely damped dorsalis pedis artery waveform distal to common iliac and superficial femoral artery occlusion. Normally, this waveform should look like Figure 3-3, C. Acceleration is severely delayed, and a large amount of flow is present throughout diastole, consistent with severe ischemia.

internal and external carotid arteries, which have low and moderate pulsatility, respectively. Pulsatility is also of value within the liver for differentiating among the portal veins, hepatic veins, and hepatic arteries, as discussed in Chapter 30.

LAMINAR AND DISTURBED FLOW

Blood generally flows through arteries in an orderly way, with blood in the center of the vessel moving faster than the blood at the periphery. This flow pattern is described as *laminar*, because the movement of blood is in parallel lines.[1,2,4,14,15] When flow is laminar, the great majority of blood cells are moving at a uniform speed, and the Doppler spectrum shows a thin line that outlines a clear space called the *spectral window* (Figure 3-7).*

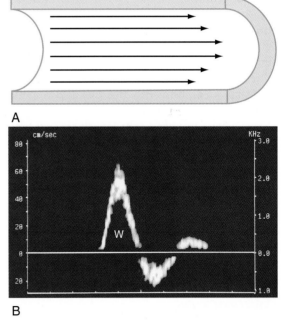

A

B

FIGURE 3-7 Laminar flow. **A,** Illustration of parallel lines of blood cell movement. **B,** Doppler spectrum during laminar flow. At all times, the blood cells are moving at similar velocities. As a result, the spectrum is a thin line that encloses a well-defined black "window" *(W)*.

In *disturbed flow,* the movement of blood cells is less uniform and orderly than in laminar flow. Disturbed flow is manifested as spectral broadening or filling in of the spectral window.[1,2,4,15-19] The *degree* of spectral broadening

---

*The term *plug flow* is actually more precise for this spectral pattern, as discussed in Chapter 1, but the term *laminar* is used throughout this text, in keeping with common convention.

is proportionate to the *severity* of the flow disturbance, as illustrated in Figure 3-8. Although disturbed blood flow often indicates vascular disease, it must be recognized that flow disturbances also occur in normal vessels. Kinks, curves, and arterial branching may produce flow disturbances, as illustrated quite vividly in the carotid bulb, where a prominent area of reversed flow is a normal occurrence[11,20,21] (Figure 3-9). In addition, a spurious disturbed flow appearance may be created in normal arteries through the use of a large sample volume that encompasses both the slow-flow area near the vessel wall and more rapid flow at the vessel center.[16-19] The Doppler spectrum, in such cases, appears broadened because both the high-velocity flow at the vessel center and the slow flow at the periphery of the vessel are encompassed by the wide sample volume.

VOLUME FLOW

Modern duplex instruments are capable of measuring the volume of blood flowing through a vessel (volume flow).[1,2,30-32] This is done by measuring the average flow velocity across the entire lumen (slow peripheral flow and high central flow) through several cardiac cycles while simultaneously measuring the vessel diameter, which is converted mathematically into cross-sectional area. Knowing the average velocity and the vessel area, it is an easy matter for the Doppler instrument to calculate the blood flow (in mL/min), and this is done automatically by the ultrasound instrument. Although the ability to calculate volume flow has been available on duplex instruments for more than 20 years and measurement accuracy appears satisfactory, issues of reproducibility have kept volume flow measurements from routine use in a clinical setting.[†]

DIAGNOSIS OF ARTERIAL OBSTRUCTION

Now that we have covered the basic concepts of Doppler spectral analysis, we can turn to the "heart of the matter," namely, how to use Doppler spectral analysis to diagnose arterial obstruction. Five main categories of information are used in this process: (1) increased stenotic zone velocity, (2) disturbed flow in the poststenotic

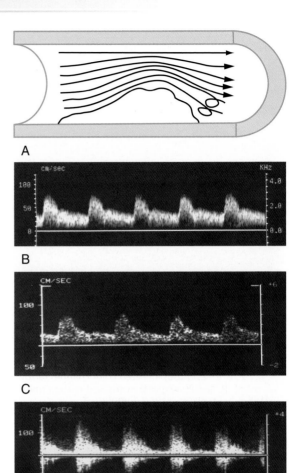

A

B

C

D

FIGURE 3-8 Disturbed flow. **A,** Disturbed flow illustration. **B,** Minor flow disturbance is indicated by spectral broadening at peak systole and through diastole. **C,** Moderate flow disturbance causes fill-in of the spectral window. **D,** Severe flow disturbance is characterized by spectral fill-in, poor definition of spectral borders, and simultaneous forward and reversed flow. The audible Doppler signal has a loud, gruff character when flow is severely disturbed.

zone, (3) proximal pulsatility changes, (4) distal pulsatility changes, and (5) indirect effects of obstruction, such as collateralization.[‡] These categories are summarized in Table 3-1, and each is discussed in the following sections.

INCREASED STENOTIC ZONE VELOCITY

The term *stenotic zone* refers to the narrowed portion of the arterial lumen. For determining the severity of arterial stenosis, the single most

---

[†]References 4-9,14-16,30,31,33,34.

[‡]References 2,4-10,13,15-19,22-27,29,33,35.

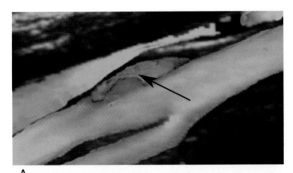

A

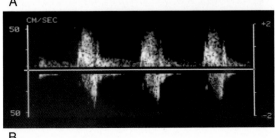

B

FIGURE 3-9 Normal bifurcation flow disturbance. **A,** Flow reversal in the bulbous portion of the common and internal carotid arteries causes localized color changes (*arrow,* blue color). **B,** Simultaneous forward and reverse flow is evident in the bulbous region on the Doppler spectrum.

TABLE 3-1 Spectral Features of Arterial Obstruction
Local effects
Elevated flow velocity in the stenotic lumen
Poststenotic flow disturbance
Proximal (upstream) pulsatility changes
Increased pulsatility
Decreased velocity overall, due to decreased flow
Distal (downstream) pulsatility changes
Slowed systolic acceleration
Broad systolic peak
Increased diastolic flow (reduced peripheral resistance)
Decreased velocity overall
Secondary (collateral) effects
Increased size, velocity, and volume flow in collateral vessels
Reversed flow in collateral vessels
Decreased pulsatility (flow resistance) in collateral vessels

valuable Doppler finding is increased velocity in the stenotic zone. Flow velocity is increased in the stenotic zone because blood must move more quickly if the same volume is to flow through the narrowed lumen as through the larger, normal lumen. The increase in stenotic zone velocity is directly proportional to the severity of luminal narrowing.

Three stenotic zone velocity measurements are commonly used to determine the severity of arterial stenoses (Figure 3-10): (1) *peak systolic velocity* (also called peak systole), which is the highest systolic velocity within the stenosis; (2) *end-diastolic velocity* (also called end diastole), which is the highest end-diastolic velocity; and (3) the *systolic velocity ratio,* which compares peak systole in the stenosis with peak systole proximal to the stenosis (in a normal portion of the vessel).

Peak systole in the stenotic zone is the first Doppler parameter to become abnormal as an arterial lumen becomes narrowed. The region of maximum velocity within the stenotic zone may be quite small, and for that reason, the sonographer must "search" the stenotic lumen with the sample volume to locate the highest flow velocity. If the highest flow velocity is overlooked, the degree of stenosis may be underestimated. As shown in Figure 3-11, peak systole rises steadily

with progressive narrowing, but ultimately the flow resistance becomes so high (at greater than 80% diameter reduction) that peak systole falls to normal or even subnormal levels. This drop in velocity can cause the unwary to underestimate the severity of a high-grade stenosis. Low flow velocity in a very high grade stenosis may also lead to false diagnosis of arterial occlusion if the velocity is so low that Doppler signals are not detected.

The end-diastolic velocity (end diastole) in the stenotic zone generally remains normal with less than 50% (diameter) narrowing, as there is no pressure gradient across the stenosis in diastole. With moderate stenosis (50%-70% diameter reduction), however, a pressure gradient exists throughout diastole, and end-diastolic velocity is elevated in proportion to stenosis severity. With severe stenosis (>70% reduction in diameter), a substantial pressure gradient exists throughout diastole, and diastolic velocities are high. Furthermore, with progression of stenosis severity, end-diastolic velocity increases at a greater rate, proportionately, than the peak systolic velocity, and as a result, the *difference* between peak systolic and end-diastolic velocity decreases. End-diastolic velocity, therefore, is a particularly good marker for severe stenosis.[9]

The *systolic velocity ratio,* as defined previously, is an additional important parameter for the diagnosis of arterial stenosis. This parameter is used to compensate for patient-to-patient hemodynamic

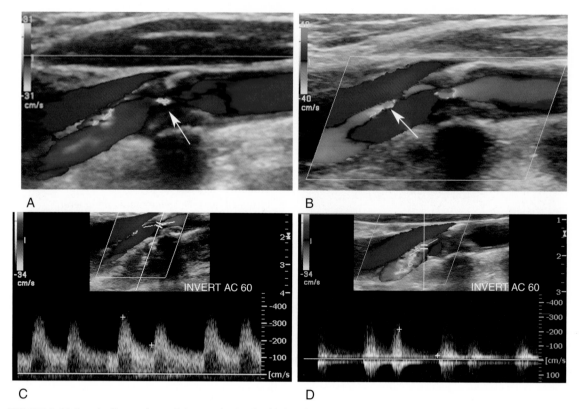

FIGURE 3-10 Local effects of arterial stenosis. **A,** The high velocities present in the narrowed portion of the arterial lumen generate an area of color aliasing *(arrow)* within the stenotic lumen. **B,** Disturbed flow in the poststenotic area generates a mixture of colors *(arrow).* **C,** Doppler spectrum analysis shows markedly elevated flow velocity, with a peak systolic velocity of 370 cm/sec and end-diastolic velocity of 164 cm/sec. **D,** Severe flow disturbance is evident in the poststenotic region, as indicated by simultaneous forward and reverse flow, spectrum fill-in, and poor definition of the spectrum margins.

variables, such as cardiac function, heart rate, blood pressure, and arterial compliance. Tachycardia, for instance, tends to increase peak systole in the stenotic zone, whereas poor myocardial function may decrease peak systole. The systolic velocity ratio allows the patient to act as his or her own physiologic "standard," because peak systole in the stenotic zone is compared with peak systole in a normal arterial segment (e.g., the common carotid artery). The systolic velocity ratio is used clinically in a number of circumstances, including the measurement of internal carotid, renal, and extremity artery stenoses.

POSTSTENOTIC FLOW DISTURBANCE

The poststenotic zone is the region immediately beyond an arterial stenosis in which disorganized or "disturbed" flow occurs. The demonstration of disturbed flow is an important diagnostic feature. To understand why flow is disturbed in the poststenotic region, envision the flow stream from the stenotic lumen suddenly spreading out in the much larger, poststenotic zone, causing the laminar flow pattern to be lost and the flow to become disorganized, which generates a disturbed Doppler spectral pattern, as illustrated in Figures 3-8 and 3-10, *B.* In some cases, frank swirling movements (or turbulence) occur in the poststenotic zone, producing simultaneous forward and reverse flow on the Doppler spectrum. The maximal flow disturbance occurs within 1 cm beyond the stenosis,[16] and in very severe stenoses, soft tissues adjacent to this portion of the artery may vibrate, causing a "visible bruit" on color Doppler images, as illustrated later in this chapter. Approximately 2 cm beyond the stenosis, the flow disturbance becomes less violent and spectral broadening diminishes. An orderly, laminar flow pattern may be reestablished within 3 cm beyond the stenosis,[4,16] but this distance is variable.

Poststenotic flow disturbances can be visually graded,[2,4,6,9,15-19] as shown in Figure 3-8. In

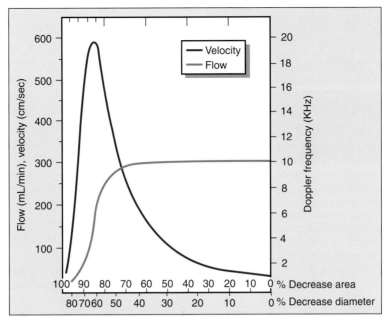

FIGURE 3-11 Relationship among velocity, flow, and lumen size. This graph refers specifically to internal carotid artery stenosis, but the principles illustrated apply to stenoses in other arteries throughout the body. Note that peak systolic velocity in the stenotic internal carotid lumen (labeled *velocity*) increases exponentially as the lumen diameter decreases (from right to left). The highest velocities correspond to approximately 70% diameter reduction. With greater stenosis severity, peak systolic velocity falls off rapidly to zero (because of rapidly increasing flow resistance). In contrast to velocity, volume flow (labeled *flow*) remains stable until the lumen diameter is reduced by about 50%. With further reduction in lumen size, volume flow falls off very rapidly to zero. Finally, note the relationship of percent diameter and area reduction, as shown at the base of the figure. Fifty percent diameter reduction equals about 70% area reduction, and 70% diameter reduction equals about 90% area reduction! *(Modified from Spencer MP: Full capability Doppler diagnosis. In Spencer MP, Reed JM, editors: Cerebrovascular evaluation with Doppler ultrasound, The Hague, Netherlands, Martinus Nijhoff, 1981, p. 213, with kind permission from Kluwer Academic Publishers.)*

general, minimal and even moderate flow disturbances are of little diagnostic value, because they may occur in both normal and abnormal vessels. Severe flow disturbance, however, generally does not occur in normal vessels and is an important sign of high-grade arterial narrowing or other arterial pathology such as an intimal flap, dissection, or an arteriovenous fistula. Severe flow disturbances are "beacons" indicating the presence of arterial disease. Whenever a severe flow disturbance is detected, the sonographer should search carefully for an adjacent stenosis or other vascular lesion. In some cases, the stenosis may be obscured by plaque calcification (preventing direct ultrasound visualization), and in such instances, poststenotic disturbed flow may be the only sign of significant arterial narrowing.

PROXIMAL PULSATILITY CHANGES

Arterial obstruction causes increased pulsatility (as defined previously) in portions of the artery proximal to (upstream from) the stenosis, and

this finding, therefore, may be very important diagnostically. The classic example of this phenomenon occurs with severe internal carotid artery obstruction, which causes the Doppler spectrum in the common carotid artery to have high-pulsatility features rather than the normal low-pulsatility pattern (Figure 3-12). To understand why pulsatility is increased proximal to a stenosis, imagine that blood flowing in the common carotid artery is being propelled toward a "valve" in the internal carotid artery that is 90% or 100% closed rather than wide open. How do you think the velocity waveform will appear in the common carotid artery? First, you can imagine that in systole, flow will go forward for only a brief moment and will then slow abruptly; therefore, the systolic peak will be sharp and narrow. Second, there will be relatively little flow in diastole, because intra-arterial pressure will be insufficient to force blood through the closed valve. Third, back-pressure from the blockage may cause a brief flow reversal early in diastole, equivalent to

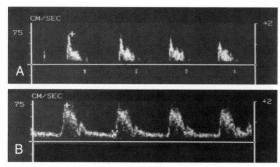

FIGURE 3-12 Increased common carotid artery pulsatility due to internal carotid artery occlusion. **A,** A high-resistance flow pattern is evident in this common carotid artery, consisting of sharp systolic peaks, diastolic flow reversal, and absence of flow throughout most of diastole. The ipsilateral internal carotid artery was occluded. **B,** The contralateral common carotid artery shows normal flow features.

the reflected wave seen in normal extremity arteries. Finally, flow velocity in the common carotid artery will be low throughout the entire cardiac cycle because the closed valve will reduce blood flow overall. The increase in pulsatility proximal to a stenosis may be lessened in the presence of collateral flow. For instance, abnormal common carotid pulsatility may be absent, in spite of a high-grade internal carotid stenosis, if a large volume of collateral flow occurs via the external carotid artery. In such cases, collateral vessels provide an alternative, low-resistance pathway for blood flow and decrease the level of pulsatility.

DISTAL PULSATILITY CHANGES

Doppler waveform abnormalities seen distal to a stenosis (downstream) also have considerable value in the diagnosis of arterial stenosis. As noted previously in the section on acceleration, the flow velocity in a normal, wide-open artery increases abruptly in systole, and the systolic peak is reached quickly (see Figure 3-5, A). In contrast, the Doppler waveform distal to a *severe* arterial obstruction has a "damped" appearance (see Figure 3-5, B and C), which means that the systolic acceleration is slowed, the systolic peak is rounded, the maximum systolic velocity is lower than normal, and diastolic flow is increased. The terms *pulsus tardus* and *pulsus parvus* ("tardus parvus") are also used to describe these damped, post-obstructive waveforms. *Tardus* refers to delayed arrival of the systolic peak, and *parvus* refers to overall low velocity. There are three causes for the pulsus tardus and parvus appearance. First, it

can be imagined that blood is being "squeezed" slowly through the obstructed lumen (or tiny collaterals), rather than "flying" along a broad tube. Therefore, it takes longer to reach peak velocity in systole, and systolic acceleration is reduced. Second, flow velocity is low, because less blood is moving through the obstructed vessel. This makes the Doppler waveform smaller than normal overall. Finally, ischemic distal tissues are "begging" for blood, with capillary beds wide open. The resultant decrease in peripheral resistance allows blood to flow throughout diastole, even in vessels that normally would not have diastolic flow (e.g., extremity arteries). The net effect of all three factors is the damped (also called *dampened*) waveform appearance described previously. The importance of this waveform shape cannot be overstated, since it clearly indicates the presence of arterial obstruction proximal to the Doppler examination site. Unfortunately, these "tardus parvus" waveforms are not always identified distal to a significant stenosis or occlusion. In other words, the presence of these damped waveforms is very specific but less sensitive for significant inflow disease.

Waveform damping due to proximal obstruction may be assessed visually, but it also is possible to quantify damping by measuring the acceleration time or acceleration index and with pulsatility indices described previously in this chapter.

SECONDARY (COLLATERAL) EFFECTS

The final diagnostic features of arterial obstruction of diagnostic importance are flow changes in collateral vessels. Arterial obstruction commonly alters flow in collateral channels that may be near to or distant from the site of obstruction. These flow alterations include increased velocity, increased volume flow, reversed flow direction, and pulsatility changes. For example, the external carotid artery may become an important collateral vessel in the event of ipsilateral or contralateral internal carotid stenosis or occlusion. Likewise, the vertebral artery may become a collateral source of arm perfusion in cases of subclavian artery obstruction. In such cases, blood flow may reverse in the ipsilateral vertebral artery and flow may be substantially increased in the contralateral vertebral artery, accompanied, in turn, by increased vessel size and flow velocity.

Secondary manifestations of arterial obstruction can be important diagnostically for the following reasons: (1) they may indicate that an obstructive lesion exists that would not be apparent otherwise, for example, when reversed vertebral flow calls attention to subclavian stenosis; (2) the location of collaterals roughly indicates the level of obstruction; and (3) secondary flow changes provide some data, albeit limited, about the adequacy of the collateral system circumventing an obstructive lesion. Such changes are of particular importance in transcranial Doppler applications, as considered in Chapter 12.

COLOR FLOW ULTRASOUND IMAGING

One of the more remarkable developments in ultrasound instrumentation is color flow ultrasound imaging, which superimposes a blood flow image on a standard gray-scale ultrasound image, permitting visual assessment of blood flow. Color flow imaging is an essential component of ultrasound vascular diagnosis, and for that reason, the proper use of this modality is very important. Color flow has certain idiosyncrasies and limitations that can cause significant diagnostic error if the sonographer has insufficient understanding of this modality and its applications. Therefore, it is worthwhile to review this subject.

PRINCIPLES OF COLOR FLOW IMAGING

There are three methods of generating color flow images, color Doppler, time-domain imaging, and power Doppler. We generally lump these together under the general term *color flow*, but the more specific terms *color Doppler* and *power Doppler* also are commonly used.

Color Doppler Imaging

Gray-scale ultrasound instruments use only two pieces of information from each echo that returns from the patient's body: the distance from the echo to the transducer (determined by the time of flight of the ultrasound pulse) and the strength of the echo. The echo signal typically contains other information, such as a Doppler frequency shift, but this information is disregarded. Color Doppler instruments[36-40] utilize the Doppler shift information, in addition to time of flight and amplitude information, to illustrate blood flow in color, as shown in Figure 3-13. For each echo shown on the color Doppler image, the instrument makes five determinations:

1. *How long has it taken for the sound beam to travel to and from the site of the echo?* As is the case in

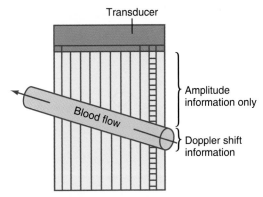

FIGURE 3-13 Color Doppler instrumentation. Stationary reflectors generate only amplitude information and are represented in shades of gray. Moving reflectors generate a Doppler frequency shift and are shown in color. Different colors can be used to show flow toward the transducer (increased Doppler-shifted frequency) and away from the transducer (decreased Doppler-shifted frequency).

all ultrasound machines, this "time of flight" of the ultrasound beam indicates the distance of the echo reflector from the transducer.

2. *How strong is the echo?* The strength or amplitude of the ultrasound signal determines how brightly the echo is displayed on the image, both for the gray-scale and the color Doppler components.

3. *Is a Doppler frequency shift present?* If so, the echo is represented in color; if not, it is represented in shades of gray.

4. *What is the magnitude of the Doppler frequency shift?* The magnitude of the Doppler shift is proportionate to the blood flow velocity and the Doppler angle (shown in Figure 3-2). Different frequency levels are shown on the image as different color shades or hues.

5. *What is the direction of the Doppler shift?* The instrument determines whether flow is toward or away from the transducer by noting whether the echo has a higher or lower frequency than the ultrasound beam sent out from the transducer. A higher Doppler frequency means flow is (relatively) toward the transducer, and a lower Doppler frequency means flow is away from the transducer. It is customary to show flow in one direction in blue and flow in the other direction in red. However, the operator can select other color schemes, if desired.

You should note that both the direction of flow and the velocity of flow (Doppler shift) are shown on the color Doppler image (Figure 3-14). This can be done in two ways. With the shifting

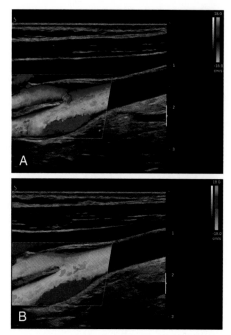

FIGURE 3-14 Color flow schemes. A variety of color schemes are used in color Doppler instruments. **A,** With this scheme, progressive increase in the frequency shift changes the image color from red to pink to white, or from dark blue to light blue to white, depending on the flow direction. **B,** With this scheme, the color changes from red to yellow or from blue to green.

hue method, different colors are used to represent different frequency levels (e.g., with increasing frequency/velocity, the color shifts through blue, green, yellow, and white). With the changing shade method, the same color is shown, but the color gets lighter as the frequency increases (e.g., through dark red, light red, pink, and, finally, white). Some sonologists prefer the shifting hue method, believing that it more clearly represents changes in the frequency shift and may demonstrate aliasing more clearly, as considered later.

Time-Domain Color Flow Imaging

The color flow images generated with the time-domain method[41] look like the flow images produced with the Doppler method previously described, but these color flow techniques are actually quite different. In the time-domain method, the ultrasound instrument identifies clusters of echoes (called *speckle*) within the ultrasound image and notes how far these clusters move on successive ultrasound pulses. By repeatedly "testing" echo clusters for movement, the instrument recognizes regions where flow is present. Flow direction and flow velocity

are ascertained directly with the time-domain method, by noting which way and how fast the clusters move.[41] Time-domain flow imaging is not widely used by ultrasound equipment manufacturers. The most commonly used color flow methods are color Doppler and power Doppler.

Power Doppler Flow Imaging

The third method of color flow imaging is used widely in vascular diagnosis and is called *power Doppler flow imaging*, or *power Doppler*, for short. As its name implies, this is a Doppler method, but it differs from standard color Doppler imaging, previously described, in that the *power* or intensity of the Doppler signal is measured and mapped in color, rather than the Doppler frequency shift, per se.[42] Stated differently, the instrument determines how strong the Doppler shift is at all locations within the image field and displays locations where the strength of the Doppler signal exceeds a threshold level (Figure 3-15). The term *power*, as used here, has the same meaning as in "Doppler power spectrum," as described earlier in this chapter. Compared with standard color Doppler imaging, power Doppler[42] is said to be more sensitive in detecting blood flow and less dependent on the Doppler angle. These advantages mean that smaller vessels and vessels with slow flow rates can be imaged; furthermore, even tissue perfusion can be assessed, to a limited degree. The enhanced sensitivity of power Doppler imaging is derived from more extensive use of the dynamic range of the Doppler signal than is possible with standard color Doppler imaging. More of the dynamic range can be used, because noise that would overwhelm the standard color Doppler image can be assigned a uniform background color (e.g., light blue). Hence, anything that represents noise is blue (Figure 3-15, *C*), and anything that represents flow is another color (usually gold). Furthermore, power Doppler imaging is not affected by aliasing. Even the aliased (wrapped-around) portion of the signal (see Chapter 2) has power and can be displayed as flow. Newer units allow color/power imaging that combines the directionality of color Doppler with the sensitivity of power Doppler.

Power Doppler imaging has one additional advantage that makes it especially valuable for use with ultrasound echo-enhancing agents (see Chapter 4). Power Doppler imaging is less subject to *blooming* than standard color

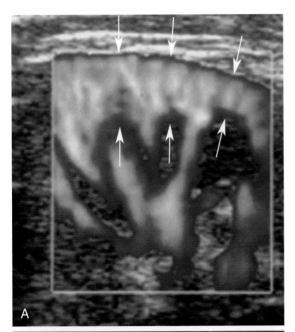

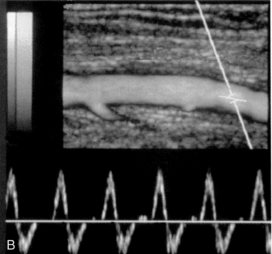

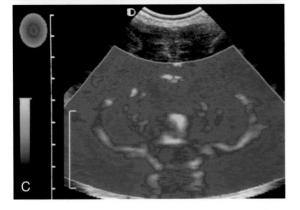

FIGURE 3-15 Power Doppler illustrations. **A,** Renal vessels are seen with striking detail, including small vessels in the renal cortex *(arrows)*. Note the absence of flow direction information; all vessels are yellow even though flow in some vessels is toward the cortex (arteries) and in others is toward the renal hilum (veins). **B,** Quantitative spectral information can be obtained in the power Doppler mode. **C,** This power Doppler image of the cranial vasculature uses a blue background, which enhances flow detection because noise is converted to a uniform blue color. With color Doppler, noise would blur the margins of the vessels.

Doppler imaging. Blooming is the spread of color outside of the blood vessel that occurs when the amplification of the Doppler signal is too great. Blooming is a particular problem when an echo-enhancing agent (ultrasound contrast agent) is used to improve the detection of blood flow. Intravenous injection of the echo-enhancing agent greatly increases the Doppler signal intensity, causing overamplification and severe blooming. With power Doppler imaging, blooming does *not* occur, owing to the way that the flow–no flow determination is made.[42] Power Doppler imaging, therefore, may be the preferred method for ultrasound imaging with echo enhancement.

In spite of its potential advantages over color Doppler, power Doppler has two major limitations. First, the frame rate may be slower than color Doppler, which renders this imaging method less valuable for rapidly moving vessels, rapidly moving patients (especially children), and areas subject to respiratory or cardiac motion. Second, power Doppler does not provide flow direction information! (Remember, the power of the Doppler signal is imaged, not the Doppler shift, per se.) Without measuring the Doppler shift, the flow direction cannot be determined.

ADVANTAGES OF COLOR FLOW IMAGING

Leaving the technical details behind, let us consider color flow imaging from a clinical perspective: Where does color flow help, and where does it have problems? Stated differently, what are the capabilities and limitations of color flow ultrasound?

Technical Efficiency

Perhaps the greatest advantage of color flow imaging is technical efficiency. When moving blood is encountered, the vessel "lights up," even if the vessel is too small to be resolved on the gray-scale image. Because vessels stand out in vivid color, they may be located and followed much more easily than with gray-scale instruments. Furthermore, basic judgments about blood flow can be made relatively easily with color flow imaging. The sonographer can quickly determine the presence of flow, the direction of flow, and the existence of focal flow disturbances. These capabilities have expanded the applications of duplex sonography. For example, with color flow imaging, it is possible to quickly examine long vascular segments, such as a vascular bypass graft, with relative ease. Furthermore, color flow imaging facilitates examination of vessels that are difficult to study with gray-scale imaging, such as the calf veins and the renal arteries.

Assistance in Sorting Out Abdominal Anatomy

Another advantage of color flow imaging is simplified differentiation between vascular and non-vascular structures, which is particularly useful in the abdomen. From a radiologist's perspective, one of the most obvious applications is sorting out porta hepatis anatomy. The bile ducts, which do not exhibit flow, may be differentiated visually from the porta hepatis vessels; moreover, the hepatic artery and portal vein may be differentiated visually by their flow characteristics.

Flow Assessment in the Entire Lumen

A major advantage of color flow imaging is the depiction of blood flow throughout entire vascular segments, rather than only within the Doppler sample volume. Because flow features are visible over a large area, localized flow abnormalities are readily apparent and are less likely to be overlooked than with gray-scale duplex methods. The sonographer is immediately made aware of the location of any flow abnormality, which speeds up the examination and permits rapid assessment of long segments of vessels for obstruction and other pathology.

Visual Measurement of Vascular Lumen

As compared with gray-scale ultrasound, color flow imaging makes it easier to define the residual lumen in stenotic or dilated vessels,[43,44] permitting visual (non-Doppler) measurement of patent segments (Figure 3-16). Direct, visual stenosis measurement remains problem prone, however, because of vessel tortuosity, color

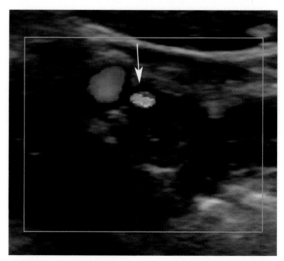

FIGURE 3-16 Enhanced residual lumen estimation. The residual lumen (*arrow*) is clearly visualized in this color flow image, potentially enhancing measurement accuracy.

blooming, off-axis measurements, and acoustic shadows from calcified plaque.

Differentiation of Severe Stenosis and Occlusion

The ability of color flow imaging, and especially power Doppler, to detect low-velocity flow in a tiny residual lumen facilitates the differentiation between occlusion of an artery and near occlusion with a "trickle" of residual flow (Figure 3-17). Personal experience suggests that color flow imaging is of value in this regard, and studies of the carotid arteries have shown improved results for detecting flow in near-occluded internal carotid arteries.[45,46]

LIMITATIONS OF COLOR FLOW IMAGING

So much for the advantages of color flow imaging, most of which quickly become obvious with use. Now to the limitations, which can have adverse diagnostic consequences if they are not understood by the sonographer. Many of the limitations listed here also occur with three-dimensional (3D) color flow imaging, which is discussed later in this chapter.

Flow Information is Qualitative

It is most important to recognize that color flow information is *qualitative* and not quantitative.[36-41] There are three reasons for this.

First, *the color flow image is based on the average Doppler shift* within the vessel, rather than the *peak* Doppler shift. Recall that quantitative Doppler spectrum measurements are based on the peak

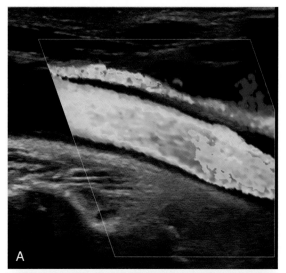

FIGURE 3-17 Small residual lumen. The tiny residual lumen in this internal carotid artery (ICA) would not be visible without color flow imaging. CCA, common carotid artery.

Doppler shifts, not the average shift. The average Doppler shift is *not* helpful for actually putting a number on a stenosis; you need the peak values. Furthermore, the average Doppler shift is lowered by flow disturbances (turbulence).

The second reason that color flow information is qualitative is *the lack of Doppler angle correction*. We previously indicated the importance of Doppler angle correction for accurate spectral Doppler measurements. It is easy to understand, therefore, that lack of angle correction is a significant contribution to the qualitative nature of the color flow image. Colors coded for high velocity may be seen in a vessel that is diving steeply away from the transducer when the velocities in that vessel are not actually very high.

Finally, *color flow information shows only a few frequency levels*. Color flow imaging is, in essence, a visual form of Doppler spectrum analysis, but it is a very crude form in which only a few large frequency "steps" are visible. These few steps provide only a general sense of altered flow velocity.

Because color flow images are qualitative, Doppler spectrum analysis (pulsed Doppler) must still be used to derive quantitative flow data (Figure 3-18). However, quantitative flow data can be derived from the color flow display with some time-domain color flow imaging systems, but these instruments are not widely used.

Low Pulse Repetition Frequencies and Frame Rates

A tremendous amount of data must be processed by the color flow instrument to generate each pixel (picture element) and each image frame. Processing these data takes time, which

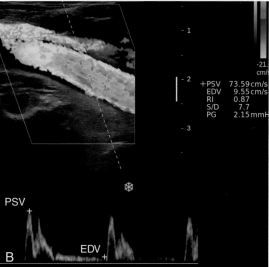

FIGURE 3-18 Color flow information is qualitative, not quantitative. **A,** It appears that the flow velocity is elevated in this carotid artery because there is aliasing artifact in the lumen of the vessel. **B,** Angle-corrected spectral Doppler measurement shows that the peak systolic velocity is not elevated (73.59 cm/sec).

may significantly degrade both the gray-scale and color Doppler images. This problem results principally from reduction of the pulse repetition frequency (PRF) (the number of pulses sent out per second) and the frame rate (the number of times per second that the monitor image is renewed). B-flow imaging, discussed later, is not subject to these image-resolution limitations.

Image degradation during color flow operation occurs in the following forms: (1) loss of spatial resolution; (2) a greater tendency for

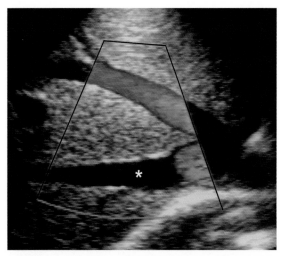

FIGURE 3-19 Spurious absence of flow. It appears that flow is absent in the right hepatic vein *(asterisk)* because this vessel is perpendicular to the color Doppler line of sight.

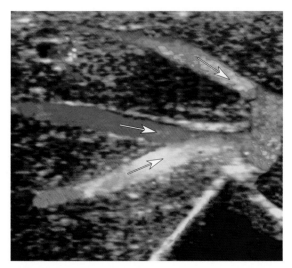

FIGURE 3-20 Color flow direction is relative to the transducer. Two of the hepatic veins are blue and one is red, implying that the flow direction in the red vessel is opposite that in the blue vessels. Flow actually is toward the inferior vena cava *(arrows)* in all of the vessels, but flow in the red vessel is *relatively* toward the transducer (top of image), whereas flow in the other vessels is *relatively* away from the transducer.

Doppler aliasing, which can cause spurious representation of high-velocity flow; (3) diminished temporal resolution, limiting the ability to visualize rapidly moving cardiac or vascular events (for example, cardiac valve motion may be less clearly seen with color flow scanning than with gray-scale scanning); and (4) visible image flicker when the frame rate falls below 15 frames/sec. (At that point, the human eye no longer "blurs" the ultrasound images into a moving picture.)[47]

Blood Flow Detection is Angle Dependent

Blood flow is not detected with color Doppler devices in vessels that are perpendicular to the ultrasound beam. (Color and spectral Doppler devices are similar in this respect.) A false-positive diagnosis of vascular occlusion may occur if a vessel is approximately perpendicular to the ultrasound beam, as shown in Figure 3-19. This is a particularly severe problem with curved array transducers. (Try imaging vessels with a curved array, and you will see what we mean.)

Flow Direction is Arbitrary

It is crucial to remember that the color of the vessel on the color flow image is *not* an absolute indication of flow direction. The color is assigned relative to the transducer (Figure 3-20; see Figure 3-14). The operator may reverse the color scheme (e.g., arteries blue, veins red) simply by reversing the orientation of the transducer or by pushing a button. To determine the true direction of flow,

the operator must closely observe the orientation of the vessel of interest relative to the transducer, check the direction of flow with pulsed Doppler, or refer to a vessel in which the flow direction is known (such as the aorta, if you are working in the abdomen).

COLOR MAY OBSCURE VASCULAR PATHOLOGY

If the instrument controls are improperly adjusted, the color flow information tends to "bloom" into the surrounding gray-scale image (Figure 3-21). Important vascular pathology, including plaque and venous thrombus, may be obscured by blooming. The absence of blooming is a desirable feature of B-flow imaging, as mentioned later.

COLOR FLASH

With color flow imaging, anything within the field of view that moves relative to the transducer is shown in color. In the abdomen, peristaltic motion, cardiac motion, or transmitted pulsations from great vessels may generate blotches of color on the ultrasound image called *color flash*, which can obscure large portions of the field of view, including structures of interest. The color flash problem is particularly apparent in the upper abdomen because of heart motion.

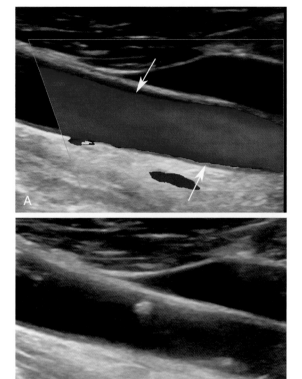

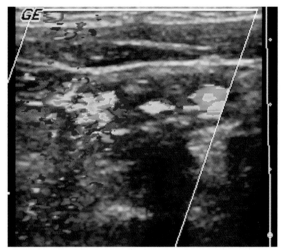

FIGURE 3-22 Visible bruit. Soft-tissue vibrations cause a montage of color adjacent to this stenotic internal carotid artery.

FIGURE 3-21 Color obscures plaque. **A,** Color blooming obscures carotid plaques *(arrows)*. **B,** The plaque is seen optimally with color flow turned off.

THE STRANGE CASE OF THE VISIBLE BRUIT

The *visible bruit* is a peculiar, but useful, flow phenomenon (Figure 3-22) that can be seen with color flow imaging.[48] A montage of color is seen within the soft tissues adjacent to the blood vessel as a result of vibration of the vessel wall and surrounding soft tissues. The wall vibration, in turn, is caused by a severe flow disturbance within the vessel. Low-level frequencies are produced in the adjacent soft tissues that receive a color assignment by the instrument. The visible bruit is associated particularly with arteriovenous fistulas but is also encountered with arterial stenoses and pseudoaneurysms.

A visible bruit suggests severe arterial stenosis, but caution is advised in interpreting this finding, because severe flow disturbances may sometime occur in the absence of significant stenosis. The term *visible bruit* is a misnomer, because a bruit is a sound and is not visible. Nonetheless, we like this term because the tissue vibration seen with color flow imaging also causes the bruit to be heard with a stethoscope.

OPTIMIZING COLOR FLOW IMAGE QUALITY

The color flow image is derived from relatively weak reflections from red blood cells. Because of the weakness of these echoes, the ability to demonstrate flow with ultrasound is particularly sensitive to instrument settings. The following technical tricks, summarized in Table 3-2, should be tried when it is difficult to obtain an adequate color flow image. The same procedures are applicable to 3D color flow imaging.

1. *Velocity range:* Consider whether the instrument is set for the proper velocity range. If the instrument is set to detect arterial velocities, it is not sensitive to venous velocities, or vice versa. Adjust the PRF or the velocity range to a level appropriate for the vessel of interest.
2. *Doppler angle:* Remember that the Doppler angle profoundly affects the color flow image. The strength of the color flow image diminishes as the Doppler angle approaches 90°; that is, the ultrasound beam is perpendicular to the blood vessel. So, when flow is absent in a vessel, ask, "Do I have an appropriate Doppler angle?" If not, move the color flow box or the transducer to improve the Doppler angle.
3. *Field of view:* Consider the depth of field shown on the image. Use only as much depth as you need! Greater depth requires a longer round-trip time for the ultrasound pulses,

TABLE 3-2 What to Check When You Cannot Detect Blood Flow
Velocity range (PRF)
Doppler angle
Field of view
Color box size
Color gain
Power Doppler
Color priority
Thump control
Wall filter
Is flow too slow?

PRF, pulse repetition frequency.

decreasing the PRF and the number of pulses per square centimeter of tissue and increasing the signal-processing time. The net result is diminished ability to display flow (as well as gray-scale image degradation).

4. *Color box size:* Consider the size of the color box. For the same reasons that were stated previously for *field of view*, pulse-echo information becomes increasingly "diluted" as the color box is enlarged. It is best to use a small color box, especially when examining vessels deep within the body.

5. *Power and gain:* Determine if the output power of the instrument, the time-compensated gain, and the color gain are optimal. Insufficient power or gain can result in inadequate color flow information.

6. *Color priority:* Consider whether the gray-scale versus color priority is adjusted correctly. Most (if not all) color flow instruments permit the operator to determine whether the gray-scale or color image is given more attention. If the gray-scale image is prioritized, then the color image suffers, and vice versa. If you are having trouble detecting flow, shift the image processing priority toward color.

7. *Thump control:* See if the thump control is eliminating too much color flow information. *Thump control* refers to electronic filtering that removes color artifacts generated by the heart or vascular pulsations. Thump control is not needed in smaller peripheral vessels and should be set as low as is practical.

8. *Wall filter:* Check the wall filter setting. If the wall filter is set too high, low-frequency signals generated by low-velocity flow are eliminated. The wall filter is designed to eliminate

low-frequency noise, but if it is set too high, it also eliminates flow information. This is not a problem with high-velocity flow, but it may be a major problem for detection of venous flow or for evaluating small parenchymal arteries.

9. *Very slow flow:* Finally, remember that flow might be present that simply is too slow for color flow visualization. Power Doppler or spectral Doppler may be more sensitive to the presence of slow flow than standard color Doppler imaging, and it may be useful to switch to these modalities when a vessel appears occluded.

THREE-DIMENSIONAL VASCULAR IMAGING

Advances in computer technology and transducer design have made 3D ultrasound imaging a reality[49-53] (Figure 3-23). Although the reconstruction algorithms utilized with current 3D ultrasound units are not as sophisticated as those used for computed tomography or magnetic resonance imaging, they are adequate for clinical use, and the utilization of 3D ultrasound continues to grow. Most studies have concentrated on obstetric, cardiac, and gynecologic applications. There are few clinical studies that have evaluated vascular applications of 3D ultrasound. Areas of current investigation include the carotid bifurcation and carotid stenosis, endovascular applications, intracranial vascular disease, remodeling in bypass grafts, and abdominal aortic aneurysms.

Three-dimensional presentation of ultrasound data can be performed with commercially available ultrasound systems. Off-line graphics workstations can also be utilized to generate, view, and store 3D data sets. These data sets may be obtained by combining stacks of two-dimensional slices to generate a volume of tissue. More recently, 3D ultrasound information can be obtained directly, through the acquisition of a volume of data generated by sweeping, tilting, or rotating the transducer across the area of interest.

There are several options for review of 3D data. The images can be displayed as a set of sequential images that can be reviewed manually, with the use of a trackball or keyboard. Multiple planes, including axial, sagittal, and coronal images, can be displayed simultaneously for comparison. In addition, the information may be viewed as a volume-rendered data set, emphasizing different

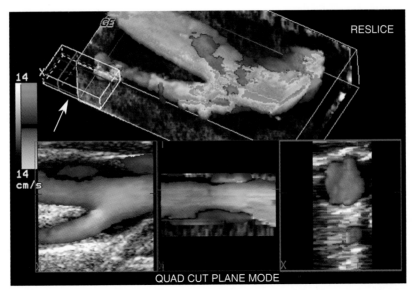

FIGURE 3-23 Three-dimensional ultrasound image. The large image at the top is shaded to display the three dimensionality inherent in this carotid bifurcation image. The three boxes at the bottom show different two-dimensional perspectives, based on the stored three-dimensional data. Orientation is provided by the navigator *(arrow)*. The colored borders around the two-dimensional images correspond to the planes of section seen in the navigator.

tissue or blood flow characteristics. Interactive review of the data allows the examiner to rotate the volume in any plane or section, scroll through individual slices, and subtract superficial or unwanted information. Real-time 3D examination (also known as four-dimensional imaging) is currently available on clinical ultrasound units. Future software modifications will allow virtual fly-through examination of blood vessels in real time.

The advantages of 3D ultrasound include the ability to obtain anatomic views not possible with two-dimensional imaging. The examiner can reformat the volume of image data in different imaging planes to extract information obscured by overlying tissue or artifacts. In addition, a surface (or transparent) display of the data can be obtained. Off-line review of patient data sets is also available. Recalculation of velocity measurements and assessment of different imaging planes for arterial stenosis, after the patient has left the ultrasound area, is available on current systems.

There are several limitations that have slowed widespread acceptance of 3D ultrasound. Reformatting and analysis of the 3D data is time consuming. Artifacts related to motion, scatter, attenuation, and color flash seriously degrade the quality of the 3D Doppler information. Current workstations that allow the analysis of 3D ultrasound data are expensive and do not always

interface with current picture-archiving systems. Finally, it is also difficult to store and retrieve 3D ultrasound information with some picture-archiving system technology.

B-MODE FLOW IMAGING

B-mode flow imaging[54-56] (B-flow for short) is one of the newer methods for flow imaging available on medical ultrasound instruments. As the name implies, B-flow shows blood flow with the gray-scale, or B-mode, image and is not a Doppler method. Both the flowing blood and the surrounding stationary structures are shown in shades of gray (Figure 3-24). For B-flow imaging, digitally encoded wide-band pulses are transmitted and reflected from the moving blood cells. The returning echoes are decoded and filtered to increase sensitivity for the detection of moving scatterers and to distinguish blood from tissue. Since this is not a Doppler technique, no velocity or frequency information is provided, and spectrum analysis does not apply. This is a purely visual, nonquantitative method of showing blood flow.

Probably the most useful aspect of B-flow is the precise definition of the boundary between flowing blood and the vessel wall. Because this is not a Doppler imaging method, the problems of blooming and overamplification of the flow signals, cited previously, do not apply. In addition,

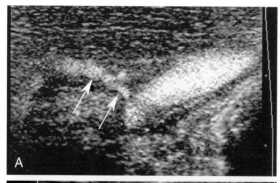

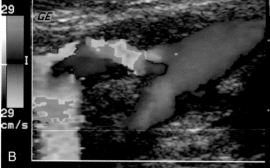

FIGURE 3-24 B-flow ultrasound. **A,** This long axis B-flow image accurately shows the size of the stenotic internal carotid artery lumen *(arrows)*. **B,** The lumen size is greatly exaggerated by color flow imaging due to blooming and other artifacts.

the B-flow technique does not degrade the spatial or temporal resolution of the B-mode image, as is the case with color flow imaging. Thus, the tendency of color Doppler to obscure the vessel wall and plaque is eliminated. In superficial arteries, such as the carotid arteries, the presence, extent, and severity of plaque in arteries is shown more clearly with B-flow than with color Doppler or even standard B-mode sonography. Potentially, B-flow may clarify the depiction of irregular plaque surfaces resulting from plaque ulceration, which would contribute significantly to its value for carotid artery imaging. In the venous system, small deep vein thrombi are well demonstrated with B-flow as filling defects that can be distinguished from flowing blood. Venous insufficiency and incompetent valves are also easily seen with this technique. Finally, B-flow is useful for demonstrating complex flow states, as seen with bypass grafts, arteriovenous fistulas, pseudoaneurysms, and dialysis grafts, where color Doppler artifacts may obscure flow information.

Because B-flow relies on the amplification of very weak echoes from red blood cells, it is limited by ultrasound attenuation, which restricts the

depiction of deep vessels, especially those in which blood is moving rapidly. B-flow, therefore, works particularly well with superficial vascular imaging.

REFERENCES

1. Wells PNT, Skedmore R: Doppler developments in the last quinquennium, *Ultrasound Med Biol* 11:613–623, 1986.
2. Taylor KJW, Holland S: Doppler ultrasound: part I. Basic principles, instrumentation, and pitfalls, *Radiology* 174:297–307, 1990.
3. Hutchison KJ, et al: A comparison of Doppler ultrasonic waveforms processed by zero crossing and spectrographic techniques in the diagnosis of peripheral arterial disease, *Angiology* 32:277–289, 1981.
4. Reneman RS, Spencer MP: Local Doppler audio spectra in normal and stenosed carotid arteries in man, *Ultrasound Med Biol* 5:1–11, 1979.
5. Johnston KW, et al: Cerebrovascular assessment using a Doppler carotid scanner and real-time frequency analysis, *J Clin Ultrasound* 9:443–449, 1981.
6. Brown PM, et al: A critical study of ultrasound Doppler spectral analysis for detecting carotid disease, *Ultrasound Med Biol* 8:515–523, 1982.
7. Zwiebel WJ: Color duplex imaging and Doppler spectrum analysis: principles, capabilities, and limitations, *Semin Ultrasound CT MR* 11:84–96, 1990.
8. Zwiebel WJ, Knighton R: Duplex examination of the carotid arteries, *Semin Ultrasound CT MR* 11:97–135, 1990.
9. Bluth EI, et al: Carotid duplex sonography: a multicenter recommendation for standardized imaging and Doppler criteria, *Radiographics* 8:487–506, 1988.
10. Feigenbaum H: Doppler color flow imaging, *Heart Dis Update* 2:25–50, 1988.
11. Zierler RE, et al: Noninvasive assessment of normal carotid bifurcation hemodynamics with color flow ultrasound imaging, *Ultrasound Med Biol* 13:471–476, 1987.
12. Middleton WD, Foley WD, Lawson TL: Flow reversal in the normal carotid bifurcation: color Doppler flow imaging analysis, *Radiology* 167:207–210, 1988.
13. Spencer MP: Frequency spectrum analysis in Doppler diagnosis. In Zwiebel WJ, editor: *Introduction to vascular ultrasonography*, ed 2, Philadelphia, 1986, WB Saunders, pp 53–80.
14. Smith JJ, Kampine JP: The peripheral circulation and its regulation. In Smith JJ, Kampine JP, editors: *Circulatory physiology: the essentials*, Baltimore, 1980, Williams & Wilkins.
15. Baker D: Application of pulsed Doppler techniques, *Radiol Clin North Am* 18:79–103, 1980.
16. Douville Y, Johnston KW, Kassam M: Determination of the hemodynamic factors which influence the carotid Doppler spectral broadening, *Ultrasound Med Biol* 11:417–423, 1985.
17. Campbell JD, Hutchison KJ, Karpinski E: Variation of Doppler ultrasound spectral width in the post-stenotic velocity field, *Ultrasound Med Biol* 15:611–619, 1989.
18. Merode TV, et al: Limitations of Doppler spectral broadening in the early detection of carotid artery disease due to the size of the sample volume, *Ultrasound Med Biol* 9:581–586, 1983.
19. Knox RA, et al: Empirical findings relating sample volume size to diagnostic accuracy in pulsed Doppler cerebrovascular studies, *J Clin Ultrasound* 10:227–232, 1982.

20. Ku DN, et al: Hemodynamics of the normal human carotid bifurcation: in vitro and in vivo studies, *Ultrasound Med Biol* 11:13–26, 1985.
21. Phillips DJ, et al: Flow velocity patterns in the carotid bifurcations of young, presumed normal subjects, *Ultrasound Med Biol* 9:39–49, 1983.
22. Nimura Y, et al: Studies on arterial flow patterns: instantaneous velocity spectrums and their phasic changes with directional ultrasonic Doppler technique, *Br Heart J* 36:899–907, 1974.
23. Rutherford RB, Kreutzer EW: Doppler ultrasound techniques in the assessment of extracranial arterial occlusive disease. In Nicolaides AN, Yao JST, editors: *Investigation of vascular disorders*, London, 1981, Churchill Livingstone.
24. Rutherford RB, Hiatt WR, Kreutzer EW, The use of velocity wave form analysis in the diagnosis of carotid artery occlusive disease, *Surgery* 82:695–702, 1977.
25. Nicolaides AN, Angelides NS: Waveform index and resistance factor using directional Doppler ultrasound and a zero crossing detector. In Nicolaides AN, Yao JST, editors: *Investigation of vascular disorders*, London, 1981, Churchill Livingstone.
26. Gosling RG: Doppler ultrasound assessment of occlusive arterial disease, *Practitioner* 220:599–609, 1978.
27. Kotval PS: Doppler waveform parvus and tardus, *J Ultrasound Med* 8:435–440, 1989.
28. Pourcelot L: Applications cliniques de l'examen Doppler transcutane. In Peronneau P, editor: *Velocimetrie Ultrasonore Doppler*, vol 34, Paris, 1974, INSERM, pp 780–785.
29. Stuart B, et al: Foetal blood velocity waveforms in normal pregnancy, *Br J Obstet Gynaecol* 87:780–785, 1980.
30. Avasthi PS, et al: A comparison of echo-Doppler and electromagnetic renal blood flow measurements, *J Ultrasound Med* 3:213–218, 1984.
31. Gill RW: Measurement of blood flow by ultrasound: accuracy and sources of error, *Ultrasound Med Biol* 11:625–641, 1985.
32. Burns PN, Jaffe CC: Quantitative flow measurements with Doppler ultrasound: techniques, accuracy, and limitations, *Radiol Clin North Am* 23:641–657, 1985.
33. Fei DY, et al: Flow dynamics in a stenosed carotid bifurcation model. Part I: basic velocity measurements, *Ultrasound Med Biol* 14:21–31, 1988.
34. Chang BB, et al: Hemodynamic characteristics of failing infrainguinal in situ vein bypass, *J Vasc Surg* 12:596–600, 1990.
35. Spencer MP: Full capability Doppler diagnosis. In Spencer MP, Reed JM, editors: *Cerebrovascular evaluation with Doppler ultrasound*, The Hague, Netherlands, 1981, Martinus Nijhoff, p 213.
36. Switzer DF, Nanda NC: Doppler color flow mapping, *Ultrasound Med Biol* 11:403–416, 1985.
37. Merritt CRB: Doppler blood flow imaging: integrating flow with tissue data, *Diagn Imaging* 11:146–155, 1986.
38. Powis RL: Color flow imaging: understanding its science and technology, *J Diagn Med Sonograph* 4:236–245, 1988.
39. Carroll BA: Carotid sonography: pitfalls and color flow, *Appl Radiol* 10:15–21, 1988.
40. Nelson TR, Pretorius DH: The Doppler signal: where does it come from and what does it mean? *Am J Roentgenol* 151:439–447, 1988.
41. Gardiner W, Fox MD: Color flow ultrasound imaging through the analysis of speckle motion, *Radiology* 172:866–868, 1989.
42. Murphy KJ, Rubin JM: Power Doppler: it's a good thing, *Semin Ultrasound* 18:13–21, 1997.
43. Erickson SJ, et al: Stenosis of the internal carotid artery: assessment using color Doppler imaging compared with angiography, *Am J Roentgenol* 152:1299–1305, 1989.
44. Polak JF, et al: Internal carotid artery stenosis: accuracy and reproducibility of color-Doppler assisted duplex imaging, *Radiology* 173:793–798, 1989.
45. Chang YJ, et al: Common carotid artery occlusion: evaluation with duplex sonography, *Am J Neuroradiol* 16:1099–1105, 1995.
46. Lee DH, et al: Duplex and color Doppler flow sonography of occlusion and near occlusion of the carotid artery, *Am J Neuroradiol* 17:1267–1274, 1996.
47. Powis RL, Powis WD: *A thinker's guide to ultrasonic imaging*, Baltimore, 1984, Urban & Schwarzenberg, pp 345–364.
48. Middleton WD, Erickson S, Melson GL: Perivascular color artifact: pathologic significance and appearance on color Doppler ultrasound images, *Radiology* 171:647–652, 1989.
49. Delcker A, Schurks M, Polz H: Development and applications of 4-D ultrasound (dynamic 3-D) in neurosonology, *J Neuroimaging* 9:229–234, 1999.
50. Delcker A, Diener HC: Quantification of atherosclerotic plaques in carotid arteries by 3-D ultrasound, *Br J Radiol* 67:672–678, 1994.
51. Leotta DF, et al: Remodeling in peripheral vein graft revisions: serial study with three-dimensional ultrasound imaging, *J Vasc Surg* 37:798–807, 2003.
52. Nelson TR, et al: Feasibility of performing a virtual patient examination using three-dimensional ultrasonographic data acquired at remote locations, *J Ultrasound Med* 20:941–952, 2001.
53. Pretorius DH, et al: Three-dimensional ultrasound in obstetrics and gynecology, *Radiol Clin North Am* 39:499–521, 2001.
54. Umemura A, Yamada K: B-mode flow imaging of the carotid artery, *Stroke* 32:2055–2057, 2001.
55. Furuse J, et al: Visualization of blood flow in hepatic vessels and hepatocellular carcinoma using B-flow sonography, *J Clin Ultrasound* 29:1–6, 2001.
56. Pellerito JS: Current approach to peripheral arterial sonography, *Radiol Clin North Am* 3:553–567, 2001.

VASCULAR APPLICATIONS OF ULTRASOUND CONTRAST AGENTS

4

DANIEL A. MERTON, BS, RDMS, FSDMS, FAIUM, and LAURENCE NEEDLEMAN, MD

INTRODUCTION

The clinical applications of gray-scale ultrasound (US), spectral Doppler, and color flow imaging are quite impressive. Nevertheless, there are situations where the ability to obtain diagnostically adequate data using these conventional US modes is limited. This is particularly true for the evaluations of deep-lying vessels (because of signal attenuation), the detection of slow-moving blood flow, and the ability to detect blood flow signals in small vessels. The sensitivity of ultrasound equipment and the recognized operator dependency of US can also impact the results of sonographic examinations.

Intravenous (IV) ultrasound contrast agents (UCAs) have been shown to improve the evaluation of blood flow in both large and small vessels, as well as in the cardiac chambers. Although in the United States UCAs are approved only for echocardiographic indications by the Food and Drug Administration (FDA), in other parts of the world the use of contrast-enhanced ultrasound imaging (CEUS) has been established as a valuable imaging procedure for a variety of clinical applications.

When UCAs were first introduced, their primary application was as a "rescue tool" to salvage nondiagnostic conventional US examinations. Used in this capacity, the addition of UCAs has been shown to reduce or eliminate some of the current limitations of US and Doppler blood flow imaging. Recent advances in diagnostic US equipment have resulted in "contrast-specific" US technologies that markedly improve the capabilities of the modality and expand its already impressive range of clinical applications.

TYPES OF ULTRASOUND CONTRAST AGENTS

For more than two decades intravenously administered agitated saline has been utilized for "bubble study" echocardiography examinations.[1] Hand agitation of saline results in the formation of microbubbles. After injection into a peripheral vein, the microbubbles increase the reflectivity of the blood in the right heart (and right-to-left intracardiac shunts when present), and this can easily be detected with gray-scale and Doppler US modes. However, agitated saline cannot be used to evaluate the left heart chambers or the systemic circulation because the microbubbles do not normally cross the pulmonary circulation and reach the left cardiac chambers.

Commercially available UCAs are nontoxic, have microbubbles that are small enough to traverse the pulmonary capillary beds (i.e., <8 μm in size) but large enough to reflect US signals. They are also stable enough to provide multiple recirculations, which results in several minutes of contrast enhancement after an IV bolus injection. Most UCA microbubbles contain heavy gases (e.g., sulfur hexafluoride or SF6, or fluorocarbons) that improve microbubble longevity after administration.[2] Microbubble stability is provided by the shell, which is most commonly composed of phospholipids, surfactants, and other compounds. Table 4-1 lists UCAs that are FDA approved in the United States and their approved indications, and Table 4-2 lists UCAs that are commercially available elsewhere in the world. Several reports have confirmed that when used appropriately UCAs have very acceptable safety profiles.[3,4]

VASCULAR AGENTS

Vascular or "blood-pool" UCAs enhance Doppler flow signals by adding more and stronger acoustic scatterers in the blood.[5] This results in improved detection of blood flow signals from vessels that are often difficult to assess (e.g., the intracranial vessels, renal arteries, and small capillaries within organs). When used with "contrast-specific" imaging modes (see later), UCAs also improve gray-scale US visualization of flowing blood and increase the echogenicity of contrast-containing tissues.

In general, after IV administration, vascular UCAs remain in the body's vascular spaces. When the microbubbles break down or are ruptured, the components of the microbubble shell are metabolized or eliminated by the body and the gas is exhaled.[2]

TISSUE-SPECIFIC AND TARGETED AGENTS

Tissue-specific UCAs differ from blood-pool UCAs in that these agents are designed to attach to or enter the cells of specific tissues. UCAs have been developed to target plaque and thrombus.[6] By actively attaching to the particular target, the UCA increases the echogenicity of the surface.

These microbubble agents may attach to fibrin, platelets, or other components of thrombi.[7] The presence of thrombus associated with a plaque as determined by CEUS might alter patient management and therapy. Some tissue-specific UCAs can be used to improve the detection of blood flow, as well as enhance the echogenicity of targeted tissue.

Sonazoid (GE Healthcare, Oslo, Norway) contains microbubbles that are targeted to the reticuloendothelial system.[8] This agent has been used to improve detection of liver lesions in humans and for lymphatic applications in animal models.[9] Tissue-specific UCAs target specific types of tissues, and their behavior is predictable so they can be classified as molecular imaging agents.[10]

THERAPEUTIC UCAs

Numerous investigators are attempting to develop UCAs that can be used for therapeutic applications. Typically, therapeutic UCAs have a specific ligand or other binding moiety attached to their shell. The ligand targets a receptor on the surface of a specific cell or tissue so that the UCA attaches to the surface. The microbubble can simply contain a gas or also contain a drug. The delivery of acoustic energy with ultrasound causes disruption or cavitation of the microbubble and the delivery of simple mechanical energy to the surface of the tissue or, if the microbubble contains a drug, also liberates the drug contained by the microbubble to the tissue.

Thrombus-binding UCAs are an example of such an application. A microbubble bound to

TABLE 4-1 UCAs that are Approved by the U.S. Food and Drug Administration*	
Agent, Manufacturer	**Approved Indication(s)**
Optison™, GE Healthcare, Princeton, NJ	Left ventricular opacification / endocardial border definition (LVO/EDB)
Definity®, Lantheus Medical Imaging, N. Billerica, MA	LVO/EDB
Imagent®, IMCOR Pharmaceuticals, Inc., San Diego, CA	LVO/EDB (Imagent is not currently being marketed.)

*This information is considered accurate as of June, 10, 2011. The status of ultrasound contrast agents in the United States is subject to change.

TABLE 4-2 UCAs that are Commercially Available Outside the United States*		
Agent, Manufacturer	**Countries**	**Approved Indications**
Optison™, GE Healthcare, Chalfont St. Giles, UK	European Union	Left ventricular opacification / endocardial border definition (LVO/EDB)
SonoVue®, Bracco Imaging S.p.A., Milan, Italy	European Union, Norway, Switzerland, China, Singapore, Hong Kong, South Korea, Iceland, India, Canada	LVO/EBD, breast, liver, portal vein, extracranial carotid, peripheral arteries (macrovascular, microvascular)
		Approved in Canada for LVO/EBD and diagnostic assessment of vessels
Definity®, Lantheus Medical Imaging, N. Billerica, MA	Canada, Mexico, Israel, New Zealand, India, Australia	LVO/EBD, liver, kidney
	European Union, Korea, Singapore, United Arab Emirates	Approved in these countries only for LVO/EBD
Sonazoid®, Daiichi Pharmaceutical Co., Ltd, Tokyo, Japan (Manufactured and distributed in partnership with GE Healthcare)	Japan	Focal liver lesions

*This information is considered accurate as of June, 10, 2011. The status of ultrasound contrast agents around the world is subject to change.

thrombus is insonated and made to collapse, thereby liberating mechanical energy on the thrombus surface. This can help fragment the thrombus. Additional research is being performed using thrombus-targeting UCAs in patients receiving a thrombolytic agent so that insonation with the US beam further enhances thrombolysis (referred to as "sonothrombolysis").[11,12]

Other therapeutic UCAs are being developed for IV drug delivery to treat a variety of abnormalities, including coronary neointimal hyperplasia and malignancies.[13] The use of therapeutic UCAs for diseases such as blood clots and certain ischemic strokes shows promise.[14]

UCA ADMINISTRATION

Typically, contrast is administered in small (<3 mL) IV bolus injections via a peripheral vein. This provides several minutes of enhancement. If additional contrast enhancement is required, a second administration can be performed. UCAs can also be administered via slow IV infusion to provide prolonged enhancement.[15] The additional enhancement time provided by the infusion of contrast is useful for difficult or time-consuming examinations. Infusion of Definity (Lantheus Medical Imaging, N. Billerica, MA) has been approved by the FDA for echocardiographic applications.[16]

CONTRAST-SPECIFIC ULTRASOUND TECHNOLOGIES

Although conventional gray-scale US and Doppler flow imaging can be used for CEUS, the results are not ideal and artifacts can be encountered.[17] Investigations have been focused on ways to exploit the interactions between US energy and contrast microbubbles in order to improve the clinical utility of CEUS. These investigations have resulted in the development of "contrast-specific" imaging modes such as harmonic imaging, intermittent imaging, and flash-echo imaging. Because the clinical utility of UCAs is greatly improved by the use of these contrast-specific modes, their use is now required during UCA clinical trials and highly preferred when performing clinical CEUS examinations.[18]

HARMONIC IMAGING

When subjected to the acoustic energy present in the US imaging field, UCA microbubbles oscillate in size (i.e., they get larger and smaller). The reflected echoes from the oscillating microbubbles contain energy components at the fundamental frequency (i.e., the transmitted frequency) and at higher and lower harmonics (subharmonics).[19] In harmonic imaging (HI) mode, the US system is configured to receive only echoes at a particular harmonic frequency of the transmit frequency (e.g., 7.0 MHz for a 3.5 MHz transducer).[20,21] When UCAs are imaged with HI mode, the received harmonic echoes from the oscillating microbubbles have a higher signal-to-noise ratio than would be provided by using fundamental US so that regions with microbubbles are more easily appreciated on the resulting gray-scale CEUS image.

Wide-band HI is a recent advance in HI-mode technology (also referred to as phase-inversion HI and pulse-inversion HI) that employs processing algorithms designed to preferentially display echoes arising from contrast microbubbles and suppress echoes arising from body tissues.[22] This imaging technique uses a sequence of two ultrasound pulses that are identical in frequency and amplitude but the second pulse is 180 degrees out of phase with the first pulse. When the two pulses encounter a linear reflector (e.g., body tissue), the resultant echoes cancel one another out, but when the two pulses strike a nonlinear reflector (e.g., contrast microbubble), the harmonic components of the signals combine to result in a signal of higher intensity. Thus, wide-band HI provides a way to better differentiate areas with and without contrast microbubble and has the potential to display blood flow in real-time using gray-scale US, thus obviating the need to use Doppler modes (Figure 4-1). Some

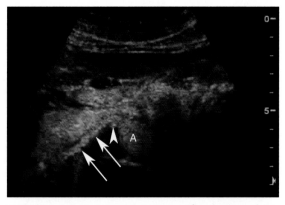

FIGURE 4-1 Transverse contrast-specific ultrasound image of the aorta *(A)* and right renal artery *(arrows)* demonstrates a normal-caliber renal artery and no indication of stenosis. Echogenic plaque *(arrowhead)* is present near the ostium. *(Courtesy of Hans-Peter Weskott, MD, Klinikum Region Hannover, Hannover, Germany.)*

scanners can also perform contrast-specific three-dimensional (3D) imaging. Harmonic Doppler US modes (e.g., harmonic power Doppler imaging [PDI], power modulation imaging) have also been developed.[22]

LOW MECHANICAL INDEX IMAGING AND INTERMITTENT IMAGING

The energy present within the ultrasound beam can cause microbubble destruction during CEUS examinations.[23] Microbubble destruction decreases contrast enhancement by a UCA and therefore decreases the possible clinical utility of the UCA. This must be taken into consideration when using UCAs. One relatively easy way of avoiding this problem is to lower the acoustic output power (i.e., decrease the mechanical index [MI]).

In some cases the intentional destruction of contrast microbubbles in the imaging field is used as a diagnostic tool. For example, CEUS is first used to confirm the presence of contrast material in the target tissue followed by the application of higher acoustic output power (e.g., color Doppler imaging [CDI]) to destroy the microbubbles. After the microbubbles are destroyed, the return of contrast material into the tissue is observed using low-MI CEUS imaging (Figure 4-2). This method can be used to evaluate the rate of re-fill of blood flow (i.e., "reperfusion") in normal tissues such as the myocardium or skeletal muscles, or to assess neovascularity for tumor characterization.[24-26]

Intermittent imaging is another method to reduce microbubble destruction.[22] In this mode, the system is gated to transmit and receive data at predetermined time intervals (e.g., one pulse every second) or is triggered on a specific portion of the electrocardiogram (e.g., the r wave). Intermittent imaging allows additional microbubbles to enter the field so there is an even greater increase in reflectivity of the contrast-containing vessel or tissue than is possible by continuous real-time imaging. An obvious disadvantage to intermittent imaging is the lack of real-time data. However, there are US systems that provide a dual-image display with high-MI intermittent imaging on one display and low-MI real-time data shown on the other. Several reports have described the clinical potential of using the combination of UCAs and contrast-specific intermittent imaging modes.[27-29]

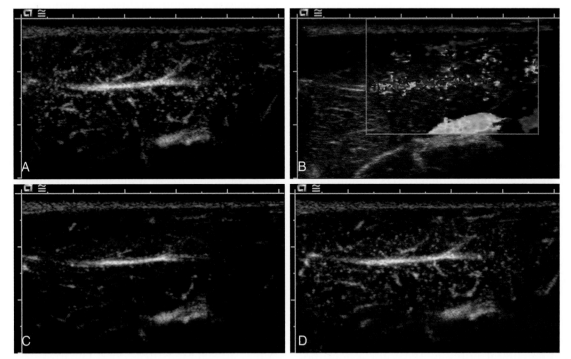

FIGURE 4-2 CEUS demonstration of re-fill of contrast-containing blood flow in skeletal muscle. Contrast-enhanced blood flow is identified in the leg muscle **(A)** using low (0.18) mechanical index (MI) contrast-specific imaging. Color Doppler imaging (CDI) with an MI of 1.9 **(B)** is used to rupture the contrast microbubbles. Progressive re-fill of contrast-containing blood flow is demonstrated using low-MI CEUS at 5 s **(C)** and 19 s **(D)** after bubble destruction.

QUANTIFICATION OF CONTRAST ENHANCEMENT

The use of UCAs provides quantification capabilities that cannot be obtained using conventional US, such as the ability to assess contrast dynamics (e.g., time to peak enhancement and duration of enhancement), measure changes in signal intensity over time (i.e., time-intensity curves), and compare the transit time (i.e., wash-in, wash-out) of contrast-containing blood through organs and tumors.[30-32] Ultrasound systems are available that have on-board calculation packages that can be used to quantify the unique data obtained when UCAs are administered.

ARTIFACTS

The use of UCAs can result in unique imaging artifacts. When imaged with conventional color flow imaging modes, UCAs can cause excessive signal enhancement that causes the display of color Doppler signals beyond the vessel walls.[17] This "color blooming" artifact is easily recognized and can usually be eliminated by reducing the color gain setting, increasing the pulse-repetition frequency, or otherwise reducing color sensitivity.

UCAs can also cause artifacts on spectral Doppler displays. For example, contrast-enhanced spectral Doppler waveforms may demonstrate spectral broadening that was not present before contrast administration, whereas microbubble destruction can cause high-intensity spikes on the spectral display. Several reports have indicated that contrast enhancement can increase the peak velocity displayed on Doppler spectral waveforms.[33-35] Although this artifact does not affect pulsatility indices or velocity ratios, it should be considered when spectral Doppler is used during contrast-enhanced US examinations. It is also important to recognize that noncontrast Doppler US velocity criteria commonly used to indicate disease may not be appropriate for CEUS examinations.

CLINICAL APPLICATIONS OF UCAS

The use of CEUS has been investigated for virtually all clinical applications of diagnostic sonography.[36-41]

The clinical utility of UCAs for echocardiographic examinations is well established, and UCAs are routinely utilized to improve endocardial border definition (EBD) and to assess regional wall motion. Contrast-enhanced echocardiography is also used to improve the detection of intracardiac thrombus, to assess anatomic abnormalities, and for stress echocardiography.[42-44]

Vascular applications of CEUS include evaluation of the cerebrovascular system, peripheral vessels, and abdominal and retroperitoneal vasculature.[45-47] Although qualitative assessments can be performed with conventional color flow imaging modes after contrast administration, more commonly, contrast-specific imaging modes are employed.

CEREBROVASCULAR APPLICATIONS

The use of UCAs for the evaluation of the cerebrovascular system includes the intracranial and extracranial blood vessels. The use of CEUS for evaluations of the carotid arteries and other relatively large vessels has the potential to permit direct assessments of the functional lumen and plaque morphology in a manner similar to other imaging modalities such as arteriography and computed tomographic angiography (Figure 4-3).

Extracranial Vessels

Several investigators have used CEUS in an attempt to solve the vexing problem of distinguishing carotid occlusion from pseudo-occlusion.[48,49] Furst and colleagues[48] evaluated 20 patients with angiographically proven internal carotid artery pseudo-occlusions. This was compared to a control group of 13 patients with occlusion. Sensitivity and specificity were 70% and 92%, respectively, for unenhanced color Doppler, which increased to 83% and 92%, respectively, when Levovist (Schering AG, Berlin, Germany) enhanced CDI was used. The sensitivity and specificity for contrast-enhanced PDI were 94% and 100%, respectively, but this was not significantly improved over conventional PDI with a 95% sensitivity and 92% specificity.

More recently, Kono and associates[50] used wide-band harmonic gray-scale CEUS to image carotid stenoses. In 20 patients, Optison (GE Healthcare, Princeton, NJ) was injected by multiple boluses of 0.5 to 1.0 mL (up to the maximum allowable dose of 8.7 mL). Gray-scale images were obtained in long and short axis and the degree of stenosis measured using the North American Symptomatic Carotid Endarterectomy Trial (NASCET) technique. In 10 patients who underwent angiography, the correlation coefficient between CEUS and arteriography was 0.988

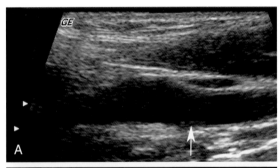

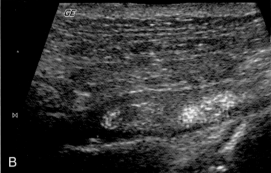

FIGURE 4-3 Contrast-enhanced ultrasound imaging (CEUS) demonstration of a carotid artery dissection and occlusion. Conventional ultrasound (US) of the carotid bulb **(A)** demonstrates minimal wall thickening *(arrow)*. The CEUS image **(B)** demonstrates contrast in the common carotid artery but contrast abruptly stops producing a rounded leading edge. The hemorrhage from the dissection is anechoic, which explains the false-negative findings on conventional US. *(Courtesy of Philip J. Bendick, PhD, William Beaumont Hospital, Royal Oak, MI.)*

(p <0.001). In 2 patients, calcifications obscured the vessel lumen.

Hammond and co-workers[51] also used CEUS in an attempt to differentiate internal carotid artery stenoses from occlusions. This group compared the diagnostic accuracy of CEUS with contrast-enhanced magnetic resonance angiography (CE-MRA) and time-of-flight magnetic resonance angiography (MRA) using digital subtraction angiography as a reference standard in 31 patients who had suspected carotid occlusion on conventional US. The authors concluded that no additional imaging is required when occlusion is confirmed by either CEUS or CE-MRA.

A published study by Pfister and associates[52] described the use of conventional Doppler US, 3D US (with and without a UCA and contrast-enhanced B-flow imaging [GE Healthcare, Waukesha, WI]) for the evaluation of internal carotid artery stenosis. The authors studied 25 patients and found that contrast-enhanced 3D B-flow had a 93% correlation with surgical findings. The use

of 3D CEUS was especially valuable in cases of circular calcifications and severe stenoses and to improve assessment of internal carotid artery plaque morphology.

Intracranial Applications

Sonographic assessment of the intracranial vasculature is often limited by the small size of the intracranial vessels, poor acoustic windows, and signal attenuation through the calvaria. The addition of UCAs during transcranial Doppler (TCD) studies has the ability to improve evaluations of intracranial blood flow.

Specific indications for transcranial CEUS include assessments of patients with venous thromboses or arterial occlusions or stenoses and for evaluation of brain tumors.[53-55] Droste and colleagues[56] evaluated 47 patients with color flow imaging and pulsed Doppler with spectral analysis before and after injection of the contrast agent SonoVue (Bracco Imaging S.p.A., Milan, Italy). Contrast-enhanced TCD significantly improved the number of intracranial vessel segments that could be evaluated: only 26 middle cerebral arteries could be assessed with conventional TCD as compared to 65 following contrast administration.

Evaluation of Plaque and Vessel Wall

Recently investigators have begun to use CEUS to characterize vessel walls and to study preclinical disease as assessed by intima-media thickness (IMT) and endothelial dysfunction. CEUS is being investigated for IMT measurement in order to better define the wall of the carotid artery and to determine the blood-vessel interface with greater precision[57] (Figure 4-4). Endothelial injury and atherosclerotic lesions are being studied in experimental models.[58,59]

The use of CEUS to evaluate blood flow in the vasa vasorum and carotid artery plaque neovascularization is a promising area of investigation.[60-63] Plaque neovascularization is predominantly derived from the arterial wall vasa vasorum. Changes to the vascular morphology of the vessel wall precede the development of obvious plaque and luminal narrowing, and these early vascular changes can be identified using CEUS (see Figure 4-4). The use of CEUS for the evaluation of carotid artery plaque neovascularity is an active area of research and may become a valuable noninvasive method to identify patients who are at increased risk for cardiovascular events.

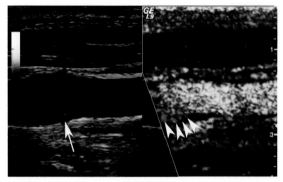

FIGURE 4-4 Improved delineation of the carotid lumen and detection of plaque neovascularization in the carotid artery vasa vasorum. This dual image display demonstrates the conventional ultrasound (US) image on the left and a contrast-specific image on the right. An area of plaque *(arrow)* is suggested on the conventional US image. Contrast-enhanced blood flow is seen within the functional lumen of the carotid artery and vessels within the vasa vasorum *(arrowheads)* consistent with plaque neovascularization. *(Courtesy of Steven Feinstein, MD, Rush University Medical Center, Chicago, IL.)*

PERIPHERAL ARTERIAL APPLICATIONS

Atherosclerotic plaque is a common cause of acoustic shadowing that limits visualization of vessel walls and hampers blood flow detection during US evaluations of the peripheral arteries. Although CEUS typically cannot overcome problems related to acoustic shadowing, the use of CEUS has been found to improve detection of flow distal to the shadowed area (i.e., "run-off" studies) so that a tight stenosis can be differentiated from a complete occlusion. The use of CEUS can also provide information regarding blood flow into the limbs (see Figure 4-2).

The ability of CEUS to serve as a rescue tool for nondiagnostic conventional Doppler evaluations has been confirmed in several studies. Langholz and associates[64] studied 33 patients with iliac or lower extremity arterial disease. All of the CEUS examinations were considered adequate in answering the diagnostic question, and the use of CEUS was particularly helpful to improve visualization of blood flow in the iliac arteries despite the presence of overlying bowel gas.

Spinazzi and Llull[65] reported on the use of SonoVue in a variety of body areas, including peripheral arteries (58 patients), extracranial carotid arteries (59 patients), intracranial arteries (78 patients), and abdominal/retroperitoneal vessels (55 patients). Subjects had an unenhanced US scan that was not fully diagnostic, and all 192 CEUS evaluations were compared to a reference standard. Patients underwent color or power Doppler imaging followed by spectral Doppler utilizing one of four doses of contrast agent. For extracranial carotid and peripheral arteries, the percentage of agreement with the reference standard was significantly improved as compared to unenhanced US. The best results were with the highest dose (2.4-mL bolus), where the agreement improved from 31% to 69%.

Several recent reports have described the use of CEUS for the assessment of patients with peripheral artery disease (PAD). Lindner and colleagues[66] studied 26 controls and 39 symptomatic PAD patients to determine if CEUS could help determine the severity of arterial disease. The investigators performed CEUS with patients at rest and after 2 minutes of exercise. Compared to control subjects, patients with PAD had lower skeletal muscle blood flow as detected with CEUS immediately after exercise and lower flow reserve. The group concluded that CEUS could be used to determine the severity of PAD.

A report by Duerschmied and co-workers[67] described the use of CEUS to evaluate calf muscle perfusion and vascular collateralization in patients with PAD. These authors found that CEUS could improve detection of perfusion deficits as well as the degree of arterial collateralization in symptomatic PAD patients.

PERIPHERAL VENOUS APPLICATIONS

The use of compression sonography is highly effective for the evaluation of patients with suspected deep venous thrombosis (DVT). Thus, only a few early reports have been published that describe the use of UCAs for peripheral venous applications.[68,69]

Puls and colleagues[69] used Levovist in 31 patients who had suspected DVT and at least one vein segment that was inadequately imaged with CDI. Baseline CDI was inadequate in 43 of 279 vessel segments, and contrast-enhancement was seen in 40 of these 43 segments. Of the 27 vein segments that were confirmed to have DVT on venography, 18 were detected on baseline imaging whereas CEUS identified 25. Three iliac vein thromboses were identified with CEUS, but only one was detected at baseline and five of the seven additional DVTs detected with CEUS were below the knee. The diagnostic accuracy increased from 60% (26 of 43 vein segments) before contrast administration to 86% (37 of 43 vein segments) with CEUS.

ABDOMINAL AND RETROPERITONEAL APPLICATIONS

The use of CEUS has been investigated for a wide variety of abdominal applications, including the evaluation of the aorta and its branches, the portal venous system, and the abdominal organs.[70] CEUS has been investigated for the evaluation of organ perfusion (including transplant organs) and for tumor characterization.

Renal Artery Stenosis

US detection of renal artery stenosis (RAS) is challenging. The renal arteries are deep and can be tortuous, which makes their sonographic evaluation challenging and time consuming. Ultrasonic visualization of the renal vessels is also limited by overlying bowel and patient obesity. Published reports suggest that the addition of a UCA can improve sonographic evaluations of patients with suspected RAS by improving the ability to localize and assess blood flow in the main renal arteries and intrarenal branch vessels, as well as reducing examination time[71,72] (see Figure 4-1).

Missouris and colleagues[71] investigated intrarenal waveforms following administration of Levovist in 21 subjects. Examination time was reduced from 25 minutes using unenhanced US to 14 minutes with CEUS. Compared to the unenhanced US studies, the use of CEUS improved sensitivity (from 85% to 94%) and specificity (from 79% to 88%).

A study published in 2011 described the use of Levovist-enhanced US for the evaluation of RAS as compared with conventional CDI in 120 hypertensive patients.[73] Angiography was performed in the 40 patients who had RAS diagnosed by one of the two US techniques (RAS was identified with CDI in 33 cases and with CEUS in 38). Angiography confirmed RAS in all 38 patients diagnosed by CEUS, suggesting that CEUS has sensitivity, specificity, and accuracy levels similar to those of angiography. There were six false-negative and two false-positive CDI studies.

Mesenteric Applications

Gray-scale and Doppler US evaluation of the superior mesenteric, celiac, and inferior mesenteric arteries can be limited by poor visualization of the vessels, inadequate Doppler beam-to-vessel angles, and other factors. The use of CEUS has been shown to be a valuable addition to conventional US to assess the mesenteric vessels

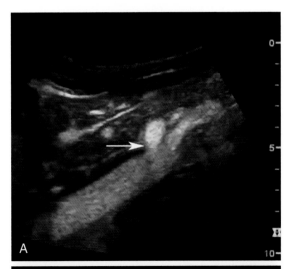

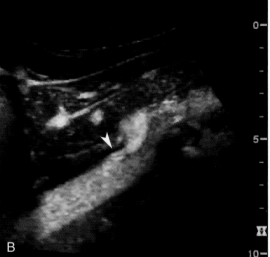

FIGURE 4-5 Contrast-enhanced ultrasound imaging (CEUS) demonstration of the celiac artery in a patient who has median arcuate ligament syndrome. The longitudinal view of the aorta during deep inspiration **(A)** demonstrates a normal celiac artery *(arrow)*. However, during expiration **(B)** the origin of the celiac artery is compressed and displaced inferiorly by the median arcuate ligament *(arrowhead)*. The use of real-time CEUS provides a means to assess these dynamic events to facilitate the diagnosis of median arcuate ligament syndrome. *(Courtesy of Hans-Peter Weskott, MD, Klinikum Region Hannover, Hannover, Germany.)*

(Figure 4-5). Blebea and associates[74] evaluated 17 patients before and after infusion of Definity and compared their results to angiography. Stenosis or occlusion was detected with CEUS in 81% of the vessels studied compared to just 55% with unenhanced US. The improvement of CEUS over conventional US was most evident in the celiac and mesenteric arteries, but the results did not reach statistical significance.

Hepatic Applications

Aside from echocardiography, the most common application of UCAs is for liver lesion detection and characterization.[75,76] Studies have determined that the sensitivity of CEUS for characterization of focal liver lesions is comparable to that of contrast-enhanced computed tomography (CT) or magnetic resonance imaging (MRI).[77] However, the use of CEUS for these applications is beyond the scope of this chapter.

Contrast-enhanced US has been shown to improve the detection of hepatic blood flow in normal subjects as well as patients with liver disease and portal hypertension (PHT).[78-80] Sonographic examinations for PHT include qualitative assessment of blood flow with color flow imaging to identify the presence and direction of flow in the splenic, superior mesenteric, and main portal veins, as well as the intrahepatic portal and hepatic veins. The use of UCAs would be expected to improve the detection of low-velocity blood flow in the portal venous system in patients with PHT. These low-velocity signals can be difficult to detect using conventional sonography. Contrast-enhanced US may also improve the detection of portosystemic collaterals. Additionally, CEUS has been used effectively for assessment of transjugular intrahepatic portosystemic shunt (TIPS).[81]

Sellars and associates[80] used Levovist to study both normal volunteers and patients with cirrhosis. Doppler flow signals from the portal vein were enhanced in all cases after administration of Levovist. This study compared the duration of enhancement provided by a bolus administration to that of three different infusion rates (slow, medium, and fast). A bolus delivery provided the shortest duration of contrast enhancement, whereas the slow infusion technique provided the longest duration. Contrast-enhancement persisted for a mean duration of 113 seconds after a bolus injection when compared to as much as 569 seconds during a slow infusion.

Published reports have described CEUS-detectable alterations in blood flow transit time through the hepatic parenchyma of patients with diffuse and focal liver disease when compared to normal controls.[82] Transit-time analysis of contrast-enhanced blood flow through the liver has also been investigated in an attempt to identify hemodynamic changes that result from the presence of metastases.[83,84]

Organ Transplants

Sonography is often employed as a first-line examination in the immediate postsurgical period to evaluate renal, hepatic, and pancreatic transplants, as well as for serial studies to assess organ viability. Conventional sonography is useful in the evaluation of blood flow within the organ but does not have an adequate level of sensitivity to detect flow at the microvascular level (i.e., tissue perfusion). When a vascular abnormality is suspected, angiography or contrast-enhanced CT or MRI may be necessary to obtain a definitive diagnosis.[85] However, angiography is invasive, CT requires ionizing radiation, and administration of contrast media required for these examinations may be contraindicated in renal-compromised patients.

CEUS has been shown to improve the assessment of blood flow in the arteries and veins that supply the transplant, the host vessels to which these vessels are anastomosed, as well as the parenchyma of transplanted organs (Figure 4-6). CEUS has also been found to improve the ability to detect ischemic regions within native and transplanted organs.[86-88]

Sindhu and colleagues[89] reported on the use of CEUS to evaluate the hepatic arteries of 31 liver transplant patients who had parvus tardus Doppler waveforms and compared the results to arteriography or follow-up US. They reported that CEUS could have obviated the need for arteriography in approximately 63% of studies.

The use of UCA provides an additional means to evaluate and quantify blood flow to and within transplanted organs. Kay and co-workers[90] evaluated 20 consecutive renal transplant patients for overall perfusion and regional variations in perfusion. All patients were studied within 7 days of transplantation. A bolus injection of SonoVue was administered, and the kidney was imaged with low-MI CEUS for 1 minute following injection. Time-intensity curves were generated for three areas (cortex, medullary pyramid, and interlobar artery) in the upper, mid, and lower poles. Parameters of time-intensity curves included contrast arrival time, time to peak enhancement, peak intensity, gradient of the slope, and the area under curve. There was good interobserver agreement for all values measured from the cortex and medulla, but poor interobserver correlation for the vascular values. Renal perfusion as determined by CEUS correlated with the transplant estimated

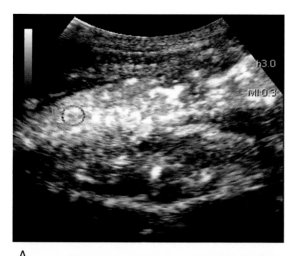

A

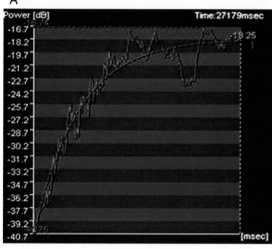

B

FIGURE 4-6 Contrast-enhanced ultrasound imaging (CEUS) evaluation of a pancreatic transplant. CEUS **(A)** demonstrates enhancement throughout the gland. Quantitative enhancement data from the region of interest *(red circle)* is provided by the time-intensity curve **(B)**, which demonstrates changes in signal intensity (vertical axis) over time (horizontal axis). *(Courtesy of Antonio Sergio Marcelino, MD, Sirio-Libanes Hospital and Cancer Institute of University of Sao Paulo, Sao Paulo, Brazil.)*

glomerular filtration rate at 3 months after transplantation. The investigators concluded that estimates of transplant perfusion as quantified by CEUS may be of future benefit in transplant recipients and potentially utilized as a prognostic tool.

Aortic Graft and Stent Surveillance

The use of CEUS is gaining attention as a viable alternative to other diagnostic imaging examinations used to evaluate patients after endovascular aneurysm repair of abdominal aortic aneurysms.[47,91,92] Postsurgical surveillance of

these patients is required to detect endoleaks when present, and patients need to be followed for months or even years after endovascular aneurysm repair. Administration of a UCA provides several minutes of enhancement, so the graft can be evaluated over time to detect both fast-flowing and slow-flowing endoleaks. This is an advantage over CT since the postcontrast CT scans are acquired for up to three phases to limit ionizing radiation exposure and decrease cumulative radiation exposure. CEUS can also provide information regarding the precise location of the endoleak and differentiate between type 1 and type 2 endoleaks (Figure 4-7).

Bendick and colleagues[93] reported excellent results using Optison to improve detection of endoleaks. Six endoleaks were detected using unenhanced US, and delayed-phase CT identified eight. All eight leaks were detected using CEUS, and the addition of UCA to the examination allowed the investigators to determine if the leaks were type 1 or 2. Additionally, two proximal attachment leaks not seen on CT were seen with CEUS and were subsequently confirmed by angiography. In another study Giannoni and associates[91] used CEUS for surveillance of 30 patients who had aortic stent-grafts and compared the CEUS results to either computed tomographic angiography (CTA) or MRA. All endoleaks detected by CTA or MRA were detected by CEUS, yielding a 100% sensitivity.

Emerging Applications

The use of conventional sonography is rapidly being embraced by a large number of "emerging users," including anesthesiologists, rheumatologists, emergency department personnel, and others. Published reports suggest that CEUS holds promise for indications such as the evaluation of trauma patients (i.e., to better identify active bleeding and organ damage) and assessment of the vascularity in and around tendons and joints to identify early signs of inflammation as well as to monitor therapy.[94-96] The clinical utility of CEUS will likely become established as a valuable diagnostic tool for these and other new applications.

CONCLUSIONS

Two UCAs are currently being marketed in the United States: Optison and Definity. However, as of this writing they are FDA approved only for

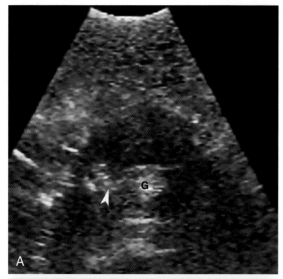

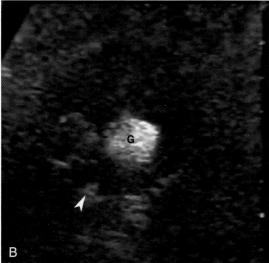

FIGURE 4-7 Evaluations of endovascular aortic aneurysm repair grafts. Transverse contrast-enhanced ultrasound (US) image **(A)** demonstrates blood flow in the graft *(G)* and a small area of contrast-containing blood flow entering the aneurysm sac *(arrowhead)* consistent with a type 1 endoleak. This leak was present only during systole but was readily visualized with real-time contrast-enhanced ultrasound imaging (CEUS). In another patient **(B)**, CEUS demonstrates contrast-enhanced blood flow in the graft *(G)* and a very small amount of flow from a lumbar vessel into the aneurysm sac *(arrowhead)* consistent with a type 2 endoleak. *(Courtesy of Philip J. Bendick, PhD, William Beaumont Hospital, Royal Oak, MI.)*

echocardiographic applications. In the future, additional agents and/or clinical applications of existing agents are likely to become available. UCAs have been shown to salvage nondiagnostic US examinations and render them diagnostic. The use of UCAs has also lead to new US applications that were not possible without their use.

UCAs have been shown to improve the detection of blood flow signals in large and small vessels throughout the body, as well as to improve the sonographic detection and characterization of tumors, areas of inflammation, and varied pathologies in many areas throughout the body. Improvements in US technology that exploit the acoustic behavior of contrast microbubbles are further expanding the clinical capabilities of contrast-enhanced sonography. The use of CEUS is expected to increase as the clinical utility of sonography is increasingly recognized.

REFERENCES

1. Lang RM, Mor-Avi V: Clinical utility of contrast-enhanced echocardiography, *Clin Cardiol* 29(9 Suppl 1):I15–I25, 2006.
2. Wheatley MA: Composition of contrast microbubbles: basic chemistry of encapsulated and surfactant-coated bubbles. In Goldberg BB, Raichlen JS, Forsberg F, editors: *Ultrasound contrast agents*, ed 2, London, 2001, Martin Dunitz Ltd, pp 3–13.
3. Wei K, et al: The safety of Definity and Optison for ultrasound image enhancement: a retrospective analysis of 78,383 administered contrast doses, *J Am Soc Echocardiogr* 11:1202–1206, 2008.
4. Dijkmans PA, et al: Safety and feasibility of real time adenosine myocardial contrast echocardiography with emphasis on induction of arrhythmias: a study in healthy volunteers and patients with stable coronary artery disease, *Echocardiography* 26(7):807–814, 2009.
5. Forsberg F: Physics of ultrasound contrast agents. In Goldberg BB, editor: *Ultrasound contrast agents*, London, 1997, Martin Dunitz Ltd, pp 9–20.
6. Unger EC, et al: In Goldberg BB, Raichlen JS, Forsberg F, editors: *Ultrasound contrast agents*, ed 2, London, 2001, Martin Dunitz Ltd., pp 337–345.
7. Takeuchi M, et al: Enhanced visualization of intravascular and left atrial appendage thrombus with the use of a thrombus-targeting ultrasonographic contrast agent (MRX-408A1); in vivo experimental echocardiographic studies, *J Am Soc Echocardiogr* 12:1015–1021, 1999.
8. Arita J, et al: Correlation between contrast-enhanced intraoperative ultrasound using Sonazoid and histologic grade of resected hepatocellular carcinoma, *AJR Am J Roentgenol* 196(6):1314–1321, 2011.
9. Goldberg BB, et al: Contrast-enhanced ultrasound imaging of sentinel lymph nodes after peritumoral administration of Sonazoid in a melanoma tumor animal model, *J Ultrasound Med* 30(4):441–453, 2011.
10. Miller JC, Thrall JH: Clinical molecular imaging, *J Am Coll Radiol* 1:4–23, 2004.
11. Laing ST, McPherson DD: Cardiovascular therapeutic uses of targeted ultrasound contrast agents, *Cardiovasc Res* 83(4):626–635, 2009.
12. Molina CA, et al: Transcranial ultrasound in clinical sonothrombolysis (TUCSON) trial, *Ann Neurol* 66(1): 28–38, 2009.

13. Porter R, Xie F: Targeted drug delivery using intravenous microbubbles. In Goldberg BB, Raichlen JS, Forsberg F, editors: *Ultrasound contrast agents*, ed 2, London, 2001, Martin Dunitz Ltd., pp 347–352.

14. Unger EC, et al: Therapeutic applications of microbubbles, *Eur J Radiol* 2:160–168, 2002.

15. Albrecht T, et al: Prolongation and optimization of Doppler enhancement with a microbubble US contrast agent by using continuous infusion: preliminary experience, *Radiology* 207:339–347, 1998.

16. Lantheus Medical Imaging: prescribing information. http://www.definityimaging.com/prescribing_info.html. Accessed June 6, 2011.

17. Forsberg F, et al: Artifacts in ultrasound contrast agent studies, *J Ultrasound Med* 13:357–365, 1994.

18. Greenbaum L, et al: American Institute of Ultrasound in Medicine recommendations for contrast-enhanced liver ultrasound imaging clinical trials, *J Ultrasound Med* 26:705–716, 2007.

19. Forsberg F, et al: Breast lesions: imaging with contrast-enhanced sub-harmonic US: initial experiences, *Radiology* 244:718–726, 2007.

20. Forsberg F, et al: Gray-scale and color Doppler flow harmonic imaging with proteinaceous microspheres, *Radiology* 197(P):403, 1995.

21. Kono Y, Mattrey RT: Harmonic imaging with contrast microbubbles. In Goldberg BB, Raichlen JS, Forsberg F, editors: *Ultrasound contrast agents*, ed 2, London, 2001, Martin Dunitz Ltd., pp 37–46.

22. De Jong N, et al: Contrast-specific imaging methods. In Goldberg BB, Raichlen JS, Forsberg F, editors: *Ultrasound contrast agents*, ed 2, London, 2001, Martin Dunitz Ltd., pp 25–36.

23. Harvey CJ, et al: Acoustic emission imaging. In Goldberg BB, Raichlen JR, Forsberg F, editors: *Ultrasound contrast agents: basic principles and clinical applications*, ed 2, London, 2001, Martin Dunitz Ltd., pp 71–80.

24. Wei K, et al: Quantification of myocardial blood flow with ultrasound induced destruction of microbubbles administered as a constant venous infusion, *Circulation* 97:473–483, 1998.

25. Hope SD, Chin CT, Burns PB: Perfusion imaging with pulse inversion Doppler and microbubble contrast agents: in vivo studies of the myocardium, *Proceedings of IEEE Ultrasonics Symposium* 1:597–600, 1998.

26. Blomley MJK, et al: Improved imaging of liver metastases with stimulated acoustic emission in the late phase of enhancement with the US contrast agent SH U 508A: early experience, *Radiology* 210:409–416, 1999.

27. Sirlin CB, et al: Effect of gated US acquisition on liver and portal vein contrast enhancement, *Radiology* 201(P):158, 1996.

28. Wei K, et al: Quantification of renal blood flow with contrast-enhanced ultrasound, *J Am Coll Cardiol* 37(4):1135–1140, 2001.

29. Hudson JM, Karshafian R, Burns PN: Quantification of flow using ultrasound and microbubbles: a disruption replenishment model based on physical principles, *Ultrasound Med Biol* 35(12):2007–2020, 2009.

30. Blomley MJ, et al: Liver microbubble transit time compared with histology and Child-Pugh score in diffuse liver disease: a cross sectional study, *Gut* 52(8):1188–1193, 2003.

31. Kishimoto N, et al: Renal blood flow measurement with contrast-enhanced harmonic ultrasonography: evaluation of dopamine-induced changes in renal cortical perfusion in humans, *Clin Nephrol* 59(6):423–428, 2003.

32. Hudson JM, Karshafian R, Burns PN: Quantification of flow using ultrasound and microbubbles: a disruption replenishment model based on physical principles, *Ultrasound Med Biol* 35:2007–2020, 2009.

33. Needleman L, et al: US contrast does not change canine renal Doppler pulsatility indices, *Radiology* 209(P):461, 1998.

34. Gutberlet M, et al: Do ultrasonic contrast agents artificially increase maximum Doppler shift? in vivo study of human common carotid arteries, *J Ultrasound Med* 17(2):97–102, 1998.

35. Kroger K, Massalha K, Rudofsky G: The use of the echo-enhancing agent Levovist does not influence the estimation of the degree of vascular stenosis calculated from peak systolic velocity ratio, diameter reduction and cross section area reduction, *Eur J Ultrasound* 8(1):17–24, 1998.

36. Lencioni R, editor: *Enhancing the role of ultrasound with contrast agents*, Milan, 2006, Springer-Verlag.

37. Quaia E, editor: *Contrast media in ultrasonography: basic principles and clinical applications*, Berlin, 2005, Springer-Verlag.

38. Zamorano JL, Fernandez MA: *Contrast echocardiography in clinical practice*, Milan, 2004, Springer-Verlag.

39. Albrecht T, et al: *Contrast-enhanced ultrasound in clinical practice: liver, prostate, pancreas, kidney and lymph nodes*, Milan, 2005, Springer-Verlag.

40. Liu JB, et al: Contrast-enhanced ultrasound imaging. In McGahan JP, Goldberg BB, editors: *Diagnostic ultrasound: a logical approach*, ed 2, New York, 2008, Informa Healthcare, pp 39–62.

41. Abramowicz JS: Ultrasound contrast media; has the time come in obstetrics and gynecology? *J Ultrasound Med* 24:517–531, 2005.

42. Grayburn PA, Raichlen JS: Evaluation of the heart at rest. In Goldberg BB, Raichlen JR, Forsberg F, editors: *Ultrasound contrast agents: basic principles and clinical applications*, ed 2, London, 2001, Martin Dunitz Ltd., pp 143–154.

43. Nathan S, Feinstein SB: Evaluation of the heart during exercise and pharmacologic stress. In Goldberg BB, Raichlen JR, Forsberg F, editors: *Ultrasound contrast agents: basic principles and clinical applications*, ed 2, London, 2001, Martin Dunitz Ltd., pp 155–164.

44. Lopes LR, et al: The usefulness of contrast during exercise echocardiography for the assessment of systolic pulmonary pressure, *Cardiovasc Ultrasound* 13(6):51, 2008.

45. Needleman L, Merton DA: Imaging of peripheral vascular pathology. In Goldberg BB, Raichlen JS, Forsberg F, editors: *Ultrasound contrast agents: basic principles and clinical applications*, ed 2, London, 2001, Martin Dunitz Publishing, pp 267–276.

46. Robbin ML: The utility of contrast in the extra-cranial carotid ultrasound examination. In Goldberg BB, Raichlen JR, Forsberg F, editors: *Ultrasound contrast agents: basic principles and clinical applications*, ed 2, London, 2001, Martin Dunitz Ltd., pp 239–252.

47. Pfister K, et al: Contrast harmonic imaging ultrasound and perfusion imaging for surveillance after endovascular abdominal aneurysm repair regarding detection and characterization of suspected endoleaks, *Clin Hemorheol Microcirc* 43:119–128, 2009.

48. Furst G, et al: Reliability and validity of noninvasive imaging of internal carotid artery pseudo-occlusion, *Stroke* 30(7):1444–1449, 1999.

49. Droste DW, et al: Ultrasound contrast enhancing agents in neurosonology: principles, methods, future possibilities, *Acta Neurol Scand* 102(1):1–10, 2000.

50. Kono Y, et al: Carotid arteries: contrast-enhanced US angiography–preliminary clinical experience, *Radiology* 230(2):561–568, 2004.

51. Hammond CJ, et al: Assessment of apparent internal carotid occlusion on ultrasound: prospective comparison of contrast-enhanced ultrasound, magnetic resonance angiography and digital subtraction angiography, *Eur J Vasc Endovasc Surg* 35(4):405–412, 2008.

52. Pfister K, et al: Pre-surgical evaluation of ICA-stenosis using 3D power Doppler, 3D color coded Doppler sonography, 3D B-flow and contrast enhanced B-flow in correlation to CTA/MRA: first clinical results, *Clin Hemorheol Microcirc* 41(2):103–116, 2009.

53. Kunz A, et al: Echo-enhanced transcranial color-coded duplex sonography in the diagnosis of cerebrovascular events: a validation study, *AJNR Am J Neuroradiol* 27:2122–2127, 2006.

54. Bogdahn U, Holscher T, Schlachetzki F: Transcranial color-coded duplex sonography (TCCS). In Goldberg BB, Raichlen JR, Forsberg F, editors: *Ultrasound contrast agents: Basic principles and clinical applications*, ed 2, London, 2001, Martin Dunitz Ltd., pp 253–265.

55. Droste DW: Clinical utility of contrast-enhanced ultrasound in neurosonology, *Eur Neurol* 59(Suppl 1):2–8, 2008.

56. Droste DW, et al: Benefit of echocontrast-enhanced transcranial arterial color-coded duplex ultrasound, *Cerebrovasc Dis* 20(5):332–336, 2005.

57. Feinstein SB, Voci P, Pizzuto F: Noninvasive surrogate markers of atherosclerosis, *Am J Cardiol* 89(5A):31C–43C, 2002.

58. Sirlin CB, et al: Contrast-enhanced B-mode US angiography in the assessment of experimental in vivo and in vitro atherosclerotic disease, *Acad Radiol* 8(2):162–172, 2001.

59. Villanueva FS, Wagner WR, Klibanov AL: Targeted ultrasound contrast agents: identification of endothelial dysfunction. In Goldberg BB, et al: *Ultrasound Contrast Agents: basic principles and clinical applications*, London, 2001, Martin Dunitz, pp 353–365.

60. Shah F, et al: Contrast-enhanced ultrasound imaging of atherosclerotic carotid plaque neovascularization: a new surrogate marker of atherosclerosis? *Vasc Med* 12(4):291–297, 2007.

61. Magnoni M, et al: Contrast-enhanced ultrasound imaging of periadventitial vasa vasorum in human carotid arteries, *Eur J Echocardiogr* 10:260–264, 2009.

62. Coli S, et al: Contrast-enhanced ultrasound imaging of intraplaque neovascularization in carotid arteries: correlation with histology and plaque echogenicity, *J Am Coll Cardiol* 52(3):223–230, 2008.

63. Staub D, et al: Vasa vasorum and plaque neovascularization on contrast-enhanced carotid ultrasound imaging correlates with cardiovascular disease and past cardiovascular events, *Stroke* 4(1):41–47, 2010.

64. Langholz J, et al: Contrast enhancement in leg vessels, *Clin Radiol* 51:31–34, 1996.

65. Spinazzi A, Llull JB: Diagnostic performance of SonoVue-enhanced color duplex sonography of vascular structures, *Acad Radiol* 9(Suppl 1):S246–S250, 2002.

66. Lindner JR, et al: Limb stress-rest perfusion imaging with contrast ultrasound for the assessment of peripheral arterial disease severity, *JACC Cardiovasc Imaging* 1(3):343–350, 2008.

67. Duerschmied D, et al: Simplified contrast ultrasound accurately reveals muscle perfusion deficits and reflects collateralization in PAD, *Atherosclerosis* 202(2):505–512, 2009.

68. Vorwerk D, et al: Dynamic contrast medium-aided ultrasound cavography in patients with a caval filter, *Ultraschall Med* 1:146–149, 1990.

69. Puls R, et al: Signal-enhanced color Doppler sonography of deep venous thrombosis in the lower limbs and pelvis, *J Ultrasound Med* 18:185–190, 1999.

70. Oka MA, Rubens DJ, Strang JG: Ultrasound contrast agent in evaluation of abdominal vessels, *J Ultrasound Med* 20:S84, 2001.

71. Missouris CG, et al: Non-invasive screening for renal artery stenosis with ultrasound contrast enhancement, *J Hypertens* 14(4):519–524, 1996.

72. Needleman L: Review of a new ultrasound contrast agent- EchoGen emulsion, *Appl Radiol* 26(S):8–12, 1997.

73. Ciccone MM, et al: The clinical role of contrast-enhanced ultrasound in the evaluation of renal artery stenosis and diagnostic superiority as compared to traditional echo-color-Doppler flow imaging, *Int Angiol* 30(2):135–139, 2011.

74. Blebea J, et al: Contrast enhanced duplex ultrasound imaging of the mesenteric arteries, *Ann Vasc Surg* 16(1):77–83, 2002.

75. EFSUMB Study Group: Guidelines and good clinical practice recommendations for contrast enhanced ultrasound (CE-US) – Update 2008, *Ultraschall Med* 29:28–44, 2008.

76. Burns P, Wilson S: Focal liver masses: enhancement patterns on contrast-enhanced images - concordance of US scans with CT scans and MR images, *Radiology* 242:162–174, 2007.

77. Trillaud H, et al: Characterization of focal liver lesions with SonoVue® enhanced sonography: international multicenter-study in comparison to CT and MRI, *World J Gastroenterol* 15(30):3748–3756, 2009.

78. Albrecht T, et al: Non-invasive diagnosis of hepatic cirrhosis by transit-time analysis of an ultrasound contrast agent, *Lancet* 353:1579–1583, 1999.

79. Lee KH, et al: Contrast-enhanced dynamic ultrasonography of the liver: optimization of hepatic arterial phase in normal volunteers, *Abdom Imaging* 28(5):652–656, 2003.

80. Sellars ME, et al: Infusions of microbubbles are more cost-effective than bolus injections in Doppler studies of the portal vein: a quantitative comparison of normal volunteers and patients with cirrhosis, *Radiology* 217(P):396, 2000.

81. Skjoldbye B, et al: Doppler ultrasound assessment of TIPS patency and function- the need for echo enhancers, *Acta Radiol* 39:675–679, 1998.

82. Leen E, et al: Contrast enhanced Doppler perfusion index: detection of colorectal liver metastases, *Radiology* 209(P):292, 1998.

83. Hohmann J, et al: Hepatic transit time analysis using contrast-enhanced ultrasound with BR1: a prospective study comparing patients with liver metastases from colorectal cancer with healthy volunteers, *Ultrasound Med Biol* 35(9):1427–1435, 2009.

84. Zhou JH, et al: Haemodynamic parameters of the hepatic artery and vein can detect liver metastases: assessment using contrast-enhanced ultrasound, *Br J Radiol* 81(962):113–119, 2008.

85. Karamehic J, et al: Ultrasonography in organs transplantation, *Med Arh* 58(1 Suppl 2):107–108, 2004.

86. Benozzi L, et al: Contrast-enhanced sonography in early kidney graft dysfunction, *Transplant Proc.* 41(4):1214–1215, 2009.

87. Boggi U, et al: Contribution of contrast-enhanced ultrasonography to nonoperative management of segmental ischemia of the head of a pancreas graft, *Am J Transplant* 9(2):413–418, 2009.

88. Faccioli N, et al: Contrast-enhanced ultrasonography of the pancreas, *Pancreatology* 9(5):560–566, 2009:4.

89. Sidhu PS, et al: Microbubble ultrasound contrast in the assessment of hepatic artery patency following liver transplantation: role in reducing frequency of hepatic artery arteriography, *Eur Radiol* 14(1):21–30, 2004.

90. Kay DH, et al: Ultrasonic microbubble contrast agents and the transplant kidney, *Clin Radiol* 64(11):1081–1087, 2009.

91. Giannoni MF, et al: Contrast-enhanced ultrasound for aortic stent-graft surveillance, *J Endovasc Ther* 10(2):208–217, 2003.

92. Iezzi R, et al: Endoleaks after endovascular repair of abdominal aortic aneurysm: value of CEUS, *Abdom Imaging* 35(1):106–114, 2010.

93. Bendick PJ, et al: Efficacy of ultrasound scan contrast agents in the noninvasive follow-up of aortic stent grafts, *J Vasc Surg* 37(2):381–385, 2003.

94. Valentino M, et al: Contrast-enhanced ultrasonography in blunt abdominal trauma: considerations after 5 years of experience, *Radiol Med* 114(7):1080–1093, 2009.

95. Weskott HP: Emerging roles for contrast-enhanced ultrasound, *Clin Hemorheol Microcirc* 40(1):51–71, 2008.

96. Backhaus M: Ultrasound and structural changes in inflammatory arthritis: synovitis and tenosynovitis, *Ann N Y Acad Sci* 1154:139–151, 2009.

Cerebral Vessels

THE ROLE OF ULTRASOUND IN THE MANAGEMENT OF CEREBROVASCULAR DISEASE

5

ANDREI V. ALEXANDROV, MD, and CLOTILDE BALUCANI, MD

Successful implementation of systemic reperfusion therapy for acute ischemic stroke and the need to implement treatment quickly to improve outcomes have led clinicians to look for ways to image the brain and vessels more efficiently. From this perspective, ultrasound for the evaluation of cerebrovascular disease has evolved from a simple screening test for detecting significant carotid stenosis into a method to evaluate the extracranial and intracranial circulation, perform real-time physiologic assessment, and monitor reperfusion.

Carotid duplex and transcranial duplex/Doppler are noninvasive, not reliant on ionizing radiation, relatively inexpensive, and available worldwide. Despite advances in magnetic resonance and computed tomography (CT) imaging, there will always be patients who cannot undergo or repeatedly receive these tests. Thus, it is essential for stroke clinicians to know how to perform and interpret cerebrovascular ultrasound as an alternative or follow-up vascular imaging tool.

In the "acute stroke scenario," carotid Doppler and transcranial Doppler evaluation can be considered as an extension of the neurologic examination because these tests enable clinicians to confirm the vascular origin of patient symptoms, detect the abnormality, and localize the involved vessels.

Transcranial Doppler (TCD) in particular provides a wealth of information, including real-time bedside assessment of pathophysiologic changes in patients with cerebrovascular disease, including monitoring of thrombus dissolution or reocclusion, collateral development, and cerebral embolization, as well as the progress of therapies.[1-15]

Cerebrovascular ultrasound can be used for rapid detection and quantification of the severity of arterial occlusive disease, thus facilitating patient selection for reperfusion therapies, invasive angiography, and urgent interventional treatment, and for assessment of the short- and long-term prognosis. No other imaging method in wide use today offers the same potential for continuous real-time monitoring of arterial blood flow. In addition, ultrasound waves can have a therapeutic effect through the transmission of mechanical energy directly to the soft tissues. The therapeutic application of ultrasound has been shown to augment residual blood flow and to speed up thrombolysis, allowing acute stroke patients to recover more rapidly.[16-17]

Prerequisites to a successful practice of cerebrovascular ultrasound include knowledge of anatomy, physiology of cardiovascular and nervous systems, fluid dynamics, and pathologic changes in a variety of cerebrovascular disorders, as well as basics of ultrasound physics and instrumentation. The accuracy of the practice of ultrasound (both performance and interpretation) varies between practitioners of different skill, knowledge, and experience. Besides credentialing, constant learning and improvement through consistent application, local validation of ultrasound testing and interpretation, and continuing quality improvement are the keys to successful practices.[18]

It is also desirable that each neurovascular ultrasound laboratory validates its own diagnostic criteria in order to reduce variability and improve consistency of ultrasound interpretation. This requirement in the United States is endorsed by the Intersocietal Commission for Accreditation of Vascular Laboratories (ICAVL)[19] (www.icavl.org).

This chapter will describe cerebrovascular ultrasound scanning protocols and criteria for interpretation and illustrate how ultrasound provides information helpful in stroke patient management.

Clinicians who perform and interpret cerebrovascular ultrasound typically use it to do the following:

- Differentiate normal from diseased vessels and quantify the degree of the arterial stenosis and plaque burden

- Identify the disease process, including acute occlusions or dissections in the major extracranial and intracranial vessels, including lesions amenable to interventional treatment (LAITs)
- Identify collateral flow pattern and flow direction for assessing the ability of collateral circulation to maintain cerebral blood flow
- Detect, localize, and quantify cerebral embolism, particularly in the context of intraoperative monitoring of carotid revascularization procedures
- Detect and grade right-to-left shunts
- Assess recanalization and reocclusion with thrombolysis
- Monitor and even augment thrombolysis
- Predict stroke risk in sickle cell disease (SCD)
- Identify subclavian steal syndrome
- Evaluate cerebrovascular autoregulation or vasomotor reactivity
- Identify intracranial steal and reversed Robin Hood syndrome
- Detect and monitor arterial spasm
- Identify hyperemia
- Indirectly detect excessive intracranial pressure and assess cerebral circulatory arrest

Finally, ICAVL recommends consistent use of and adherence to standardized scanning protocols. This helps identify common sources of error in the accuracy of ultrasound testing compared to other modalities and eliminate systematic sources of error through quality improvement.[19] Published examples of extracranial carotid, vertebral, and intracranial ultrasound protocols are available.

This chapter will focus on interpretation and clinical significance of a variety of cerebrovascular findings.

CAROTID ATHEROSCLEROTIC DISEASE: CLINICAL IMPLICATIONS OF EARLY DETECTION

Up to 15% of cerebral infarctions are associated with embolic debris and thrombi originating from atherosclerotic plaques at the carotid bifurcation.[20] The risk for stroke in patients with carotid atherosclerosis is closely associated with the severity of luminal stenosis. For asymptomatic patients with less than 75% stenosis, the yearly risk for stroke is less than 1%, but this risk increases to 2% to 5% for patients with stenosis greater than 75%.[21,22] The risk is much higher in symptomatic patients (i.e., those who have had previous transient ischemic attacks or strokes) at 10% in the first year for those with severe lesions, with risk rising to 30% to 35% over the next 5 years.[23]

On the other hand, carotid atherosclerotic disease is one of the major potentially preventable causes of stroke. Three pivotal studies (the North American Symptomatic Carotid Endarterectomy Trial [NASCET], the European Carotid Surgery Trial [ECST], and the Veteran Affairs Cooperative Studies Program Trial) have clearly shown the benefits of carotid endarterectomy (CEA) compared with medical treatment in recently symptomatic patients with severe carotid stenosis.[24-26] The pooled analysis of these three trials showed significant benefits of surgery in the group with severe stenosis (70%-99% stenosis in NASCET; absolute risk reduction of 16%, $P <.001$) after 5 years of follow-up.[27] In patients with mild stenosis (50% or less in NASCET), the risks incurred during CEA outweighed the benefits of surgery.[27] Patients with moderate stenosis (50%-69% in NASCET) still benefitted from surgery, although the overall gains were more modest than in patients with severe stenosis, with an absolute risk reduction of 4.6% after 5 years.[27] In asymptomatic carotid artery disease, the efficacy of CEA is also poorly defined. Results from the Asymptomatic Carotid Atherosclerosis Study (ACAS) showed a 47% relative reduction in the risk for ipsilateral stroke and perioperative death in patients randomized to surgery despite a 5-year risk for ipsilateral stroke without the operation of only 11%.[28] The UK Medical Research Council Asymptomatic Carotid Surgery Trial (ACST) Collaborative Group confirmed a modest benefit of CEA in asymptomatic patients who were younger than 75 years and who had at least 70% carotid stenosis on ultrasound: immediate CEA halved the net 5-year stroke risk from about 12% to about 6%.[29] There is a growing body of evidence from observational and epidemiologic studies that the risk for subsequent stroke in patients with carotid stenosis is highest in the first few weeks after onset of transient ischemic attacks (TIAs) or minor strokes, and this risk declines rapidly thereafter.[30-32] This finding implies a short time window for effective stroke prevention, necessitating the rapid identification of patients with substantial carotid stenosis and the swift initiation of medical treatment or revascularization procedures.

Furthermore, during the last decade, several clinical trials have tested and compared the efficacy and safety of different carotid revascularization procedures. Carotid stenting has emerged as a safe alternative to CEA, leading to safely treating patients with carotid artery disease who have contraindications to surgery or when surgery is not a suitable rescue. One of the largest randomized stroke prevention trials ever, the Carotid Revascularization Endarterectomy vs Stenting Trial (CREST) took place at 117 centers in the United States and Canada over a 9-year period. The overall safety and efficacy of the two procedures was largely the same with equal benefits for both men and for women, and for patients who had previously had a stroke and for those who had not.[33] It appears that CEA could be more beneficial in older patients, whereas stenting is associated with higher likelihood of periprocedural strokes. These findings should be interpreted with caution. First, confidence intervals on procedure benefit vs age were wide, and secondly the definitions of myocardial infarction (more common after CEA) and stroke were not the same in terms of clinical significance and severity. Overall, both procedures offered similar secondary stroke recurrence rates and remained viable options for stroke prevention.[33]

The availability of different therapeutic strategies along with the need to act quickly make ultrasound a perfect tool to identify candidates for revascularization procedures.

The mainstay of carotid imaging is, therefore, to enable accurate prediction of the severity of stenosis expressed as clinically relevant ranges of the NASCET study[34] and to facilitate delivery of treatment within a short time window.[30]

The association between carotid stenosis, stroke risk, and the effectiveness of endarterectomy was originally established using digital subtraction angiography (DSA).

Randomized trials[24,25,28] used DSA as the diagnostic test to measure the degree of carotid stenosis expressed as the percentage *linear diameter* reduction of the internal carotid artery (ICA) determined by specific methods. To apply these methods, only one view of the narrowest residual lumen (*d*) should be selected and the measurement sites (*n*) should be chosen

differently for each method (Figure 5-1). The stenosis is calculated using the formula

$$\text{ICA Diameter Reduction} = (1 - d/n) \times 100\% \quad (5\text{-}1)$$

where *d* and *n* are the diameter measurements made in mm.

The *North American (N) method* is also called the *NASCET method* or the *"distal" degree of stenosis.* It is recommended by the National Quality Forum in the United States as a mandatory component for reporting carotid angiographic studies, and uses the distal ICA diameter as the denominator *n.*

Major advantages of this method are the availability of validated diagnostic criteria for ultrasound screening, and consistent prognostic data regarding the risk for stroke and benefit of CEA. On the other hand, underestimation of the degree of carotid stenosis by 15% to 25% compared to other angiographic methods and area estimates should be taken into account, as well as an estimated interobserver variability of up to 30% for the values determined for the same angiogram.

The *European (E) method,* or the *"local" degree of stenosis,* requires drawing an imaginary outline of

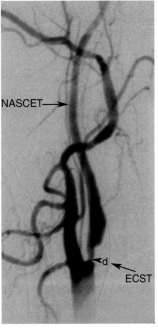

FIGURE 5-1 The North American (NASCET) and European (ECST) methods of measuring carotid stenosis; NASCET and ECST identify the denominator (n) measurement sites. d, diameter of the smallest residual lumen on a single angiographic plane; ECST, European Carotid Surgery Trial; NASCET, North American Symptomatic Carotid Endarterectomy Trial.

the ICA bulb to estimate the normal dimensions of the vessel at the site of the tightest narrowing. Although there is no objective way to decide where exactly the normal vessel wall is supposed to be on the DSA image, the E method has a good reproducibility between the experienced observers and provides stenosis values closer to anatomic stenosis than the N method. For instance, a 70% N stenosis is equal to 84% E stenosis and 90% area stenosis. This is largely due to the fact that the ICA bulb diameter estimate is greater than the diameter of the distal ICA in the normal vessel and its segment beyond the stenosis.

Like the N method, the E method is in wide use and gives consistent prognostic data regarding the risk for stroke and benefit of CEA. The E method has good reproducibility despite the subjective nature of the bulb diameter estimation, but this depends on the interpreter's experience. In the United States, national pay-for-performance quality requirements indicate that an ultrasound (and angiography) report should specifically refer to the NASCET range or percent stenosis. DSA is an invasive, potentially hazardous, labor- and time-intensive, and expensive technique.[35] The risk for groin hematoma has been reported as high as 8% in large series, although these hematomas rarely cause considerable morbidity or delay hospital discharge.[36] DSA requires skilled operators and is usually done by specialists at neurovascular centers; it remains less readily available to community physicians, and this may cause delays in management of patients with an acute cerebrovascular presentation.

Delay in access is a problem given the impetus to treat patients with TIAs or minor strokes rapidly in the first 1 or 2 days after the event, when the risk for subsequent cerebrovascular accident is the highest.[37] Thus, DSA—the historical gold standard in carotid luminal stenosis assessment—has now mostly been replaced by noninvasive carotid imaging techniques such as carotid Doppler ultrasound and magnetic resonance angiography (MRA), or at least less-invasive techniques such as computed tomographic angiography (CTA) or contrast-enhanced MRA. These noninvasive imaging modalities are now widely available, although access for patients varies between hospitals. Most centers now consider noninvasive techniques, alone or in combination, to be sufficiently accurate to replace DSA in the routine assessment of carotid disease.

This approach is supported by a recent meta-analysis[38] in which the use of noninvasive diagnostic strategies enables more patients to receive endarterectomy more quickly than does the use of DSA, together with the evidence that *rapid access to sensitive noninvasive carotid imaging prevents most strokes*, thereby producing a greater net benefit.[39]

CAROTID STENOSIS MEASURED BY ULTRASOUND

Noninvasive carotid ultrasound can be used to evaluate the carotid system from the proximal part of the common carotid artery (CCA) in the low neck up to the submandibular or distal part of the ICA in the upper neck. Carotid duplex is able to detect and quantify stenotic lesions in the extracranial carotid system and help in the selection of patients amenable for revascularization therapies. In addition to carotid stenosis grading, ultrasonography also has a role to play in evaluating additional aspects of carotid lesions that are associated with increased risk of stroke, such as plaque surface and texture as well as the presence of tandem or bilateral lesions.

Using B-mode imaging, a normal arterial wall can be visualized, and the presence of early stages of carotid atherosclerosis can be detected, including the intima-media thickness (IMT), fatty streak or soft plaques, and small nonstenosing plaques (Figure 5-2). It has been suggested that a thick (i.e., >1 mm) IMT complex is strongly predictive of future vascular events.[40-43]

In our opinion, IMT should be routinely checked during carotid ultrasound assessment and reported when it is abnormally thick. In our laboratory, this represents the value of IMT greater than or equal to 1 mm. We anticipate the future availability of standardized measurement methods with cutoffs for reporting IMT values as validated in large prospective studies. The percentage diameter reduction of the vessel due to the plaque protruding into the vessel lumen can be measured on the longitudinal views in the absence of shadowing. When an atherosclerotic plaque is detected on a B-mode image, its presence, location length, texture, and surface should be described in the final report.[44]

Plaques longer than 2 cm, particularly those with extensive shadowing, may lead to difficulties in the grading severity of carotid artery stenosis.

Most importantly, the report should also say if the *distal end of the plaque* has or has not been clearly visualized. The reason is that a plaque extending beyond the B-mode imaging range in the neck makes the lesion not entirely accessible

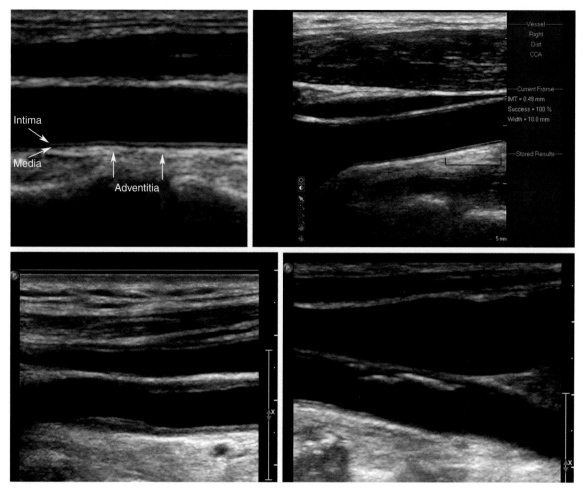

FIGURE 5-2 Normal intima-media thickness (IMT) appearance *(top left),* IMT measurement example *(top right),* fatty streak *(bottom left),* and a homogenous hyperechoic nonstenosing plaque *(bottom right).*

to the surgeon during endarterectomy. In other words, if the distal end of the plaque is not visualized, the plaque likely extends beyond the jaw level. This may lead to a cross-clamp being placed across the plaque during the endarterectomy procedure and its incomplete removal. Along with the B-mode visualization of a lesion and a decision whether it is less or greater than 50% diameter reduction, the three major Doppler velocity parameters should be reported and analyzed in terms of prediction of the NASCET range of the stenosis. These main parameters are the following:

- Peak systolic velocity (PSV)—determined from the spectrum obtained at the point of maximal narrowing
- End-diastolic velocity—determined from the spectrum obtained at the point of maximal narrowing
- Peak systolic velocity ratio—which compensates for interpatient and instrumentation variability

The PSV is mainly a function of the radius of the residual lumen as well as the length of the stenosis and the cardiac output.[45-47] It represents the best single predictor of the stenosis severity.[48] A variety of circulatory conditions influence the flow volume (FV) and velocity in the CCA and the ICA. In practice, individual variations of PSV and their influence on grading carotid stenosis can be reduced if the highest PSVs in the ICA and CCA are used to calculate the ICA/CCA PSV ratio. A multidisciplinary panel of experts was invited by the Society of Radiologists in Ultrasound to attend a 2002 consensus conference on diagnostic criteria to grade carotid stenosis with duplex ultrasound.[34] The consensus panel determined a set of criteria most suitable for grading a focal (short and unilateral) stenosis in the proximal ICA (Table 5-1).

As the degree of the stenosis increases, the PSV increases as well as the ICA/CCA ratio. However, when the resistance across the stenosis starts

TABLE 5-1 The Society of Radiologists in Ultrasound Consensus Criteria for Carotid Stenosis

Stenosis Range	ICA PSV	ICA/CCA PSV Ratio	ICA EDV	Plaque
Normal	<125 cm/sec	<2.0	<40 cm/sec	None
<50%	<125 cm/sec	<2.0	<40 cm/sec	>50% diameter reduction
50%-69%	125-230 cm/sec	2.0-4.0	40-100 cm/sec	≥50% diameter reduction
70%-near occlusion	>230 cm/sec	>4.0	>100 cm/sec	≥50% diameter reduction
Near occlusion	May be low or undetectable	Variable	Variable	Significant, detectable lumen
Occlusion	Undetectable	N/A	N/A	Significant, no detectable lumen

From Grant EG, et al: Carotid artery stenosis: Gray-scale and Doppler US diagnosis–Society of Radiologists in Ultrasound Consensus Conference, *Radiology* 229:340–346, 2003.
CCA, common carotid artery; EDV, end-diastolic velocity; ICA, internal carotid artery; N/A, not applicable; PSV, peak systolic velocity.

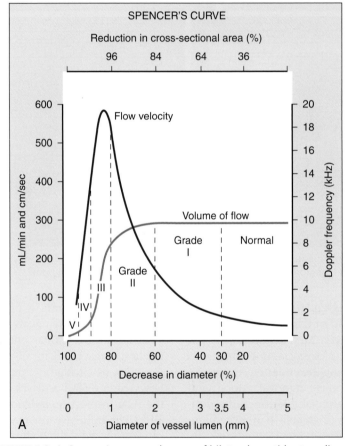

FIGURE 5-3 **A,** Spencer's curve and a case of bilateral carotid artery disease.

to impede the velocity, causing its paradoxical decrease, these lesions are often termed hemodynamically significant (Figure 5-3). Severe stenotic lesions cause a poststenotic drop in the FV at 80% or greater diameter stenosis as shown by Spencer's curve[45] (developed for axis-symmetric and focal stenoses) (see Figure 5-3, *A*). The development of such a significant blood pressure gradient occurs with the lesions "on the other side" of Spencer's curve (see Figure 5-3, *B*, right ICA),

where the volume of blood flow is decreased through the lesion and requires compensation via distal vasodilatation and development of collaterals.

Hemodynamically significant ICA lesions are usually in the 80% to 99% diameter reduction range by the NASCET method or appear as elongated stenoses of variable diameter reduction, tandem lesions, near occlusions, or occlusions. Note that FV starts to drop at 70% narrowing

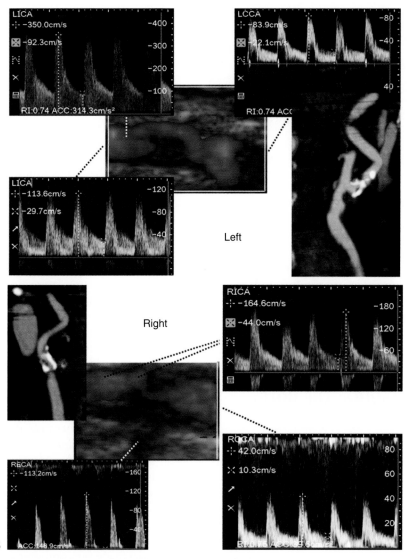

FIGURE 5-3, cont'd **B,** The left internal carotid artery (ICA) has findings consistent with greater than 70% NASCET stenosis and collateralization of flow (PSV >230 cm/sec, ICA/CCA PSV ratio <4). This places the stenosis in the grade II category on Spencer's curve on the left. A severe (>90%) stenosis of the right ICA places the stenosis on the "other" side of Spencer's curve (grade IV). Note the high-resistance right CCA waveform with a PSV decrease as compared to the left side. CCA, common carotid artery; NASCET, North American Symptomatic Carotid Endarterectomy Trial; PSV, peak systolic velocity.

according to Spencer's curve but it becomes significant at 80% diameter reduction (see Figure 5-3, A). Often, these lesions can be discovered only by using indirect criteria for grading carotid stenosis that include both extracranial and intracranial ultrasound studies.

The indirect criteria for hemodynamically significant carotid stenosis include the following:

- Decreased end-diastolic velocity (EDV) in the CCA and/or ICA in the presence of a distal lesion
- Color flow findings such as narrow and elongated residual lumen
- Internalization of the external carotid artery (ECA; low resistance and high-velocity flow in the extracranial ECA) and reversed flow direction in the ophthalmic artery (OA)
- Anterior cross-filling via anterior communicating artery (ACoA)
- Posterior communicating artery (PCoA) flow
- Increased flow pulsatility in the unilateral CCA
- Decreased flow pulsatility in the unilateral middle cerebral artery (MCA)
- Abnormal flow acceleration and pulsatility transmission index (unilateral MCA)

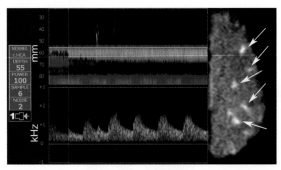

FIGURE 5-4 On the left, real-time artery-to-artery embolus shown on power motion transcranial Doppler (spike on top tracing and change in velocity on bottom tracing). On the right, a typical diffusion-weighted brain imaging shows scattered embolic strokes (arrows).

These findings can also be accompanied by evidence of microembolism, particularly in the acute phase of cerebral ischemia when tandem ICA/MCA lesions and artery-to-artery embolization are common (Figure 5-4).

IDENTIFYING VULNERABLE CAROTID PLAQUES: THE ROLE OF ULTRASOUND

Selection for carotid revascularization therapies in recently symptomatic patients with severe carotid stenosis is largely determined by assessing the degree of luminal stenosis.[49] However, there are patients who are asymptomatic or have moderate symptomatic stenoses in whom the choice between revascularization or medical intervention is less clear and for whom better methods of risk stratification are needed.[50]

This has led many investigators to search for markers of plaque vulnerability, instability, or thromboembolic potential as complementary to the degree of the luminal stenosis in stroke risk prediction.[51] Certain morphologic features of carotid plaques are increasingly believed to be one of those markers that could carry further prognostic information, and early recognition of these plaques features may identify a high-risk subgroup of patients who might particularly benefit from aggressive interventions.[52] Histologic analysis of CEA specimens suggests that vulnerable plaques are characterized by a large lipid-rich necrotic core, a thin overlying fibrous cap, an inflammatory infiltrate, neovasculature growth, and intraplaque hemorrhage.[53,54] Ultrasound imaging can directly display the plaque texture and surface that would

be reflective of these processes. B-mode imaging is ideally suited to determine whether or not atherosclerotic plaques are acoustically homogeneous or heterogeneous (Figure 5-5).

Depending on its echo-reflective property, a so-called "vulnerable" or "unstable" plaque is a plaque that appears predominately hypoechoic (echolucent) (Figure 5-6)—where echoes are uniform throughout all regions of the plaque—with irregular surface and possibly containing a thrombus attached to its ruptured surface. Clearly homogeneous plaques are most likely to be purely cellular in nature with little evidence of becoming complex (when calcifications, significant cholesterol deposition, or hemorrhage appear). Homogenous plaques are commonly associated with intimal hyperplasia.

A heterogeneous plaque has mixed areas of brightness and variations in texture. The presence of an acoustically heterogeneous plaque signifies that the atherosclerotic process has become complicated. A heterogeneous plaque, without acoustic shadowing, most commonly signifies a fibro-fatty lesion, whereas the presence of calcifications usually leads to shadowing. Echolucent plaques are thought to be more vulnerable than echo-rich plaques, because they contain more soft tissue (lipid and hemorrhage), whereas echo-rich plaques are primarily composed of fibrous tissue and calcifications.

Visual evaluation of plaque echogenicity has only fair reproducibility, whereas objective characterization is more reliable and less observer dependent.[56] Ultrasound images can be evaluated objectively by computer-assisted gray-scale median (GSM) measurements[55]; however, even computer-assisted GSM measurements assess only the median brightness of the entire plaque. Regional instability, such as hemorrhage, may exist within a plaque even with a high GSM value. This may explain why there is no consensus yet on which GSM threshold value is most sensitive to distinguish vulnerable from stable plaques. A stratified gray-scale measurement of carotid plaque echogenicity[57] or pixel segmentation with tissue mapping[58] may be a better method to characterize plaque composition. Another limitation of conventional B-mode imaging in evaluating plaques is that interpretation of images may be hampered by artifacts. This can be minimized by applying real-time compound ultrasound imaging, which uses multiple scanning angles to improve image quality.

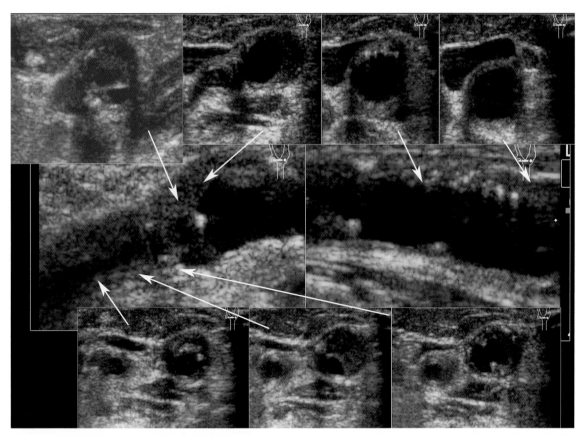

FIGURE 5-5 Composite longitudinal *(middle frames)* and transverse B-mode images *(top and bottom frames)* of a complex heterogeneous plaque. *Arrows* point to location of the corresponding cross-sectional images.

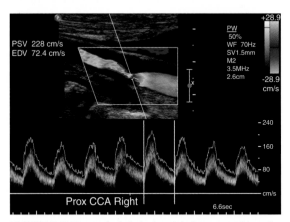

FIGURE 5-6 Hypoechoic (echolucent) plaque causing a significant internal carotid artery stenosis. Note the Doppler velocity tracing with a narrow spectral window, indicating that the sample site is at the point of maximal narrowing.

Indeed, compared to conventional B-mode imaging, real-time compound ultrasound imaging is superior for determining plaque echogenicity, possible surface irregularities, and vessel wall demarcation with good reproducibility and high interobserver agreement.[59] Another aspect of atherosclerotic plaque imaging that has been studied is its irregularity. Irregular carotid plaque surface has shown to be an independent predictor of ischemic stroke, increasing the risk nearly threefold.[60,61] The exact mechanisms between irregular plaque surface and the occurrence of ischemic stroke are not yet clear. Plaque surface irregularity may represent a potential embolic source but may also be a general marker of the severity of atherosclerosis in intracranial small vessels. Recently emerged as important markers of plaque instability and higher stroke risk are microembolic signals and diminished vasomotor capacity on TCD.[62,63] Both these phenomena can be detected and evaluated by ultrasound (see later). Furthermore, ultrasound can show the presence of tandem lesions in the carotid circulation that point to a high stroke risk. Published series have suggested that tandem lesions do not affect hemodynamics as a simple summation of separate degrees of stenosis.[64,65] Tandem lesions and an increased risk for perioperative stroke should be considered when carotid revascularization is planned.[66]

PITFALLS OF CAROTID DUPLEX

- Only 15% to 25% of all strokes are attributable to a significant carotid stenosis.
- When there is high bifurcation, the carotid bulb and distal ICA cannot be fully visualized.
- A shadow longer than 2 cm can preclude sampling the highest-velocity jet and underestimate stenosis severity.
- With tandem and bilateral lesions, current criteria are unable to identify hemodynamic significance of the disease.
- ICA lesions distal to the accessible segments cannot be evaluated.
- Vertebral artery (VA) assessment is limited in patients with suspected vertebrobasilar disease, particularly intracranial vessels.

All of these circumstances pinpoint the need for a combined assessment of carotid duplex with transcranial Doppler or duplex (our fast-track insonation protocol is shown later).

ASSESSMENT FOLLOWING CAROTID ENDARTERECTOMY AND CAROTID STENTS

An important goal of the evaluation procedures following carotid revascularization is to rule out stenosis recurrence (or restenosis). B-mode imaging of carotid arteries reconstructed after CEA [67] can show changes in the vessel wall consistent with sutures, patches, stent material, early intimal proliferation, or late atherosclerotic plaque formation (Figure 5-7).

Placement of a stent in the carotid artery alters its biomechanical properties, which may cause an increase in the ultrasound velocity measurements in the absence of a technical error or residual stenotic disease. Adjustment of the velocity criteria to identify a significant restenosis is needed.[68,69]

Of note, the specific velocity cutoffs have been recently proposed by AbuRahma and colleagues[69] for detecting in-stent restenosis of 30% or more, 50% or more, and 80% or more as follows: PSVs of 154, 224, and 325 cm/sec, respectively. PSV can increase throughout the patent stent area up to 150 cm/sec (the adopted cutoff in our laboratory). In addition to any velocity increase across the stent, we use at least a 2:1 ratio within the stent or to present and poststent segmental values to identify any degree of restenosis.

Obviously, the presence of an intrastent intimal proliferation, plaque formation, or thrombus is needed to diagnose restenosis.

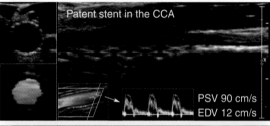
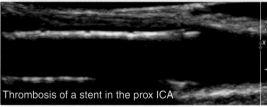

FIGURE 5-7 Carotid artery stents. *Upper images,* patent stent; *bottom image,* in-stent thrombus. CCA, common carotid artery; EDV, end-diastolic velocity; ICA, internal carotid artery; PSV, peak systolic velocity.

Our criteria for *stent deformity or restenosis* that include some previously published findings[69-71] include the following:

- B-mode evidence for equal to or greater than 30% narrowing of the stent/vessel lumen (note that if a calcified plaque is present outside the stent with parallel walls, it may produce shadowing and false impression of vessel narrowing)
- Focal velocity increase at the point of maximal narrowing greater than 150 cm/sec and stenotic to prestenotic (pre-stent) PSV ratio of 1:≥2
- Additional evidence of plaque or thrombus formation at the site of stent deformity or at the proximal or distal ends of the stent (note that low velocities and high-resistance waveforms can be found with a subtotal obstruction of the stent)

Our criteria for stent or postsurgical thrombosis or occlusion include the following:

- B-mode evidence of hypoechoic or hyperechoic filling of the reconstructed vessel lumen (Figure 5-7) (A "crescent moon" appearance of an intraluminal thrombus without significant velocity and waveform changes could also be diagnostic and will be discussed in detail in the section on arterial occlusion.)
- An abnormal residual flow signal (i.e., stenotic, blunted, minimal, or reverberating) at the longitudinal view of the reconstructed vessel or just proximal to a flow void zone
- High-resistance prereconstructed vessel or CCA signals

CAROTID ARTERY OCCLUSION AND DISSECTION

With current ultrasound technologies, one could be uncertain of the diagnosis of a *complete* (particularly acute or "fresh" vs chronic [Figure 5-8]) carotid artery occlusion. When a patient appears to have a complete occlusion at a first-ever carotid ultrasound examination, the "benefit of the doubt" could be given by reporting "occlusion or 99% stenosis" or "near occlusion." If there is a minimal residual lumen and flow in the distal ICA, this can change patient management (i.e., revascularization may be possible). In these circumstances the diagnostic accuracy of ultrasound in differentiation of complete occlusion from subtotal stenosis may be improved with contrast agents, and sensitive flow-imaging techniques[72] and other imaging modalities are required to obtain confirmation of findings.

Our criteria for carotid artery occlusion[73-75] are as follows:

1. Absent flow signal in the distal ICA on flow imaging and spectral analysis
2. High-resistance "stump" waveform with absent or reversed end-diastolic flow just proximal to the flow void area or structural lesion in the ICA
3. Drumbeat sounds of lesion motion and vessel wall covibration (usually systolic spikes of low frequency)
4. Decreased arterial wall pulsations on real-time B-mode imaging compared to the contralateral side
5. Delayed systolic flow acceleration, blunting of the MCA waveform, or evidence of flow diversion to a branching vessel (i.e., ECA), and/or collateralization of flow via OA, ACoA, or PCoA

In the absence of a structural lesion in the proximal ICA and bifurcation, the absence or reversal of the diastolic flow in these segments should raise high suspicion of a distal ICA occlusion.

In a patient with new-onset stroke symptoms, or a recent TIA, ultrasound can detect an *acute thrombosis or an embolus in the ICA.*[76,77] This can be suspected in the following instances:

- Flow signal void over a lesion with hypoechoic or anechoic intraluminal appearance (possible fresh clot on B-mode) (see Figure 5-8)
- "Crescent moon" appearance of the residual lumen on color flow imaging, indicating that

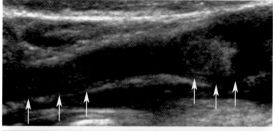
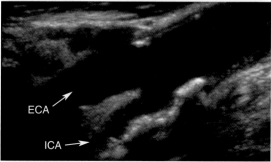

FIGURE 5-8 Acute *(top)* thromboembolic internal carotid artery (ICA) occlusion. Note intima-media thickness preservation between mixed echogenic parts of a thrombus *(arrows)*, and normal ICA lumen size. Chronic *(bottom)* ICA occlusion with vessel collapse and fibrosis. ECA, external carotid artery.

the hypoechoic structure is an intraluminal inclusion
- High velocity in the ECA or contralateral vessels, indicating flow diversion (in cases of flow-limiting thrombi)
- Presence of intracranial collaterals (in cases of flow-limiting thrombi)
- Microemboli found in the MCA on the side of the ICA lesion and symptoms

An acute thrombosis associated with carotid plaque usually shows an underlying atheroma that may be hyperechoic and have shadowing, whereas an acute embolus from the cardiac source may appear mostly hypoechoic and mobile.[76-79] *Carotid artery dissection* can be detected sonographically directly in the CCA or proximal ICA, or indirectly for the distal ICA due to its common location at the entrance to the skull (Figure 5-9). The sonographer should focus on finding an intimal flap and hemodynamic effects of an upstream lesion.[80,81]

Carotid dissection can be suspected with the following findings:

- Intimal flap is visualized in the carotid artery with abnormal flow waveforms (differentiate B-mode artifacts caused by jugular vein walls, its valves, or other bright reflectors) (see Figure 5-9, *bottom*).

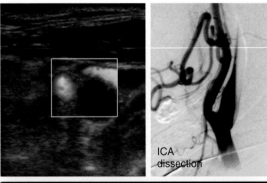

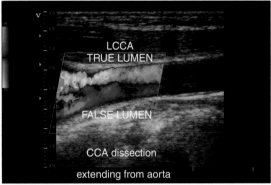

FIGURE 5-9 Internal carotid artery (ICA; *top*) and common carotid artery (CCA; *bottom*) dissections.

- High-resistance pulsatile flow signals are found proximal to hemodynamically significant dissections without evidence for an atheromatous lesion (see Figure 5-9, *bottom*).
- Two waveforms are identified, reflecting flow through the true and false lumens.
- Reversed OA or other intracranial collaterals could be found.
- Microemboli could be found in the MCA on the side of the suspected dissection.
- If a dissection is found in the CCA, suspect its origin in the aortic arch and check other proximal precerebral vessels.

Noninvasive diagnosis of ICA dissection is difficult since most of these lesions have variable locations, often involving the distal ICA at the entrance to the skull. The diagnosis is often based on indirect evidence of the distal ICA lesion and may be impossible until the dissection becomes hemodynamically significant or descends to the field of insonation. Patient history often points to trauma, neck manipulation, neck pain, episodes of excessive coughing or sneezing with respiratory infection, and the like.

Dissections can recanalize, and this process can be monitored with ultrasound. Ultrasound criteria for recanalization of previously dissected carotid artery include the following:

- Recovery of end-diastolic flow in the distal ICA (low-resistance flow) or proximal to the lesion
- Return of normal systolic flow acceleration in the MCA without collateralization of flow
- Return of normal siphon and OA signals

Note that recanalization of dissected vessels may be only partial with persistent findings of the proximal high-resistance flow signatures, distal delay in systolic acceleration, and retained collaterals. The only change could be appearance or augmentation of the diastolic flow to and through the lesion.

VERTEBRAL ARTERY STENOSIS OR OCCLUSION

Compared to carotid imaging, fewer validation studies are available for detection and quantification of the VA lesions.[82,83] VA stenosis occurs more often in V_3-V_4 segments followed by the origin of the VA (V_0), and midcervical section (V_1-V_2). Direct assessment of the V_3 segment with ultrasound is not possible.[84]

Therefore, the diagnosis of vertebral obstruction at this level is based on indirect findings: proximal signs (i.e., increased flow pulsatility and different waveforms between two sides) or distal signs (poststenotic turbulence, blunted waveform).

Our diagnostic criteria for *VA stenosis* (Figure 5-10) include the following:

1. Focal significant PSV increase with the ratio of the stenotic to the pre- or poststenotic peak systolic velocities ≥2 (usually the highest PSV exceeds 100 cm/sec to reach any significance of this finding)
2. When detectable, the presence of a structural lesion on B-mode, or turbulence, spectral narrowing, or additional abnormal waveforms on Doppler at the site of the lesion
3. Indirect prestenotic or poststenotic signs (abnormal pulsatility and waveforms)

Our criteria for VA stenoses do not include a PSV cutoff since tortuosity of the proximal VA segment, compensatory velocity increase with ICA lesions, and VA dominance may produce relatively high velocities.

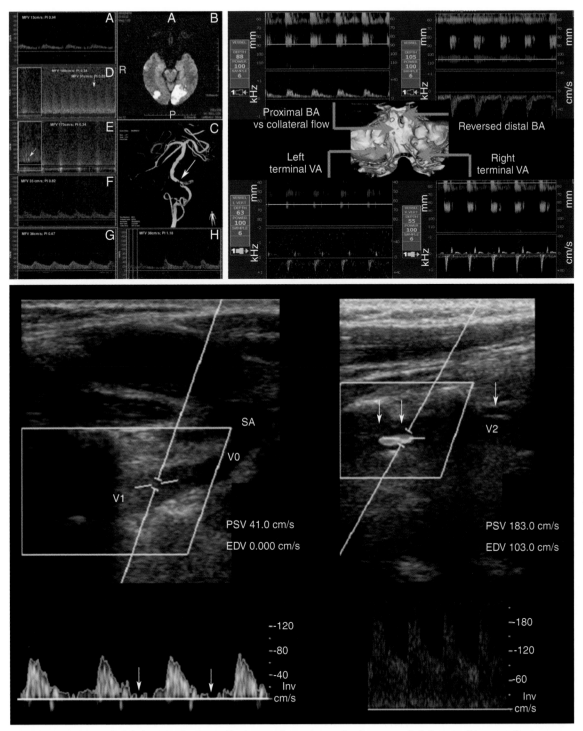

FIGURE 5-10 Example of the terminal vertebral stenosis as shown in the upper left insert of images (*large arrow, stenosis on arteriogram*). On the upper right insert, bilateral terminal vertebral artery (VA) occlusions with reversal of the basilar artery (BA) flow. The lower inserts show a high-grade proximal VA stenosis with a high-resistance *(arrow)* preobstructive flow *(left image)* and a velocity jet *(double arrows)* across the lesion *(right image)*. EDV, end-diastolic velocity; PSV, peak systolic velocity.

TABLE 5-2 Normal Depth, Direction, and Mean Flow Velocities at Assumed Zero Degree Angle of Insonation of the Arteries of the Circle of Willis

Artery	Depth (mm, Adults)	Direction	Children*	Adults
M_2 MCA	30-45	Bidirectional	<170 cm/sec	<100 cm/sec
M_1 MCA	45-65	Toward	<170 cm/sec	<100 cm/sec
A_1 ACA	62-75	Away	<150 cm/sec	<100 cm/sec
A_2 ACA†	45-65	Toward	N/A	<80 cm/sec
ICA siphon	60-65	Bidirectional	<130 cm/sec	<70 cm/sec
OA	40-60	Toward	Variable	variable
PCA	55-70	Bidirectional	<100 cm/sec	<60 cm/sec
BA	80-100+	Away	<100 cm/sec	<60 cm/sec
VA	45-80	Away	<80 cm/sec	<50 cm/sec

ACA, anterior cerebral artery; BA, basilar artery; ICA, internal carotid artery; MCA, middle cerebral artery; N/A, not available; OA, ophthalmic artery; PCA, posterior cerebral artery; VA, vertebral artery.
*Values are given for children with sickle cell anemia.
†A_2 ACA can be found through the frontal windows with transcranial color coded duplex sonography (TCCS) in select patients.

Our diagnostic criteria for *VA occlusion* are as follows:

- Flow void area and absent pulsed Doppler signals in a segment or entire VA stem
- Hypoechoic vessel lumen (acute and subacute occlusion)
- Hyperechoic vessel lumen (chronic occlusion)
- Abnormal residual flow waveforms on TCD with intracranial VA occlusion

NORMAL INTRACRANIAL FLOW FINDINGS

When performing and interpreting transcranial Doppler or duplex examinations, sound, waveform appearance, blood flow direction, actual velocity, and pulsatility measurements should be considered (Table 5-2).

Our criteria for normal TCD examination (Figures 5-11 and 5-12) include the following:

- Good windows of insonation
- Direction of blood flow and depths of insonation
- The difference between blood flow velocities in the homologous arteries is less than 30%: 15% is attributable to the difference in angle of insonation and another 15% to breathing cycles. However, posterior cerebral and vertebral arteries may have 50% to 100% difference because of dominance, hypoplasia, and tortuous course. Similarly, M_2 and M_1 MCAs may have up to 100% variation in velocity depending on tortuosity.
- A normal M_1 MCA mean flow velocity (MFV) does not exceed 170 cm/sec in

children with SCD and 100 cm/sec in adults free of anemia.

- A normal velocity ratio: MCA is greater than or equal to anterior cerebral artery (ACA), which is greater than or equal to siphon, which is greater than or equal to posterior cerebral artery (PCA), which is greater than or equal to basilar artery (BA), which is greater than or equal to VA. Velocity values can be equal between these arterial segments or sometimes exceed by 5 to 10 cm/sec (i.e., ACA > MCA, or BA > MCA), likely due to the angle of insonation or common anatomic variations.
- Patients free of hypertension while breathing room air have a positive EDV of approximately 25% to 50% of the PSV values and a low-resistance pulsatility index of Gosling and King (PI)[85] of 0.6 to 1.1 in all intracranial arteries. A high-resistance flow pattern (PI >1.2) is seen in the OAs only.
- High-resistance flows (PI >1.2) can be found in patent cerebral arteries with aging, chronic hypertension, and increased cardiac output and during hyperventilation.

The range of PI, described by Gosling and King,[85] that can be found in the arteries supplying the brain is calculated as follows:

$$PI = PSV - EDV / MFV \qquad (5\text{-}2)$$

Note that wide variations in the velocity and pulsatility of flow can be found under normal and abnormal circulatory conditions.

Besides PI, the resistance to flow can be expressed using the resistivity index (RI) described

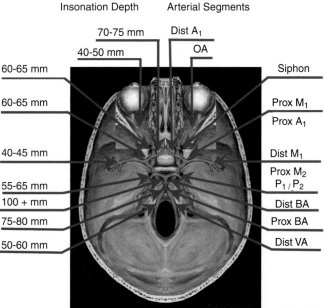

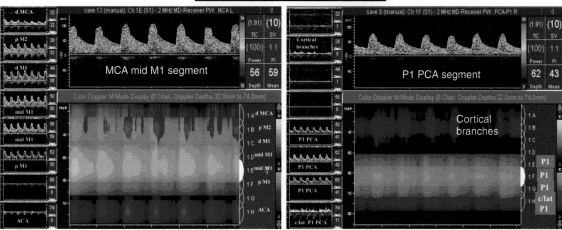

FIGURE 5-11 Transcranial Doppler: insonation depths, arterial segments for detection, and samples of the normal findings through the temporal window (segments labeled for each waveform detected). BA, basilar artery; Dist, distal; MCA, middle cerebral artery; OA, ophthalmic artery; PCA, posterior cerebral artery; Prox, proximal; VA, vertebral artery.

by Pourcelot.[86] This index is calculated as the ratio of (PSV − EDV) / PSV with normal values below 0.75. There is a controversy about which index better describes the resistance to flow since PI may be more influenced by cardiac output whereas RI is more reflective of the distal resistance.[87]

INTRACRANIAL ATHEROSCLEROTIC DISEASE

Intracranial atherosclerotic disease is now recognized as a serious risk factor carrying the highest risk for stroke recurrence.[88]

It is more prevalent in Asian, Hispanic, and African American populations. Patients who have had a stroke or TIA attributed to stenosis (50%-99%) of a major intracranial artery face a 12% to 14% risk for subsequent stroke during the 2-year period after the initial ischemic event, despite treatment with antithrombotic medications. The annual risk for subsequent stroke may exceed 20% in high-risk groups.[88] The recent emphasis on identification of stenoses greater than or equal to 50% and greater than or equal to 70% prompted reevaluation of the previous criteria and development of new ones (Table 5-3).[89]

MIDDLE CEREBRAL ARTERY STENOSIS

Primary findings for any significant MCA stenosis (i.e., > 50% diameter reduction) include a focal significant MFV increase (MFV >100 cm sec) (Figure 5-13), or PSV increase (PSV >140 cm/sec), or interhemispheric MFV difference of 1:2 in adults free of abnormal circulatory conditions.[90-92] A stenosis greater than or equal to 70% in the MCA could produce higher velocities,

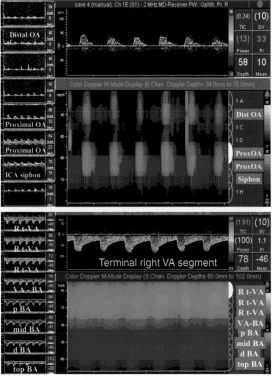

FIGURE 5-12 Normal orbital and foraminal findings on transcranial Doppler. VA, vertebral artery.

and in our laboratory we use an MFV cutoff of 120 cm/sec or greater (Figure 5-13). This velocity increase should further be associated with a ratio to a homologous segment of 1:4 or higher.

With MCA stenoses "on the other side" of Spencer's curve, a paradoxical flow velocity decrease can be found in the presence of findings such as flow diversion that indicates hemodynamic significance of a lesion. A proximal M_2-distal M_1 MCA stenosis is present if the velocity increase is found at 30 to 45 mm. A proximal M_1 MCA stenosis is usually found at 45- to 65-mm depths in adults.[93,94]

Chimowitz and colleagues[95] in the prospective part of the Warfarin-Aspirin Symptomatic Intracranial Disease (WASID) study adopted criteria that the MCA MFV equal to or greater than 100 cm/sec indicates M_1 MCA diameter reduction of 50% or more. An algorithm was developed on how to measure intracranial stenosis on DSAs. A recent meta-analysis of available studies indicated that the 100 cm/sec cutoff yielded a mean weighted average sensitivity of 100% and specificity of 97%.[92]

To improve the predictive value of any chosen velocity threshold, we use the ratio with a homologous or proximal MCA segment.[91] There is an increased interest in defining the most severe intracranial stenoses because these patients have the highest risk for stroke recurrence, and novel stenting technologies are now being tested as an adjunct to the best medical therapy for secondary stroke prevention.

If anemia, congestive heart failure, and other circulatory conditions associated with elevated or decreased velocities are present, then a focal MFV difference greater than or equal to 30% between neighboring or homologous arterial segments

TABLE 5-3 Maximum Mean Flow Velocity Thresholds at Assumed Zero Angle of Insonation for a Focal (≥50%) Intracranial Arterial Stenosis on TCD

Artery	Depth (mm)	MFV (cm/sec)	MFV ≥50% Stenosis	MFV≥70% Stenosis
M1-M2 MCA	30-65	≥100	≥100 cm/sec (use 1:2 ratio)	≥128 cm/sec (1:4 ratio)
A1 ACA	60-75	≥100	N/A	N/A
ICA siphon	60-65	≥70	≥90 cm/sec (use 1:2 ratio)	≥128 cm/sec (1:4 ratio)
PCA	60-72	≥50	N/A	N/A
BA	80-100+	≥60	≥80 cm/sec (use 1:2 ratio)	≥119 cm/sec (1:4 ratio)
VA	40-80	≥50	≥80 cm/sec (use 1:2 ratio)	≥119 cm/sec (1:4 ratio)

ACA, anterior cerebral artery; BA, basilar artery; ICA, internal carotid artery; MCA, middle cerebral artery; MFV, mean flow velocity; N/A, not available; PCA, posterior cerebral artery; VA, vertebral artery.

Prestenosis   DSA   Stenosis

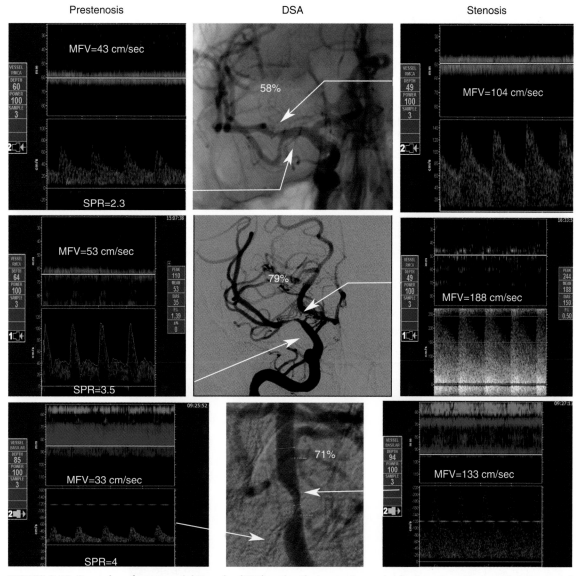

FIGURE 5-13 Examples of transcranial Doppler (TCD) and catheter angiography findings in patients with intracranial atherosclerosis. Percent stenosis represents measurements of diameter reduction. DSA, digital subtraction angiography; MFV, mean flow velocity; SPR, stenotic-prestenotic velocity ratio on TCD.

should be applied to see if the velocity increase reaches any significance. Adult patients with anemia or hyperthyroidism often have MCA mean flow velocities in the range of 60 to 110 cm/sec. In children with SCD an MCA MFV up to 170 cm/sec is considered normal.

A stenosis in the MCA may also be suspected if indirect flow disturbances are detected by TCD. These important additional findings may include the following:

- Turbulence or disturbed flow distal to the stenosis or presence of characteristic flow voids on power motion mode display, indicating a low-frequency bidirectional turbulent flow during systole
- An increased unilateral ACA MFV, indicating compensatory flow diversion
- A low-frequency noise produced by nonharmonic covibrations of the vessel wall and musical murmurs due to harmonic covibrations producing pure tones
- Microembolic signals found in the distal MCA

If FVs are increased throughout the M_1 MCA stem, the differential diagnosis includes MCA stenosis, terminal ICA or siphon stenosis, hyperemia or compensatory flow increase in the presence of contralateral ICA stenosis, ACA occlusion, or incorrect vessel identification.

MCA SUBTOTAL STENOSIS OR NEAR OCCLUSION

A critical stenosis or obstruction with near-occlusive thrombus or an embolus can produce a focal FV decrease or a "blunted" MCA waveform with slow or delayed systolic acceleration, slow later-systolic flow deceleration, low velocities, and MFV MCA less than ACA or any other intracranial artery (Figure 5-14). Decreased or minimal flow velocities with slow systolic acceleration can be found as a result of a tight elongated MCA stenosis or thrombus causing near occlusion. These focal lesions should be differentiated from a proximal ICA obstruction that can also produce delayed flow acceleration in the MCA. The minimal, blunted, or dampened waveforms are common in patients with acute ischemic stroke, particularly in

those presenting with hyperdense MCA signs on noncontrast CT scan or a flow gap on MRA.

A false-positive diagnosis of MCA subtotal stenosis can occur because of problems with vessel identification and a suboptimal angle of insonation. Incorrect probe angulation and shallow insonation usually lead to these errors. To confirm the presence of a flow-limiting lesion, branching vessels need to be evaluated. Note that an M_1-M_2 MCA subtotal stenosis is usually accompanied by flow diversion to the ACA (Figure 5-14) and/or compensatory flow increase in the PCA, indicating transcortical collateralization of flow.[96,97]

ANTERIOR CEREBRAL ARTERY (ACA)

Primary findings in an ACA stenosis include a focal significant ACA FV increase (ACA > MCA) and/or ACA MFV greater than or equal to 100 cm/sec, and/or a 30% or greater difference between the proximal and distal ACA segments, and/or a 30% or greater difference compared to the

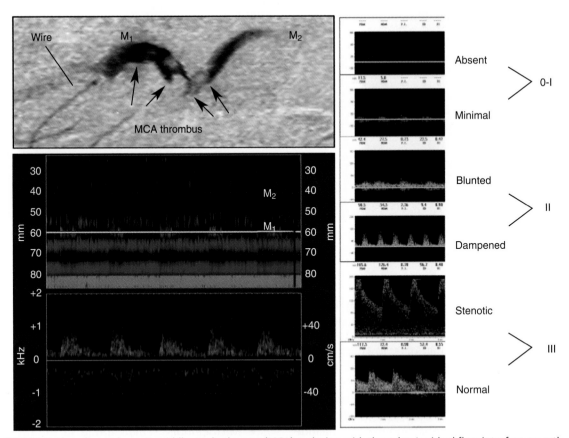

FIGURE 5-14 *Left panels:* acute middle cerebral artery (MCA) occlusion with thrombus/residual flow interface on catheter angiography shown on the upper image and high-resistance residual flow signals in the proximal MCA leading to low-resistance flow in the anterior cerebral artery (on power motion Doppler; *middle panel*). *Lower left panel:* Doppler spectral waveform of MCA. *Right panel:* Thrombolysis in Brain Ischemia (TIBI) classification of the residual flow signals and the names of the flow grades/waveforms.

contralateral ACA. Collateralization via the ACoA can be excluded by a normal contralateral ACA flow direction and the absence of stenotic signals at 75 mm (i.e., midline). Usually an A_1 ACA stenosis can be detected at 60 to 75 mm.

The differential diagnosis includes anterior cross-filling due to a proximal carotid artery disease. Additional findings may include turbulence and flow diversion into the MCA and/or compensatory flow increase in the contralateral ACA.

Decreased or minimal flow velocities at the A_1 ACA origin may indicate a suboptimal angle of insonation from the unilateral temporal window, an atretic or tortuous A_1 ACA segment, and A_1 ACA near occlusion. Since the A_2 ACA segment cannot be assessed directly by TCD, its obstruction can be suspected only if a high-resistance flow is found in the distal dominant A_1 ACA segment (70-75 mm).

Common errors include incorrect vessel identification (terminal ICA vs ACA), velocity underestimation (suboptimal angle of insonation, poor window, weak signals), and inability to differentiate a collateral flow from the stenosis.

TERMINAL ICA AND ICA SIPHON

The ICA siphon and parasellar and supraclinoid ICA segments are difficult to examine in their entirety since they navigate through bones. An orbital examination may reveal stenotic flow directed toward or away from the probe at 55 to 65 mm in adults with signals often traceable to 70 mm. The terminal ICA bifurcation is located at 60 to 75 mm from the transtemporal window. A terminal ICA/siphon stenosis produces a focal significant MFV increase, ICA is greater than MCA, and/or an ICA MFV greater than or equal to 70 cm/sec, and/or a 30% or greater difference between arterial segments.[98] The higher the focal velocity increase, the more likely TCD findings need to be confirmed by other imaging modalities. However, TCD velocity is more sensitive to mild and moderate degrees of intracranial stenosis, and correlative angiograms may still be negative despite the presence of significant disease.

The differential diagnosis includes moderate proximal ICA stenosis and/or compensatory flow increase with contralateral ICA stenosis. Additional findings in the presence of an ICA stenosis may include turbulence, blunted unilateral MCA, OA MFV increase, and/or flow reversal with low pulsatility. The ICA siphon MFVs may decrease

because of siphon near occlusion (a blunted siphon signal), or distal obstruction (i.e., MCA occlusion or increased ICP).

Common errors include vessel identification such as MCA vs terminal internal carotid artery via transtemporal approach, or ACA vs ICA with deep (>65 mm) transorbital insonation, and consequently collateralization of flow via anterior cross-filling misinterpreted as an arterial stenosis. In the absence of temporal windows, these findings may be the only, yet confusing, indicators of significant carotid disease.

POSTERIOR CEREBRAL ARTERY

A PCA stenosis produces a focal significant FV increase resulting in a PCA MFV greater than ACA or ICA; and/or a PCA MFV equal to or greater than 50 cm/sec in adults.[93,99] The PCA signals are usually located at 55 to 65 mm, the top of the basilar can be found at 70 to 80 mm, the P_1 segment is directed toward the probe, and the contralateral P_1 and unilateral P_2 segments are directed away from the probe.

Additional findings may include turbulence and a compensatory flow increase in the MCA.

The differential diagnosis includes collateral flow via the posterior communicating artery (PCoA) either toward the posterior circulation in the case of basilar artery occlusion or toward the anterior circulation in the case of MCA, terminal internal carotid artery or tandem extracranial ICA/MCA occlusions, and siphon stenosis. Of note, PCoA is a tortuous artery, and its flow direction on TCD does not necessarily indicate presence of a lesion vs collateralization. Using TCD imaging, it may be possible to differentiate PCA stenosis from collateralization of flow using the PSV.[93,100] Common sources of error include unreliable vessel identification, the presence of an arterial occlusion, and a top-of-the-basilar stenosis.

BASILAR ARTERY

Primary findings in the presence of a BA stenosis include a focal significant velocity increase where a BA MFV is greater than MCA or ACA or ICA, and/or MFV BA is greater than or equal to 60 cm/sec in adults, and/or 30% or greater difference between arterial segments.[93,101-104]

The findings of a recent study have indicated that a BA stenosis of 50% or greater can be more reliably identified when BA MFV exceeds 80 cm/sec and when the stenotic-to-normal MFV ratio is greater than or equal to 2. To detect intracranial vertebrobasilar stenosis of 70% or more, we use MFV greater than 110 cm/sec and a ratio of 4 (see Figures 5-10 and 5-13).

Although the depth range for basilar segments varied among previous studies, it is also dependent on the size of the neck and skull and the technical skills of the operator. Insonation of the distal BA can be accomplished with failure rates far less than 30%. At our laboratory, we aim to detect the distal BA in practically all subjects using the following depth criteria. The proximal BA is located at 75 mm or deeper, the mid-BA segment is located at 90 mm, and the distal BA is found at 100+ mm in most adults. The differential diagnosis includes a terminal VA stenosis if elevated velocities are found proximally (i.e., 70-80 mm). If elevated velocities are found throughout the BA stem, the differential diagnosis includes compensatory flow velocity increase. With the latter, velocities in at least one of the VAs are also elevated.

Basilar artery subtotal stenosis or near occlusion produces a focal FV decrease (≤30% difference between arterial segments and/or BA < VA), resulting in a blunted waveform. The differential diagnosis includes a fusiform (dolicho-ectatic) BA with or without thrombus since an enlarged vessel diameter may reduce flow velocities. If the end-diastolic flow is absent, the differential diagnosis includes BA occlusion or tortuosity with branch insonation at a suboptimal angle.

Additional findings may include the following:
- Turbulence and disturbed signals distal to the stenosis
- Compensatory flow increase in VAs and posterior inferior cerebellar arteries, indicating cerebellar collateralization
- Collateral supply via PcomA to PCA and reversed distal BA (see the discussion of collateral patterns).

Common sources of error include tortuous basilar ("not found" does not always mean obstructed), elongated BA obstruction, and distal BA lesions that were not reached by TCD insonation or identified because of flow presence to the superior cerebellar arteries, producing false-negative results. In cases of distal BA occlusions, transtemporal insonation of the top of the basilar using characteristic power motion-mode Doppler (PMD) flow signatures may be a valuable alternative for the identification of distal BA pathology and monitoring of recanalization. Application of power Doppler, ultrasound contrast, and duplex imaging may help detect flow in the distal basilar segment, confirm tortuosity, and identify distal branches. Also, a collateral flow from the posterior to anterior circulation in the presence of carotid lesions may increase flow velocity changes associated with mild stenosis and/or tortuosity. In the case of flow collateralization, the dominant VA velocities are also increased.

Finally, reversed flow in the BA (typically low-resistance) moving toward the probe at depths of 80 to 100 mm in the absence of antegrade basilar flow signals during suboccipital insonation is diagnostic of proximal BA occlusion with retrofilling the distal BA through the PcomA. The origin of the collateral flow in the anterior circulation can be confirmed with carotid artery tapping that can be transmitted to the reversed BA flow.

TERMINAL VERTEBRAL ARTERY

Primary findings with intracranial VA stenosis include a focal significant velocity increase where MFV VA is greater than BA, and/or MFV VA is greater than or equal to 50 cm/sec in adults, and/or there is a difference of 30% or more between the VAs or their segments. Similar to what is seen with BA stenoses, the higher the focal velocity increase, the greater the chance that angiography will show a significant stenosis. This correlation may worsen if angiography is performed days after stroke onset since the degree of a stenosis seen with a prior TCD examination can decrease because of continuing recanalization at the site of the lesion. The main problem with detecting and grading VA stenoses with TCD is that these vessels are often affected by multiple, diffuse, or elongated lesions and the resulting velocity may not necessarily be high.

An occlusion of the terminal VA may also present as a high-resistance (PI ≥ 1.2) flow in one of the VAs proximal to the obstruction, and/or a blunted or minimal flow signal, including those with reverberating pattern.

The terminal VA is found through the suboccipital window at 40 to 75 mm depending on the size of the neck and skull. To detect intracranial stenoses of 50% or greater, the PSV criteria were also developed for angle-corrected duplex ultrasound of the vertebral and other intracranial arteries.[105]

The findings of a recent study have indicated that a VA stenosis greater than or equal to 50% can be more reliably identified when VA MFV exceeds

80 cm/sec and when the stenotic-to-normal MFV ratio is greater than or equal to 2 (Figure 5-10). The cutoff of 80 cm/sec for detecting greater than 50% stenosis in the vertebrobasilar system was also adopted by the investigators of the Stroke Outcomes and Neuroimaging of Intracranial Atherosclerosis (SONIA) trial.[106]

The differential diagnosis includes proximal BA or contralateral terminal VA stenoses and a compensatory flow increase in the presence of a contralateral VA occlusion or carotid stenosis.[107]

Additional findings may include the following:

- Turbulence or disturbed flow signal distal to the stenosis
- A compensatory flow increase in the contralateral VA or its branches (cerebellar collaterals)
- Low BA flow velocities (hemodynamically significant lesion, hypoplastic contralateral VA) and low-resistance flow distal to stenoses (compensatory vasodilatation)
- The presence of distal embolization in BA or cerebellar collaterals (detectable elevated velocity in posterior inferior cerebellar artery or other cerebellar arteries)

Common sources of error include a compensatory flow increase due to hypoplastic contralateral VA, low velocities in both VAs due to suboptimal angle of insonation, extracranial VA stenosis or occlusion with well-developed muscular collaterals, elongated VA stenosis/hypoplasia, and incorrect vessel identification (i.e., posterior inferior cerebellar artery).

ARTERIAL OCCLUSION AND RECANALIZATION MONITORING

The *Thrombolysis in Brain Ischemia (TIBI) flow grading system* was developed to grade the severity of acute arterial obstructions and determine the residual flow at the thrombus-blood interface (Figure 5-14). In analogy to the Thrombolysis in Myocardial Infarction (TIMI)[11,12,108] flow grades, TIBI waveforms were developed for TCD to predict intracranial vessel patency, and this flow grading system was recently validated against invasive angiography with simultaneous TCD monitoring and intracranial catheter contrast injections. In short, TIBI grades parallel TIMI grades: absent and minimal waveforms predict a complete TIMI 0-1 occlusion, blunted and dampened waveforms correlate with persisting or partial occlusions with TIMI 2 flow, and stenotic and

normal waveforms indicate complete recanalization with TIMI 3 reperfusion with or without a residual stenosis. TIBI flow grades can be used to detect and quantify the revascularization process because these waveforms reflect the beginning, speed, timing, and completeness of recanalization. Since TIBI waveforms also reflect an overall resistance to flow through changes in velocities during each cardiac cycle, they also are predictive of tissue reperfusion and TIMI flow grades. Recently this important difference between a proximal recanalization and tissue reperfusion became a focus of scrutiny in acute interventional trials for stroke.[109] A similar flow grading system was recently suggested for reporting transcranial duplex studies.[110]

COLLATERAL PATTERNS AND FLOW DIRECTION

Understanding flow dynamics to and around an occlusion is important since the majority of patients still arrive beyond the current time window for reperfusion therapies or continue to have persisting occlusions despite treatment. Ultrasound can provide insights into how arterial blood flow is redistributed and how it responds to certain stimuli. The intracranial collateral channels are "dormant" under normal circulatory conditions. A collateral channel opens when a pressure gradient develops between the two anastomosing arterial systems.

TCD can detect some of these collateral pathways.[111-113]

1. Anterior cross-filling via the ACoA
2. PCoA
3. Reversed OA
4. Reversed BA (see Figure 5-10).

Collateral flow is directed from the donor to the recipient vessels. When present, collateral flow patterns rarely imply anatomic variants. Most often, detection of a collateral implies the presence of a flow-limiting (i.e., "hemodynamically significant") lesion or an anatomic variant proximal to the recipient arterial system and the origin of the collateral channel.

The direction of flow indicates which arterial system is the donor (the source of flow) and which is the recipient (the collateral flow destination). TCD provides information on functioning collateral channels and direction of collateral flow. An expanded battery of TCD parameters may be used to refine the evaluation of the severity of ICA lesions, particularly when multiple lesions are found or the applicability of other tests is limited due to the presence of the distal ICA lesions.

ANTERIOR COMMUNICATING ARTERY

Collateral flow through ACoA cannot be reliably distinguished from the neighboring A_1 and A_2 ACA segments because of the relatively small size of the ACoA as compared to a size of the ultrasound sample volume. Therefore, we report findings consistent with the anterior cross-filling via ACoA as opposed to the velocity and direction of flow in the ACoA itself. Sometimes a high-velocity jet with bruit can be found at midline depth, highly suggestive of flow interception through the ACoA. Even under these circumstances, other flow findings pointing to collateralization of flow should be found since focal velocity elevations can be present with an arterial stenosis as well as collaterals.

ANTERIOR CROSS-FILLING

- Elevated A_1 ACA MFVs on the donor side presenting as ACA greater than MCA and/or donor ACA MFVs more than 1.2 times greater than contralateral ACA
- Possible stenotic-like flow at 72 to 78 mm directed away from the donor side
- A normal or low MFV in A_1 ACA of the recipient side with or without A_1 flow reversal

The differential diagnosis includes distal A_1 ACA stenosis and compensatory flow increase if one of the A_1 segments is atretic. Identification of the reversed A_1 segment depends on the skill of the operator. With retrograde filling of the ICA siphon, the terminal ICA can have bidirectional flow. Thus, flow away from the probe (i.e., toward the siphon) can be mistaken for a normal A_1 ACA flow direction. A clue to the differential diagnosis is that flow velocities tend to be higher the closer one insonates to the donor site. Some advocate CCA compression or vibration to aid decision making.

POSTERIOR COMMUNICATING ARTERY

PCoA connects the posterior and anterior cerebral arterial systems and can be detected by TCD since it usually has a considerable length of greater than 5 mm and a favorable angle of insonation. When functioning, it may be detected as a flow signal consistently present at varying depths from 55 to 70 mm via the transtemporal approach. Under normal conditions, this area

has no detectable flow when the sonographer switches from the ICA bifurcation posteriorly to locate the PCA (with depth usually set around 60-64 mm). The direction of flow in PCoA corresponds to collateralization: anterior to posterior collateral flow is directed away from the probe, whereas the posterior to anterior collateral flow is directed toward the probe. Flow direction, however, can be misleading due to tortuosity of PCoA. Without imaging, vessel identification is difficult since the PCoA and PCA are prone to anatomic variations.

In collateralization via PCoA flow signals directed either away or toward the probe with posterior angulation of the transducer over the temporal window are consistently found at 55 to 70 mm. The velocity range is similar to or higher than those detected in the M_1 MCA and ICA bifurcation (anterior to posterior collateral flow) or basilar artery (posterior to anterior collateral flow). A possible stenotic-like flow signal may be found at 55 to 70 mm with similar probe angulation. Elevated velocities can also be found all the way to the top of the basilar artery (up to 75-80 mm via transtemporal approach), and in the P_2 PCA segment (usually with additional transcortical collaterals). The differential diagnosis includes terminal ICA or PCA stenoses.

Of note, collateralization of flow via PCoA carries the systolic flow acceleration signature from the donor site. The posterior-to-anterior circulation flow could have a slight delay in systolic flow acceleration similar to that seen in the vertebral arteries, whereas anterior-to-posterior collaterals often have a more vertical upstroke similar to that in the ICAs.

REVERSED OPHTHALMIC ARTERY BLOOD FLOW

The primary findings are an abnormal OA signal that includes low pulsatility flow directed primarily away from the probe via the transorbital window at 40 to 60 mm depth. Check vessel identification since an ICA siphon flow signal can be taken in the presence of low-velocity OA signals.

Additional findings may include no substantial difference in MFVs detected in the OA and siphon; high velocities in the ICA siphon, suggesting either a high-grade proximal ICA and/or siphon stenosis; and no flow signals at depths greater than 60 mm, suggesting an ICA occlusion proximal to the OA origin.

REVERSED BASILAR ARTERY BLOOD FLOW

Reversed BA blood flow arises from either a functional PCoA or through cerebellar collaterals. Its presence can explain the lack of marked patient symptoms and the relatively favorable outcome of proximal BA occlusion.

We use the following criteria to identify the reversed BA:

- Detectable flow toward the probe in the BA (low-resistance flow at depths of 80-110 mm)
- Absence of the antegrade low-resistance basilar flow signals during suboccipital insonation except abnormal TIBI flow grades 0 to 3, indicating a proximal BA obstruction
- Anterior circulation flow origin at the top of the basilar demonstrated by vertical systolic flow acceleration similar to that in the ICAs, as well as a response to the common carotid tapping

Of note, carotid tapping should be performed with caution, preferably after the extracranial ultrasound examination has confirmed the absence of significant stenosis or hypoechoic plaques in the carotid arteries.

IDENTIFICATION OF LESIONS AMENABLE TO INTERVENTION IN ACUTE STROKE

An acute intracerebral arterial occlusion is an emergency that can often benefit from urgent therapeutic intervention. It is a dynamic process that may start with partial obstruction to flow and lead to occlusion due to thrombus propagation. Reocclusion and sometimes spontaneous recanalization may also happen.

An acute arterial occlusion is often caused by a thrombus that either develops over a preexisting atheroma or lodges from an embolic source in a normal artery segment. Both scenarios are considered a "lesion amenable to intervention."[114-131]

Given the short time interval, just as "time is brain," so "time is clot." The faster the lesion is identified, the better the chances of a successful therapeutic strategy. Ultrasound allows identification of LAITs in stroke patients at the bedside.

Ultrasound testing can be performed at the bedside using a *fast-track insonation protocol* combining TCD with extracranial carotid duplex (see later) in the emergency department to facilitate rapid and timely administration of TPA.[9]

The key ultrasound findings for the diagnosis of a lesion amenable to intervention with thrombolysis (TPA) include the following:

- One of four abnormal TIBI waveforms in the vessel supplying a territory affected by ischemia; and
- Evidence of flow diversion or collateralization to compensate for this lesion (see Figure 5-14).

In the absence of flow diversion or collateralization, other findings can point to the presence of thrombus and its location, such as increased velocities consistent with the presence of a stenosis, embolic signals, and blood flow pulsatility changes in vessels proximal and distal to the suspected obstruction. With these criteria, a non–image-guided Doppler ultrasound can identify thrombus location with an accuracy exceeding 90% for the MCA and ICA. When combined with carotid duplex sonography, TCD can achieve practically 100% agreement with urgent catheter angiography in confirming the presence of a thrombotic lesion in hyperacute stroke patients.

The *combined neurovascular ultrasound examination* is done at the bedside, often with a portable device and the operator standing behind the patient headrest. The examination is guided by the clinical findings. It starts with TCD, since an acute occlusion responsible for the neurologic deficit is likely located intracranially. Extracranial carotid/vertebral duplex may reveal an additional lesion often responsible for an intracranial flow disturbance. Fast-track insonation is adapted to the localization of patient symptoms.

CLINICAL DIAGNOSIS OF CEREBRAL ISCHEMIA IN THE ANTERIOR CIRCULATION

Step 1: Transcranial Doppler

1. If time permits, begin insonation on the *non-affected side* to establish the temporal window, normal MCA waveform (M_1 depth 45-65 mm, M_2 30-45 mm), and velocity for comparison to the affected side.
2. If short on time, start on the *affected side*: first assess MCA at 50 mm. If no signals are detected, increase the depth to 62 mm. If an antegrade flow signal is found, reduce the depth to trace the MCA stem or identify the worst residual flow signal. Search for possible flow diversion to the ACA, PCA, or M_2 MCA. Evaluate and compare waveform shapes and systolic flow acceleration.

3. Continue on the *affected side* (transorbital window). Check flow direction and pulsatility in the OA at depths of 40 to 50 mm, followed by ICA siphon at depths of 55 to 65 mm.
4. If time permits or in patients with pure motor or sensory deficits, evaluate BA (depth 80-100+ mm) and terminal VA (40-80 mm).

Step 2: Carotid/Vertebral Duplex

1. Start on the *affected side* in transverse B-mode planes followed by a color or power-mode sweep from proximal to distal carotid segments. Identify CCA and its bifurcation on B-mode and color flow lumens.
2. Document if ICA (or CCA) has a lesion on B-mode with a corresponding disturbance on Doppler flow images. In patients with concomitant chest pain, evaluate CCA as close to its origin as possible.
3. Perform angle-corrected spectral velocity measurements in the mid to distal CCA, ICA, and ECA.
4. If time permits or in patients with pure motor or sensory deficits, examine the cervical portion of the vertebral arteries (longitudinal B-mode, color or power mode, spectral Doppler) on the *affected side.*
5. If time permits, perform transverse and longitudinal scanning of the arteries on the *nonaffected side.*

CLINICAL DIAGNOSIS OF CEREBRAL ISCHEMIA IN THE POSTERIOR CIRCULATION

Step 1: Transcranial Doppler

1. Start suboccipital insonation at 75 mm (VA junction), and identify BA flow at 80 to 100+ mm.
2. If abnormal signals are present at 75 to 100 mm, find the terminal VA (40-80 mm) on the nonaffected side for comparison, and evaluate the terminal VA on the affected side at similar depths.
3. Continue with a transtemporal examination to identify the PCA (55-75 mm) and possible collateral flow through the PCoA (check both sides).
4. If time permits, evaluate both MCAs and ACAs (60-75 mm) for possible compensatory velocity increase as an indirect sign of BA obstruction.

Step 2: Vertebral/Carotid Duplex Ultrasound

1. Start on the affected side by locating the CCA in the longitudinal B-mode plane, and turn the transducer downward to visualize the typical acoustic shadowing caused by the transverse processes of the midcervical vertebrae.
2. Apply color or power modes and spectral Doppler to identify flow in the VA segments between vertebral bodies.
3. Follow the VA course to its origin, and obtain Doppler velocity spectral waveforms. Perform similar examination on the other side.
4. If time permits, perform bilateral duplex examination of the CCA, ICA, and ECA.

EFFICACY

This combined neurovascular ultrasound examination can identify lesions amenable to intervention in over 90% of patients eligible for reperfusion therapies and in over 40% of patients with TIAs or spontaneously resolved symptoms.

These ultrasound protocols can quickly identify a lesion that is likely responsible for the onset of stroke symptoms, grade its severity, locate it, and identify the probable pathogenic mechanism, in minutes and at the bedside.

MONITORING THROMBOLYTIC THERAPY WITH ULTRASOUND

Delaying TPA therapy beyond 4.5 hours after symptom onset in favor of using more sophisticated imaging methods than a noncontrast CT is not clinically justifiable since TPA efficacy decreases with time and the first noticeable improvement of blood flow to the brain occurs at a median time of 17 minutes after a TPA bolus is administered.[132-141] Median time to completion of recanalization is 35 minutes after bolus administration, and those patients who complete recanalization before the end of the first hour of TPA infusion are 3.5 times more likely to achieve favorable outcome at 3 months.

Spontaneous complete recanalization of an MCA occlusion occurs at a rate of approximately 6% per hour during the first day after symptom onset.[133-140] Systemic TPA doubles the chance of complete MCA recanalization rate to almost 13% during the first hour of treatment (partial and complete recanalization rate is 50% with systemic TPA) (Figure 5-15).

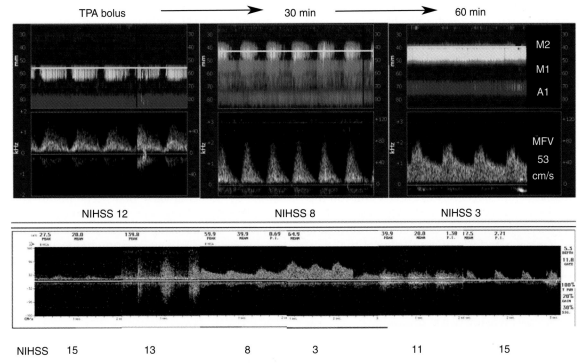

FIGURE 5-15 Arterial recanalization and reocclusion during systemic tissue plasminogen activator (TPA) administration for an acute ischemic stroke. *Upper images:* Complete early middle cerebral artery recanalization; NIHSS, National Institutes of Health Stroke Scale scores of the severity of the neurologic deficit indicating dramatic clinical recovery. *Lower images:* Early recanalization followed by reocclusion with corresponding NIHSS scores indicating clinical deterioration following improvement during TPA infusion. MFV, mean flow velocity.

The likelihood of early complete recanalization of an M_2 MCA occlusion with systemic TPA is 44%. It is 30% for an M_1 MCA occlusion, 27% for a tandem MCA/ICA occlusion, and less than 6% for a terminal ICA occlusion.[135] Patients with persisting proximal occlusions have only a 10% chance of complete recovery by 3 months. This information can be used to discuss additional intra-arterial reperfusion procedures to lyse or remove thrombus with a catheter even after full-dose intravenous TPA.

Real-time TCD monitoring can detect early arterial reocclusion (see Figure 5-15). This can affect 15% to 25% of TPA-treated patients, more commonly those with partial or incomplete initial recanalization or with a large atheromatous burden in the affected arterial segment. Arterial reocclusion accounts for two-thirds of the patients who experience neurologic deterioration following improvement with TPA therapy. Although intracranial arterial reocclusion can occur before or during TPA administration, the majority of these events happen after discontinuation of TPA infusion. On average, reocclusion occurs at 65 minutes

after bolus administration. After early reocclusion, there is a 33% chance of a favorable neurologic outcome at 3 months, compared to 50% in patients with stable early recanalization.[136,137]

Early complete recanalization is closely associated with dramatic clinical recovery[138-140] and is thought to be the mechanism responsible for improved stroke outcomes. Therefore, any means of facilitating early recanalization would be expected to result in a faster and more complete recovery from stroke. This goal can be achieved by the application of ultrasound-enhanced thrombolysis.

ULTRASOUND-ENHANCED THROMBOLYSIS

Experimental models have clearly shown over the past 30 years that ultrasound energy facilitates the activity of fibrinolytic agents within minutes of being applied to an environment where thrombus- and blood-containing thrombolytic agents are present.[142-153]

The mechanisms of ultrasound-enhanced thrombolysis include improved drug transport, reversible alteration of the structure of fibrin, and increased TPA binding to fibrin over wide frequency ranges.

Although kilohertz frequencies penetrate better and cause less heating than those in the megahertz ranges, a combination of TPA with an experimental kilohertz delivery system resulted in excessive risk for intracerebral hemorrhage (ICH) in stroke patients.

We used diagnostic 2-MHz TCD to evaluate acute stroke patients and reported an unexpectedly high rate of complete recanalization and a dramatic clinical recovery when TPA infusion was continuously monitored with TCD. The analysis of phase I clinical results allowed us to determine the sample size for a phase II clinical trial that, besides studying the safety of TCD monitoring, was powered to demonstrate 20% difference in the primary end point of complete recanalization within 2 hours after TPA bolus administration.

The CLOTBUST trial (Combined Lysis of Thrombus in Brain ischemia using transcranial Ultrasound and Systemic TPA) was a phase II multicenter randomized clinical trial (Houston, Barcelona, Edmonton, Calgary).[154] All patients with acute ischemic stroke were treated with 0.9 mg/kg intravenous TPA within 3 hours of symptom onset. All patients had an MCA occlusion on pretreatment TCD and were randomized to continuous monitoring with TCD (target group) or placebo monitoring (control). Safety end point was symptomatic ICH. Primary combined activity end point was complete recanalization on TCD or dramatic clinical recovery to a total National Institutes of Health Stroke Scale (NIHSS) score of 3 or less, or improvement by 10 or more NIHSS points within 2 hours of TPA bolus administration. Secondary end points included outcomes at 3 months by the modified Rankin score (mRS).

All projected 126 patients received TPA and were randomized 1:1 to continuous monitoring (median NIHSS 16) or control (median NIHSS 17). Age, occlusion location (M_1-MCA or M_2-MCA) on TCD, and time to TPA bolus were similar. Symptomatic ICH occurred in 3 target patients and 3 controls; difference in risk is not significant (0.0%; 95% CI, –0.07%, 0.07%). Complete recanalization or dramatic clinical recovery within 2 hours after TPA bolus (primary end point) was observed in 31 (49%, target) vs 19 (30%, control), $P = 0.03$. At 3 months, 22 (41.5%, target) and 14 (28%, control) patients achieved favorable outcomes (mRS 0-1), NS. In

stroke patients treated with intravenous TPA, continuous TCD monitoring of intracranial occlusion safely augmented TPA-induced arterial recanalization and was coupled with early dramatic clinical recovery (25% target vs 8% control, $P=0.02$) at 2 hours after treatment onset.[154] The CLOTBUST trial showed that TCD has a positive biological activity that aided systemic thrombolytic therapy and provided clinical evidence of ultrasound-enhanced thrombolysis in humans.

Based on these findings, we believe that ultrasound can improve existing therapies for ischemic stroke by inducing early brain reperfusion and complete arterial segment recanalization, which can lead to dramatic clinical recoveries. Our international collaborative group has focused on testing the ability of ultrasound-activated gaseous microspheres to further amplify TPA activity.[155]

GASEOUS MICROSPHERES AND SONOLYSIS

Molina and associates pioneered coupling commercially available microspheres with TCD for treatment of acute stroke patients. The group compared the CLOTBUST target arm to a 2-MHz continuous TCD monitoring combined with Levovist air microspheres (Schering AG, Germany). Investigators demonstrated that at 2 hours after recombinant tissue-type plasminogen activator (rt-PA) bolus the rt-PA+TCD+Levovist group achieved a 55% sustained recanalization rate compared to 38% in the rt-PA+TCD group of the CLOTBUST trial.[156]

Since then, several studies have reported findings with different commercially available microspheres and confirmed higher recanalization rates with the addition of microspheres.[157-159] The safety and feasibility of infusion of new and more stable C_3F_8 (perflutren lipid) microspheres in patients treated with ultrasound-enhanced thrombolysis have recently been reported.[160]

In a pilot clinical trial of perflutren lipid microspheres,[160] microspheres permeated to areas with no pretreatment residual flow[161] in 75% of patients, and in 83%, residual flow velocity improved at a median of 30 minutes from the start of microsphere infusion (range, 30 sec-120 min) by a median of 17 cm/sec, or 118% above pretreatment values. No symptomatic ICH (sICH) was found in either the target (rt-PA+2-MHz TCD monitoring+ microspheres) or in the control group (rt-PA+2-MHz TCD monitoring).

Moreover, microspheres were moving at velocities higher than surrounding residual red blood cell flow in patients with MCA occlusions (39.8±11.3 cm/sec vs 28.8±13.8 cm/sec, $P <0.001$). As a sign of efficacy, perflutren lipid microspheres, TCD, and rt-PA completely lysed 50% of proximal MCA occlusions. This compares favorably to concurrent and historic controls receiving rt-PA alone.[162] Most recently, a multicenter microspheres dose escalation study called TUCSON (*Transcranial Ultrasound in Clinical Sonothrombolysis*)[163] was completed. Stroke patients with pretreatment proximal intracranial occlusions on TCD were randomized (2:1 ratio) to rt-PA with perflutren lipid microspheres (MRX-801) infusion over 90 minutes (cohort 1 1.4 mL, cohort 2 2.8 mL) and continuous TCD insonation, while controls received rt-PA and brief TCD assessments. The primary safety end point was sICH within 36 hours post-TPA. Among 35 patients (cohort 1= 12, cohort 2 =11, controls =12), no sICH occurred in cohort 1 and controls, while 3 (27%, with 2 fatal) sICHs occurred in cohort 2 ($P = 0.028$). Sustained complete recanalization rates at the end of TCD monitoring were 67% cohort 1, 46% cohort 2, and 33% controls ($P = 0.255$). The median time to any recanalization tended to be shorter in cohort 1 (30 minutes, interquartile range [IQR] = 6) and cohort 2 (30 minutes, IQR = 69) compared to controls (60 minutes, IQR = 5; $P = 0.054$). Although patients with sICH had similar screening and pretreatment systolic blood pressure (SBP) levels in comparison to the rest, higher SBP levels were documented in sICH patients at 30 minutes, 60 minutes, 90 minutes, and 24 to 36 hours following rt-PA bolus.[163]

Although the study was stopped halfway by the sponsor for administrative reasons, this trial showed that perflutren lipid microspheres can be safely administered with rt-PA at the first dose tier, confirming the previous pilot study results. The rates of recanalization and clinical recovery tended to be higher in both microspheres dose tiers compared to controls.[163]

However, it should be noted that sustained complete recanalization rates at the end of TCD monitoring were higher in cohorts 1 and 2 without reaching statistical significance ($P = 0.255$). Similarly, the differences between groups in terms of functional outcomes were not significant ($P = 0.167$). In agreement with previous studies, the addition of microspheres to rt-PA with ultrasound monitoring should achieve a 50% complete recanalization rate for proximal intracranial occlusions. In a recent meta-analysis[162] a combination of rt-PA and transcranial ultrasound in the low MHz range with or without gaseous microspheres safely doubled the chance of rt-PA–induced recanalization.

Ribo and associates[164] studied the safety and efficacy of local microspheres administration during intra-arterial thrombolysis and continuous TCD monitoring for MCA recanalization: after no recanalization was achieved with rt-PA, nine patients underwent intra-arterial (IA)-rescue procedures with addition of microspheres, suggesting that the combination of ultrasound and intra-arterial microspheres with rt-PA may be a strategy to enhance the thrombolytic effect of TPA and increase recanalization rates.

Enhancing the efficacy of TPA, the only approved systemic therapy for stroke, is a desirable goal. It seems that microspheres administration combined with the application of ultrasound energy offer a promising therapeutic approach to achieve this target.

Microspheres combined with the application of ultrasound energy may be an effective treatment strategy that can complement the current intravenous–intra-arterial approaches to recanalize thrombi resistant to fibrinolysis alone. Improvements in ultrasound and microspheres-assisted stroke therapies may require the replacement of experienced sonographers that need to be available for around-the-clock emergency situations with an operator-independent device that could reliably deliver ultrasound energy in the right location to activate microspheres and induce recanalization in restless stroke patients. Making this technology available to all emergency departments would facilitate health care delivery and promote phase III clinical trials of ultrasound-enhanced thrombolysis.

SPECIFIC TCD APPLICATIONS IN CEREBROVASCULAR DISEASES

TCD AND SICKLE CELL DISEASE

Sickle cell disease (SCD) is an autosomal recessive disorder associated with thrombotic occlusions of the large intracranial arteries. Young children with SCD are at a very high risk for stroke.[165,166] The internal carotid or the middle and anterior cerebral arteries are affected in the majority of SCD patients, thereby explaining the moyamoya pattern of collateral vessels that is sometimes seen.[165-169]

Transfusion therapy is very effective in the prevention of first and recurrent ischemic strokes in children with SCD[165-171] and decreases the risk for stroke to about 10%.

Since the associations between disease severity and survival are strikingly variable and treatment options burdensome, numerous investigations have tried to identify risk factors and develop prediction models to improve treatment strategies.

Adams and co-workers[172] in 1998 demonstrated the utility of TCD in primary stroke prevention, where abnormally increased TCD velocities predict stroke.

Flow velocities TCD criteria for SCD used in the Stroke Prevention Trial in Sickle Cell Anemia (STOP) are the following[172]:

- MFV of up to 170 cm/sec—normal
- MFV of 171 to 199 cm/sec—conditional
- MFV of equal to or greater than 200 cm/sec—abnormal

An MFV of 200 cm/sec or greater is accompanied by a stroke risk of 40% within the next 3 years. In these patients transfusion therapy, with reduction of hemoglobin S to less than 30% of total hemoglobin, lowers this risk by 70% compared with standard care alone.

TCD allows detection and quantification of relevant large intracranial artery stenosis[172-175] and reduces the need for cerebral angiography and the small associated risk for worsening SCD. TCD has shown its validity as a screening tool to assess stroke risk in children 2 to 16 years of age with SCD.

An optimal timing to rescreen children with SCD and normal TCD is not yet established, but a repeat TCD examination every 6 months seems to be reasonable.

CEREBRAL EMBOLIZATION AND DETECTION OF RIGHT-TO-LEFT SHUNTS

Ultrasound can detect, quantify, and localize experimentally induced emboli in real time,[176] and TCD can document this process in vivo (Figure 5-16).[177-179] TCD has an established clinical value to monitor stroke patients with presumed cardiac, arterial, or paradoxical sources for brain embolization. Identification of microembolic signals (MESs) may suggest potential sources of embolism (e.g., heart chambers and septum, aortic arch, arterial stenosis or dissection, circulating emboli with infection or fat embolism). It can also be used to monitor carotid and

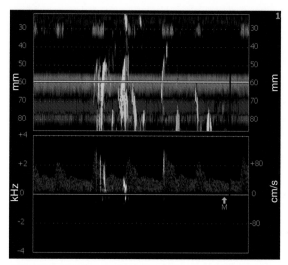

FIGURE 5-16 Microembolic signals in the middle cerebral artery and anterior cerebral artery on PMD TCD. PMD, power motion-mode Doppler; TCD, transcranial Doppler.

cardiac surgery, angioplasty/stenting, and intra-arterial rescue procedures in acute stroke.

Most MESs detected by TCD are asymptomatic since the size of the particles producing them is usually comparable to or even smaller than the diameter of brain capillaries.[180] Strict standards should be followed when an interpreter documents and reports microemboli on TCD.[181]

The gold standard for MES identification still remains the online interpretation of real-time, videotaped, or digitally stored Doppler flow signals.[182]

The spectral recording should be obtained with minimal gain at a fixed angle of insonation with a small (<10 mm) sample volume. The probe should be maintained with a fixation device during at least 0.5 to 1 hour of monitoring. The use of a two-channel device with simultaneous registration and a prolonged monitoring period may improve the yield of the procedure. Multigated or multirange registration at different insonation depths may improve differentiation of embolic signals from artifacts. Using multiple channels may increase the chance of detection during the same period of time.

According to the International Cerebral Hemodynamics Society definition,[183] the MESs have the following characteristics (Figure 5-16, spectral Doppler, *bottom*):

- Random occurrence during the cardiac cycle
- Brief duration (usually <0.1 second)
- High intensity (>3 dB over background)
- Primarily unidirectional signals (if fast Fourier transformation is used)
- Audible component

TABLE 5-4 Criteria for Counting Embolic Signals on Spectral Display of a Single-Channel Transcranial Doppler (TCD) and on M-Mode Display of Power Motion-Mode Doppler (PMD) (see Figure 5-16, Upper Image of PMD Display)

Criterion	TCD	PMD
1	Transient, lasting 0.3 sec	The "embolic signature" is visible at least 3 dB higher than the highest spontaneous PMD display of background blood flow signal.
2	≥3dB higher intensity than that of the highest background flow signal	The embolic signature reflects motion in one direction at a minimum spatial extent of 7.5 mm and a minimum temporal extent of 30 msec. An MCA embolic signature is required to move toward the probe, with a positively sloped track (see Figure 5-16). An ACA embolic signature moves away from the probe, with a negatively sloped track (see Figure 5-16).
3	Unidirectional	The embolic signature must traverse a specific depth determined by the highest intensity of the insonated artery to avoid repeated counting of the same embolus.
4	Accompanied by snap, chip, or moan on the audible output	N/A

From The International Cerebral Hemodynamics Society Consensus Statement: *Stroke* 26:1123, 1995 and Saqqur M, et al: Improved detection of microbubble signals using power M-mode Doppler, *Stroke* 35:e14–e17, 2004.
ACA, anterior cerebral artery; MCA, middle carotid artery; N/A, not applicable.

Contrast PMD recordings of the cervical submandibular extracranial ICA and the BA have been shown to be at least as sensitive and specific as the traditional MCA method in detecting right-to-left shunts (RLSs), suggesting its possible utility in patients with poor transcranial ultrasonic bone windows (Table 5-4).[184,185]

Spencer and colleagues[186] compared the sensitivity of PMD TCD and single-gate TCD to detect contrast bubble emboli through RLS during transcatheter patent foramen ovale closure. The authors documented that significantly more emboli were detected using PMD than with single-gate TCD. Based on their findings, they developed a six-level logarithmic scale (Spencer's logarithmic scale, SLS) for the grading of RLS (Table 5-5). SLS grades III to V were shown to be highly sensitive and specific in predicting whether a functional patent foramen ovale was present on transesophageal echocardiography and whether it can be confirmed with catheterization. Their findings showed that Spencer's grades III to V criteria have a higher positive predictive value in detecting large and functional RLS than the International Consensus Criteria (ICC) (60% vs 32%). Our group has recently prospectively compared the SLS to the ICC for the grading of RLS.[187] Our findings confirmed the advantages of using SLS criteria since they offer a broader range for grading shunt conductance while being as sensitive as ICC but more

TABLE 5-5 Spencer's Logarithmic Scale for Grading Right-to-Left Shunt During Bilateral Middle Cerebral Artery Monitoring (Count of Embolic Tracks Is Performed on PMD Display)

Grade	Number of Embolic Tracks
0	0
I	1-10
II	11-30
III	31-100
IV	100-300
V	>300

From Spencer MP, et al: Power M-mode transcranial Doppler for diagnosis of patent foramen ovale and assessing transcatheter closure, *J Neuroimaging* 14:342–349, 2004.

specific to detect large shunts. In our study, the use of SLS grade III or higher for quantification of RLS decreased by more than 50% the number of false-positive TCD diagnoses to predict large RLS on transesophageal echocardiography.

SUBCLAVIAN STEAL SYNDROME

Subclavian steal is a hemodynamic condition of reversed flow in one VA to compensate for a proximal hemodynamic lesion in the unilateral subclavian artery.[188,189] Thus, blood flow is diverted or "stolen" from the brain to feed the arm. Subclavian steal is usually an accidental finding since it rarely produces neurologic symptoms. If the patient is asymptomatic, it is called subclavian

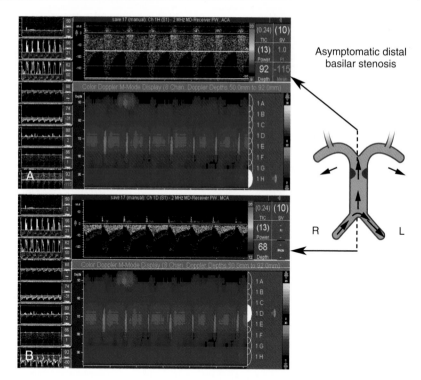

Asymptomatic distal basilar stenosis

FIGURE 5-17 Inccidental finding of an asymptomatic basilar artery stenosis **(A)** and subclavian steal phenomen on (partly reversed subclavian artery blood flow) **(B)** in a stroke patient with anterior circulation symptoms confirmed by magnetic resonance imaging. Doppler spectra show an alternating flow signal consistent with subclavian steal phenomenon present at rest. L, left; MCA, middle cerebral artery; R, right.

steal phenomenon, and it usually indicates a widespread atherosclerosis in aortic branches. If symptoms of vertebrobasilar ischemia are present, it is called subclavian steal syndrome.

Subclavian steal is well studied with ultrasound.[190-205] When steal is present at rest, the main findings include a difference in blood pressure between arms of 20 mm Hg or more and, usually, systolic flow reversal (alternating flow signal [Figure 5-17] or absent diastolic flow) in the "stealing" VA as well as a low resistance flow in the donor artery. Right-to-left subclavian steal is found in 85% of cases due to the anatomic differences in the origin of these arteries.

If the blood pressure difference between the arms is 10 to 20 mm Hg and the steal waveforms are not present at rest, or flow reversal is incomplete, the hyperemia test should be performed to provoke the steal and to augment flow reversal. The cuff should be inflated to higher than systolic blood pressure values, and flow reduction to the arm should be maintained about 1 to 1.5 minutes (maximum 3 minutes, if tolerated by patient). This duration of arterial compression produces ischemia in the arm. The cuff should be quickly released, and any augmentation of flow should be monitored by TCD. Once the cuff is released, the blood flow enters tissues with increased metabolic demand produced by a short

period of ischemia. Greater demand for blood flow augments the steal, and alternating flow can be visualized for a short period of time in the recipient VA. Recent studies have shown that subclavian steal phenomenon can be easily identified by alternating flow signatures on a motion mode display.

CEREBRAL VASOMOTOR REACTIVITY, BREATH-HOLDING INDEX

A variety of tests were introduced to evaluate intracranial hemodynamics using the phenomenon of vasomotor reactivity, including carbon dioxide reactivity with TCD, acetazolamide testing with TCD, cerebral blood flow scanning techniques, and the breath-holding index (BHI).[206-209]

The latter is the simplest way of challenging vasosmotor reactivity if a patient is compliant and capable of holding his/her breath for 30 seconds. This index is calculated using the MFVs obtained by TCD before breath holding (baseline) and at the end of 4 seconds of breathing after 30 seconds of breath holding:

$$BHI = \frac{\frac{MFV_{end} - MFV_{baseline}}{MFV_{baseline}} \times 100}{\text{Seconds of breath holding}} \quad (5\text{-}3)$$

The patient should be able to hold breath voluntarily for at least 24 seconds, preferably 30 seconds. BHI values of less than 0.69 are predictive of risk for stroke in patients who have asymptomatic severe ICA stenoses and symptomatic occlusions.

BHI is not as quantifiable as achieved carbon dioxide levels, and it requires patient cooperation, but BHI does not require any gas-monitoring equipment or intravenous injections. BHI may represent a screening test in the outpatient clinic to identify patients who have impaired vasomotor reactivity.

REVERSED ROBIN HOOD SYNDROME

Neurologic deterioration can occur in about 15% of acute stroke patients.[210-212]

Reocclusion of the artery, progression of edema, and cardiovascular instability can lead to extension of the ischemic area of the brain and cause worsening of the patient's neurologic status.[213-215] However, these long-recognized mechanisms do not account for all cases of neurologic deterioration or symptom recurrence. The natural way to compensate for an acute arterial occlusion is to steal blood flow, and this concept has been well known in cardiology since the 1960s. Once a feeding vessel is blocked, arteries and arterioles distal to it dilate to decrease resistance and attract blood flow. This mechanism provides an incentive for the blood flow to travel a longer pathway through collaterals to reach areas distal to an occlusion. Therefore, tissues distal to an occlusion steal blood from normally perfused areas.

Counterintuitively, the same collateral pathways that are recruited to compensate for a lesion can serve as pathways for transient decreases in blood flow and steal from malperfused tissues. This can occur when normal vessels outside of the ischemic zone dilate more that those within this region. Changes in cerebral hemodynamics can be detected in real time using TCD, and several groups, including ours, deployed this modality to determine predictors of neurologic deterioration. We observed paradoxical decreases in flow velocity during episodes of hypercapnia in vessels supplying ischemic areas of the brain at the time of expected velocity increase in nonaffected vessels.[216]

Hypercapnia triggered vasodilatation more effectively in normal vessels, thus producing arterial blood flow steal toward the path of least resistance. The steal magnitude was linked to severity of neurologic worsening in acute stroke patients.[216,217] We termed this reversed Robin Hood for analogy with "rob the poor to feed the rich."[216] In the first documented cases of the reversed Robin Hood syndrome, neurologic worsening was more pronounced in patients with sleep apnea, a condition that elevates carbon dioxide levels and effectively causes hypercapnia. This can trigger a perfect storm of worsening symptoms and tissue damage in an acute stroke patient. Apnea correction can reduce the chances of new vascular events.

Our recently developed criterion for detection of this hemodynamic steal phenomenon with TCD[216,217] is as follows:

- MFV decrease in the affected vessel at the time of hypercapnia-induced velocity increase in the normal MCA

The steal magnitude (SM, %) is quantified as the maximum negative percent velocity reduction during breath holding:

$$SM = [(MFVm - MFVb) / MFVb] \times 100, \quad (5\text{-}4)$$

where m is the minimum MFV and b is the baseline MFV.

Steal is considered present when SM is negative (i.e., SM<0) in the affected vessel. After the steal is documented on TCD, reversed Robin Hood syndrome is suspected if new or recurrent neurologic worsening by 2 or more NIHSS points is observed without concurrent changes in blood pressure or arterial patency. TCD can show reversed Robin Hood syndrome in 7% and hemodynamic steal in 14% of patients with acute cerebral ischemia.[218]

Interestingly, the factors associated with the steal and clinical syndrome included younger age, large-vessel atheromatous disease, persisting proximal arterial occlusion, and daytime sleepiness. The presence of detectable collaterals such as ACoA, PCoA, and reversed OA are also more common in patients with reversed Robin Hood syndrome. This is counterintuitive, but a functional major collaterals channel can act as a "double-edge sword": it can deliver sufficient blood flow to tissues distal to an arterial occlusion and also deprive those tissues of blood flow if a pressure gradient across the channel changes unfavorably. The reversed Robin Hood syndrome may provide a missing link between acute thromboembolic occlusion, hypoventilation, and sleep apnea and may identify patients for early noninvasive ventilatory correction and brain perfusion augmentation through blood pressure and FV manipulations.

REFERENCES

1. Liepsch D: Principles and models of hemodynamics. In Hennerici M, Mearis S, editors: *Cerebrovascular Ultrasound: theory, practice, and future developments,* Cambridge, 2001, Cambridge University Press, pp 27–28.
2. von Reutern GM, Budingen HJ: *Ultrasound diagnosis of cerebrovascular Disease* Stuttgart, 1993, Georg Thieme Verlag, 56-62.
3. Toole JF: *Cerebrovascular disorders* ed 4, New York, 1990, Raven Press, 28-49.
4. Perktold K, Karner G: Computational principles and models of hemodynamics. In Hennerici M, Mearis S, editors: *Cerebrovascular Ultrasound: theory, practice, and future developments,* Cambridge, 2001, Cambridge University Press, pp 63–76.
5. Glagov S, et al: Morphogenesis of the atherosclerotic plaque. In Hennerici M, Mearis S, editors: *Cerebrovascular Ultrasound: theory, practice, and future developments,* Cambridge, 2001, Cambridge University Press, pp 117–133.
6. von Reutern GM, Budingen HJ: *Ultrasound diagnosis of cerebrovascular Disease* Stuttgart, 1993, Georg Thieme Verlag, 76-80.
7. Lindegaard KF, et al: Assessment of intracranial hemodynamics in carotid artery disease by transcranial Doppler ultrasound, *J Neurosurg* 63: 89–898, 1985.
8. Hennerici M, Rautenberg W, Schwartz A: Transcranial Doppler ultrasound for the assessment of intracranial arterial flow velocity—Part I. Examination technique and normal values, *Surg Neurol* 27:439–448, 1987.
9. Chernyshev OY, et al: Yield and accuracy of urgent combined carotid/transcranial ultrasound testing in acute cerebral ischemia, *Stroke* 36(1):32–37, 2005 Jan. Epub 2004 Nov 29.
10. Adams RJ, et al: Transcranial Doppler correlation with cerebral angiography in sickle cell disease, *Stroke* 23:1073–1077, 1992.
11. Otis SM, Ringelstein EB: The transcranial Doppler examination: Principles and applications of transcranial Doppler sonography. In Tegeler CH, Babikian VL, Gomez CR, editors: *Neurosonology,* St Louis, 1996, Mosby, pp 140–155.
12. Babikian V, et al: Transcranial Doppler validation pilot study, *J Neuroimaging* 3:242–249, 1993.
13. Bragoni M, Feldmann E: Transcranial Doppler indices of intracranial hemodynamics. In Tegeler CH, Babikian VL, Gomez CR, editors: St Louis, 1996, Mosby, pp 129–139.
14. Alexandrov AV, et al: Practice standards for transcranial Doppler ultrasound: Part I–test performance, *J Neuroimaging* 17:11–18, 2007.
15. Sharma VK, et al: Role of transcranial Doppler ultrasonography in evaluation of patients with cerebrovascular disease, *Curr Neurol Neurosci Rep* 7:8–20, 2007.
16. Tsivgoulis G, et al: Validation of transcranial Doppler with computed tomography angiography in acute cerebral ischemia, *Stroke* 38:1245–1249, 2007.
17. Tsivgoulis G, et al: Association of pretreatment ASPECTS scores with tPA-induced arterial recanalization in acute middle cerebral artery occlusion, *J Neuroimaging* 18:56–61, 2008.
18. Alexandrov AV, Tegeler CH: Diagnostic criteria for transcranial Doppler sonography: a model for quality assurance and laboratory accreditation, *Vascular Ultrasound Today* 4:1–24, 1999.
19. ICAVL: *Accreditation material,* Columbia, MD 2009. http://www.icavl.org.
20. Fairhead JF, Mehta Z, Rothwell PM: Population-based study of delays in carotid imaging and surgery and the risk of recurrent stroke, *Neurology* 65:371–375, 2005.
21. Autret A, et al: Stroke risk in patients with carotid stenosis, *Lancet* 1:888–890, 1987.
22. Hertzer NR, et al: Surgical versus non-operative treatment of asymptomatic carotid stenosis. 290 patients documented by intravenous angiography, *Ann Surg* 204:163–171, 1986.
23. Dennis MS, et al: A comparison of risk factors and prognosis for transient ischemic attacks and minor ischemic strokes, The Oxfordshire Community Stroke Project, *Stroke* 20:1494–1499, 1989.
24. Randomised trial of endarterectomy for recently symptomatic carotid stenosis: final results of the MRC European carotid surgery trial (ECST), *Lancet* 351:1379–1387, 1998.
25. Barnett HJ, et al: Benefit of carotid endarterectomy in patients with symptomatic moderate or severe stenosis, North American Symptomatic Carotid Endarterectomy Trial Collaborators, *N Engl J Med* 339:1415–1425, 1998.
26. Mayberg MR, et al: Carotid endarterectomy and prevention of cerebral ischemia in symptomatic carotid stenosis, Veterans Affairs Cooperative Studies Program 309 Trialist Group, *JAMA* 266:3289–3294, 1991.
27. Rothwell PM, et al: Analysis of pooled data from the randomised controlled trials of endarterectomy for symptomatic carotid stenosis, *Lancet* 361:107–116, 2003.
28. Executive Committee for the Asymptomatic Carotid Atherosclerosis Study: Endarterectomy for asymptomatic carotid artery stenosis, *J Am Med Assoc.* 273:1421–1428, 1995.
29. Halliday A, et al: Prevention of disabling and fatal strokes by successful carotid endarterectomy in patients without recent neurological symptoms: randomised controlled trial, *Lancet* 363:1491–1502, 2004.
30. Rothwell PM, et al: Endarterectomy for symptomatic carotid stenosis in relation to clinical subgroups and timing of surgery, *Lancet* 363:915–924, 2004.
31. Lovett JK, et al: Very early risk of stroke after a first transient ischemic attack, *Stroke* 34:e138–e140, 2003.
32. Rothwell PM: Does transient ischemic attack deserve emergency care? *Nat Clin Pract Neurol* 2:174–175, 2006.
33. Brott G, et al: Stenting versus endarterectomy for treatment of carotid-artery stenosis, *N Engl J Med* 363:11–23, 2010.
34. Grant EG, et al: Carotid artery stenosis: Gray-scale and Doppler US diagnosis–Society of Radiologists in Ultrasound Consensus Conference, *Radiology* 229:340–346, 2003.
35. U-King-Im J, et al: Contrast-enhanced MR angiography vs intra-arterial digital subtraction angiography for carotid imaging: activity-based cost analysis, *Eur Radiol* 14:730–735, 2004.
36. Willinsky RA, et al: Neurologic complications of cerebral angiography: prospective analysis of 2,899 procedures and review of the literature, *Radiology* 227:522–528, 2003.
37. Rothwell PM, et al: Effect of urgent treatment of transient ischaemic attack and minor stroke on early recurrent stroke (EXPRESS study): a prospective population-based sequential comparison, *Lancet* 370:1432–1442, 2007.

38. Wardlaw JM, et al: Accurate, practical and cost-effective assessment of carotid stenosis in the UK, *Health Technol Assess* 10: 1–182, 2006.
39. Wardlaw JM, et al: Carotid artery imaging for secondary stroke prevention: both imaging modality and rapid access to imaging are important, *Stroke* 40(11):3511–3517, 2009 Nov. Epub 2009 Sep 3.
40. Lorenz MW, et al: Prediction of clinical cardiovascular events with carotid intima-media thickness: a systematic review and meta-analysis, *Circulation* 115(4):459–467, 2007 Jan 30. Epub 2007 Jan 22. Review.
41. Polak JF: Carotid intima-media thickness: An early marker of cardiovascular disease, *Ultrasound Q* 25(2):55–61, 2009 Jun.
42. Touboul PJ, et al: Mannheim carotid intima-media thickness consensus (2004-2006). An update on behalf of the Advisory Board of the 3rd and 4th Watching the Risk Symposium, 13th and 15th European Stroke Conferences, Mannheim, Germany, 2004, and Brussels, Belgium, 2006, *Cerebrovasc Dis* 23(1):75–80, 2007. Epub 2006 Nov 14.
43. O'Leary DH, Polak JF: Intima-media thickness: a tool for atherosclerosis imaging and event prediction, *Am J Cardiol* 90(10C):18L–21L, 2002 Nov 21. Review.
44. Johnson JM, et al: Natural history of asymptomatic carotid plaque, *Arch Surg* 120:1010–1012, 1985.
45. Spencer MP, Reid JM: Quantitation of carotid stenosis with continuous wave (C-W) Doppler ultrasound, *Stroke* 10:793–798, 1979.
46. Bendick PJ: Hemodynamics of arterial narrowing and occlusion, *J Vasc Tech* 18:235–240, 1994.
47. Alexandrov AV, et al: Correlation of peak systolic velocity and angiographic measurement of carotid stenosis revisited, *Stroke* 28:339–342, 1997.
48. Hunink MG, et al: Detection and quantification of carotid artery stenosis: Efficacy of various Doppler velocity parameters, *AJR Am J Roentgenol* 160(3):619–625, 1993 Mar.
49. Wardlaw JM, et al: Non-invasive imaging compared with intraarterial angiography in the diagnosis of symptomatic carotid stenosis: A meta-analysis, *Lancet* 367:1503–1512, 2006.
50. Demarco JK, Rutt BK, Clarke SE: Carotid plaque characterization by magnetic resonance imaging: review of the literature, *Top Magn Reson Imaging* 12:205–217, 2001.
51. Brant-Zawadzki MN, Chappell FM, Wardlaw JM: *Barking Up the Wrong Straw Man Radiology* 253:570, November 1, 2009.
52. U-King-Im JM, Young V, H Gillard J: Carotid-artery imaging in the diagnosis and management of patients at risk of stroke, *Lancet Neurol* 8(6):569–580, June 2009.
53. Spagnoli LG, et al: Extracranial thrombotically active carotid plaque as a risk factor for ischemic stroke, *JAMA* 292:1845–1852, 2004.
54. Redgrave JN, et al: Histological assessment of 526 symptomatic carotid plaques in relation to the nature and timing of ischemic symptoms: the Oxford Plaque Study, *Circulation* 113:2320–2328, 2006.
55. de Bray JM, et al: Reproducibility in ultrasonic characterization of carotid plaques, *Cerebrovasc Dis* 8:273–277, 1998.
56. Sabetai MM, et al: Reproducibility of computer-quantified carotid plaque echogenicity: can we overcome the subjectivity? *Stroke* 31:2189–2196, 2000.
57. Sztajzel R, et al: Stratified gray-scale median analysis and color mapping of the carotid plaque: correlation with endarterectomy specimen histology of 28 patients, *Stroke* 36:741–745, 2005.
58. Lal BK, et al: Noninvasive identification of the unstable carotid plaque, *Ann Vasc Surg* 20:167–174, 2006.
59. Kern R, et al: Characterization of carotid artery plaques using real-time compound B-mode ultrasound, *Stroke* 35:870–875, 2004.
60. Prabhakaran S, et al: Carotid plaque surface irregularity predicts ischemic stroke: the northern Manhattan study, *Stroke* 37:2696–2701, 2006.
61. Kitamura A, et al: Carotid intima-media thickness and plaque characteristics as a risk factor for stroke in Japanese elderly men, *Stroke* 35:2788–2794, 2004.
62. King A, Markus HS: Doppler embolic signals in cerebrovascular disease and prediction of stroke risk: a systematic review and meta-analysis, *Stroke* 40(12):3711–3717, 2009 Dec. Epub 2009 Oct 22. Review.
63. Aaslid R: Cerebral autoregulation and vasomotor reactivity, *Front Neurol Neurosci* 21:216–228, 2006. Review.
64. Rouleau PA, et al: Carotid artery tandem lesions: frequency of angiographic detection and consequences for endarterectomy, *AJNR Am J Neuroradiol* 20:621–625, 1999.
65. Day AL, Rhoton AL, Quisling RG: Resolving siphon stenosis following endarterectomy, *Stroke* 11:278–281, 1980.
66. Guppy KH, et al: Hemodynamics of in-tandem stenosis of the internal carotid artery: when is carotid endarterectomy indicated? *Surg Neurol* 54:145–152, 2000.
67. Roederer GO, et al: Post-endarterectomy carotid ultrasonic duplex scanning concordance with contrast angiography, *Ultrasound Med Biol* 9:73–78, 1983.
68. Robbin ML, et al: Carotid artery stents: early and intermediate follow-up with Doppler US, *Radiology* 205:749–756, 1997.
69. AbuRahma AF, et al: Carotid duplex velocity criteria revisited for the diagnosis of carotid in-stent restenosis, *Vascular* 15:119–125, 2007.
70. AbuRahma AF, et al: Optimal carotid duplex velocity criteria for defining the severity of carotid in-stent restenosis, *J Vasc Surg* 48:589–594, 2008.
71. AbuRahma AF, et al: Effect of contralateral severe stenosis or carotid occlusion on duplex criteria of ipsilateral stenoses: comparative study of various duplex parameters, *J Vasc Surg* 22:751–761, 1995.
72. Ferrer JM, et al: Use of ultrasound contrast in the diagnosis of carotid artery occlusion, *J Vasc Surg* 31:736–741, 2000.
73. Schneider PA, et al: Effect of internal carotid artery occlusion on intracranial hemodynamics. Transcranial Doppler evaluation and clinical correlation, *Stroke* 19:589–593, 1988.
74. Muller M, et al: Transcranial Doppler ultrasound in the evaluation of collateral blood flow in patients with internal carotid artery occlusion: correlation with cerebral angiography, *AJNR Am J Neuroradiol* 16:195–202, 1995.
75. AbuRahma AF, et al: The reliability of color duplex ultrasound in diagnosing total carotid artery occlusion, *Am J Surg* 174:185–187, 1997.
76. Kimura K, et al: Duplex carotid sonography in distinguishing acute unilateral atherothrombotic from cardioembolic carotid artery occlusion, *AJNR Am J Neuroradiol* 18:1447–1452, 1997 Sep.

77. Kimura K, et al: Oscillating thromboemboli within the extracranial internal carotid artery demonstrated by ultrasonography in patients with acute cardioembolic stroke, *Ultrasound Med Biol* 24:1121–1124, 1998.

78. Lee TH, et al: Carotid ultrasonographic findings in intracranial internal carotid artery occlusion, *Angiology* 44:607–613, 1993.

79. Sharma VK, et al: Thrombotic occlusion of the common carotid artery (CCA) in acute ischemic stroke treated with intravenous tissue plasminogen activator (TPA), *Eur J Neurol* 14:237–240, 2007.

80. Baumgartner RW, et al: Carotid dissection with and without ischemic events: local symptoms and cerebral artery findings, *Neurology* 57:827–832, 2001.

81. Beletsky V, Norris JW: Spontaneous dissection of the carotid and vertebral arteries, *N Engl J Med* 345:467, 2001.

82. De Bray JM, et al: Transcranial Doppler ultrasonic examination in vertebro-basilar circulatory pathology [in French], *Mal Vasc* 14:202–205, 1989.

83. Bartels E, Fuchs HH, Flugel KA: Duplex ultrasonography of vertebral arteries: examination, technique, normal values, and clinical applications, *Angiology* 43(3 Pt 1):169–180, 1992.

84. Bartels E: *Color-Coded Duplex Ultrasonography of the Cerebral Vessels* Stuttgart, 1999, Schattauer p.118.

85. Gosling RG, King DH: Arterial assessment by Doppler-shift ultrasound, *Proc R Soc Med* 67:447–449, 1974.

86. Pourcelot L: *Applications cliniques de l'examen Doppler transcutane. Les colloques de l'Institute national de la Sante et de la Recherche medicale*, 1974, INSERM. 213-240.

87. Michel E, Zernikow B: Gosling's pulsatility index revisited, *Ultrasound Med Biol* 24:597–599, 1998.

88. Qureshi AI, et al: Intracranial atherosclerotic disease: an update, *Ann Neurol* 66(6):730–738, 2009 Dec. Review.

89. Qureshi AI, et al: *J Neuroimaging. Consensus conference on intracranial atherosclerotic disease: rationale, methodology, and results* 19(Suppl 1):1S–10S, 2009 Oct.

90. Arenillas JF, et al: Progression and clinical recurrence of symptomatic middle cerebral artery stenosis: a long-term follow-up transcranial Doppler ultrasound study, *Stroke* 32:2898–2904, 2001.

91. Felberg RA, et al: Screening for intracranial stenosis with transcranial Doppler: the accuracy of mean flow velocity thresholds, *J Neuroimaging* 12:9–14, 2002.

92. Navarro JC, et al: The accuracy of transcranial Doppler in the diagnosis of middle cerebral artery stenosis, *Cerebrovasc Dis* 23:320–325, 2007.

93. Alexandrov AV: Transcranial Doppler sonography: principles, examination technique and normal values, *Vascular Ultrasound Today* 3:141–160, 1998.

94. Aaslid R: *Transcranial Doppler Sonography,* Wien, 1986, Springer Verlag, 39-59.

95. Chimowitz MI, et al: The Warfarin-Aspirin Symptomatic Intracranial Disease Study, *Neurology* 45:1488–1493, 1995.

96. Alexandrov AV, et al: Yield of transcranial Doppler in acute cerebral ischemia, *Stroke* 30:1604–1609, 1999.

97. Alexandrov AV, et al: Intracranial clot dissolution is associated with embolic signals on transcranial Doppler, *J Neuroimaging* 10:27–32, 2000.

98. Demchuk AM, et al: Specific transcranial Doppler flow findings related to the presence and site of arterial occlusion with transcranial Doppler, *Stroke* 31:140–146, 2000.

99. Tsivgoulis G, et al: Applications and advantages of power motion-mode Doppler in acute posterior circulation cerebral ischemia, *Stroke* 39:1197–1204, 2008.

100. Kimura K, et al: Evaluation of posterior cerebral artery flow velocity by transcranial color-coded real-time sonography, *Ultrasound Med Biol* 26:195–199, 2000.

101. Ringelstein EB: Ultrasonic diagnosis of the vertebro-basilar system. II. Transnuchal diagnosis of intracranial vertebrobasilar stenoses using a novel pulsed Doppler system [in German], *Ultraschall Med* 6:60–67, 1985.

102. Droste DW, et al: Echocontrast enhanced transcranial colour-coded duplex offers improved visualization of the vertebrobasilar system, *Acta Neurol Scand* 98:193–199, 1998.

103. Postert T, et al: Power-based versus conventional transcranial color-coded duplex sonography in the assessment of the vertebrobasilar-posterior system, *J Stroke Cerebrovasc Dis* 6:398–404, 1997.

104. Ribo M, et al: Detection of reversed basilar flow with power-motion Doppler after acute occlusion predicts favorable outcome, *Stroke* 35:79–82, 2004.

105. Baumgartner RW, Mattle HP, Schroth G: Assessment of >50% and <50% intracranial stenoses by transcranial color-coded duplex sonography, *Stroke* 30:87–92, 1999.

106. Stroke Outcomes and Neuroimaging of Intracranial Atherosclerosis (SONIA) Trial Investigators: Stroke Outcome and Neuroimaging of Intracranial Atherosclerosis (SONIA): design of a prospective, multicenter trial of diagnostic tests, *Neuroepidemiology* 23:23–32, 2004.

107. Oder B, et al: Hypoplasia, stenosis and other alterations of the vertebral artery: does impaired blood rheology manifest a hidden disease? *Acta Neurol Scand* 97:398–403, 1998.

108. Comparison of invasive and conservative strategies after treatment with intravenous tissue plasminogen activator in acute myocardial infarction: results of the thrombolysis in myocardial infarction (TIMI) phase II trial, The TIMI Study Group. *N Engl J Med* 320(10):618–627, 1989 Mar 9.

109. Tsivgoulis G, et al: Association of pretreatment ASPECTS scores with tPA-induced arterial recanalization in acute middle cerebral artery occlusion, *J Neuroimaging* 18:56, 2008.

110. Nedelmann M, et al: Consensus recommendations for transcranial color-coded duplex sonography for the assessment of intracranial arteries in clinical trials on acute stroke, *Stroke* 40(10):3238–3244, 2009 Oct. Epub 2009 Aug 6.

111. Bass A, et al: Comparison of transcranial and cervical continuous-wave Doppler in the evaluation of intracranial collateral circulation, *Stroke* 21:1584–1588, 1990.

112. Schneider PA, et al: Noninvasive assessment of cerebral collateral blood supply through the ophthalmic artery, *Stroke* 22:31–36, 1991.

113. Rutgers DR, et al: A longitudinal study of collateral flow patterns in the circle of Willis and the ophthalmic artery in patients with a symptomatic internal carotid artery occlusion, *Stroke* 31:1913–1920, 2000.

114. The National Institutes of Neurological Disorders and Stroke rt-PA Stroke Study Group: Tissue plasminogen activator for acute ischemic stroke, *N Engl J Med* 333:1581–1587, 1995.

115. Hacke W, et al: Thrombolysis with alteplase 3 to 4.5 hours after acute ischemic stroke, *N Engl J Med* 359:1317–1329, 2008.

116. The IMS: Study Investigators. Combined intravenous and intra-arterial recanalization for acute ischemic stroke: the interventional management of stroke study, *Stroke* 35:904–912, 2004.

117. Fieschi C, et al: Clinical and instrumental evaluation of patients with ischemic stroke within six hours, *J Neurol Sci* 91:311–322, 1989.

118. del Zoppo GJ, et al: Recombinant tissue plasminogen activator in acute thrombotic and embolic stroke, *Ann Neurol* 32:78–86, 1992.

119. Halsey JH Jr: Prognosis of acute hemiplegia estimated by transcranial Doppler ultrasonography, *Stroke* 19:648–649, 1988.

120. Zanette EM, et al: Comparison of cerebral angiography and transcranial Doppler sonography in acute stroke, *Stroke* 20:899–903, 1989.

121. Ringelstein EB, et al: Type and extent of hemispheric brain infarctions and clinical outcome in early and delayed middle cerebral artery recanalization, *Neurology* 42:289–298, 1992.

122. Alexandrov AV, Bladin CF, Norris JW: Intracranial blood flow velocities in acute ischemic stroke, *Stroke* 25:1378–1383, 1994.

123. Toni D, et al: Early spontaneous improvement and deterioration of ischemic stroke patients. A serial study with transcranial Doppler ultrasonography, *Stroke* 29:1144–1148, 1998.

124. Kaps M, Link A: Transcranial sonographic monitoring during thrombolytic therapy, *Am J Neuroradiol* 19:758–760, 1998.

125. Alexandrov AV, et al: The yield of transcranial Doppler in acute cerebral ischemia, *Stroke* 30:1605–1609, 1999.

126. Alexandrov AV, et al: Speed of intracranial clot lysis with intravenous TPA therapy: sonographic classification and short term improvement, *Circulation* 103:2897–2902, 2001.

127. Demchuk AM, et al: Thrombolysis in Brain Ischemia (TIBI) TCD flow grades predict clinical severity, early recovery and mortality in intravenous TPA treated patients, *Stroke* 32:89–93, 2001.

128. Demchuk AM, et al: Specific transcranial Doppler flow findings related to the presence and site of arterial occlusion with transcranial Doppler, *Stroke* 31:140–146, 2000.

129. Alexandrov AV, et al: Intracranial clot dissolution is associated with embolic signals on transcranial Doppler, *J Neuroimaging* 10:27–32, 2000.

130. Burgin WS, et al: Transcranial Doppler ultrasound criteria for recanalization after thrombolysis for middle cerebral artery stroke, *Stroke* 31:1128–1132, 2000.

131. Martínez-Sánchez P, et al: Update on ultrasound techniques for the diagnosis of cerebral ischemia, *Cerebrovasc Dis* 27(Suppl 1):9–18, 2009. Epub 2009 Apr 3. Review.

132. Hacke W, et al: Association of outcome with early stroke treatment: pooled analysis of ATLANTIS, ECASS, and NINDS rt-PA stroke trials, *Lancet* 363(9411):768–774, 2004 Mar 6.

133. Labiche LA, Malkoff M, Alexandrov AV: Residual flow signals predict complete recanalization in stroke patients treated with TPA, *J Neuroimaging* 13:28–33, 2003.

134. Alexandrov AV, et al: Ultrasound-enhanced systemic thrombolysis for acute ischemic stroke, *N Engl J Med* 351:2170–2178, 2004.

135. Saqqur M, et al: Site of arterial occlusion identified by transcranial Doppler (TCD) predicts the response to intravenous thrombolysis for stroke, *Stroke* 38:948–954, 2007.

136. Alexandrov AV, Grotta JC: Arterial re-occlusion in stroke patients treated with intravenous tissue plasminogen activator, *Neurology* 59:862–867, 2002.

137. Molina CA, et al: Predictors of early arterial reocclusion after tPA-induced recanalization, *Stroke* 35:250, 2004. [abstract].

138. Alexandrov AV, et al: High rate of complete recanalization and dramatic clinical recovery during TPA infusion when continuously monitored by 2 MHz transcranial Doppler monitoring, *Stroke* 31:610–614, 2000.

139. Christou I, et al: Timing of recanalization after TPA therapy determined by transcranial Doppler correlates with clinical recovery from ischemic stroke, *Stroke* 31:1812–1816, 2000.

140. Felberg RA, et al: Early dramatic recovery during IV-TPA infusion: clinical pattern and outcome in acute MCA stroke, *Stroke* 33:1301–1307, 2002.

141. Rha JH, Saver JL: The impact of recanalization on ischemic stroke outcome: a meta-analysis, *Stroke* 38:967–973, 2007.

142. Trubestein R, et al: Thrombolysis by ultrasound, *Clin Sci Mol Med* 51:697–698, 1976.

143. Tachibana K, Tachibana S: Ultrasonic vibration for boosting fibrinolytic effects of urokinase in vivo, *Thromb Haemost* 46:211, 1981. [abstract].

144. Lauer CG, et al: Effect of ultrasound on tissue-type plasminogen activator-induced thrombolysis, *Circulation* 86:1257–1264, 1992.

145. Blinc A, et al: Characterization of ultrasound-potentiated fibrinolysis in vitro, *Blood* 81:2636–2643, 1993.

146. Kimura M, et al: Evaluation of the thrombolytic effect of tissue-type plasminogen activator with ultrasound irradiation: in vitro experiment involving assay of the fibrin degradation products from the clot, *Biol Pharm Bull* 17:126–130, 1994.

147. Akiyama M, et al: Low-frequency ultrasound penetrates the cranium and enhances thrombolysis in vitro, *Neurosurgery* 43:828–832, 1998.

148. Suchkova V, et al: Enhancement of fibrinolysis with 40-kHz ultrasound, *Circulation* 98:1030–1035, 1998.

149. Behrens S, et al: Low-frequency, low-intensity ultrasound accelerates thrombolysis through the skull, *Ultrasound Med Biol* 25:269–273, 1999.

150. Spengos K, et al: Acceleration of thrombolysis with ultrasound through the cranium in a flow model, *Ultrasound Med Biol* 26(5):889–895, 2000 Jun.

151. Behrens S, et al: Transcranial ultrasound-improved thrombolysis: diagnostic vs therapeutic ultrasound, *Ultrasound Med Biol.* 27(12):1683–1689, 2001 Dec.

152. Daffertshofer M, Hennerici M: Ultrasound in the treatment of ischaemic stroke, *Lancet Neurol* 2:283–290, 2003.

153. Polak JF: Ultrasound energy and the dissolution of thrombus, *N Engl J Med* 351:2154–2155, 2004.

154. Alexandrov AV, et al: Ultrasound-enhanced systemic thrombolysis for acute ischemic stroke, *N Engl J Med* 351:2170–2178, 2004.

155. Alexandrov AV, et al: Ultrasound enhanced thrombolysis for acute ischemic stroke: phase I findings of the CLOTBUST trial, *J Neuroimaging* 14:113–117, 2004.

156. Molina CA, et al: Microbubble administration accelerates clot lysis during continuous 2-MHz ultrasound monitoring in stroke patients treated with intravenous tissue plasminogen activator, *Stroke* 37(2):425–429, 2006.

157. Larrue V, et al: Transcranial ultrasound combined with intravenous microbubbles and tissue plasminogen activator for acute ischemic stroke: a randomized controlled study, *Stroke* 38:472, 2007. [abstract].

158. Perren F, et al: Microbubble potentiated transcranial duplex ultrasound enhances IV thrombolysis in acute stroke, *J Thromb Thrombolysis* 25:219–223, 2008.

159. Rubiera M, et al: Do bubble characteristics affect recanalization in stroke patients treated with microbubble-enhanced sonothrombolysis? *Ultrasound Med Biol* 34:1573–1577, 2008.

160. Alexandrov AV, et al: A pilot randomized clinical safety study of sonothrombolysis augmentation with ultrasound-activated perflutren-lipid microspheres (μS) for acute ischemic stroke, *Stroke* 39:1464–1469, 2008.

161. Sharma VK, et al: Quantification of microspheres (μS) appearance in brain vessels: implications for residual flow velocity measurements, dose calculations and potential drug delivery, *Stroke* 39:1476–1481, 2008.

162. Tsivgoulis G, et al: Safety and efficacy of ultrasound-enhanced thrombolysis: a meta-analysis of randomized and non-randomized studies, *Stroke* 41:280–287, 2010.

163. Molina CA, et al: Transcranial ultrasound in clinical sonothrombolysis (TUCSON) trial, *Ann Neurol* 66:28–38, 2009.

164. Ribo M, et al: Intra-arterial administration of microbubbles and continuous 2-MHz ultrasound insonation to enhance intra-arterial thrombolysis, *J Neuroimaging* 20:224–227, 2010.

165. Adams RJ: Stroke prevention and treatment in sickle cell disease, *Arch Neurol* 58(4):565–568, 2001 Apr. Review.

166. Adams RJ: Big strokes in small persons, *Arch Neurol* 64(11):1567–1574, 2007 Nov. Review.

167. Bunn HF: Pathogenesis and treatment of sickle cell disease, *N Engl J Med* 337(11):762–769, 1997 Sep 11. Review.

168. Buchanan GR, et al: Sickle cell disease, *Hematology Am Soc Hematol Educ Program* 35–47, 2004. Review.

169. Steinberg MH: Sickle cell anemia, the first molecular disease: overview of molecular etiology, pathophysiology, and therapeutic approaches, *ScientificWorldJournal* 8:1295–1324, 2008 Dec 25. Review.

170. Adams RJ, et al: Cerebral infarction in sickle cell anemia: Mechanism based on CT and MRI, *Neurology* 38(7):1012–1017, 1988 Jul.

171. Pegelow CH, et al: Risk of recurrent stroke in patients with sickle cell disease treated with erythrocyte transfusions. *J Pediatr* 126(6):896–899, 1995 Jun.

172. Adams RJ, et al: Prevention of a first stroke by transfusions in children with sickle cell anemia and abnormal results on transcranial Doppler ultrasonography, *N Engl J Med* 339(1):5–11, 1998 Jul 2.

173. Adams RJ, Brambilla D: Optimizing Primary Stroke Prevention in Sickle Cell Anemia (STOP 2) Trial Investigators. Discontinuing prophylactic transfusions used to prevent stroke in sickle cell disease, *N Engl J Med* 353(26):2769–2778, 2005 Dec 29.

174. Adams RJ: TCD in sickle cell disease: an important and useful test, *Pediatr Radiol* 35(3):229–234, 2005 Mar. Epub 2005 Feb 10. Review.

175. Miller ST, et al: Silent infarction as a risk factor for overt stroke in children with sickle cell anemia: a report from the Cooperative Study of Sickle Cell Disease, *J Pediatr* 139(3):385–390, 2001 Sep.

176. Spencer MP, et al: Experiments on decompression bubbles in the circulation using ultrasonic and electromagnetic flowmeters, *J Occup Med* 11:238–244, 1969.

177. Padayachee TS, et al: Transcranial measurement of blood velocities in the basal cerebral arteries using pulsed Doppler ultrasound: a method of assessing the Circle of Willis, *Ultrasound Med Biol* 12:5–14, 1986.

178. Deverall PB, et al: Ultrasound detection of micro-emboli in the middle cerebral artery during cardiopulmonary bypass surgery, *Eur J Cardiothorac Surg* 2:256–260, 1988.

179. Spencer MP, et al: Detection of middle cerebral artery emboli during carotid endarterectomy using transcranial Doppler ultrasonography, *Stroke* 21:415–423, 1990.

180. Spencer MP: The detection of cerebral emboli using Doppler ultrasound: In Newell DW, Aaslid R, editors: *Transcranial Doppler*, New York, 1992, Raven Press, pp 52–58.

181. Ringelstein EB, et al: Consensus on microembolus detection by TCD. International Consensus Group on Microembolus Detection, *Stroke* 29:725–729, 1998.

182. Cullinane M, et al: Evaluation of new online automated embolic signal detection algorithm, including comparison with panel of international experts, *Stroke* 31:1335–1341, 2000.

183. The International Cerebral Hemodynamics Society Consensus Statement: *Stroke* 26:1123, 1995.

184. Saqqur M, et al: Improved detection of microbubble signals using power M-mode Doppler, *Stroke* 35:e14–e17, 2004.

185. Topcuoglu MA, Palacios IF, Buonanno FS: Contrast M-mode power Doppler ultrasound in the detection of right-to-left shunts: utility of submandibular internal carotid artery recording, *J Neuroimaging* 13:315–323, 2003.

186. Spencer MP, et al: Power M-mode transcranial Doppler for diagnosis of patent foramen ovale and assessing transcatheter closure, *J Neuroimaging* 14:342–349, 2004.

187. Lao AY, et al: Detection of Right-to-Left Shunts: Comparison between the International Consensus and Spencer Logarithmic Scale Criteria, *J Neuroimaging* 18:402–406, 2008.

188. Toole JF: *Cerebrovascular Disorders*, ed 4, New York, Raven Press.

189. Voigt K, Kendel K, Sauer M: Subclavian steal syndrome. Bloodless diagnosis of the syndrome using ultrasonic pulse echo and vertebral artery compression [in German], *Fortschr Neurol Psychiatr Grenzgeb* 38:20–33, 1970.

190. Reutern GM, Budingen HJ, Freund HJ: The diagnosis of obstructions of the vertebral and subclavian arteries by means of directional Doppler sonography [in German], *Arch Psychiatr Nervenkr* 222:209–222, 1976.

191. Yoneda S, et al: Subclavian steal in Takayasu's arteritis. A hemodynamic study by means of ultrasonic Doppler flowmetry, *Stroke* 8:264–268, 1977.

192. Pourcelot L, et al: Contribution of the Doppler examination to the diagnosis of subclavian steal syndrome [in French], *Rev Neurol (Paris)* 133:309–323, 1977.

193. Walker DW, Acker JD, Cole CA: Subclavian steal syndrome detected with duplex pulsed Doppler sonography, *AJNR Am J Neuroradiol* 3:615–618, 1982.

194. Ringelstein EB, Zeumer H: Delayed reversal of vertebral artery blood flow following percutaneous transluminal angioplasty for subclavian steal syndrome, *Neuroradiology* 26:189–198, 1984.

195. Ackerstaff RG, et al: Ultrasonic duplex scanning in atherosclerotic disease of the innominate, subclavian and vertebral arteries. A comparative study with angiography, *Ultrasound Med Biol* 10:409–418, 1984.

196. Pokrovskii AV, et al: Ultrasonic angiography in the diagnosis of lesions of the brachiocephalic branches of the aorta, *Kardiologiia* 25:82–86, 1985.

197. Kuperberg EB, IuL Grozovskii, Agadzhanova LP: Functional test of reactive hyperemia in the diagnosis of the vertebro-subclavian steal syndrome using ultrasonic dopplerography [in Russian], *Zh Nevropatol Psikhiatr Im S S Korsakova* 86:28–34, 1986.

198. Bornstein NM, Norris JW: Subclavian steal: A harmless haemodynamic phenomenon? *Lancet* 2:303–305, 1986.

199. Ackermann H, Diener HC, Dichgans J: Stenosis and occlusion of the subclavian artery: ultrasonographic and clinical findings, *J Neurol* 234:396–400, 1987.

200. Ackermann H, et al: Ultrasonographic follow-up of subclavian stenosis and occlusion: natural history and surgical treatment, *Stroke* 19:431–435, 1988.

201. Klingelhofer J, et al: Transcranial Doppler ultrasonography of carotid-basilar collateral circulation in subclavian steal, *Stroke* 19:1036–1042, 1988.

202. Bornstein NM, Krajewski A, Norris JW: Basilar artery blood flow in subclavian steal, *Can J Neurol Sci.* 15:417–419, 1988.

203. Lunev DK, et al: Cerebrovascular disorders in various types of the subclavian steal syndrome [in Russian], *Zh Nevropatol Psikhiatr Im S S Korsakova* 91:10–14, 1991.

204. Nicholls SC, Koutlas TC, Strandness DE: Clinical significance of retrograde flow in the vertebral artery, *Ann Vasc Surg* 5:331–336, 1991.

205. de Bray JM, et al: Effect of subclavian syndrome on the basilar artery, *Acta Neurol Scand* 90:174–178, 1994.

206. Markus HS, Harrison MJ: Estimation of cerebrovascular reactivity using transcranial Doppler, including the use of breath-holding as the vasodilatory stimulus, *Stroke* 23(5):668–673, 1992 May.

207. Ringelstein EB, Van Eyck S, Mertens I: Evaluation of cerebral vasomotor reactivity by various vasodilating stimuli: Comparison of CO2 to acetazolamide, *J Cereb Blood Flow Metab* 12(1):162–168, 1992 Jan.

208. Müller M, et al: Assessment of cerebral vasomotor reactivity by transcranial Doppler ultrasound and breath-holding. A comparison with acetazolamide as vasodilatory stimulus, *Stroke* 26(1):96–100, 1995 Jan.

209. Gur AY, Bornstein NM: TCD and the Diamox test for testing vasomotor reactivity: clinical significance, *Neurol Neurochir Pol* 35(Suppl. 3):51–56, 2001. Review.

210. Toni D, et al: Progressing neurological deficit secondary to acute ischemic stroke: a study on predictability, pathogenesis, and prognosis, *Arch Neurol* 52:670–675, 1995.

211. Dávalos A, et al: Neurological deterioration in acute ischemic stroke: potential predictors and associated factors in the European cooperative acute stroke study (ECASS) I, *Stroke* 30:2631–2636, 1999.

212. Grotta JC, et al: Clinical deterioration following improvement in the NINDS rt-PA Stroke Trial, *Stroke* 32:661–668, 2001.

213. Kasner SE, et al: Predictors of fatal brain edema in massive hemispheric ischemic stroke, *Stroke* 32:2117–2123, 2001.

214. Toni D, et al: Early spontaneous improvement and deterioration of ischemic stroke patients. A serial study with transcranial Doppler ultrasonography, *Stroke* 29:1144–1148, 1998.

215. Baracchini C, et al: The quest for early predictors of stroke evolution: Can TCD be a guiding light? *Stroke* 31:2942–2947, 2000.

216. Alexandrov AV, et al: Reversed Robin Hood syndrome in acute ischemic stroke patients, *Stroke* 38:3045–3048, 2007.

217. Tsivgoulis G, et al: Reversed Robin Hood syndrome: Correlation of neurological deterioration with intracerebral steal magnitude, *Stroke* 39:725, 2008. [Abstract].

218. Alexandrov AV, et al: Prevalence and risk factors associated with reversed Robin Hood syndrome in acute ischemic stroke, *Stroke* 40:2738–2742, 2009.

NORMAL CEREBROVASCULAR ANATOMY AND COLLATERAL PATHWAYS

6

JOSEPH F. POLAK, MD, MPH, and JOHN S. PELLERITO, MD, FACR, FSRU, FAIUM

The vascular system of the human brain differs significantly, both anatomically and physiologically, from other organs in the body. Although it accounts for only 2% of the body weight, the brain receives 15% of the cardiac output and consumes 20% of the body's oxygen supply in the basal state.[1]

Cerebral arteries are little influenced by sympathetic nerves, unlike other arteries, but they are markedly affected by chemical changes in the blood, especially changes in local carbon dioxide and oxygen levels.[2,3]

Obstructive lesions of the cerebrovascular system can produce a wide array of neurologic symptoms. Clinicians must attempt to identify the exact areas involved in the disease process; however, this is often made difficult by individual variability in the cerebral vasculature. Indeed, the extent of clinical symptoms is entirely dependent on the ability of the collateral circulation to maintain adequate cerebral perfusion. Therefore, understanding the normal and collateral anatomy and the mechanisms of cerebral blood flow is essential to the diagnosis of obstructive disease in the cerebrovascular system.

This chapter addresses the anatomic and physiologic principles that influence the investigation of the vascular supply to the brain. It is important to stress the significance of appreciating the hemodynamics of the brain. Individuals vary considerably in their ability to compensate for alterations in cerebral blood flow, and the clinician must be aware of the effect of collateral pathways on local delivery of blood supply and neurologic symptoms.

As new treatment modalities become available for both extracranial and intracranial pathologies, a basic appreciation of normal anatomy, congenital variations, and collateral vascular pathways is extremely important. Endovascular treatment with angioplasty and stenting are now being used frequently to treat intracranial atherosclerotic

disease, coiling for aneurysm disease, and thrombolysis for acute stroke. Implementation of these interventions requires an extensive knowledge of the extracranial and intracranial vascular anatomy.

VASCULAR ANATOMY

The brain is supplied directly by four vessels: the two internal carotid arteries and the two vertebral arteries. Any discussion of the cerebrovascular system must begin at the origins of these vessels, because obstructive disease, stenoses, ulcerative plaques, aneurysms, or anomalies anywhere in these arteries may produce a stroke or symptoms of vascular insufficiency.

The blood supply for the central nervous system[1,4,5] derives from the three great vessels arising from the aortic arch in the superior mediastinum—the brachiocephalic, the left common carotid, and the left subclavian arteries (Figure 6-1). The brachiocephalic artery travels upward, slightly posterior from the arch to the right of the neck for its 4- to 5-cm length, dividing into the right common carotid artery and the right subclavian artery at the upper border of the right sternoclavicular junction. The left common carotid artery ascends from the arch and passes beneath the left sternoclavicular joint. Neither common carotid has collateral branches, but each divides into the internal and external carotid arteries at the level of the upper border of the thyroid cartilage.

The internal carotids supply most of the anterior circulation to the cerebrum (Figure 6-2). In their cervical portion, the internal carotid arteries may be relatively straight or may take a tortuous course as they travel to the base of the skull. With the exception of very rare anomalies, there are no branches of the internal carotid arteries in the neck. As they proceed intracranially, the internal carotid arteries give rise to the caroticotympanic branches in the petrous bone, the

128

meningohypophyseal branches in the cavernous sinus region, and the ophthalmic arteries immediately distal to the cavernous sinus. Eight millimeters beyond the clinoid process, within the dura mater, the internal carotid arteries give rise to the posterior communicating arteries, which join with the posterior cerebral arteries. Further cephalad, the internal carotid arteries divide into the middle and anterior cerebral arteries and give rise posteriorly to the anterior choroidal arteries.

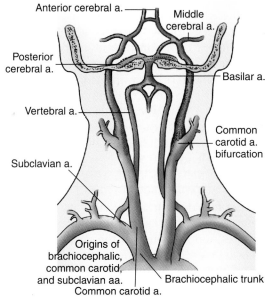

Anterior cerebral a.
Middle cerebral a.
Posterior cerebral a.
Basilar a.
Vertebral a.
Common carotid a. bifurcation
Subclavian a.
Origins of brachiocephalic, common carotid, and subclavian aa.
Common carotid a.
Brachiocephalic trunk

FIGURE 6-1 Extracranial cerebrovascular anatomy showing major arterial pathways to the brain. a., artery; aa., arteries.

The external carotid arteries normally supply no blood to the brain. However, several of their branches can become important collateral pathways if occlusion occurs in the internal carotid or vertebral arteries. The branches of the external carotid artery are the ascending pharyngeal, the superior thyroid, the lingual, the external maxillary, the occipital, the facial, the posterior auricular, the internal maxillary, the transverse facial, and the superficial temporal arteries. The external carotid branches most vital to collateral circulation are those in communication with the ophthalmic artery and those that interconnect between the muscular branches of the occipital and vertebral arteries (Figure 6-3).

The posterior circulation to the brain is supplied in large part by the vertebral arteries. They arise from the subclavian arteries. The vertebral arteries lie within the foramina transversarium of the upper cervical vertebrae and wind anteriorly into the subarachnoid space at the side of the medulla oblongata at the level of the atlanto-occipital interspace. They proceed cephalad and anteriorly until they reach the pontomedullary level, where they join to form the basilar artery. Four branches arise from the basilar artery as it courses upward before dividing into the posterior cerebral arteries. Branches of the basilar artery supply the entire pons and the superior and anterior aspects of the cerebellum. Branches of the vertebral arteries supply the medulla and the interior surface of the cerebellum.

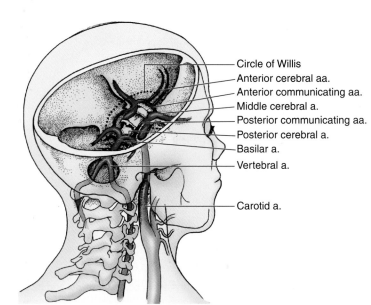

Circle of Willis
Anterior cerebral aa.
Anterior communicating aa.
Middle cerebral a.
Posterior communicating aa.
Posterior cerebral a.
Basilar a.
Vertebral a.
Carotid a.

FIGURE 6-2 Intracranial cerebrovascular anatomy showing anastomotic connections of the circle of Willis. Note that the principal blood supply to intracranial structures is through the carotid arteries. a., artery; aa., arteries.

The cerebral branches of the internal carotid and vertebral arteries are joined at the base of the brain by an arterial circle known as the circle of Willis, the most important element of the intracranial collateral circulation and also a common site of aneurysm formation. It is a hexagonal arrangement of arteries composed of the anterior, middle, and posterior cerebral arteries, which are joined together by the anterior and posterior communicating arteries (see Figure 6-2). Under normal circumstances, there is little mixing of blood through the communicating arteries. However, in instances of arterial occlusion of the carotid or vertebrobasilar arteries, this circle opens to function as a vital collateral pathway (see later).

Component arteries of the circle of Willis can vary greatly in size, and there are at least nine congenital variations in the structure of the circle (Figure 6-4). The most common anomalies involve the absence or hypoplasia of one or both communicating arteries. An anomalous origin of the posterior cerebral artery from one or both internal carotid arteries has also been commonly encountered. Anomalies in the anterior portion of the circle are less commonly found, although among these, absence or hypoplasia of the proximal segment of the anterior cerebral artery between the internal carotid and anterior communicating arteries is more common. The most

important variants in terms of decreasing collateral potential are those in which the anterior or posterior communicating arteries are absent or atretic. These conditions may isolate the anterior and posterior circulations or the left and right hemispheric carotid territories.

Normal arch formation is shown in Figure 6-5, A. Anomalous formations can occur in the extracranial circulation, most commonly involving the origins of the carotid and vertebral arteries. Most frequent is a sharing or close association between the origin of the brachiocephalic artery with the left common carotid artery, also called bovine arch, with two variants: less often (5%–7%), the left common carotid artery may arise from the brachiocephalic artery (Figure 6-5, B) or have a shared origin with the brachiocephalic artery, with a prevalence of approximately 20% (Figure 6-5, C). An anomalous origin of the left vertebral artery on the aortic arch between the left common carotid and subclavian arteries has a low prevalence of 0.5% to 1% (Figure 6-5, D). Rarely, the right subclavian artery may have an aberrant origin on the aortic arch. Other abnormalities may occur in the cervical region, such as agenesis of the internal carotid arteries, but these are rare. Abnormalities in the vertebral arteries are usually limited to variations in size between the left and right, referred to as vertebral artery dominance.

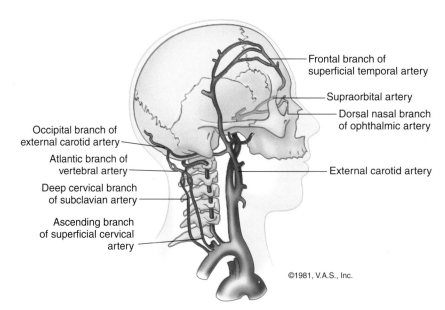

Occipital branch of external carotid artery

Atlantic branch of vertebral artery

Deep cervical branch of subclavian artery

Ascending branch of superficial cervical artery

Frontal branch of superficial temporal artery

Supraorbital artery

Dorsal nasal branch of ophthalmic artery

External carotid artery

©1981, V.A.S., Inc.

FIGURE 6-3 Extracranial cerebrovascular anatomy. Note the anastomotic connections between the external and internal carotid arteries and among the occipital, cervical, and vertebral arteries.

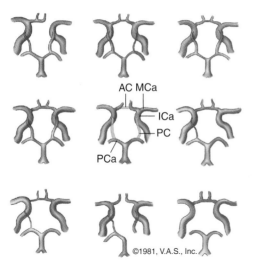

FIGURE 6-4 Nine of the possible configurations of the circle of Willis, the most important cerebrovascular collateral pathway. The center drawing depicts one configuration in which there is no communication between the anterior (AC) and posterior (PC) circulation due to atretic anterior and posterior communicating arteries. ICa, internal carotid artery; MCa, middle cerebral artery; PCa, posterior cerebral artery.

CEREBRAL HEMODYNAMICS

Before discussing the potential collateral pathways in the cerebrovascular system, it is best to explain the dynamics of cerebral blood flow[1,4] to help gain an appreciation of the importance of collateralization.

Despite the brain's large apportionment of the body's blood supply (15% of the cardiac output), there is little circulatory reserve because of the brain's high metabolic rate. Furthermore, the brain has no significant oxygen or glucose stores, making it entirely dependent on the vascular system for maintenance.[1,4] This is why even short episodes of interrupted cerebral flow can bring on symptoms of cerebral dysfunction, and cellular death can occur within 3 to 8 minutes of vascular failure.

Extrinsically, cerebral blood flow varies with the effective arterial perfusion pressure. Adequate perfusion relies on systemic blood pressure, cardiac output, and blood volume. Within the

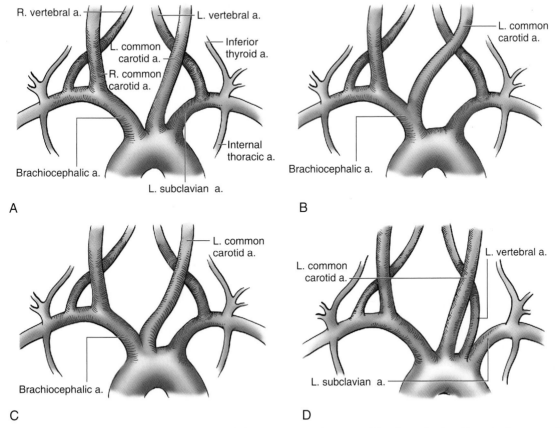

FIGURE 6-5 A, Normal arch configuration. **B,** Left common carotid artery arising from the brachiocephalic artery. **C,** Sharing or close association of the origin of the brachiocephalic artery with the left common carotid artery. **D,** Anomalous origin of the left vertebral artery on the aortic arch between the left common carotid and subclavian arteries. a., artery; L., left; R., right.

range of fluctuation possible for these extrinsic factors, blood flow can be modulated by a group of intrinsic factors that control cerebral vascular resistance. Among these factors are intracranial pressure, arterial oxygen tension, carbon dioxide tension, blood viscosity, and vascular tone. Although the cerebral vessels are supplied with nerves, there has been little evidence that they play a significant role in controlling blood flow. Oxygen and carbon dioxide concentrations play the greatest roles in modulating cerebrovascular resistance, with carbon dioxide being the more significant factor.[2,3]

Variations in cerebral blood gas concentrations serve to provide consistent blood flow within a wide range of systemic pressures and also provide local control to areas with varying demands.[3] For instance, if the brain requires more oxygen than is being supplied, it produces more carbon dioxide. This increase in carbon dioxide causes vasodilatation and increases blood flow until enough oxygen has been supplied to reduce the carbon dioxide concentration. This effect can happen either globally or locally.

Compensatory cerebral vasodilatation is also the mechanism that maintains cerebral blood flow when cerebral perfusion pressure drops as a person assumes an upright position. However, if the circulation is compromised by atherosclerotic disease, compensation may be insufficient, leading to symptoms of regional or diffuse hypoxia or anoxia.

COLLATERALIZATION

The vital role of collateral circulation in arterial occlusion has been appreciated for more than a century, but its involvement in cerebrovascular occlusive disease has become an increasingly important consideration as treatment of extracranial and intracranial pathologies has become more common. The advent of angiography[6-8] certainly improved our understanding of treatment options and, more recently, other diagnostic techniques such as duplex ultrasound, four-vessel selective arch intracranial angiography, magnetic resonance angiography, and computed tomographic angiography have all provided us with a better appreciation of the existence and importance of collateral pathways. Clinicians evaluating symptoms of cerebrovascular insufficiency or other pathologies must be aware of the extent of (or lack of) collateral circulation as they prepare

for modern interventional procedures. For example, when contemplating carotid stenting with embolic protection, one must consider the condition of the contralateral internal carotid artery and its contribution to the intracranial circulation (Figure 6-6). In the presence of contralateral internal carotid artery occlusion, the cerebral protection device most likely should be one that permits continued flow on the ipsilateral side during the procedure. Similarly, clamping of the carotid artery during endarterectomy will stop blood flow to the ipsilateral hemisphere if the circle of Willis is incomplete.

It was once believed that arteries in the brain were end arteries, but it is now known that capillary and precapillary anastomoses are common.[9] To appreciate these collateral pathways better, it should be noted that there are two types of arterial branches supplying the brain. The more important types in terms of neuronal function and nutrient supply for the central nervous system are the penetrating arteries. However, it is the diffuse circumferential or superficial arteries that spread over the entire surface of the cervical hemispheres, brain stem, and spinal cord through which collateral circulation takes place. The circle of Willis and the major arterial trunks are included in this superficial system.

The routes for intracranial collateral circulation can be divided into three categories: large interarterial connections, intracranial-extracranial anastomoses, and small interarterial communications. The major pathway is the circle of Willis, providing communication between the two carotid arteries or between the basilar artery and the right or left carotid artery. As described earlier, the anatomic variations possible within this arterial circle are normally of little importance unless occlusion in one of the cervical vessels occurs, demanding collateral blood flow.

Second only to the circle of Willis in importance are the complex intracranial-extracranial or prewillisian anastomoses. Perhaps the best-known prewillisian anastomosis is that between the external and internal carotid arteries, through the orbital and ophthalmic arteries. Other external-to-internal carotid collaterals include the meningohypophyseal and caroticotympanic branches. Additional important prewillisian anastomoses may be encountered clinically, including the following: (1) the occipital branch of the external carotid artery in communication with the atlantic branch of the vertebral artery; (2) the deep

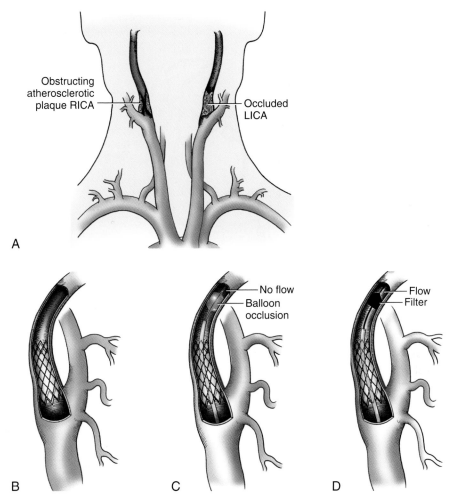

FIGURE 6-6 A, Obstructing atherosclerotic plaque in the right internal carotid artery and an occluded left internal carotid artery. **B**, Proposed treatment is internal carotid artery stenting with embolic protection. **C**, Balloon occlusive device eliminates flow. **D**, Filter device permits flow while trapping emboli and is probably a better choice in this case. LICA, left internal carotid artery; RICA, right internal carotid artery.

cervical and ascending cervical branches of the subclavian artery connecting with branches of the lower vertebral artery, the atlantic branch of the upper vertebral artery, and the occipital branch of the internal carotid artery; and (3) the external carotid arteries communicating across the midline. Also included in the prewillisian group is the rete mirabile or "wonderful net" of transdural anastomoses across the subdural space from the dural arteries to arteries on the surface of the brain.

Of lesser importance are the leptomeningeal collaterals forming the meningeal border zone network. These connect the terminal cortical branches of the main cerebral arteries across the border zones along each vascular territory. Although these are not major collateral pathways, they may be sufficiently developed to interfere

with the diagnosis of cerebrovascular insufficiency. Indeed, arterial occlusions may not become symptomatic because of adequate perfusion by the leptomeningeal anastomoses in the portion of the thrombosed artery's distribution. Similarly, excellent collateral flow around a thrombosed cortical vessel may induce rapid clearing of a neurologic deficit, leading the clinician to believe an extracranial occlusive process is involved.

It should be noted that there are no effective anastomotic pathways between neighboring cerebral artery branches, deep penetrating arteries, or the superficial and deep branches of the cerebral arteries.

The opening of collateral pathways is dependent largely on the age of the individual and the time sequence of occlusion. In older individuals, collateral pathways are more likely to be

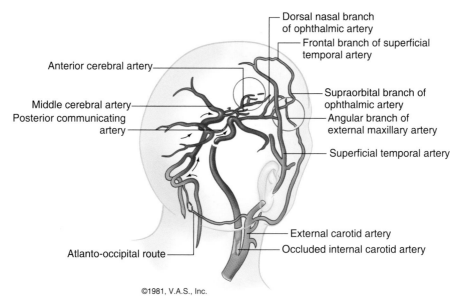

©1981, V.A.S., Inc.

FIGURE 6-7 Major external carotid and vertebral collateral pathways associated with internal carotid artery occlusion.

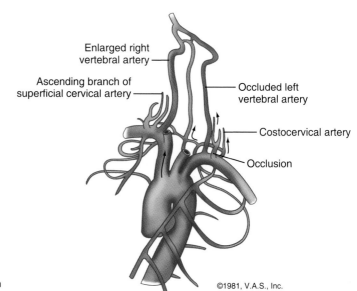

©1981, V.A.S., Inc.

FIGURE 6-8 Major collateral pathways in vertebral artery occlusion.

hypoplastic or involved in the atherosclerotic process. Even collateral vessels of sufficient luminal size are often not able to adapt rapidly enough to sudden occlusions, such as from embolism. Hence, collateral flow has a better chance of developing adequately in persons with slowly evolving atherosclerotic occlusions. When multiple atherosclerotic lesions are present, the adequacy of the collateral channels may be greatly lessened. Also affecting the adequacy of a collateral bed are the availability of multiple rather than single collateral sources and the pathologic conditions of the vessels, reducing their capacity for dilatation.

Extracranially, there are numerous cervicocranial collaterals. Occlusion of an internal carotid produces collateral circulation to the carotid siphon through the external carotid and ophthalmic arteries (Figure 6-7). The anterior and middle cerebral arteries in this case are also supplied from the opposite anterior cerebral artery and the posterior cerebral artery through the anterior and posterior communicating arteries. In the case of vertebral occlusion near its origin (Figure 6-8), flow is shunted to the thyrocervical and costocervical trunks, with compensatory enlargement of the opposite vertebral artery. Collateral circulation

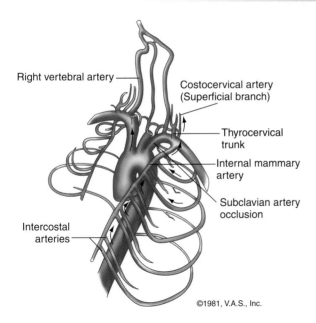

Right vertebral artery

Costocervical artery
(Superficial branch)

Thyrocervical
trunk

Internal mammary
artery

Subclavian artery
occlusion

Intercostal
arteries

©1981, V.A.S., Inc.

FIGURE 6-9 Major collateral pathways in proximal subclavian artery occlusion.

arising from occlusion of large branches of the aortic arch is through the intercostal and internal mammary arteries to the subclavian, and then through the branches of the thyrocervical and costocervical trunks to the vertebral and carotid arteries (Figure 6-9).

Historically, a number of procedures have been used to judge collateral flow. The simplest method of estimating intracranial collateral potential was a 5-minute common carotid compression test. Today, though, with the advent of angiography and magnetic resonance angiography techniques, such procedures are rarely used. The ability to actually visualize collateral flow in pathologic conditions and create a "road map" for interventional correction has changed diagnosis and treatment considerably.

CONCLUSIONS

The arterial system of the human brain, when afflicted by obstructive lesions, can produce a wide range of symptoms that are often nonspecific. The severity and character of these symptoms will vary as a function of basic arterial anatomy, variants of normal, and the arterial segment(s) affected by the obstructive lesion(s). The physician must also be cognizant of cerebral hemodynamics and the presence of the effect of collateral pathways on cerebral hemodynamics in order to appropriately interpret Doppler ultrasound findings and arrive at an accurate diagnosis. Modern treatments using endoluminal technologies have accentuated the need for a better understanding of vascular anatomy, its variations, and collateral pathways.

This chapter has presented a review of normal cerebrovascular anatomy and commonly encountered anomalies, with a discussion of hemodynamics and the development of collateral branches. Commonly encountered extracranial and intracranial collateral pathways have been reviewed while emphasizing their clinical significance.

REFERENCES

1. Stephens R, Stilwell D: *Arteries and veins of the human brain*, Springfield, IL, 1969, Charles C. Thomas.
2. Aaslid R: Cerebral autoregulation and vasomotor reactivity, *Front Neurol Neurosci* 21:216–228, 2006.
3. Madden JA: The effect of carbon dioxide on cerebral arteries, *Pharmacol Ther* 59:229–250, 1993.
4. McVay C: *Anson and McVay surgical anatomy*, Philadelphia, PA, 1984, WB Saunders.
5. Standring S: *Gray's anatomy, the anatomical basis of clinical practice*, Philadelphia, 2009, Churchill Livingstone, Elsevier.
6. Fields W, et al: *Collateral circulation of the brain*, Baltimore, 1965, Williams & Wilkins.
7. Henderson RD, et al: Angiographically defined collateral circulation and risk of stroke in patients with severe carotid artery stenosis. North American Symptomatic Carotid Endarterectomy trial (NASCET) group, *Stroke* 31:128–132, 2000.
8. Kim JJ, et al: Regional angiographic grading system for collateral flow: correlation with cerebral infarction in patients with middle cerebral artery occlusion, *Stroke* 35:1340–1344, 2004.
9. Van den Bergh R, Vander Eecken H: Anatomy and embryology of cerebral circulation. In Luyendijk W, editor: *Progress in Brain Research*, vol 30, Amsterdam, 1968, Elsevier, pp 1–26.

NORMAL FINDINGS AND TECHNICAL ASPECTS OF CAROTID SONOGRAPHY

7

JOSEPH F. POLAK, MD, MPH

ULTRASOUND APPEARANCE OF THE NORMAL CAROTID ARTERY WALLS

The wall of every artery is composed of three layers: intima, media, and adventitia. The innermost layer abutting the lumen is the *intima*, or endothelial lining of the artery. The middle layer is the *media*, which contains a preponderance of connective tissue (common carotid artery [CCA]) with an increasing proportion of smooth muscle cells (internal carotid artery [ICA]). This layer is responsible for most of the structural strength and stiffness of the artery. The outer layer is the *adventitia*, which is composed of connective tissue.

All three layers can be visualized on ultrasound images (Figure 7-1). The two transition zones between the lumen and the intima and between the media and adventitia produce two parallel echogenic lines, with an intervening zone of low echoes that corresponds to the media. The transition between media and adventitia also corresponds to the external elastic lamina as seen on pathologic studies. The thickness of the intima cannot be directly imaged from the ultrasound image since it typically measures 0.2 mm or less and is below the resolution of transcutaneous ultrasound.[1] What is seen is due to the reflection of the ultrasound beam at the lumen-intima interface. This is better appreciated on the far wall than for the near wall of the CCA.[2] There is a close correlation between histology and ultrasound-based measurements of the intima-media thickness.[1,3]

The intimal reflection should be straight, thin, and parallel to the adventitial layer. Significant undulation and thickening of the intima indicate more advanced changes due to atherosclerosis (see Chapter 8) or, rarely, fibromuscular hyperplasia. After endarterectomy, the lumen-intima interface is less prominent at the surgical site because the intima has been removed.

On transverse sections, clear visualization of the lumen-intima interface indicates that the image plane is perpendicular to the vessel axis. The lumen-intima interface is best seen on longitudinal images when the image plane passes through the center of the artery and the ultrasound beam forms a 90-degree incident angle with the wall interfaces (Figure 7-2; see Video 7-1).

The carotid bulb is a functional definition describing the widened portion of the distal CCA extending to the junction of the external and internal carotid arteries (the flow divider; Figure 7-3). The carotid sinus originates along the medial wall of the proximal ICA where it is adjacent to the external carotid artery (ECA). The carotid bulb spans the junction of the internal and external carotid arteries and blends into the dilatation of the sinus along the lateral aspect (opposite the flow divider) of the proximal ICA. The true ICA has parallel walls above (distal to) the sinus. The degree to which the carotid arteries widen at the carotid bulb varies from one individual to another. Usually the widening is slight, but some normal individuals have capacious carotid bulbs that may harbor large plaques in the absence of significant carotid stenosis. The CCA is an elastic artery, whereas the ICA is a muscular artery.[4] The region of the ICA sinus is of mixed characteristics between a muscular and an elastic artery.[5]

NORMAL BLOOD FLOW CHARACTERISTICS

In normal common carotid arteries that are relatively straight, blood flow is *laminar*, meaning that blood cells move in parallel lines with the central blood cells moving faster than the more peripheral blood cells. The distribution of blood flow velocity across the diameter of the artery follows a parabolic pattern (see Chapter 1) with slower

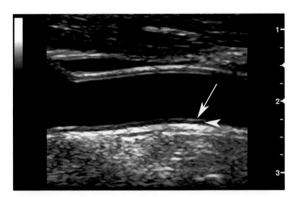

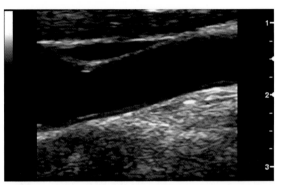

FIGURE 7-1 Normal arterial wall anatomy. This longitudinal image of the common carotid artery demonstrates a sharp line (specular reflection) that emanates from the intimal surface *(arrow)*. The black (relatively echolucent) region peripheral to this reflection represents the media of the artery *(arrowhead)*. The outermost echogenic (white) area is the adventitia of the artery. This blends into the also echogenic periadventitial region.

FIGURE 7-2 Off-axis view of the carotid wall. The angle between ultrasound beam and the walls of the common carotid artery are not perpendicular. This leads to a loss of the key lumen-intima interface.

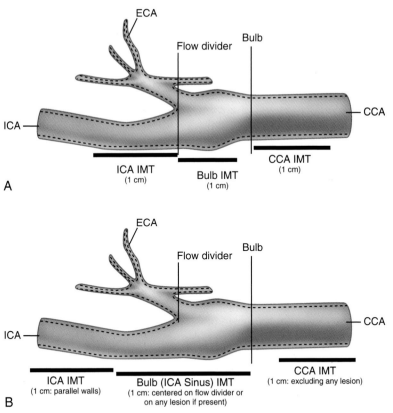

FIGURE 7-3 Anatomy of the carotid bifurcation; intima-media thickness (IMT) protocol. **A,** This diagram shows the key landmarks of the carotid artery bifurcation. The bulb is defined as being the zone of dilatation of the common carotid artery (CCA) to the level of the flow divider (the junction of internal carotid artery [ICA] and external carotid artery [ECA]). The flow divider is also the location of the carotid body and the adjacent nerve complex of the carotid sinus. The lines define the location where IMT measurements are made in one of the protocols used in epidemiologic studies. **B,** This diagram shows a more typical anatomic definition of the carotid bifurcation. The ICA is a muscular artery with parallel walls and lies just above the carotid artery sinus. The lateral wall of the carotid artery sinus (inferior wall on the diagram) is a transition between the elastic CCA and the muscular ICA.

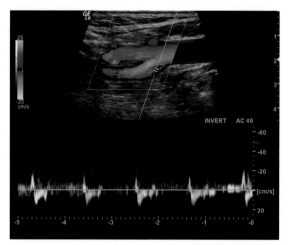

FIGURE 7-4 Long-axis view of the carotid bifurcation. The blue area in the carotid bulb and proximal internal carotid artery represents the normal flow reversal zone. The Doppler spectrum sampled at this site is shown at the bottom of the image and demonstrates the complex flow pattern with some red cells moving forward and others backward.

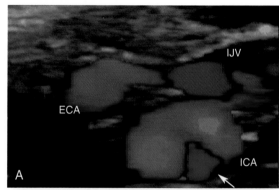

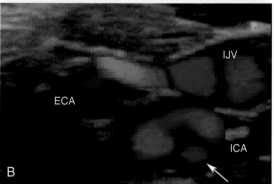

FIGURE 7-5 Flow reversal. **A,** This transverse video shows the zone of flow reversal (blue; *arrow*) in the proximal internal carotid artery (ICA) at peak systole. The ICA (located inferiorly and to the right) is typically larger than the external carotid artery (located to the left and upward; ECA). The structure above these two branches is a partly collapsed internal jugular vein (IJV). **B,** This transverse video shows the zone of flow reversal (blue; *arrow*) in the proximal ICA at end diastole. The ICA (located inferiorly and to the right) is typically larger than the ECA (located to the left and upward). The structure above these two branches is a partly collapsed IJV. Blood flow signals are not as strong as at peak systole.

velocities near the vessel wall and faster velocities near the center. Blood flow is not always laminar in nondiseased vessels since the artery segment has to be straight in order for the conditions of laminar flow to apply. Tortuous segments, kinks, or areas of branching disrupt the normal laminar flow pattern. The most noteworthy normal flow disturbance occurs at the carotid bifurcation (Figures 7-4 and 7-5; see Video 7-2), where a zone of blood flow reversal is established in the CCA bulb and proximal ICA.[6-8] The size of the zone of flow separation appears to be related to anatomic factors, including the diameter of the artery lumen and the angle between the ICA and the ECA.

The features of the common, external, and internal carotid spectral Doppler waveforms are distinct from each other, and changes in the Doppler tracings can offer clues as to the presence of occlusive disease. The pulsatile contour of Doppler waveforms can be used to distinguish the ICA and ECA. The ECA has a very pulsatile appearance during systole and early diastole that is due to reflected arterial waves from its branches. The ICA demonstrates less pulsatility. The CCA shares the appearance of both waveforms. The diastolic component of the waveform also shows typical differences with the ICA having the highest diastolic component, the external the lowest, and the CCA an appearance somewhere in the middle. These features are illustrated in Figure 7-6.

The normal range of velocities in the carotid branches varies as a function of age. The younger patient has higher blood flow velocities, likely a reflection of a higher cardiac output. ICA velocities decrease with age, reaching typical values between 60 and 90 cm/sec for ages 60 years and above.[9,10] Blood flow velocities vary with physiologic state of the individual, being higher with exercise than at rest. For this reason, the carotid examination should be conducted after the patient has been at rest for 5 to 10 minutes. Peak systolic velocities in the CCA tend to parallel the values in the ICAs. In addition, on average, the common carotid blood flow velocity in the low neck is 10 to 20 cm/sec higher than near the bifurcation.[11] This observation is of considerable importance, as the measured peak systolic

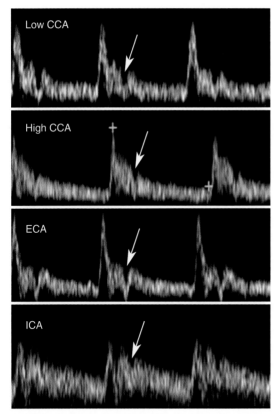

FIGURE 7-6 Normal carotid artery Doppler waveforms. *low CCA*: Waveforms in the very low common carotid artery (CCA) show some pulsatility due to the closeness of their origin or to the angle made as the carotid enters the neck. There is a moderate amount of blood flow throughout diastole. *high CCA*: Waveforms in the common carotid artery close to the bifurcation show moderately broad systolic peaks and a moderate amount of blood flow throughout diastole. *ECA*: External carotid artery (ECA) waveforms have sharp systolic peaks, pulsatility due to reflected waves from its branches, and relatively little flow in diastole as compared to the internal carotid artery (ICA). *ICA*: The ICA waveforms have broad systolic peaks and a large amount of flow throughout diastole. The *arrows* indicate the dicrotic notch, the transition from systole to diastole.

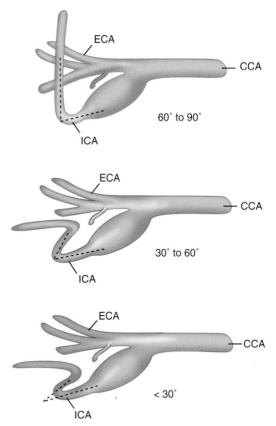

FIGURE 7-7 Coils and kinks. This diagram summarizes a classification system for different degrees of carotid artery coiling and kinking. Coils are considered a variant of normal that can lead to significant kinks over time due to aging and exposure to elevated blood pressure. CCA, common carotid artery; ECA, external carotid artery; ICA, internal carotid artery.

velocity ratio (ICA peak systolic velocity/CCA peak systolic velocity; see Chapter 9) will depend on the location where velocities are sampled in the CCA. The CCA peak systolic velocity should therefore be obtained before the beginning of the bulb, ideally 2 to 4 cm below. Since the ultrasound transducer typically measures 4 cm, it can be used to help locate this point by placing one end at the level of the bulb and sampling at the mid transducer, or approximately 2 cm below the beginning of the bulb. The mean peak systolic velocity in the ECA is reported as being 77 cm/sec in normal individuals, and the maximum velocity does not normally exceed 115 cm/sec. Considerable patient-to-patient variability occurs in ECA flow velocity in normal individuals because pulsatility varies considerably from one person to another since some individuals have a sharply spiked systolic peak, while others have a more blunted peak. As discussed in Chapter 3, the Doppler spectral waveforms are almost always altered in the region of the bulb (see Figure 7-4), a reflection of the complex flow dynamics that occur at this location.[6]

Peak systolic ICA velocities as high as 120 cm/sec have been reported in some normal adults, but these values are exceptional, and an ICA velocity exceeding 100 cm/sec should be viewed as potentially abnormal in older individuals. Elevated velocities can be seen in normal carotid arteries that diverge from a straight line and become curved. These elevated velocities are also associated with different degrees of coiling of the artery ultimately leading to kinking. Examples of a classification of carotid kinks[12] is shown in Figure 7-7. The sharp kinks (30 degrees or less) are likely to cause marked, and therefore pathologic, pressure drops (see Video 7-3). Blood flow velocities can therefore be artificially elevated as the blood flows into and out of the curved segment. Values up to 150 cm/sec

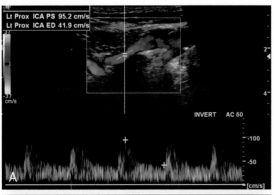

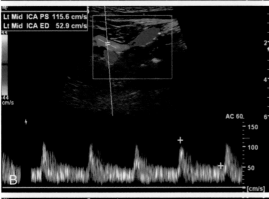

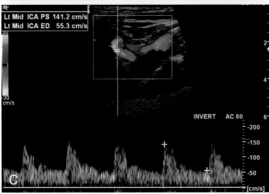

FIGURE 7-8 Elevated velocity in a coiling internal carotid artery. The Doppler waveform shows high velocities of 141 cm/sec simply due to the curvature of the internal carotid artery distally **(C)** but not in the proximal curve **(B)** with peak velocity of 116 cm/sec. Compare these values to the peak velocity of 95 cm/sec in the more proximal straight segment **(A)**. Peak systolic velocity values of up to 150 cm/sec can be seen and considered non-pathologic.

can be seen without a significant lesion being present (Figure 7-8). Carotid coils are likely due to genetic factors.[13] However, with time and exposure to elevated blood pressures, these artery segments may develop significant kinking requiring surgical intervention.[14,15]

In any situation where blood flow velocities are elevated, the sonographer should ask the following questions: (1) Is there a lesion in the carotid? (2) Is the vessel curved? (3) Is the cardiac output elevated? (4) Is there a technical error such as the angle correction is greater than 60 degrees or the angle correction is not in the direction of blood flow? The presence of an elevated blood pressure without an increased cardiac output should not significantly elevate the blood flow velocities in the carotid branches.

VESSEL IDENTITY

A key element of the examination is to correctly distinguish the internal from the external carotid artery. The ICA should be the larger of the two branches since it takes 70% to 80% of the net blood flow from the CCA. It is also typically located superficial to the ECA from a posterolateral imaging approach.[16] All of the findings listed in Table 7-1 are useful for distinguishing between the ICA and ECA. The ICA has a low-resistance flow pattern, whereas the ECA has a high-resistance pattern. If the identity of the carotid bifurcation branches is uncertain, moving the Doppler sample volume back and forth between the two branches helps distinguish internal from external carotid arteries. A transverse sweep of the bifurcation may also help distinguish these vessels. The ECA is the only one with branches, although these can be hard to visualize (Figure 7-9). Because of this, the greatest reliance is given to performing a "temporal tap" maneuver. The maneuver consists of placing a finger in front of the ear and feeling the pulse of the preauricular branch of the superficial temporal artery. The latter is a branch of the ECA. The operator then rapidly applies intermittent pressure on the artery. This rapid application of intermittent pressure alters the pressure in the external carotid system and results in easily seen oscillations on the Doppler tracing (Figure 7-10). The temporal tap maneuver has a slight effect on the ICA spectral tracing that decreases with distance from the bifurcation. In the ECA, the oscillations should increase in magnitude as one

TABLE 7-1 Features That Identify the External and Internal Carotid Arteries

Features	External Carotid Artery	Internal Carotid Artery
Size	Usually smaller of the two	Usually larger of the two
Branches	Always	Very rarely (case reports)
Orientation	Proceeds anteriorly toward the face	Proceeds deep and slightly posteriorly toward the mastoid
Doppler characteristics	High resistance	Low resistance
Response to temporal tap	Well-perceived oscillations	Poorly perceived to absent oscillations

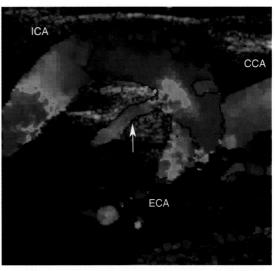

FIGURE 7-11 Anomalous internal carotid artery (ICA) branch. Branches from the cervical ICA are extremely rare *(arrow)*. Location varies, but it is normally within the first few centimeters from the origin of the artery. CCA, common carotid artery; ECA, external carotid artery.

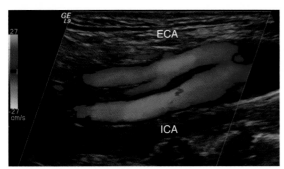

FIGURE 7-9 External carotid branch. This color Doppler image shows the external carotid artery (ECA) with its branches as compared to the internal carotid artery (ICA).

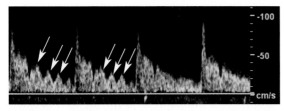

FIGURE 7-10 Temporal artery tapping identifies the external carotid artery. The sonographer rapidly pressed and released his or her finger on the location of the pre-auricular branch of the temporal artery. This "temporal tap" maneuver generates sharp deflections *(arrows)* on the external carotid artery waveform.

progresses away from the bifurcation. Differences in ECA and ICA pulsatility are also manifested in the color Doppler image (see Video 7-2). Blood flow is more consistent throughout the cardiac cycle in the ICA than in the ECA. As a result,

color intensity *varies less* from diastole to systole in the internal carotid whereas it appears to flicker in the external carotid. On occasion, ICA occlusions can cause hypertrophy of an external carotid branch that can mimic the appearance of an ICA. Use of the temporal tap will confirm that the vessel is part of the ECA system.

There are rare instances of branches arising from the ICA (Figure 7-11). The location of these branches can vary from near the bifurcation to a few centimeters above. Typically, they consist of ascending pharyngeal branches that anastomose with the ECA. They can maintain patency of the distal ICA when there is a proximal occlusion.[17,18]

EXAMINATION PROTOCOL

An examination protocol should be established within each vascular laboratory to ensure that carotid sonography is performed consistently, comprehensively, and accurately. The ultrasound protocols described here are generic. These techniques may be modified to match the needs of specific patients or vascular laboratories. In all cases, however, the protocol should meet or exceed the standards established by the *American Institute of Ultrasound in Medicine,** the*

---

*American Institute of Ultrasound in Medicine, 14750 Sweitzer Lane, Suite 100, Laurel, MD 20707; http://www.aium.org.

Intersocietal Commission for the Accreditation of Vascular Laboratories,[†] or the *American College of Radiology.*[‡]

INSTRUMENTATION

The carotid duplex examination should be performed only with appropriate instrumentation. The current standard of practice in the United States includes the following equipment: (1) high-frequency (5 MHz or above) transducers with short focal distances designed for near-field work; (2) color Doppler imaging; (3) duplex ultrasound with angle correction capabilities; and (4) Doppler spectral waveform analysis. Power Doppler imaging is recommended to assess low flow states and possible occlusions. Harmonic imaging is recommended to improve resolution and reduce artifacts.

PATIENT POSITION

We examine the carotid arteries with the patient in the supine position and with the examiner seated at the patient's head. This is the most ergonomically sensible position since the sonographer's elbow is supported. Exposure of the neck is achieved by having the patient drop the ipsilateral shoulder as far as possible and turning his or her head away from the side being examined. Do not hesitate to vary the position of the head and neck during the examination to facilitate visualization of the vessels. Be creative!

TRANSDUCER POSITION

Several transducer positions are used to examine the carotid arteries in long-axis (longitudinal) planes, as illustrated in Figure 7-12. Selective short-axis (transverse) views of the carotid arteries are obtained from an anterior, lateral, or posterolateral approach, depending on which best shows the vessels (see Figure 7-12, *A*). Generally, the posterolateral and far-posterolateral (see Figure 7-12, *B* and *C*) positions are most useful for showing the carotid bifurcation and the ICA, but,

in some cases, an anterolateral approach (see Figure 7-12, *D*) works best.

The *far* posterolateral approach often provides the best images of the distal reaches of the ICA. To use this view effectively, it is necessary to turn the patient's head far to the contralateral side and to place the transducer posterior to the sternocleidomastoid muscle (see Figure 7-12, *C*). Neophyte sonographers generally have difficulty imaging the ICA, because they fail to approach the vessel from a sufficiently posterior location. Varying these positions may also be helpful during the examination of very calcified vessels in order to find the flow stream.

CAROTID ARTERY VERSUS JUGULAR VEIN

The CCA lies immediately adjacent and deep to the internal jugular vein. The two are easily distinguished from each other. Blood flow in the carotid artery is toward the head and pulsatile, whereas blood flow in the jugular vein is toward the feet and has typical venous flow features (low velocity, undulating flow pattern, "windstorm" sound). The caliber of the carotid artery is fairly uniform, whereas the caliber of the jugular vein varies markedly from moment to moment, in response to respiration. Finally, the carotid arteries are thick walled, and a distinct intimal reflection is visible. The jugular vein wall is thin (invisible), and the vein collapses with slight pressure from the transducer.

IMAGE ORIENTATION

Consistent with internationally accepted conventions, we orient longitudinal images with the patient's head on the left side of the image. Likewise, transverse images generally are oriented as if viewed from the patient's feet, with the patient's right side on the left side of the image. Optional labeling of the structures is useful, especially on the transverse views.

RECORDING

Most studies consist of a set of static images taken at specific locations. Many ultrasound instruments can record short video clips, often in conjunction with digital picture archiving and communication systems (PACS). These clips are very helpful for illustrating dynamic features of the carotid

[†]Intersocietal Commission for the Accreditation of Vascular Laboratories, 6021 University Boulevard, Suite 500, Ellicott City, MD 21043; http://www.icavl.org.
[‡]American College of Radiology, 1891 Preston White Drive, Reston, VA 20191; http://www.acr.org.

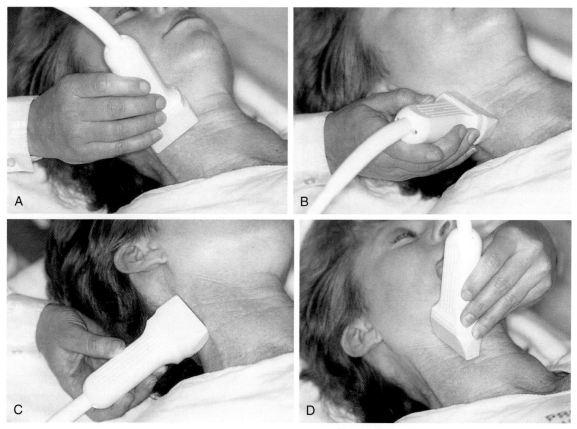

FIGURE 7-12 Transducer positions for duplex carotid ultrasound examination: **A,** This position is used to perform a transverse sweep from the clavicle to the angle of the jaw. **B,** The posterolateral projection is approximately 45 degrees from the horizontal and is a "default" position of the transducer. **C,** The far posterolateral is an ancillary projection that is occasionally used to visualize the distal internal carotid artery. **D,** The anterolateral projection can sometimes help visualization in patients with very thick necks.

examination. In Western nations, digital picture archiving computer systems are now in common use for recording ultrasound images. The use of film, transparency or emulsion, remains common, mostly due to financial issues.

The examination is conducted in a systematic fashion:

We start with the right carotid artery and then go to the left. All segments of the examination are recorded in sequence, beginning with the CCA and proceeding into the ICA and then the ECA. With this patterned approach, images are recorded in an orderly, predictable way, which greatly simplifies interpretation of the studies. The patterned recording approach, furthermore, reduces the potential for errors of omission and potential diagnostic errors.

Velocity data and sonographer notes can be stored on a worksheet that is filed permanently in the vascular laboratory. This is becoming less commonplace in a PACS environment since

blood flow velocity data (derived from spectrum analysis) can be recorded on a chart in the ultrasound device (Figure 7-13) with room for key notations concerning plaque location and severity. A dictated report is included in the hospital chart and is transmitted to the referring clinician.

THE EXAMINATION SEQUENCE

According to a generic protocol, a typical carotid examination follows these steps:

1. **Step 1.** *Get oriented!* The best way to do this is to place the transducer in a transverse plane and to slowly sweep the probe from the level of the clavicle upward to the jaw (see Figure 7-12, *A*). This can be done in a gray-scale mode and with color Doppler imaging. This scan is used to obtain an overall evaluation of carotid anatomy and to plan for possible additional interrogation at sites of obvious pathology.

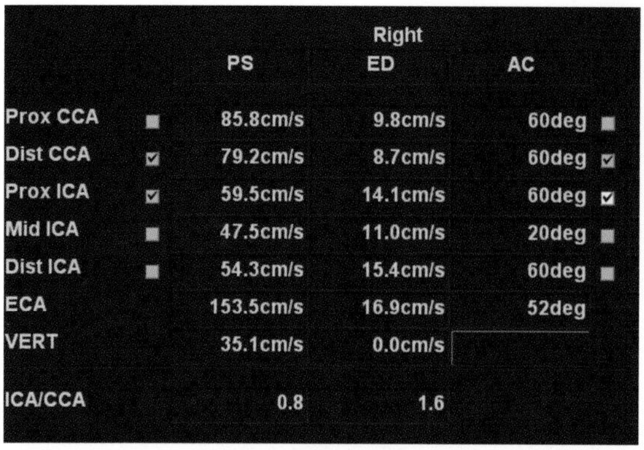

		Right		
	PS	**ED**	**AC**	
Prox CCA	▪	85.8cm/s	9.8cm/s	60deg ▪
Dist CCA	☑	79.2cm/s	8.7cm/s	60deg ☑
Prox ICA	☑	59.5cm/s	14.1cm/s	60deg ☑
Mid ICA	▪	47.5cm/s	11.0cm/s	20deg ▪
Dist ICA	▪	54.3cm/s	15.4cm/s	60deg ▪
ECA		153.5cm/s	16.9cm/s	52deg
VERT		35.1cm/s	0.0cm/s	
ICA/CCA		0.8	1.6	

FIGURE 7-13 Record of Doppler velocities. Example of a digital record of the Doppler velocities acquired at multiple levels during a carotid examination. Peak systolic (PS) and end-diastolic (ED) velocities are recorded, as well as the angle correction (AC).

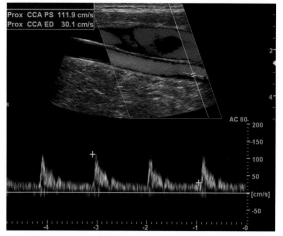

FIGURE 7-14 Proximal common carotid artery (CCA) velocity measurement. The CCA is clearly visualized; the Doppler sample volume is central in the artery and as low in the neck as possible.

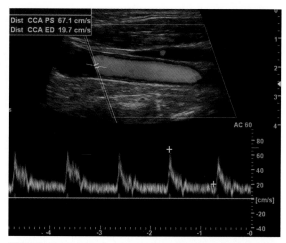

FIGURE 7-15 Distal common carotid artery (CCA) velocity measurement. The CCA is clearly visualized; the Doppler sample volume is central in the artery and below the carotid bulb. The Doppler sample might have to be obtained a bit lower in the CCA, by approximately 2 cm, if velocity ratios are going to be used to make a diagnostic decision.

2. **Step 2**. Choose the transducer position that best displays the carotid vessels in a longitudinal view. Generally, the posterolateral approach, as shown in Figure 7-12, *B,* is most advantageous.

3. **Step 3**. *Survey the common carotid artery with color Doppler imaging and record a velocity spectrum* from the CCA low in the neck (Figure 7-14). A recording site that is free of disease is preferred. Record a second waveform close to the bifurcation (Figure 7-15), and the following points should be noted: (1) the measurement point should be 2 to 4 cm below the carotid bulb (if using the peak systolic velocity ratio for diagnosis); (2) care should be taken that the sample

volume is squarely within the center of the vessel; and (3) the Doppler angle must be sufficient (60 degrees or less) to accurately measure the peak systolic velocity (see Chapter 3). These conditions are extremely important, as improper sampling of the CCA may artificially raise or lower the peak systolic velocity, in turn skewing the systolic velocity ratio used to estimate ICA narrowing (see Chapters 3 and 9). The result could be inaccurate diagnosis of clinically significant carotid narrowing. Many laboratories will also acquire an image in the mid CCA.

4. **Step 4**. *Survey the carotid bifurcation with color flow imaging, and repeat the process with transverse images.* The purpose of this survey is to confirm the patency of the arteries, to identify and localize plaque and associated flow abnormalities, and to define the junction of the ECA and ICA (so that plaque location can be determined correctly).

5. **Step 5**. *Confirm the identity of the ICA and ECA by their Doppler spectral signatures (see Figure 7-6), by anatomic features summarized in Table 7-1, and by performing the temporal tap maneuver (see Figure 7-10).* The proper identification of the branch vessels is essential since an ECA stenotic lesion is usually not subject to treatment, whereas significant ICA stenoses are usually treated. A color Doppler image of the proximal ECA and

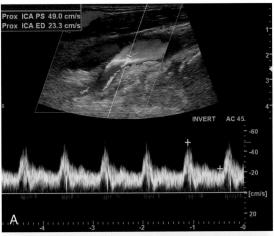

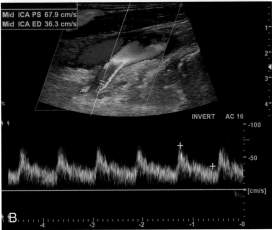

FIGURE 7-16 Internal carotid artery evaluation. **A,** The proximal internal carotid artery may have some distortion due to the proximity to the bifurcation and the carotid sinus. **B,** The more distal internal carotid artery has the more typical Doppler waveform appearance.

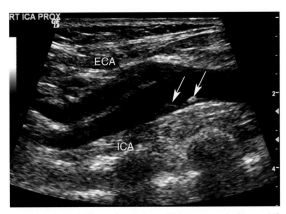

FIGURE 7-17 Bifurcation image. This gray-scale (B-mode) image shows the internal and external carotid arteries. It is useful for localizing plaque *(arrows).* ECA, external carotid artery; ICA, internal carotid artery.

The "tuning fork" view simultaneously shows both the ECA and the ICA (Figures 7-9 and 7-17) and is very useful for localizing plaque. Unfortunately, this view frequently cannot be achieved (because of an unfavorable orientation of the carotid bifurcation). An alternative is to tilt the transducer back and forth and identify the point where the internal and external carotid arteries originate.

7. **Step 7.** When a stenosis is present, *record angle-corrected velocity spectra in the stenosis* (as discussed in Chapter 3) and also obtain color Doppler images that illustrate the location and length of the stenosis, as well as the flow disturbances present in the prestenotic and poststenotic regions. If possible, confirm the degree of luminal narrowing on cross-sectional images. Video clips of the color flow and spectral components can provide dynamic information of value to the interpreting physician.

8. **Step 8.** *Evaluate vertebral artery flow,* as discussed in Chapter 11. Record a longitudinal image of the portion of each vertebral artery between the transverse processes of the vertebral bodies and representative Doppler spectral waveform, including measurement of the peak systolic velocity.

9. **Step 9.** *Assessment of subclavian artery blood flow,* to detect stenosis or occlusion of these vessels, is optionally done in many institutions. This examination is recommended when reversal of flow is noted in the vertebral artery to document the cause of "subclavian steal." Each subclavian artery is imaged in the long axis, from either a

ICA should be recorded. Duplex images of the proximal and distal ICA should be recorded (Figure 7-16). Many laboratories will also record a set of two or three longitudinal images along the course of the ICA.

6. **Step 6.** With the survey completed and the identity of the ICA and ECA confirmed, *scrutinize significant areas of plaque formation,* documenting the location and thickness of plaque, the degree of luminal reduction, and other plaque features (as discussed in subsequent chapters). Transverse images are used to subjectively assess plaque thickness and luminal narrowing. Gray-scale images often show plaque features better than color Doppler images because color may overwrite the gray-scale information.

supraclavicular approach or a transpectoral approach (see Chapter 15). This can be done at the beginning or the end of the ipsilateral carotid examination. A representative Doppler spectral waveform is recorded for each vessel. These waveforms should show a high-resistance flow pattern with a triphasic waveform. A low-resistance or damped pattern, and lack of pulsatility, suggest stenosis or occlusion proximal to the point of Doppler examination. In some cases, a subclavian stenosis may be visualized directly. In such instances, color Doppler images of the stenosis should be recorded, and Doppler spectral measurement should be obtained just proximal to, in, and distal to the stenosis, in the same manner as for carotid stenosis.

REFERENCES

1. Wong M, et al: Ultrasonic-pathological comparison of the human arterial wall. Verification of intima-media thickness, *Arterioscler Thromb* 13:482–486, 1993.
2. Wendelhag I, et al: Ultrasound measurement of wall thickness in the carotid artery: fundamental principles and description of a computerized analysing system, *Clinl Physiol* 11:565–577, 1991.
3. Pignoli P, et al: Intimal plus medial thickness of the arterial wall: a direct measurement with ultrasound imaging, *Circulation* 74:1399–1406, 1986.
4. Gomes CR, Chopard RP: A morphometric study of age-related changes in the elastic systems of the common carotid artery and internal carotid artery in humans, *Eur J Morphol* 41:131–137, 2003.
5. Meyerson SB, Hall JL, Hunt WE: Intramural neural elements in components of the carotid bifurcation. A histological basis for differential function, *J Neurosurg* 34:209–221, 1971.
6. Ku DN, et al: Pulsatile flow and atherosclerosis in the human carotid bifurcation. Positive correlation between plaque location and low oscillating shear stress, *Arteriosclerosis* 5:293–302, 1985.
7. Middleton WD, Foley WD, Lawson TL: Flow reversal in the normal carotid bifurcation: color Doppler flow imaging analysis, *Radiology* 167:207–210, 1988.
8. Polak JF, et al: Pulsed and color Doppler analysis of normal carotid bifurcation flow dynamics using an in-vitro model, *Angiology* 41:241–247, 1990.
9. Homma S, Sloop GD, Zieske AW: The effect of age and other atherosclerotic risk factors on carotid artery blood velocity in individuals ranging from young adults to centenarians, *Angiology* 60:637–643, 2009.
10. Zbornikova V, Lassvik C: Duplex scanning in presumably normal persons of different ages, *Ultrasound Med Biol* 12:371–378, 1986.
11. Meyer JI, et al: Common carotid artery: variability of Doppler US velocity measurements, *Radiology* 204:339–341, 1997.
12. Metz H, et al: Kinking of the internal carotid artery, *Lancet* 1:424–426, 1961.
13. Del Corso L, et al: Tortuosity, kinking, and coiling of the carotid artery: expression of atherosclerosis or aging? *Angiology* 49:361–371, 1998.
14. Koskas F, et al: Stenotic coiling and kinking of the internal carotid artery, *Ann Vasc Surg* 7:530–540, 1993.
15. Oliviero U, et al: Prospective evaluation of hypertensive patients with carotid kinking and coiling: an ultrasonographic 7-year study, *Angiology* 54:169–175, 2003.
16. Trigaux JP, Delchambre F, Van Beers B: Anatomical variations of the carotid bifurcation: implications for digital subtraction angiography and ultrasonography, *Br J Radiol* 63:181–185, 1990.
17. Littooy FN, et al: Anomalous branches of the cervical internal carotid artery: two cases of clinical importance, *J Vasc Surg* 8:634–637, 1988.
18. Bowen JC, et al: Anomalous branch of the internal carotid artery maintains patency distal to a complete occlusion diagnosed by duplex scan, *J Vasc Surg* 26:164–167, 1997.

ULTRASOUND ASSESSMENT OF CAROTID PLAQUE

8

EDWARD I. BLUTH, MD, FACR

The role of characterization of plaque as part of the duplex carotid examination is becoming more important as the significance and relationship of "vulnerable" plaque or unstable plaque relative to stroke become better understood. While the degree of stenosis, as defined by increased systolic and diastolic internal carotid artery (ICA) velocities and abnormal ICA/common carotid artery (CCA) ratios, is still of great importance, other parameters, particularly the character of carotid plaque, are beginning to be considered more significant when choosing the type and method of carotid intervention.[1-3]

Stroke, as a result of atherosclerotic disease, is the third leading cause of death in the United States. Approximately 20% to 30% of strokes are thought to be the result of ischemia from severe flow-limiting stenosis due to atherosclerotic disease involving the extracranial carotid arteries.[4] It is also estimated that 80% of strokes are thromboembolic in origin, with carotid plaque as the embolic source.[3]

Embolism, not flow-limiting stenosis, is the most common cause of transient ischemic attacks (TIAs). Fewer than half of patients with documented TIAs have hemodynamically significant stenoses. It is important to identify, therefore, atherosclerotic lesions that may contain hemorrhage or ulceration that can serve as a nidus for emboli that cause both TIAs and stroke and in particular, low-grade atherosclerotic lesions containing hemorrhage that might otherwise be ignored.[5] Polak and colleagues[6] have shown that plaque, particularly hypoechoic (heterogeneous) plaque, is an independent risk factor for developing a stroke. Of patients with hemispheric symptoms, 50% to 70% demonstrate hemorrhagic or ulcerated plaque. Significantly, plaque analysis of carotid endarterectomy specimens has implicated intraplaque hemorrhage as an important factor in the development of neurologic symptoms.[7-14]

Plaque characterization, performed appropriately, can be useful in determining which patients are at greatest risk for embolic stroke as a result of identifying "vulnerable" or unstable plaque.

EARLY PLAQUE DETECTION: INTIMA-MEDIA THICKENING

Atherosclerotic plaque is initially revealed sonographically by an increase in the combined thickness of the intima and media layers and subsequently by echogenic material that encroaches on the arterial lumen.[15-23]

Homma and colleagues[22] found that the normal intima-media thickness in the CCA—as measured in areas void of plaque—increases linearly with age, from a mean of 0.48 mm at age 40 years to 1.02 mm at age 100 years, following the formula (0.009 × age in years) + 0.116 mm. In addition to age-related change, intima-media thickness also increases in response to early plaque formation; thus, the intima-media measurement can be used in clinical settings as a marker for cardiovascular risk as well as in research.[17,19-21,23-27]

In literature reports, the intima-media thickness has been measured variously in the tubular and bulbous portions of the CCA and in the proximal ICA. Typically, longitudinal images are used that clearly depict the intimal reflection and the media. The cut points for intima-media thickness between normal and abnormal populations have varied among reported studies; therefore, it is difficult to establish a single cut point that defines abnormality. In addition, the age-related variance described previously must be considered. It is a reasonable assumption, however, that an intima-media thickness of 0.9 mm or more is abnormal and is likely to be associated with sonographically visible plaque. Please note that older studies tended to include areas of visible plaque in the measurements of intima-media thickness, which is no longer recommended: The intima-media thickness measurement should not include grossly visible plaque.

Thickening of the intima-media complex implies occult plaque formation, but plaque may, of course, be seen directly with ultrasound when it achieves sufficient size to protrude into the carotid artery lumen. Small carotid artery plaques are very commonly present in individuals older than 50 years,[20-22,25,27] and the prevalence of plaque increases with age to a high of 80% for men between 80 and 100 years old. (The prevalence is somewhat lower for women.) Because of their prevalence, the significance of small carotid plaques is uncertain. Large and potentially dangerous plaques are not common, with a reported incidence in large population-based studies of 2% or less for men and women 50 years and older.[20]

The interobserver variation for plaque detection ranges from fair to good among reported studies.[24-27,28] The causes of such variation include the technologists' skill level, ultrasound image quality, failure to examine the same vascular segment, lack of a uniform definition of findings indicating the presence of plaque, lack of careful technique and uniform accepted protocols for evaluating plaque, lack of combining both the sagittal and transverse images in assessing plaque characteristics, and inappropriately attempting to characterize plaque when using color and power imaging modes. With improvements in instrumentation and methods, interobserver variation may be expected to improve with time, but technical diligence and quality assurance methods are required to ensure accurate plaque detection and assessment.

METHODOLOGY OF PLAQUE CHARACTERIZATION

Plaque is evaluated most accurately with gray scale, without the use of color or Doppler imaging. The patient should be studied carefully to determine plaque location, extent, thickness, severity, and texture, as well as to assess luminal narrowing.[29] Plaque should always be studied, scanned, and evaluated in both the transverse and sagittal projections (Figure 8-1).[14,30] Both views are necessary because plaque is irregular and may not be completely included in the sagittal view. A properly obtained transverse view ensures that the full plaque is being studied and is therefore the most important view in gray-scale plaque assessment. In describing plaque extent, the observer should report the location and in which vessels the plaque is present (CCA and/or ICA) and the approximate length. Severity refers to the thickness of plaque and the degree of luminal narrowing. This is more difficult to define sonographically because plaque varies in thickness from one location to another. The best means for assessing carotid plaque thickness is

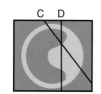

Transverse view of homogeneous plaque

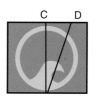

Transverse view of heterogeneous plaque

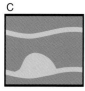

C

Sagittal view of homogeneous plaque

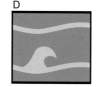

D

Sagittal view of homogeneous plaque falsely appearing as heterogeneous

A

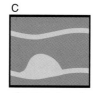

C

Sagittal view of heterogeneous plaque falsely appearing as homogeneous

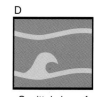

D

Sagittal view of heterogeneous plaque

B

FIGURE 8-1 Line diagrams showing the value of obtaining both transverse and sagittal images when characterizing plaque. In the sagittal plane, images can be obtained that would falsely simulate homogeneous plaque (**A;** *line C*) or heterogeneous plaque (**B,** *line D*). Correlation in both planes is necessary to be certain that the plaque is characterized correctly. *(From Bluth EI. Evaluation and characterization of carotid plaque. Semin Ultrasound CT MR18:57–65, 1997. Reprinted with permission.)*

from *transverse* (short-axis) images, which most accurately show the maximum thickness of the plaque and the resultant degree of luminal narrowing. Assessment of luminal narrowing or stenosis should always be performed in conjunction with pulsed Doppler velocity criteria. Plaque severity can be grossly overestimated or underestimated when using longitudinal images alone.

When reporting plaque severity, it is suggested to use generic terms, such as *minimal, moderate,* and *severe*. In evaluating texture, careful assessment must be made to estimate the degree of sonolucency within the plaque with gray-scale imaging. Most importantly, great care and effort must be taken to evaluate the plaque in the transverse as well as the sagittal projection. We have found it most useful to initially assess the plaque to determine the severity, so that we can correlate with the Doppler assessment that follows. Then, we employ the use of color, power, and Doppler spectral analysis to grade the degree of stenosis.

CHARACTERIZATION OF PLAQUE: HOMOGENEOUS OR HETEROGENEOUS

Two major methods are used to characterize plaque: the homogeneous-heterogeneous terminology[9,14,29-34] (Bluth classification) and the International Classification System.[7,35] The classification

systems use different terminology to describe plaque morphology. The International Classification System describes the plaque as either uniformly or predominately sonolucent (hypoechoic) or echogenic (hyperechoic). The Bluth classification utilizes heterogeneous as greater than 50% sonolucent (hypoechoic) and homogeneous to describe plaque that is greater than 50% echogenic (hyperechoic). The systems correlate to one another: a Bluth heterogeneous plaque corresponds to types 1 and 2 of the international system and a Bluth homogeneous plaque corresponds to types 3 and 4. Type 5 of the international system refers to plaque that cannot be classified because of calcifications or poor visualization (Table 8-1).

An important focus of these classification schemes is determining the degree of sonolucency within the visualized plaque. With international type 1 plaque, the appearance is uniformly and completely (90% or more) sonolucent. With type 2, the plaque is greater than 50% sonolucent but contains echogenic areas (Figure 8-2). The surface may be either smooth or irregular. International type 3 plaque has less than 50% sonolucency; in other words, primarily echogenic. Type 4 plaque is uniformly and completely echogenic. A Bluth homogeneous plaque is inclusive of all plaque that is less than 50% sonolucent and includes plaque that is uniformly echogenic but also contains plaque with some small sonolucent areas (Figure 8-3). The surface of the plaque is always

TABLE 8-1 **Plaque Classification Systems**			
	International		**Bluth**
TYPE 1	Uniformly sonolucent	Heterogeneous	Predominantly sonolucent (>50%)
TYPE 2	Predominantly sonolucent (>50%)	Heterogeneous*	>50% sonolucent <50% echogenic Calcification may be present
TYPE 3	Predominantly echogenic (>50%)	Homogeneous*	>50% echogenic <50% sonolucent Calcification may be present
TYPE 4	Uniformly echogenic	Homogeneous	Uniformly echogenic
TYPE 5†	Unclassified due to poor visualization; calcifications causing inadequate visualization	Report as unable to classify†	

Editor's note: The terms *heterogeneous* and *homogeneous* as used in the Bluth classification do not correspond to the common use of these terms. For most vascular laboratories, homogeneous represents an even echo pattern and heterogeneous a mixed echo pattern. For example, the international classification would then be reformulated as follows:
Type 1: Uniformly sonolucent or homogeneous (> 90% low echoes)
Type 2: Predominantly sonolucent (>50%) or heterogeneous (predominantly low echoes)
Type 3: Predominantly echogenic (>50%) or heterogeneous (predominantly high echoes)
Type 4: Uniformly echogenic or homogeneous (> 90% high echoes).
*Calcifications can be present, but plaque is classified in areas seen.
†For plaque partially visualized, classification should be performed on the basis of the region seen.

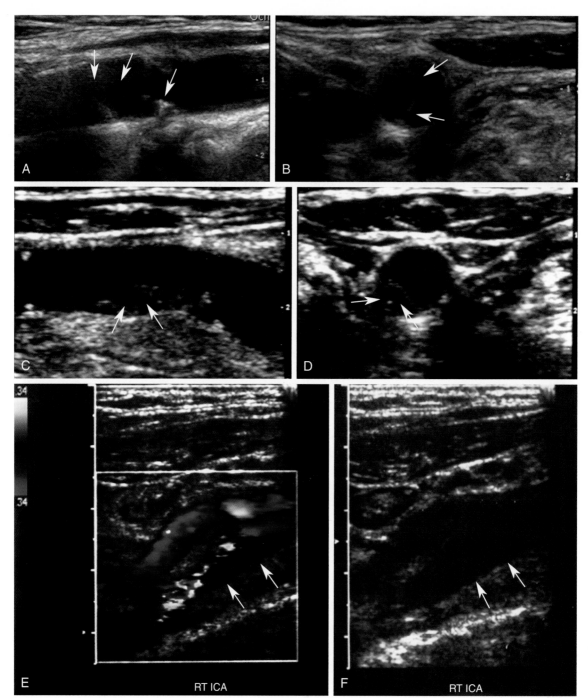

FIGURE 8-2 Heterogeneous plaque. Sagittal **(A)** and transverse **(B)** images of the internal carotid artery (ICA), showing almost completely sonolucent plaque *(arrows),* consistent with heterogeneous plaque (type 1). Note smooth plaque surface. Sagittal **(C)** and transverse **(D)** images of the ICA showing focal sonolucent areas *(arrows)* within the plaque greater than 50% of volume, corresponding to heterogeneous plaque (type 2). Note the irregular surface of the plaque. Sagittal **(E)** image of the ICA, showing heterogeneous sonolucent plaque *(arrows)* most evident on color flow duplex imaging by the small displaced residual lumen. The plaque is completely sonolucent (type 1) and indicative of acute hemorrhage. On the gray-scale image alone **(F),** plaque may be easily overlooked because of the degree of sono-lucency. However, the color flow Doppler images showing the displaced residual lumen enable the correct diagnosis.

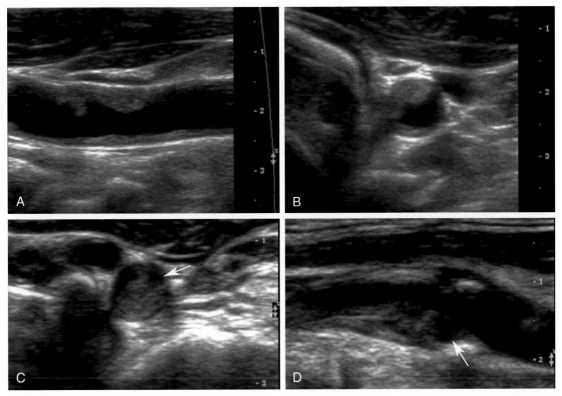

FIGURE 8-3 Homogenous plaque. Homogeneous plaque (type 4) in sagittal **(A)** and transverse **(B)** orientation. Note the uniform echo texture. Homogeneous plaque (type 3) in sagittal **(C)** and transverse **(D)** orientation. Note the focal hypoechoic area within the plaque *(arrow)* estimated to be less than 50% of plaque volume.

smooth. Calcifications can be seen in either of the plaque types and are not part of the classification scheme in determining heterogeneous or homogeneous plaque. Type 5 in the international system defines calcifications in the plaque that obscure proper assessment.

Plaque types 1 and 2, are believed to be associated with intraplaque hemorrhage and/or ulceration and are considered unstable, "vulnerable," and subject to abrupt increases in plaque size following hemorrhage or embolization.[30,31,33,36,37] Types 1 and 2 plaque are typically found in symptomatic patients with stenoses that are greater than 70% of diameter (see Figure 8-2). However, this type of plaque can also be seen in patients with a low degree of stenosis. Types 3 and 4 plaque are generally composed of fibrous tissue and/or calcification. These types of plaque are generally more benign, stable plaques that are common in asymptomatic individuals (see Figure 8-3). Echogenic (homogeneous) plaques are much more commonly identified than sonolucent (heterogeneous) plaques, occurring in 80% to 85% of patients examined.

Sonography has been shown in multiple studies to accurately determine the presence or absence of intraplaque hemorrhage (sensitivity, 90% to 94%; specificity, 75% to 88%).* Therefore, if examiners carefully follow the appropriate methodology and classification system, they can be confident in advising patients and referring physicians about the stability or potential "vulnerability" of the plaque identified. In centers where accuracy has been proven, plaque characterization is now being considered as a key component in determining therapeutic plans and interventions.

PLAQUE PATHOGENESIS

The exact pathophysiologic explanation and mechanism for the development and progression of carotid plaque are not completely understood. Some contend that atherosclerosis and plaque buildup are responses to injury that are mediated (or directed) by the endothelial cells that line the

*References 7,13,32,33,38,39.

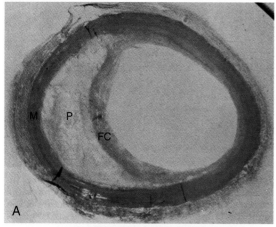

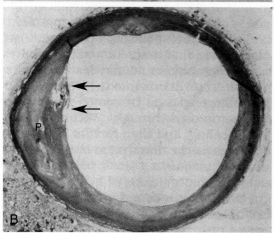

FIGURE 8-4 Plaque histology. **A,** Microscopic section of an uncomplicated plaque. The fibrous cap *(FC)* is intact, and the plaque contents *(P)* are homogeneous *(M,* media). **B,** Microscopic section of a complicated plaque. The fibrous cap is ruptured, and an area of cavitation is present *(arrows).* The plaque contents *(P)* are heterogeneous. *(From O'Leary D, Glagov S, Zarins C, et al. Carotid artery disease. In Rifkin MD, Charboneau JW, Laing FC, editors:* Ultrasound 1991: special course syllabus, *77th Scientific Assembly and Annual Meeting, Oak Park, IL, RSNA Publications, 1991, pp 189–200. Reproduced with the kind permission of Daniel O'Leary, MD.)*

arteries.[28,40-43] Three processes occur in the course of plaque formation. First, lipids from the blood accumulate in the subendothelium. Secondly, the lipid material is ingested by macrophages, forming foam cells, so named because of their foamy microscopic appearance. Finally, smooth muscle cells migrate from the muscular layer to the subendothelial layer and become transformed into fibroblasts. These form a collagenous (fibrous) matrix within the plaque and also form a fibrous cap on the luminal side of the plaque, below the intimal layer. Up to this point, the plaque structure is stable (Figure 8-4).

Recent evidence that inflammation plays an important pathogenic role in the evolution of plaque has been increasing.[1,40] Ongoing inflammation causes the breakdown of foam cells and other components of plaque and leads to the accumulation of inflammatory debris. The inflammatory process disrupts the structure of the plaque, weakens the fibrous cap, and extends to the intima. Histologic studies have also demonstrated that stable plaques are characterized by a chronic inflammatory infiltrate, whereas an active inflammatory process is noted at the surface and cap in vulnerable and ruptured plaques.[1,44] This active inflammatory process may cause disruption of the fibrous cap and the endothelium, which may directly cause embolization of material through the shedding of plaque contents into the bloodstream. Intraplaque hemorrhage appears to be associated with the breakdown of plaque and the disruption of the fibrous cap. Embolization is also caused by the adherence of platelets or thrombus to denuded plaque surface. This material is subsequently shed into the bloodstream and ultimately to the brain, where it may occlude cerebral arteries and cause ischemia or infarction.

In addition, the presence of adventitial vasa vasorum, intimal angiogenesis, and plaque neovascularization has been described and confirmed by histologic studies as another important predictor of instability in atheromatous lesions in cerebrovascular and cardiovascular patients.[1] Angiogenesis has been shown to be present regularly within atherosclerotic plaques, and atheroma vulnerability and symptomatic carotid disease have been associated with an increased number of microvessels that may be responsible for intraplaque hemorrhage when these small, newly generated, and vulnerable vessels rupture within the plaque.[1,45-47] As such, angiogenesis is thought to be an important cellular response to inflammation.

Evidence has also been uncovered in recent years suggesting that bacterial infection may play a role in plaque formation.[48-50] Perhaps in the future bacterial infection may be shown to cause the inflammatory angiogenesis response. Additional research into this concept is needed.

Central to current thinking about plaque evolution, however, is the concept that stable, uncomplicated plaque tends to be transformed into complicated and vulnerable plaque through acute and chronic inflammation and an injury process that includes plaque necrosis and hemorrhage.[40,43,51-54]

Furthermore, it appears that repeated cycles of injury and repair occur in many plaques. Hence, large plaques tend to be complicated histologically, whereas small plaques tend to be uncomplicated. However, as a result of inflammation and injury, plaque can change and become more complicated over time. Surveillance is therefore necessary. In the future, with continued research, the role of infection, inflammation, and mechanical disruption should emerge as factors affecting the development and stability of carotid plaque. At the present time, it appears that intraplaque hemorrhage and plaque necrosis may be identified by the sonolucent appearance within the plaque using standard high-resolution gray-scale imaging.

NEW METHODOLOGIES

Concerns about interobserver variability led to the development of less-subjective methods of plaque assessment, first reported by El Atrozy and associates[55] and subsequently refined by others.[56-61] These methods measure the sonographic or gray-scale density of plaque, which in turn is expressed either as a median gray-scale/density level, called the gray-scale median (GSM), for the entire plaque or as the difference between the highest and lowest values within a plaque. These methods provide an objective, measurable value that describes plaque echogenicity, eliminating the subjectivity of visual plaque assessment. Evidence demonstrates that interobserver variability is good to excellent with these techniques, especially when ultrasound instrument adjustment is standardized. Reports of excellent correlation of GSM and symptomatology also have been published. Reiter and colleagues[62] have developed a GSM level for echolucency of plaque after standardizing and adjusting the B-mode images. They obtained standardized GSM levels for asymptomatic patients with greater than 30% stenosis and identified that increasing echolucency (lower GSM) of carotid plaques over a 6- to 9-month interval is predictive of major cardiovascular events affecting coronary, peripheral, and cerebrovascular circulation. However, they found that absolute GSM levels were not associated with a specific risk.[48] The difficulty with this GSM method is the need for off-line computer equipment to analyze plaque gray-scale or optical density levels. Such assessment is time consuming, and the necessary equipment is currently available only in a research setting. It is likely, however, that in the future a measurement

package designed to evaluate plaque echogenicity could be incorporated into ultrasound instrumentation, facilitating clinical application.

Another new methodology used to assess and characterize plaque morphology is three-dimensional ultrasound. Seabra and Sanches[63] have described an algorithm based on graft cuts to improve the segmentation of potential foci of instability across the carotid plaque obtained from noiseless reconstructed volumes. They postulate that this methodology will make it easier to characterize plaque by computing local indicators obtained from noiseless reconstructed volumes containing the plaque.

Acoustic radiation force impulse imaging has recently been described as a new method to ascertain the vulnerability of a plaque to rupture.[64] This technique assesses the mechanical forces of plaque in excised vessels. Fibrous plaque and calcified regions were associated with very low displacements relative to the surrounding tissue, whereas relatively large displacements were observed in soft, lipid-filled regions. This methodology has the potential to add a new dimension to the characterization of plaque.

Both magnetic resonance imaging (MRI) and computed tomography (CT) have also been recently used to successfully and accurately characterize plaque and to grade stenosis.[65-70] Saba and colleagues[71,72] have recently shown good agreement in assessing homogeneous and heterogeneous plaque types (and the international system plaque types) between ultrasound echo-color Doppler and multidetector-row CT angiography.[71,72] However, they also reported poor agreement in the evaluation of plaque ulceration.[72] Recently, the ability to combine the complementary information provided by three-dimensional MRI and ultrasound carotid imaging via nonrigid registration techniques has been reported; this may lead to better carotid assessment.[73]

However, considering the increased cost of MRI and CT, the radiation associated with CT, and the greater accessibility of ultrasound instrumentation, ultrasound remains the most appropriate method for plaque characterization. However, in patients with extensive calcification obscuring visualization (type 5 plaque), which cannot be classified with ultrasound, perhaps MRI, CT, or a fused variant could be used. Enhancements in examination methodology and patient selection are areas that will receive continued study.

ULTRASOUND CONTRAST AND PLAQUE CHARACTERIZATION

Recently there has been interest in applying ultrasound contrast agents to plaque characterization. Ultrasound contrast has been used to better define plaque morphology, assess the margins and extent of plaque, and detect intraplaque angiogenesis.[1,47] In particular, contrast carotid ultrasound has been shown to identify adventitial vasa vasorum and plaque neovascularization. It has been suggested that these immature vessels leak toxic and inflammatory plasma components into the extracellular matrix of the media/intima. This increase in plasma volume reduces vessel wall oxygen diffusion, enhancing further angiogenesis and plaque inflammation, and ultimately plaque instability and rupture. Vicenzini and co-workers[1] have shown that microbubbles diffuse easily in the fibrous tissue of carotid plaques that histologically correspond to newly generated vessels, thus confirming that plaques undergo angiogenesis that could be related to progression and remodeling. Interestingly, the microbubble diffusion appears to have been oriented from the external adventitial layers toward the intimal lumen. Vicenzini postulates that this supports the theory that intraplaque hemorrhage and ulcerations can be related to the rupture of newly formed intraplaque microvessels, which, as they are immature and have a thin wall, are submitted to local triggering factors such as mechanical forces and shear stress. Owen and colleagues[47] have reported that symptomatic patients have greater plaque inflammation than asymptomatic patients, as demonstrated by the flow patterns after injected contrast. Thus, contrast could be useful not only to determine unstable or "vulnerable" plaque but also to follow nonsevere carotid stenosis with stable plaque to look for interval change, as well as to determine whether medical treatment is being effective in reducing angiogenesis or other inflammatory changes. Contrast ultrasound represents a new approach to better define plaque "vulnerability" and cerebrovascular risk (Figure 8-5). Further work in this area is required, representing a new opportunity to extend the usefulness of ultrasound.

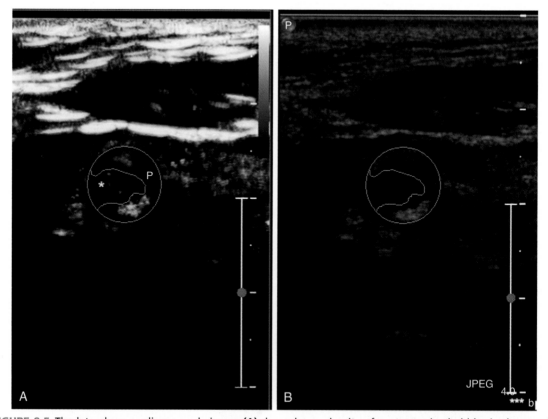

FIGURE 8-5 The late-phase nonlinear mode image **(A)** shows lower density of contrast microbubbles in the carotid lumen (*) compared with that inside the carotid plaque (P). Corresponding fundamental mode image **(B)** delineates the carotid plaque and lumen. *(Image courtesy of Professor Edward Leen and Dr. David Owen of Imperial College London, UK.)*

ULCERATION

Gray-scale ultrasound has been unsuccessful in consistently and reliably identifying ulcerated plaque.[36,72,74] However, virtually all ulcerated plaques that are accurately identified fit into the heterogeneous pattern and as such are recognized as potentially unstable.[14,30,36,75] Findings suggestive of plaque ulceration include a focal depression or break in the plaque that causes an irregular surface or an anechoic area within the plaque that extends to the plaque surface without an intervening echo between the vessel lumen and the anechoic plaque region. Recent studies also demonstrate that color and power Doppler ultrasound may improve sonographic identification of plaque ulceration. Color or power Doppler ultrasound or B-flow imaging (a proprietary non-Doppler imaging technique) may demonstrate slow-moving eddies of color within an anechoic region in plaque, which would suggest ulceration.[75] The demonstration of these flow vortices was 94% accurate in predicting ulcerative plaque at surgery in one study.[76] Saba and colleagues[72] reported sensitivity for identifying ulcerations of 37.5% for ultrasound compared to 93.75% for multidetector CT. However, preliminary studies suggest that the use of ultrasound contrast agents may improve the ability to identify plaque surface characteristics and thereby define ulcerations more accurately.[1] Further studies reporting the efficacy of ultrasound contrast in the identification of ulcerations are needed.

CONCLUSIONS

Carotid plaque characterization can be accurately performed with standard existing equipment by carefully optimizing the gray-scale parameters and studying plaque in the transverse as well as sagittal projections. Adhering carefully to either the homogeneous/heterogeneous or international classification systems is necessary. Special attention should be given to the degree of sonolucency within the plaque, best seen in the transverse images. The author prefers to use the homogeneous/heterogeneous terminology, but these two parameters can be split into four and the International Classification System used. Heterogeneous or types 1 and 2 plaque are potentially unstable and are "vulnerable," histologically correlating to plaque with intraplaque hemorrhage. When classified, plaque type should

be taken into consideration when choosing a therapeutic course of action. With the introduction of ultrasound contrast agents, a more accurate assessment of plaque stability or vulnerability may be possible. As a result, ultrasound will play an essential role in identifying those who are at risk for cerebrovascular events. At the present time, a carefully performed ultrasound gray-scale examination is a vital and integral component of duplex carotid ultrasound examination and should be performed on all those sent for evaluation of the extracranial carotid arteries.

REFERENCES

1. Vicenzini E, et al: Imaging of carotid plaque angiogenesis, *Cerebrovasc Dis* 27(Suppl 2):48–54, 2009.
2. Rothwell PM, et al: Carotid Endarterectomy Trialists' Collaboration. Analysis of pooled data from the randomised controlled trials of endarterectomy for symptomatic carotid stenosis, *Lancet* 361:107–116, 2003.
3. Fontenelle LJ, Simper SC, Hanson TL: Carotid duplex scan versus angiography in evaluation of carotid artery disease, *Am Surg* 60:864–868, 1994.
4. Endarterectomy for asymptomatic carotid artery stenosis: Executive Committee for the Asymptomatic Carotid Atherosclerosis Study, *JAMA* 273:1421–1428, 1995.
5. Carroll BA: Carotid sonography, *Radiology* 178:303–313, 1991.
6. Polak JF, et al: Hypoechoic plaque at US of the carotid artery: an independent risk factor for incident stroke in adults aged 65 years or older. Cardiovascular Health Study, *Radiology* 208:649–654, 1998. Erratum in: Radiology 209: 288–291, 1998.
7. Langsfeld M, Gray-Weale AC, Lusby RJ: The role of plaque morphology and diameter reduction in the development of new symptoms in asymptomatic carotid arteries, *J Vasc Surg* 9:548–557, 1989.
8. Leahy AL, et al: Duplex ultrasonography and selection of patients for carotid endarterectomy: plaque morphology or luminal narrowing? *J Vasc Surg* 8:558–562, 1988.
9. Reilly LM, et al: Carotid plaque histology using real-time ultrasonography. Clinical and therapeutic implications, *Am J Surg* 146:188–193, 1983.
10. Persson AV, Robichaux WT, Silverman M: The natural history of carotid plaque development, *Arch Surg* 118:1048–1052, 1983.
11. Lusby RJ, et al: Carotid plaque hemorrhage. Its role in production of cerebral ischemia, *Arch Surg* 117:1479–1488, 1982.
12. Edwards JH, et al: Atherosclerotic subintimal hematoma of the carotid artery, *Radiology* 133:123–129, 1979.
13. Imparato AM, Riles TS, Gorstein F: The carotid bifurcation plaque: pathologic findings associated with cerebral ischemia, *Stroke* 10:238–245, 1979.
14. Bluth E, Carroll B: The extracranial cerebral vessels. In Rumack CM, Wilson SR, Charboneau JW, et al, editors: *Diagnostic Ultrasound*, ed 4, St. Louis, MO, 2011, Elsevier.
15. Streifler JY, Benavente OR, Fox AJ: The accuracy of angiographic detection of carotid plaque ulceration: results from the NASCET study [abstract], *Stroke* 22:149, 1991.

16. Pignoli P, et al: Intimal plus medial thickness of the arterial wall: a direct measurement with ultrasound imaging, *Circulation* 6:1399–1406, 1986.

17. Poli A, et al: Ultrasonographic measurement of the common carotid artery wall thickness in hypercholesterolemic patients. a new model for the quantitation and follow-up of preclinical atherosclerosis in living human subjects, *Atherosclerosis* 70:253–261, 1988.

18. Riley WA, et al: Reproducibility of noninvasive ultrasonic measurement of carotid atherosclerosis: the asymptomatic carotid artery plaque study, *Stroke* 23:1062–1068, 1992.

19. Bond MG, et al: Detection and monitoring of asymptomatic atherosclerosis in clinical trials, *Am J Med* 86:33–36, 1989.

20. Ebrahim S, et al: Carotid plaque, intima media thickness, cardiovascular risk factors, and prevalent cardiovascular disease in men and women: The British Regional Heart Study, *Stroke* 30:841–850, 1999.

21. Sun Y, et al: Carotid atherosclerosis, intima media thickness and risk factors—an analysis of 1781 asymptomatic subjects in Taiwan, *Atherosclerosis* 164:89–94, 2002. Erratum in: Atherosclerosis 176:205, 2004.

22. Homma S, et al: Carotid plaque and intima-media thickness assessed by B-mode ultrasonography in subjects ranging from young adults to centenarians, *Stroke* 32:830–835, 2001.

23. Sakaguchi M, et al: Equivalence of plaque score and intima-media thickness of carotid ultrasonography for predicting severe coronary artery lesion, *Ultrasound Med Biol* 29:367–371, 2003.

24. Li R, et al: Reproducibility of extracranial carotid atherosclerotic lesions assessed by B-mode ultrasound: the atherosclerosis risk in communities study, *Ultrasound Med Biol* 22:791–799, 1996. Erratum in: Ultrasound Med Biol 23:797, 1997.

25. Salonen R, et al: Prevalence of carotid atherosclerosis and serum cholesterol levels in eastern Finland, *Arteriosclerosis* 8:788–792, 1988.

26. Sutton-Tyrrell K, et al: Measurement variability in duplex scan assessment of carotid atherosclerosis, *Stroke* 23:215–220, 1992.

27. Prati P, et al: Prevalence and determinants of carotid atherosclerosis in a general population, *Stroke* 23:1705–1711, 1992.

28. Gibbons GH, Dzau VJ: The emerging concept of vascular remodeling, *N Engl J Med* 330:1431–1438, 1994.

29. Bluth EI, et al: Carotid duplex sonography: a multicenter recommendation for standardized imaging and Doppler criteria, *Radiographics* 8:487–506, 1988.

30. Bluth EI: Evaluation and characterization of carotid plaque, *Semin Ultrasound CT MR* 18:57–65, 1997.

31. Merritt CR, Bluth EI: The future of carotid sonography, *AJR Am J Roentgenol* 158:37–39, 1992.

32. Bluth EI, Kay D, Merritt CR, et al: Sonographic characterization of carotid plaque: detection of hemorrhage, *AJR Am J Roentgenol* 146:1061–1065, 1986.

33. Merritt CRB, Bluth EI: Ultrasonographic characterization of carotid plaque. In Labs KH, editor: *Diagnostic Vascular Ultrasound*, London, 1991, Hodder & Stoughton.

34. Bluth EI: B-mode evaluation and characterization of carotid plaque. In Tegeler CH, Babikian VL, Gomez CR, editors: *Neurosonology*, St. Louis, MO, 1996, Mosby-Year Book, pp 62–67.

35. Geroulakos G, et al: Characterization of symptomatic and asymptomatic carotid plaques using high-resolution real-time ultrasonography, *Br J Surg* 80:1274–1277, 1993.

36. Bluth EI: Extracranial carotid arteries: Intraplaque hemorrhage and surface ulceration, *Minerva Cardioangiol* 46:81–85, 1998.

37. Bluth EI: Plaque morphology as a risk factor for stroke, *JAMA* 284:177, 2000.

38. Sterpetti AV, et al: Ultrasonographic features of carotid plaque and the risk of subsequent neurologic deficits, *Surgery* 104:652–660, 1988.

39. Weinberger J, et al: Atherosclerotic plaque at the carotid artery bifurcation. Correlation of ultrasonographic imaging with morphology, *J Ultrasound Med* 6:363–366, 1987.

40. Libby P: Atherosclerosis: The new view, *Sci Am* 286:46–55, 2002.

41. Ross R, Glomset JA: The pathogenesis of atherosclerosis (first of two parts), *N Engl J Med* 295:369–377, 1976.

42. Ross R, Glomset JA: The pathogenesis of atherosclerosis (second of two parts), *N Engl J Med* 295:420–425, 1976.

43. O'Leary D, et al: Carotid artery disease. In Rifkin MD, Charboneau JW, Laing FC, editors: *Ultrasound 1991: Special Course Syllabus, 77th Scientific Assembly and Annual Meeting*, Oak Park, IL, 1991, RSNA Publications, pp 189–200.

44. Spagnoli LG, et al: Extracranial thrombotically active carotid plaque as a risk factor for ischemic stroke, *JAMA* 292:1845–1852, 2004.

45. Mofidi R, et al: Association between plaque instability, angiogenesis and symptomatic carotid occlusive disease, *Br J Surg* 88:945–950, 2001.

46. Fleiner M, et al: Arterial neovascularization and inflammation in vulnerable patients: early and late signs of symptomatic atherosclerosis, *Circulation* 110:2843–2850, 2004.

47. Owen D, et al: The use of contrast-enhanced ultrasound to detect inflammation with the carotid atherosclerotic plaque in humans. RSNA Annual Meeting December 2, 2009. Chicago, IL.

48. Neureiter D, Heuschmann P, Stintzing S, et al: Detection of *Chlamydia pneumoniae* but not of *Helicobacter pylori* in symptomatic atherosclerotic carotids associated with enhanced serum antibodies, inflammation and apoptosis rate, *Atherosclerosis* 168:153–162, 2003.

49. Ezzahiri R, et al: *Chlamydia pneumoniae* infection induces an unstable atherosclerotic plaque phenotype in LDL-receptor, ApoE double knockout mice, *Eur J Vasc Endovasc Surg* 26:88–95, 2003.

50. Sessa R, et al: *Chlamydia pneumoniae* DNA in patients with symptomatic carotid atherosclerotic disease, *J Vasc Surg* 37:1027–1031, 2003.

51. O'Donnell TF Jr, et al: Correlation of B-mode ultrasound imaging and arteriography with pathologic findings at carotid endarterectomy, *Arch Surg* 120:443–449, 1985.

52. Lusby RJ, et al: Carotid plaque hemorrhage. Its role in production of cerebral ischemia, *Arch Surg* 117:1479–1488, 1982.

53. Reilly LM: Importance of carotid plaque morphology. In Bernstein EF, editor: *Vascular Diagnosis*, St. Louis, 1993, Mosby, pp 333–340.

54. Bassiouny HS, et al: Juxtalumenal location of plaque necrosis and neoformation in symptomatic carotid stenosis, *J Vasc Surg* 26:585–594, 1997.

55. Elatrozy T, et al: The effect of B-mode ultrasonic image standardisation on the echodensity of symptomatic and asymptomatic carotid bifurcation plaques, *Int Angiol* 17:179–186, 1998.

56. el-Barghouty N, et al: The identification of the high risk carotid plaque, *Eur J Vasc Endovasc Surg* 11:470–478, 1996.

57. Droste DW, et al: Comparison of ultrasonic and histo-pathological features of carotid artery stenosis, *Neurol Res* 19:380–384, 1997.

58. Hatsukami TS, et al: Carotid plaque morphology and clinical events, *Stroke* 28:95–100, 1997.

59. Biasi GM, et al: Computer analysis of ultrasonic plaque echolucency in identifying high risk carotid bifurcation lesions, *Eur J Vasc Endovasc Surg* 17:476–479, 1999.

60. Ciulla MM, et al: Assessment of carotid plaque composition in hypertensive patients by ultrasonic tissue characterization: A validation study, *J Hypertens* 20:1589–1596, 2002.

61. Mayor I, et al: Carotid plaque: Comparison between visual and grey-scale median analysis, *Ultrasound Med Biol* 29:961–966, 2003.

62. Reiter M, et al: Increasing carotid plaque echolucency is predictive of cardiovascular events in high-risk patients, *Radiology* 248:1050–1055, 2008.

63. Seabra J, Sanches J: Three-dimensional labeling of vulnerable regions in carotid plaques using Graph-Cuts, *Conf Proc IEEE Eng Med Biol Soc* 2008:3150–3153, 2008.

64. Dahl JJ, et al: Acoustic radiation force impulse imaging for noninvasive characterization of carotid artery atherosclerotic plaques: A feasibility study, *Ultrasound Med Biol* 35:707–716, 2009.

65. Nederkoorn PJ, et al: Carotid artery stenosis: Accuracy of contrast-enhanced MR angiography for diagnosis, *Radiology* 228:677–682, 2003.

66. Nandalur KR, et al: Composition of the stable carotid plaque: Insights from a multidetector computed tomography study of plaque volume, *Stroke* 38:935–940, 2007.

67. Porsche C, et al: Evaluation of cross-sectional luminal morphology in carotid atherosclerotic disease by use of spiral CT angiography, *Stroke* 32:2511–2515, 2001.

68. Saam T, et al: The vulnerable, or high-risk, atherosclerotic plaque: Noninvasive MR imaging for characterization and assessment, *Radiology* 244:64–77, 2007.

69. Bouwhuijsen Q, et al: Atherosclerotic carotid plaque composition in a healthy elderly population: The Rotterdam Study. RSNA Annual Meeting December 2, 2009. Chicago, IL.

70. Ota H, Zhu D, Demarco JK: Carotid intraplaque hemorrhage is associated with enlargement of lipid-rich necrotic core and plaque volume over time: in vivo 3T MRI prospective study. RSNA Annual Meeting December 2, 2009. Chicago, IL.

71. Saba L, et al: Multidetector-row CT angiography in the study of atherosclerotic carotid arteries, *Neuroradiology* 49:623–637, 2007.

72. Saba L, et al: Vulnerable plaque: Detection of agreement between multi-detector-row CT angiography and US-ECD, *Eur J Radiol* 77:509, 2011.

73. Nanayakkara ND, et al: Nonrigid registration of three-dimensional ultrasound and magnetic resonance images of the carotid arteries, *Med Phys* 36:373–385, 2009.

74. Bluth EI, et al: The identification of ulcerative plaque with high resolution duplex carotid scanning, *J Ultrasound Med* 7:73–76, 1988.

75. Stahl JA, Middleton WD: Pseudoulceration of the carotid artery, *Ultrasound Med* 11:355–358, 1992.

76. Ballard JL, et al: Cost-effective evaluation and treatment for carotid disease, *Arch Surg* 132:268–271, 1997.

ULTRASOUND ASSESSMENT OF CAROTID STENOSIS

9

EDWARD G. GRANT, MD, and MICHELLE MELANY, MD

The identification of carotid stenosis is perhaps the most essential of all functions of the cerebrovascular ultrasound examination. While the majority of stenotic lesions occur in the proximal internal carotid artery (ICA), other sites in the carotid system may be involved and may or may not be the cause of significant neurologic events. Up to 30% of all major hemispheric events (stroke, transient ischemic attack [TIA], or amaurosis fugax) are thought to originate from disease at the carotid bifurcation.[1] However, stenoses in other areas of the carotid arteries may be equally significant, including lesions in the distal ICA (an area not typically visible on routine carotid ultrasound), the common carotid artery (CCA), or on the right in the innominate artery (IA). Stenoses of the external carotid artery (ECA) are not typically of clinical import but should also be identified as they may account for the presence of a bruit on clinical examination and should be known to the surgeon at the time of carotid endarterectomy (CEA).

A number of large, well-controlled, multicenter trials both in North America and Europe have confirmed the effectiveness of CEA in preventing stroke in patients with stenoses at the ICA origin compared to optimized medical therapy. The North American Symptomatic Carotid Endarterectomy Trial (NASCET) has shown CEA resulted in an absolute reduction of 17% in stroke at 2 years when compared with medical therapy in symptomatic patients with 70% or greater stenosis.[2] The NASCET also reported improvement in outcome with CEA in patients in the 50% to 69% lesion category, although the amount of improvement was far less than in those with higher-grade stenoses.[3] The Asymptomatic Carotid Atherosclerosis Study (ACAS) also showed a reduction in stroke in asymptomatic patients with 60% or greater lesions, but, like the moderate range of stenoses in the NASCET, there was only a 5.8% reduction in stroke risk over 5 years.[4] Other studies, both here and abroad, have confirmed the benefit of CEA and have validated the role of this procedure in reducing the risk for future stroke.[5,6] However, with the advent of statin therapy, trials comparing CEA with medical management have been undertaken, and how this newer nonsurgical treatment will eventually affect management remains to be seen.

As technology has improved and confidence in imaging has grown, the ultrasound examination has assumed an increasingly important role in the selection of patients for CEA. In many facilities, ultrasound is the only imaging technique used. In others, magnetic resonance angiography (MRA) or computed tomographic angiography (CTA) may be performed in combination with sonography in cases where significant luminal narrowing is identified on the ultrasound or the results are equivocal. While the ultimate imaging algorithm remains to be determined, the role of conventional angiography as a diagnostic technique has markedly decreased except when carotid stent placement is considered.

The evaluation of ICA stenosis will be emphasized in this chapter because it has been extensively studied and is strongly associated with TIA and stroke. The diagnosis of stenotic disease affecting other parts of the carotid system may be clinically important and will form part of this chapter as well.

ICA STENOSIS

With the development of duplex Doppler in the early 1980s, a number of investigators reported excellent results using sonography in diagnosing carotid stenoses,[7-10] but ultrasound only gradually became the primary technique for carotid evaluation that it is today. While the role of ultrasound in the evaluation of carotid stenosis evolved and its technical attributes improved (increasing gray-scale resolution, addition of color Doppler in the late 1980s), contrast angiography remained the gold standard and was extensively employed in many institutions for decades. Most of the large studies describing the effectiveness of CEA, in fact, relied on angiography as the gold standard. Similarly, most studies in which the degree of carotid stenosis was characterized using ultrasound relied on carotid angiography as well. Before 1991, when the results of the NASCET trial were released, most angiographic studies characterized the severity of stenosis by measuring the size of the residual lumen and comparing it as a percentage to the size of the original vessel lumen. Although this is an appropriate method in most vessels, there are several unique features of the proximal ICA that render this measurement technique problematic in this vessel. To begin with, on all conventional angiographic studies, the original lumen is not actually seen. Although this is not a major problem in peripheral arteries when the original lumen is visible on both sides of a stenosis, lesions at the origin of the ICA typically do not have a "normal" lumen on both sides. The estimation of the original lumen is further complicated by the presence of a normal but highly variable region of dilatation, the carotid bulb. The difficulty in estimating the exact location of the original lumen of the proximal ICA, in fact, introduced a great degree of interobserver error in estimating the degree of ICA stenosis. To avoid interobserver error, the participants of the NASCET[2] and ACAS[4] studies published in 1991 and 1995, respectively, devised a different method: comparing the smallest residual luminal diameter to the luminal diameter of the "normal" ICA distal to the stenosis (Figure 9-1).

While the so-called NASCET method may not truly reflect the degree of luminal narrowing at the site of stenosis, this method has the advantage of minimizing interobserver error.[11] One should be aware that the European Carotid Surgery Trial (ECST) study[5] continued to rely on the conventional method of stenosis measurement, and, although both confirmed the effectiveness of CEA, their methods of measurement of ICA stenosis were quite different. In general, for a given diameter of a residual lumen, the calculation of percent stenosis tends to be significantly higher using the pre-NASCET measurement method in comparison to the NASCET method. The NASCET technique is currently the standard

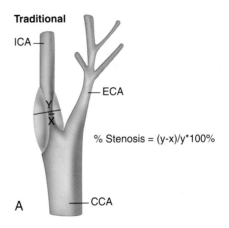

Traditional

$$\% \text{ Stenosis} = (y\text{-}x)/y*100\%$$

A

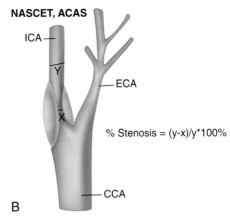

NASCET, ACAS

$$\% \text{ Stenosis} = (y\text{-}x)/y*100\%$$

B

FIGURE 9-1 Methods of measuring the degree of internal carotid artery (ICA) stenosis at contrast angiography. **A,** Older or so-called University of Washington method compares residual lumen *(X)* to original luminal diameter *(Y).* Both measurements are taken at the level of the stenosis itself. **B,** North American Symptomatic Carotid Endarterectomy Trial (NASCET) method compares residual lumen *(X)* to distal normalized lumen *(Y).* Because the original lumen is unable to be seen on a contrast angiogram, the exact location is difficult to determine, leading to a great deal of interobserver error. ACAS, Asymptomatic Carotid Atherosclerosis Study; CCA, common carotid artery; ECA, external carotid artery. *(Reprinted with permission from Scoutt LM, Grant EG: Carotid ultrasound. In Angtuaco TL, Hamper UM, Ralls PW, et al, editors:* Practical sonography for the radiologist: categorical course syllabus 2009, *Leesburg, VA, 2009, American Roentgen Ray Society, pp 99–111.)*

on which the large clinical North American studies were based and should be used to make clinical decisions about which patients undergo CEA. As such, Doppler thresholds taken from studies that did not use the NASCET method of measurement should not be used. Values from more recent evaluations[12-23] are strongly advised unless your facility has its own internally validated thresholds.

DOPPLER PARAMETERS

Innumerable Doppler parameters have been proposed to characterize ICA stenosis. These include both absolute angle-adjusted velocity measurements and various ratios. Currently, most laboratories rely on two or more of the three following measurements: peak systolic velocity (PSV), the ratio of peak systolic velocity in the ICA to that in the ipsilateral distal CCA (VICA/VCCA), and end-diastolic velocity (EDV). PSV is by far the most commonly used as it is easily obtained and highly reproducible. Statistically, however, all three perform about equally. In our own study, we found PSV and VICA/VCCA performed almost identically with regard to the identification of ICA stenoses greater than or equal to 70% when compared with angiography (Figure 9-2). EDV was slightly less accurate.[13] Other authors have not found EDV to be any less accurate than the other two parameters.[24] While statistics would suggest that one could choose any of these three parameters and produce equal results, when considering an individual patient, one must account for the fact that there is a great deal of variation of absolute velocity across any population. For that reason, the addition of ratio measurements to PSV may identify those who, for hemodynamic reasons (e.g., hypertension, low cardiac output, tandem lesions), fall outside the expected norm for either PSV or EDV. Low cardiac output, for example, may diminish a patient's ability to generate expected velocities for a given degree of stenosis, and a ratio may actually be more reflective of the true degree of vessel narrowing. Conversely, velocities in the ICA contralateral to a high-grade stenosis or occlusion may be spuriously high if the vessel is the major supplier of collateral blood flow around the circle of Willis,[25-27] and, again, the ratio value should be strongly considered in arriving at a diagnosis. An important technical point to be made when calculating the VICA/VCCA is that the denominator *must* be obtained from the distal CCA approximately 2 cm proximal to the bifurcation. While there is no reason for this other than convention, a study by Lee and colleagues[28] showed that, in most patients, the systolic velocity decreases in the CCA as one goes from proximal to distal within the vessel. Therefore, if the CCA velocity for the ratio is obtained from the proximal portion of the artery, the ratio may be spuriously low, potentially causing an underestimation of the degree of stenosis based on this parameter.

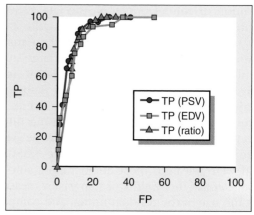

FIGURE 9-2 Receiver operating characteristic (ROC) curve for an ultrasound test to detect 70% or greater internal carotid artery (ICA) stenosis evaluating three Doppler ultrasound parameters: peak systolic velocity (PSV; *green circles*), end-diastolic velocity (EDV; *blue squares*), and the ratio of peak systolic velocity in the ICA to that in the ipsilateral distal common carotid artery (VICA/VCCA; *red triangles*). The vertical axis shows the number of true positives (TP). The horizontal axis shows the number of false positives (FP). This was based on a population of 266 carotid vessels from our institution. All three parameters perform well; PSV and VICA/VCCA are essentially identical. EDV performs slightly inferiorly.[13]

Hathout and associates[29] recently proposed an interesting approach to ICA ratio measurements whereby the authors constructed a ratio of the highest PSV at the site of the stenosis and compared it to the distal normalized velocity in the same vessel. Because it mimics the method of measurement used in the NASCET trial, the authors called it the "sonographic NASCET index." Given that the two velocity values are taken from the actual vessel involved by the stenosis, the authors postulated and indeed showed that this method produced superior results in characterizing the degree of ICA stenosis when compared to more commonly applied Doppler parameters. While the commonly used systolic velocity ratio (VICA/VCCA) performs well, the denominator is obtained from the CCA, which can potentially be affected by extraneous factors such as disease in the bulb and/or ECA.

PSV may also be falsely elevated in tortuous vessels. This is likely related to both a true increase in velocity as blood accelerates around a curve as well as difficulty in assigning a correct Doppler angle. Hence, if the ICA is extremely tortuous, one should use caution when making the diagnosis of an ICA stenosis on the basis of increased Doppler parameters alone without observing narrowing of the vessel lumen on gray-scale and/ or color flow imaging and poststenotic turbulence on the spectral Doppler tracing. In general, one should always consider the gray-scale and color Doppler appearance of the vessel in question (so called plaque burden) and visual estimates of vessel narrowing to determine if all diagnostic features (both visual and velocity data) of a stenosis are in alignment. Simply using a "cookbook" style of application of Doppler velocity thresholds may lead to significant diagnostic errors.

DOPPLER THRESHOLDS

Numerous thresholds were published before NASCET,[7-10] and, as mentioned earlier, these older studies invariably used angiographic measurements that were not performed using the NASCET method as their gold standard and are, therefore, not directly applicable to the estimation of the degree of ICA stenosis in use today. A review of the post-NASCET literature on ICA stenosis,[12-23] however, yields a remarkably wide range of recommended values to diagnose a given degree of ICA stenosis regardless of the parameters evaluated. All of these investigations have generated Doppler thresholds using angiographic measurements derived using the NASCET technique. The method of measurement of the gold standard is, therefore, not a factor in this variation. Many attribute the wide variation in published threshold values to what has been called "interlaboratory variation"—or inherent differences that are found when comparing one facility to another, such as different scan or measurement technique, interobserver variability of the Doppler examination,[30] or even equipment.[31] Certainly, it is well known that older Doppler units were prone to inconsistency, but that appears to have been largely overcome with improved technology. Other sources of variation in Doppler results may be related to patient population/referral patterns, disease prevalence, the mix of symptomatic versus asymptomatic patients, and the use of varied operative thresholds.

While actual differences in results when comparing one laboratory to another undoubtedly account for some of the variation in published thresholds, the most significant factor is probably the variation in statistical methods of selection of Doppler criteria. For this reason, it is important to understand how individual investigators arrived at their conclusions. Most authors have chosen Doppler thresholds based on an acceptable level of peak accuracy, sensitivity, or specificity, or some combination of the three. It is probably worth pointing out that in none of these studies did the authors actually attempt to diagnose a specific degree of stenosis, rather they sought to choose threshold values that would differentiate those arteries with an angiographically proven percent stenosis that was above or below a specified degree of severity. For example, they investigated the ability of a threshold to differentiate between vessels having greater or less than 70% stenosis.

Review of several articles where receiver operating characteristic (ROC) data are available[13,15] reveals that peak accuracy of Doppler for differentiating lesions above or below a certain degree of stenosis remains remarkably constant over a broad range of velocities and ratios and is, therefore, a relatively poor method of choosing a threshold. While this fact may at first appear counterintuitive, if Doppler can simply differentiate those patients with hemodynamically normal ICAs (Doppler values are not affected until the degree of stenosis reaches approximately 50%) from those with vessel narrowing, one automatically begins with an accuracy that is equivalent to the number of normal patients. Even in a laboratory with a large referral population, the majority of patients/vessels will not have significant stenoses. Choosing a threshold based on an acceptable level of sensitivity or specificity has the advantage over simple peak accuracy of being associated with a predictable clinical effect, in that it reflects the number of false positives or negatives produced by a given threshold. Unfortunately, reviewing the actual ROC data from a study done at our institution (Table 9-1), one can see that there is no obvious cut-off value; sensitivity simply decreases gradually as the threshold value is raised (more patients with operative lesions are missed), while specificity gradually increases (fewer patients are sent to surgery or correlative imaging unnecessarily). In situations in which there is a large benefit (e.g., stroke risk reduction) from CEA (≥70% stenosis in symptomatic patients), one would logically choose high sensitivity (a lower threshold velocity). Conversely, in patients with low benefit from CEA (50%–69% stenosis in symptomatic patients or ≥60% stenosis in asymptomatic patients), specificity should be favored over sensitivity. The decision

TABLE 9-1 Receiver Operating Characteristic Data from 202 Patients Showing Changes in Peak Systolic Velocity (PSV) Sensitivity, Specificity, and Accuracy for the Diagnosis of Angiographically Proven Stenoses of 70% or Greater. As Threshold Levels are Raised, Sensitivity Gradually Decreases While Specificity Increases. There is No Obvious "Cut Point" to Indicate an Ideal Threshold. Of Note, Accuracy Remains Relatively Flat Over the Entire Spectrum of Possible Threshold Values, Indicating that Alone, It is a Poor Choice for Selection of a Threshold.[13]			
PSV/Averaged Data			
PSV 70%	**Sensitivity**	**Specificity**	**Accuracy**
100	100	82.8	85
125	100	87.6	89.2
150	96.1	90.5	91.2
175	96.1	92.5	93
200	92.2	95.1	94.7
225	86.3	95.7	94.5
250	70.6	96.8	93.5
275	66.7	97.1	93.2
300	60.8	97.4	92.7
350	41.2	98.6	91.2
400	33.3	99.4	91

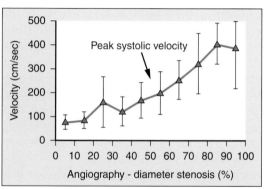

FIGURE 9-3 Graph demonstrating the relationship between average peak systolic velocity (PSV; y-axis) and percent luminal narrowing as determined by contrast angiography using North American Symptomatic Carotid Endarterectomy Trial (NASCET) method of measurement (x-axis). Average PSV clearly increases with increasing severity of angiographically determined stenosis. Error bars show one standard deviation about mean. Note marked overlap in adjacent categories of stenosis. This overlap shows that velocity measurements are not able to differentiate between 10% gradations in stenosis. Given the degree of overlap, only widely differing degrees of stenosis can be confidently differentiated by Doppler alone. *(Reprinted with permission from the Radiological Society of North America from Grant EG, et al: Ability to use duplex US to quantify internal carotid stenoses: fact or fiction?* Radiology *214:247–252, 2000.)*

by an author to favor sensitivity versus specificity has undoubtedly been *the major factor* in variation of recommended Doppler values in the literature.

Most ultrasound facilities approach the ultrasound diagnosis of ICA stenosis by stratifying the degree of vessel narrowing into relatively broad categories rather than attempting to predict the exact degree of stenosis. Several studies have shown that, indeed, the average PSV and VICA/VCCA ratio rise in direct proportion to the severity of stenosis as determined by angiography.[3,32] However, the standard deviations around each of these average velocity values are quite large, suggesting that Doppler cannot predict the exact degree of vessel narrowing. This makes the use of diagnostic strata necessary (Figure 9-3). We feel strongly that the diagnostic strata proposed by the Consensus Conference of the Society of Radiologists in Ultrasound (SRU) (0%–49%, 50%–69%, and ≥70%–95%) represent practical values that are clinically relevant and in keeping with the thresholds used in the NASCET trial.[2,34]

In addition to choosing optimal Doppler parameters and stratifying the degree of stenosis,

there is also considerable confusion about the choice of Doppler thresholds in diagnosing ICA stenosis. It should be obvious that there is no single perfect method for choosing Doppler thresholds with regard to characterizing the degree of stenosis in the ICA. Ideally, in a given noninvasive testing facility, one should develop thresholds based on angiographically correlated Doppler data. Few, if any, laboratories can do this today because the number of angiograms has dropped dramatically in recent years. In laboratories with such internally validated thresholds, one should continue to use them and be very wary about any proposed change. In laboratories without the ability to obtain angiographic correlation now or in the past, the numbers provided by the SRU consensus conference provide reasonable values that can be applied in almost any situation[34] (Table 9-2) and have been adopted by a large number of laboratories. These values have recently been validated against angiography and produced a sensitivity of 95.3% and specificity of 84.4%.[24] The SRU consensus data represent a compromise between sensitivity and specificity, with

TABLE 9-2 Results of Society of Radiologists in Ultrasound Consensus Conference on the Diagnosis of Internal Carotid Artery Stenosis

	ICA PSV (cm/sec)	Plaque/Diameter	ICA/CCA PSV Ratio	ICA EDV (cm/sec)
Normal	<125	None	<2.0	<40
<50%	<125	<50%	<2.0	<40
50%-69%	125-230	≥50%	2.0-4.0	40-100
≥70% to near occlusion	>230	≥50%	>4.0	>100
Near occlusion	High, low, or undetectable	Visible	Variable	Variable
Total occlusion	Undetectable	Visible, no detectable lumen	N/A	N/A

Modified from Grant EG, et al: Carotid artery stenosis: gray-scale and Doppler US diagnosis—Society of Radiologists in Ultrasound Consensus Conference, *Radiology* 229:340–346, 2003.
CCA, common carotid artery; EDV, end-diastolic velocity; ICA, internal carotid artery; PSV, peak systolic velocity.

emphasis on the former, and are based on the outcomes of the large clinical trials referred to earlier (Figures 9-4 and 9-5).

OCCLUSION VERSUS NEAR OCCLUSION OF THE ICA

Patients who have an occluded ICA have an incidence of stroke that is similar to that of the general population and is, therefore, relatively low. This is likely because the source of emboli created by a stenotic lesion is no longer present and because most patients recruit sufficient blood flow across the Circle of Willis from the contralateral ICA to maintain sufficient intracranial blood flow despite the absence of the contribution of the ipsilateral ICA. From a treatment standpoint, it should also be obvious that CEA is not technically possible in an occluded artery as there is no focal lesion to remove. Nearly occlusive lesions, on the other hand (which have also been variously termed subtotal occlusions, pseudo-occlusions, preocclusions, or string signs), have a highly significant incidence of stroke of approximately 11% per year,[2] roughly equivalent to that of 70% to 90% ICA stenoses. The differentiation between total and near occlusion is, therefore, essential because occlusions are not operative lesions whereas near occlusion, in most cases, should be treated surgically.

The definition of an occluded vessel is quite straightforward: cessation or blockage of flow anywhere along its course. In the ICA, this most commonly occurs at or near the bifurcation, but can occur distally, usually in the intracranial portion of the ICA. Regardless, as stated earlier, these patients are not operative candidates. For the definition of a near occlusion of the ICA one really has to go back to the angiographic literature where this phenomenon was first described. While near occlusion is typically a very severe form of ICA stenosis, the unique feature is the collapse or decreasing size of the ICA lumen beyond the area of stenosis. This is likely due to extremely decreased flow in the lumen. In some cases, the apparent decrease in luminal diameter may be accentuated by pooling of the small amount of contrast that passes beyond the stenosis in the posterior portion of the vessel, making it appear smaller angiographically than it really is. By definition, near occlusion is diagnosed when the ICA lumen is smaller than the ipsilateral ECA. Physiologically, flow is so diminished that delayed imaging may be necessary as normal timing of the angiogram would only show contrast in the ECA. An interesting feature of a near occlusion is that NASCET measurement methods cannot be applied because the so-called normal lumen has decreased in size and would render the degree of narrowing less than it really is. By convention, these lesions are usually classified as greater than 95%.

The sonographic characteristics of ICA occlusion are well known, but several different appearances may be encountered. In the classic case, the occluded lumen will be plainly visible as an anechoic/hypoechoic region occupying the entire vessel, and no spectral, color, or power Doppler signals will be seen within the lumen (Figure 9-6). Often, internal areas of echogenic or calcified plaque can be identified within the occluded lumen. In some cases, the occluded vessel cannot be identified distinctly, and the diagnosis of ICA occlusion is made on the basis of finding a single vessel at the bifurcation. When occlusion

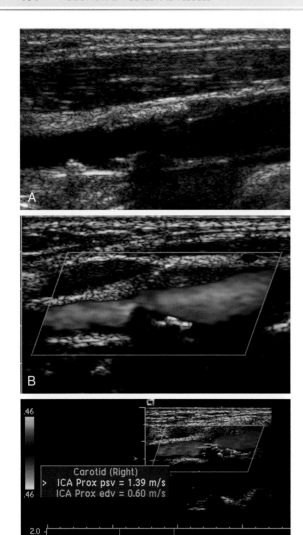

FIGURE 9-4 Moderate (50%–69%) internal carotid artery (ICA) stenosis in an asymptomatic 73-year-old man, before coronary artery bypass surgery. **A,** Gray-scale image shows a moderate amount of soft and calcific plaque in the right carotid bulb, extending into the proximal ICA. **B,** Color Doppler image suggests a greater degree of stenosis than was apparent on the gray-scale image. **C,** Spectral Doppler suggests a 50% to 69% stenosis based on mildly elevated peak systolic velocity (PSV; 139 cm/sec) and end-diastolic velocity (EDV; 60 cm/sec). Systolic ratio was also elevated to 2.4.

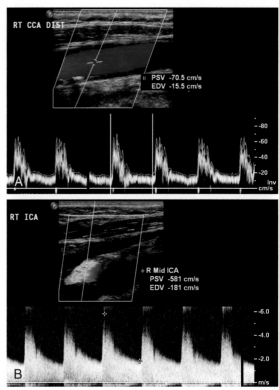

FIGURE 9-5 Severe (70% or greater) internal carotid artery (ICA) stenosis in a 66-year-old man with history of multiple transient ischemic attacks referable to the right hemisphere. **A,** Spectral Doppler image of the distal right common carotid artery (CCA) demonstrates a peak systolic velocity (PSV) of 70.5 cm/sec. **B,** Color Doppler image from the ipsilateral ICA shows a dense calcific plaque with posterior acoustic shadowing beyond which is an area of intense aliasing suggesting elevated velocities. Spectral Doppler image confirms marked velocity elevation: PSV = 581 cm/sec, end-diastolic velocity (EDV) = 181 cm/sec, systolic ratio = 8.2.

of the ICA presents in this way, it can be complicated by the presence of large ECA collaterals, which can be mistaken for the ICA. Fortunately, given the anatomic detail provided by color Doppler using current equipment, this should be a relatively uncommon pitfall. In case of doubt, the sonographer should consider documenting the response to the temporal tap maneuver since the patent external carotid artery should show a strong response to the maneuver. Often a patent stump remains at the ICA origin, and, in most cases, the occluded area can be found easily as the stump rarely extends far beyond the origin of the vessel. In this situation, one can often identify a region of bidirectional flow in the stump using color Doppler because forward flow is reflected backwards by the occluding thrombus/plaque. An additional feature of ICA occlusion is the finding of "externalized" or high-resistance flow patterns in the ipsilateral CCA. Because all flow in the CCA is directed into the ECA, the spectral pattern in the CCA reflects its end organ (the musculature of the head and neck), and a high-resistance pattern is found.

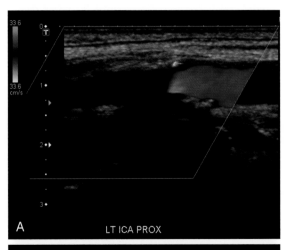

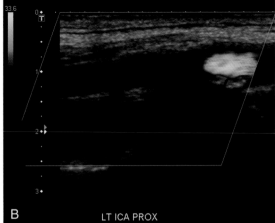

FIGURE 9-6 Internal carotid artery (ICA) occlusion in a 65-year-old woman with recent history of stroke. **A,** Color Doppler imaging shows anechoic proximal ICA lumen with complete absence of color. **B,** Power Doppler with its increased sensitivity further suggests occlusion, because no residual lumen is depicted. Magnetic resonance angiography (not shown) confirmed occlusion of the ICA.

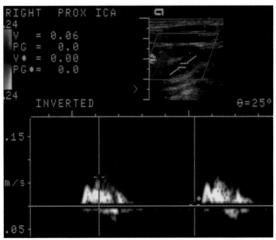

FIGURE 9-7 Distal internal carotid artery (ICA) occlusive disease in a 55-year-old man with right hemispheric transient ischemic attacks. Spectral Doppler image shows extremely low peak systolic velocity (PSV; 6 cm/sec) and absent diastolic flow. These findings suggest a severe distal obstructive lesion. Note relative absence of plaque at the bifurcation. Magnetic resonance angiography (not shown) confirmed high-grade stenosis at the carotid siphon.

Externalization of the CCA may not occur if the ECA is serving as a major collateral around the ICA occlusion. In this scenario, the ECA will produce low-resistance waveforms that will be reflected back into the CCA. The vast majority of occlusions distal to the ICA origin occur at the carotid siphon. This area is obviously not included in the typical carotid examination. Distal lesions may be identified by transcranial Doppler,[35] although most authorities currently lean toward CTA or MRA for imaging the intracranial vasculature. Although distal lesions are not directly visualized by the carotid Doppler examination, they can be implied if diastolic flow is absent in the proximal ICA and the PSV is low when compared to the opposite side (Figure 9-7). Absent diastolic flow in the ICA is always abnormal. In addition to distal occlusion, the differential should include ICA dissection and markedly increased intracranial pressure.

As noted earlier, the imaging characteristics of carotid occlusion are relatively straightforward. Unfortunately, one cannot be completely confident with this diagnosis using ultrasound alone as a minute, residual channel may be present and missed even using the most sensitive scan technique. A review of existing studies shows that the residual lumen in patients with near occlusions was not identified by ultrasound in 15% to 30% of cases.[36,37] For this reason, the sonographer must search diligently for a residual lumen. One should maximize color sensitivity and use power Doppler, if available. Several studies have now demonstrated that the addition of a sonographic contrast agent can greatly increase sensitivity when trying to depict a nearly occlusive lesion.[37,38] Both of these referenced studies have shown 100% success in differentiating between nearly and totally occlusive lesions. Because of the lack of sensitivity of noncontrast Doppler ultrasound, if a complete occlusion is suspected at or near the bifurcation and a sonographic contrast study is not performed, MRA or CTA should be employed to confirm its presence.

In our experience,[36] nearly occlusive lesions identified with imaging may be divided into two groups. About 75% will have a focal, very severe

FIGURE 9-8 Near occlusion of left internal carotid artery (ICA) with focal lesion in a 79-year-old man with history of previous left hemispheric stroke. **A,** Color Doppler image of left ICA origin shows a very narrowed stream of flow when compared to the size of the surrounding plaque/original lumen. **B,** Extensive scanning failed to demonstrate the expected high-speed jet of flow. Maximum peak systolic velocity found was 53 cm/sec. **C,** Magnetic resonance angiography confirms the presence of a typical focal nearly occlusive lesion. Note extremely narrowed lumen, essentially to the point of absence of signal *(arrows)*. Distal ICA is much smaller than the contralateral ICA and is smaller than the ipsilateral external carotid artery.

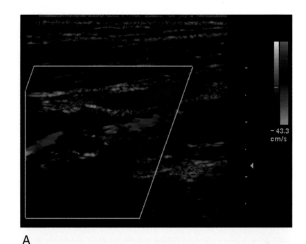

A

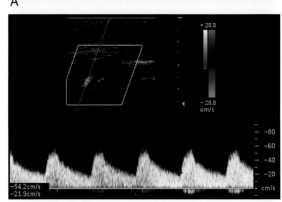

B

stenosis with varying degrees of collapse of the ICA lumen distal to the stenosis. Sonographically, the majority of these lesions will have an appearance similar to other high-grade lesions. Failure to diagnose these stenoses can occur in cases where the lesion is so severe that the PSV is actually in the mid-range stenotic or even normal. In the case of nearly occlusive lesions, one must often base the diagnosis on the visual appearance at color or power Doppler rather than spectral Doppler parameters (Figure 9-8). These lesions are also treated in a manner similar to more typical ICA stenoses, by CEA or stenting, depending on the practice pattern of the treating surgeon. Although the majority of nearly occlusive lesions are actually very severe focal stenoses with distal collapse, approximately 25% actually have diffuse, severe narrowing of the ICA and no focal stenosis at any point along the course of the vessel (Figure 9-9). Such "string lesions," as we have called them (to differentiate them from the more common focal lesions), may be very difficult to identify at sonography and are often the nearly occlusive lesions that are mistaken for complete occlusion. These lesions may require MRA or CTA to depict the lumen and the full extent of the vessel narrowing. The underlying pathology of these string lesions is poorly understood. Some investigators believe that these may represent chronic dissections. Given the diffuse nature of these lesions, CEA is not possible as there is no focal stenosis to remove or open. These string lesions, however, may be the source of emboli and recurrent TIAs. In these cases, ligation of the ICA may be the best alternative, since such a diffusely and severely narrowed ICA contributes little to the overall perfusion of the brain.

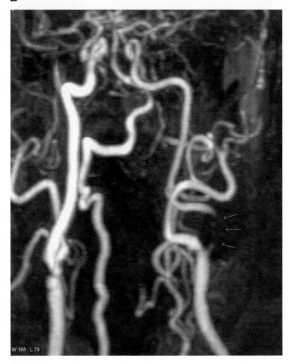

C

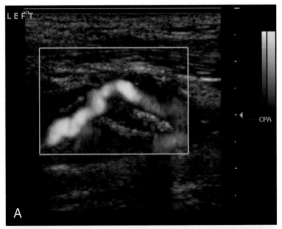

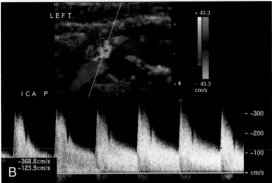

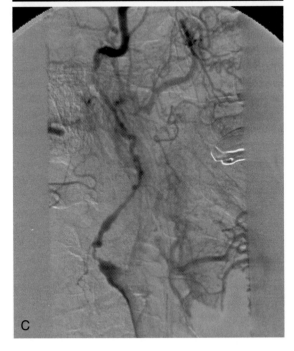

FIGURE 9-9 Near occlusion of internal carotid artery (ICA) with diffuse disease in a 71-year-old man with worsening transient ischemic attacks. **A,** Power Doppler image demonstrates diffusely narrowed lumen with unusual pattern of wall irregularity. Lumen measured between 2 and 3 mm in transverse diameter. Note size discrepancy between residual and original lumen, which is largely occupied by plaque. **B,** Spectral evaluation demonstrates high-velocity flow throughout visualized cervical ICA with peak systolic velocity of 328 cm/sec. No focal area of velocity elevation was found. **C,** Angiogram confirms presence of diffusely narrowed and irregular ICA lumen that filled in a delayed fashion. Vessel was patent throughout. *(From El-Saden S, Grant EG, Hathout GM, et al: Imaging of the internal carotid artery: the dilemma of total versus near total occlusion,* Radiology *221:301–308, 2001.)*

THE COMMON CAROTID ARTERY

In most patients, the origin of the right CCA can be identified as it arises from the innominate artery in the supraclavicular fossa. The left CCA, however, originates directly from the aorta, and its proximal portion is too caudal to be seen with sonography. The normal spectral pattern in the CCA is a low-resistance artery because the majority of blood is directed toward the ICA in the normal patient. As described above, loss of diastolic flow in the CCA is abnormal and, though not specific, may be associated with ICA occlusion because all blood is then directed to the ECA. Relatively high resistance waveforms may be seen in the proximal CCA and are likely the result of its proximity to the aorta. In these situations, increasing diastolic flow is typically identified as one proceeds distally in the CCA. Similarly, velocities in the CCA often decrease as one proceeds from proximal to distal.[28] Thus, in keeping with previously published studies,[7] one must always obtain CCA measurements for the VICA/VCCA ratio approximately 1 to 2 cm proximal to the carotid bulb in order to obtain consistent and comparable ratio measurements. One should never use velocities obtained in the carotid bulb because PSV will drop as diameter increases.

Scattered, smooth, fibrofatty plaques are quite common in the CCA. Significant stenoses are infrequent in this vessel but do occur and may be the cause of hemispheric symptoms. We have found ICA stenoses to be approximately 15 to 20 times more common than those in the CCA. Although the vast majority of CCA lesions are secondary to atherosclerosis, patients with previous trauma, fibromuscular dysplasia, Takayasu's arteritis, or a history of head and neck irradiation have an increased incidence of CCA stenosis. In many of these cases, vascular abnormalities present as elongated and often bizarre stenoses.

There are few published criteria for characterizing CCA lesions, probably due to the relative rarity of these stenoses and the fact that PSV throughout the CCA is not constant. A recent article by Slovut and colleagues[39] showed that a PSV of greater than 182 cm/sec was the most accurate value for diagnosing 50% or greater stenosis with a sensitivity of 64% and specificity of 88%. Sensitivity, specificity, and accuracy of carotid duplex were higher when the stenosis was located in the mid or distal aspects of the CCA (sensitivity 76%, specificity 89%). However, given the known inconsistency of PSV in the CCA as one proceeds distally, the use of this parameter does not seem advisable in our opinion and the use of systolic velocity ratios proximal to and in, or immediately distal to, a stenosis seems far more practical. Unfortunately, to the best of our knowledge, there are no correlative studies on which to base threshold values. As is often applied to stenotic disease elsewhere in the body, we rely on a doubling of the velocity to suggest a moderate stenosis and a fourfold increase in velocity or greater to suggest a greater than 70% lesion (Figure 9-10). In our experience, one can more reliably use gray-scale measurements to estimate the degree of stenosis in the CCA than in the ICA. This is likely due to the larger size and deeper location of the CCA, which places it more optimally in the focal zone of the transducer.

An area of potential diagnostic difficulty in the diagnosis of CCA stenoses is the origin of the left carotid artery. As mentioned above, this area is not seen sonographically because of its location in the chest, but stenoses may occur at this site and be responsible for hemispheric symptoms. The diagnosis of left CCA origin stenoses, therefore, can only be implied based on Doppler abnormalities from the *visualized* portions of the CCA. In general, any striking asymmetry of flow velocities in which the left is lower than the right should be viewed with suspicion. Unfortunately, there is minimal literature available to give quantifiable parameters on how large this asymmetry should be before being considered abnormal, and mild to moderate variations between the right and left CCA velocity are common. In a series published some years ago, the authors found that

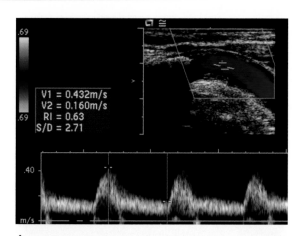

A

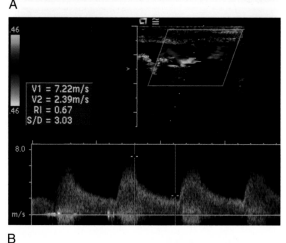

B

FIGURE 9-10 Left common carotid artery (CCA) stenosis in a 65-year-old man with dizziness and history of prior neck irradiation for squamous cell carcinoma. **A,** Color/spectral Doppler image from mid left CCA shows calcific plaque. Proximal to the plaque, peak systolic velocity (PSV) was 43 cm/sec. **B,** Progressive, irregular narrowing was encountered as scan progressed distally. Area of focal aliasing produced maximum PSV of 722 cm/sec. Magnetic resonance angiography confirmed severe stenosis involving much of the mid and distal left CCA with extremely irregular walls (not shown).

the normal ipsilateral to contralateral CCA ratio should be between 0.7 and 1.3.[40] In general, any patient with spiky, turbulent flow or a tardus-parvus CCA waveform, or patients with left CCA PSV less than 50 cm/sec in whom PSV in the right CCA is considerably higher should be viewed with suspicion and the left CCA/right CCA ratio calculated. MRA and CTA can depict the origins of the great vessels from the aorta well and should be considered in any patient in whom there is a suspicion of a proximal left CCA lesion.[41]

In our experience, CCA occlusion should be readily and definitively diagnosed with ultrasound.

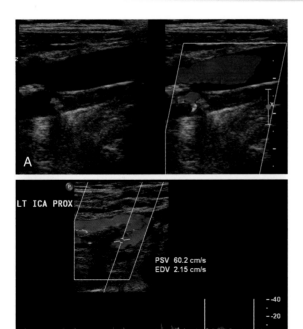

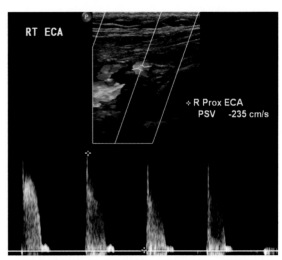

FIGURE 9-12 External carotid artery (ECA) stenosis in a 71-year-old woman with a right neck bruit. Imaging of the proximal right ECA shows a sharp waveform with absent diastolic flow typical of the ECA. Peak systolic velocity (PSV) was 235 cm/sec. Internal carotid artery was normal. Spectral Doppler criteria for grading ECA stenoses have not been published, but this likely represents a moderate degree of stenosis.

FIGURE 9-11 Common carotid artery (CCA) occlusion with patent internal carotid artery (ICA) and external carotid artery (ECA) in a 72-year-old man with dizziness. **A,** Gray-scale imaging suggests occlusion of left ICA. Vessel lumen is filled with inhomogeneous plaque. Color Doppler image confirms absence flow in CCA. Note small size of vessel compared to adjacent jugular vein. **B,** Color Doppler image at bifurcation demonstrates two patent vessels. Flow in the ECA is depicted in blue and directed toward the bifurcation (positive Doppler shift on the Doppler spectrum). Flow in the ICA proceeds in the opposite direction (toward the head) and is depicted in red.

However, it is essential to scan the bifurcation of these patients because, in up to 25% of patients, the ICA and ECA will remain patent.[42] For this to occur, flow in one of the vessels must be reversed. In almost all cases, it will be the ECA, with its rich supply of potential collaterals that reverses and provides blood to the ICA. This interesting phenomenon produces dramatic pictures on color Doppler examination, with one vessel displayed in red and the other in blue (Figure 9-11).

THE EXTERNAL CAROTID ARTERY

The ECA supplies the muscles of the face and neck and, as such, is typically a high-resistance artery with relatively less diastolic flow than the ipsilateral ICA. The ECA is also easily differentiated from the ICA by the presence of branches,

the first of which is typically the superior thyroidal artery. The ECA has received less attention than its neighbor, the ICA, for obvious reasons: it is not associated with stroke, and stenoses are far less common in the ECA when compared to the ICA. While the precise characterization of ECA stenoses is of little value, stenoses may be the cause for a bruit in the neck and should at least be described in the carotid ultrasound report. The values typically used to grade stenoses of the ICA do not apply to the ECA, and, to the best of our knowledge, there are no published criteria for ECA stenoses. Given the lack of clinical import and threshold values, trying to quantify ECA lesions is probably not worthwhile. For practical reasons we tend to simply state that the vessel is stenotic and classify the lesion as mild, moderate, or severe (Figure 9-12). The ECA may serve as an important source of collateral flow in patients with severe stenoses or occlusion of the ICA. In such cases flow in the ECA may convert to a low-resistance waveform and could be confused with the normally low-resistance ICA.[43,44]

THE INNOMINATE ARTERY

Occlusive disease of the innominate or brachiocephalic artery is relatively unusual but may cause a wide range of significant symptoms. In the study of Brunhölzl and von Reutern,[45] the authors identified only 20 cases among 30,000 patients; however, their study relied only on non-invasive testing. Older angiographic investigations indicate that IA lesions account for as many as 2.5% to 4 % of atherosclerotic lesions of the extracranial and intracranial cerebral arteries,[45,46] but this incidence included minor degrees of stenosis that would be unlikely to produce either clinical symptoms or the hemodynamic alterations necessary to produce an abnormal Doppler study. The IA gives rise to both the right CCA and the right subclavian artery. The latter in turn gives off the right vertebral artery. Given this huge vascular distribution, compromise of the IA can produce symptoms related to both the anterior (e.g., cerebral hemispheric strokes, TIAs) and posterior (cerebellar and brain stem strokes, dizziness) cerebral circulation, as well as symptoms of arm ischemia. Patients with significant IA disease also often have stenotic lesions elsewhere in the right circulation such as the ICA origin, which may complicate localization of the offending lesion.

The potential for numerous and varied collateral pathways, as well as concurrent stenosis elsewhere, in patients with severe IA disease explains the observation that waveform abnormalities (e.g., flow reversal, mid-systolic deceleration) do not affect all vessels in the right carotid/vertebral systems equally. It also likely explains the poor correlation between the severity of angiographically measured stenosis and the severity of the Doppler waveform abnormalities. Furthermore, it is likely that the sonographic abnormalities associated with IA disease are not static and change as new collaterals are recruited. Although Brunhölzl and von Reutern[45] proposed a classification system of IA stenosis based on multiple subjective Doppler criteria, our experience[47] is more in keeping with that of Schwend and co-workers,[48] who felt that the variability in Doppler findings was more reflective of collateral circulatory patterns than the severity of IA stenosis. Although we did not find good correlation between Doppler abnormalities and the degree of angiographically measured stenosis of the IA, our study suggests that the degree of stenosis must be relatively high to produce demonstrable alterations on a Doppler examination. Among the patients in our study, all had stenoses that were greater than 70% at angiography.[47]

The physiologic alterations associated with significant occlusive disease of the IA appear to

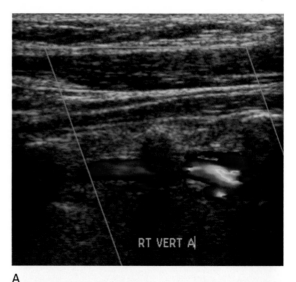

A

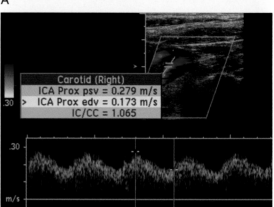

B

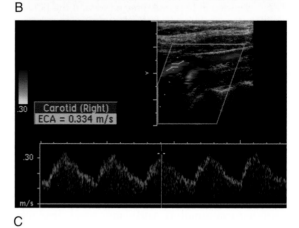

C

FIGURE 9-13 Innominate artery stenosis in a 65-year-old woman with left hemiparesis. **A,** Color Doppler image of the right vertebral artery shows reversed flow. **B,** Right internal carotid artery waveforms have a subtle mid-systolic deceleration and abundant diastolic flow. **C,** External carotid artery also shows an abnormal, low-resistance flow pattern and a tardus-parvus waveform. Magnetic resonance angiography confirmed severe stenosis of the innominate artery (not shown).

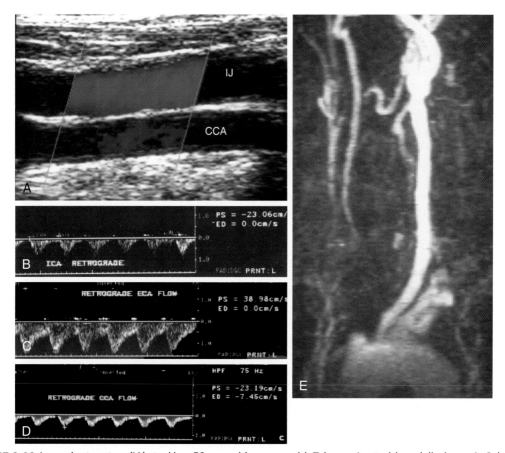

FIGURE 9-14 Innominate artery (IA) steal in a 56-year-old woman with Takayasu's arteritis and dizziness. **A,** Color Doppler image of the right common carotid artery shows reversal of flow direction. Common carotid artery (CCA) flow is displayed in the same color as the adjacent jugular vein. **B** to **D,** Spectral Doppler shows reversed flow in all three vessels of the right carotid system (CCA, external carotid artery [ECA], and internal carotid artery). Note the low-resistance flow pattern in the ECA. **E,** Magnetic resonance angiography reveals complete occlusion of the IA immediately beyond its origin. *(From Grant EG, et al: Innominate artery occlusive disease: sonographic findings, AJR Am J Roentgenol 186:394–400, 2006.)*

present a specific and readily identifiable constellation of findings at Doppler ultrasound. These alterations are secondary to compromise of blood flow in the subclavian artery and are similar to the findings in subclavian steal in that reversal of flow (either complete or partial) in the right vertebral artery is an essential part of the complex. Unlike findings in classic subclavian steal, lesions of the IA are located proximal to the subclavian artery and produce alterations in the flow patterns of the right carotid system as well as the vertebral system. Review of the literature on the subject[46,47,49] reveals that the vertebral artery appears to be affected preferentially over the carotid, with complete reversal of vertebral artery flow found in the majority of patients. The degree to which the carotid circulation is involved is more variable. Doppler abnormalities range from

subtle, mid-systolic deceleration, the "bunny rabbit sign,"[50] in one or more of the carotid branches (Figure 9-13) to the rare finding of complete reversal of flow in all carotid arteries (Figure 9-14), the "innominate steal phenomenon."[51-53] Killen and Gobbel,[54] in fact, termed preservation of antegrade flow in the right carotid system at the expense of the vertebral artery as "carotid recovery." Although the physiologic basis for this phenomenon has not been thoroughly explained, it is likely that flow is more readily diverted across the vertebrobasilar junction than across the Circle of Willis. Severely tardus-parvus waveforms in the carotid arteries should also be viewed with suspicion in any patient with reversed flow in the right vertebral artery and should suggest IA stenosis.

As mentioned in the section dealing with stenoses of the CCA, marked asymmetry between the PSV in the right and left CCA is abnormal. In the case of decreased velocity in the right CCA, an IA lesion should be considered. The normal ratio between the right and left CCA PSV should be between 0.7 and 1.3.[40] In our series of patients with IA lesions, the average right to left velocity ratio was 3.4 with a range of 1.7 to 5.7.[47] All patients in our series, therefore, fell outside the normal range. As is the case with lesions of the left CCA origin, MRA and CTA perform well in the evaluation of IA lesions and should be considered for confirmation and characterization of any suspected IA stenotic or occlusive disease.[41]

SUMMARY

This chapter provides an overview of key elements of the Doppler waveforms that are altered by carotid artery stenotic lesions. Knowledge of the typical alterations in blood flow patterns can help identify the presence of carotid artery pathologies located at the level of the bifurcation, intracranially, or at the origin of the great vessels.

REFERENCES

1. Eisenberg R, et al: Relationship of transient ischemic attack and angiographically demonstrable lesions of the carotid artery, *Stroke* 8:483–486, 1977.
2. North American Symptomatic Carotid Endarterectomy Trial Collaborators: Beneficial effect of carotid endarterectomy in symptomatic patients with high-grade carotid stenosis, *N Engl J Med* 325:445–453, 1991.
3. Barnett HJM, et al: Benefit of carotid endarterectomy in patients with symptomatic moderate or severe stenosis, *N Engl J Med* 339:1415–1425, 1998.
4. Executive Committee for the Asymptomatic Carotid Atherosclerosis Study: Endarterectomy for asymptomatic carotid artery stenosis, *JAMA* 273:1421–1428, 1995.
5. European Carotid Surgery Trialists' Collaborative Group: MRC European Carotid Surgery Trial: Interim results for symptomatic patients with severe (70-99%) or with mild (0–29%) carotid stenosis, *Lancet* 337:1235–1243, 1991.
6. Hobson RW, et al: Efficacy of carotid endarterectomy for asymptomatic carotid stenosis, *N Engl J Med* 328:221–227, 1993.
7. Garth K, et al: Duplex ultrasound scanning of the carotid arteries with velocity spectrum analysis, *Radiology* 147:823–827, 1983.
8. Jacobs N, et al: Duplex carotid sonography: criteria for stenosis, accuracy, and pitfalls, *Radiology* 154:385–391, 1985.
9. Blackshear W Jr, et al: Carotid artery velocity patterns in normal and stenotic vessels, *Stroke* 11:67–71, 1980.
10. Dreisbach JN, et al: Duplex sonography in the evaluation of carotid artery disease, *AJNR Am J Neuroradiol* 4:678–680. 20, 1983.
11. Gagne PJ, et al: Can the NASCET technique for measuring carotid stenosis be reliably applied outside the trial? *J Vasc Surg* 24:449–456, 1996.
12. Hunink MGM, et al: Detection and quantification of carotid artery stenosis: efficacy of various Doppler parameters, *AJR Am J Roentgenol* 160:619–625, 1993.
13. Grant EG, et al: Doppler sonographic parameters for detection of carotid stenosis: is there an optimum method for their selection? *AJR Am J Roentgenol* 172:1123–1129, 1999.
14. Moneta GL, et al: Screening for asymptomatic internal carotid artery stenosis: duplex criteria for discriminating 60% to 99% stenosis, *J Vasc Surg* 21:989–994, 1995.
15. Moneta GL, et al: Correlation of North American Symptomatic Carotid Endarterectomy Trial (NASCET) angiographic definition of 70% to 99% internal carotid artery stenosis with duplex scanning, *J Vasc Surg* 17:152–159, 1993.
16. Carpenter JP, et al: Determination of sixty percent or greater carotid artery stenosis by duplex Doppler ultrasonography, *J Vasc Surg* 22:697–705, 1995.
17. Carpenter JP, et al: Determination of duplex Doppler ultrasound criteria appropriate to the North American Symptomatic Carotid Endarterectomy Trial, *Stroke* 27:695–699, 1996.
18. Neale ML, et al: Reappraisal of duplex criteria to assess significant carotid stenosis with special reference to reports from the North American Symptomatic Carotid Endarterectomy Trial and the European Carotid Surgery Trial, *J Vasc Surg* 20:642–649, 1994.
19. Hood DB, et al: Prospective evaluation of new duplex criteria to identify 70% internal carotid artery stenosis, *J Vasc Surg* 23:254–262, 1996.
20. Browman MW, et al: Duplex ultrasonography criteria for internal carotid stenosis of more than 70% diameter: angiographic correlation and receiver operating characteristic curve analysis, *Can Assoc Radiol J* 46:291–295, 1995.
21. Wilterdink JL, et al: Performance of carotid ultrasound in evaluating candidates for carotid endarterectomy is optimized by an approach based on clinical outcome rather than accuracy, *Stroke* 27:1094–1098, 1996.
22. Derdeyn CP, Powers WJ: Cost-effectiveness of screening for asymptomatic carotid artery disease, *Stroke* 27:1944–1950, 1996.
23. Jahromi AS, et al: Sensitivity and specificity of color duplex ultrasound measurement in the estimation of internal carotid artery stenosis: A systematic review and meta-analysis, *J Vasc Surg* 41:962–972, 2005.
24. Braun RM, et al: Ultrasound imaging of carotid artery stenosis: application of the society of radiologists in ultrasound consensus criteria to a single institution clinical practice, *Ultrasound Q* 24:161–166, 2008.
25. AbuRahma AF, et al: Effect of contralateral severe stenosis or carotid occlusion on duplex criteria of ipsilateral stenoses: comparative study of various duplex parameters, *J Vasc Surg* 22:751–762, 1995.
26. Busuttil SJ, et al: Carotid duplex overestimation of stenosis due to severe contralateral disease, *Am J Surg* 172:144–148, 1996.
27. Beckett WW Jr, et al: Duplex Doppler sonography of the carotid artery: false-positive results in an artery contralateral to an artery with marked stenosis, *AJR Am J Roentgenol* 155:1091–1095, 1990.
28. Lee VS, et al: Variability of Doppler US measurements along the common carotid artery: effects on estimates of internal carotid arterial stenosis in patients with angiographically proved disease, *Radiology* 214:387–392, 2000.

29. Hathout GM, et al: Sonographic NASCET index: a new Doppler parameter for assessment of internal carotid artery stenosis, *AJNR Am J Neuroradiol* 26:68–75, 2005.

30. Tessler FN, et al: Inter- and intra-observer variability of Doppler peak velocity measurements: an in-vitro study, *Ultrasound Med Biol* 16:653–657, 1990.

31. Howard G, et al: An approach for the use of Doppler ultrasound as a screening tool for hemodynamically significant stenosis (despite heterogeneity of Doppler performance): A multicenter experience, *Stroke* 27:1951–1957, 1996.

32. Bluth EI, et al: Carotid duplex sonography: a multi-center recommendation for standardized imaging and Doppler criteria, *Radiographics* 8:487–506, 1988.

33. Grant EG, et al: The ability of spectral Doppler to quantify internal carotid stenoses: fact or fiction? *Radiology* 214:247–252, 2000.

34. Grant EG, et al: Carotid artery stenosis: gray-scale and Doppler US diagnosis — Society of Radiologists in Ultrasound Consensus Conference, *Radiology* 229:340–346, 2003.

35. Valaikiene J, et al: Transcranial color-coded duplex sonography for detection of distal internal carotid artery stenosis, *AJNR Am J Neuroradiol* 29:347–353, 2008.

36. El-Saden S, et al: Imaging of the internal carotid artery: the dilemma of total versus near total occlusion, *Radiology* 221:301–308, 2001.

37. Ferrer JM, et al: Use of ultrasound contrast in the diagnosis of carotid artery occlusion, *J Vasc Surg* 31:736–741, 2000.

38. Ohm C, et al: Diagnosis of total internal carotid occlusions with duplex ultrasound and ultrasound contrast, *Vasc Endovascular Surg* 39:237–243, 2005.

39. Slovut DP, et al: Detection of common carotid artery stenosis using duplex ultrasonography: a validation study with computed tomographic angiography, *J Vasc Surg* 51(1):65–70, 2010.

40. Vaisman U, Wojciechowski M: Carotid artery disease: new criteria for evaluation by sonographic duplex scanning, *Radiology* 158:253–255, 1986.

41. Randoux B, et al: Proximal great vessels of aortic arch: comparison of three-dimensional gadolinium enhanced MR angiography and digital subtraction angiography, *Radiology* 229:697–707, 2003.

42. Dashefsky SM, et al: Total occlusion of the common carotid artery with patent internal carotid artery. Identification with color flow Doppler imaging, *J Ultrasound Med* 10:417–421, 1991.

43. Rohren EM, et al: A spectrum of Doppler waveforms in the carotid and vertebral arteries, *AJR Am J Roentgenol* 181:1695–1704, 2003.

44. AbuRahma AF, et al: The reliability of color duplex ultrasound in diagnosing total carotid artery occlusion, *Am J Surg* 174:185–187, 1997.

45. Brunhölzl CH, von Reutern GM: Hemodynamic effects of innominate artery occlusive disease. Evaluation by Doppler ultrasound, *Ultrasound Med Biol* 15:201–204, 1989.

46. Hass WK, et al: Joint study of extracranial arterial occlusion, *JAMA* 203:961–968, 1968.

47. Grant EG, et al: Innominate artery occlusive disease: sonographic findings, *AJR Am J Roentgenol* 186:394–400, 2006.

48. Schwend RB, et al: Carotid steal syndrome: a case study, *J Neuroimaging* 5:195–197, 1995.

49. Mozersky DJ, et al: Hemodynamics of innominate artery occlusion, *Ann Surg* 123–127, 1973 Aug.

50. Kliewer MA, et al: Vertebral artery Doppler waveform changes indicating subclavian steal physiology, *AJR Am J Roentgenol* 174:815–819, 2000.

51. Patesi F, et al: The innominate steal, *Vasc Dis* 5:214–225, 1968.

52. Blakemore WS, et al: Reversal of blood flow in the right vertebral artery accompanying occlusion of the innominate artery, *Ann Surg* 161:353, 1964.

53. Verlato F, et al: Diagnosis of high-grade stenosis of innominate artery, *Angiology* 44:845–851, 1993.

54. Killen DA, Gobbel WG: Subclavian steal-carotid recovery phenomenon, *J Thorac Cardiovasc Surg* 50:421–426, 1965.

CAROTID OCCLUSION, UNUSUAL PATHOLOGIES, AND DIFFICULT CAROTID CASES

10

JOHN S. PELLERITO, MD, FACR, FSRU, FAIUM, and JOSEPH F. POLAK, MD, MPH

In this chapter we review rare or uncommon carotid artery pathologies. Although these cases are part of the differential diagnosis of carotid artery disease, a sonographer is unlikely to see many if any of these cases during a typical year.

We emphasize the typical appearance and Doppler characteristics of these uncommon and rare cases.

CAROTID OCCLUSION

Distinguishing a complete carotid artery occlusion from a subtotal carotid artery occlusion is one of the most important differential diagnoses made during a carotid evaluation. The finding of carotid occlusion carries significant clinical implications since this diagnosis precludes therapeutic options, including endarterectomy and stent placement. The diagnosis requires careful evaluation of the occluded segment as well as the inflow and outflow vessels. Review of the technical parameters must be performed to avoid pitfalls and misdiagnosis. Absence of blood flow in the carotid artery may be related to low-flow state, poor Doppler sensitivity, limited visualization of the carotid artery, near-total occlusion, or carotid occlusion.[1-4] In this section, we review the findings and pitfalls associated with confirming the presence of a carotid artery occlusion.

Atherosclerosis is by far the most common cause of carotid artery occlusion, but fibromuscular dysplasia and arterial dissection (discussed later) are additional causes. Patients may be acutely symptomatic or asymptomatic during presentation. Most occlusions in the carotid system occur in the internal carotid artery (ICA), but occlusion also may occur in the common carotid artery (CCA) or external carotid artery (ECA). The incidence of CCA occlusion occurs approximately one-tenth as often as ICA occlusion[5] but is sufficiently common to be seen in a typical community-based vascular practice. CCA occlusion is frequently accompanied by stroke or other neurologic events but may also be encountered in the absence of neurologic symptoms.[5] The ICA may remain patent in spite of CCA occlusion (Figure 10-1), because collateral supply to the ICA develops through the ipsilateral or contralateral ECA branches. Flow reverses in the collateral ECA branches and remains cephalad in the ICA.

Optimization of transducer frequency and position is important to assess the carotid vessels. Careful optimization of the color, power, and pulsed Doppler is essential for the correct diagnosis. The color gain, color velocity scale, or pulse repetition frequency (PRF) and color wall filter must be optimized for slow flow to assess for patency. Similarly, the pulsed Doppler gain, PRF, and wall filter must be adjusted to detect blood flow in the vessel. Thorough interrogation of the vessel lumen with an ample sample volume is required.

Carotid occlusion is recognized on Doppler studies as the absence of blood flow in the carotid artery with color, power, and pulsed Doppler. No flow is seen on the spectral (pulsed Doppler) display at low PRF settings. Remember, pulsed Doppler is more sensitive than color Doppler for the detection of slow- or low-velocity flow. Do not mistake the highly damped arterial flow signals for venous flow. (Check the flow direction.) Finally, look at the occluded vessel from several transducer approaches, including the transverse plane, before concluding that flow is absent. Echogenic material may be seen filling the lumen of the artery in subacute or chronic occlusion. Fresh thrombus is hypoechoic and may require increased gray-scale settings to visualize. The vessel may be small in size in a chronic occlusion. Prominent collateral vessels may be seen from ECA branches.

There are important secondary signs of ICA occlusion. Besides the absence of flow on Doppler

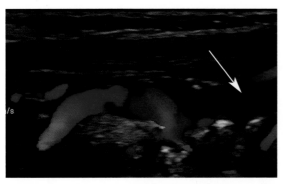

FIGURE 10-1 Common carotid artery occlusion. A color Doppler image shows absence of blood flow in the common carotid artery (*arrow*). Flow is identified in the internal carotid artery, which is supplied from the external carotid artery.

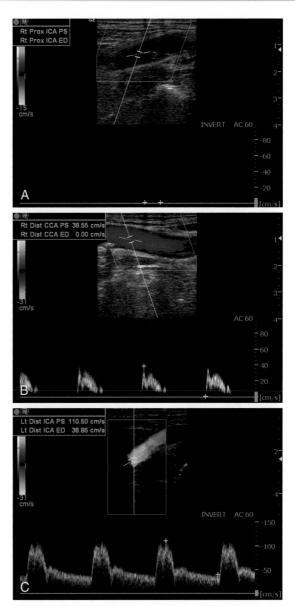

FIGURE 10-2 Internal carotid artery (ICA) occlusion. **A,** No flow is present in the ICA, and the vessel is filled with minimally echogenic material. **B,** High-resistance, low-velocity flow is noted in the common carotid artery, consistent with outflow obstruction. **C,** Slightly elevated velocities are seen in the contralateral ICA, consistent with compensatory flow.

examination, a pulsatile or rocking flow pattern is seen in the distal CCA proximal to the site of occlusion. This is related to antegrade blood flow striking the obstructing segment in systole and reversing in diastole. The Doppler waveforms obtained in the CCA show a low-velocity, high-resistance waveform with decreased, absent, or reversed flow in diastole (Figure 10-2). Increasing resistance is usually noted in the distal CCA, closer to the occlusion, because of outlet obstruction. There may be increased, low-resistance flow in the ECA as collaterals attempt to increase blood flow on the ipsilateral side. This is called "internalization of the ECA" and reflects collateral flow to the brain. Increased flow velocities may be seen in the contralateral ICA with ipsilateral ICA stenosis or occlusion. This is referred to as "compensatory flow of the contralateral ICA" and is another mechanism to increase blood flow to the brain.

False-positive diagnoses may occur when the artery is obscured by acoustic shadowing, when image quality is poor, when Doppler signals are weak, and especially when the vessel is nearly occluded and only a "trickle" of flow is present in near-total occlusion of the artery. A near occlusion of the ICA often produces the angiographic "string sign" (Figure 10-3). It is important to realize that the apparent small caliber of the arterial lumen represented by the "string" of contrast is an artifact. The string sign results from puddling of the slow-moving contrast agent in the dependent (posterior) portion of the arterial lumen with the patient supine. The distal lumen may in fact be widely patent, and the stenosis localized at the ICA origin.

Distinguishing carotid occlusion from high-grade carotid stenosis can be a challenging task for the sonographer or sonologist. Low flow in a near-total occlusion may be difficult to detect with preset Doppler parameters and requires optimization of color, power, and pulsed Doppler settings. The use of power Doppler imaging is recommended because of its sensitivity to low flow rates, and studies using color or power

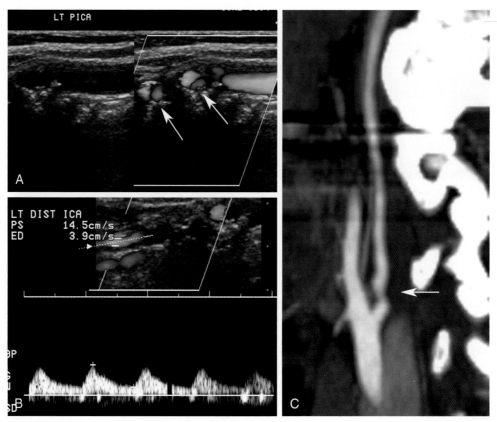

FIGURE 10-3 Near occlusion of the internal carotid artery (ICA). **A,** Irregular plaque and discontinuous color flow is noted on the gray-scale and color Doppler images of the proximal left ICA consistent with severe narrowing of the vessel. At first glance, it appears that the ICA is occluded, but with diligent scanning, flow is identified by focal areas of color. **B,** There is extension of plaque into the distal ICA on the color Doppler display, indicating diffuse disease. Pulsed Doppler of the ICA shows extremely low flow velocity and tardus-parvus waveforms consistent with severe inflow abnormality. **C,** Computed tomographic angiography demonstrates a tight narrowing in the proximal ICA consistent with a high-grade stenosis.

Doppler[6,7] report close to 100% sensitivity and specificity in the diagnosis of near occlusion of the ICA. To attain this level of accuracy, however, several technical details must be followed. First, adjust the instrument to detect minimum flow velocity. The PRF should be as low as possible, and the low-frequency filter should be minimized so that low-frequency signals are not excluded. Second, obtain the best possible view of the occluded vessel and scrutinize the lumen for any hint of blood flow. Remember that the view chosen should optimize the Doppler angle of the color flow image. Toggling between color and power Doppler is helpful especially when motion artifacts are a problem. Third, interrogate the visualized segments of the carotid artery with spectral Doppler. The signals obtained may be very weak, so high Doppler gain settings are needed.

CAROTID ARTERY DISSECTION

Arterial dissection refers to the entry of blood into the wall of the artery, separating the layers of the wall and creating a false lumen through which blood flows.[8-14] For blood to enter the wall and cause dissection, there must be a rent in the intima, which may be caused by violent trauma, iatrogenic trauma, or an underlying weakness of the muscular layer that allows the intima to tear. The location at which the wall layers separate varies. In some cases, only the intima is dissected from the wall, while in other cases, portions of the media or the media and adventitia may delaminate. Thus, the thickness of the membrane separating the true and false lumens varies. Dissection through the adventitial layer may allow pseudoaneurysm formation adjacent to the artery.

Arterial dissection produces a false lumen that may be blind-ended or may reconnect with the true lumen at a site distal to the point of dissection. A blind-ended false lumen can thrombose (occlude) and bulge into the true lumen, causing stenosis or occlusion. Blood continues to flow in the false lumen if its distal end reconnects with the true lumen. Following carotid dissection, embolization or reduced flow may cause thrombosis of intracranial vessels and brain damage. Less commonly, pseudoaneurysm occurs when dissection extends to the serosal or periadventitial layer of the carotid artery.

Carotid artery dissection usually originates in the aortic arch and extends only to the carotid bifurcation, but dissection can extend into the ICA. Three to seven percent of aortic arch dissections are complicated by stroke or transient cerebral ischemia.[12-14] Common carotid extension most commonly occurs with ascending arch dissection (Stanford's type A), which usually is related to atherosclerotic disease but also may be caused by elastic tissue degeneration, as seen with Marfan's or Ehlers-Danlos syndrome. Stanford's type B dissection, occurring distal to the aortic arch, usually does not affect the carotid arteries. Considering that neurologic symptoms are uncommon when carotid dissection extends from the aortic arch, carotid dissection is occasionally an incidental finding at carotid sonography.

Carotid dissection may also originate within the ICA, usually beginning at the skull base.[8,10] This dissection may occur either spontaneously or following trauma. Some "spontaneous" dissections may not really be spontaneous and may actually result from nonviolent trauma, such as unusually strenuous exercise or rapid neck motion. In some cases, the precipitating trauma may be unrecognized by the patient. Arterial pathology may also lead to atraumatic ICA dissection, including fibromuscular dysplasia (FMD), Marfan's syndrome, cystic medial necrosis, and Ehlers-Danlos syndrome. Unlike CCA dissection, the false lumen of ICA dissection is almost always occluded by thrombus.

Seventy percent of spontaneous ICA dissections or those following minimal trauma occur in patients 35 to 50 years of age, with an equal incidence in men and women. Systemic hypertension is present in one of three cases and is considered a predisposing factor. Presentation includes headache, neck and facial pain, hemispheric ischemic symptoms, and cranial nerve palsy. Seventy percent of ICA dissections resolve with mild or no neurologic deficit, but 25% of patients suffer disabling neurologic consequences and 5% of cases are fatal.[8,10] Spontaneous restoration of ICA flow occurs in many cases of high-grade stenosis or occlusion through retraction of the thrombus in the false lumen, relieving compression of the true lumen. Therapies employed for carotid dissection are usually antithrombotic and antihypertensive medications.

Carotid dissection resulting from violent trauma most commonly originates with direct injury to the ICA, either from stretching of the artery across cervical spine structures or from direct arterial compression by cervical spine elements or the mandible.[11,13] Trauma causes a rent in the intima and an injury that weakens the underlying wall structure, permitting delamination. Serious neurologic consequences are more common with traumatic carotid dissection than with atraumatic dissection.[10]

The ultrasound findings associated with common carotid dissection[9,10,12] may be dramatic when the intima is separated from the rest of the wall and flutters in the flow stream with each cardiac cycle (Figure 10-4). Severe flow disturbances are caused by the flapping intima (Figure 10-5). However, if the tissue between the true and false lumens is thick, the intervening membrane is stiffer and dissection is indicated simply by duplication of the carotid lumen on color Doppler.

The classic sonographic presentation of ICA dissection is a smooth, tapering stenosis (Figure 10-6) occurring in a patient who is younger than the typical patient with atherosclerotic stenosis (i.e., <50 years of age). Regardless of age, however, consider dissection in any patient with a smooth, tapering ICA stenosis *without visible atherosclerotic plaque*. In other cases of ICA dissection, the sonographic findings may be subtle and easily overlooked. The ICA lumen may be *normal* in the area just above the bifurcation if dissection beginning at the skull base does not extend down to the point of sonographic visualization. In such instances, the only detectable abnormality is increased flow resistance seen in the Doppler waveforms and possibly reduced flow velocity overall due to distal ICA obstruction. In some cases, a thin intimal flap may not be appreciated during color Doppler examination because of color-blooming artifact. That is, the color will write over the thin flap, and only the color flow disturbance is seen. The flap is

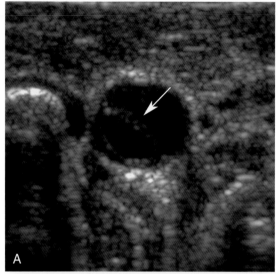

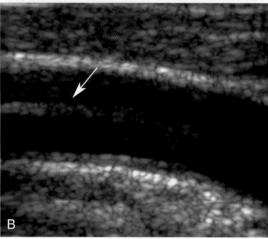

FIGURE 10-4 Common carotid artery (CCA) dissection. **A,** This short-axis, gray-scale image shows an intimal flap (*arrow*) in the lumen of the CCA. **B,** Long-axis gray-scale image of the CCA also shows the intimal flap (*arrow*).

better seen when the examiner turns off the color display and examines the vessel with gray-scale imaging. Another presentation is ICA *occlusion* with no apparent cause. Again, the absence of atherosclerotic plaque or youthful presentation should suggest the diagnosis of dissection.

When carotid dissection is recognized, the sonographer should obtain the following information. First, the extent of dissection should be ascertained, which in turn may indicate whether dissection originated in the aortic arch or the ICA. Second, the presence, direction, and characteristics of flow in the true and false lumen are documented. Third, the patency of the ECA and ICA is determined, and Doppler waveforms from both vessels are analyzed to assess the status of

the ICA circulation and the presence of ECA collateralization. Finally, if dissection causes stenosis, the degree of narrowing should be evaluated both visually (color flow) and with Doppler velocity measurements. Further evaluation with conventional arteriography, magnetic resonance angiography, or computed tomographic angiography is usually performed to appreciate the full extent of dissection.

CAROTID PSEUDOANEURYSM

A pseudoaneurysm, or false aneurysm, is a vascular mass that results from a hole in the arterial wall with circulating blood flow that is confined by soft tissue and hematoma. A true aneurysm is one in which the artery walls are intact but stretched. Carotid pseudoaneurysms[15-22] most often result from violent trauma (usually penetrating) but also occur iatrogenically from attempted percutaneous jugular vein catheterization or during therapeutic/diagnostic arteriography. Additional causes are carotid dissection or pathologies that weaken the arterial wall, such as vasculitis, fibrous dysplasia, Marfan's syndrome, and Ehlers-Danlos syndrome.

Iatrogenic and posttraumatic pseudoaneurysms are usually accompanied by considerable ecchymosis or other trauma-associated findings. Pseudoaneurysms caused by nonpenetrating trauma, arterial diseases, or catheterization may present only with a palpable, and usually pulsatile, mass, neck pain, or cranial nerve palsy. Neurologic symptoms of any kind, including cerebral ischemia/stroke, are reported in 40% of cases, and these may be accompanied by imaging evidence of cerebral infarction. Perhaps the most dramatic consequence of carotid pseudoaneurysm is rupture and life-threatening soft tissue hemorrhage, but this occurs only rarely. Until recently, therapy for carotid pseudoaneurysm has been surgery, but clinically stable lesions may now be treated nonsurgically with covered wall stents.

Sonographically, carotid pseudoaneurysms are spherical perivascular lesions into which blood is seen to circulate from the carotid artery (Figure 10-7). The size of the lesion is variable, as is the relative proportion of thrombus and circulating blood within the pseudoaneurysm. Some pseudoaneurysms may be largely thrombosed, with only a small amount of blood flow. Other lesions may show large areas of swirling blood flow with little thrombus. In all cases, however, a to-and-fro

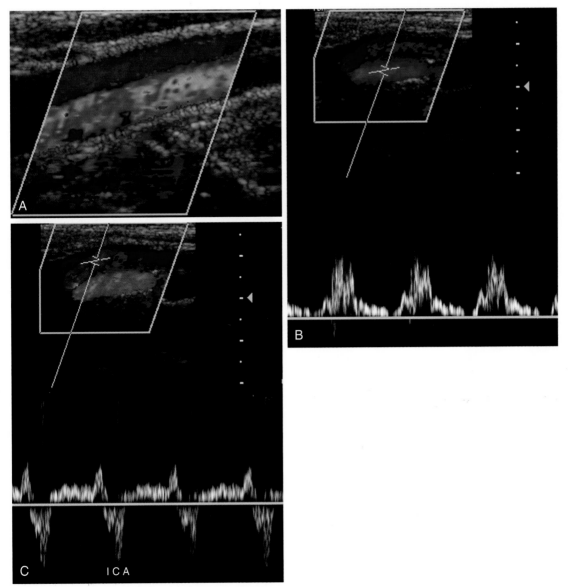

FIGURE 10-5 Common carotid artery dissection. **A,** This long-axis, color flow image shows division of the common carotid artery into two lumens. In this case, the dissection membrane was thick and moved very little with each arterial pulse. **B,** Doppler waveforms in the bottom lumen have continuous forward flow throughout the cardiac cycle, suggesting that this is the true lumen. **C,** To-and-fro flow is present in the top lumen, suggesting it is the false lumen.

flow pattern should be seen in the neck of the pseudoaneurysm on spectral Doppler examination, similar to pseudoaneurysms found in the groin. The distance of the pseudoaneurysm from the carotid artery also is variable, and the length of the "neck" connecting the two varies from one case to another. The diameter of the neck also varies. It is likely that pseudoaneurysms with short, fat necks and large arterial openings are more worrisome clinically than those with long, skinny necks, but no data have been collected to support this assumption.

In assessing a pseudoaneurysm sonographically (carotid or elsewhere), the following information should be gathered: (1) the size and location of the lesion; (2) the presence of to-and-fro flow in the pseudoaneurysm neck, confirming that the lesion is indeed a pseudoaneurysm; (3) the length and diameter of the neck; and (4) the proportion of thrombus and flowing blood. The latter two findings are potentially important, as they may influence the choice of therapy. A small pseudoaneurysm with little flow and a long, thin neck may safely occlude spontaneously and

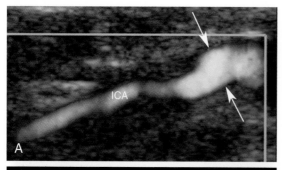

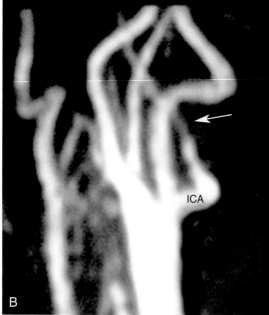

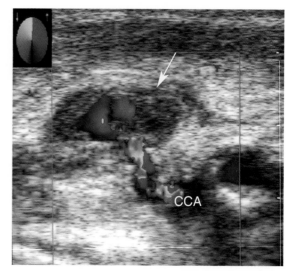

FIGURE 10-7 Carotid pseudoaneurysm. Color flow examination shows a pseudoaneurysm (*arrow*) connected with the common carotid artery (CCA) by a thin neck.

FIGURE 10-6 Spontaneous internal carotid artery (ICA) dissection. **A,** The ICA abruptly tapers from its normal size (*arrows*) at its origin. It is smoothly narrowed throughout its length (power Doppler image). **B,** Magnetic resonance angiography in the same patient shows diffuse narrowing of the ICA (*arrow*) beyond its origin, consistent with dissection.

require no therapy. Follow-up Doppler sonography is used to follow pseudoaneurysms to assess for thrombosis or interval growth.

CAROTID ARTERIOVENOUS FISTULA

A fistula is an opening that connects two epithelialized structures. In the case of an arteriovenous fistula (AVF),[15-22] communication occurs between an artery and a vein. An AVF almost always results from trauma, either violent or iatrogenic. The most likely site of occurrence is between the femoral artery and vein, because this is a common location for vascular catheterization, but AVFs can occur elsewhere, including

the carotid artery. In carotid fistulas, the cause may be blunt trauma, penetrating trauma, or attempted jugular vein catheterization. Because the carotid artery and the internal jugular vein lie side-by-side, they are subject to AVF formation, but a fistula may occur with other neck veins as well. Clinical findings associated with carotid AVF include visible neck trauma; ecchymosis; a palpable hematoma; a palpable or audible thrill; and a dilated, hyperdynamic draining vein. High-output cardiac failure may occur with large fistulas. Treatment is surgical (ligation) or interventional (covered wall stent).

The ultrasound hallmark of an arteriovenous fistula (Figure 10-8) is turbulent and, in some cases, pulsatile venous flow. The turbulence often is powerful and dramatic, and on color flow imaging, it may generate a "visible color bruit" adjacent to the vein, caused by vibration of surrounding soft tissues. A high-velocity jet is usually identified between the carotid artery and jugular vein at the site of the arteriovenous communication. However, visualization of the fistula is not always possible because the opening may be small, or turbulent effects may obscure the fistula. In the absence of these findings, the diagnosis of arteriovenous fistula should be questioned. With large AVFs, high-volume venous flow is apparent, as indicated by high-Doppler-velocity measurements. Ancillary findings that may accompany an AVF include soft tissue fluid (ecchymosis), a hematoma, or a pseudoaneurysm.

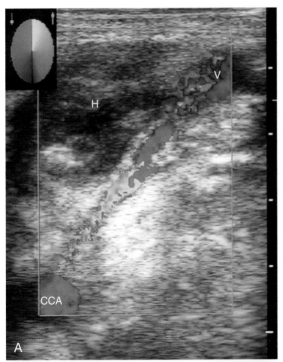

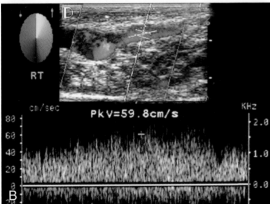

FIGURE 10-8 Carotid arteriovenous fistula. **A,** This transverse color flow image shows a lengthy tract connecting the common carotid artery (CCA) with a superficial vein (V). A soft tissue hematoma (H) also is visible. **B,** Doppler interrogation of the draining vein shows turbulent, high-velocity flow (almost 60 cm/sec).

Fibromuscular Dysplasia

FMD[23-25] is a disorder of unknown etiology that affects medium-sized arteries. Women are affected by the disease three times more commonly than men, and the disorder usually presents in adults 25 to 50 years old. Although familial association is reported in 11% of cases, FMD is not a genetic disorder in strict terms. The renal arteries are the most common site for FMD, with the internal carotid artery a distant second. Other medium-sized arteries are occasionally involved. The most common presenting clinical symptom in FMD patients is systemic hypertension, caused by renal artery stenosis. With carotid involvement, transient cerebral ischemia is the usual presentation, although stroke can also occur. About 30% of FMD patients have aneurysms of the intracranial cerebral arteries; hence, an additional presentation may be cerebral hemorrhage.

FMD is a dysplastic disorder, not degenerative or inflammatory. The pathologic process is overgrowth of smooth muscle cells and fibrous tissue within the arterial wall. In the most common form, seen in 85% of cases, the media is primarily involved, and in the remaining cases, either the adventitia or the intima is the primary site. The medial form has a characteristic "string-of-beads" angiographic appearance (Figure 10-9, C) caused by alternating areas of medial fibroplasia and focal aneurysmal dilatation. Sonographically, this classic FMD form produces a series of ridges in the arterial wall (usually the ICA), as shown in Figure 10-9, A. This may be best seen with power Doppler imaging. However, there are two other imaging presentations of FMD: a long, tubular ICA stenosis or asymmetric ICA outpouching. In all cases, however, the ICA is selectively involved, and the affected area tends to be relatively distal in the ICA.

When FMD exhibits the classic "string-of-beads" appearance, differentiation from other carotid pathology generally is not difficult. The "long stenosis" presentation is a different story, however. This form is not specific and may be mistaken for atherosclerosis or dissection. The latter is particularly problematic, as ICA dissection is said to complicate about 20% of FMD cases. Differentiation from atherosclerosis generally is on the basis of age, as FMD usually presents at a younger age than does atherosclerosis, and location, since lesions due to FMD occur 1 cm or more above the carotid bifurcation. The absence of calcified plaque also suggests the diagnosis of FMD. Many cases of FMD will require correlation with arteriography, magnetic resonance angiography, or computed tomographic angiography for confirmation or definitive diagnosis.

Carotid Body Tumor

The normal carotid body is a tiny ovoid structure 1 to 1.5 mm in size located in the adventitia of the carotid bifurcation. The function of

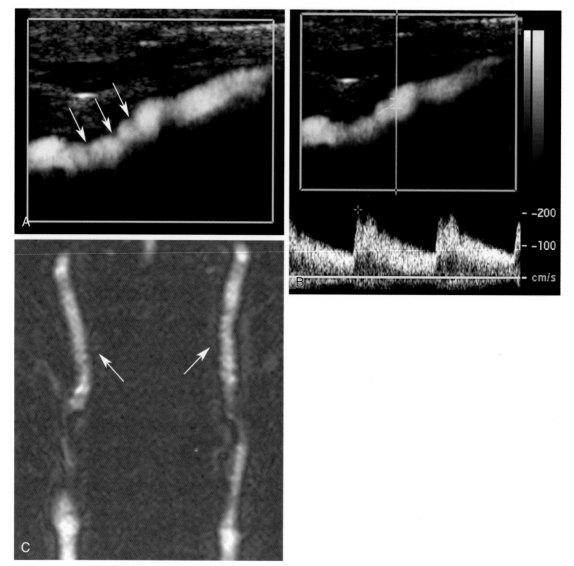

FIGURE 10-9 Carotid fibromuscular dysplasia. **A,** This power Doppler image shows a series of ridges (*arrows*) along the lumen of the internal carotid artery characteristic of fibromuscular dysplasia. **B,** Spectral Doppler shows moderate flow disturbance and elevation of flow velocity (about 200 cm/sec). **C,** Magnetic resonance angiography shows the classic ridged appearance in both internal carotid arteries (*arrows*).

the carotid body is not well understood, but it is a component of the autonomic nervous system that participates in the control of arterial pH, blood gas levels, and blood pressure.[11]

Carotid body tumors[11,26,27] are paragangliomas of relatively low malignant potential that arise in the carotid body. The most common presentation is a palpable neck mass with headache. Neck pain is the second most common presentation. These are rare tumors, and up to 25% are initially thought to be enlarged lymph nodes before surgical biopsy (which can lead to substantial hemorrhage of these highly vascular tumors). Although the malignant potential of

carotid body tumors is small, resection is standard therapy to prevent local adverse effects, such as laryngeal nerve palsy and invasion of the carotid arteries. Untreated, they may cause carotid stenosis or occlusion or may result in carotid rupture. Local recurrence occurs in 6% of cases and distant metastasis in 2% of cases.

On sonographic examination, carotid body tumors are highly vascular masses nestled within the "crotch" of the carotid bifurcation, as seen in Figure 10-10. In some cases, the tumor may encase or surround the ECA or ICA, causing stenosis or potentially complicating surgical excision. It is useful, therefore, to assess the relationship of

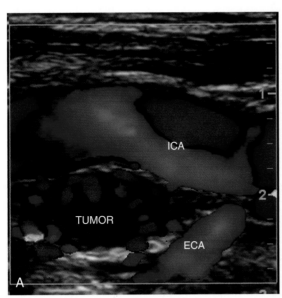
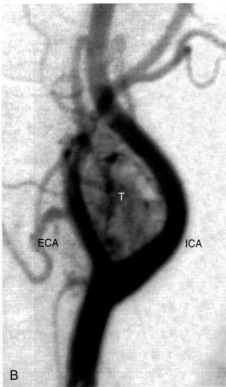

FIGURE 10-10 Carotid body tumor. **A,** This longitudinal color flow image shows a homogeneous, hypoechoic tumor (*TUMOR*), which splays the internal carotid artery (ICA) and external carotid artery (ECA) branches. Blood flow *(color areas)* was easily detected in the tumor. **B,** Carotid arteriography in the lateral projection shows the highly vascular nature of the mass (*T*).

the tumor to the bifurcation vessels. Ultrasound may also be used to follow the growth of small tumors if surgery is not anticipated (e.g., in an older adult with limited life expectancy or a poor surgical candidate). Arteriography is usually performed preoperatively, and the tumor may be embolized angiographically through ECA feeders to reduce vascularity in anticipation of surgery.

DIFFICULT CAROTID CASES

The editors of this text have, over the years, encountered cases that have surprised and challenged us or others. Our goal here is to present examples of some tricky cases so that, hopefully, the readers of this text will recognize the pertinent features of these cases.

CASE 1

Introduction

This 68-year-old man presented with a right cervical bruit. Doppler evaluation demonstrates high velocities approaching 500 cm/sec in the right ICA. Elevated velocities are noted in the left common and internal carotid arteries. These findings are shown in Figure 10-11. Please review this information and determine the severity of the left ICA stenosis.

Analysis

Elevated peak systolic velocity (PSV; 496 cm/sec) and end-diastolic velocity (185 cm/sec) are consistent with greater than 80% stenosis of the proximal right ICA. At first glance, the PSV (172 cm/sec) in the left ICA suggests a 50% to 69% stenosis, but notice that the color flow image is normal and does not suggest that level of narrowing. The PSV in the distal left CCA is 132 cm/sec. If you calculate the PSV ratio (ICA/CCA), you get 1.3, which is well below the 2.0 level usually seen with narrowing of 50% or more. The reason for the spuriously high velocities is the contralateral ICA stenosis. The PSV in the CCA is well above the normal level, which rarely surpasses 100 cm/sec. This phenomenon is called *compensatory flow* through the normal or less

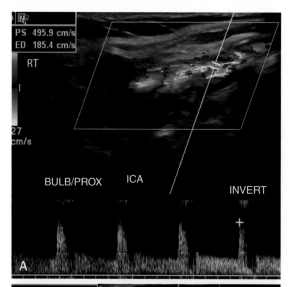

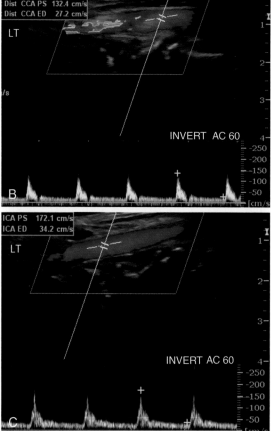

FIGURE 10-11 Case 1. **A,** Right internal carotid artery (ICA) color flow image with spectral display. **B,** Left distal common carotid artery (CCA) color image with Doppler spectrum. **C,** Left ICA color image with Doppler spectrum.

severely involved carotid artery. The carotid artery opposite the high-grade stenosis or occlusion demonstrates increased PSVs, which appear out of proportion to the degree of narrowing identified on gray-scale and color Doppler examination. The systolic velocity ratio (ICA/CCA) performs better, therefore, than the ICA PSV alone in grading stenosis severity. In this case, the left carotid vessels are serving as collaterals that make up for diminished right carotid blood flow. The higher volume of blood flow skews all velocities upward in the left carotid system, including the ICA stenosis velocity. One important clue to the diagnosis of compensatory flow is elevation of PSVs throughout the entire contralateral CCA and ICA.

Diagnosis

High-grade (greater than 80%) stenosis of the right proximal ICA and less than 50% left ICA stenosis with increased flow velocity due to collateralization (compensatory flow).

Points to Remember

1. High-flow states, regardless of cause, increase PSV, possibly causing overestimation of stenosis severity.
2. Always look at the "big picture," not just an isolated velocity measurement. Review all the velocity measurements for each carotid artery. Think about what is happening in the entire carotid/vertebral system, and remember that altered flow physiology in one vessel may affect Doppler findings in other vessels.
3. Always consider the systolic velocity ratio when you diagnose stenosis severity. This is particularly valuable for high- and low-flow states.
4. Always compare the spectral Doppler, gray-scale, and color flow findings. If they do not correspond, ask yourself, "Does this make sense?"

CASE 2

Introduction

This 78-year-old man presented with a transient ischemic attack. Doppler waveforms for review include the right CCA near its origin and bilateral ICAs (Figure 10-12). What side is the abnormality on? Why are the waveforms abnormal? The right vertebral artery waveform is also submitted for your analysis. How do you put this study together? Where must the lesion be for all the findings to make sense?

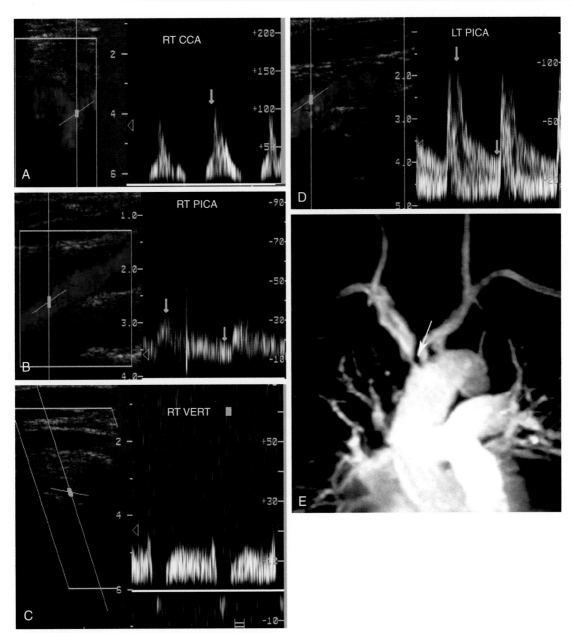

FIGURE 10-12 Case 2. **A,** Right common carotid artery (CCA) Doppler spectrum obtained near its origin. **B,** Right proximal internal carotid artery (PICA) Doppler spectrum. **C,** Right vertebral artery (VERT) Doppler spectrum. **D,** Left proximal internal carotid artery (PICA) Doppler spectrum. **E,** Magnetic resonance angiography demonstrates innominate artery stenosis (*arrow*).

Analysis

Note that all of the Doppler waveforms on the right side are damped and of lower velocity. The left ICA is normal in appearance and velocity. This pulsus parvus (poor amplitude) and tardus (late upstroke) appearance always indicates that you are downstream from a stenosis. Because the findings are unilateral, they indicate that the stenosis is on the right only.

The vertebral artery waveform is biphasic, usually indicating a subclavian lesion. In this case, to account for all the findings, the lesion should be in the proximal, nonvisualized segment of the arterial tree and must be involving the innominate artery since this is the only vessel that would produce flow abnormalities in both the carotid and vertebral arteries on the right.

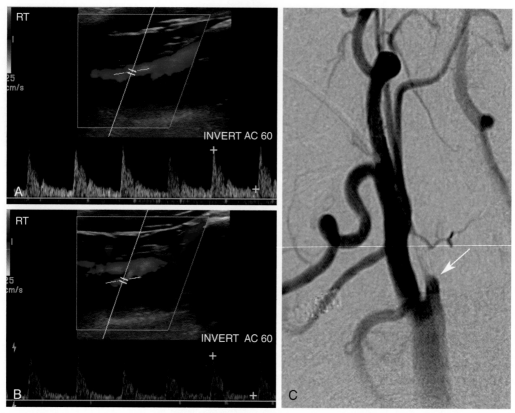

FIGURE 10-13 Case 3. **A** and **B,** Right carotid bifurcation branches. **C,** Right carotid arteriogram. Arrow indicates the stump of the occluded internal carotid artery.

Diagnosis

High-grade, innominate artery stenosis.

Points to Remember

Important arterial pathology may exist that is outside the range of direct carotid visualization (either proximal or distal). Such pathology is revealed only by Doppler findings.

1. Always compare the waveform shape and Doppler velocity measurements from both carotid arteries side to side. Differences may not be as obvious as in this case, but even subtle differences should be treated as suspicious.
2. Stenoses occur at the aortic origin of the brachiocephalic arteries. The most frequent sites are the innominate, left common carotid, and left subclavian arteries.
3. Biphasic flow in the vertebral artery suggests a subclavian lesion ("subclavian steal"). If the flow abnormalities include the ipsilateral right carotid arteries, think innominate lesion.

CASE 3

Introduction

This 73-year-old woman suffered a right hemispheric stroke. Take a look at the Doppler signals derived from the right carotid bifurcation branches (Figure 10-13, *A* and *B*). Decide which is the ICA and which is the ECA *before* you look at the angiogram in the same figure (Figure 10-13, *C*).

Analysis

The right ICA is occluded, but this fact was missed by the inexperienced sonographer and sonologist involved with this case. It is easy, in retrospect, to understand why this misdiagnosis occurred. The two Doppler waveforms shown in Figure 10-13 are virtually identical because they both are from ECA branches. Unfortunately, the similarity of the waveforms was not appreciated. In addition, the sonographer did not tap on the superficial temporal artery. If she had, the fact that both vessels were, in fact, ECA branches may have been apparent.

The pulsatility of the Doppler waveforms is another observation that might have prevented this error. Both waveforms are *more* pulsatile than normally seen in the ICA.

Finally, an anatomic factor contributing to the error was the inability to identify the occluded ICA. Over time, the occluded ICA may become fibrotic and blend into the surrounding tissues.

Diagnosis

ICA occlusion.

Points to Remember

1. The Doppler signals in the ICA and ECA should always sound different, and the waveforms should always look different.
2. The sonographer should "tap" (use a finger to rapidly press and release the palpable pulse) the preauricular branch of the superficial temporal artery in front of the ear to identify the ECA, and the resulting Doppler spectrum should be recorded as part of each carotid ultrasound examination.
3. If you cannot decide if one bifurcation vessel is the ECA and the other is the ICA, *do not guess!* It is better to say that you are unsure than to make a diagnostic error. When in doubt, our sonographers label the carotid branches A and B, rather than ECA and ICA, and we, the physicians, take it from there. Basically, we have two options: bring the patient back and look for ourselves, or refer the patient for another imaging study such as magnetic resonance or computed tomographic angiography.
4. Misidentification of the ICA and ECA can be very important in cases of stenosis. Patient management may be inappropriate if an ECA stenosis is attributed to the ICA or vice versa. (In the case presented here, the misdiagnosis did not affect clinical management, as the ICA was occluded.)

CASE 4

Introduction

A screening carotid ultrasound was ordered on this 55-year-old man before cardiac surgery. With gray-scale and color flow imaging, only a few small plaques were seen in the cervical portions of the carotid arteries. Please review the Doppler waveform findings shown in Figure 10-14 and make a diagnosis.

Analysis

The Doppler waveforms are uniformly damped with a tardus-parvus appearance, and flow velocity is low in all areas, indicating a "global" physiologic disorder. The two principal considerations are aortic valve disease and poor myocardial function. In this case, the patient was awaiting aortic valve replacement for severe aortic stenosis. Had the problem been severe aortic insufficiency, a to-and-fro flow pattern with diastolic reversal might be seen in the Doppler waveforms.

Diagnosis

Aortic valve stenosis causing global damping of carotid Doppler waveforms.

Points to Remember

1. Global low velocity and damping are usually caused by aortic valve disease or poor myocardial function. Tardus-parvus waveforms suggest proximal stenosis, obviously involving the thoracic aorta since all branches are affected.
2. Cardiac function can profoundly affect carotid Doppler findings. If this patient had a carotid stenosis, velocities in the stenosis would have been substantially lower than in an individual without heart disease. As in the case of compensatory flow (see Case 1), the ICA/CCA systolic velocity ratios approximate the level of disease better than ICA peak velocity used independently.
3. Always consider the "global" view of cardiovascular physiology when interpreting carotid ultrasound studies.

CASE 5

Introduction

This 58-year-old man presented with syncope. Look at the findings presented in Figure 10-15, and grade the left ICA lesion.

Assessment

Color Doppler imaging of the left ICA demonstrates an area of aliasing consistent with increased velocities and focal stenosis. The PSV in the mid ICA is 158 cm/sec. No focal plaque or significant luminal narrowing is seen in this region of the vessel. The PSV in the distal CCA is 79 cm/sec. The ICA/CCA ratio is 2:1. The velocity measurements and ratio suggest a 50% to 69%

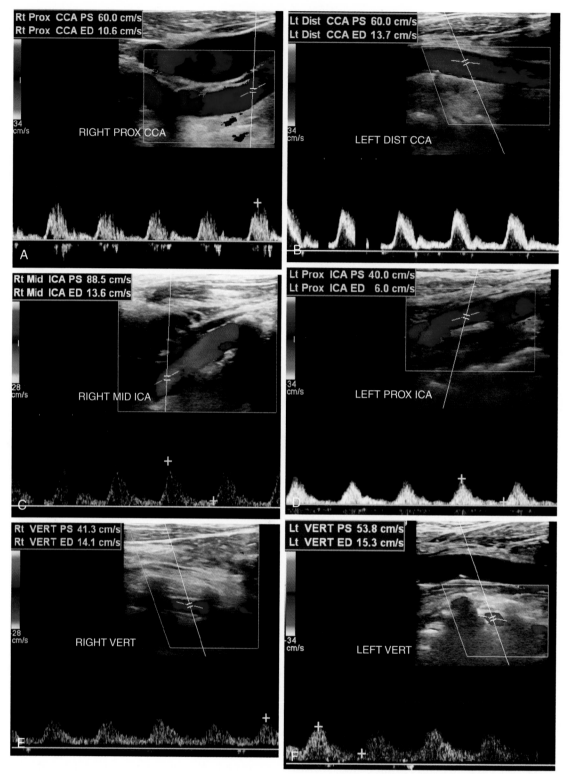

FIGURE 10-14 Case 4. **A** and **B,** Right and left common carotid artery (CCA) Doppler spectra. **C** and **D,** Right and left internal carotid artery (ICA) Doppler spectra. **E** and **F,** Right and left vertebral artery (VERT) samples.

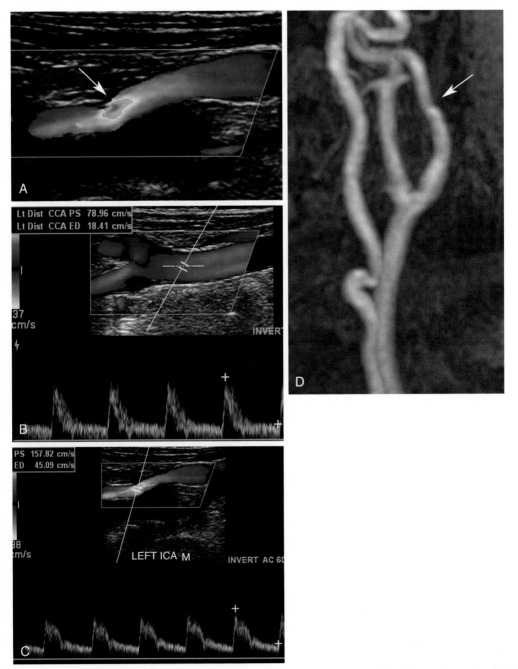

FIGURE 10-15 Case 5. **A,** Color Doppler image of the left internal carotid artery (ICA). **B,** Color and pulsed Doppler images of the left common carotid artery (CCA). **C,** Color image and pulsed Doppler waveforms of the left ICA. **D,** Magnetic resonance angiogram of the left carotid artery.

stenosis of the left ICA. No plaque or increased velocity is seen in the right carotid artery.

The confusing thing about this case is the increased velocity in the mid ICA without corresponding plaque. This is not a typical location for atherosclerotic disease. Moreover, the vessel takes a turn at the site of aliasing, suggesting tortuosity or kinking. Magnetic resonance imaging/magnetic resonance angiography was performed as part of the syncope workup.

Diagnosis

Kinking of the mid portion of the ICA, confirmed at magnetic resonance angiography.

Points to Remember

1. Most stenoses of the ICA occur at the bifurcation and proximal segments of the ICA.
2. Stenosis is usually characterized by luminal narrowing and plaque.
3. Focal elevation in velocity can occur in a region of vessel tortuosity or kinking.
4. Consider correlation with another study when there is discordance between diagnostic criteria.

CASE 6

Introduction

This 70-year-old patient presents with a right cerebrovascular accident. Color Doppler imaging demonstrates no evidence of focal stenosis in the left CCA or ICA (Figure 10-16). Pulsed Doppler reveals low-velocity flow in the ICA with a normal systolic upstroke. Can you determine the location of the lesion?

Assessment

Gray-scale evaluation of the CCA and ICA reveals no evidence of significant atherosclerotic plaque. Color Doppler demonstrates a homogeneous flow pattern in the ICA without focal aliasing to suggest a stenosis. Pulsed Doppler reveals normal velocity in the CCA with abnormally elevated resistance and a normal upstroke consistent with an outflow lesion. Waveforms from the ICA show a marked decrease in PSV and increasing resistance with a normal systolic upstroke, also consistent with distal disease.

Diagnosis

Significant stenosis of the supraclinoid ICA, confirmed at magnetic resonance angiography.

Points to Remember

1. Unusually low velocities in the ICA without significant plaque may be related to an inflow or outflow lesion. Check the contralateral side to assess for normal or abnormal flow. If the flow abnormality is bilateral, consider cardiac disease or aortic lesion.
2. Low-velocity, low-resistance flow with a damped (tardus-parvus) appearance usually indicates an inflow lesion.
3. Low-velocity, high-resistance flow with a normal systolic upstroke is highly suggestive of an outflow lesion.

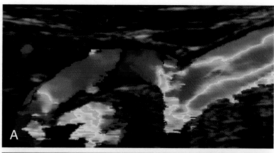

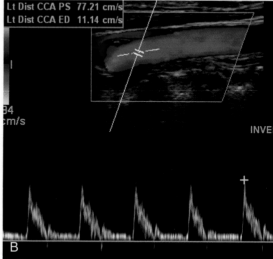

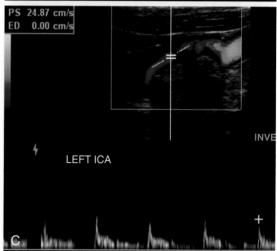

FIGURE 10-16 Case 6. **A,** Color Doppler image of the left internal carotid artery (ICA). **B,** Pulsed Doppler waveforms of the left common carotid artery (CCA). **C,** Pulsed Doppler samples of the left ICA.

REFERENCES

1. Middleton WD, Foley WD, Lawson TL: Color flow Doppler imaging of carotid artery abnormalities, *AJR Am J Roentgenol* 150:419–425, 1988.
2. Erickson SJ, et al: Color Doppler evaluation of arterial stenoses and occlusions involving the neck and thoracic inlet, *Radiographics* 9:389–406, 1989.

3. Hallam MJ, Reid JM, Cooperberg PL: Color flow Doppler and conventional duplex scanning of the carotid bifurcation: Prospective, double-blinded correlative study, *AJR Am J Roentgenol* 152:1101–1105, 1989.

4. Steinke W, Kloetzsch C, Hennerici M: Carotid artery disease assessed by color Doppler flow imaging: Correlation with standard Doppler sonography and angiography, *AJR Am J Roentgenol* 154:1061–1068, 1998.

5. Chang YJ, et al: Common carotid artery occlusion: Evaluation with duplex sonography, *AJNR Am J Neuroradiol* 16:1099–1105, 1995.

6. Lee DH, et al: Duplex and color Doppler flow sonography of occlusion and near occlusion of the carotid artery, *AJNR Am J Neuroradiol* 17:1267–1274, 1996.

7. Mattos MA, et al: Identifying total carotid occlusion with colour flow duplex scanning, *Eur J Vasc Surg* 6:204–210, 1992.

8. Petro GR, et al: Spontaneous dissection of the cervical internal carotid artery: Correlation of arteriography, CT, and pathology, *AJNR Am J Neuroradiol* 148:393–398, 1987.

9. Hennerei M, Steinke W, Rautenberg W: High-resistance Doppler flow pattern in extracranial carotid dissection, *Arch Neurol* 46:670–672, 1989.

10. Provenzale JM: Dissection of the internal carotid and vertebral arteries: Imaging features, *AJR Am J Roentgenol* 165:1099–1104, 1995.

11. Cottrell ED, Smith LL: Management of uncommon lesions affecting the extracranial vessels. In Rutherford RB, editor: *Vascular Surgery*, vol II, Philadelphia, 1995, WB Saunders, pp 1622–1636.

12. Zielin´ski T, et al: Persistent dissection of carotid artery in patients operated on for type A acute aortic dissection—carotid ultrasound follow-up, *Int J Cardiol* 70:133–139, 1999.

13. Sturzenegger M, et al: Ultrasound findings in carotid artery dissection: analysis of 43 patients, *Neurology* 45:691–698, 1995.

14. Walker PJ, Sarris GE, Miller DC: Peripheral vascular manifestations of acute aortic dissection. In Rutherford RB, editor: *Vascular Surgery*, vol II, Philadelphia, 1995, WB Saunders, pp 1087–1102.

15. El-Sabrout R, Cooley DA: Extracranial carotid artery aneurysms: Texas Heart Institute experience, *J Vasc Surg* 31:702–712, 2000.

16. Kuzniec S, et al: Diagnosis of limbs and neck arterial trauma using duplex ultrasonography, *Cardiovasc Surg* 6:358–366, 1998.

17. Munera F, et al: Penetrating neck injuries: helical CT angiography for initial evaluation, *Radiology* 216:356–362, 2000.

18. Takeuchi Y, et al: Differential diagnosis of pulsatile neck masses by Doppler color flow imaging, *Ann Otol Rhinol Laryngol* 104:633–638, 1995.

19. Needleman L, Nack TL: Vascular and nonvascular masses, *J Vasc Technol* 18:299–306, 1994.

20. Goldberg BB: Iatrogenic femoral arteriovenous fistula: Diagnosis with cold Doppler imaging, *Radiology* 170:749–752, 1989.

21. Biffl WL, et al: Treatment-related outcomes from blunt cerebrovascular injuries: Importance of routine follow-up arteriography, *Ann Surg* 235:699–706, 2002.

22. Redekop G, Marotta T, Weill A: Treatment of traumatic aneurysmal and arteriovenous fistulas of the skull base by using endovascular stents, *J Neurosurg* 95:412–419, 2001.

23. Moore WS: *Vascular surgery: a comprehensive review*, ed 6, Philadelphia, 1999, WB Saunders, 142–143, 295, 306–307.

24. Van Damme H, Sakalihasan N, Limet R: Fibromuscular dysplasia of the internal carotid artery: Personal experience with 13 cases and literature review, *Acta Chir Belg* 99:163–168, 1999.

25. Stewart MT, et al: The natural history of carotid dysplasia, *J Vasc Surg* 3:305–310, 1986.

26. Rao AB, et al: Paragangliomas of the head and neck: Radiologic-pathologic correlation, *Radiographics* 19:1605–1632, 1999.

27. Muhm M, et al: Diagnostic and therapeutic approaches to carotid body tumors: Review of 24 patients, *Arch Surg* 132:279–284, 1997.

ULTRASOUND ASSESSMENT OF THE VERTEBRAL ARTERIES

PHILLIP J. BENDICK, PhD

The relationship between carotid atherosclerotic disease and lateralizing symptoms of cerebrovascular ischemia, such as transient ischemic attacks, amaurosis fugax, and stroke, is well established, and carotid endarterectomy has been shown to be effective in the management of selected groups of these patients. However, no consistently successful diagnostic and management techniques are available for those patients who present with a more confusing clinical picture of nonlocalizing symptoms of transient cerebral ischemia, such as blurred vision, ataxia, vertigo, syncope, or generalized extremity weakness. It can be difficult to determine whether the symptoms arise from carotid artery thromboembolic disease, generalized ischemia resulting from carotid or vertebrobasilar artery occlusive disease (or both), or some factor not directly related to the cerebral vasculature, such as cardiac disease.[1-5] Symptomatology of posterior circulation ischemia is typically multiple and varied, and the potential contribution of vertebrobasilar insufficiency may be difficult to evaluate (Box 11-1). Although treatment of vertebral artery disease can be a successful and relatively safe procedure, the selection of appropriate patients for such reconstruction can be confounded by the previously mentioned diagnostic uncertainties, as well as by the fact that symptoms of posterior circulation ischemia frequently improve following carotid artery endarterectomy or reconstruction.[6,7]

Angiography, performed on the basis of the patient's clinical history data, historically has been the definitive diagnostic procedure to identify significant vertebrobasilar obstructive lesions.[8,9] The use of duplex ultrasound as a primary diagnostic technique for the diagnosis of vertebrobasilar insufficiency has been limited. Routine evaluation of the vertebral arteries is an accreditation requirement for extracranial cerebrovascular examinations by the Intersocietal Commission for the Accreditation of Vascular Laboratories,* as well as other accrediting organizations, but this assessment typically is limited to the presence or absence of flow and flow direction. Standard textbooks have limited reference to the vertebral arteries; for example, in Strandness's textbook[10] on vascular disorders, only two paragraphs of the entire chapter on extracranial arterial disease deal with the vertebral arteries, and then only to discuss qualitative waveform evaluation.

Duplex ultrasound has been shown to be an effective noninvasive technique for the evaluation of the extracranial segments of the vertebral arteries.[11-13] Adequate imaging and quantitative spectral Doppler velocity data can be obtained from a portion of the midsegment of the extracranial vertebral arteries in more than 98% of patients and vessels.[14,15] It is possible to collect imaging and spectral Doppler velocity data from the origin of the right vertebral artery in more than 80% of patients and from the origin of the left vertebral artery in approximately two-thirds of patients. The sections below describe appropriate duplex ultrasound evaluation techniques, the qualitative and quantitative data that can be obtained, and the interpretation and possible clinical significance of these results.

EXAMINATION TECHNIQUES

Because most hemodynamically significant lesions of the vertebral arteries occur at their origin (Region V1, defined as the segment from the origin of the vertebral artery to its entrance into the foramen of the transverse process, which occurs at the level of the sixth cervical vertebra in approximately 90% of cases), it would seem that this would be the logical site to begin the duplex ultrasound examination. Anatomically, however,

---

*6021 University Boulevard, Suite 500, Ellicott City, MD 21043; www.icavl.org.

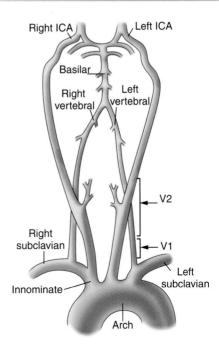

FIGURE 11-1 Normal cerebrovascular anatomy. The approximate locations of the V1 and V2 segments of the vertebral artery are shown. ICA, internal carotid artery.

this approach can be technically difficult (if not technically impossible) in as many as one-third of patients, because visualization of the origin of the vertebral artery may be obstructed by the clavicle, which interferes with the necessary probe position. Occasionally (in 3%–5% of cases) the left vertebral artery originates directly from the aorta. In addition, as the first major branch of the subclavian artery, the vertebral artery origin may be markedly tortuous, making proper angle correction for velocity measurements very difficult. Finally, the origin and proximal segment of the vertebral artery may be confused with other large branches arising from the proximal subclavian artery, such as the thyrocervical trunk.

A more reliable approach to assessment of the vertebral arteries is to initially evaluate the vessel near its midsegment, or Region V2 (the segment of the vertebral artery that courses cranially through the foramina to the transverse process of the axis). (Figure 11-1) This segment of vessel is typically quite straight, with minimal tortuosity; does not have any significant taper or diameter changes; has no immediately adjacent blood vessels, except the vertebral vein; and has no significant branching segments that would make flow velocity measurements unreliable. In addition, Region V2 of the vertebral arteries is only rarely involved with atherosclerotic obstructive disease. Further distally, the vertebral artery may be interrogated using a suboccipital approach and transcranial Doppler techniques, but Region V3

(the segment that extends from the artery's exit at the axis to its entrance into the spinal canal) and Region V4 (extending from the point of perforation of the dura to the origin of the basilar artery) are generally inaccessible to duplex ultrasound during an extracranial cerebrovascular examination.

Imaging of Region V2 is most easily accomplished by first obtaining a good longitudinal view of the mid–common carotid artery at the approximate level of the third through fifth cervical vertebrae. Once this image has been obtained, a slight lateral rocking motion of the probe will bring the vertebral artery into view (see Video 11-1). The vertebral artery is readily identified by the prominent anatomic landmarks of the transverse processes of the cervical spine, which appear as bright echogenic lines in the image, beyond which deeper-lying tissues are obscured by acoustic shadowing (Figure 11-2). Between these anechoic, rectangular-shaped regions of acoustic shadowing lies an anechoic band representing the vertebral artery, as seen with grayscale sonography. Color flow Doppler imaging helps to identify the vertebral artery by the pulsatile pattern of color flow within the anechoic band. The color flow image also distinguishes the vertebral artery from the adjacent vertebral

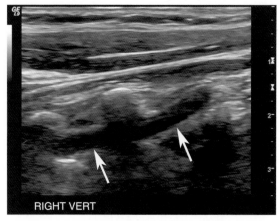

FIGURE 11-2 Normal vertebral artery. Longitudinal gray-scale image of a normal vertebral artery segment *(arrows)* at the approximate level of C3 to C5 (Region V2) showing the acoustic shadowing from the adjacent bony transverse processes of the spine.

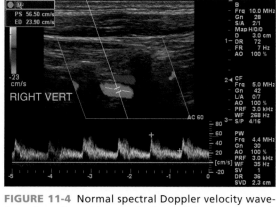

FIGURE 11-4 Normal spectral Doppler velocity waveform from the midsegment of a vertebral artery. Peak systole is well defined, with a peak systolic velocity (PSV) of 56 cm/sec. Sustained antegrade flow is present throughout the cardiac cycle, similar to the normal flow patterns in the internal carotid artery.

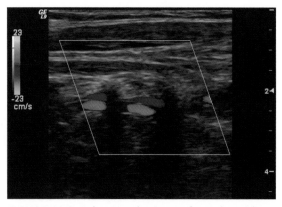

FIGURE 11-3 Color Doppler image from the midsegments of a normal vertebral artery and vein, with the artery color coded red (flow from right to left, toward the brain) and the vertebral vein color coded blue. Note the dropout of color Doppler flow signals in the regions of acoustic shadowing caused by the transverse processes of the spine.

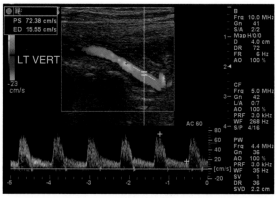

FIGURE 11-5 Color and spectral Doppler image at the origin of a normal vertebral artery. The overall waveform has a sharp systolic upstroke and is characteristic of low-resistance flow; note that peak systole is mildly exaggerated relative to end diastole (compare to Figure 11-4) secondary to the local hemodynamic effects at a site of vessel branching.

vein (Figure 11-3), but typically the gray-scale image, with its anatomic landmarks, is sufficient for identifying the vertebral artery. Once an image of the artery has been obtained, the spectral Doppler sample volume can be placed in midvessel (Figure 11-4) to obtain qualitative and quantitative data for the evaluation of local hemodynamics. If these data appear abnormal, the vertebral artery can be followed back toward its origin as far as possible (Figure 11-5), using combined gray-scale and color Doppler imaging, to assess flow hemodynamics in the proximal segment of the artery.

VERTEBRAL ARTERY HEMODYNAMICS: QUALITATIVE ASSESSMENT

NORMAL FINDINGS

Qualitatively, the spectral Doppler velocity waveform in the vertebral artery should appear as a scaled-down version of the normal flow signal in the internal carotid artery, since both directly supply the low-resistance intracranial vascular system. The waveform should have a well-defined systolic peak with sustained flow throughout diastole, as seen in Figure 11-4. There is wide variability in the absolute peak systolic velocity in normal patients, with a range of 20 cm/sec to 60 cm/sec.[13] Up to three-quarters of all patients have a dominant vertebral artery, which demonstrates larger size and higher flows than the contralateral side, most often occurring on the left side.

ELEVATED VELOCITY AND STENOSIS

Abnormalities in vertebral artery flow hemodynamics caused by stenotic lesions can be detected readily from the spectral Doppler waveform characteristics and flow velocity data. The few prevalence and natural history studies on atherosclerotic stenosis of the vertebral artery that are available show that the vast majority of these lesions, greater than 90%, occur at the origin.[16] Visible narrowing on color flow examination accompanied by high-velocity color aliasing and the mosaic pattern characteristic of poststenotic disturbed flow are findings indicating vertebral artery stenosis. The confirmatory evidence is high-velocity flow documented with spectral Doppler measurements. No velocity criteria are available to define the severity of vertebral artery stenoses; however, more than a focal doubling of velocity implies a greater than 50% diameter reduction. Ultrasound diagnosis of stenosis at the vertebral artery origin is complicated by the frequent occurrence of considerable tortuosity in the proximal 1 to 2 cm of the vertebral artery (Figure 11-6). Because of tortuosity, disturbed flow is commonly seen in the nonstenotic proximal vertebral artery, and kinking of the vessel may occur, generating elevated flow velocities. Tortuosity also may render angle-corrected Doppler velocity measurements unreliable. Considering these problems, ultrasound assessment of origin stenoses of the vertebral arteries must be considered qualitative. If damped flow signals are present distal to the stenosis, then one can be reasonably confident that the lesion is hemodynamically significant. Otherwise, the findings must often be regarded as suggestive of hemodynamic significance, and confirmation must be sought with angiography. Correct diagnosis is important, as modern surgical and interventional techniques have made it possible to repair most proximal vertebral artery stenoses with good success.

There are a number of other hemodynamic conditions that might lead to abnormally strong or highly accelerated flow patterns in the vertebral arteries. The most common was mentioned earlier, namely, the presence of a dominant

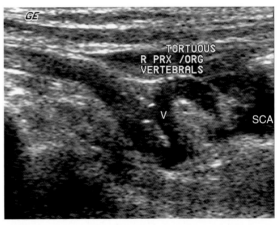

FIGURE 11-6 Longitudinal gray-scale image of the origin of a normal vertebral artery. Note the tortuosity of the proximal segment (Region V1) of the artery. PRX/ORG, origin and proximal segments of the vertebral artery.

vertebral artery, most often seen on the left side. Significantly increased vertebral artery velocities also may be seen when one or both vertebral arteries are the compensatory mechanism for occlusive disease elsewhere in the cerebrovascular system (Figure 11-7). This may be a consequence of occlusion or near occlusion of an internal carotid artery or the contralateral vertebral artery, or it may represent compensatory flow from a subclavian steal in the contralateral vertebral artery. Rarely, high-velocity turbulent flow patterns may be detected in the midsegment of a vertebral artery because of extrinsic compression from the bony spine (often associated with changes in head or neck position, frequently referred to as "bow hunter's syndrome"), luminal narrowing secondary to vasculitis, or because of a mid–vertebral artery atherosclerotic stenosis. Vertebral artery dissection is not commonly associated with elevated flow velocities in the absence of significant narrowing in either the true or the false lumen (Figures 11-8 and 11-9).

ABSENCE OF FLOW

The absence of a flow signal in a vertebral artery that is adequately imaged is diagnostic of a vertebral artery occlusion, similar to other blood vessels. Although the occlusion is typically at the origin of the artery, there may be a segmental occlusion, and this should be verified whenever possible by more proximal evaluation of the vertebral artery, as close to the origin as can be accomplished.

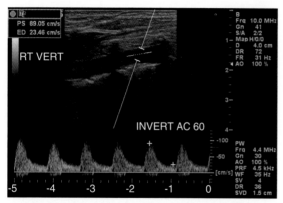

FIGURE 11-7 Compensatory vertebral artery flow. Elevated right vertebral artery flow (peak systolic velocity [PSV]; 89 cm/sec) is evident in a patient with a left ICA occlusion.

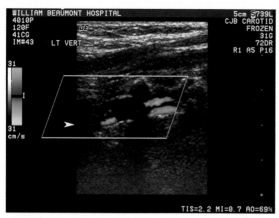

FIGURE 11-8 Color Doppler image of a vertebral artery dissection with color visualized in both the true and false lumens.

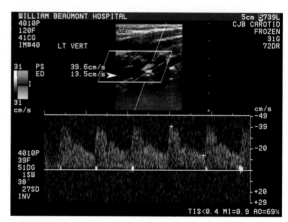

FIGURE 11-9 Color and spectral Doppler image of a vertebral artery dissection with essentially normal flow characteristics noted in the true lumen. The Doppler waveform shows low-resistance characteristics, and peak systolic velocity (PSV; 39.6 cm/sec) is in the normal range.

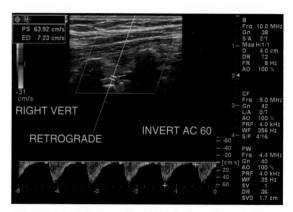

FIGURE 11-10 Reversed vertebral flow. The color Doppler image and the spectral Doppler velocity signal show reversed flow in the vertebral artery throughout the cardiac cycle secondary to subclavian steal.

FLOW REVERSAL

A more common finding than absence of flow in the vertebral artery is reversed flow, or subclavian steal. This is a simple diagnosis to make with duplex ultrasound because retrograde vertebral artery flow is seen throughout the cardiac cycle (Figure 11-10), although one must be careful not to confuse the pulsatile flow signal in the vertebral vein with reversed vertebral artery flow. In 90% of cases, reversed vertebral flow (due to subclavian steal) occurs on the left side. In patients with subclavian steal, it should also be possible to document abnormal flow velocity waveforms in the distal segment of the affected subclavian artery (Figure 11-11). When vertebral flow reversal is seen on the right side, it is important to determine whether the source of the steal is the subclavian artery, which affects only vertebral

artery flow, or the innominate artery, which has a significant effect on both the right common carotid and vertebral arteries. Typically, patients with subclavian steal also have a systolic pressure difference greater than 15 to 20 mm Hg between the normal and affected arms. An additional finding may be increased vertebral artery size and strong compensatory flow contralateral to the subclavian steal; because of the great degree of variability in normal vertebral artery size and flow velocity cited previously, however, this finding is not diagnostic as an isolated observation.

Frequently, in cases of subclavian steal, there may be a subclavian artery obstruction at its origin that is hemodynamically significant but not so severe as to cause a complete reversal of flow in the ipsilateral vertebral artery. The changing

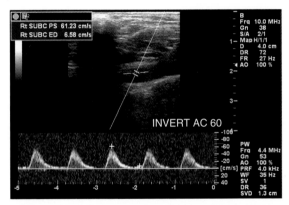

FIGURE 11-11 Doppler findings in subclavian steal. Spectral Doppler velocity signal from the distal subclavian artery in the patient with subclavian steal shown in Figure 11-10. The waveform is monophasic with a delayed systolic upstroke, and damped, characteristic of severe proximal obstruction at the origin of the subclavian artery.

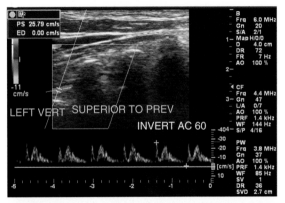

FIGURE 11-12 Vertebral waveform abnormalities ipsilateral to early subclavian steal. This spectral Doppler vertebral signal shows early systolic deceleration. The point of minimum flow, where the spectral trace hits the zero-flow baseline, occurs at peak systole, when the pressure drop across the subclavian artery stenosis is maximum.

balance of hemodynamic forces during the cardiac cycle causes systolic flow deceleration in the vertebral artery (Figure 11-12), which if severe enough, is manifest as bidirectional flow (Figure 11-13). During peak systole, a significant pressure drop occurs across the subclavian artery stenosis in association with a high-velocity flow jet. At the same time, normal systolic pressure is present in the contralateral vertebral artery and basilar artery. As a result, there is a net pressure gradient, from distal to proximal, across the vertebral artery on the side of the subclavian stenosis, which causes deceleration during systole or even transient reversal of flow. During the diastolic phase of the cardiac cycle, flow velocities across the subclavian artery lesion are diminished and no significant pressure drop occurs across the stenosis; thus, during diastole, the net pressure gradient within the affected vertebral artery is essentially normal and produces antegrade flow with diminished absolute flow velocities.

When the balance of hemodynamic forces produces a bidirectional flow pattern, the overall effect is a net volume blood flow in the vertebral artery that is very small, on the order of only a few milliliters per minute. This net flow may be either antegrade or retrograde, and angiographically, the low flow rate may result in nonvisualization of the vertebral artery, mimicking occlusion.[17]

DIMINISHED FLOW

In those patients with a dominant vertebral artery, the nondominant, anatomically small vertebral artery may demonstrate flow characteristics

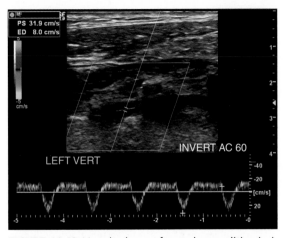

FIGURE 11-13 Vertebral waveform abnormalities ipsilateral to progressive subclavian steal. This spectral Doppler vertebral signal shows bidirectional flow. In this case, the subclavian stenosis is severe enough to cause transient reversal of flow during peak systole, with diminished but antegrade flow during diastole.

of increased vascular resistance, with diminished flow velocities at peak systole and throughout diastole. In more severe cases of a hypoplastic, atretic (less than 2-mm lumen diameter) vertebral artery, which can occur in up to 15% of patients,[18] vascular resistance over the course of the vessel may be so elevated that the spectral Doppler waveform takes on characteristics of a near total distal occlusion (i.e., an absence of detectable diastolic flow; Figure 11-14). Severe, proximal vertebral artery obstructive disease also may be responsible for diminished vertebrobasilar system flow and cerebrovascular symptoms.

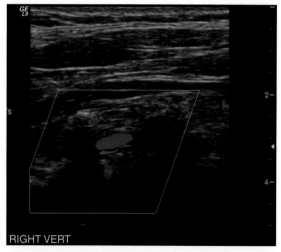

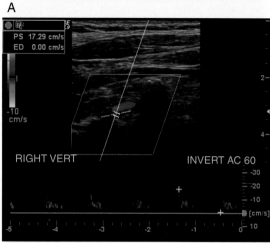

FIGURE 11-14 Atretic vertebral artery. **A,** Color Doppler sagittal image of an atretic vertebral artery (lumen diameter less than 2 mm) shown in red, with the adjacent vertebral vein (color coded blue) clearly seen. **B,** Diminished flow (peak systolic velocity [PSV]; 17 cm/sec) in this anatomically small vertebral artery. The spectral Doppler velocity waveform exhibits characteristics of a high-resistance flow signal, with absence of diastolic flow, caused by the increased vascular resistance of the small vessel lumen.

In such cases, the spectral Doppler velocity waveform exhibits a tardus-parvus waveform, characteristic of damping, a waveform with delayed onset of a rounded, poorly defined systolic peak, poor antegrade flow during diastole, and significantly diminished velocities throughout the cardiac cycle (Figure 11-15). If damped Doppler waveforms are seen in a vertebral artery, a careful duplex ultrasound examination of the proximal segment and origin of the affected vertebral artery should be conducted to identify the site

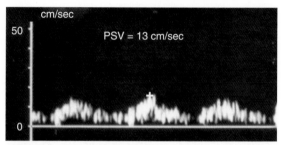

FIGURE 11-15 Diminished flow in mid–vertebral artery secondary to a proximal stenosis. The velocity waveform shows the classic tardus-parvus shape, with a rounded, poorly defined systolic peak and diminished velocities throughout the cardiac cycle. (Peak systolic velocity [PSV] is 13 cm/sec.)

and severity of any obstructive lesion that may be present.

VERTEBRAL ARTERY HEMODYNAMICS: QUANTITATIVE ASSESSMENT

In addition to the qualitative evaluation of vertebral artery flow hemodynamics, it is possible to quantitate volume flows in the vertebrobasilar arterial system. This may provide clinically helpful information in some cases, as many of the posterior circulation symptoms are thought to represent ischemia, unlike the thromboembolic nature of most carotid artery territory symptoms. Technically, the ability to calculate vertebral artery volume flow is present on most duplex ultrasound instruments. It requires a combination of spectral Doppler velocity data, from which a time-averaged velocity for a complete cardiac cycle can be calculated, and a measurement of the vessel lumen diameter, from which cross-sectional area can be calculated. These two measurements can be combined to give volume flow in milliliters per minute. Measurement accuracy approaches approximately ±10% in a vessel segment such as the mid–vertebral artery, which is relatively straight and nontapering and is without significant branches at the measurement site.[19,20] Our own experience has shown that it is technically possible to measure volume flow in more than 99% of vertebral arteries (1491 of 1500 consecutive patients). As with peak systolic velocities, patients with normal physiology show a wide variation in volume flows, ranging from less than 75 mL/min to more than 150 mL/min. When both vertebral arteries are considered together, however, the normal total (right plus left) vertebral artery flow is approximately

200 mL/min or greater. Patients with nonlocalizing cerebrovascular symptoms suggestive of posterior circulation ischemia are much more likely to have overall diminished (<200 mL/min) vertebrobasilar system flow than asymptomatic patients or those with lateralizing, hemispheric symptoms. This is particularly true if there is only minimal or no obstructive disease in the carotid artery systems, thus identifying a group of symptomatic patients with potentially true posterior circulation ischemia secondary to poor vertebrobasilar system hemodynamics. The clinical importance of a finding of diminished vertebrobasilar flow depends on the underlying cause of poor flow and whether it can be remedied. Causes of diminished vertebrobasilar flow include bilateral hypoplastic vertebral arteries, poor cardiac output, and intracranial occlusion of the distal vertebral or basilar artery. Qualitative assessment of the spectral Doppler velocity flow waveform can be used to diagnose distal vertebral or basilar occlusion, because the absolute velocities in both systole and diastole are likely to be severely diminished because of elevated distal vascular resistance, particularly at end diastole. If an intracranial lesion is suspected as the underlying cause of diminished vertebral flow waveforms, this can be effectively evaluated by angiography, as newer technologies allow angioplasty and stenting of the basilar artery.

CORRELATIVE IMAGING WITH MAGNETIC RESONANCE ANGIOGRAPHY AND COMPUTED TOMOGRAPHIC ANGIOGRAPHY

While duplex ultrasound has replaced conventional angiography in most cases for the diagnosis of carotid artery atherosclerotic disease and management decisions regarding carotid endarterectomy, the duplex ultrasound findings are often corroborated by computed tomographic angiography (CTA) or magnetic resonance angiography (MRA). The same can be said for evaluation of the vertebral arteries as these techniques continue to evolve (Figure 11-16). Vertebral artery stenosis and extrinsic vertebral arterial compression by the bony structures in Regions V2 and V3 are readily detected, particularly with contrast enhancement and three-dimensional image reconstruction.[21,22] In addition, phase-contrast MRA measures actual vertebral artery flows and directly assesses

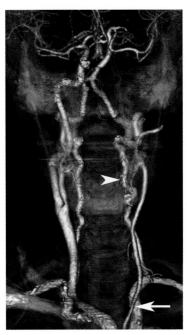

FIGURE 11-16 Computed tomographic angiography of the aortic arch and great vessels. Three-dimensional reconstruction shows the anatomic relationships of the vessels with shading for lumen, wall calcification, and surrounding bony structures. Note the hypoplastic left common carotid artery *(arrow)* and severe innominate artery disease with a large dominant left vertebral artery *(arrowhead)*.

vertebrobasilar arterial hemodynamics.[23] From a cost-effective perspective, duplex ultrasound remains the initial best choice for vertebral artery evaluation, but if there are equivocal ultrasound findings, contrast-enhanced three-dimensional CTA or MRA may be needed to acquire the necessary diagnostic information. In particular, when duplex ultrasound findings suggest vertebral artery obstructive disease at a site not accessible to direct imaging, such as an inaccessible vertebral artery origin or a high-resistance flow waveform characteristic of more distal (Regions V3 or V4) disease, these techniques are able to visualize the region of interest with minimal invasiveness. The limitations of MRA for the vertebral arteries are much the same as those for the carotid arterial system. Not all patients are candidates for magnetic resonance procedures because of metallic implants or an inability to cooperate fully for the examination. The percentage of such patients increases with increasing age; unfortunately, so does the incidence of cerebrovascular disease involving the vertebrobasilar system. Signal dropout in regions of severe flow turbulence,

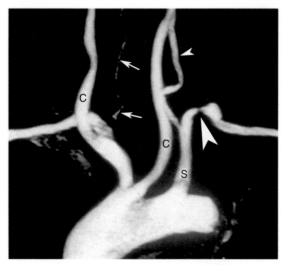

FIGURE 11-17 Magnetic resonance angiography (MRA) of the vertebral arteries. MRA of the aortic arch shows both proximal common carotid arteries *(C)* and the proximal left vertebral artery *(small arrowhead)*. The right vertebral artery *(arrows)* is hypoplastic with severely diminished flow and, consequently, is not well seen. Note the stenosis of the left subclavian artery *(S) (large arrowhead)* and poststenotic dilatation. Because this stenosis lies beyond the vertebral origin, it would not affect vertebral artery flow.

such as that distal to a stenosis or in a region of very slow flow, as might be seen in a hypoplastic vessel, also limit the diagnostic capability of MRA in some cases (Figure 11-17). CTA provides high-resolution images of the posterior circulation in patients without contraindications to iodinated contrast material or impaired renal function. Current reconstruction algorithms allow subtraction of soft tissue and osseous structures to provide high-definition views of the extracranial and intracranial circulations.

TREATMENT OF DISEASE

Multiple large clinical trials have shown the benefits of carotid endarterectomy for stenotic, atherosclerotic lesions in appropriately selected patients, and more recent trials are designed to extend therapeutic management to angioplasty and stenting. Similar data for revascularization of vertebral artery stenoses is lacking. The wide variety of presenting symptoms of posterior circulation ischemia can make appropriate patient selection challenging, and these patients often present with a mixture of both carotid and vertebral artery disease. Yet in those patients presenting with transient symptoms of posterior

circulation ischemia, the 5-year stroke risk is between 20% and 35% and the stroke-associated mortality is approximately 25% higher than that for carotid territory strokes. Surgical centers of excellence have reported good results for direct vertebral arterial reconstruction, either a vertebral artery transposition or vertebral artery bypass, with outcomes comparable to carotid endarterectomy.[24] There are no data to suggest, however, that these results are widely generalizable. Recent studies have looked at angioplasty and stenting of vertebral artery stenoses, with good early technical success.[25-27] These reports have tended to be small clinical series with relatively short follow-up and have shown complication rates similar to carotid artery stenting but with a higher early (2-year) restenosis rate of 25% to 35%. Larger comparative trials also looking at the long-term outcome of best medical therapy will be needed to establish the clinical efficacy of these procedures in stroke prevention.

CONCLUSIONS

Duplex ultrasound provides a very reliable noninvasive technique for the evaluation of the vertebral arteries. Arterial flow hemodynamics can be evaluated qualitatively by assessing the presence or absence of flow, flow direction, and the characteristics of the spectral Doppler flow waveform itself for relative systolic/diastolic flows and systolic flow deceleration. In addition, quantitative volume flow measurements can be made in the vertebral arteries for those patients with symptoms of possible or suspected posterior circulation ischemia. Overall evaluation of vertebral artery hemodynamics provides useful clinical information in (1) assessing the hemodynamic status of the entire extracranial cerebrovascular system, (2) assessing the pathways and adequacy of compensatory collateral flows in patients with significant obstructive disease, (3) potentially identifying a subgroup of patients whose clinical presentation may be related strictly to the posterior circulation, and (4) identifying flow abnormalities in the vertebrobasilar system secondary to lesions that can be addressed and corrected surgically or with other interventional techniques, similar to what is presently done for carotid territory lesions. Well-designed clinical trials are needed to determine the indications for and the effectiveness of these interventions in stroke prevention.

REFERENCES

1. Fisher CM, et al: Atherosclerosis of the carotid and vertebral arteries—extracranial and intracranial, *J Neuropathol Exp Neurol* 24:455–476, 1965.
2. Castaigne P, et al: Arterial occlusions in the vertebrobasilar system, *Brain* 96:133–154, 1973.
3. Ford JJ, et al: Carotid endarterectomy for nonhemispheric transient ischemic attacks, *Arch Surg* 110:1314–1317, 1975.
4. Ferro JM, et al: Diagnosis of stroke by the nonneurologist: a validation study, *Stroke* 29:1106–1109, 1998.
5. Savitz SI, Caplan LR: Vertebrobasilar disease, *N Engl J Med* 352:2618–2626, 2005.
6. Malone JM, et al: Combined carotid vertebral vascular disease, *Arch Surg* 115:783–785, 1980.
7. Bogousslavsky J, Regli F: Vertebrobasilar transient ischemic attacks in internal carotid artery occlusion or tight stenosis, *Arch Neurol* 42:64–68, 1985.
8. Pritz MB, et al: Vertebral artery disease: radiologic evaluation, medical management, and microsurgical treatment, *Neurosurgery* 9:524–530, 1981.
9. Imparato AM, et al: Cervical vertebral angioplasty for brain stem ischemia, *Surgery* 90:842–852, 1981.
10. Strandness DE Jr: Extracranial artery disease. In Strandness DE, editor: *Duplex scanning in vascular disorders*, ed 2, New York, 1993, Raven Press, pp 113–157.
11. Ackerstaff RGA, et al: Ultrasonic duplex scanning in atherosclerotic disease of the innominate, subclavian and vertebral arteries: a comparative study with angiography, *Ultrasound Med Biol* 10:409–418, 1984.
12. Bendick PJ, Jackson VP: Evaluation of the vertebral arteries with duplex sonography, *J Vasc Surg* 3:523–530, 1986.
13. Bendick PJ, Glover JL: Hemodynamic evaluation of vertebral arteries by duplex ultrasound, *Surg Clin North Am* 70:235–244, 1990.
14. Ackerstaff RGA, et al: Ultrasonic duplex scanning of the prevertebral segment of the vertebral artery in patients with cerebral atherosclerosis, *Eur J Vasc Surg* 2:387–393, 1988.
15. Kuhl V, et al: Color-coded duplex ultrasonography of the origin of the vertebral artery: normal values of flow velocities, *J Neuroimaging* 10:17–21, 2000.
16. Moufarrij NA, et al: Vertebral artery stenosis: long-term follow-up, *Stroke* 15:260–263, 1984.
17. Bendick PJ: Duplex examination. In Berguer R, Caplan LR, editors: *Vertebrobasilar arterial disease*, St. Louis, 1992, Quality Medical Publishers, pp 93–103.
18. Cloud GC, Markus HS: Diagnosis and management of vertebral artery stenosis, *Q J Med* 96:27–34, 2003.
19. Bendick PJ, Glover JL: Vertebrobasilar insufficiency: evaluation by quantitative duplex flow measurements, *J Vasc Surg* 5:594–600, 1987.
20. Hoyt K, et al: Accuracy of volumetric flow rate measurements: an in vitro study using modern ultrasound scanners, *J Ultrasound Med* 28:1511–1518, 2009.
21. Sylaja PN, et al: Prognostic value of CT angiography in patients with suspected vertebrobasilar ischemia, *J Neuroimaging* 18:46–49, 2008.
22. Provenzale JM, Sarikaya B: Comparison of test performance characteristics of MRI, MR angiography, and CT angiography in the diagnosis of carotid and vertebral artery dissection: a review of the medical literature, *AJR Am J Roentgenol* 193:1167–1174, 2009.
23. Guppy KH, et al: Hemodynamic evaluation of basilar and vertebral artery angioplasty, *Neurosurgery* 51:327–333, 2002.
24. Berguer R, et al: Surgical reconstruction of the extracranial vertebral artery: management and outcome, *J Vasc Surg* 31:9–18, 2000.
25. Coward LJ, et al: Long-term outcome after angioplasty and stenting for symptomatic vertebral artery stenosis compared with medical treatment in the Carotid and Vertebral Artery Transluminal Angioplasty Study (CAVATAS): a randomized trial, *Stroke* 38:1526–1530, 2007.
26. Eberhardt O, et al: Stenting of vertebrobasilar arteries in symptomatic atherosclerotic disease and acute occlusion: case series and review of the literature, *J Vasc Surg* 43:1145–1154, 2006.
27. Compter A, et al: VAST: Vertebral Artery Stenting Trial. Protocol for a randomised safety and feasibility trial, *Trials* 9:65, 2008.

ULTRASOUND ASSESSMENT OF THE INTRACRANIAL ARTERIES

12

DARIUS G. NABAVI, MD; MARTIN A. RITTER, MD; SHIRLEY M. OTIS, MD;
and E. BERND RINGELSTEIN, MD

In 1965, Miyazaki and Kato[1] first reported the use of continuous-wave Doppler ultrasound for the assessment of extracranial cerebral vessels. Despite its rapid development in other medical fields, this technique was not applied to the intracranial vessels until 1982. At that time, Aaslid and colleagues[2] developed a transcranial Doppler (TCD) device with a pulsed-wave sound emission of 2 MHz that could successfully penetrate the skull and accurately measure blood flow velocities in the basal arteries and the circle of Willis. With the introduction of TCD, it became possible to record intracranial blood flow velocity directly, and TCD became an important noninvasive method for assessing cerebral hemodynamics and for evaluating intracranial cerebrovascular disease. The continuous development and refinement of ultrasonography during the past two decades lead to a broad spectrum of clinical TCD applications. The introduction of transcranial color-coded duplex sonography (TCCS) into clinical use was an important technical refinement. TCCS combines B-mode imaging with frequency-based color flow imaging and Doppler sonography.[3] By means of TCCS, direct on-line visualization of the basal cerebral arteries and their flow directions became possible, allowing for angle-corrected measurements of blood flow velocities at defined depths. Subsequently, power-based[4] and three-dimensional TCCS[5] were added, and ultrasound contrast agents were introduced,[6] further enhancing the diagnostic capability of this innovative technique[7] (see Chapter 4).

Ultrasound contrast agents have likewise provided the opportunity to detect right-to-left cardiac shunts[8] and to perform perfusion studies of the brain parenchyma based on indicator dilution principles.[9]

The detection of microembolic signals (MESs) by means of TCD constitutes another developmental landmark by allowing the noninvasive estimation of microemboli reaching the intracranial arteries.[10]

A recent development of transcranial ultrasonography, the therapeutic use of ultrasound-assisted thrombolysis (sonothrombolysis),[11] has opened a new era of *neurovascular* ultrasound.

This chapter provides an overview of the main technical and clinical aspects of intracranial ultrasonography and briefly introduces the latest technical and clinical developments.

EXAMINATION TECHNIQUES

GENERAL PREREQUISITES

Two prerequisites should be fulfilled before performing a TCD examination: (1) the status of the extracranial arteries has to be known, and (2) the patient needs to rest comfortably to avoid major fluctuations in blood carbon dioxide levels and movement artifacts. In addition, two main anatomic considerations must be dealt with by the examiner: (1) the ultrasonic "windows" through which the ultrasound beam can penetrate the skull are often limited or difficult to identify; and (2) the arteries at the base of the skull vary greatly in respect to size, course, development, and site of access.[12-15] The transmission of ultrasound signals through the cranium has been extensively studied.[16,17] It depends on the skull structure, which consists of three layers, each of which influences ultrasound transmission in different ways. Grolimund[17] has performed a number of in vitro experiments showing that a wide range of energy loss occurs in different skull samples, and that the energy loss varies greatly from one location to another and among individuals. In no case was the power measured behind the skull greater than 35% of the transmitted power. It was further shown that the skull can provide the effect of an acoustic lens, and that refraction or distortion of the beam depends more on the variation of bone thickness than on the angle of insonation.

TCD AND TCCS DEVICES

Transcranial ultrasound applications require a large signal-to-noise ratio. This is one of the reasons why the available transcranial instruments have a lower bandwidth, and, therefore, a larger and less-defined sample volume than most other pulsed Doppler devices. Commercial TCD systems mostly use a 2-MHz, pulsed, range-gated Doppler device with good directional resolution. TCCS is performed with 1.8- to 3.6-MHz phased-array sector transducers. Further instrumental requirements are (1) transmitting powers ranging between 10 and 100 mW/cm/sec, (2) adjustable Doppler gate depth, (3) pulse repetition frequency up to 20 kHz, (4) focusing of the ultrasonic beam at a distance of 40 to 60 mm from the probe, and (5) on-line display of the time-averaged velocity and peak systolic velocity (PSV; "envelope") derived from spectral analysis of the ultrasonic signals. Several commercially available TCD machines are equipped with special headbands or helmets to enable continuous monitoring.

ULTRASONIC WINDOWS

Four main ultrasound approaches have been described to insonate the intracranial arteries: the transtemporal, transorbital, suboccipital (i.e., transforaminal), and submandibular approaches,[18,25] as illustrated in Figure 12-1. An extensive nomenclature has been developed for describing the segments of the intracranial cerebral arteries, and this terminology is used in this chapter. If you are unfamiliar with cerebral artery nomenclature, please refer to Figure 12-2.

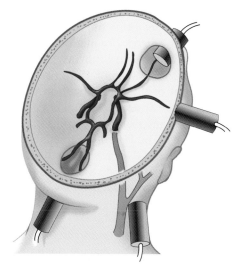

FIGURE 12-1 Relationship of ultrasonic probes to the available ultrasound windows within the skull and to the basal cerebral arteries.

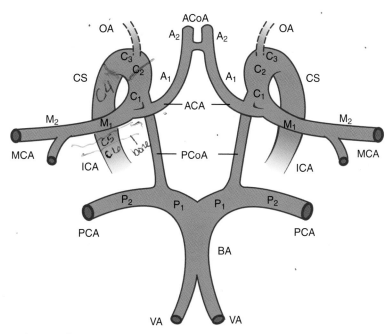

FIGURE 12-2 Nomenclature of the basal cerebral arteries of the circle of Willis. ACA, anterior cerebral artery (segments A_1, A_2); ACoA, anterior communicating artery; BA, basilar artery; CS, carotid siphon (segments C_1-C_3); ICA, internal carotid artery; MCA, middle cerebral artery (segments M_1, M_2); OA, ophthalmic artery; PCA, posterior cerebral artery (segments P_1, P_2); PCoA, posterior communicating artery; VA, vertebral artery.

Transtemporal Approach

The probe is placed on the temporal aspect of the head, cephalad to the zygomatic arch and immediately anterior and slightly superior to the tragus of the ear conch (Figure 12-3, position *1*). This is usually the most promising examination site.

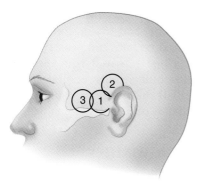

FIGURE 12-3 Available temporal ultrasonic windows and probe placement. *1,* Preauricular position; *2,* posterior window; *3,* anterior window. The probe should first be placed in the preauricular region to identify the middle cerebral artery. Very subtle meander-like movements of the probe should be performed in each position. If position *1* is not successful, position *2* should be tried next, before position *3* is chosen.

A more posterior window immediately cephalad and slightly dorsal to the first one (Figure 12-3, position *2*) may be more appropriate in a minority of cases, especially for insonation of the P_2 segment of the posterior cerebral arteries (PCAs). In some patients, a more frontally located temporal ultrasonic window may be present (Figure 12-3, position *3*). By using these transtemporal approaches, the beam can be angulated anteriorly or posteriorly relative to the corresponding probe positions on the opposite side of the head. The *anterior* orientation of the beam allows for the insonation of the M_1 and M_2 segments of the middle cerebral arteries (MCAs), the C_1 segment of the carotid siphon (CS), the A_1 segment of the anterior cerebral artery (ACA), and often the anterior communicating artery (Figure 12-4, *A*). The *posteriorly* angulated beam insonates the P_1 and P_2 segments of the PCA, the top of the basilar artery (BA), and the posterior communicating arteries (Figure 12-4, *B*).

Transorbital Approach

Components of the anterior cerebral circulation may be evaluated by placing the transducer against the closed eyelid.[13] To avoid damage to

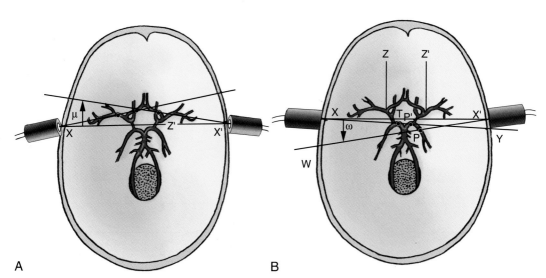

A   B

FIGURE 12-4 Position of the probe in the temporal region to insonate the anterior and posterior parts of the circle of Willis. **A,** Line *X-X'* indicates a frontal plane that runs through the regular placement of the probe on either side and, simultaneously, perpendicular to the sagittal midline of the skull. *Z'* indicates the site of the intracranial internal carotid artery bifurcation. The *X'-Z'* distance is 63 ± 5 mm. The angle μ is the angle with which the probe is aimed more anteriorly toward the middle cerebral artery and anterior cerebral artery segments. This angle was found to be 6 ± 1.1 degrees. **B,** The angle ω indicates the angle with which the beam is directed more posteriorly to insonate the top *(T)* of the basilar artery (BA) and the P_1 segments *(P')* on both sides. This angle was found to be 4.6 ± 1.2 degrees. The BA bifurcation could be insonated at depths of 78 ± 5 mm, corresponding to the distance *X-T* or *X'-T*, respectively. *Y* indicates the fictional point at which the pathway of the beam then transits the contralateral skull—that is, approximately 2 to 3 cm behind the external acoustic meatus. The P_2 segments *(P)* can also be insonated if the beam is directed even more posteriorly and slightly caudally (line *X'-P*). *W* lies approximately 5 cm behind the contralateral external acoustic meatus.

the lenses of the eyes, the power of the ultrasound transmission has to be reduced. The ophthalmic artery can usually be insonated at depths of 45 to 50 mm, whereas the C_3 segment (anterior knee of the CS) is normally met at insonation depths of 60 to 65 mm (Figure 12-5, A). At slightly greater insonation depths of 70 to 75 mm, the C_2 segment shows flow away from the probe (upward deflection), and the C_4 segment shows flow toward the probe (downward deflection). These flow directions apply only when the beam is nearly sagittal (slight medial obliquity) and enters the skull through the supraorbital or infra-orbital fissures. Typical insonation depths and velocities are shown in Figure 12-5, B. The trans-orbital approach is much less established and validated than the transtemporal or suboccipital approach.

Suboccipital (Transforaminal) Approach

The suboccipital (transforaminal) approach is essential for screening the distal vertebral artery (VA; V4 segment) and the BA throughout its entire length. The probe is placed exactly between the posterior margin of the foramen magnum and the palpable spinous process of the first cervical vertebra, with the beam aimed at the bridge of the nose (Figure 12-6, A).[2] The insonation depth is set at 65 mm, and the right and left VAs are tracked individually from this (deepest) point back toward the foramen magnum, using progressively smaller insonation depths (from 65 down to 35 mm). As the depth decreases, the sound beam is angled more and more sharply toward the side of the head. The extradural part of the VA, on the posterior arch of the atlas

(V3 segment), can also be screened. Flow is toward the transducer in this segment. The BA can be tracked cephalad from the point at which the VAs unite. The superior end of the BA is reached at a depth of approximately 95 to 125 mm. Flow in the intradural VAs and the BA is normally directed away from the probe. Typical insonation depths and flow velocities are shown in Figure 12-6, B.

Submandibular Approach

The submandibular approach completes the examination in that the retromandibular and more distal extradural parts (C_5-C_6 segments) of the internal carotid artery (ICA) can be evaluated. This particular examination is a useful complement to extracranial studies, because it facilitates the detection of ICA dissection and chronic ICA occlusion with abundant collateralization through the external carotid artery. With the transducer positioned as shown in Figure 12-7, A, the beam is directed slightly medially and posteriorly. The ICA can regularly be tracked to a depth of 80 to 85 mm, at which point it bends medioanteriorly to form the CS. Typical insonation depths and flow velocities are shown in Figure 12-7, B.

DIAGNOSTIC APPROACH

Basic TCD Examination

In general, it is most convenient to start with transtemporal insonation, to identify the MCA on either side at an insonation depth of 50 to 55 mm, and then to track the ipsilateral arterial network, step by step, in various directions.

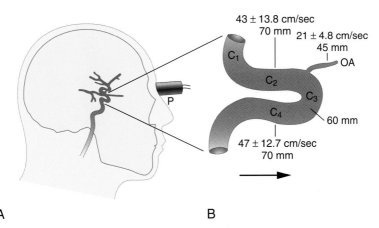

A   B

FIGURE 12-5 Insonation of the ophthalmic artery and carotid siphon by the transorbital approach. **A,** Probe (P) location and relationship to the ophthalmic artery and carotid siphon. **B,** Representative insonation depths and normal flow values within various segments of the carotid siphon (C_1-C_4) and ophthalmic artery (OA).

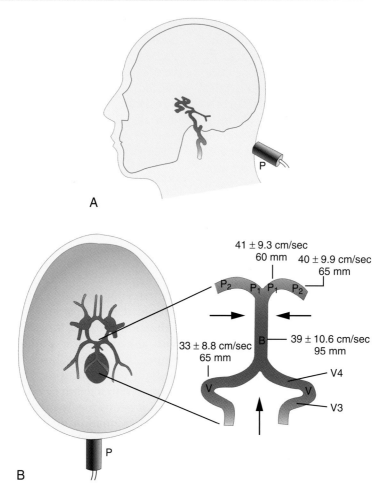

FIGURE 12-6 **A,** Transcranial Doppler examination of the vertebral system by the suboccipital approach. **B,** Representative insonation and normal flow values within the distal vertebral arteries (V) and the basilar trunk (B). The P₁ and P₂ velocities are measured transtemporally. P, probe.

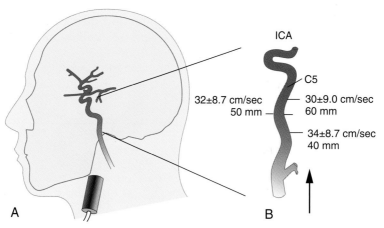

FIGURE 12-7 **A,** Transcranial Doppler examination of the petrous portion of the internal carotid artery (ICA) by the submandibular approach. The ICA can be traced from depths of 25 to 80 mm, corresponding to the C₅ segment of the ICA. **B,** Representative insonation depths and normal flow values within the distal intracranial ICA.

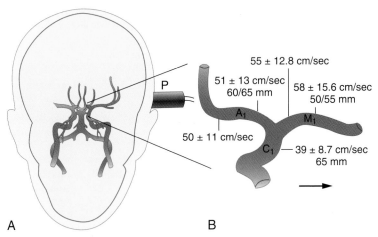

FIGURE 12-8 Typical transtemporal distances and velocities for the anterior cerebral artery and the middle cerebral artery. **A,** The beam axis is in line with the C_1, M_1, and A_1 segments of the cerebral vessels. **B,** Representative insonation depths and flow velocities are illustrated.

Proof of traceability of the MCA is necessary for its unequivocal identification. This is also true for other arteries at the base of the brain. *Traceability* refers to the fact that the MCA (and usually other arteries) can be tracked in incremental steps from a more shallow insonation depth (35 mm) to deeper sites (55 mm) without changes in the character of the flow profile and flow direction. When tracking the MCA medially (65-70 mm), an abrupt change in flow direction (away from, rather than toward the probe) indicates insonation of the A_1 segment of the ACA. Flow signals *toward* the probe at this depth usually emanate from the CS at its junction with the MCA. Typical depths and flow velocities are shown in Figure 12-8.

By angling the beam more posteriorly from a transtemporal approach, the P_1 segment of the PCA can be picked up most readily at an insonation depth of 65 to 70 mm. The PCA can then be tracked to the top of the BA (75 mm) and from there to the contralateral PCA (80-85 mm) (see Figure 12-4, *B*). The two criteria of traceability (i.e., the display of bilateral blood flow at the junction with the BA and the change of flow direction within the contralateral PCA) are very important features for identifying the PCAs without compression tests.

After the completion of the examination from *both* temporal windows, additional information may be obtained through the orbital, suboccipital, or submandibular pathways. The vessels that are accessible from these sites, as well as the techniques for identifying these vessels, were described previously. A protocol for TCD examination is presented in Table 12-1.

TCCS Examination

TCCS is now a well-established diagnostic method, allowing direct noninvasive imaging of intracranial vascular structures.[3,19] This visual approach provides for more rapid and reliable vessel identification, permitting exact localization of the Doppler sample volume, and shortening the examination time.[19,20] This technique has evolved rapidly over the past years and includes not only vascular (i.e., arterial and venous) imaging but also imaging of the brain parenchyma. Usually the transtemporal and suboccipital approaches are used for TCCS examinations. No systematic data exist for the submandibular approach. The transorbital TCCS investigation has been performed chiefly by ophthalmologists until now, and thus systematic data are mainly available in ophthalmologic journals.[21]

For transtemporal insonation, the probe is positioned axially along the orbitomeatal line and the hypoechoic, butterfly-shaped midbrain is visualized as an anatomic landmark at a depth of 6 to 8 cm. From this perspective, the circle of Willis can then easily be depicted (Figure 12-9). For the suboccipital approach, the hypoechoic foramen magnum and the hyperechoic clivus serve as the anatomic landmarks, with both VAs located at their lateral edges (Figure 12-10). The origin of the BA can also be visually identified in most cases at a depth of 75 to 95 mm. Generally, the reference depths of the target vessels

TABLE 12-1 Transcranial Doppler Protocol: Identification Criteria and Normal Flow Velocities

Position of Probe	Arterial Segment	Insonation Depth Range (mm)	Reference Depth (mm)	Normal Flow Velocity (Mean ± SD) (cm/sec)	Main Features for Identification of Vessel Segment
Transtemporal	MCA	30-60	50	55 ± 12 (60)	M_1: Insonation depth 50 mm; traceability forward and backward; flow toward probe; slightly anterior angulation of beam
	M_1	45-60	50	55 ± 12	
	ACA	60-75	70	50 ± 11 (50)	Insonation depth; flow away from probe; traceability with slight anterior angulation of beam; for clear-cut differentiation from carotid siphon
	C_1 (C_2) (carotid siphon transtemporal approach)	60-70	65	39 ± 9 (40)	Insonation depth; relatively low flow velocity compared to M_1 segment; slightly anterior and caudal angulation of beam; flow toward probe
	P_1 (posterior cerebral artery)	60 (55)-75	70	39 ± 10 (40)	Insonation depth; flow toward probe (ipsilateral P_1); traceability to top of basilar and contralateral P_1; slightly posterior and caudal angulation of beam; relatively low flow velocity compared with M_1 segment
	P_1 and $P_{1'}$ (top of basilar)	70-80	75	40 ± 10	Insonation depth; bidirectional flow; traceability backward and forward; angulation of beam
	P_2 (PCA)	60-65	65	40 ± 10 (40)	Flow away from probe; placement of probe; posterior angulation of probe; modulation by opening and closing eyes
Suboccipital	Extradural distal vertebral artery	40-55	50	34 ± 8 (35)	Suboccipital placement of probe; insonation depth; strongly lateral angulation of beam; flow toward probe
	Intradural distal vertebral artery	60-95 (100)	70	38 ± 10 (35)	Insonation depth Beam aimed at bridge of nose or slightly laterally; traceability forward and backward
	Basilar trunk	70 (65)-115 (120)	95 (100, if possible)	41 ± 10 (40)	Insonation depth; flow away from probe; often slight increase of flow velocity compared to vertebral artery; traceability of vertebrobasilar axis
Ophthalmic	C_2 (carotid siphon, transorbital approach)	65-80	70	41 ± 11 (45)	Sagittal or slightly oblique angulation of beam; flow away from beam; flow away from probe; insonation depth
	C_3 (carotid siphon, transorbital approach)	65 (60)	65	(bidirectional, not measured)	Bidirectional signal; sagittal angulation of beam; insonation depth

TABLE 12-1 Transcranial Doppler Protocol: Identification Criteria and Normal Flow Velocities—cont'd

Position of Probe	Arterial Segment	Insonation Depth Range (mm)	Reference Depth (mm)	Normal Flow Velocity (Mean ± SD) (cm/sec)	Main Features for Identification of Vessel Segment
	C_4 and distal part of C_5 (carotid siphon, transorbital approach)	65-80 (85)	70	47 ± 14 (45)	Sagittal or slightly oblique and caudal angulation of beam; flow toward probe; insonation depth
	Ophthalmic artery	35-55	45	21 ± 5 (20)	Insonation depth; flow toward probe
	Contralateral A_1 (ACA; transorbital approach, ancillary approach if lack of temporal window)	75-80	Not defined	Measurements in a few cases only	Strongly oblique angulation of beam through optic canal; flow toward probe; compression test necessary for differentiation from carotid siphon and MCA
Submandibular	C_6 and retromandibular segment of ICA extradural ICA; submandibular)	35-80 (85)	60	30 ± 9 (30)	Flow away from probe; medial angulation of beam; insonation depth

ACA, anterior cerebral artery; ICA, internal cerebral artery; MCA, middle cerebral artery; PCA, posterior cerebral artery; SD, standard deviation.

are similar to the values given previously for TCD examination. TCCS also allows for the examination of cerebral venous sinuses and large basal cerebral veins, although this has not become part of the clinical routine.

Vessel Identification

The primary TCD parameters for identifying the cerebral arteries are the following:
1. Insonation depth
2. Direction of blood flow at insonation depth
3. Flow velocity (mean flow velocity and systolic or diastolic peak flow velocity)
4. Probe position (e.g., temporal, orbital, suboccipital, submandibular)
5. Direction of the ultrasonic beam (e.g., posterior, anterior, caudad, cephalad)
6. Traceability of vessels

Compression of the extracranial carotid arteries, as a means for intracranial vessel identification, has gradually been excluded from the clinical routine because of the low, but definite,

risk for cerebral embolism.[22,23] This is especially the case since the advent of TCCS used in conjunction with ultrasound contrast agents, because the identification of the major cerebral arteries and their collateral pathways is possible, for the most part, without compression maneuvers. Carotid compression should be definitely avoided in patients with extracranial atheromatous disease.

Blood Flow Velocity Measurements

The mean blood flow velocities of various arterial segments, and their age dependency, are shown in Tables 12-2 and 12-3.[24] Normal flow velocity values in adults show little variation among different investigators.[14,25-27] The highest velocities are almost always found in the MCA or the ACA. The PCAs and BAs have lower Doppler shifts than the MCA in normal subjects. The same pattern has not been noted, however, in cerebral blood flow studies, in which flow is measured in cubic centimeters per second. Two explanations have been offered for this discrepancy between velocity and volume flow: (1) The measurement sites

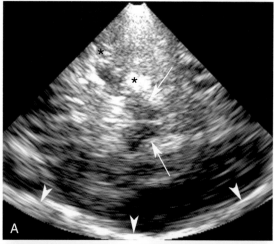

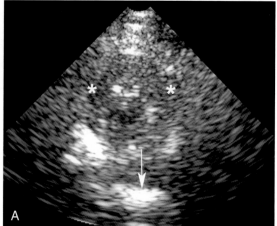

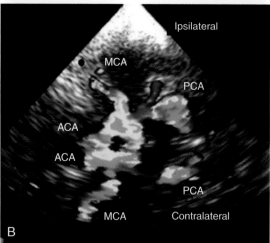

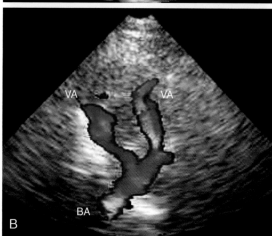

FIGURE 12-9 Illustration of a typical transtemporal transcranial color-coded duplex sonography (TCCS) examination. **A,** For initial spatial orientation, the examination is started with a large-scale, B-mode cranial view, which is usually achieved at a depth of 14 to 17 cm. Visualization of the hyperechoic contralateral skull *(arrowheads)* proves the presence of adequate transcranial ultrasound penetration. If the hypoechoic, butterfly-shaped midbrain *(arrows)* and the hyperechoic sphenoid bone *(asterisks)* can be visualized, then the correct insonation plane has been achieved. **B,** For the color-mode examination, the insonation depth is reduced to 8 to 10 cm; the precommunicating (P_1) and postcommunicating (P_2) segments of the posterior cerebral artery (PCA) can be visualized as they follow the edge of the midbrain. More anteriorly, the sphenoidal (M_1) and the insular (M_2) parts of the middle cerebral artery (MCA), and the precommunicating (A_1) part of the anterior cerebral artery (ACA) can be depicted. In rare cases, and with excellent bone insonation conditions (as illustrated), the entire circle of Willis can be displayed. The distal part of the internal carotid artery (ICA) is also assessable with the probe tilted downward.

FIGURE 12-10 Illustration of a typical suboccipital (or transforaminal) transcranial color-coded duplex sonography (TCCS) examination. **A,** For initial spatial orientation, the examination is started with a large-scale, B-mode cranial view, which is usually achieved at a depth of 11 to 13 cm. Visualization of the hypoechoic foramen magnum *(asterisks)* and the hyperechoic clivus *(arrow)* proves the adequacy of transcranial ultrasound penetration. **B,** For the color-mode examination, the insonation depth is usually reduced to 8 to 11 cm, visualizing segments (V4) of both vertebral arteries (VAs) as they follow the edges of the foramen magnum. The Y-shaped conjunction of the VAs with the basilar artery (BA) is usually located close to the clivus. Note, however, that the origin of the BA is highly variable and all three arteries are not always visible within the same insonation plane.

TABLE 12-2 Normal Values of Mean Blood Velocity for Arteries* (Transtemporal Approach)

Age (yr)	Mean Blood Velocity (cm/sec)		
	MCA (M1)	ACA (A1)	PCA (P1)
10-29	70 ± 16.4	61 ± 14.7	55 ± 9.0
30-49	57 ± 11.2	48 ± 7.1	42 ± 8.9
50-59	51 ± 9.7	46 ± 9.4	9 ± 9.9
60-70	41 ± 7.0	38 ± 5.6	36 ± 7.9
Insonated depth (mm)	50-55	60-65	60-65

*Measurements for the middle (MCA), anterior (ACA), and posterior (PCA) cerebral arteries according to age.

TABLE 12-3 Normal Values of Mean Blood Velocity for Arteries* (Suboccipital Approach)

Age (yr)	Mean Blood Velocity (cm/sec)		
	PCA (P1)	BA	VA
10-29	54 ± 8.0	46 ± 11	45 ± 9.8
30-49	40 ± 8.5	38 ± 8.6	34 ± 8.2
50-59	39 ± 10.1	32 ± 7.0	37 ± 10.0
60-70	35 ± 11.1	32 ± 6.7	35 ± 7.0
Insonated depth (mm)	60-65	85-90	60-65

*Measurements for the posterior cerebral (PCA), basilar (BA), and vertebral (VA) arteries according to age.

may be different[28] or (2) more probably, different velocities occur as a compensatory mechanism to keep volume flow constant in arteries of different size.[25] Thus, velocities are slower in large vessels and faster in small ones. Normal angle-corrected blood flow velocity values using TCCS have likewise been established and are only slightly higher than those obtained with TCD.[20,29] The TCD documentation of decreasing flow velocities with increasing age[20,27] correlates well with age-related changes in cerebral blood flow[28] and underlines the validity and sensitivity of TCD and TCCS data as a semiquantitative estimate of cerebral blood flow.

Functional Reserve Testing

Transcranial Doppler is an ideal functional test for detecting rapid changes in cerebral perfusion, because the technique provides excellent resolution of flow velocity changes occurring over time. Functional tests are predominantly aimed at the evaluation of the reserve mechanism of the cerebral vasculature, using various stimuli such as hypocapnia or hypercapnia, shift in the pH by acetazolamide, increased or reduced systemic arterial pressure, and hypoxia. The CO_2 (carbon dioxide) dilatory effect is mainly restricted to the peripheral arterial vascular bed, particularly the small cortical vessels.[28] With changing CO_2 concentrations, the

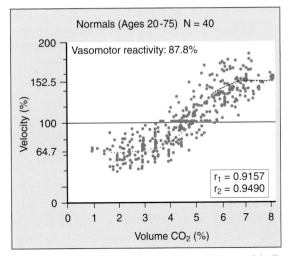

FIGURE 12-11 Vasomotor reactivity in 40 normal individuals (ages 20-75 years). Blood flow velocity changes are shown during carbon dioxide (CO_2)-induced hypercapnia *(upper curve)* and hypocapnia *(lower curve)*. The average change was 87.8% (52.5% and 35.3% hypercapnia and hypocapnia, respectively). *(From Ringelstein EB, Sievers C, Ecker S, et al: Noninvasive assessment of CO_2-induced cerebral vasomotor response in normal individuals and patients with internal carotid artery occlusions, Stroke 19:964, 1988. Copyright © American Heart Association.)*

relationship between flow velocity and volume flow within a large cerebral artery is linear,[30] provided that the CO_2 level does not directly affect the diameter of the large proximal arterial segment.[31]

Velocities measured from the MCA with changing CO_2 concentrations show a biasymptotic, S-shaped curve (Figure 12-11).

A "preserved" vasomotor reserve implies that a drop in perfusion pressure can be counterbalanced by vasodilatation of cortical arterioles to maintain sufficient cortical blood supply. The vasomotor reserve may become exhausted if the resistance vessels in brain areas with low perfusion pressure are already maximally dilated.[30-33] In this state, the resistance vessels are refractory to any further vasodilatory stimuli, and hypercapnia cannot increase blood flow. This condition may be critical, because ischemic brain injury can occur if the perfusion pressure is further reduced for any reason. Measurements of the vasomotor reserve capacity are useful in evaluating the hemodynamic impact of extracranial occlusive carotid disease.

The pulsatility index, as defined by Gosling (see Chapter 3), reflects the resistance in the peripheral vascular bed and has been suggested as a sensitive index of diastolic runoff—that is, with increased peripheral vasodilatation, diastolic runoff is expected to increase and the pulsatility index to decrease.[34] However, in a large series of patients with carotid artery occlusion, the pulsatility index appeared to be much poorer for predicting the intracranial hemodynamic situation than the vasomotor reserve capacity.[35]

DIAGNOSTIC PARAMETERS FOR SPECIFIC CLINICAL APPLICATIONS

INTRACRANIAL STENOSIS AND OCCLUSION

The detection of carotid siphon (CS) stenosis using TCD was first reported in 1986 by Spencer and Whisler,[13] who used similar criteria to those used for carotid bifurcation disease. Since then, a number of authors have reported similar findings for the CS and have extended TCD applications to other brain arteries.[36-39] The most obvious clinical advantage of ultrasound is the rapid screening of the acute stroke patient for intracranial vessel obstruction. Normal TCD findings in stroke patients have considerable clinical impact.

Definition of Stenosis With TCD

The following are typical TCD features of circumscribed stenosis of a large basal cerebral artery (Figure 12-12): (1) increased flow velocity; (2) disturbed flow (spectral broadening and enhanced systolic and low-frequency echo components); and (3) covibration phenomena (vibration of vessel wall and surrounding soft tissue).[25,35] It is unclear whether the PSV (>120-160 cm/sec) or the mean systolic velocity (>80-120 cm/sec) should be used as a threshold value.[39] With a mean velocity value of 100 cm/sec, a sensitivity of 100%, and a specificity of 97.9%, as well as positive and negative predictive values of 88.8% and 94.9%, were reported in detecting intracranial stenoses with a diameter of 50% or more.[38] For the vertebrobasilar system, a threshold of more than 2 kHz peak systolic Doppler shift showed a sensitivity of 80% and a specificity of 97% in detecting stenoses of 50% or more.[37] Most authors agree that, in comparison with the contralateral vessel segment, a relative increase in PSV of more than 30% is suspicious for hemodynamically significant stenosis, and a relative increase of more than 50% indicates a definite intracranial artery stenosis.

Definition of Occlusion With TCD

Basal cerebral artery occlusion can be detected by three observations: (1) the absence of arterial signals at an expected depth; (2) the presence of signals in vessels that communicate with the occluded artery; and (3) altered flow in communicating vessels, indicating collateralization. For example, occlusion of the MCA is diagnosed from the lack of an MCA signal in the presence of flow signals from other vessels (i.e., the PCA, the ACA, or the distal CS). This combination of findings also confirms that the temporal window is satisfactory. In a recent study, TCD showed a sensitivity of 83% and a specificity of 94.4%, with an overall accuracy of 91.6%, in the detection of intracranial vessel occlusion.[40] In accordance with the well-established, angiography-based Thrombolysis in Myocardial Infarction (TIMI) criteria in cardiology, Demchuk and colleagues[41] have proposed the so-called Thrombolysis in Brain Ischemia (TIBI) criteria for the TCD-based classification of the MCA status during and after thrombolysis. The TIBI scale, ranging from 0 (MCA occlusion) to 5 (normal MCA), is given in Table 12-4. In acute stroke patients undergoing thrombolytic therapy, the TIBI criteria were found to be accurate in the prediction of the clinical outcome.[42]

Pitfalls and Diagnostic Accuracy

Noninvasive demonstration of intracranial arterial stenosis and occlusion is a valuable clinical tool, but various errors can occur: (1) lack

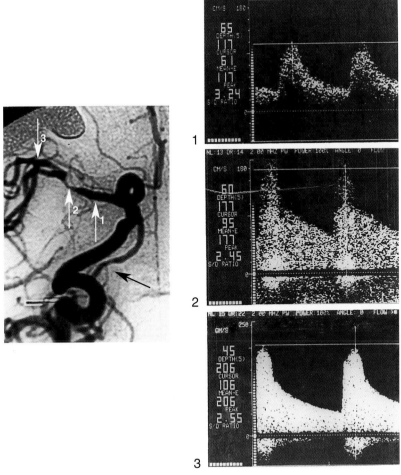

FIGURE 12-12 Middle cerebral artery stenosis and associated transcranial Doppler changes: *(1)* normal proximal flow; *(2)* increased systolic and diastolic peak velocity and spectral broadening (turbulent flow) at the center of the stenosis; *(3)* distal turbulent flow.

of flow signal due to an inadequate temporal window, (2) misinterpretation of hyperdynamic collateral channels[34] or arteriovenous malformation (AVM) feeders[25,43] as stenosis, (3) displacement of arteries because of a space-occupying lesion, (4) misinterpretation of physiologic variables in the circle of Willis,[25] (5) misdiagnosis of vasospasm as stenosis,[44] and (6) misinterpretation of reactive hyperemia following spontaneous recanalization as stenosis.[45] In most of these situations, however, the velocity increases are generally seen *throughout* the course of the involved arteries, which distinguishes these conditions from the typically *localized* areas of increased velocity resulting from stenosis.

Diagnostic accuracy of TCD in the VA-BA system remains a particular problem. Difficulties with VA-BA diagnosis result from the following: (1) the normal flow and the size of the vessels are highly variable; (2) the location and course of the arteries are unpredictable; (3) often the junction of the VAs cannot reliably be identified; (4) absence of the VA flow signal on one side may not represent disease (e.g., so-called posterior inferior cerebellar artery [PICA]-ending anomaly in severe VA hypoplasia); and (5) occlusion of one VA or a "top of the basilar" occlusion does not necessarily lead to relevant flow abnormalities.[46]

Detection of Intracranial Stenosis and Occlusion With TCCS

For TCCS, usually the angle-corrected PSV is used as the main parameter for the definition of intracranial stenosis. In 1999, Baumgartner

TABLE 12-4 **TIBI Criteria for TCD Monitoring of the MCA Recanalization During and After Thrombolytic Therapy[41]**

TIBI Score	Status of the MCA Flow	TCD Criteria
0	Occlusion	• No flow signal
1	Near occlusion or minimal residual flow	• Early systolic low-flow signal • No diastolic flow signal
2	Strongly reduced	• Reduced systolic and diastolic velocity • Flattened early systolic increment • Pulsatility index <1.2
3	Moderately reduced	• Normal systolic increment • Pulsatility index >1.2 • Relative reduction of blood flow velocity of >30% as compared with the contralateral side
4	Stenotic signal	• Mean blood flow velocity >80 cm/sec or relative increase of velocity >30% as compared with the contralateral side • Detection of turbulent flow
5	Normal signal	• Side-to-side difference of blood flow velocity <30% • Comparable values of pulsatility index

MCA, middle cerebral artery; TCD, transcranial Doppler; TIBI, Thrombolysis in Brain Ischemia.

TABLE 12-5 **Threshold Values of Angle-Corrected Peak Systolic Velocity (PSV) for the Detection of Intracranial Stenoses of ≥50% With TCCS[47]**

Vessel	PSV Cutoff (cm/sec)	Sensitivity (%)	Specificity (%)	Positive Predictive Value (%)	Negative Predictive Value (%)
MCA	≥220	100	100	100	100
ACA	≥155	100	100	100	100
PCA	≥145	100	100	100	91
BA	≥140	100	100	100	100
VA	≥120	100	100	100	100

ACA, anterior cerebral artery; BA, basilar artery; MCA, middle cerebral artery; PCA, posterior cerebral artery; VA, vertebral artery.

and co-workers[47] published the results of the largest TCCS validation study yet on the detection of intracranial stenosis. Table 12-5 gives the cutoff values of PSV for the different intracranial arteries. These values show excellent accuracy for the identification of stenoses of 50% or greater diameter reduction. Cutoff values ranged from 220 cm/sec for the MCA to 120 cm/sec for the VA. The TCCS accuracy in the detection of stenoses between 30% and 50% (diameter reduction) showed a high negative predictive value (100%) but only a moderate positive predictive value, ranging from 73% to 100%. The latter results can be explained by the weak hemodynamic effects of low-grade stenosis. Others have used much lower cutoff values of 120 cm/sec or more PSV, or a side-to-side difference of more than 30 cm/sec, for

the definition of TCCS-based intracranial stenosis.[48] Video 12-1 and Figure 12-13 show an example of a high-grade MCA stenosis in a young man.

TCCS diagnosis of an intracranial artery occlusion is based on the absence of flow signals using both the color and the spectral Doppler modes (Figure 12-14). In some cases, the occluded arterial segment appears slightly hyperechoic on B-mode imaging. In contrast to the TCD technique, the use of the correct insonation site and the presence of an adequate insonation window can be easily confirmed with TCCS. Diagnostic confidence of TCCS for intracranial vessel occlusion is up to 100%[49,50] and can be further supported by the use of ultrasound contrast agents.[51,52] Video 12-2 and Figure 12-15 illustrate a case of acute MCA occlusion and insufficient

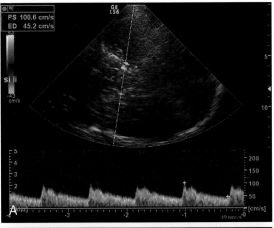

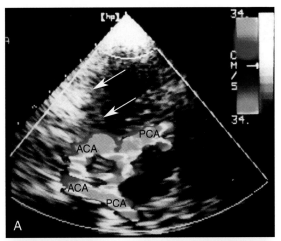

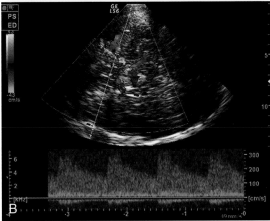

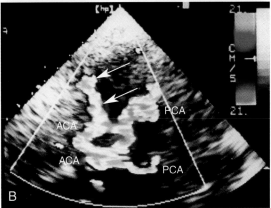

FIGURE 12-13 An axial insonation plane through the temporal bone window. **A,** Prestenotic flow signal of the MCA. **B,** Doppler waveform at the stenosis (300 cm/sec).

FIGURE 12-14 Middle cerebral artery (MCA) occlusion and recanalization detected with transcranial color-coded duplex sonography (TCCS). **A,** Typical finding of a proximal MCA occlusion, with echocontrast-enhanced TCCS (Levovist) in an acute stroke patient. Note the excellent visualization of both posterior cerebral arteries (PCAs) around the midbrain and both anterior cerebral arteries (ACAs) as well. No flow is present within the presumed course of the MCA using both the color mode *(arrows)* and the Doppler spectral mode (not shown). (Compare this image with Figure 12-7, *B.*) **B,** Several days later, spontaneous MCA recanalization has occurred, with the entire MCA *(arrows)* depicted with contrast-enhanced TCCS.

bone window in an older adult woman with acute stroke, whereas Figure 12-16 shows evidence of severe vertebrobasilar occlusive disease.

In a multicenter trial, the feasibility and validity of TCCS, in conjunction with ultrasound contrast agents, for the detection of intracranial steno-occlusive disease has been convincingly shown.[48] A recent meta-analysis of 25 studies proved the early vessel status to be highly predictive of the clinical outcome in patients suffering from acute stroke.[53] The main parameters and criteria for the use of TCCS in acute stroke trials have now been defined.[54]

ASSESSMENT OF THE EFFECTS OF EXTRACRANIAL OCCLUSIVE DISEASE

In addition to directly assessing the basilar cerebral arteries, an additional important clinical application of TCD is evaluation of the hemodynamic effects of *extracranial* vascular disease on the *intracranial* circulation.

Carotid Stenosis or Occlusion

Significant changes occur in the intracranial circulation because of the reduced perfusion pressure caused by extracranial flow-limiting disease. With ICA obstruction of 80% or more, the ipsilateral MCA velocity and the pulsatility index generally decrease as a result of vasodilatation in the distal arterial circulation ipsilateral to the obstruction.[30,35] Increased velocities and turbulence are encountered and usually indicate

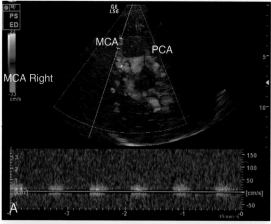

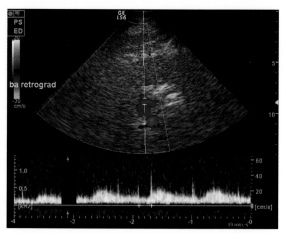

FIGURE 12-16 The probe is in a suboccipital position and directed in an axial plane, slightly angulated upward (transnuchal approach; see Figure 12-10). The Doppler waveform shows reversed direction of blood flow and decreased pulsatility in the basilar artery.

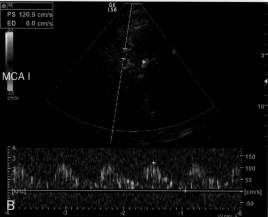

FIGURE 12-15 A, Preserved blood flow in the posterior cerebral artery (PCA) ipsilateral to a middle cerebral artery (MCA) occlusion and, following the administration of contrast material, the typical "blooming" effect that occurs if the gain settings are not adjusted. **B,** Only short flashes of red are visible in the ipsilateral (right) MCA. The M_1 segment is functionally occluded by Doppler waveform evaluation (Thrombolysis in Brain Ischemia [TIBI] 1,) made from the right temporal bone window. By contrast, Doppler blood flow signals in the left MCA as imaged from the left temporal bone window are normal **(B).**

collateralization. The identification of collateral flow in patients with extracranial carotid disease is possible with TCD[12,14,55] and TCCS.[56] Four main collateral pathways can be distinguished: (1) via the anterior communicating artery (ACoA), (2) via the posterior communicating artery (PCoA), (3) via the ophthalmic artery, and (4) via ipsilateral leptomeningeal arteries. Because the small communicating arteries are not always visible with TCCS,[56] indirect hemodynamic signs of the involved arteries are of considerable importance for identifying and localizing collateralization.

Sonographic criteria for intracranial collateralization are given in Table 12-6. In general, the more sonographic criteria that are present, the more confident is the TCCS diagnosis of collateralization. Video 12-3 and Figure 12-17 illustrate findings in two patients with ICA occlusions and their respective intracranial collateral pathways.

Evaluation of hemodynamic disturbances within the carotid artery–MCA pathway is of particular interest in patients with subtotal ICA obstruction, both unilateral and bilateral. Although the predominant mechanism of stroke is thromboembolism, rather than a low-flow effect, a small subgroup of patients experience transient ischemic attacks, permanent stroke, or progressive ischemic eye disease caused by critically reduced blood flow.[57,58] This subgroup of patients may benefit from recanalization surgery, including external carotid–internal carotid bypass. The identification of these individuals is based on the detection of an exhausted cerebral vascular reserve, which can be assessed through TCD measurement of the CO_2 responsiveness of the cerebral arteries.[30]

Vertebrobasilar System

The subclavian steal mechanism is the classic paradigm for studying hemodynamic disturbances in the human vertebrobasilar system. In case of severe obstruction of the proximal subclavian artery on either side, blood to the affected arm will flow retrograde through the ipsilateral

TABLE 12-6 Sonographic Criteria for TCD and TCCS for the Detection of Intracranial Collateralization in Case of Severe Extracranial Artery Disease[56]	
Collateral Pathway	TCD/TCCS Criteria
ACoA	• Retrograde and increased flow in $ACA_{ipsilateral}$ • Orthograde and increased flow in $ACA_{contralateral}$ • Strong turbulences in the region of the AcoA (mostly with TCCS)
PCoA	• Direct visualization of the PCoA (TCCS) • Increased velocity in P_1 segment of the $PCA_{ipsilateral}$ • Velocity ratio of P_1/P_2 segment of the $PCA_{ipsilateral}$ >1.5 • Velocity ratio of $P_{1ipsilateral}/P_{1contralateral}$ >1.5 • Increased velocity within the BA (and sometimes VAs)
Ophthalmic artery	• Retrograde flow in ipsilateral ophthalmic artery • Additional findings in extracranial ultrasonography (e.g., reduced pulsatility index within ipsilateral external carotid artery)
Leptomeningeals	• Increased velocity in the entire ipsilateral PCA ($P_{1ipsilateral} = P_{2ipsilateral}$) • Increased velocity in $ACA_{contralateral}$ without retrograde flow within $ACA_{ipsilateral}$

ACA, anterior cerebral artery; ACoA, anterior communicating artery; BA, basilar artery; PCA, posterior cerebral artery; PCoA, posterior communicating artery; TCCS, transcranial color-coded duplex sonography; TCD, transcranial Doppler; VA, vertebral artery.

VA and be "stolen" from the contralateral vertebral and sometimes basilar artery. Rapid flow changes caused by any type of VA blood flow restriction can be measured directly within the BA. Under resting conditions, blood flow within the BA is almost never critically impaired, even if the subclavian steal is continuous. If the contralateral feeding VA is also diseased (or hypoplastic), however, BA blood flow may become reduced, may demonstrate a to-and-fro flow pattern within each cardiac cycle, or may even be reversed. During hyperemia testing of the stealing arm, blood flow velocity and direction of flow within the basilar trunk may become more or less affected (Figure 12-18). BA blood flow is very resistant to any critical changes resulting from the subclavian steal mechanism. Actually, the subclavian steal, as such, is a benign condition, and even in patients with vertebrobasilar stroke or transient ischemic attack, most symptoms are caused by cerebral microangiopathy rather than large artery flow disturbances.[12] Subclavian artery disease, however, is a strong indicator of coexisting coronary artery disease and future cardiac death.

MONITORING OF CEREBRAL VASOSPASM

Monitoring of vasospasm using TCD is a well-recognized tool in the clinical management of patients suffering from subarachnoid hemorrhage.[14,44] There is a close correlation between increased flow velocities within the spastic basal arteries (MCA, PCA, ACA) and the severity of the subarachnoid hemorrhage.[59,60] This correlation is valid with respect to the size and extent of the subarachnoid clot, the clinical state of the patient, and the angiographically documented severity of spasm (if the Doppler shift is greater than 3 kHz or 120 cm/sec). The side with the more severe flow changes on TCD examination corresponds to the predominant location of the blood clot and the presumed site of the aneurysm. A steep increase in blood flow velocity (>20 cm/sec/day) within the first few days after the bleed is associated with a poor prognosis. Usually, an MCA velocity exceeding 200 cm/sec in patients with vasospasm is associated with a critical reduction in cerebral blood flow (Table 12-7). The time course of the development of vasospasm is also of clinical interest. In general, vasospasm occurs from 4 to 14 days following subarachnoid hemorrhage, but a TCD-detectable increase in velocity often precedes the onset of symptoms by hours to days.

Recent data indicate that TCCS is likewise useful for vasospasm detection, using the criteria previously defined with TCD.[19,61,62] In some patients, TCCS may directly visualize the aneurysm,[62-64] depending on its localization and size and the experience of the examiner. The minimum-size aneurysm that can be detected is reported to be greater than 6 to 8 mm.[60] Due to the availability of other noninvasive angiographic techniques (e.g., computed tomography and magnetic resonance angiography), however, TCCS has not become a routine diagnostic modality in the search for aneurysms.[65]

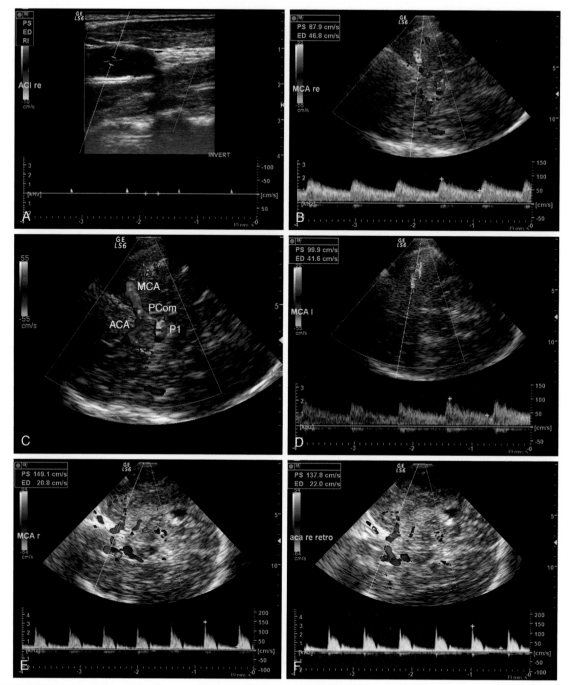

FIGURE 12-17 Doppler studies from a young man with thrombotic occlusion of his right internal carotid artery (ICA) are shown first. **A,** A blunted/absent Doppler waveform blood flow pattern in the ICA. Intracranially, this carotid occlusion is well collateralized: color Doppler signals and Doppler waveforms in the middle cerebral artery (MCA) appear normal **(B)**. Blood flow signals **(C)** in the anterior cerebral artery (ACA) are retrograde (red, should be blue), the posterior communicating artery (PCom) is also visible (color filled and reversed), and the P_1 segment is hyperperfused (aliasing effect). The blood flow profiles and velocities of the ipsilateral MCA **(A)** and the contralateral MCA **(D)** show no significant difference, confirming good collateral flow. In a second case, a middle-age man presents with occlusion of the right ICA. His MCA is also occluded distally. Blood flow profiles show increased pulsatility in the MCA **(E)** and in the retrogradely perfused ACA **(F),** also suggestive of a distal MCA occlusion.

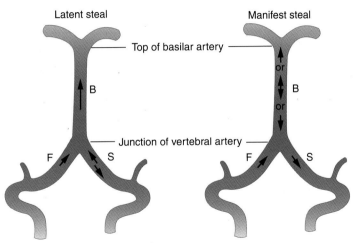

FIGURE 12-18 Schematic representation of flow conditions in various vertebrobasilar vessel segments in patients with the subclavian steal mechanism. With latent steal, flow in the feeding (contralateral) vertebral artery *(F)* is increased during brachial hyperemia and is normal in the basilar artery trunk *(B)*. By contrast, the blood column shows an alternating flow direction in the stealing vertebral artery *(S)*. During manifest steal, blood flow in the stealing vertebral artery *(S)* is continuously reversed. This either has no effect on basilar artery blood flow or causes alternating or reverse flow within the basilar artery trunk. During transcranial Doppler examination, each of the three vessel segments can be clearly differentiated by means of their characteristic flow changes during brachial hyperemia.

TABLE 12-7 Clinical Relevance of Increased Middle Cerebral Artery Flow Velocities After Subarachnoid Hemorrhage

Middle Cerebral Artery Flow Velocity	Time-Averaged Peak Velocity (Mean; cm/sec)	Clinical Consequences
Normal or nonspecifically increased	≤80	Should be observed further
Subcritically accelerated	>80-120	Moderate vasospasm; preventive therapy indicated
Critically accelerated	>120-140	Severe vasospasm; consequent treatment necessary
Highly critical flow acceleration	>140	Severe vasospasm; delayed ischemic deficit highly probable

Modified from Harders A: *Neurosurgical applications of transcranial Doppler sonography,* New York, 1986, Springer-Verlag.

INTRAOPERATIVE MONITORING

Another ostensibly important application of TCD is intraoperative monitoring. The unique advantages of TCD, in comparison with other relative cerebral blood flow measurement techniques, are its complete noninvasiveness and its potential for detecting rapid alterations of blood supply on a real-time basis. TCD monitoring delivers direct, immediate information regarding cerebral perfusion, thus anticipating potential hazards or permitting rapid modification of therapy. TCD monitoring has been used during carotid endarterectomy, open heart surgery with cardiopulmonary bypass, and intensive care

therapy.[12,66] In most studies, the M_1 segment of the MCA is insonated at a depth of 50 to 55 mm. TCD monitoring can be performed either with repeated examinations at extremely short intervals or continuously, using a headband to hold the transducer in place.

Most experience with TCD monitoring has been accumulated during *carotid endarterectomy.*[67-69] It has been shown that MCA flow is affected far less during intraoperative clamping of the carotid artery than expected, raising the possibility that shunts are inserted too often. An MCA velocity of more than 10 cm/sec during clamping has been associated with adequate

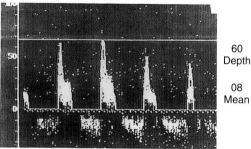
Middle cerebral artery

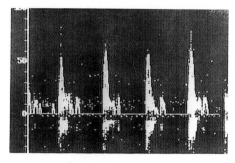
Common carotid artery

FIGURE 12-19 Brain death. Transcranial Doppler changes are noted in the left middle cerebral and extracranial common carotid arteries. The characteristic reflux phenomenon seen during late systole is demonstrated.

collateral circulation.[69] It has further been shown that the amount of microembolization detected with TCD during the dissection and wound closure is predictive of postoperative stroke.[69] This on-line acoustic feedback from TCD, indicating cerebral microembolism, had a direct influence on the surgical technique.[70]

Transcranial Doppler monitoring during *open heart surgery* has revealed a number of disturbances in cerebral blood flow that result from extracorporeal bypass (a pumping technique that severely alters blood flow physiology).[66] Brain damage and perioperative stroke may occur during extracorporeal bypass. TCD measurements have thrown considerable doubt on the theory that such injury is caused by critical *hypoperfusion*. On the contrary, accidental cerebral *hyperperfusion* may play a more decisive role, as well as air microemboli and loss of cerebral autoregulation. In addition, the frequency of cerebral microemboli detected with TCD during open heart surgery correlates with the degree of neuropsychologic deficit.[71,72]

INTENSIVE CARE UNIT MONITORING

Transcranial Doppler is a useful technique for monitoring critically ill patients in the intensive care unit.[73] Eligible patients are predominantly those with raised intracranial pressure (e.g., after head injury) and those with severe cerebrovascular occlusive disease, including cervical artery dissections.[74,75] Monitoring may also be informative, and possibly beneficial, for the patient's outcome in high- and low-pressure hydrocephalus and in low-flow states associated with extracranial occlusive disease, myocardial failure, or valvular disease, as well as impending brain death. TCD monitoring may provide further information about the pathophysiology of various abnormal conditions that affect intensive care patients

and ultimately may be helpful for therapy. In a recent multicenter study, the use of TCD modified the diagnostic and therapeutic management in 36% of critically ill patients.[76] Although Aaslid and Lindegaard[77] have proposed certain parameters of the TCD profile that are likely to reflect the cerebral perfusion pressure, and thus also the intracranial pressure, these parameters have not yet been validated. Only a few TCCS studies have been conducted concerning critical care applications.[78]

BRAIN DEATH

The accurate diagnosis of brain death has become more important in view of the ethical issues that surround the transplantation field. Determination of brain death was for a long time based on three parameters: (1) clinical criteria, (2) electroencephalographic criteria, and (3) angiographic demonstration of absent intracranial circulation.[79] The arrest of intracranial flow results in a characteristic reflux phenomenon in the basal cerebral arteries during late systole. This to-and-fro movement is easily noted in the TCD flow velocity waveform[77] (Figure 12-19). In several large clinical studies, TCD findings correlated perfectly with ancillary diagnostic tests to confirm brain death, with neither false-positive nor false-negative findings.[80,81] Therefore, in proper hands, TCD constitutes an accepted and reliable noninvasive diagnostic test to confirm brain death by demonstrating the stoppage of the cerebral circulation.[82]

ARTERIOVENOUS MALFORMATIONS AND FISTULAS

Although an AVM is a developmental abnormality, the arteries and veins involved in supplying blood to the AVM are anatomically normal and are the usual arteries supplying the region of the brain where the AVM is located. These arteries, which exclusively or partially feed AVMs, can unequivocally be identified with TCD by means of their significant flow abnormalities—that is, increased flow velocity, reduced pulsatility, and reduced responsiveness to CO_2.[83] In a consecutive series, more than 80% of large- to medium-sized AVMs were detected, but more than 60% of smaller AVMs were missed with TCD.[84] TCCS also allows the direct visualization of the AVM.[19,63] For TCCS, a similar diagnostic sensitivity of 80% in the identification of AVMs was reported.[85] In addition to AVMs, other types of intracranial arteriovenous shunts can be detected with TCD and TCCS, such as carotid siphon–cavernous sinus fistulas or dural fistulas.[19,86]

CEREBRAL VENOUS THROMBOSIS AND INTRACEREBRAL HEMORRHAGE

Studies on healthy volunteers indicate that cerebral sinuses and veins can be visualized in 50% to 90% of cases, depending on the vessel segment examined.[87] Preliminary data suggest that cerebral venous thrombosis can be diagnosed using TCCS.[88] Ultrasonographic criteria are (1) abnormal elevation of blood flow velocities within intracranial sinuses and veins and (2) direct visualization of cerebral sinuses with decreased or absent flow. In a recent study in patients suffering from thrombosis of cerebral sinuses and veins, monitoring of venous hemodynamics was a significant predictor of the long-term outcome.[89] Direct visualization of the intracranial sinuses, however, requires significant expertise and, generally, the use of ultrasound contrast agents.

TCCS studies have shown that a sharply demarcated, hyperechogenic area within the brain tissue in stroke patients is indicative of intracerebral hemorrhage.[19,90] Although sensitivity and specificity values were as high as 94% and 95% in 133 consecutive stroke patients with sufficient temporal bone windows,[91] TCCS still cannot replace computed tomographic or magnetic resonance brain imaging in this cohort of patients. In a recent study, hemorrhagic transformation following thrombolytic therapy of acute stroke could be detected with a sensitivity of 90%.[92] Thus, ultrasound can serve as a complementary bedside technique to noninvasively monitor acute stroke patients and their treatment effects but cannot replace radiologic brain imaging techniques as a prerequisite for thrombolytic therapy.

NEW DEVELOPMENTS

MICROEMBOLIC SIGNALS (MES)

The first reports on *gaseous* microemboli detected with ultrasound were published by Spencer and colleagues[93] in 1969 and were associated with decompression sickness and open heart surgery. More than 20 years later, this approach became the focus of clinical interest when the same group detected MES (also termed high-intensity transient signals [HITS]) for the first time with TCD in a patient undergoing carotid endarterectomy.[94] Surprisingly, MES occurred during the preparation time, before the artery was opened, indicating that the MES represented *solid* emboli arising from the arteriosclerotic plaque. Since then, numerous experimental and clinical studies have been published concerning MES, including two consensus statements.[10,95] The latter provide internationally accepted definitions of MES and cover major issues involving TCD instrumentation and software systems. The consensus opinions state that a microembolic TCD signal must (1) be short in duration (<300 msec), (2) be at least 3 dB above the background signal, (3) be mainly unidirectional within the Doppler spectrum, and (4) produce a characteristic sound ("chirp," "snap," "moan"). Typical MESs detected with TCD are illustrated in Figure 12-20. It has been shown that the emboli underlying MESs are usually too small to elicit clinical symptoms. Nevertheless, there is now overwhelming evidence that MESs possess clinical and prognostic relevance in patients with various sources of cardiac, arterial, or extracorporeal brain embolism.[96-100] Several studies have shown that the amount of detected microemboli is a marker of stroke risk on an individual basis, thus serving as a valuable surrogate parameter in clinical trials.[100] In part, they also permit the monitoring of treatment efficacy.[101] The recent introduction of sophisticated MES detection software has considerably improved the monitoring procedure and its diagnostic confidence. Thus, MES detection represents a useful tool for improving the stratification of individuals prone to cerebral embolic events and for evaluating new primary and secondary prevention strategies (Table 12-8). However, the procedure is still time

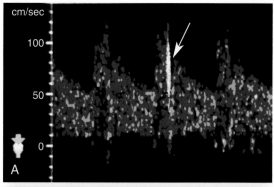

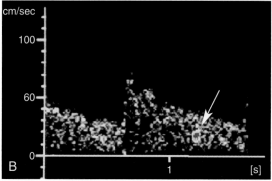

FIGURE 12-20 Illustrative examples of typical microembolic signals (MESs), detected with transcranial Doppler (TCD), in a patient with artificial heart valves. These appear randomly within the systolic **(A)** or the diastolic **(B)** phase of the Doppler spectrum *(arrows)*. The origin of the MES and the maximum intensity elevation are always located within the Doppler spectrum; however, with strong MES intensity gradients (mostly seen with systolic MES), the upper edges—and, rarely, also the lower edges—of the signal may run off the flow spectrum. Note that the intensity of the background TCD signal has to be decreased for MES monitoring (as seen) to allow for effective MES identification.

consuming and needs the continuous presence of a human observer. This limits the routine use of this technique.

ULTRASOUND PERFUSION IMAGING

The introduction of ultrasound contrast agents opened the possibility of ultrasound-mediated measurement of tissue perfusion, based on fundamental indicator-dilution principles.[102] This made it possible to monitor the tissue perfusion of the brain in patients suffering from cerebrovascular disease almost noninvasively and at the bedside. With the use of harmonic imaging techniques, it recently has been shown that contrast enhancement is visible using transcranial B-mode ultrasound imaging, permitting transtemporal brain perfusion mapping.[9] In the first

clinical series reported on acute stroke patients, a positive correlation was found between TCCS-derived brain perfusion maps and incident brain infarction.[103,104] Ultrasound perfusion measurements have been made with bolus tracking, a technique that uses indicator-dilution principles to track signal intensity after the injection of a bolus of contrast agent. It is unreliable because ultrasound energy can destroy some of the microbubbles, thereby violating the underlying premise of the indicator-dilution approach.[105] An alternative approach, using refill kinetics during a *constant infusion* of an ultrasound contrast agent has proven to be useful for brain perfusion measurements.[106] Recent technologic developments have enabled automated brain perfusion measurements and have already been evaluated in the clinical setting[107] (Figure 12-21). The low spatial resolution of TCCS systems used for ultrasound-based brain perfusion measurements is a limitation that may be overcome in the future. The restricted brain volume that can be investigated through the temporal bone (one plane, limited access to ipsilateral cortical tissue, limited signal from contralateral side due to energy loss) might be impossible to circumvent. At present, ultrasound perfusion imaging is still in the preclinical stage, with ongoing studies trying to determine which of the two techniques (bolus approach versus refill kinetics) is superior in generating reproducible perfusion maps of the brain.

SONOTHROMBOLYSIS

In 1942, Lynn and co-workers[108] showed for the first time that focused, in vivo ultrasound can induce selective tissue damage without affecting the surrounding areas. It is now well known that tissue insonation may lead to various physiochemical tissue reactions, such as heating and denaturation, microstreaming effects, release of free radicals, and alterations of blood cells and coagulation, already being used in clinical medicine.[11] The ability of ultrasound to augment the dissolution of thrombus was first reported in 1989 by Kodo.[109] This capability has been verified in numerous experimental studies using in vitro and animal models.[110,111] It has been shown that the insonation of thrombus alone[112] or in combination with fibrinolytic agents[113] significantly accelerates the thrombolytic process. This effect has been termed *ultrasound-assisted thrombolysis* or *sonothrombolysis*. Using a variety of ultrasound frequencies (20 kHz-3 MHz) and intensities

TABLE 12-8 Amount and Clinical Relevance of Intracranially Circulating Microemboli Detected by TCD[93-101]

Clinical Collective	Prevalence of Microembolic Signals (Range; %)	Prognostic Impact	Remarks
Normal probands	0	-	
Acute ischemic stroke	9-71	(+)	Higher MES load early after stroke Positive correlation to cause of stroke Subgroup of studies showed correlation with short-term risk for recurrent stroke
Carotid artery stenosis		+	MES-positive patients showed higher rate of cerebral ischemia
Asymptomatic	2-29		More MES with higher degree of stenosis
Symptomatic	18-100		
Intracranial artery stenosis		+	MES-positive patients showed slightly higher rate of cerebral ischemia
Asymptomatic	0		More MES with short latency to recent symptoms
Symptomatic	22-75		
Acute dissection of brain-supplying arteries	36-75	(+)	In one study positive correlation of MES prevalence to risk for recurrent cerebral ischemia
Aortic source of embolism	13-48	-	Minor correlation to plaque thickness
Prosthetic heart valves	69-100	-	High prevalence of cavitation-induced gaseous microemboli without clinical or prognostic impact No correlation to intensity of antihemostatic treatment
Left ventricular assist devices	28-100	(+)	In part correlation of MES prevalence to risk for recurrent cerebral ischemia No correlation to intensity of antihemostatic treatment
Atrial fibrillation (AF)	15-40	(+)	Higher MES prevalence in valvular than in nonvalvular AF Higher MES prevalence in symptomatic AF and in patients with recent cerebral ischemia
Interventions on brain-supplying arteries	38-100	-	Mostly very high MES numbers without clinical or prognostic impact
Open heart surgery	82-100	(+)	Weak correlation of intraoperative MES load to postoperative neuropsychologic deficits

MES, microembolic signal; TCD, transcranial Doppler.
Prognostic impact: - denotes no evidence; (+) minor/inconsistent evidence; + clear evidence that has been confirmed and reproduced in several studies.

(3 mW-8 W/cm²), a clear dose relationship of this phenomenon has been demonstrated.[110] It is now believed that not *macrostructural* (e.g., clot disruption) but rather *microstructural* alterations (e.g., dysconfiguration of fibrin molecules) are mainly responsible for the sonothrombolytic effect, via a microcavitation process. In addition to several clinical studies in patients suffering from acute coronary syndromes, the first reports on successful sonothrombolysis in acute stroke patients have appeared.[114,115] Sonothrombolysis is a very exciting, novel tool that may increase the efficacy of the purely pharmacologic approach of thrombolysis in acute stroke. Acceleration of intracranial vessel recanalization could reduce final cerebral infarct size and therefore improve the long-term outcome[115,116] of stroke patients. Recent studies indicate that the use of echo-contrast-enhanced agents can further enhance the effect of sonothrombolysis via microbubble-induced cavitation.[117,118] Establishing this bedside technique as a *therapeutic* tool could revolutionize the entire field of acute stroke treatment. However, safety issues concerning

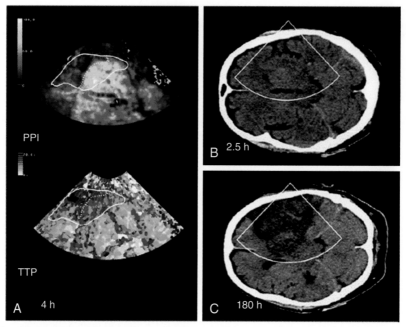

FIGURE 12-21 The figure shows corresponding axial planes of the computed tomographic (CT) scan and the ultrasound perfusion imaging of a 70-year-old patient with middle cerebral artery infarction (National Institutes of Health Stroke Scale [NIHSS]: 12). **A,** Ultrasound perfusion studies were done following a 2.5-mL Sonovue bolus injection as contrast agent. Ultrasound perfusion studies are presented as pixelwise peak intensity (PPI) and time to peak intensity (TTP) maps. PPI is coded as 0% to 100%, TTP as 0 to 20 seconds (color coded as levels of blue). CT scans were obtained 2.5 hours **(B)** and 180 hours **(C)** after symptom onset. The corresponding field of view of the ultrasound perfusion studies is projected as a white frame over the CT scans.

TABLE 12-9 Main Indications for Vascular TCD and TCCS in Clinical and Experimental Settings

1. Detection of intracranial stenoses and occlusions in the major basal arteries
2. Evaluation of intracranial hemodynamic effects and collateral flow of extracranial occlusive disease (e.g., occlusions, subclavian steal)
3. Monitoring of intracranial vessel recanalization in acute stroke
4. Monitoring of intracranial cerebral hemodynamics
   a. After subarachnoid hemorrhage (e.g., presence and severity of vasospasms)
   b. In patients with increased intracranial pressure (e.g., on the intensive care unit)
   c. During and after extracranial revascularization procedures (e.g., carotid endarterectomy, carotid angioplasty)
   d. Before and during neuroradiologic interventions (e.g., balloon occlusion) for presence of collateral pathways
   e. During open heart surgery
   f. In evolution of brain death
5. Detection and quantification of cerebral circulating microemboli
6. Detection and quantification of right-to-left shunts
7. Functional tests
   a. Stimulation of intracranial arterioles with carbon dioxide or other vasoactive drugs (e.g., assessing vasomotor reserve capacity)
   b. Language lateralization (e.g., before neurosurgery)
   c. External stimulation of visual cortex
8. Still in the developmental stage
   a. Brain perfusion imaging
   b. Ultrasound-assisted thrombolysis

TCCS, transcranial color-coded duplex sonography; TCD, transcranial Doppler.

the risk for intracerebral hemorrhage are under investigation.

CONCLUSIONS

Through continuous refinements and technical innovations during the past three decades, transcranial ultrasound is no longer limited to the sonographic measurement of blood flow velocities. Today, transcranial ultrasound offers multimodal, high-resolution, and real-time imaging of the brain's structure and vasculature. Using modern equipment and a variety of ultrasound modalities, information can be acquired about anatomy, hemodynamic status, and function of the central nervous system and its supplying arteries and veins (Table 12-9). Nevertheless, TCD and TCCS remain portable, easy-to-access, dynamic, highly reliable, and reproducible techniques in clinical medicine that support various therapeutic decisions. Noninvasiveness further advocates the use of TCD as a monitoring tool, particularly during surgical or neurointerventional procedures. Overall, transcranial ultrasound with TCD and TCCS has revolutionized our understanding of cerebrovascular disease, and these modalities now are key in the diagnostic workup of cerebrovascular disorders. In most countries, TCD and TCCS are in the hands of physicians and technicians with neurologic background who deal appropriately and carefully with its capabilities and limitations. However, we must be aware that all these methods require *sufficient knowledge*, *practical skills*, and *technical expertise*. In other words, we have to ensure continuous education and adequate training in the fascinating field called *neurosonology*.

REFERENCES

1. Miyazaki M, Kato K: Measurement of cerebral blood flow by ultrasonic Doppler technique, *Jpn Circ J* 29:375, 1965.
2. Aaslid R, Markwalder T-M, Norris H: Noninvasive transcranial Doppler ultrasound recording of flow velocity in basal cerebral arteries, *J Neurosurg* 57:769, 1982.
3. Bogdahn U, et al: Transcranial color-coded real-time sonography in adults, *Stroke* 21:1680, 1990.
4. Bude RO, Rubin JM, Adler RS: Power versus conventional color Doppler sonography: Comparison in the depiction of normal intrarenal vasculature, *Radiology* 192:777, 1994.
5. Klötzsch C, et al: Contrast-enhanced three-dimensional transcranial color-coded sonography of intra-cranial stenoses, *AJNR Am J Neuroradiol* 23:208, 2002.
6. Otis S, Rush M, Boyajian R: Contrast-enhanced transcranial imaging. Results of an American phase-two study, *Stroke* 26:203, 1995.
7. Nabavi DG, et al: Diagnostic benefit of echocontrast enhancement for the insufficient transtemporal bone window, *J Neuroimaging* 9:102, 1999.
8. Jauss M, Zanette E: Detection of right-to-left shunt with ultrasound contrast agent and transcranial Doppler sonography, *Cerebrovasc Dis* 10:490, 2000.
9. Wiesmann M, Seidel G: Ultrasound perfusion imaging of the human brain, *Stroke* 31:2421, 2000.
10. Ringelstein EB, et al: Consensus on microembolus detection by TCD. International Consensus Group on Microembolus detection, *Stroke* 29:725, 1998.
11. Francis CW, Behrens S: Ultrasonic thrombolysis. In Hennerici M, Meairs S, editors: *Cerebrovascular Ultrasound. Theory, Practice and Future Developments*, Cambridge, UK, 2001, Cambridge University Press.
12. Ringelstein EB: A practical guide to transcranial Doppler sonography. In Weinberger J, editor: *Noninvasive Imaging of Cerebral Vascular Disease*, New York, 1989, AR Liss, p 75.
13. Spencer MP, Whisler D: Transorbital Doppler diagnosis of intracranial arterial stenosis, *Stroke* 17:916, 1986.
14. Aaslid R, Markwalder TM, Nornes H: Noninvasive transcranial Doppler ultrasound recording of flow velocity in the basal cerebral arteries, *J Neurosurg* 57:769, 1982.
15. Arnolds B, von Reutern GM: Transcranial Doppler sonography: Examination technique and normal reference values, *Ultrasound Med Biol* 12:115, 1986.
16. White DN, Curry GR, Stevenson RJ: The acoustic characteristics of the skull, *Ultrasound Med Biol* 4:225, 1978.
17. Grolimund P: Transmission of ultrasound through the temporal bone. In Aaslid R, editor: *Transcranial Doppler Sonography*, New York, 1986, Springer-Verlag, p 10.
18. Aaslid R, editor: *Transcranial Doppler Sonography*, New York, 1986, Springer-Verlag, p 39.
19. Baumgartner RW: Transcranial color duplex sonography in cerebrovascular disease: A systematic review, *Cerebrovasc Dis* 16:4, 2003.
20. Schöning M, Buchholz R, Walter J: Comparative study of transcranial color duplex sonography and transcranial Doppler sonography in adults, *J Neurosurg* 78: 776–784, 1993.
21. Greenfield DS, Heggerich PA, Hedges TR III: Color Doppler imaging of normal orbital vasculature, *Ophthalmology* 102:1598–1605, 1995.
22. Mast H, Ecker S, Marx P: Cerebral ischemia induced by compression tests during transcranial Doppler sonography, *Clin Investig* 71:46, 1993.
23. Khaffaf N, et al: Embolic stroke by compression maneuver during transcranial Doppler sonography, *Stroke* 25:1056, 1994.
24. Otis S, Ringelstein EB: Transcranial Doppler sonography. In Bernstein ED, editor: *Noninvasive Diagnostic Techniques in Vascular Disease*, St. Louis, 1990, CV Mosby, p 59.
25. Ringelstein EB, et al: Transcranial Doppler sonography. Anatomical landmarks and normal velocity values, *Ultrasound Med Biol* 16:745–761, 1990.
26. Hennerici M, et al: Transcranial Doppler ultrasound for the assessment of intracranial arterial flow velocity— Part I. Examination technique and normal values, *Surg Neurol* 27:439, 1987.
27. Grolimund P, Seiler RW: Age dependence of the flow velocity in the basal arteries—a transcranial Doppler ultrasound study, *Ultrasound Med Biol* 14:191, 1988.

28. Frackowiak RSJ, Lenzi GL, Jones T: Quantitative measurements of cerebral blood flow and oxygen metabolism in man using 15-oxygen and positron emission tomography. Theory, procedure and normal values, *J Comput Assist Tomogr* 4:727, 1980.

29. Baumgartner RW, et al: A validation study on the intraobserver reproducibility of transcranial color-coded duplex sonography velocity measurements, *Ultrasound Med Biol* 20:233, 1994.

30. Ringelstein EB, et al: Noninvasive assessment of CO_2-induced cerebral vasomotor response in normal individuals and patients with internal carotid artery occlusions, *Stroke* 19:963, 1988.

31. Huber P, Handa J: Effect of contrast material, hypercapnia, hyperventilation, hypertonic glucose and papaverine on the diameter of the cerebral arteries—angiographic determination in man, *Invest Radiol* 2:17, 1987.

32. Markwalder TM, et al: Dependency of blood flow velocity in the middle cerebral artery on end-tidal carbon dioxide partial pressure—a transcranial ultrasound Doppler study, *J Cereb Blood Flow Metab* 4:368, 1984.

33. Ringelstein EB, Otis SM, Schneider PA: Noninvasive assessment of CO_2-induced cerebral vasomotor reactivity. Comparison with rCBF findings during 133-xenon inhalation measurement, *J Cereb Blood Flow Metab* 1: 161, 1989.

34. Gosling RG, King DH: Processing arterial Doppler signals for clinical data. In De Vlieger M, editor: *Handbook of Clinical Ultrasound*, New York, 1978, John Wiley & Sons.

35. Ley-Pozo J, Willmes K, Ringelstein EB: Relationship between pulsatility indices of Doppler flow signals and CO_2-reactivity within the middle cerebral artery in extracranial occlusive disease, *Ultrasound Med Biol* 16:763, 1990.

36. Niederkorn R, Neumayer K: Transcranial Doppler sonography: A new approach in the noninvasive diagnosis of intracranial brain artery disease, *Eur Neurol* 26:65, 1987.

37. de Bray JM, et al: Detection of vertebrobasilar intracranial stenoses: Transcranial Doppler sonography versus angiography, *J Ultrasound Med* 16:213, 1997.

38. Felberg RA, et al: Screening for intracranial stenosis with transcranial Doppler: The accuracy of mean flow velocity thresholds, *J Neuroimaging* 12:9, 2002.

39. Rorick MB, Nichols FT, Adams RJ: Transcranial Doppler correlation with angiography in detection of intracranial stenosis, *Stroke* 25:1931, 1994.

40. Demchuk AM, et al: Accuracy and criteria for localizing arterial occlusion with transcranial Doppler, *J Neuroimaging* 10:1, 2000.

41. Demchuk AM, et al: Thrombolysis in brain ischemia (TIBI) transcranial flow grades predict clinical severity, early recovery, and mortality in patients treated with intravenous tissue plasminogen activator, *Stroke* 32:89, 2001.

42. Saqqur M, et al: CLOTBUST Investigators. Residual flow at the site of intracranial occlusion on transcranial Doppler predicts response to intravenous thrombolysis: A multi-center study, *Cerebrovasc Dis* 27:5, 2009.

43. Schwartz A, Hennerici M: Noninvasive transcranial Doppler ultrasound in intracranial angiomas, *Neurology* 36:626, 1986.

44. Aaslid R, et al: Evaluation of cerebrovascular spasm with transcranial Doppler ultrasound, *J Neurosurg* 60:37, 1984.

45. Ringelstein EB, et al: Type and extent of hemispheric brain infarctions and clinical outcome in early and delayed middle cerebral artery recanalization, *Neurology* 42:289, 1992.

46. Brandt T, et al: CT angiography and Doppler sonography for emergency assessment in acute basilar artery ischemia, *Stroke* 30:606, 1999.

47. Baumgartner RW, Mattle HP, Schroth G: Assessment of ≥50% and <50% intracranial stenoses by transcranial color-coded duplex sonography, *Stroke* 30:87, 1999.

48. Gerriets T, et al: DIAS I: Duplex-sonographic assessment of the cerebrovascular status in acute stroke. A useful tool for future stroke trials, *Stroke* 31:2342, 2000.

49. Seidel G, Kaps M, Gerriets T: Potential and limitations of transcranial color-coded sonography in stroke patients, *Stroke* 26:2061, 1995.

50. Kenton AR, et al: Comparison of transcranial color-coded sonography and magnetic resonance angiography in acute stroke, *Stroke* 28:1601, 1997.

51. Nabavi DG, et al: Potential and limitations of echocontrast-enhanced ultrasonography in acute stroke patients: A pilot study, *Stroke* 29:949, 1998.

52. Postert T, et al: Contrast-enhanced transcranial color-coded real-time sonography: A reliable tool for the diagnosis of middle cerebral artery trunk occlusion in patients with insufficient temporal bone window, *Stroke* 29:1070, 1998.

53. Stolz E, et al: Can early neurosonology predict outcome in acute stroke?: A metaanalysis of prognostic clinical effect sizes related to the vascular status, *Stroke* 39:2355, 2008.

54. Nedelmann M, et al: Consensus recommendations for transcranial color-coded duplex sonography for the assessment of intracranial arteries in clinical trials on acute stroke, *Stroke* 40:3238, 2009.

55. Anzola GP, et al: Transcranial Doppler sonography and magnetic resonance angiography in the assessment of collateral hemispheric flow in patients with carotid artery disease, *Stroke* 26:214, 1995.

56. Baumgartner RW, et al: Transcranial color-coded duplex sonography in the evaluation of collateral flow through the circle of Willis, *AJR Am J Neuroradiol* 18: 127, 1997.

57. Caplan LR, Sergay S: Positional cerebral ischemia, *J Neurol Neurosurg Psychiatry* 39:385, 1976.

58. Ringelstein EB, et al: The pathogenesis of strokes from internal carotid artery occlusion: Diagnostic and therapeutic implications, *Stroke* 14:867, 1983.

59. Harders A, Gilsbach JM: Time course of blood velocity changes related to vasospasm in the circle of Willis measured by transcranial Doppler ultrasound, *J Neurosurg* 66:718, 1987.

60. Seiler RW, et al: Cerebral vasospasm evaluated by transcranial ultrasound correlated with clinical grade and CT-visualized subarachnoid hemorrhage, *J Neurosurg* 64:594, 1986.

61. Proust F, et al: Usefulness of transcranial color-coded sonography in the diagnosis of cerebral vasospasm, *Stroke* 30:1091, 1999.

62. Becker G, et al: Diagnosis and monitoring of subarachnoid hemorrhage by transcranial color-coded real-time sonography, *Neurosurgery* 28:814, 1991.

63. Martin PJ, et al: Intracranial aneurysms and arteriovenous malformations: Transcranial colour-coded sonography as a diagnostic aid, *Ultrasound Med Biol* 20:689, 1994.
64. Wardlaw JM, Cannon JC, Sellar RJ: Use of color power transcranial Doppler sonography to monitor aneurysmal coiling, *AJNR Am J Neuroradiol* 17:864, 1996.
65. Klötzsch C, Harrer JU: Cerebral aneurysms and arteriovenous malformations, *Front Neurol Neurosci* 21:171, 2006.
66. von Reutern GM, et al: Transcranial Doppler ultrasonography during cardiopulmonary bypass in patients with severe carotid stenosis or occlusion, *Stroke* 19:674, 1989.
67. Schneider PA, et al: Transcranial Doppler monitoring during carotid arterial surgery, *Surg Forum* 38:333, 1987.
68. Padayachee TS, et al: Monitoring middle cerebral artery blood velocity during carotid endarterectomy, *Br J Surg* 73:98, 1986.
69. Ackerstaff RG, et al: Association of intraoperative transcranial Doppler monitoring variables with stroke from carotid endarterectomy, *Stroke* 31:1817, 2000.
70. Jansen C, et al: Carotid endarterectomy with transcranial Doppler and electroencephalographic monitoring: A prospective study in 130 operations, *Stroke* 24:665, 1993.
71. Barbut D, et al: Determination of size of aortic emboli and embolic load during coronary artery bypass grafting, *Ann Thorac Surg* 63:1262, 1997.
72. Braekken SK, et al: Association between intraoperative cerebral microembolic signals and postoperative neuropsychological deficit: Comparison between patients with cardiac valve replacement and patients with coronary artery bypass grafting, *J Neurol Neurosurg Psychiatry* 65:573, 1998.
73. Alvarez del Castillo M: Monitoring neurologic patients in intensive care, *Curr Opin Crit Care* 7:49, 2001.
74. Babikian VL, et al: Transcranial Doppler sonographic monitoring in the intensive care unit, *J Intensive Care Med* 6:36, 1991.
75. Dittrich R, et al: Polyarterial clustered recurrence of cervical artery dissection seems to be the rule, *Neurology* 69:180–186, 2007.
76. Grupo de Trabajo de Neurointensivismo y Trauma de la Sociedad Espanola de Medicina Intensiva, Critica y Unidades Coronarias (SEMICYUC); Grupo de Trabajode Neurologia Critica de la Societat Catalana de Medicina Intensiva i Critics (SOCMIC): Clinical use of transcranial Doppler in critical neurological patients. Results of a multicenter study, *Med Clin (Barc)* 120:241, 2003.
77. Aaslid R, Lindegaard KF: Cerebral hemodynamics. In Aaslid R, editor: *Transcranial Doppler Sonography*, New York, 1986, Springer-Verlag, p 60.
78. Shiogai T, et al: Morphological and hemodynamic evaluations by means of transcranial power Doppler imaging in patients with severe head injury, *Acta Neurochir Suppl (Wien)* 71:94, 1998.
79. Black PM: Brain death. Medical progress, *N Engl J Med* 299:338, 1978.
80. Ducrocq X, et al: Brain death and transcranial Doppler: Experience in 130 cases of brain dead patients, *J Neurol Sci* 160:41, 1998.
81. Zurynski Y, et al: Transcranial Doppler ultrasound in brain death: Experience in 140 patients, *Neurol Res* 13:248, 1991.
82. Wijdicks EF: The diagnosis of brain death, *N Engl J Med* 344:1215, 2001.
83. Diehl RR, et al: Blood flow velocity and vasomotor reactivity in patients with arteriovenous malformations: A transcranial Doppler study, *Stroke* 25:1574, 1994.
84. Mast H, et al: Transcranial Doppler ultrasonography in cerebral arteriovenous malformations. Diagnostic sensitivity and association of flow velocity with spontaneous hemorrhage and focal neurological deficit, *Stroke* 26:1024, 1995.
85. el-Saden SM, et al: Transcranial color Doppler imaging of brain arteriovenous malformations in adults, *J Ultrasound Med* 16:327, 1997.
86. Sommer C, et al: Noninvasive assessment of intracranial fistulas and other small arteriovenous malformations, *Neurosurg* 30:522–528, 1992.
87. Stolz E, et al: Transcranial color-coded duplex sonography of intracranial veins and sinuses in adults. Reference data from 130 volunteers, *Stroke* 30:1070, 1999.
88. Stolz E, Kaps M, Dorndorf W: Assessment of intracranial venous hemodynamics in normal individuals and patients with cerebral venous thrombosis, *Stroke* 30:70, 1999.
89. Stolz E, et al: Intracranial venous hemodynamics is a factor related to a favorable outcome in cerebral venous thrombosis, *Stroke* 33:1645, 2002.
90. Seidel G, Kaps M, Dorndorf W: Transcranial color-coded duplex sonography of intracerebral hematomas in adults, *Stroke* 24:1519, 1993.
91. Maurer M, et al: Differentiation between intracerebral hemorrhage and ischemic stroke by transcranial color-coded duplex-sonography, *Stroke* 29:2563, 1998.
92. Seidel G, et al: Sonographic evaluation of hemorrhagic transformation and arterial recanalization in acute hemispheric ischemic stroke, *Stroke* 40:199, 2009.
93. Spencer MP, et al: The use of ultrasonics in the determination of arterial aeroembolism during open-heart surgery, *Ann Thorac Surg* 8:489, 1969.
94. Spencer MP, et al: Detection of middle cerebral artery emboli during carotid endarterectomy using transcranial Doppler ultrasonography, *Stroke* 21:415, 1990.
95. Consensus Committee of the Ninth International Cerebral Hemodynamic Symposium: Basic identification criteria of Doppler microembolic signals, *Stroke* 26:1123, 1995.
96. Droste DW, Ringelstein EB: Detection of high intensity transient signals (HITS): How and why? *Eur J Ultrasound* 7:23, 1998.
97. Nabavi DG, Sliwka U: Mikroembolusdetektion mittels transkranieller Dopplersonographie, *Klin Neurophysiol* 30:275, 1999.
98. Ritter MA, et al: Prevalence and prognostic impact of microembolic signals in arterial sources of embolism. A systematic review of the literature, *J Neurol* 255:953, 2008.
99. King A, Markus HS: Doppler embolic signals in cerebrovascular disease and prediction of stroke risk: A systematic review and meta-analysis, *Stroke* 40:3711, 2009.
100. Markus HS, et al: Dual antiplatelet therapy with clopidogrel and aspirin in symptomatic carotid stenosis evaluated using Doppler embolic signal detection. The Clopidogrel and Aspirin for Reduction of Emboli in Symptomatic Carotid Stenosis (CARESS) trial, *Circulation* 111:2233–2240, 2005.
101. Goertler M, et al: Rapid decline of cerebral microemboli of arterial origin after intravenous acetylsalicylic acid, *Stroke* 30:66–69, 1999.

102. Meier P, Zierler KL: On the theory of the indicator-dilution method for measurement of blood flow and volume, *J Appl Physiol* 6:731, 1954.

103. Federlein J, et al: Ultrasound evaluation of pathological brain perfusion in acute stroke using second harmonic imaging, *J Neurol Neurosurg Psychiatry* 69:616, 2002.

104. Meyer K, et al: Harmonic imaging in acute stroke: Detection of a cerebral perfusion deficit with ultrasound and perfusion MRI, *J Neuroimaging* 13:166, 2003.

105. Lassen NA, Perl W: *Tracer kinetic methods in medical physiology*, New York, 1979, Raven Press.

106. Rim SJ, et al: Quantification of cerebral perfusion with "Real-Time" contrast-enhanced ultrasound, *Circulation* 20:2582, 2001.

107. Maciak A, et al: Automatic detection of perfusion deficits with Bolus Harmonic Imaging, *Ultraschall Med* 29:618, 2008.

108. Lynn JG, et al: A new method for the generation and use of focused ultrasound in experimental biology, *J Gen Physiol* 26:179, 1942.

109. Kudo S: Thrombolysis with ultrasound effect, *Tokyo Med J* 104:1005, 1989.

110. Ishibashi T, et al: Can transcranial ultrasonication increase recanalization flow with tissue plasminogen activator? *Stroke* 33:1399, 2002.

111. Eggers J, Ossadnik S, Seidel G: Enhanced clot dissolution in vitro by 1.8-MHz pulsed ultrasound, *Ultrasound Med Biol* 35:523, 2009.

112. Rosenschein U, et al: Ultrasound imaging-guided non-invasive ultrasound—thrombolysis: Preclinical results, *Circulation* 102:238, 2000.

113. Lauer CG, et al: Effect of ultrasound on tissue-type plasminogen activator-induced thrombolysis, *Circulation* 86:1257, 1992.

114. Alexandrov AV, et al: High rate of complete recanalization and dramatic clinical recovery during tPA infusion when continuously monitored with 2-MHz transcranial Doppler monitoring, *Stroke* 31:610, 2000.

115. Eggers J, et al: Effect of ultrasound on thrombolysis of middle cerebral artery occlusion, *Ann Neurol* 53:797, 2003.

116. Eggers J, et al: Sonothrombolysis with transcranial color-coded sonography and recombinant tissue-type plasminogen activator in acute middle cerebral artery main stem occlusion: Results from a randomized study, *Stroke* 39:1470, 2008.

117. Alexandrov AV, et al: A pilot randomized clinical safety study of sonothrombolysis augmentation with ultrasound-activated perflutren-lipid microspheres for acute ischemic stroke, *Stroke* 39:1464, 2008.

118. Molina CA, et al: Microbubble administration accelerates clot lysis during continuous 2-MHz ultrasound monitoring in stroke patients treated with intravenous tissue plasminogen activator, *Stroke* 37:425, 2006.

Extremity Arteries

ARTERIAL ANATOMY OF THE EXTREMITIES

13

GREGORY M. KECK, MD; JOHN S. PELLERITO, MD, FACR, FSRU, FAIUM;
and JOSEPH F. POLAK, MD, MPH

The evaluation of arterial disease of the extremities requires knowledge of vascular anatomy. This chapter provides this basic information for the upper and lower extremities. Normal anatomy, common variants, and major collateral routes[1-6] are illustrated, primarily by representative arteriograms. The chapter is formatted as a series of captioned illustrations, with the bulk of the instructional material contained within the figure captions.

It is increasingly common for arterial anatomy and pathology to be depicted noninvasively in a clinical setting with computed tomography or magnetic resonance imaging. Image quality with these modalities approaches that of catheter angiography. Because conventional arteriography remains the gold standard, angiographic images are used in this chapter, as they best depict anatomic detail.

The following terms are used to describe extremity anatomy in this chapter. The *arm* is the portion of the upper extremity between the shoulder and elbow. The *forearm* is the portion between the elbow and wrist. The *thigh* is the portion of the lower extremity between the hip and knee, and the *calf* is the portion between the knee and ankle.

UPPER EXTREMITY

NORMAL FEATURES

The normal arterial anatomy of the upper extremity is depicted graphically in Figure 13-1. Figures 13-2 to 13-5 are detailed arteriographic views of

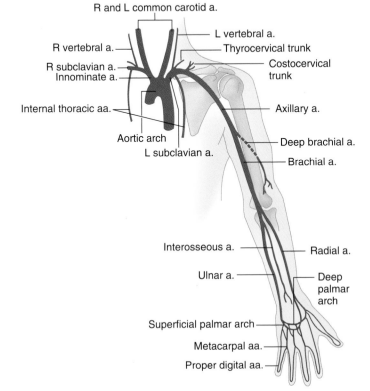

FIGURE 13-1 Arterial anatomy of the upper extremity. Note that the internal thoracic arteries (internal mammary arteries), which are tributaries of the subclavian arteries, are used commonly for coronary artery bypass. The deep palmar arch arises from the radial artery, and the superficial palmar arch arises from the ulnar artery. These arches may or may not communicate with each other. a., artery; aa., arteries; L, left; R, right.

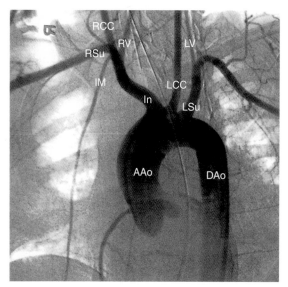

FIGURE 13-2 The aortic arch connects the ascending aorta (AAo) with the descending aorta (DAo). Three great vessels originate from the aortic arch; the innominate artery (In) originates on the right side of the arch, followed by the left common carotid artery (LCC) and the left subclavian artery (LSu). The innominate artery divides into the right common carotid artery (RCC) and the right subclavian artery (RSu). The right and left vertebral arteries (RV, LV) originate from the subclavian arteries, even though this is not apparent on the right side of this illustration. The internal mammary artery (IM) also arises from the subclavian artery.

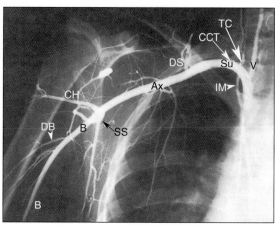

FIGURE 13-3 The subclavian artery (Su) becomes the axillary artery (Ax) at the lateral margin of the first rib. The axillary artery, in turn, becomes the brachial artery (B) after crossing the inferolateral margin of the teres major muscle.[3] The thyrocervical (TC) and costocervical (CCT) trunks are noteworthy branches of the subclavian artery, because they may be mistaken for the vertebral artery (V) during duplex examination. The multiple branches that supply the scapular musculature serve as collaterals when the subclavian or innominate arteries are obstructed. CH, circumflex humeral artery; DB, deep brachial artery; DS, dorsal scapular artery; IM, internal mammary artery; SS, subscapular artery.

FIGURE 13-4 Arterial anatomy (A) and osseous landmarks (B) at the elbow. The brachial artery (B) divides at the elbow, forming the radial (R) and ulnar (U) arteries. The interosseous artery (I) is a branch of the ulnar artery, which in some individuals continues to the wrist. RR, recurrent radial artery; UR, ulnar recurrent artery.

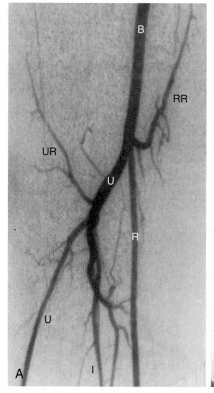

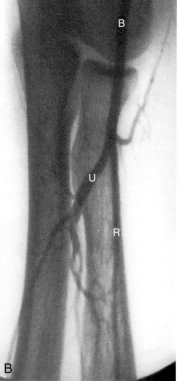

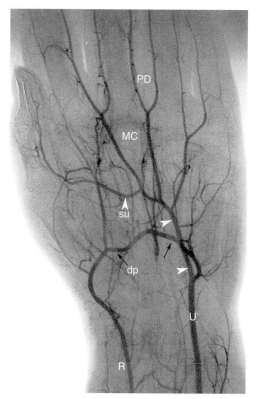

FIGURE 13-5 The radial artery (R) terminates in the deep palmar arch (dp; *black arrows*). The ulnar artery (U) terminates in the superficial palmar arch (su; *white arrowheads*). Communicating vessels usually connect the deep and superficial arches, as shown here. The metacarpal (MC; also called the common palmar digital artery or dorsal metacarpal artery) and proper palmar digital (PD) arteries are branches of the superficial and deep arches.

specific regions of the upper extremity arterial tree, beginning at the aorta and extending to the digits. These figures should be reviewed carefully, because their legends provide the instructional content.

ANATOMIC VARIANTS

Many anatomic variants can occur in the arterial tree of the upper extremities. The more commonly encountered variants are presented in Table 13-1.[1-3] Familiarity with these variants can prevent confusion and error during duplex examination. An example of an upper extremity anatomic variant is presented in Figure 13-6.

COLLATERAL ROUTES

Many of the tributaries seen in Figures 13-1 to 13-6 may serve as collaterals when the main arterial trunks of the upper extremity are blocked.

The following is a summary of the more common collateral routes.[2]
1. Obstruction of the proximal subclavian or brachiocephalic arteries
   a. Collateral flow from cranial and/or neck arteries to the subclavian artery distal to the obstruction (e.g., subclavian steal phenomenon)
   b. Collateral flow from pelvic, abdominal wall, and thoracic wall arteries to the subclavian artery distal to the obstruction
2. Obstruction of the distal subclavian or axillary arteries
   a. Collateral flow from the thoracic wall or shoulder region to the axillary artery distal to the obstruction
3. Obstruction of the brachial artery or its branch vessels
   a. Collateral flow from the distal arm to the proximal forearm
   b. Collateral flow from the midarm to the distal arm and/or forearm
   c. Retrograde flow filling the palmar arches of the hand

Figure 13-7 shows an example of collateralization in response to radial artery occlusion.

LOWER EXTREMITY

NORMAL ANATOMY

The lower extremity arterial tree begins at the aortic bifurcation, and this portion of the vasculature is included in this chapter. For details concerning abdominal vascular anatomy, see Chapter 26. The major arteries of the lower extremity are illustrated graphically in Figure 13-8. Figures 13-9 to 13-13 are angiographic depictions of the regional arterial anatomy of the lower extremity.

ANATOMIC VARIANTS

The arterial anatomy of the lower extremity is fairly constant. Anatomic variations that may be encountered occasionally are presented in Table 13-2.[4] The relative infrequency of these variations is also cited in this table.

COLLATERAL ROUTES

Multiple variations are possible in the collateral routes that circumvent lower extremity arterial obstruction. The following is an outline of the more common collateral pathways.[4,5] It is important for vascular laboratory personnel to

TABLE 13-1 Arterial Variants of the Upper Extremity		
Structure	Variant	Frequency of Occurrence in the Population (%)
Aortic arch and great vessels	Common origin of the right brachiocephalic and left common carotid arteries	22
	Left vertebral artery origin directly from the aorta	4-6
	Common origin of both common carotid arteries	<1
Arm and forearm	Radial artery origin from the axillary artery	1-3
	Early division of the brachial artery: 1. High origin of the radial artery (Figure 13-6) 2. Accessory (duplicated) brachial artery	19
	Ulnar artery origin from the brachial or axillary artery	2-3
	Low origin (5-7 cm below elbow joint) of ulnar artery	<1
	Persistent median artery	2-4

be familiar, in general terms, with the more commonly seen collateral pathways, as illustrated in Figures 13-14 through 13-18:

1. Distal aorta or bilateral common iliac artery obstruction
   a. Collateral flow from thoracic and abdominal wall arteries to pelvic arteries distal to the obstruction
   b. Collateral flow from arteries of the bowel to pelvic arteries distal to the obstruction
   c. Collateral flow from lumbar arteries to pelvic arteries distal to the obstruction
2. Unilateral common iliac artery obstruction
   a. Collateral flow from contralateral iliac and/or femoral arteries to arteries of the pelvis or thigh distal to the obstruction
   b. Collateral pathways as just mentioned, with supply to the ipsilateral pelvic arteries
3. External iliac and common femoral artery obstruction
   a. Collaterals arising primarily from ipsilateral pelvic arteries or contralateral pelvic and/or femoral arteries to supply arteries of the proximal thigh distal to the obstruction
   b. Previously mentioned pathways also possibly involved to varying degrees

4. Deep femoral artery obstruction
   a. Collateral flow from proximal ipsilateral pelvic arteries, contralateral pelvic arteries, and/or contralateral femoral arteries to the deep femoral artery distal to the obstruction
   b. Collateral flow from the distal superficial femoral or popliteal arteries to the distal deep femoral artery
5. Superficial femoral or popliteal artery obstruction
   a. Collateral flow from the deep femoral artery to the distal superficial femoral artery or to the popliteal artery
   b. Collateral flow from the distal superficial femoral artery to the popliteal artery or to the proximal trifurcation vessels in the calf
   c. Collateral flow from the proximal to distal popliteal artery and/or popliteal artery to trifurcation vessels
6. Obstruction of trifurcation arteries
   a. Collateral flow from patent proximal calf branches to distal arteries in the lower leg or ankle
   b. Collateral flow from distal peroneal branches to distal anterior or posterior tibial arteries

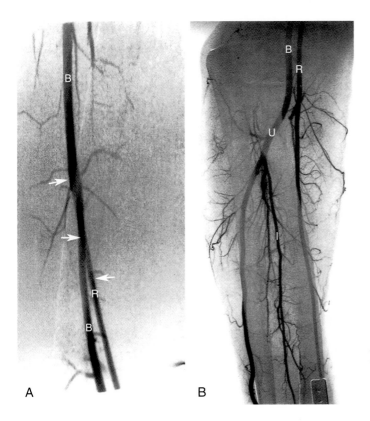

A   B

FIGURE 13-6 High origin of the radial artery. Arteriograms of the arm **(A)** and forearm **(B)** demonstrate a high origin of the radial artery (R; *arrows*) at the level of the mid-humerus. B, brachial artery; I, interosseous artery; U, ulnar artery.

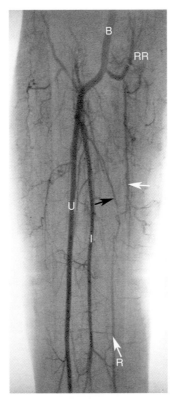

FIGURE 13-7 Collateral circulation in radial artery occlusion. The distal portion of the radial artery (R; *large arrow*) is primarily filled in a retrograde manner from the superficial and deep palmar arches (not shown). Antegrade collateral supply also is provided by the recurrent radial artery (RR; *white arrows*) and by the interosseous artery (I; *black arrow*). B, brachial artery; U, ulnar artery.

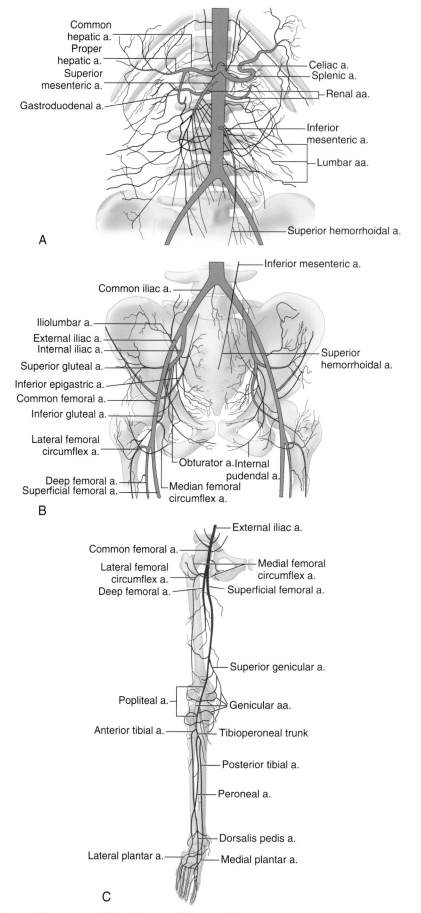

FIGURE 13-8 Arterial anatomy of the abdomen **(A)**, pelvis **(B)**, and lower extremity **(C)**. a., artery; aa., arteries.

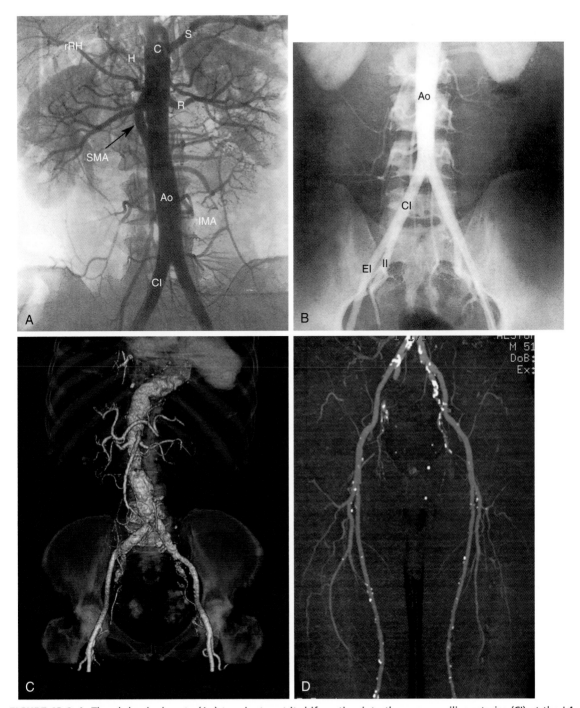

FIGURE 13-9 A, The abdominal aorta (Ao) terminates at its bifurcation into the common iliac arteries (CI) at the L4 vertebral level. **B,** The common iliac arteries divide at the lumbosacral junction into the internal (II) and external iliac (EI) arteries. The internal iliac artery (also called the hypogastric artery) supplies the pelvic viscera and musculature. The branches of this artery become important collateral routes, as seen in other figures. The external iliac artery is continuous with the common femoral artery at the inguinal ligament, as shown in Figure 13-10. **C,** Three-dimensional, volume-rendered (VR) computed tomographic (CT) angiogram of the aorta and iliofemoral arterial segment. **D,** Maximum intensity projection (MIP) of CT angiogram of the iliofemoral segments demonstrates focal calcifications in the patent vessels.

Continued

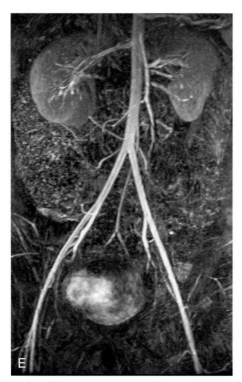

FIGURE 13-9, cont'd E, Gadolinium-enhanced magnetic resonance angiogram (MRA) of the aorta, iliac, and femoral segments. The anatomy is dramatically illustrated by three-dimensional reconstruction methods. C, celiac artery; H, hepatic artery; IMA, inferior mesenteric artery; R, left renal artery; rRH, replaced right hepatic artery; S, splenic artery; SMA, superior mesenteric artery.

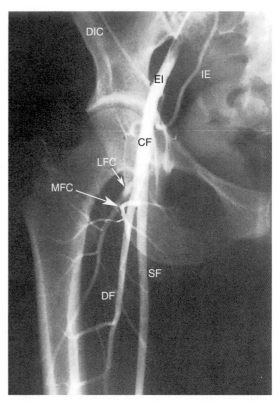

FIGURE 13-10 The external iliac artery (EI) is continuous with the common femoral artery (CF), which is a short segment (about 4 cm long). The common femoral artery bifurcates, forming the superficial (SF) and deep (DF) femoral arteries. A prominent branch, called the lateral femoral circumflex artery (LFC), arises dorsally, just before the common femoral artery divides. The superficial femoral artery continues throughout the thigh without major branches. The deep femoral artery, also called the profunda femoris artery, has multiple muscular branches. The proximal muscular branches communicate with the pelvic arteries, and the distal branches communicate with tributaries of the popliteal artery at the knee. Thus, the deep femoral artery is an important collateral route, for both iliac and superficial femoral artery occlusion. DIC, deep iliac circumflex artery; IE, inferior epigastric artery; MFC, medial femoral circumflex artery.

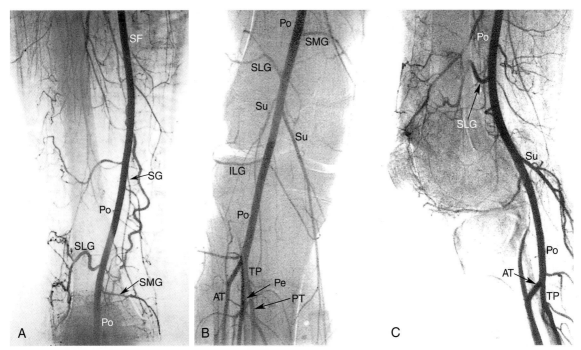

FIGURE 13-11 Anteroposterior **(A, B)** and lateral **(C)** views of the superficial femoral and popliteal arteries. In the distal portion of the thigh, the superficial femoral artery (SF) enters the adductor canal and becomes the popliteal artery (Po). This junction is also marked by the supreme genicular artery (SG). The popliteal artery passes behind the knee and ends, in most individuals, by bifurcating into the anterior tibial artery (AT) and the tibioperoneal trunk (TP). The genicular and sural arteries are important collateral routes for both superficial femoral and popliteal arterial obstruction. ILG, inferior lateral genicular artery; Pe, peroneal artery; PT, posterior tibial artery; SLG, superior lateral genicular artery; SMG, superior medial genicular artery; Su, sural artery.

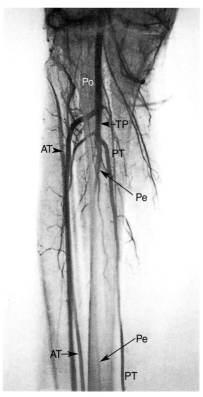

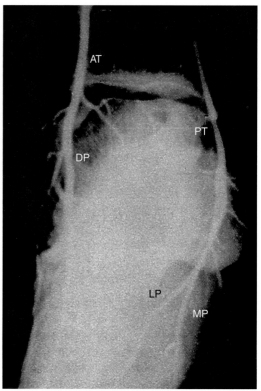

FIGURE 13-12 The anterior tibial artery (AT) courses anterolaterally from its origin and passes through the interosseous membrane. It then courses along the anterolateral aspect of the leg to the foot. The tibioperoneal trunk (TP) is of variable length and usually bifurcates into the peroneal (Pe) and posterior tibial (PT) arteries. The peroneal artery, also seen in Figure 13-11, *B*, extends down the leg to just above the ankle. The posterior tibial artery continues along a posteromedial course to the foot. Po, popliteal artery.

FIGURE 13-13 Oblique view of the right foot. The anterior tibial artery (AT) courses onto the dorsum of the foot, where it becomes the dorsalis pedis artery (DP). The posterior tibial artery (PT) passes behind the medial malleolus and shortly thereafter bifurcates, forming the medial plantar (MP) and lateral plantar (LP) arteries. The plantar arch of the foot is formed by the union of the lateral plantar artery with the plantar metatarsal branch (not shown) of the dorsalis pedis artery. The plantar arch gives rise to the metatarsal and digital branches.

TABLE 13-2 Arterial Variants of the Lower Extremity	
Variant	**Frequency of Occurrence in the Population (%)**
Duplication of the superficial femoral artery	Rare
High bifurcation of the popliteal artery	~4
High bifurcation of the popliteal artery, with the peroneal arising from the anterior tibial artery	~2
Normal-level bifurcation of the popliteal artery, with the peroneal arising from the anterior tibial artery	Rare
Absent posterior tibial artery; may have distal reconstitution at the level of the ankle by way of the peroneal artery	1-5
Hypoplasia or aplasia of the anterior tibial artery with resultant absence of dorsalis pedis pulse	4-12
Anomalous location of the dorsalis pedis artery	8

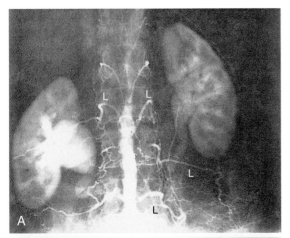

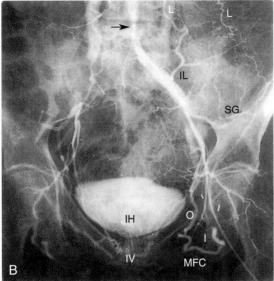

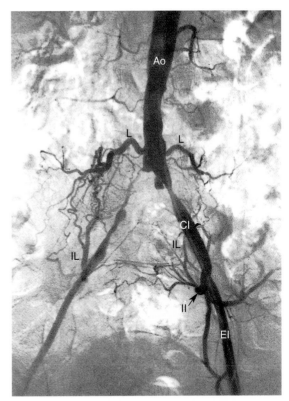

FIGURE 13-15 Right common iliac artery occlusion and left common iliac artery (CI) stenosis are circumvented by lumbar (L) collaterals, which communicate with ilio-lumbar (IL) branches of the internal iliac artery (II). The internal iliac artery, in turn, restores flow to the external iliac (EI) artery. Ao, aorta.

FIGURE 13-14 Aortic and iliac obstruction—superior **(A)** and inferior **(B)** segments. The site of a severe aortic stenosis is indicated by the *black arrow* in **B**. The right common iliac artery is occluded, and the left external iliac artery is severely stenotic. The following collateral routes are apparent: (1) lumbar arteries (L) → to the iliolumbar (IL) and superior gluteal (SG) arteries; (2) obturator internis artery (O) → to the median femoral circumflex artery (MFC), circumventing the left external iliac obstruction; (3) inferior hemorrhoidal (IH) and inferior vesicle (IV) branches across the pelvis from the left to the right internal iliac system (circumventing the right common iliac occlusion).

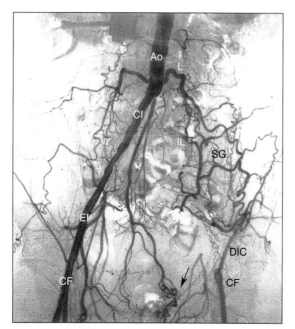

FIGURE 13-16 Hemorrhoidal collaterals (*arrow*) are of particular interest in this illustration. These branches of the inferior mesenteric artery illustrate the potential for collateralization from arteries that supply the gut. Prominent lumbar (L) → to gluteal (IL, SG) collaterals are evident on the left side. Ao, aorta; CF, common femoral artery; CI, common iliac artery; DIC, deep iliac circumflex artery; EI, external iliac artery; IL, iliolumbar artery; SG, superior gluteal artery.

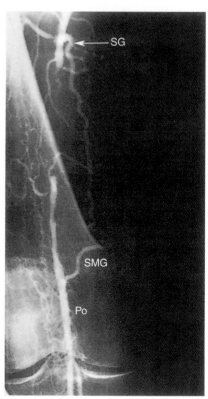

FIGURE 13-17 Occlusion of the proximal popliteal artery (Po) is circumvented by genicular collaterals (supreme genicular, SG → to superior medial genicular, SMG).

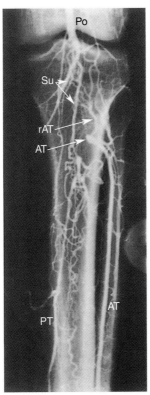

FIGURE 13-18 Distal popliteal (Po) artery occlusion is circumvented as follows: (1) sural (Su) and small muscular branches → to the recurrent anterior tibial artery (rAT), which supplies the anterior tibial artery (AT); (2) sural (Su) and small muscular branches → to the posterior tibial artery (PT).

REFERENCES

1. Kadir S: Arteriography of the thoracic aorta. In Kadir S, editor: *Diagnostic Angiography*, Philadelphia, 1986, WB Saunders, pp 124–171.
2. Kadir S: Arteriography of the upper extremities. In Kadir S, editor: *Diagnostic Angiography*, Philadelphia, 1986, WB Saunders, pp 172–206.
3. Rose SC, Kadir S: Arterial anatomy of the upper extremity. In Kadir S, editor: *Atlas of Normal and Variant Angiographic Anatomy*, Philadelphia, 1991, WB Saunders, pp 55–95.
4. Kadir S: Arteriography of the lower extremities. In Kadir S, editor: *Diagnostic Angiography*, Philadelphia, 1986, WB Saunders, pp 254–307.
5. Stieghorst MF, Crummy AB: Lower extremity arterial anatomy and collateral routes. In Zwiebel WJ, editor: *Introduction to Vascular Ultrasonography*, ed 2, Orlando, FL, 1986, Grune & Stratton, pp 278–303.
6. Muller RF, et al: *Arteries of the abdomen, pelvis and lower extremity*, Rochester, NY, Eastman Kodak.

NONIMAGING PHYSIOLOGIC TESTS FOR ASSESSMENT OF LOWER EXTREMITY ARTERIAL DISEASE

14

MARSHA M. NEUMYER, BS, RVT, FSDMS, FSVU, FAIUM

Atherosclerosis of the peripheral arteries is recognized as a major cause of death and disability. It has been estimated that at least 8 million people in the United States alone have stenosis or occlusion of one or more of their lower limb arteries. Of this group, approximately 4 million are symptomatic, while the majority have asymptomatic disease but are at future risk for compromised ambulation, arterial ulceration, and the need for revascularization.[1,2] Compounding these facts, recent investigations suggest that 30% of smokers, diabetic patients over age 50, and those over 70 years of age have peripheral arterial disease.[3,4] As such, it is important to define test procedures that are capable of detecting and localizing arterial disease, documenting critical ischemia, determining the potential for healing, and defining the therapeutic options.

Historically, digital subtraction arteriography has been the method of choice for confirmation of arterial disease affecting the lower limb and has served as the standard for planning reconstructive surgery or endovascular procedures. This invasive procedure has an associated, albeit low, morbidity and may underestimate or overestimate the functional significance of eccentric lesions.[5-7] Digital subtraction arteriography has been supplanted in many facilities by three-dimensional magnetic resonance or computed tomographic angiography. Regardless of the procedure used, it must be recognized that none of these modalities is capable of accurately defining the functional impact of multisegmental occlusive disease on tissue perfusion.

The indirect, noninvasive assessment of extremity arteries was introduced in the 1960s as a valued mechanism for confirmation and localization of arterial disease, determination of disease severity, and definition of response to therapy.[8-14] Recognizing that significant blockage in the limb arteries resulted in reduced blood pressure and volume of blood in the tissues distal

to the obstruction, investigators used a variety of diagnostic tools to document the physiologic alterations in pressure and flow. Although some of the earlier techniques are no longer used, indirect, physiologic testing remains the primary diagnostic method for assessment of lower limb arterial disorders in the modern vascular laboratory. These nonimaging studies are complemented with duplex sonography, which provides site-specific, quantitative diagnostic information.

INSTRUMENTATION

DIRECTIONAL, CONTINUOUS-WAVE DOPPLER

Continuous-wave (CW) Doppler flowmeters can be used to detect the presence, quality, and direction of blood flow in the extremity arteries. As noted in Chapter 2, the principle of Doppler ultrasound is based on the difference between the transmitted frequency and the frequency of the returned signal (Doppler effect). When applied to blood flow this is, quite simply, the perceptible change in frequency of the sound beam proportional to the velocity of the reflected signal. This relationship is expressed in the Doppler equation

$$\Delta f = \frac{2Vf_0 \cos \theta}{c} \qquad (14\text{-}1)$$

where Δf is the Doppler shift, the number 2 represents the round-trip travel time for the sound wave, V is the velocity of the moving red cells, f_0 is the carrier Doppler frequency, $\cos \theta$ is the angle of insonation, and c is the constant for the speed of sound in soft tissue.

It can be seen from the equation that the Doppler shift is directly proportional to the blood flow velocity, the transmitting Doppler frequency, and the cosine of the angle of insonation. One of the practical disadvantages of CW Doppler is that the angle must be assumed because this is a non-imaging modality. It should also be noted that the frequency shift will increase as the cosine of the angle of insonation approaches 0 (cosine of 0 = 1) and will decrease as the angle of the sound beam to blood flow approaches the perpendicular (cosine of 90 degrees = 0). For an angle of insonation greater than 90 degrees, the Doppler shift will be negative.

As noted in earlier chapters, the depth of the vessel is inversely proportional to the transmitting frequency of the Doppler used for arterial interrogation. Given this, transmitting frequencies in the range of 5 to 10 MHz are most commonly used for evaluation of the lower extremity arterial system, with the lower-frequency CW transducers used for examination of deeper vessels such as the common femoral artery.

CW Doppler utilizes two crystals: one crystal continuously transmits sound waves, while the other continuously receives the returned signals from all moving targets within its path. These signals are summed and may be projected audibly or represented as an analog display. Care must be taken to avoid contamination of the arterial signal with signals from superimposed venous flow and to ensure that arterial phasicity and pulsatility are accurately represented by optimizing the transmit frequency, angle of insonation, gain, and analog display.

A normal, resting peripheral artery will demonstrate both forward and reverse flow components (Figure 14-1). This multiphasic flow pattern is most often displayed as an analog tracing. The graphic display represents the average of the frequency shifts that occur over time. Using a zero-crossing detector, blood flow direction can be displayed on a strip chart recorder and retained for later qualitative analysis. This device employs a frequency-to-voltage converter. The output of the voltage is proportional to the number of zero crossings. Every time the input signal crosses through zero in a positive direction, a tag is set. The tag is reset every time the signal crosses through zero in a negative direction. The Doppler frequency is estimated based on the number of times the tag is set every second. Several important deficiencies have been associated with zero-crossing detectors. Although the display is generally acceptable, it is very dependent on the signal-to-noise ratio, amplitude of the signal, and transient response.[15] The information (mean frequency shifts) is not quantitative because the

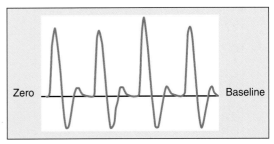

FIGURE 14-1 Continuous-wave Doppler analog waveform demonstrating a normal triphasic flow pattern. Note rapid systolic acceleration, the reverse flow component, and the forward diastolic flow phase. *(Modified from Scissons R:* Physiological testing techniques and interpretation, *North Kingstown, RI, 2003, Unetixs Educational Publishing.)*

angle of insonation is not known. Because of this, low frequency shifts (low velocities) may be overestimated and high frequency shifts (high velocities) may be underestimated.

State-of-the-art CW Doppler flowmeters can detect blood flow velocity as low as 6 cm/sec. The blood flow velocity in critically ischemic limbs with multisegmental occlusive disease may be too low to detect using this technology.[16] It may be difficult for the examiner to audibly differentiate ischemic low-velocity, minimally pulsatile, arterial flow from the returned venous signal. In such cases, alternative methods, such as those that evaluate tissue perfusion or tissue oxygen levels, may need to be employed to determine potential for healing.

Although CW Doppler is recognized as a valued tool for assessment of blood flow, its technical limitations must be considered. Distorted waveforms may be recorded unless care is taken to optimize the position and angle of the probe (Figure 14-2).

The signal may be attenuated by scar tissues or calcification of the arterial wall. Perhaps the most serious deficiency is the inability to control the sample volume depth (range ambiguity) in order to retrieve velocity information at a precise location within a designated vessel. This problem is overcome when pulsed Doppler is utilized for velocity assessment (see Chapter 17).

Continuous-Wave Doppler Analysis

As noted in Figure 14-1, a normal resting peripheral arterial signal is multiphasic with one or more diastolic components. The initial systolic forward flow is followed by rapid deceleration to a brief period of early diastolic flow reversal,

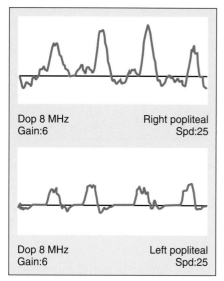

FIGURE 14-2 Continuous-wave Doppler analog wave-forms illustrating technical errors that occurred during recording. The waveforms recorded over the right popliteal artery demonstrate venous interference during the diastolic flow phase. The angle of insonation has not been optimized for recording the left popliteal waveforms, resulting in underestimation of the frequency shift and dampened, distorted waveform morphology.

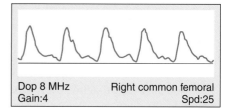

FIGURE 14-3 Continuous-wave Doppler analog wave-forms recorded over the common femoral artery in a patient with flow-reducing stenosis (>60%) in the superficial femoral artery. Note the loss of the reverse flow component.

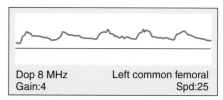

FIGURE 14-4 Continuous-wave Doppler analog wave-forms recorded over the common femoral artery in a patient with flow-reducing (>60%) iliac artery stenosis. Note the delayed systolic acceleration, loss of the reverse flow component, and delayed diastolic runoff.

resulting from high peripheral vascular resistance and a negative pressure gradient. A second phase of forward blood flow during diastole is pronounced when peripheral resistance is decreased (such as a warm limb). Diastolic blood flow can be decreased or absent during this phase when there is increased distal resistance and loss of compliance due to age-associated calcification and arterial wall stiffening. This can also be seen when the extremity is cold.

The absence of early diastolic flow reversal suggests a forward flow demand (Figure 14-3). This is most often associated with vasodilatation that occurs with flow-reducing arterial disease (>60% diameter-reducing lesions), but may result from exercise-induced vasodilatation or increased body temperature.

With intrinsic disease, arterial pressure is higher proximal to the site of narrowing and lower distally. The reduction in distal pressure is accompanied by a loss of kinetic energy distal to the stenosis. With disease progression, there is further loss of energy and pressure, which results in increased vasodilatation. When flow-limiting stenosis is proximal to the site of Doppler interrogation, the waveform will be characterized by delayed systolic upstroke as a consequence of the

increased time required for blood to bypass the stenosis through collateral channels. As severity of disease increases, vascular resistance decreases and the waveform morphology is characterized by delayed diastolic runoff (bowing to the right) and loss of amplitude (Figure 14-4).

The profile of a stenosis is characterized by the alterations in frequency shift and Doppler waveform morphology. Proximal to a severe stenosis, the waveform may appear normal if the lesion is well collateralized. When there are no collateral pathways, a "thump-like" signal with reduced amplitude, and no runoff, will be recorded (Figure 14-5).

The Doppler signal obtained directly over the stenosis will demonstrate a high frequency shift (velocity) at peak systole and loss of the early diastolic reverse flow component. A forward flow pattern is present throughout systole and diastole. The audible signal is high pitched and harsh. Immediately distal to the stenosis, the frequency shift will decrease and forward diastolic flow is present. Multisegmental disease may compromise blood flow so critically that the waveforms will be severely dampened, and may be absent, when flow is so limited that it cannot be detected by CW Doppler.

Identification of flow-limiting disease and classification of disease severity may be enhanced

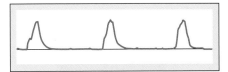

FIGURE 14-5 This CW Doppler analog waveform was obtained proximal to a severe stenosis that is poorly collateralized and demonstrates a low-amplitude, "thump-like" signal, with low, or absent, diastolic flow.

by quantitative Doppler waveform analysis. Historically, several methods of waveform analysis have been employed, including calculation of a pulsatility index (PI), inverse damping factor, pulse wave transit time, acceleration time (AT), and the Laplace transform analysis. While each of these has met with varying levels of success and acceptance, only the PI and AT have retained popularity. The peak-to-peak PI (peak 1 frequency shift – peak 2 frequency shift / mean frequency shift) relates the peak-to-peak frequency shift (velocity) to the integrated mean frequency shift (velocity) and is independent of the angle of insonation. The relationship of peak-to-peak frequency shift and the integrated mean frequency shift is illustrated in Figure 14-6.

In the normal lower limb, the PI values increase from proximal to distal. The PI of the common femoral artery is normally greater than 5 and most often is between 6 and 7, whereas the popliteal artery has a PI between 7 and 9, and the posterior tibial artery PI range is 12 to 16.[17] In the presence of a pressure-flow-reducing lesion, the reverse flow component of the Doppler waveform is absent (peak 2) and the PI decreases. Comparing their results to intra-arterial pressure measurements, Thiele and colleagues[18] demonstrated that a common femoral artery PI greater than 4 was predictive of a normal aortoiliac segment. In the absence of superficial femoral artery occlusive disease, a common femoral artery PI less than 4 was highly predictive of flow-limiting aortoiliac disease.

Hemodynamically significant disease proximal to the common femoral artery can be identified by measurement of the systolic AT on the Doppler waveform (Figure 14-7). Normally, common femoral artery systolic rise time is rapid (<122 msec). Flow velocity is slower when blood must move around an area of blockage through high-resistance collateral pathways. In such cases, the systolic rise time is extended to greater than

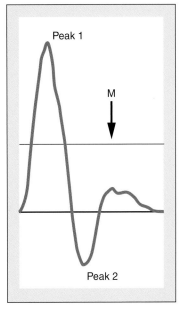

FIGURE 14-6 Diagram illustrating the relationship of the peak-to-peak frequency shift (peak 1 – peak 2) and the integrated mean frequency shift (M) for calculation of the pulsatility index (PI).

144 msec. It is important to optimize the Doppler signal and angle of insonation because false-positive results are likely when the Doppler angle is greater than 60 to 70 degrees and the waveform is dampened. The signal will also be attenuated when cardiac output is reduced.

PLETHYSMOGRAPHY

Plethysmography is a tool for recording volume changes in tissues of the limbs or digits. Most commonly, the volume changes are related to alterations in the blood flow volume that occur throughout the cardiac cycle and as a result of pressure-flow-reducing lesions in the major arteries of the lower limb. Historically, a number of plethysmographic tools have been used to examine the arterial and venous circulation of the lower extremity. Although the majority of these are still in limited use, modern vascular laboratories most often employ air-calibrated plethysmography (pulse volume recording [PVR]) and photoplethysmography (PPG).

Air-Calibrated Plethysmography

Changes in limb volume occur with passage of the arterial pulse pressure wave from the aorta into the arterial tree of the lower extremities. In systole, blood moves rapidly from the main arterial branches into the microcirculation, with a

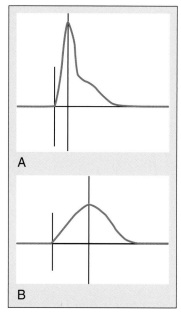

FIGURE 14-7 Diagrams illustrating the method used for determining the systolic acceleration time. **A,** The acceleration time (rise time) is the time elapsed from onset of systole to peak systole. **B,** The significant delay to peak systole in a waveform obtained distal to a flow-limiting stenosis (tardus-parvus waveform).

resultant increase in tissue perfusion and limb volume. During diastole, the pressure in the main arterial tree diminishes with subsequent reduction in limb volume. The momentary changes in limb volume can be documented with PVR. This testing modality employs pneumatic cuffs that are applied segmentally on the limbs (Figure 14-8).

The cuffs serve as sensors for arterial flow and alterations in limb volume. The cuffs are calibrated by injecting air into the cuff bladder to achieve a cuff pressure approximating 65 mm Hg and a volume sufficient to ensure that the cuff bladders are snug against the skin.[19]

During systole, air in the cuff bladder surrounding the limb segment is displaced as a consequence of limb expansion. In diastole, arterial inflow decreases and the pressure and volume of air in the cuff bladder is stabilized. These changes are sensed by a pressure transducer and translated into an analog recording that displays the amplitude and contour of the pulse wave. Although the frequency response of some devices approximates only 20 Hz, this has been shown to be sufficient for demonstration of the high-frequency components expressed in the arterial pulse pressure wave.[20]

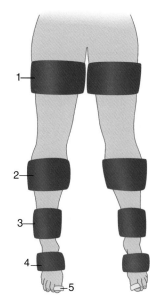

FIGURE 14-8 Application of pneumatic cuffs for lower extremity pulse volume recording.

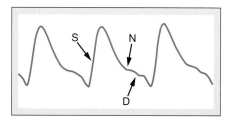

FIGURE 14-9 Pulse volume waveforms illustrating normal waveform morphology. Note rapid systolic (S) upstroke, dicrotic notch (N), and gradual diastolic (D) runoff.

Pulse Volume Waveform Analysis

The analog pulse volume wave contour parallels the intra-arterial pressure contour. The normal wave exhibits rapid systolic upstroke (anacrotic limb), a sharp systolic peak, a reflected wave (dicrotic notch) on the deceleration slope, and gradual runoff in diastole (Figure 14-9). The reflected wave signifies elevated peripheral resistance, which is expected in the normal resting muscular bed of the lower limb. Vascular resistance is reduced in response to any situation that elicits an increased flow demand (e.g., significant arterial stenosis or occlusion, exercise, or inflammation). With a pressure-flow-reducing lesion (>50%-60% diameter reduction) proximal to the recording cuff, systolic acceleration is delayed, the systolic peak becomes rounded, the dicrotic notch is absent, and the rate of runoff is reduced (Figure 14-10).

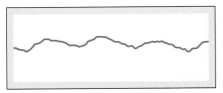

FIGURE 14-10 Pulse volume waveforms recorded distal to flow-limiting (>60%) stenosis. Note the loss of amplitude compared to a normal waveform, the delayed systolic upstroke, absence of the dicrotic notch, and delayed runoff.

The amplitude of the pulse volume recording is dependent on the total flow and pulse pressure at a given limb segment. As such, the amplitude of the pulse volume wave provides clues to the presence of hemodynamically significant disease and the extent of compensatory flow in the microcirculation. Pulse volume amplitude is normally high in the absence of pressure-flow-reducing lesions. The amplitude is reduced when there is significant arterial obstruction proximal to the segment where the pulse wave is recorded. As disease severity increases, the amplitude of the waveform decreases. These findings reflect the associated reduction in pulse pressure and tissue perfusion. As such, whenever there is a significant change in the amplitude and contour of the PVR waveform compared to the more proximal recording, flow-limiting disease should be suspected. The offending lesion may be beneath the cuff or between the two cuff levels.

In situations where there is abundant flow in the tissue bed (e.g., well-developed collaterals, arteriovenous fistulas or malformations), the pulse volume waveform will demonstrate higher amplitude compared to the more proximal waveform recordings. For example, in the absence of flow-limiting disease in the superficial femoral artery, the amplitude of the PVR waveform recorded at below-knee level will be higher than the amplitude of the thigh and ankle waveforms (Figure 14-11). This is the result of the additional volume of flow to the thigh and knee region through the profunda femoris branches and the geniculate system. Absence of the amplitude increase suggests superficial femoral artery occlusion. Distal superficial femoral artery obstruction should be suspected if the below-knee waveform demonstrates no increase in amplitude and the waveforms recorded at thigh level are normal. In addition, it should be noted that waveform amplitude can be affected by blood pressure, vasomotor tone, ventricular stroke volume, patient positioning, edema, and/or obesity.

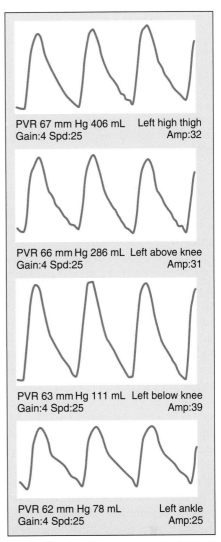

FIGURE 14-11 In the absence of proximal flow-limiting disease, the pulse volume recording waveforms from the below-knee segment of the limb will normally demonstrate increased amplitude compared to the thigh waveforms. This is the result of increased flow volume from the profunda femoris and geniculate arteries.

Photoplethysmography

Photoelectric plethysmography is used primarily for assessing the quantity of blood in the cutaneous circulation. This technology employs a light-emitting diode that transmits infrared light into the skin. A phototransistor detects the reflected signal from red blood cells coursing through the microcirculation in the tissues beneath the sensor. The changes in electrical resistance within the phototransistor are expressed as a waveform that displays signals throughout the cardiac cycle that are proportional to the number of red blood cells in the tissues.[21] The PPG sensor is attached

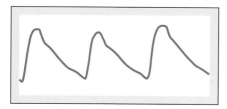

FIGURE 14-12 Normal photoplethysmographic wave-forms. Note rapid systolic rise time, the dicrotic notch, and gradual diastolic runoff.

to the skin by using clear, double-stick tape or a tension-sensitive clip that houses the sensor. It is important to avoid attachment techniques that have potential for increased pressure on the sensor (clips that are applied over the sensor and Velcro straps or tape used to secure the sensor to the skin or digit) as this will force blood away from the tissue beneath the sensor. Although, in the truest sense of the term, PPG does not measure limb or digit volume changes due to alterations in blood flow, the pulse waveform morphology closely resembles the pulse volume waveforms recorded with PVRs (Figure 14-12).

PPGs have shown value as sensors for arterial flow to facilitate measurement of digital pressures and for assessment of potential for healing wounds, ulcers, and amputation sites. The morphology of the plethysmographic waveform may be altered in situations that cause vasodilatation or vasoconstriction such as temperature variations, inflammation, or pharmacologics. It is important to note that the PPG waveforms cannot be quantitated; they yield information about tissue perfusion that is based on subjective analysis of waveform morphology.

PHYSIOLOGIC TESTING PROCEDURES

MEASUREMENT OF ARTERIAL PRESSURE

Systolic pressure normally increases as blood flows from central to peripheral arteries in the lower extremities.[22,23] In contrast, diastolic and mean pressures decrease. The augmentation of systolic pressure is in large part a consequence of differences in the arterial wall compliance between the central and peripheral arteries, the resistance to arterial flow in the muscular beds of the normal resting lower limb, the decrease in arterial diameter of the leg arteries compared to the aorta, and the effects of energy loss associated with movement of blood. Given this, assuming

the absence of significant narrowing of the subclavian and/or axillary arteries, ankle systolic blood pressures are normally equal to or greater than the central aortic pressure measured at brachial level.

When the luminal diameter of a peripheral artery is narrowed by more than 50% to 60% as a result of disease or extrinsic compression, systolic pressure is decreased distal to the site of narrowing. This hemodynamic feature provides an excellent mechanism for detection of pressure-reducing stenoses in any segment of the limb. It should be noted that peak systolic pressure may decrease with lesser degrees of arterial narrowing.[8] The reasons for this are most often apparent clinically and do not influence the interpretation of noninvasive test procedures if all diagnostic data are integrated.

Limb systolic pressures are measured using pneumatic cuffs, a sphygmomanometer, and a sensor for arterial flow distal to the pressure cuff. A variety of sensors are available, but, most commonly, CW Doppler is used to ensure a complete and accurate examination. Although pressures can be obtained by manually inflating the cuffs, physiologic examinations are facilitated by use of a commercially available system that provides all the instrumentation required for CW Doppler, pressure, and plethysmographic assessments.

In 1950, Winsor[24] demonstrated that accurate measurement of limb systolic pressure could be achieved when the width of the pneumatic cuff bladder exceeded 50% of the diameter of the limb segment that it encompassed. In more recent studies, investigators have shown that accurate noninvasive assessment of limb systolic pressures is possible when the width of the cuff bladder is at least 20% greater than the diameter of the limb beneath the cuff.[25] While this has been shown to be true in the majority of cases, it must be recognized that the variation in the girth and shape of the thigh contributes to a range of pressures in both normal patients and those with significant arterial disease. Thigh pressures tend to be overestimated because the pressure in the cuff may not be transmitted completely to the depth of the arteries in the central part of the thigh. To differentiate inflow (iliofemoral) from outflow (femoropopliteal) obstruction, Barnes[26] employed narrow (12 × 40 cm) blood pressure cuffs at high-thigh and above-knee levels. Many laboratories prefer to use a narrower cuff (17 × 40 cm) at the high-thigh level to improve differentiation of inflow and outflow lesions.

ANKLE PRESSURES AND THE ANKLE-BRACHIAL INDEX

Because systolic pressure in the tibial arteries is normally equal to or greater than the central aortic pressure, a decrease in ankle pressure compared to brachial pressure signifies the presence of flow-limiting proximal arterial disease. This simple test procedure provides an accurate, rapid means for detecting the presence of lower limb arterial disease and is predictive of disease severity.[8-11]

The systolic pressure in the brachial artery is initially measured by placing an appropriately sized blood pressure cuff around the upper arm. The cuff may be connected to a manometer that is hand-held or contained in a modular system. Using a CW Doppler probe, an arterial signal is recorded in either the brachial, radial, or ulnar artery. While the arterial signal can be recorded in any nondiseased artery distal to the cuff, the brachial artery is most commonly used as it is easily accessible and provides a brisk, audible signal. The blood pressure cuff is inflated to suprasystolic pressure, resulting in transient occlusion of the brachial artery. The cuff should be slowly deflated until the arterial signal is again noted. The systolic pressure is recorded as the pressure at which the arterial signal reappears. It is important to use a deflation rate of only 2 to 3 mm Hg per second, as a faster rate may result in underestimation of the opening arterial systolic pressure. The study is repeated using the contralateral brachial artery. While brachial systolic pressures may be symmetrical, there is often a side-to-side difference in pressure. A brachial systolic pressure gradient exceeding 20 mm Hg suggests the presence of significant narrowing of the subclavian and/or axillary arteries on the side with the lower pressure. The higher of the two arm pressures will be used in calculation of the ankle-brachial index (ABI).

The systolic pressure is then measured in the dorsalis pedis (DP) artery by applying an appropriately sized blood pressure cuff around the ankle. The arterial signal in the DP artery is recorded using a CW Doppler probe (Figure 14-13). The DP pressure is obtained in a manner identical to that used for measurement of the brachial systolic pressure. The study is repeated using the posterior tibial (PT) artery as the target (Figure 14-14). The pressures in the DP and PT are retained for calculation of the ABI.

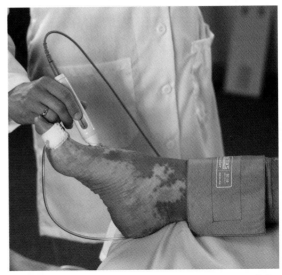

FIGURE 14-13 Technique used for measurement of the arterial pressure in the dorsalis pedis artery. Note position of ankle cuff and continuous-wave Doppler probe.

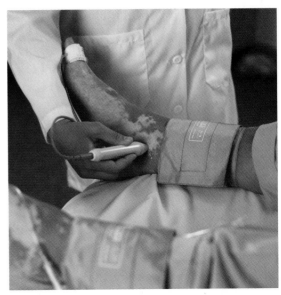

FIGURE 14-14 Technique used for measurement of the arterial pressure in the posterior tibial artery. Note position of ankle cuff and continuous-wave Doppler probe.

If critical disease in the DP and PT arteries precludes pressure measurements for these vessels, a global ankle pressure can be obtained by placing a PPG sensor on the great toe and recording the arterial signal from the digital cutaneous circulation. While this technique offers a rapid means for determining the ankle pressure, several important issues should be noted. This method obviates the ability to detect disease isolated to the DP or PT circulation; it provides the summation of

TABLE 14-1 The Relationship of the Ankle-Brachial Index (ABI) to Peripheral Arterial Disease (PAD)

Range of ABI	Level of PAD
0.9-1.3	No significant PAD
0.8-0.9	Mild PAD
0.5-0.8	Moderate PAD
<0.5	Severe PAD
<0.3	Critical PAD

pressures from the DP, PT, peroneal, and collateral arteries. In addition, the arterial microcirculation may be affected by vasoconstriction or vasodilatation as a consequence of proximal arterial disease, inflammation, changes in temperature, or medication. These factors alter the plethysmographic waveform, which may potentially impact accurate determination of arterial pressure.

A ratio of the highest ankle systolic pressure (PT or DP) to the higher of the two brachial systolic pressures is termed the *ankle-brachial index*, or ABI (alternatively called the *ankle-arm index*). Because the ankle pressures normally equal or exceed the brachial pressure, the ABI should be equal to or greater than 1.0. It has been shown that the mean value of a normal ABI is 1.11 +/- 0.10.[27] Potential for error in interpretation of the ABI is introduced if the brachial pressure exceeds 200 mm Hg or the ABI is greater than 1.3 as a result of elevated tibial artery pressure caused by calcification of the tibial arteries.

Interpretation of Ankle Pressures and the ABI

The ABI not only identifies the presence or absence of arterial occlusive disease proximal to the ankle, but also serves as a reliable marker for severity of disease. As such, determination of the ABI should be the initial test in evaluation of a patient suspected of lower limb arterial disease and compared to the clinical presentation. As noted in Table 14-1, an ABI in the range of 0.5 to 0.9 would most likely be documented in patients presenting with mild to moderate claudication. Critical ischemia, rest pain, and ankle pressures less than 40 mm Hg, are associated with multisegmental occlusive disease and, most often, an ABI less than 0.3.

It is important to recognize that a broad overlap in ankle pressures exists dependent on the clinical presentation and the patient's pain tolerance. Yao[27] reported a range of ABIs from 0.2 to 1.0 with a mean of 0.59 +/- 0.15 in patients with intermittent claudication. In patients with

ischemic rest pain, the ABI ranged from 0 to 0.65 with a mean of 0.26 +/- 0.13, while patients with gangrenous lesions had a mean ABI of 0.05 +/- 0.08. Because of the possibility of technical variation in follow-up evaluations, changes in the ABI must be 0.15 or greater to be considered clinically significant.

The absolute ankle pressure has demonstrated diagnostic value. Ischemic rest pain is unlikely in a nondiabetic patient with an absolute ankle pressure greater than 60 mm Hg. Rest pain is likely when the ankle pressure deteriorates to less than 35 mm Hg, and ischemic ulcers are unlikely to heal with an ankle pressure less than 40 to 50 mm Hg. Ischemic rest pain is unlikely in a diabetic patient with an ankle pressure greater than 80 mm Hg but is probable when the ankle pressure is less than 40 mm Hg.

Because of the overlap in ankle pressures, it is important to relate the clinical presentation to the resting pressures and ABI. For example, a patient with a resting ABI of 0.8 but complaints of 50-yard claudication would be best served diagnostically with constant-load treadmill exercise testing to differentiate true vascular claudication from pain associated with other pathology (e.g., spinal stenosis). The same would apply to a patient presenting with symptoms of claudication and a resting ABI of 1.0. As noted by Hirsch,[4] it is important to remember that the prevalence of lower limb arterial disease is disproportionate to the number of symptomatic patients.

In recent years, investigators have established an association between the ABI and cardiovascular morbidity and mortality. Sikkink and associates[28] studied 154 patients with an ABI less than 0.9 and demonstrated 5-year cumulative survival rates of only 63% in patients with an ABI less than 0.5. The Strong Heart Study assessed the association of low (0.9) and high (>1.4) ABI with risk for all-cause and cardiovascular disease mortality in American Indians.[29] Surprisingly, an ABI greater than 1.4 predicted mortality with a similar strength as an ABI less than 0.9. The investigators demonstrated that patients with peripheral arterial disease had an increased incidence of coronary events. Peripheral arterial disease was diagnosed in one-third of the men and one-quarter of the women with coronary artery disease. An ABI less than 0.67 was independently associated with cardiac events and increased the risk for cardiac death by two-thirds. While the implications

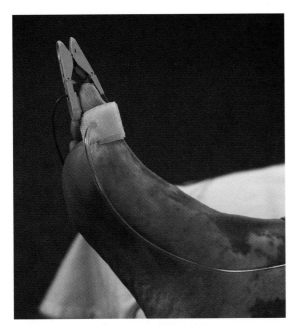

FIGURE 14-15 Toe pressures are measured by application of an appropriately sized blood pressure cuff to the base of the digit and a photoplethysmographic sensor to the tissue bed distal to the cuff.

TABLE 14-2 The Relationship of the Toe-Brachial Index (TBI) to Peripheral Arterial Disease (PAD)	
Range of TBI	Severity of PAD
≥0.8	No significant PAD
0.2-0.5	Claudication
<0.2	Rest pain

of this study are striking, it must be noted that an ABI greater than 1.4 indicates comorbid conditions such as diabetes and renal impairment.

DETERMINATION OF TOE PRESSURES

Unlike the tibial arteries, digital arteries infrequently calcify. In fact, evidence suggests that in the absence of flow-limiting proximal atherosclerotic disease, there is no significant difference in mean toe-brachial indices (TBIs) in normal diabetic and nondiabetic patients. Therefore, in cases where elevated tibial artery systolic pressures (>200 mm Hg) preclude accurate determination of the ABI, the systolic pressure in the great toe should be substituted for the tibial pressure and a TBI calculated.[30] Digital pressure measurement in the great toe requires an appropriately sized blood pressure cuff (2.5-3.0 cm) and a sensor for arterial flow (Figure 14-15).

Most commonly, PPG sensors are used, but CW Doppler flowmeters may also be employed. Normally, digital pressures are greater than 80% of the systemic pressure and a TBI equal to or greater than 0.80 would be consistent with the absence of proximal flow-reducing disease.[31] It should be noted that this value is dependent on the sensor that is chosen to detect arterial flow and the instrumentation that is used to record the digital pressure. As proximal arterial disease

increases in severity, toe pressure decreases proportionally as noted in Table 14-2.

A TBI value less than 0.5 suggests proximal arterial disease of moderate severity, while an index less than 0.2 and toe pressures less than 30 mm Hg are consistent with critical ischemia and poor potential for healing. An absolute toe pressure less than 30 to 50 mm Hg is consistent with chronic limb ischemia according to the recommendations of the Trans Atlantic Inter-society Consensus (TASC) group.[32] As noted by these authors, toe pressures are best used to predict the absence of chronic limb ischemia rather than to identify its presence.

Occlusive lesions involving the plantar or digital arteries, such as thromboangiitis obliterans or microembolism, can be identified by measurement of toe pressures and analysis of digital plethysmographic waveforms. In many cases where disease is confined to arteries distal to the ankle, the ABI will be normal.

SEGMENTAL SYSTOLIC PRESSURE MEASUREMENTS

As noted, the resting ABI identifies the presence of flow-reducing proximal limb arterial disease. It does not, however, identify the location of the offending lesions or indicate the relative significance of multisegmental obstruction. If the resting ABI and/or TBI indicate flow compromise in the proximal arterial tree, the lesion(s) can be localized by measuring systolic pressures at multiple limb levels. Most often, measurements are determined bilaterally at four levels: high thigh, above knee, below knee, and ankle (Figure 14-16, *A*).

Appropriately sized blood pressure cuffs are inflated to suprasystolic levels at each location, and CW Doppler is used to sense the presence of arterial flow in a distal artery in a manner similar to that used for measuring ankle systolic pressures. To prevent errors in pressure measurement resulting from reactive hyperemia induced by occlusive cuff pressures, the study is initiated at ankle level with subsequent progression to the more proximal cuff level.

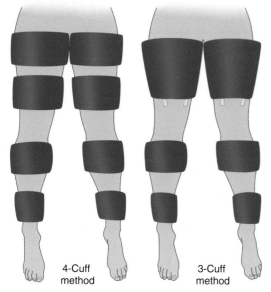

4-Cuff
method

3-Cuff
method

FIGURE 14-16 Illustration demonstrating application of blood pressure cuffs for measurement of segmental pressures. **A,** Cuffs are applied at high-thigh, above-knee, below-knee, and ankle levels when a four-cuff technique is employed. **B,** The three-cuff technique employs a broad, contoured thigh cuff.

Recognizing the potential for errors in pressure measurement associated with the cuff artifact at high thigh, many laboratories use a single thigh measurement rather than a two-cuff technique. The three-cuff method employs a broad (19 × 40 cm) contour cuff that encircles the thigh (Figure 14-16, *B*).

Using this cuff, a normal thigh pressure would equal the brachial pressure. A decrease in thigh pressure greater than 30 mm Hg compared to the systemic pressure suggests significant disease in the aortoiliac, iliofemoral, or femoropopliteal segment. Quite often, additional testing (CW Doppler, duplex sonography) is required to localize the occlusive lesions.

Interpretation of Segmental Systolic Pressure Measurements

As previously noted, limb pressures normally increase from high-thigh to ankle level with the ankle pressure remaining equal to, or greater than, the systemic pressure. In the absence of flow-limiting disease, intra-arterial pressures in the common femoral and brachial arteries are identical. Using the four-cuff technique for measuring segmental pressures, and assuming the use of appropriately sized blood pressure cuffs,

the high-thigh pressure should exceed the brachial pressure by 30 to 40 mm Hg.[33] A reduction in high-thigh blood pressure signifies arterial compromise proximal to or beneath the high-thigh cuff. A calculated high-thigh to brachial systolic pressure index can be used to identify flow-limiting aortoiliac disease. Normally, the thigh-brachial index exceeds 1.2.[34] An index between 0.8 and 1.2 signifies pressure-flow-reducing stenosis in the aortoiliac segment; an index less than 0.8 is commonly associated with iliac artery occlusion.

Pressure gradients should be greater than 20 to 30 mm Hg between each cuff level on the limb. Pressure gradients exceeding 30 mm Hg suggest stenosis of the arterial segment beneath the more proximal cuff or between cuffs. A decrease in pressure greater than 40 mm Hg between cuff levels is commonly associated with arterial occlusion. In the absence of lower extremity arterial disease, blood should flow symmetrically from the abdominal aorta into the arterial trees of the legs and segmental pressures should be comparable side-to-side. A pressure difference exceeding 20 to 30 mm Hg at the same cuff level highlights the possibility of hemodynamically significant disease on the side with the lower pressure.

Measurement variability[35] is increased when the arterial flow rate is so slow that it is difficult to differentiate arterial from venous flow. In such cases it is helpful to augment the venous flow signal by compressing the limb distally; the arterial signal will either diminish or remain unchanged. Careful attention must be given to interpretation of pressure gradients in markedly hypertensive patients, where increased gradients are occasionally documented, and in patients with low cardiac output, where the pressure gradients may be decreased.[24]

While systolic pressure measurements are a valued tool for identification of pressure-flow-reducing lesions in the lower limb, it must be noted that this test localizes disease to segments of the limb and does not accurately differentiate flow-reducing stenosis from arterial occlusion. Similar pressures may be obtained distal to critical stenoses that are poorly collateralized and arterial occlusions that are well collateralized. Segmental pressure measurements should not be obtained in limbs with arterial stents or symptoms of acute deep venous thrombosis or superficial thrombophlebitis and may be inaccurate in patients with evidence of medial calcification of the peripheral arteries.

POSTEXERCISE ANKLE PRESSURE RESPONSE

Patients with chronic peripheral arterial disease most commonly complain of intermittent claudication. This exercise-related limb pain occurs as a consequence of the inability of the collateral circulation to meet the flow demands of exercising muscle. At rest, the average blood flow to the lower limb is in the range of 300 to 500 mL/min.[22] With moderate levels of exercise, total limb blood flow must increase by more than fivefold in order to meet the metabolic demands imposed by working calf muscle. The increased blood flow is accommodated by vasodilatation of peripheral collateral resistance vessels and the muscular arterioles that control the distribution of flow to the capillary bed.[36] In the absence of disease in the vessels of the main arterial tree, the increased flow has little to no impact on the systolic pressure at ankle level. When pressure-flow-reducing lesions are present in the lower extremity arteries, blood must bypass the obstruction(s) by way of high-resistance collaterals. Surprisingly, even when multisegmental disease is present, resting blood flow may be maintained in the normal range, because of the low flow demand of resting muscle, and the compensatory decrease in vascular resistance that occurs distal to the obstructed arterial segments. During exercise, the flow rate is increased to meet the muscle demand, and a pressure gradient develops across the lesion because the collateral circulation cannot maintain distal perfusion pressures.

Constant-load treadmill exercise testing with documentation of the postexercise ankle pressure response can be used to advantage in the vascular laboratory to assess the degree of circulatory compromise associated with atherosclerotic disease. There are multiple reasons to consider treadmill exercise testing in patients with symptoms of intermittent claudication: (1) the exercise simulates the activity that produces the symptoms, (2) the severity of pain can be determined and localized to one or more limb segments, (3) it can be determined whether postexercise ankle pressures deteriorate to ischemic levels, (4) the duration of postexercise hyperemia (recovery time) can be determined, (5) true vascular claudication can be differentiated from pseudoclaudication caused by venous insufficiency or neurospinal

or musculoskeletal conditions, and (6) exercise testing has shown value for assessment of disease progression and response to therapy. While not a cardiac stress test, constant-load treadmill exercise testing is contraindicated in patients with gait disturbances, poorly controlled hypertension, and history of unstable angina, myocardial infarction, congestive heart failure, cardiac arrhythmia, or shortness of breath.

Historically, the ABI is determined at rest. The patient then exercises on a treadmill at an elevation of 12% and a constant speed of 2 mph. This elevation and speed simulate the circulatory response induced by normal ambulation. The degree of elevation and walking speed can be altered to lower levels, but it is important that the same speed and elevation are consistent for each patient for follow-up evaluations. The patient walks to the point of claudication, and ankle pressures are measured immediately after exercise and at 3-minute intervals until the pressures return to preexercise levels (Figure 14-17).

Interpretation of Treadmill Exercise Results

Normally, ankle pressures increase slightly or do not change with exercise because vasodilatation provides the required volume increase. Single-segment lesions most often result in an initial drop in pressure with return to baseline values within 3 to 5 minutes. Return to baseline pressure is delayed when multisegmental disease is present. In such cases, ankle pressures return to baseline values within 10 to 12 minutes dependent on the extent of collateral compensatory flow. A decrease in ankle pressure to 60 mm Hg or less is consistent with critical ischemia and vascular claudication. It is important to document the recovery time, the symptoms that are experienced during exercise, and the preexercise and postexercise pressures, as this information yields valuable clues to the severity of disease and the extent of collateral compensatory flow. It is important to realize that the duration of exercise may be influenced by the patient's motivation, tolerance for pain, and/or symptoms that precede claudication such as shortness of breath or back or hip pain.

It is more difficult to determine the location of arterial occlusive disease based on the postexercise ankle pressure response. Strandness and Bell[37] demonstrated that the location of disease impacted the magnitude of the pressure drop and the recovery time. A decrease in ankle

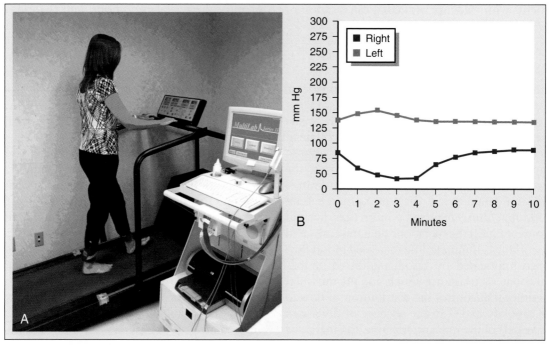

FIGURE 14-17 Treadmill exercise with postexercise ankle pressure response. **A,** The patient walks on the treadmill at a constant speed and elevation. **B,** Ankle pressures are measured immediately following exercise and at 3-minute intervals until pressures return to preexercise levels. The right leg has an abnormal pressure response, whereas the left leg has a normal response.

pressure following exercise most often indicates arterial obstruction proximal to the popliteal artery. Because the more proximal arteries supply a greater muscle mass than the distal arteries, the effect of proximal occlusive disease on ankle pressure is more pronounced. A postexercise ABI in the range of 0.9 to 0.6 is most often predictive of isolated infrapopliteal disease, whereas inflow (aortoiliac) disease reduces the distal pressures to a greater degree. Multisegmental lesions decrease the postexercise pressures dramatically, with a resulting ABI below 0.3.

REACTIVE HYPEREMIA TESTING

Some patients may not be able to perform constant-load treadmill exercise testing due to cardiopulmonary disease, amputation, or gait disturbance. In such cases, reactive hyperemia testing may be used to increase extremity blood flow and vasodilatation.

To perform the test, wide, contoured blood pressure cuffs are placed around the thighs and appropriately sized cuffs are placed at ankle level. The thigh cuffs are inflated to suprasystolic pressure (20-30 mm Hg higher than the brachial pressure) for 3 to 7 minutes to occlude the thigh

arteries. This results in local hypoxia and vasodilatation. Following cuff deflation, ankle pressures are measured at 30-second intervals for 3 to 6 minutes or until ankle pressures return to preocclusion level.

Interpretation of Reactive Hyperemia Test Results

Normally, following deflation, ankle pressures immediately decrease approximately 20% to 30% compared to the preocclusive level and return to approximately 90% of baseline within 1 minute. This is in sharp contrast to the normal response to treadmill exercise, where a postexercise drop in ankle pressure signifies flow-limiting disease. In patients with arterial occlusive disease, the deterioration in postocclusive pressure noted with reactive hyperemia testing parallels that seen following treadmill exercise, but recovery to preocclusive levels is much faster.[38] Patients with single-segment arterial disease most often demonstrate less than 50% decrease in ankle pressure, whereas those with multisegmental disease have a postocclusive decrease in pressure that exceeds 50%. Caution is warranted in the interpretation of reactive hyperemia studies, because similar

TABLE 14-3 Summary of Pressures and Indices for Assessment of Lower Extremity Arterial Disease	
Parameters	Interpretation
Ankle systolic pressure	Normally greater than brachial pressure by approximately 10%
Ankle-brachial index	Normally 0.9-1.3; critical ischemia when <0.3
High-thigh systolic pressure	Normally 30-40 mm Hg greater than brachial systolic pressure
Thigh-brachial index	Normally >1.2
Segmental pressure gradients	Normally <20-30 mm Hg between adjacent levels on same leg or between same level on two legs
Toe systolic pressure/index	Normally more than 80% of the brachial systolic pressure; toe brachial index is normally >0.8
Treadmill exercise test	Normal walking time is 5 min without symptoms; no decrease in ankle pressure after exercise (2 mph, 12% elevation)
Critical ischemia after exercise	Postexercise ankle pressure ≤60 mm Hg is consistent with critical ischemia and vascular claudication

results may be found in normal patients and those with flow-limiting arterial disease.[38]

Although infrequently utilized in the modern vascular laboratory, there are recognizable benefits associated with reactive hyperemia testing. It can be performed portably using appropriately sized blood pressure cuffs, a sphygmomanometer, and a handheld Doppler and is less time consuming than a treadmill exercise study. The major deficiency is that it does not simulate the physiologic response to exercise-associated claudication that is achieved with treadmill exercise. In addition, the test is very uncomfortable, and thigh compression should be avoided in patients with femoropopliteal bypass grafts and femoral stents.

ALTERNATIVE METHODS OF STRESS TESTING

For patients who are unable or unwilling to perform treadmill exercise or reactive hyperemia testing, other methods of stress testing have been used. These include heel raises, hall walking, plantar and dorsiflexion, and use of a pedal ergometer. While these tests elicit increased flow to the calf muscles, the exercise load cannot be standardized, and therefore they have little value for evaluation of therapeutic response or disease progression.

Pressure measurements, indices, and poststress results currently employed for the diagnosis of lower extremity arterial disease are summarized in Table 14-3.

DIAGNOSTIC ALGORITHM

The extent of peripheral arterial testing should be individualized based on the patient's presenting symptoms and clinical findings, in particular,

evidence of critical limb ischemia. In general, the patient's history and physical examination will define the clinical queries leading to a choice of either indirect, physiologic testing or duplex scanning. If the clinical queries relate to confirmation of lower limb arterial disease and definition of its location and severity, indirect, physiologic testing should be chosen as the primary testing method. If, on the other hand, there is evidence of critical limb ischemia, a pulsatile mass, or arteriovenous communication, then direct imaging should be the procedure of choice.

Keeping in mind that reimbursement and accreditation mandates require a combination of pressures and waveforms, it is helpful to have a diagnostic algorithm to follow when performing physiologic assessments (Figure 14-18).

By using a combination of pressures and plethysmographic and/or Doppler waveforms, accurate evaluations can be achieved in a time- and cost-efficient manner. The diagnostic pathway is based on the resting ankle pressures and ABI. If the ankle pressures, ABI, and Doppler waveforms recorded at ankle level are normal, but the patient presents with symptoms consistent with intermittent claudication, the next step would be constant-load treadmill exercise testing with postexercise ankle pressure measurements to unmask peripheral arterial disease. If there is an exercise-associated decrease in ankle pressure, disease location could be identified by analysis of CW Doppler waveforms recorded at the common femoral artery (PI and systolic AT) to detect flow-reducing iliac disease and at the popliteal artery (systolic AT) to identify hemodynamically significant femoropopliteal disease. If the tibial arteries are noncompressible, toe pressures should be obtained, and a TBI calculated, to identify peripheral arterial disease. Because calcification of arterial segments proximal to the ankle cannot be discounted, segmental systolic pressure measurements may be misleading. Segmental pulse volume recording could be used to detect hemodynamically significant disease in the inflow, outflow, and runoff vessels, and to define the extent of collateral compensatory flow. If the ankle pressures are abnormal, but the tibial arteries are compressible, then the pathway would lead to segmental systolic pressure measurements and treadmill exercise testing, if indicated. Color duplex sonography would be chosen to define disease location, differentiate stenosis from occlusion, detail the extent of disease, and characterize aneurysms, pseudoaneurysms, and arteriovenous fistulas.

CLINICAL APPLICATIONS

DIAGNOSIS AND FOLLOW-UP OF PATIENTS

As previously stated, physiologic testing provides an accurate, quantitative, reproducible method for identification and localization of peripheral arterial disease and for determination of

disease severity. Since the studies are noninvasive and can be repeated frequently, they afford an excellent means for follow-up of patients and for documentation of the natural history of the disease process. Systolic pressure measurements have special value in patients who present with symptoms such as spinal arthritis or musculoskeletal disorders that mimic peripheral arterial disease or coexist with it. While resting pressure measurements will quite often reveal the severity of arterial dysfunction, the pressure response to exercise is frequently required to differentiate vascular claudication from pseudoclaudication. Intermittent claudication is confirmed when the postexercise ankle pressure is less than 60 mm Hg.

In many cases, the presence and severity of lower extremity arterial disease can be determined based on the patient's medical history and physical examination. Noninvasive assessment using indirect, physiologic testing provides a baseline against which disease progression, or response to revascularization, can be measured. If revascularization has been successful, the ABI should increase, segmental pressure gradients should decrease, and the amplitude of the PVR waveforms should improve. If single-segment disease was present, revascularization should result in

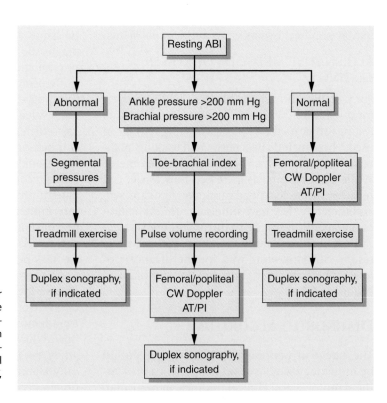

FIGURE 14-18 Diagnostic algorithm for evaluation of peripheral arterial disease using ankle-brachial index (ABI), continuous-wave (CW) Doppler waveform analysis, pulse volume recording, toe-brachial index , constant-load treadmill exercise, and duplex sonography. AT, acceleration time; PI, pulsatility index.

immediate return of ankle pressures to normal or near-normal levels. Significant decrease in the ABI (>0.15), or deterioration in the segmental pressures, PVR, and/or CW Doppler waveforms post-operatively, may suggest surgical technical error, but most often implies the presence of disease proximal or distal to the revascularized segment.

DETECTION OF DISEASE PROGRESSION

Pressure gradients become more pronounced, and the volume of flow to the distal limb more restricted, as the severity of the occlusive process increases. Follow-up physiologic studies may demonstrate more remarkable reductions in segmental pressures and significant damp-ening of the PVR and CW Doppler waveforms when compared to previous studies. As noted earlier in this chapter, studies of reproducibility of ankle pressure measurements[35] suggest that changes in the ABI greater than 0.15 are sig-nificant and indicate the likelihood of disease progression. Comparison of walking time and the extent of the postexercise decrease in ankle pressure can be used to monitor progression of known disease and to detect new-onset disease at other sites.

DETERMINING POTENTIAL FOR HEALING

Quite often physicians are faced with patients who have severe ischemia and skin lesions but who may be a poor risk for revascularization due to comorbid conditions. In other patients, arterial disease may be so extensive that recon-struction may not be possible. In 1973, Carter[39] demonstrated that measurement of distal systolic pressures could be used to predict healing of arte-rial lesions. Amputation could not be avoided in nondiabetic and diabetic patients when the ankle pressure was less than 55 mm Hg. Non-diabetic patients healed arterial lesions when the ankle pressure was greater than 55 mm Hg, but diabetic patients often failed to heal even when ankle pressures were elevated. This finding was associated with a higher incidence of medial calcinosis and severe arterial occlusive disease in the tibial vessels of the diabetic patients. Toe pressures were predictive of healing potential in the limbs of both diabetic and nondiabetic patients. Chances of healing were good when the toe pressures were greater than 30 mm Hg.

Potential for healing may also be predicted based on evaluation of tissue perfusion sur-rounding an ischemic lesion or amputation

site. Plethysmographic waveforms can be recorded in a clockwise fashion around an area of interest.

Pulsatile waveforms exhibiting rapid systolic upstroke, a dicrotic notch, and brisk runoff are found in tissues with good arterial inflow. Waveforms characterized by delayed systolic acceleration and diastolic runoff, or absence of pulsatility, suggest compromised arterial inflow and poor healing potential. As previously noted, care must be taken to consider situations that might cause local vasoconstriction or vasodilata-tion and to take this into account when interpret-ing PPG waveform morphology.

Raines and co-workers[40] demonstrated that PVR may have a valued role in determining potential for healing of below-knee amputa-tion. Patients were unlikely to heal a below-knee amputation when their calf and ankle blood pressures exceeded 65 mm Hg and 30 mm Hg, respectively, but the calf and ankle PVR were minimally pulsatile or lacked pulsatility. Con-versely, healing was likely when the calf and ankle PVR demonstrated good amplitude and normal, or near-normal, waveform morphology. Investigations also revealed that in the absence of sepsis and osteomyelitis, a toe amputation will heal if a pulsatile PVR waveform is recorded at the base of that digit. Such findings are also pre-dictive of successful healing of a transmetatarsal amputation.

PREDICTING SURGICAL OUTCOME

Systolic pressure measurements have been used to predict relief of symptoms and graft patency following arterial reconstruction. Bone and col-leagues[41] were able to predict successful outcome following aortofemoral bypass grafting when the preoperative thigh-brachial index was 0.85 or less. It was also noted that improvement may occur in patients when the index exceeds this value and in those whose disease is confined to the aortoiliac arteries. Their research also indi-cated that, compared to the preoperative value, an increase in the ABI greater than 0.1 during the first 12 hours following aortofemoral bypass strongly correlated with symptomatic improve-ment.[41] Further confirmation that aortofemoral reconstructions are most likely to be success-ful when disease is confined to the aortoiliac segments is based on the findings of others.[42] Investigators have shown that more than 90% of patients will have symptom relief following aortofemoral bypass when the preoperative ABI is greater than 0.8. Only 64% of patients experience the same degree of improvement when the ABI is less than 0.4, a value consistent with multisegmental disease.[41]

INTRAOPERATIVE AND RECOVERY ROOM MONITORING

PVR has been used historically to intraoperatively monitor the results of reconstructive arterial surgery. The presence of normal PVR waveforms immediately distal to proximal arterial revascularization in patients with femoropopliteal and tibial disease is predictive of successful revascularization. In cases where the PVR waveform amplitude has not returned to more than 50% of its preoperative value, calf and ankle pressure measurements have been used to complement the PVR tracings for verification of adequate restoration of flow.

Pulses may be difficult to palpate postoperatively in patients with known distal arterial occlusive disease or lower extremity edema. This problem may be overcome by using PVR at ankle, metatarsal, or digital level, digital PPG, or CW Doppler waveform analysis during the recovery period. Early detection of a failing reconstruction is often key to salvage. If revascularization has been successful, the amplitude of the PVR and PPG waveforms should increase, or remain stable, in the early postoperative period. Dampening of the plethysmographic waveforms and reduction in the ABI or TBI are strong indicators of a failing arterial reconstruction.

DETECTION OF AORTIC COARCTATION

A difference of 70 mm Hg or more between the brachial and ankle systolic pressures at rest can be used to detect coarctation and assess the efficacy of surgical intervention.[43] It has been shown that patients with coarctation of the thoracic aorta may not have intermittent claudication and little to no change in ankle pressure following exercise. This is most likely due to the development of extensive collateralization that provides adequate compensatory flow to the exercising muscles of the lower limb.

CONCLUSIONS

Assessment of lower extremity arteries using non-imaging, physiologic testing provides essential hemodynamic information that confirms and localizes arterial disease and allows determination of disease severity and definition of response to therapy. A diagnostic algorithm, which uses a combination of pressures and waveforms, facilitates accurate, time-efficient studies. Arterial physiologic testing may be complemented with duplex sonographic evaluations, which provide site-specific morphology information.

As with all areas of diagnostic sonography, accurate patient evaluations depend on the knowledge, experience, and expertise of the sonographer and the physician interpreter. High-quality patient care is best achieved when the studies are performed and interpreted by credentialed sonographers and physicians in accredited vascular facilities.

REFERENCES

1. Rosamond W, et al: Heart disease and stroke statistics—2008 update: a report from the American Heart Association Statistics Committee and Stroke Statistics Subcommittee. *Circulation* 117:e25–e146, 2008.
2. Marinelli MR, et al: Noninvasive testing vs. clinical evaluation of arterial disease, *JAMA* 241:2031–2034, 1979.
3. Micklin A: Peripheral arterial disease: what are we missing? *The Women's Journal* 3, 2009.
4. Hirsch AT, et al: Peripheral arterial disease detection, awareness, and treatment in primary care, *JAMA* 286(11):1317–1324, 2001.
5. Thomas M, Andrews MR: Value of oblique projections in translumbar aortography, *Am J Roentgenol* 116:187–193, 1973.
6. Crummy AB, et al: Biplane arteriography in ischemia of the lower extremity, *Radiology* 126:111–115, 1978.
7. Sethi GR, Scott SM, Takaro T: Multi-plane angiography for precise evaluation of aortoiliac disease, *Surgery* 78:154–159, 1975.
8. Carter SA: Clinical measurements of systolic pressures in limbs with arterial occlusive disease, *JAMA* 207:1869–1874, 1969.
9. Strandness DE Jr, Bell JW: Peripheral vascular disease: diagnosis and objective evaluation using mercury strain gauge, *Ann Surg* 161(suppl):1–35, 1965.
10. Sumner DS, Strandness DE: The relationship between calf blood flow and ankle blood pressure in patients with intermittent claudication, *Surgery* 65:763–771, 1969.
11. Yao JST, Hobbs JT, Irvine WT: Ankle systolic pressure measurements in arterial diseases affecting the lower extremities, *Br J Surg* 56:676–679, 1969.
12. Strandness DE, Bell JW: Ankle pressure responses after reconstructive arterial surgery, *Surgery* 59:514–516, 1966.
13. Strandness DE, et al: Ultrasonic flow detection: a useful technique in the evaluation of peripheral vascular disease, *Am J Surg* 113:311–320, 1967.
14. Pascarelli EF, Bertrand CA: Comparison of blood pressures in the arms and legs, *N Engl J Med* 270:693–698, 1964.
15. Johnston KW, Marozzo BC, Cobbold RSC: Errors and artifacts of Doppler flowmeters and their solution, *Arch Surg* 112:1335–1342, 1977.
16. Blackshear WM: Surgical indications for lower extremity arterial occlusive disease, *Part I. Curr Prob Cardiol* 6:22–32, 1981.

17. Gosling RG, et al: The quantitative analysis of occlusive peripheral arterial disease by a noninvasive ultrasonic technique, *Angiology* 22:52–55, 1971.
18. Thiele BL, et al: A systematic approach to the assessment of aortoiliac disease, *Arch Surg* 118:477–481, 1983.
19. Darling RC, et al: Quantitative segmental pulse volume recorder: a clinical tool, *Surgery* 72:873–887, 1973.
20. Raines JK: The pulse volume recorder in peripheral arterial disease. In Bernstein EF, editor: *Vascular Diagnosis*, ed 4, St. Louis, 1993, Mosby-Year Book, Inc., pp 534–543.
21. Sumner DS: Volume plethysmography in vascular disease: an overview. In Bernstein EF, editor: *Noninvasive Diagnostic Techniques in Vascular Disease*, ed 3, St. Louis, 1985, CV Mosby, pp 97–118.
22. Strandness DE, Sumner DS: *Hemodynamics for Surgeons* New York, 1975, Grune & Stratton, p. 21.
23. Taylor MG: Wave travel in arteries and the design of the cardiovascular system. In Attinger EO, editor: *Pulsatile Blood Flow*, New York, 1964, McGraw Hill.
24. Winsor T: Influence of arterial disease on the systolic blood pressure gradients of the extremity, *Am J Med Sci* 220:117, 1950.
25. Kirkendall WM, et al: Recommendation for human blood pressure determinations by sphygmomanometers: report of the sub-committee of the postgraduate education committee, American Heart Association, *Circulation* 36:980–988, 1967.
26. Barnes RW: Noninvasive diagnostic techniques and peripheral vascular disease, *Am Heart J* 97:241–258, 1979.
27. Yao JST: Hemodynamic studies in peripheral arterial disease, *Br J Surg* 57:761–766, 1970.
28. Sikkink CJ, et al: Decreased ankle/brachial indices in relation to morbidity and mortality in patients with peripheral arterial disease, *Vasc Med* 2(3):169–173, 1997.
29. Zhang Y, et al: Incidence and risk factors for stroke in American Indians: The Strong Heart Study, *Circulation* 118(15):1577–1584, 2008.
30. Toursarkissian B, et al: Noninvasive localization of infrainguinal arterial occlusive disease in diabetics, *Ann Vasc Surg* 15:73–78, 2001.
31. Carter SA, Lezack JD: Digital systolic pressures in the lower limbs in arterial disease, *Circulation* 43:905–914, 1971.
32. Kroger K, et al: Toe pressure measurements compared to ankle artery pressure measurements, *Angiology* 54(1):39–44, 2003.
33. Pascarelli EF, Bertrand CA: Comparison of blood pressures in the arms and legs, *N Engl J Med* 270:693–698, 1964.
34. Cutajar CL, Marston A, Newcombe JF: Value of cuff occlusion pressures in assessment of peripheral vascular disease, *Br J Med* 2:392–395, 1973.
35. Baker JD, Daix D: Variability of Doppler ankle pressures with arterial occlusive disease: an evaluation of ankle index and brachial ankle gradient, *Surgery* 89:134–137, 1981.
36. Sumner DS, Strandness DE Jr: The relationship between calf blood flow and ankle blood pressure in patients with intermittent claudication, *Surgery* 65:763, 1969.
37. Strandness DE Jr, Bell JW: An evaluation of the hemodynamic response of the claudicating extremity to exercise, *Surg Gynecol Obstet* 119:1237–1242, 1964.
38. Keagy BA, et al: Comparison of reactive hyperemia and treadmill tests in the evaluation of peripheral vascular disease, *Am J Surg* 142:158–161, 1981.
39. Carter SA: The relationship of distal systolic pressures to healing of skin lesions in limbs with arterial occlusive disease, with special reference to diabetes mellitus, *Scand J Clin Lab Invest* 31(suppl 128):239, 1973.
40. Raines JK, et al: Vascular laboratory criteria for the management of peripheral vascular disease of the lower extremity, *Surgery* 79:21–29, 1976.
41. Bone GE, et al: Value of segmental limb blood pressures in predicting results of aortofemoral bypass, *Am J Surg* 132:733–738, 1976.
42. Bernstein EF, Stuart SH, Fronek A: The predictive value of noninvasive testing in peripheral vascular disease. In Bernstein EF, editor: *Noninvasive Diagnostic Techniques in Vascular Disease*, St. Louis, 1982, Mosby, pp 396–403.
43. Bollinger A, Mahler F, Gruentzig A: Peripheral hemodynamics in patients with coarctation, normotensive and hypertensive arteriosclerosis obliterans of the lower limbs, *Angiology* 22:354–359, 1971.

ASSESSMENT OF UPPER EXTREMITY ARTERIAL OCCLUSIVE DISEASE

15

STEVEN R. TALBOT, RVT, FSVU

The unique structure and function of the upper extremity create challenges for the diagnosis of vascular abnormalities. Unlike the lower extremity, where atherosclerosis or thrombi are almost always the cause of symptomatic disease, upper extremity vascular problems can be more complex. Mechanical compression occurring in the troublesome thoracic outlet region, vasospasm in digital arteries, trauma-related thrombi in the hand and wrist, and embolic thrombi from the heart or from proximal arm aneurysms all must be considered when troubleshooting in the upper extremity. Hand arterial anatomy is confusing and variable and therefore requires a high level of technical expertise. Specialized probes that are capable of resolving small vessels, and displaying flow within them, are required for optimal studies. Finally, physicians and sonographers are generally out of their comfort zone when working in the arm, because arterial disease occurs less commonly in the upper extremity than in the lower extremity. Only about 5% of arterial cases involve the upper extremities.[1]

This chapter provides the basics of upper extremity arterial assessment, including

1. What to look for clinically
2. What questions to ask before getting started with testing
3. The basic anatomy of the arm and hand arteries that require examination
4. What types of noninvasive tests should be used, and in what order
5. How each examination is performed and interpreted
6. How to know when you have answered the clinical question at hand

DIAGNOSTIC WORKUP

The first steps in solving the diagnostic puzzle of hand and arm problems are to take a careful history and closely examine the fingers, hand, and arm. Both arms should be examined side by side, with attention to the following findings: Are any fingers discolored? Is there a temperature difference from one hand or finger compared with another? Are there ulcers on fingertips? Is there pain, and if so, how long has it been present? Did the pain or discomfort come on suddenly or slowly? Is the pain constant or transient? What makes the pain or discomfort better or worse? Does exposure to cold or stressful situations bring on or intensify symptoms?

CHOOSING THE RIGHT DIAGNOSTIC TOOL

Observations and historical information affect the types of tests that should be done to pinpoint the problem. Common basic noninvasive tools to investigate upper extremity arterial problems include the following:

1. Continuous-wave Doppler (with a recording device to display arterial waveforms)
2. Nonimaging physiologic tests (pulse volume recordings and segmental pressures)
3. Photoplethysmographic (PPG) sensors to detect flow in the digits
4. Color duplex imaging to directly visualize the vessels and the flow within them, and also to identify the type of pathology that is present

One or all of these tools may be needed to diagnose a given problem. For instance, if fingers are cool and discolored with exposure to cold but fine otherwise, the examination will focus on the question of whether this is a vasospastic disorder (for example, Raynaud's disease) versus a situation in which digital thrombus is present, or a combination of the two. Extensive diagnostic work will have to be done, with close attention to each finger (usually with PPG) and then some kind of cold challenge to provoke symptoms. If cold does not seem to be a factor, the cold challenge may be omitted. If the problem is positional, a baseline PPG study should be done, followed by monitoring of flow in as many different arm positions as possible. Finally, if Doppler and PPG information suggest obstruction, duplex imaging should be done to identify the cause.

Once the examiner has in mind the nature of the problem, a plan of action can be formulated for that individual. This plan may change as new information becomes available during the examination. For example, a patient with no positional symptoms turns out to have thrombus in a distal radial artery. Extra attention should then be given to the subclavian and axillary arteries,

using duplex ultrasound to check for an embolic source, such as an aneurysm or atherosclerosis. It would also be wise to have the patient go through different arm positions, with the PPG cuffs attached, to check for thoracic outlet impingement.

START WITH THE BASICS

For almost every situation where arterial disease is suspected in the upper extremity, the standard noninvasive starting point is the pulse volume recording (PVR) of arm waveforms, combined with segmental pressure measurements (Figure 15-1).

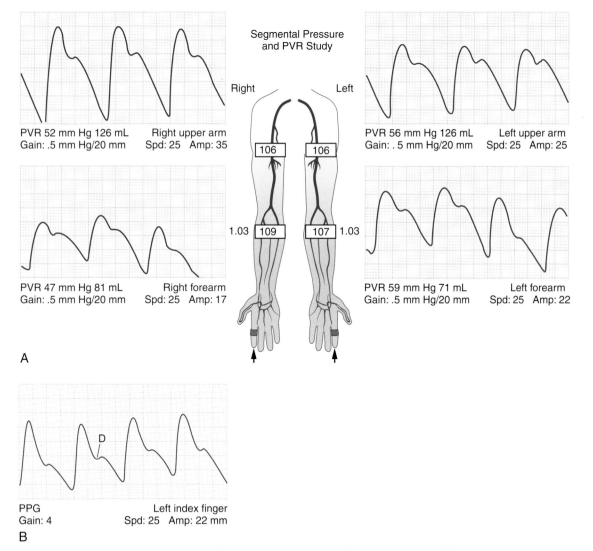

FIGURE 15-1 Normal pressures and waveforms. **A,** Upper arm and forearm (segmental) blood pressure is shown in the boxes on the illustration. The pulse volume recording (PVR) waveforms show a very short "time to peak" (from end diastole to peak systole), and a prominent dicrotic notch is present in the descending portion of the waveform. **B,** Normal *digital* photoplethysmographic (PPG) waveform shows the same features as the pneumatic, volume-based waveforms seen in part **A**. Note the dicrotic notch (D).

Continuous-wave Doppler signal assessment of the subclavian, axillary, brachial, radial, and ulnar arteries (Figure 15-2) is complementary to the segmental pressures and PVR information. If the fingers are symptomatic, PPGs (see Figure 15-1, *B*) of all digits should be obtained as well. With this simple group of tests, one can answer the basic clinical question: Is hemodynamically significant arterial obstruction present in a major arm artery?

The PVR and Doppler examinations are conducted as follows. Blood pressure cuffs are placed

about the midportion of the arm and the forearm, and PVR waveforms are taken at both levels. Then, the systolic blood pressure is measured at both levels, using the audible Doppler signal as an indication of systolic pressure. The measured blood pressures should be similar side to side, as well as from one level to the other (see Figure 15-1, *A*). A side-to-side blood pressure difference of more than 20 mm Hg or between levels, accompanied by an abnormal PVR (Figure 15-3), may indicate a hemodynamically significant lesion on the side/level with the lower pressure. This finding requires additional testing to determine the cause, usually with direct ultrasound imaging of the vessel(s) in question, as described later in this chapter.

If pressures and waveforms are normal, one can assume there is no hemodynamically significant obstruction in the arteries of the upper extremity. This observation may be an appropriate stopping point, especially if the referring physician only needs to rule out major, limb-threatening disease. It must be understood, however, that normal results of these indirect tests cannot rule out nonobstructive plaque or thrombus, aneurysm, transient mechanical compression of vessels,

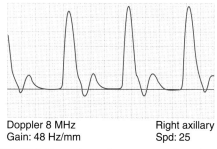

Doppler 8 MHz   Right axillary
Gain: 48 Hz/mm   Spd: 25

FIGURE 15-2 Normal continuous-wave Doppler waveforms have a high-impedance, triphasic shape characteristic of extremity arteries (with the limb at rest). Note that time to peak is very short, the systolic peak is narrow, and flow is absent in late diastole.

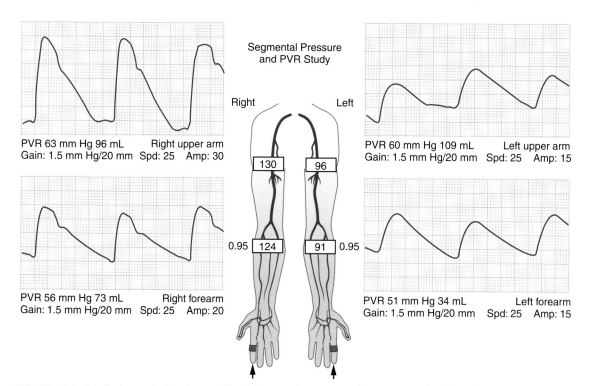

Segmental Pressure
and PVR Study

Right   Left

130   96

0.95   124   91   0.95

PVR 63 mm Hg 96 mL   Right upper arm
Gain: 1.5 mm Hg/20 mm Spd: 25   Amp: 30

PVR 56 mm Hg 73 mL   Right forearm
Gain: 1.5 mm Hg/20 mm Spd: 25   Amp: 20

PVR 60 mm Hg 109 mL   Left upper arm
Gain: 1.5 mm Hg/20 mm Spd: 25   Amp: 15

PVR 51 mm Hg 34 mL   Left forearm
Gain: 1.5 mm Hg/20 mm Spd: 25   Amp: 15

FIGURE 15-3 Subclavian occlusive disease. The right arm shows normal pressures and pulse volume recording (PVR) waveforms. On the left, the pressure measurements are more than 20 mm Hg lower than on the right, and the PVR waveforms are damped (slowed time to peak, broad waveform, absent dicrotic notch).

vasospasm, or other pathologies (such as arteritis). If any of these problems are suspected, additional testing may be required.

IS THERE A PROBLEM AT THE THORACIC OUTLET?

When a patient presents with an upper extremity circulatory problem, such as a cold, painful, or numb extremity that varies with limb positioning, a potential cause that should be identified or eliminated from the differential diagnosis early on is mechanical vascular compression at the thoracic outlet. As shown in Figure 15-4, the thoracic outlet is bounded by the clavicle, the first rib, and the scalene muscles. The thoracic outlet syndrome is a common problem, caused by impingement of the subclavian vessels and/or the brachial plexus as they leave the chest. Restriction at the thoracic outlet causes the vessels to be partially or completely compressed when the arm is in certain positions. The repeated vascular irritation over time may injure the artery or vein, leading to intimal damage or thrombus formation. Arterial emboli from thrombus formed in this area may travel distally to other parts of the upper extremity. Therefore, whenever emboli are found, one should consider that they might have originated in the subclavian or axillary arteries.

Most patients with uncomplicated thoracic outlet syndrome (without thrombus, plaque, or aneurysm) have no arm complaints unless the arm is in a certain position. The discomfort the patient experiences is likely, at least originally, to result from nerve compression, rather than transient loss of blood flow from arterial impingement. The patient describes pain or numbness and loss of sensation when the upper extremity is in a predictable and reproducible position, such as occurs with hair brushing or driving a car (with the hands in a constant position on the steering wheel). The symptoms go away soon after the arm is repositioned.

If the examiner is presented with symptoms suggesting thoracic outlet problems, the upper extremity examination should begin routinely with resting PVRs and segmental pressures, as described previously, but this assessment should be supplemented with a check for the thoracic outlet syndrome, using the following technique. The examiner has the patient sit very straight and, using continuous-wave Doppler to monitor radial or ulnar artery flow, guides the patient through maneuvers that begin with the arm abducted and externally rotated. The blood pressure cuffs are left on the arms to monitor the pulse volume waveforms during the position changes, providing the examiner with two independent indicators of the quality of blood flow in the arm as the patient moves through the provocative position changes. This can be a clumsy operation for one examiner, so two examiners should be present during this procedure, if possible. One of the examiners is positioned behind the patient and maintains gentle pressure on the patient's back with the left hand, to keep the back straight, while holding the Doppler probe used to monitor the radial or ulnar artery in the right hand. The other examiner operates the PVR device and monitors the PVR waveforms during the arm position changes. (Note: A PPG sensor attached to a finger may be used instead of continuous-wave Doppler, if desired.)

Once a good-quality Doppler signal is acquired at the radial or ulnar artery and the PVR device is adequately registering PVR waveforms, the examiner holding the Doppler probe guides the patient through the arm maneuvers. We usually start with the arm maximally abducted and externally rotated, with the shoulders pulled back as far as possible. The arm is then directed through every conceivable position, while the operators watch the PVR waveform tracing for diminished amplitude or total flattening of the waveform, accompanied by dampening or total loss of the Doppler signal. If a position is identified where such changes occur (Figure 15-5), with recovery of the signals when the arm is moved out of the position, the test is positive and indicates thoracic

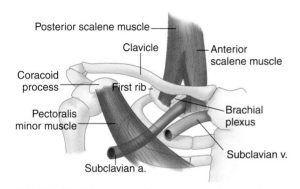

FIGURE 15-4 Thoracic outlet anatomy. The subclavian artery, brachial plexus, and subclavian vein pass through a narrow opening framed by the anterior and posterior scalene muscles, the clavicle, and the first rib. a, artery; v, vein.

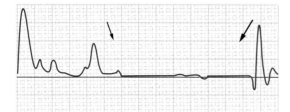

FIGURE 15-5 Thoracic outlet impingement. The Doppler signal at the radial artery goes flat *(small arrow)*, as the arm is positioned such that the subclavian artery is compressed. The signal resumes *(large arrow)* when the arm is repositioned.

outlet impingement. This arm position should be repeated, however, and the findings should be the same every time the arm is moved into the obstructing position. Care should be taken to make sure the examiner did not simply move the Doppler probe off the monitored artery during positioning, as this can be a potential source of false-positive results. If the Doppler signal disappears, yet the PVR continues to be robust, recheck the Doppler probe orientation and repeat the maneuver.

A positive result, as described previously, suggests the presence of the thoracic outlet syndrome, but many patients without symptoms may test positive when an arm is in an extreme position, such as that used for this test. This fact contributes to the controversy surrounding the use of this test alone in making the diagnosis of thoracic outlet syndrome. The diagnosis is much more solid, however, if subclavian artery stenosis is visualized with duplex imaging with the arm in the position that causes abnormal Doppler and PVR findings, or if an aneurysm is demonstrated with duplex ultrasound. The latter finding proves the occurrence of significant and repeated arterial impingement.

If Doppler signals and PVR waveforms do not diminish with various arm positions, these positions should be repeated with the head in a neutral position, with the head turned to the left, with the head to the right, with the head tilted up, and finally, with the chin on the chest. Only after every conceivable position has been tested can the examination be terminated. If all of these maneuvers fail to identify a position where flow is diminished, the test is determined to be negative for thoracic outlet impingement. This does not necessarily mean that the condition does not exist in the given patient, only that this test has been unable to identify it.

PHOTOPLETHYSMOGRAPHY OF DIGITAL FLOW EVALUATION

After flow in the arms has been checked, attention is next turned to the digits. If there are any problems such as cold, discolored, or painful fingers, arterial flow in the digits should be checked. This is commonly done with PPG sensors that are applied to the pads of the fingers. Double-stick tape is usually used to secure the PPG probe to the fingers. A normal digital PPG waveform has a rapid upstroke, a downstroke that bows toward the baseline, a dicrotic notch, and normal amplitude (see Figure 15-1, *B*). A person with normal digital arteries may have small, abnormal-looking waveforms if the extremity is cold, so care must be taken to ensure that the examination room is sufficiently warm. If there is any question of the PPG waveforms' being adversely affected by cold temperature, have the patient warm the hands with a warming blanket before testing. If good-quality, normal waveforms are present in all of the digits, the examination is complete. If the waveforms are blunted, rounded, or absent, additional testing is required.

CHECK FOR DIGITAL ARTERY THROMBUS

One of the main questions that must be answered in the event of abnormal digital PPG waveforms is whether the vessels are obstructed with thrombus, as opposed to a vasospasm problem, or whether the etiology is a combination of both. Sometimes the digital arteries are filled with intraluminal thrombus that will have originated, most likely, from a proximal artery (usually the subclavian/axillary segment) or from the heart. When the digital arteries are occluded, waveforms will be rounded (Figure 15-6, *A*), flat, or nearly flat. No amount of warming will restore the waveform contour to normal, although slight improvement may sometimes occur. Likewise, nerve block induced with local anesthesia will have little or no effect. When thrombus is suspected in the digital arteries, the palmar arches, or the arteries of the arm, duplex imaging, as described later in this chapter, may be appropriate to verify the presence and exact location of the thrombus.

CHECK FOR RAYNAUD'S DISEASE

When digits display signs of intermittent pallor, cyanosis, and rubor that is caused solely by digital arterial spasm, the condition is called

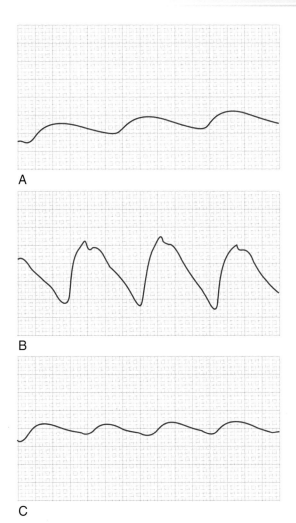

A

B

C

FIGURE 15-6 Abnormal digital photoplethysmographic waveforms. **A,** Proximal arterial obstruction—the photoplethysmographic waveforms are severely damped (widened, flattened). **B,** Raynaud's disease—mildly damped waveforms with unusually high dicrotic notch. **C,** Raynaud's phenomenon—severely damped waveforms.

Raynaud's disease (as opposed to a more serious condition called Raynaud's phenomenon, to be discussed later). Raynaud's disease usually represents an overreaction of vasomotor responses to cold or stress stimuli. Symptoms include fingers of both hands becoming virtually white as the arteries and arterioles undergo intense spasm in response to cold or stress.[2] Digital PPG waveforms may be normal or nearly normal at rest but flatten or become severely damped in response to cold stimuli or stress. The typical PPG waveform seen in this condition displays a somewhat slower upstroke than normal, along with a sharp anacrotic notch and a dicrotic notch that is located unusually high on the downslope of the

waveform (see Figure 15-6, *B*). However, a normal waveform may be seen in a patient with mild Raynaud's disease when vasospasm is aborted by warming the hand.

A cold challenge test may be helpful in identifying Raynaud's disease. This test is performed as follows. Baseline digital PPG waveforms are obtained, and the hands are immersed in ice water for 3 to 5 minutes. Waveforms are again obtained, and their return to preimmersion appearance is timed. Individuals with normal circulation will return to preimmersion levels within 10 minutes. Those with Raynaud's disease take longer, and some may not recover within a reasonable observation time unless the cycle of vasospasm is broken by warming the hand. Most patients with this condition merely need to protect the fingers from cold exposure a little more than other individuals to avoid the symptoms of Raynaud's disease. Occasionally, patients with Raynaud's disease worsen, and they develop trophic changes or ulcerations at the fingertips. However, this is seen only in patients who do not take adequate steps to protect their hands from cold exposure.

CHECK FOR RAYNAUD'S PHENOMENON

The presence of cold sensitivity complicated by fixed arterial obstruction is referred to as secondary Raynaud's phenomenon. This is a much more serious condition than Raynaud's disease, because there is vasospasm mixed with intraluminal obstruction. The fact that these two conditions are given similar names creates confusion, even among experienced examiners. *Raynaud's disease, Raynaud's phenomenon, Raynaud's syndrome, primary Raynaud's,* and *secondary Raynaud's* are all terms used—and misused—to describe these two conditions. In this chapter, we use the term *Raynaud's disease* to describe the vasospastic disorder *without intraluminal occlusion* and *Raynaud's phenomenon* to describe vasospastic disease *accompanied by* fixed arterial obstruction.[3] Regardless of the terms used, the major diagnostic challenge is to differentiate between those patients who have only vasospasm and those who have arterial obstruction as well.

PPG waveforms in a patient with Raynaud's phenomenon are more rounded in appearance than those in a patient with Raynaud's disease and may also be low in amplitude (see Figure 15-6, *C*). The waveform shape is similar to that seen with proximal arterial occlusion, and it is important to differentiate between these two etiologies with segmental pressure and Doppler, as discussed previously. When severe digital waveform abnormalities are found in the proper clinical setting, it is clear that the condition is Raynaud's phenomenon, and further assessment with hand cooling is not necessary. However, warming the hand may be useful to determine if flow to the fingers can be improved.

For those who insist on performing a cold challenge on patients with findings of Raynaud's phenomenon, it is advisable to follow the cold challenge with a pharmacologic sympathectomy, as follows. The baseline study is done first, followed by immersion of the hands in ice water for 3 to 5 minutes. The waveforms typically go flat in response to the cold challenge. Then the pharmacologic sympathectomy is performed. In such cases, a physician injects a small amount of a local anesthetic into a nerve, plexus, or ganglion to temporarily inactivate its effect on sympathetic tone. Once the local anesthetic has had a chance to act, the PPG waveforms are taken again. Major waveform improvement, above baseline levels, suggests that a permanent sympathectomy or vasodilator therapy may be helpful. If vasospasm is a major component of the problem, the hand and fingers may become very warm and the PPG waveforms may go off scale (Figure 15-7, *A*). The

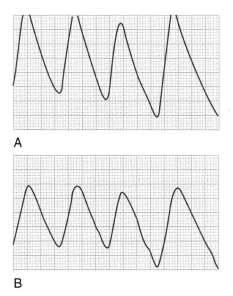

A

B

FIGURE 15-7 Vasospastic disease. **A,** The photoplethysmographic waveform of a digit is off scale after cold immersion, followed by nerve block to reopen the digital arteries. **B,** Waveform amplitude decreases after reimmersion in ice water, but the amplitude remains quite high.

hand is then reimmersed in the cold water. If the waveforms are not dampened by reimmersion (see Figure 15-7*B*), it is likely that some degree of improvement can be expected with therapy. It is not advisable to do the cold immersion test in patients with severe Raynaud's phenomenon without the ability to perform a nerve block because the maneuver can incite a severe vasospastic response that may be hard to reverse.

As noted previously, Raynaud's phenomenon represents a combination of vasospasm and arterial occlusion. Therefore, there may be a role for duplex ultrasound assessment of digital and palmar arterial patency.

WHEN TO ADD DUPLEX IMAGING

The decision as to whether duplex ultrasound imaging is necessary in the course of an upper extremity arterial examination depends on whether the indirect studies already performed have answered the clinical question at hand. If the answer is no, then duplex imaging should be performed. For example, duplex is necessary whenever the indirect tests suggest arterial obstruction. In this situation, the arm arteries are scanned to identify the exact location and severity of stenosis or occlusion. Duplex imaging can also be used to see if the problem identified by indirect tests is caused by atherosclerotic plaque or thrombus. Arterial thrombus may be treated with anticoagulants, thrombolytics, or even thrombectomy, whereas plaque is treated differently.

Duplex imaging is also used to detect an arterial aneurysm. This is an important piece of information, as an aneurysm may contain thrombus and be the source of distal arterial emboli. The subclavian and axillary arteries are the most likely areas for aneurysm formation in the arm. Repeated injury to these arteries, due to impingement at the thoracic outlet, can lead to thrombus formation, plaque formation, and even aneurysmal dilatation. For this reason, whenever there is thrombus anywhere in the arm or hand, even without indication of proximal stenosis on indirect tests, the subclavian/axillary artery region should be scanned.

DUPLEX IMAGING TECHNIQUE AND DIAGNOSTIC CRITERIA

Duplex examination of the arm arteries is similar to duplex imaging of the lower extremity. Typically, a vessel is imaged first with short-axis views to get the examiner oriented, and then the transducer is turned 90 degrees to obtain long-axis views, which are used to follow the vessels (Figure 15-8). The entire course of each major artery is imaged, including the subclavian, axillary, brachial, radial, ulnar, deep palmar arch, superficial palmar arch, and digital arteries.

Because the arm arteries are mostly superficial, high-frequency transducers can be used. Most, or sometimes all, of the arteries in the arm can be imaged with frequencies between 8 and 15 MHz. However, some areas near the clavicle may require the use of a 3- to 8-MHz transducer. Imaging of hand arteries requires very high frequencies, because these vessels are extremely small and superficial. Transducers designed for use in surgery work quite well for imaging the digital arteries, since they have a small footprint and operate at frequencies between 10 and 15 MHz.

Color flow ultrasound is used to identify blood flow within the vessels and to give the examiner an idea of the velocity and direction of flow. Pulsed-wave Doppler signals and spectral analysis are used to determine the velocity of flow at key points within the vessel (Figure 15-9). Normal, angle-corrected peak systolic velocities within the larger arm arteries, such as the subclavian and axillary arteries, generally run between 70 and 120 cm/sec. Brachial artery peak systolic velocities range from 50 to 100 cm/sec. Velocities in normal radial and ulnar arteries run between 40 and 90 cm/sec, while velocities within the palmar arches and digits are lower. Normal upper extremity Doppler waveforms are triphasic, but changes in temperature, or even maneuvers such as clenching of the fist, may dramatically change the characteristics of upper extremity waveforms, especially in and near the hand (Figure 15-10). The large arteries of the upper arm and forearm are relatively easy to identify and evaluate with ultrasound. Imaging the small arteries of the hand is very challenging for several reasons. Not

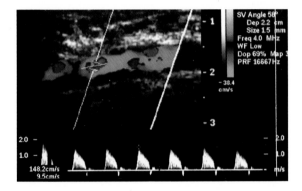

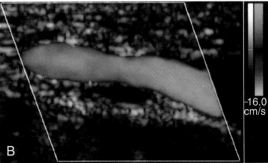

FIGURE 15-8 Typical duplex ultrasound transducer positions. **A,** The short-axis view shows the vessel in cross-section. The brachial artery (A) is seen in this color flow image, accompanied by the brachial and basilic veins (V). **B,** The long-axis view shows vessels, such as this axillary artery, along their length.

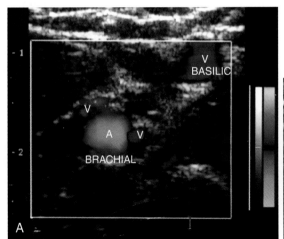

FIGURE 15-9 Pulsed-wave Doppler example. The axillary artery (AX ART) is seen in long axis with color and pulsed wave Doppler. Note that the angle-corrected velocity must be obtained with the cursor lined up with the vessel wall, and the Doppler angle must be 60 degrees or less.

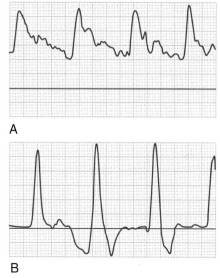

A

B

FIGURE 15-10 Environmental and muscular effects. **A,** This continuous-wave Doppler waveform was obtained from the radial artery with the hand very warm and relaxed. Note that the waveform is entirely above the baseline and it is difficult to make judgments about its triphasic pattern. **B,** This continuous-wave waveform was taken from the same vessel as in part **A,** but now the patient has his fist clenched, causing increased flow resistance. Note the dramatic change in the Doppler waveform. The triphasic, high-resistance pattern now is easily identified.

only are the vessels small, but, in addition, there are numerous anatomic variations. Furthermore, the vascular anatomy of the hand described herein is a simplified version of the actual anatomy, which includes arterial pathways beyond the scope of this chapter.[4] Nevertheless, knowledge of the anatomy shown herein is adequate to answer most of the clinical questions that are raised.

A patterned approach is required for accurate duplex ultrasound evaluation of upper extremity arteries. The ultrasound imaging protocol used in our department, as well as the relevant arterial anatomy, is illustrated in detail in Figures 15-11 to 15-19. This material is not repeated in the text; therefore, readers who are unfamiliar with upper extremity arterial ultrasound should review these figures before proceeding.

DUPLEX ULTRASOUND–DETECTED PATHOLOGY

Atherosclerotic plaque forms commonly in the subclavian and axillary arteries. The principal effect is blood flow reduction due to stenosis or

occlusion that can result in arm ischemia. Atherosclerotic obstruction of more distal arteries, such as the radial and ulnar arteries, is less common; nevertheless, distal vessels may undergo thrombosis secondary to low-flow states or atherosclerosis-related embolization.

Although stenosis of larger upper extremity arteries is most often caused by atherosclerosis, it may also be caused by vasculitis, trauma, or thoracic outlet compression. Stenosis of smaller arteries usually results from vasospastic disease or vasculitis. In the extremities, stenoses that reduce the lumen diameter by 50% or greater are flow reducing, or hemodynamically significant. Such stenoses are identified by increased velocity, poststenotic turbulence, and waveforms that are damped distal to the level of the stenosis, as shown in Figure 15-20. In addition, high-grade arterial stenosis or occlusion causes overall reduced flow velocity proximal to the point of obstruction. There are no universally accepted velocities that determine the severity of a stenosis in the arm arteries; however, when a stenosis causes the peak systolic velocity to double (compared with the prestenotic velocity), it is considered hemodynamically significant (≥50% diameter narrowing). Tighter stenoses further increase systolic and diastolic velocities.

Color Doppler imaging shows narrowing of the arterial lumen as well as altered color flow in the stenotic region consistent with elevated flow velocity and a poststenotic mosaic pattern that results from turbulent flow. With arterial occlusion, no flow is detected in the vessel lumen with color and power Doppler as well as spectral Doppler waveforms, and a damped, monophasic Doppler signal is seen distal to the area of obstruction (Figure 15-21). When occlusion is detected, it is important to determine the extent of the occluded segment and the location of arterial reconstitution by collaterals.

Arterial thrombosis may occur distal to a critical stenosis or may result from embolization, trauma, or thoracic outlet compression. The result may be occlusion or partial occlusion. Thrombus or vasculitis may be visualized directly with gray-scale imaging, but color and power Doppler imaging are useful to determine vessel patency and to assess the degree of vessel recanalization with thrombolysis (Figure 15-22). Whenever thrombus is thought to be seen in an

Text continued on p. 276.

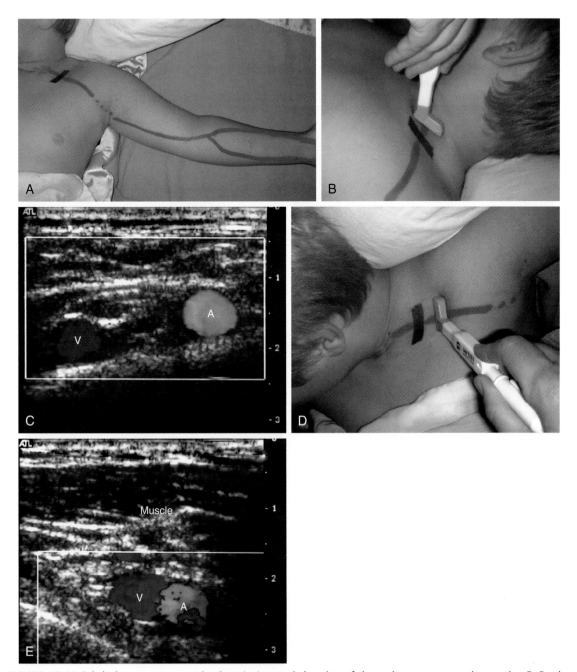

FIGURE 15-11 Subclavian segment examination. **A,** Anatomic location of the major upper extremity arteries. **B,** Duplex ultrasound imaging begins with short-axis views of the subclavian artery obtained *above* the clavicle. **C,** In the short-axis view, the artery (A) and vein (V) are identified side by side. Compression with the transducer can be used to identify the artery and vein, since the vein is more easily compressed than the artery. Visualization of the subclavian artery is difficult, at best, because of interference from the clavicle, which limits the space for the transducer and often restricts above-clavicle imaging to short-axis views. **D** and **E,** An alternative approach is to visualize the subclavian artery from an *infraclavicular* transducer position, with which the artery (A) and vein (V) are seen through the pectoral muscles, in either short- or long-axis views.

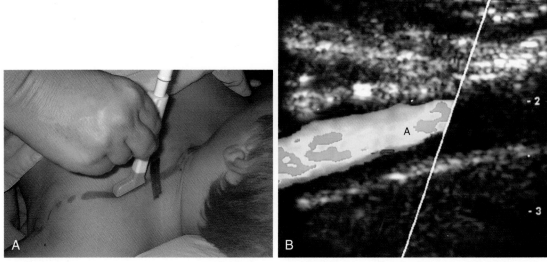

FIGURE 15-12 Long-axis subclavian examination. **A,** Once the subclavian artery is identified, rotate the transducer to visualize the artery (A) in long axis as shown in part **B.** The artery should be examined proximally and distally as far as possible for the presence of plaque, thrombus, or aneurysm. Frequently, a short segment of the proximal subclavian artery is hidden under the clavicle and cannot be examined directly.

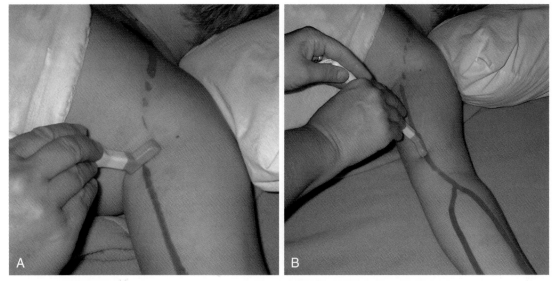

FIGURE 15-13 Axillary and brachial segment examination. At its distal end, the subclavian artery dives deeply, and at this point, the arm is raised and the probe is repositioned in the axilla to examine the axillary artery. **A,** Begin high in the axilla, with the transducer positioned for a short-axis view, and get oriented. **B,** After identifying the axillary artery, switch to a long-axis view and follow the axillary and brachial arteries down the medial side of the upper arm in the groove between the biceps and triceps muscles. The axillary artery becomes the brachial artery where it crosses the lower margin of the tendon of the teres major muscle, but this landmark is not readily identified sonographically.

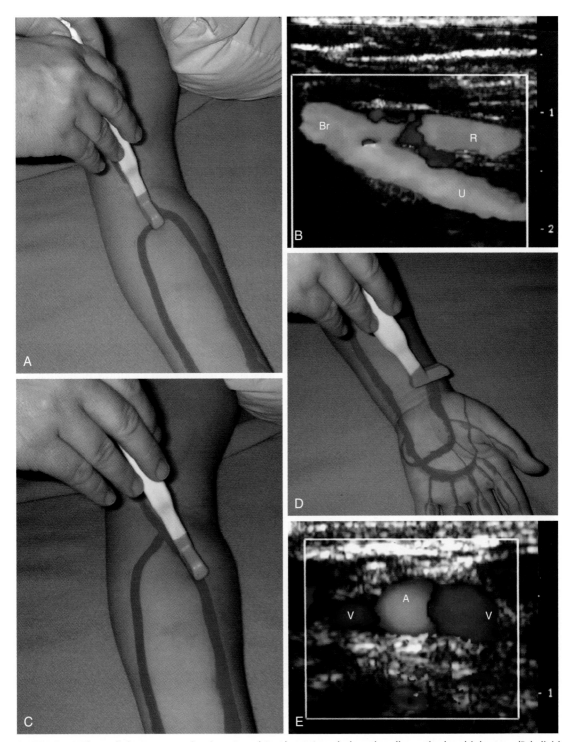

FIGURE 15-14 The radial artery examination. **A** and **B,** About 1 cm below the elbow, the brachial artery (Br) divides into the radial (R) and ulnar (U) arteries. **C,** The radial artery is examined with long-axis views throughout its course along the radial (lateral) side of the volar aspect of the forearm. **D** and **E,** When viewed in a transverse (short-axis) plane, the artery (A) is flanked by the small radial veins (V).

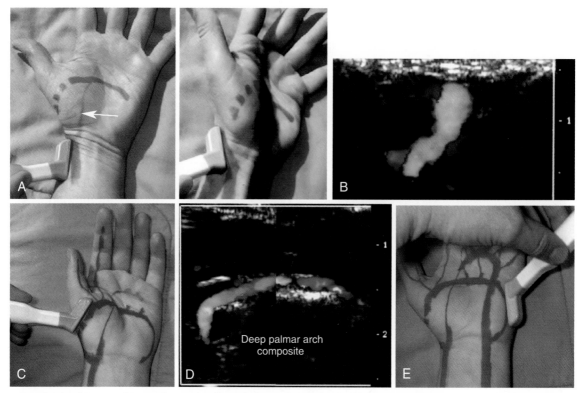

FIGURE 15-15 Deep palmar arch examination. At the wrist, radial artery anatomy gets a bit tricky. **A,** Before it enters the hand, the radial artery splits into two branches, one of which continues into the volar aspect of the hand *(arrow)* and connects with the superficial palmar arch. The main trunk of the radial artery heads posterior to the thumb before entering the palm. It is important to follow the main trunk, shown in parts **A** and **B,** by temporarily moving to the dorsal aspect of the hand. **C,** The sonographer then returns to the volar surface and follows the main trunk into the palm, where it becomes the deep palmar arch. **D,** The arch should be followed as it loops around **(E)** and connects with the ulnar artery.

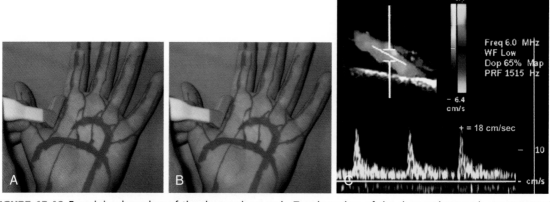

FIGURE 15-16 Examining branches of the deep palmar arch. Two branches of the deep palmar arch are commonly visualized in normal individuals. **A,** Beginning at the radial side, the first branch is the princeps pollicis, which supplies the thumb. **B,** This is followed by another small branch called the radialis indicis, which travels up the radial side of the index finger. These two vessels sometimes share a common trunk. **C,** Doppler signals in these small vessels typically are quite weak and show flow features that differ from the radial and ulnar arteries. Note that while the pattern is one of moderate resistance, flow is present through diastole. Three other small digital arteries (not shown), called the palmar metacarpals, may be seen branching from the deep palmar arch, and these eventually join the common digital arteries to supply the fingers. These arteries are usually difficult to see and follow with ultrasound.

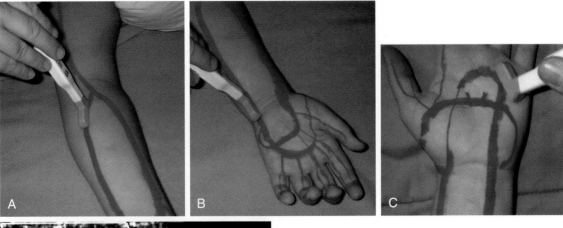

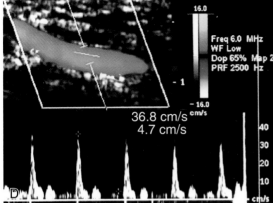

FIGURE 15-17 The ulnar artery and superficial palmar arch examination. After evaluating the radial artery and deep palmar arch, the examiner returns to the antecubital fossa to inspect the ulnar artery. **A,** After traveling deeply in the flexor muscles, the ulnar artery runs more superficially, along the volar aspect of the ulnar (medial) side of the forearm. **B,** It can be followed into the palm as a single large trunk, where it curves laterally to form the superficial palmar arch. **C,** When followed, the superficial palmar arch is seen to connect with the smaller branch of the radial artery shown in Figure 16-15, *A.* **D,** Doppler signals in the superficial palmar arch have relatively high resistance, but flow throughout diastole, similar to the deep arch.

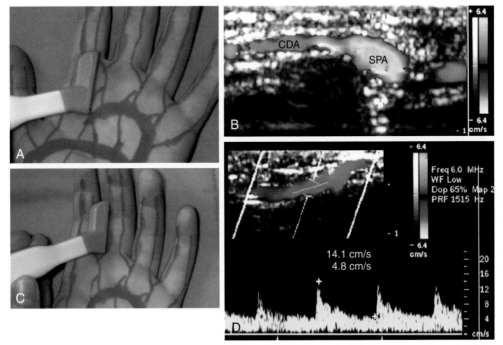

FIGURE 15-18 Digital artery examination. **A** and **B,** The principal arterial supply to digits three, four, and five is via the common digital arteries (CDA), which arise from the superficial palmar arch (SPA). **C** and **D,** These can be followed into the fingers, where each branches to form the proper digital arteries that lie on either side of the fingers. Relatively low flow resistance is evident in these vessels.

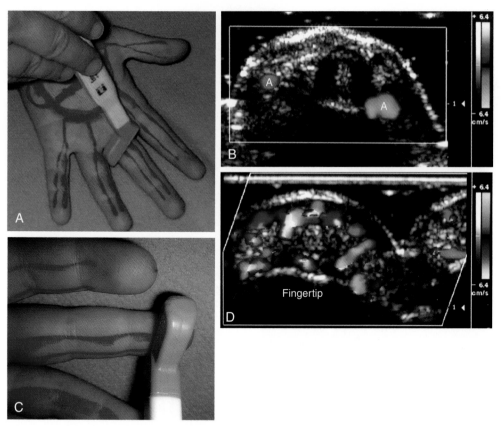

FIGURE 15-19 Proper digital artery examination. **A** and **B,** Using very high frequency transducers, the proper digital arteries (A) can be followed along the medial and lateral sides of the fingers. **C** and **D,** At the tip of each finger, the proper digital arteries join, giving off a number of small branches at the fingertips.

artery, the examiner should attempt to compress the artery using transducer pressure. If the artery is truly filled with thrombus, compression will *not* cause the artery to collapse. This is important because artifacts may be present that look like thrombus in an artery. If the artery collapses in response to compression (Figure 15-23), the suspected "thrombus" can be accurately determined to be an artifact.

Arterial aneurysms in the upper extremity are rare, but the most likely place for their occurrence is in the subclavian/axillary area. They usually occur as a result of chronic trauma, as is the case with thoracic outlet impingement, or they may occur on an idiopathic basis. Because laminated thrombus commonly forms in aneurysms, this becomes a likely source of emboli to the radial, ulnar, or hand arteries. For this reason, whenever thrombus is found in distal arteries, the subclavian/axillary arteries should be checked carefully for the presence of an aneurysm. A vessel is said to be aneurysmal when the diameter at the point of interest is at least one

and a half times the size of the artery above and below it. Most aneurysms in the arm are fusiform, as seen in Figure 15-24, rather than saccular, and for that reason, they tend to be more subtle than aneurysms in other parts of the arterial system. Localized aneurysms can also be seen in the hand, most often following repeated trauma to the ulnar artery (hypothenar hammer syndrome).

CHECK FOR VERTEBRAL-TO-SUBCLAVIAN STEAL

If a patient has a significant difference in arm blood pressure (20 mm Hg, as observed during the segmental pressure/PVR portion of the study), the duplex imaging examination should be expanded to check for vertebral-to-subclavian steal. This is a situation in which a tight stenosis or occlusion is present in the portion of the subclavian artery proximal to the ipsilateral vertebral artery. Insufficient blood flow through the obstruction causes the subclavian artery to

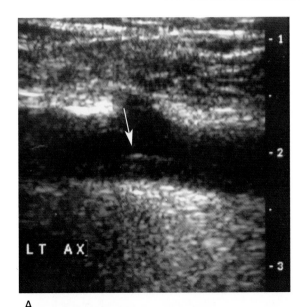

A

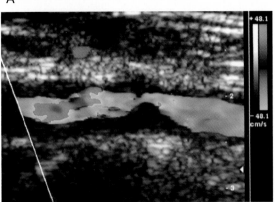

B

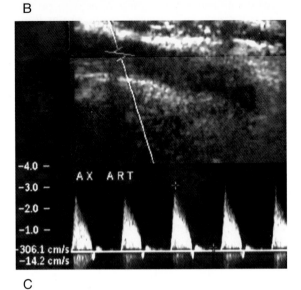

C

FIGURE 15-20 Hemodynamically significant stenosis. **A,** Plaque is seen in the axillary (LT AX) artery with B-mode imaging. **B,** Color is added to reveal the contour of the plaque and its flow effects. **C,** Pulsed Doppler is used to display the markedly increased flow velocity (306 cm/sec) in the stenosis. AX ART, axillary artery.

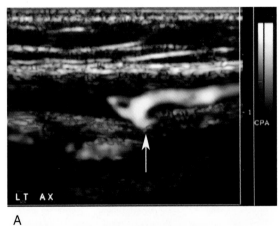

A

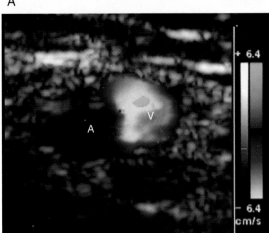

B

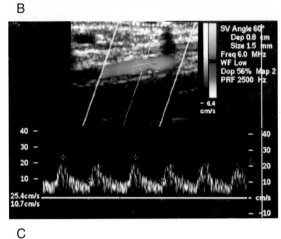

C

FIGURE 15-21 Arterial occlusion. **A** and **B,** Long- and short-axis color and power Doppler views show occlusion of an axillary artery (A). V, axillary vein. Note in part **A** that flow is reconstituted below the occlusion by a collateral *(arrow).* **C,** Below the occlusion, in the ulnar artery, Doppler waveforms are damped—monophasic, delayed time to peak, broad systolic peak, continuous diastolic flow.

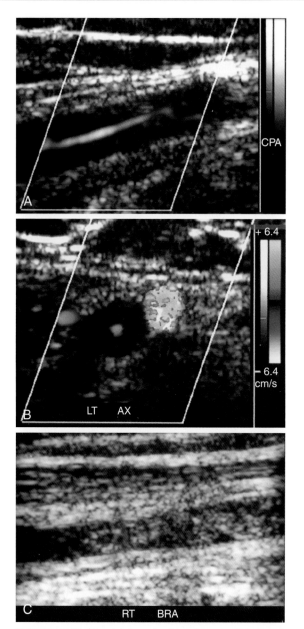

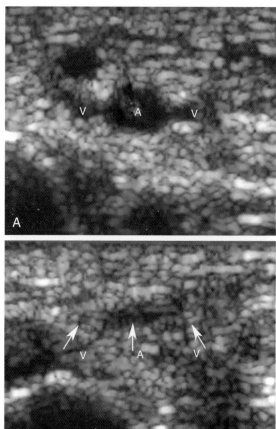

FIGURE 15-23 Artifact versus thrombus. Whenever it appears that thrombus is present in an artery (A), the vessel should be viewed in a transverse plane **(A)** and compressed with the transducer (*arrows*, part **B**). If the artery truly is thrombosed, the intraluminal thrombus will prevent it from collapsing in response to compression. However, if the artery compresses **(B)**, the examiner knows the "thrombus" was actually artifactual. V, vein.

FIGURE 15-22 Arterial thrombosis and/or vasculitis. **A** and **B,** Long- and short-axis, color flow images show faintly echogenic material throughout the axillary (AX) artery lumen, with only a small area of residual flow. The diffuseness of the occluding material and the smoothness of the residual (or recanalized) lumen favors thrombosis or vasculitis rather than atherosclerosis. **C,** In another patient, the right brachial artery (BRA) is occluded by thrombus that is more echogenic than that seen in parts **A** and **B**.

steal blood from the ipsilateral vertebral artery. Vertebral-to-subclavian steal rarely causes severe neurologic symptoms, but it may cause arterial insufficiency in the affected arm that may be clinically important. For details concerning the

pathophysiology of this condition and its clinical consequences, please see Chapter 11.

Whenever vertebral-to-subclavian steal is suspected, the examiner should check the direction of the flow in the ipsilateral vertebral artery. If flow is retrograde or undulating (to and fro), vertebral-to-subclavian steal is likely. This finding, combined with a blood pressure in the ipsilateral arm 20 mm or more lower than the opposite arm, makes a compelling case for subclavian steal. To make the case even stronger, the examiner can compare the axillary Doppler waveforms, noting that the waveforms on the side of the obstruction are more rounded and of lower

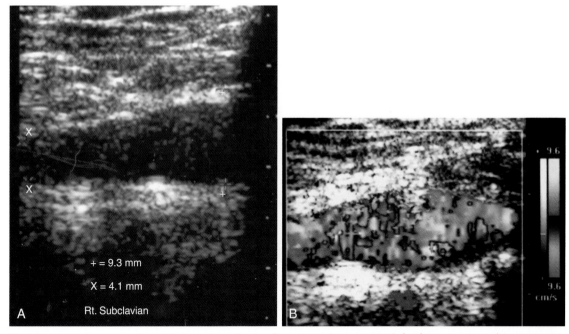

FIGURE 15-24 Aneurysm. **A** and **B,** B-mode and color flow views show a typical, fusiform aneurysm (approximately 9-mm diameter) in the subclavian/axillary segment. No thrombus is visible in this aneurysm, but aneurysms may contain thrombus that can embolize to distal vessels.

overall velocity, and they may be monophasic. The vertebral and subclavian Doppler findings are presented in detail in Chapter 11.

With diligence, the examiner can sometimes see the stenotic area of the subclavian artery directly and document the presence of stenosis, rather than occlusion. This requires angulation of the ultrasound beam deeply beneath the medial end of the clavicle. The usual features of arterial stenosis are seen (Figure 15-25). The lumen is visibly narrowed on the color flow image, with a color shift indicating elevated flow velocity. Spectral Doppler shows high-velocity systolic and diastolic flow levels in the stenotic region and turbulence distal to the stenosis. Even if the stenosis itself cannot be seen, it may be possible to detect the severe poststenotic turbulence that is invariably associated with a high-grade arterial stenosis.

Direct subclavian stenosis visualization is much more likely to be possible on the right side, as shown in Figure 15-25, than on the left, because the right subclavian artery is a branch of the innominate artery, which makes the area of stenosis much more superficial. On the right, the stenosis is generally seen in the most proximal segment of the subclavian artery,

just beyond the bifurcation of the innominate artery into the common carotid and subclavian branches.

Seeing a stenosis on the left side is much more difficult, as the subclavian artery arises from the aorta at an angle and depth that is difficult to image. This is unfortunate, considering that 85% of vertebral-to-subclavian steal cases occur on the left side.

CONCLUSIONS: ANSWERING THE CLINICAL QUESTION

This chapter is a compilation of the common physiologic and Doppler tests used to assess upper extremity arteries. Only the more frequently encountered arterial disorders affecting the upper extremities could be included. It is important to consider that any combination of the methods described herein can be used at the discretion of the ordering physician, or the examiner, to answer the clinical question at hand. Knowledge of the value of a given test in a given situation is required to ensure that a correct diagnosis is obtained. The proper combination of tests is the key to shedding light on a difficult diagnosis.

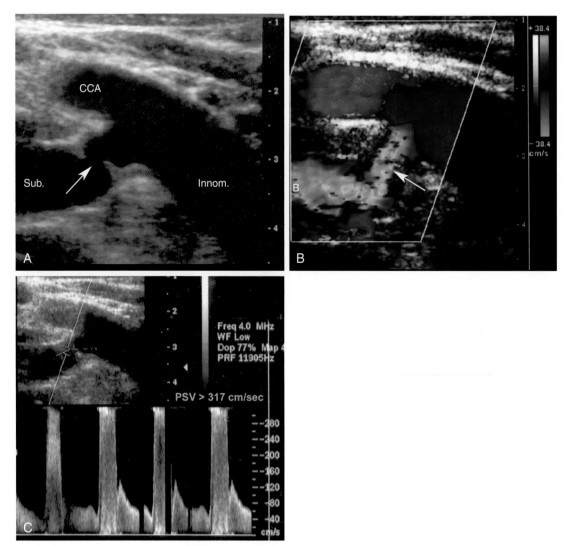

FIGURE 15-25 Subclavian stenosis. **A,** Gray-scale sonography provides a direct view of a stenosis at the origin of the subclavian artery *(arrows).* Sub, subclavian; CCA, common carotid artery; Innom, innominate artery. **B,** Color Doppler shows turbulent flow in the stenotic segment *(arrow).* **C,** Pulsed Doppler signals reveal markedly elevated flow velocity within the stenosis that cannot be measured as it exceeds the maximum velocity/frequency scale. Peak systolic velocity (PSV) exceeds 317 cm/sec.

REFERENCES

1. Zwiebel WJ: *Introduction to vascular ultrasonography*, ed 4, Philadelphia, 2000, Saunders.
2. Robbins SL: *Basic pathology*, Philadelphia, 1981, Saunders.
3. Hershey FB, Barnes RW, Sumner DS: *Noninvasive diagnosis of vascular disease*, Pasadena, 1984, Appleton Davies.
4. Crafts RC: *Textbook of human anatomy*, ed 2, New York, 1979, John Wiley and Sons.

ULTRASOUND EVALUATION BEFORE AND AFTER HEMODIALYSIS ACCESS

16

MICHELLE L. ROBBIN, MD, MS, and MARK E. LOCKHART, MD, MPH

Ultrasound can be extremely useful in the evaluation of the many problems facing the hemodialysis patient. It is a noninvasive technique that can show more vascular detail than physical examination, without the risk for phlebitis or contrast reaction from conventional venography. Current Dialysis Outcome Quality Initiative (DOQI) guidelines encourage the placement of arteriovenous fistulas (AVFs) rather than grafts, because of their greater longevity and decreased incidence of infection.[1,2] Detailed evaluation of arterial and venous anatomy before hemodialysis access improves the visualization of veins that may be suitable for native AVF placement, particularly in the patient with a history of prior failed access and/or prior placement of central catheters.

Vascular mapping before hemodialysis access also may change surgical management since the identification of a suitable efferent vein would favor the placement of an AVF rather than a graft. In addition, there is an increased likelihood of selecting the most functional vessels preoperatively, with a subsequent decrease in unsuccessful surgical explorations.[3] Vascular mapping has doubled the proportion of patients in dialysis with a fistula in our patient population.[4]

Despite preoperative vascular mapping, up to 60% of AVFs still fail to mature adequately to support hemodialysis.[5] In these patients, ultrasound can determine the potential cause of an immature AVF. It can also determine whether the AVF should be treated by the angiographer (angioplasty of a stenosis) or surgeon (AVF revision or accessory vein ligation).[6] Ultrasound is also useful in the evaluation of the patient with a hemodialysis graft, to assess for the presence of a stenosis and determine the etiology of perigraft pulsatile masses (hematoma versus pseudoaneurysm).

This chapter details hemodialysis access anatomy and the preferred order of access placement. It describes current protocols for the sonographic vascular evaluation of the end-stage renal patient, both before and after hemodialysis access placement.

BASIC CONCEPTS OF HEMODIALYSIS ACCESS

Hemodialysis is the lifeline by which the patient with end-stage renal disease eliminates excess fluid and decreases the level of various undesirable substances in the blood. The central circulation is accessed, and the blood is cleansed by diffusion across a semipermeable membrane, termed the *dialyzer*. Direct access to the circulation is accomplished by an AVF, a graft, or a central venous dialysis catheter. A native AVF is a surgically created, direct anastomosis between an artery and a vein, placed in either the forearm or upper arm. When AVF creation is not possible, an artificial graft consisting of polytetrafluoroethylene or other material may be tunneled in the superficial soft tissues of the forearm, upper arm, or upper thigh, with surgically created arterial and venous anastomoses.

During hemodialysis, two 15-gauge needles are placed into the mature AVF or graft, with the more distal needle (pointing toward the artery) carrying blood from the patient to the dialyzer. The second needle is placed more proximally (closer to the venous outflow) in the AVF or graft and returns the blood to the patient's circulation. Artery/vein configurations for the various types of AVFs and grafts are shown in Table 16-1. Figure 16-1 shows anatomic drawings of the three most common AVFs and four most common graft configurations.

Surgeons prefer to create a hemodialysis access in the nondominant arm, because the activities of daily living can be carried out with the dominant arm while the nondominant arm is healing after surgical access placement. However, most will put an AVF in the dominant arm before a graft is considered. An AVF is placed first in the

TABLE 16-1 AVF and Graft Artery/Vein Anastomoses

AVF Types	Artery	Vein
Forearm cephalic vein	Radial	Cephalic
Forearm vein transposition	Radial	Ulnar, dorsal, or volar vein
Upper arm cephalic vein	Brachial	Cephalic
Basilic vein transposition	Brachial	Basilic
Graft Types	**Artery**	**Vein**
Forearm loop	Brachial	Antecubital
Upper arm straight	Brachial	Basilic
Upper arm loop	Axillary	Axillary
Thigh graft	Common femoral/superficial femoral	Great saphenous/common femoral

AVF, arteriovenous fistula.

forearm, if the patient has suitable anatomy, and the upper arm is then "saved" for future potential dialysis access. Likewise, if an AVF cannot be placed, a forearm graft is preferred to placement of an upper arm graft. If no upper extremity graft options are available, a thigh graft is preferable to dialyzing with an indwelling venous catheter.[7] A list of the preferred order of access placement is given in Table 16-2. In general, an AVF or graft will provide higher dialysis flow rates than a tunneled catheter,[8] with a lower infection rate.[9]

DESCRIPTIVE TERMINOLOGY

The conventional way to describe vascular anatomy employs the terms *proximal* and *distal*, meaning closer and farther from the heart, respectively. We find that these terms can be confusing when used in describing dialysis access anatomy. In some circumstances, therefore, we prefer the terms *cranial* and *caudal*, meaning toward the head and toward the lower end of the body. We will use these terms in selected locations throughout this chapter, realizing that the more conventional terms are used elsewhere in this text.

VASCULAR MAPPING BEFORE HEMODIALYSIS ACCESS PLACEMENT

GENERAL PRINCIPLES

The protocol for vascular mapping before hemodialysis access placement has been previously described.[3,10] A high-resolution linear ultrasound transducer is used to evaluate the arm vessels (generally 9 MHz or higher). Gray-scale transverse plane imaging is used to identify vessels (artery and vein) and evaluate their diameter

and wall thickness. Sequential vein compression is used to assess for compressibility, indicating patency, or loss of compressibility due to acute or chronic thrombus. The depth from the skin surface of the anterior wall of the cephalic vein is measured. Color Doppler images and Doppler spectral waveforms are obtained in the longitudinal plane of vessels selected for potential vascular access.

The forearm veins and arteries are assessed to determine whether the patient is a candidate for a forearm AVF, the most desirable initial type of hemodialysis access. If vascular anatomy suitable for forearm fistula creation is not found, the upper arm vessels should be mapped. Arteries should be assessed for intimal thickening, calcification, and stenosis. The presence of significant concentric calcification should be noted, because the artery may be too calcified for successful surgical access creation. An important aspect of planning for AVF and graft creation is vessel size assessment. Minimum artery and vein diameters are shown in Table 16-3. It is important to note that upper extremity vessel mapping should be performed with the patient sitting upright, so the arm veins are dependent to the heart. This position will optimize vein diameter, along with tourniquet use. Ambient room temperature should not be cold, and warm blankets or warm compresses can be used as necessary.

FOREARM ASSESSMENT

The nondominant forearm is assessed first. The patient's arm is placed in a comfortable position on towels on top of a procedure stand (Figure 16-2) or phlebotomy chair. The internal diameter of the radial artery at the wrist should measure at least 2 mm (Figure 16-3). If the radial

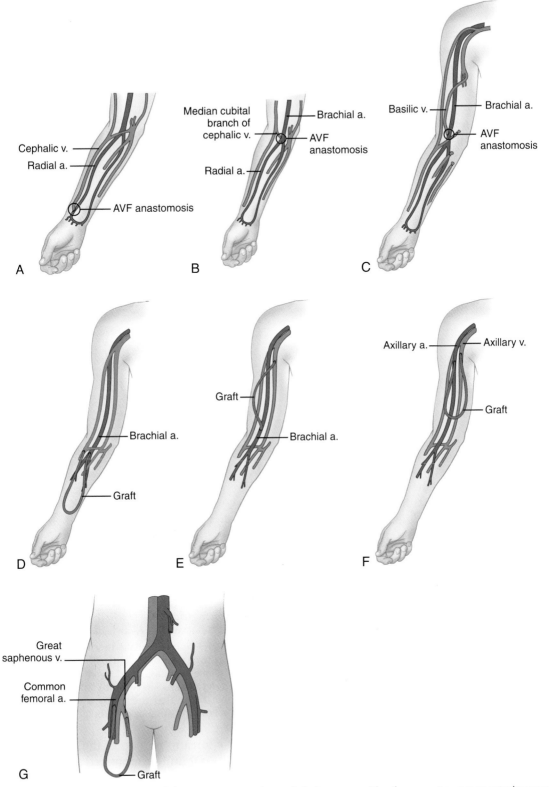

FIGURE 16-1 Anatomic drawings of the most common hemodialysis accesses. The three most common arteriovenous fistulas are radiocephalic fistula at the wrist **(A)**, brachiocephalic fistula at the antecubital fossa **(B)**, and brachiobasilic vein transposition **(C)**. The four most common grafts are forearm loop graft **(D)**, upper arm straight graft **(E)**, axillary loop graft **(F)**, and thigh graft **(G)**. AVF, arteriovenous fistula.

TABLE 16-2	Preferred Order of Access Placement

Order of Access Placement Type

1. Nondominant forearm cephalic vein fistula
2. Dominant forearm cephalic vein fistula
3. Nondominant or dominant upper arm cephalic vein fistula
4. Nondominant or dominant upper arm basilic vein transposition fistula
5. Forearm loop graft
6. Upper arm straight graft
7. Upper arm loop graft (axillary artery to axillary vein)

From Allon M, Robbin ML: Increasing arteriovenous fistulas in hemodialysis patients: problems and solutions, *Kidney Int* 62:1109–1124, 2002.

TABLE 16-3 Minimum Diameter Criteria for AVF and Graft Creation	
Vessel	**Minimum Diameter (cm)**
AVF vein	0.25
Graft vein	0.40
Artery (graft or AVF)	0.20

AVF, arteriovenous fistula.
From Silva MB, Hobson RW, Pappas PJ, et al: A strategy for increasing use of autogenous hemodialysis access procedures: impact of preoperative noninvasive evaluation, *J Vasc Surg* 27(2):307–308, 1998.

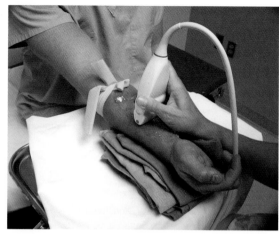

FIGURE 16-2 Proper position of arm on instrument stand for imaging of the vessels for hemodialysis planning.

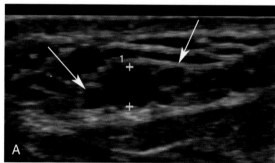

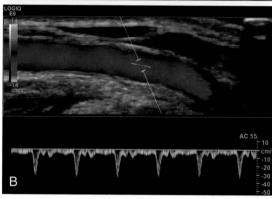

FIGURE 16-3 Normal radial artery at the wrist. **A,** Transverse gray-scale view of the radial artery shows adequate arterial diameter measuring 2.4 mm *(cursors)*. Note the small paired radial veins *(arrows)*. **B,** Color and spectral longitudinal views of the artery demonstrate normal pulsatile flow and absence of turbulent flow or aliasing.

artery internal diameter is not satisfactory within several centimeters of the wrist, the internal diameter of the ulnar artery at the wrist is measured. If the diameter of the ulnar or radial artery is not at least 2 mm in the lower third of the forearm, the forearm radial and ulnar arteries are assessed on the dominant side. If no forearm artery is satisfactory, the patient is not a candidate for a forearm AVF.

If the radial or ulnar artery at the wrist meets size criteria, the next vessel to evaluate is the cephalic vein. A tourniquet is placed moderately tightly at the midforearm. The entire distal forearm is percussed, similar to starting an intravenous line, for approximately 3 minutes. All wrist veins that measure greater than 2 mm after the 3-minute tapping are evaluated. Veins smaller than 2 mm will probably not dilate up to an adequate size. However, veins greater than 2 mm may dilate to greater than 2.5 mm with more focused tapping and/or a warm compress. Special attention is given to the cephalic vein, as this is the preferred venous outflow conduit. The cephalic vein area is assessed for the presence of a continuous vein up to the tourniquet with a diameter of at least 2.5 mm (Figure 16-4).

If the forearm portion of the cephalic vein is adequate, a tourniquet is placed at the elbow and the vein is followed in a cephalad direction to the elbow. If the vein is discontinuous or stenotic, it is not satisfactory for fistula creation. Then, a search for another adequate forearm vein should be performed. Branch points should be assessed

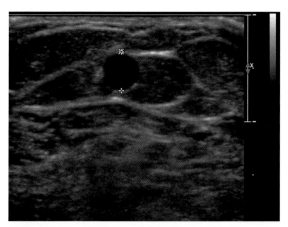

FIGURE 16-4 Normal cephalic vein at the wrist. The cephalic vein has a normal diameter measuring 3.6 mm *(cursors)* and normal depth of 3.4 mm (from skin to near wall).

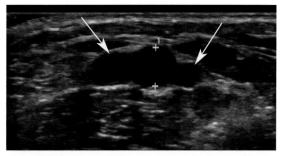

FIGURE 16-5 Normal brachial artery at the antecubital fossa. Transverse gray-scale image shows normal arterial diameter measuring 4.2 mm *(cursors)*. Note the paired brachial veins *(arrows)*.

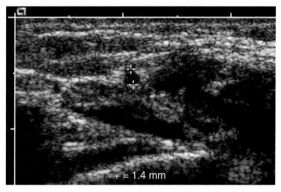

FIGURE 16-6 Small cephalic vein in the caudal upper arm. Transverse gray-scale image shows a small cephalic vein measuring 1.4 mm that does not meet 2-mm minimum diameter *(cursors)*.

carefully, because vein narrowing below 2.5 mm may occur at branch points. Following examination of the forearm, the tourniquet is moved to the axilla, and the vein of interest is followed centrally to ensure that it empties into the deep venous system. The tourniquet must be removed to evaluate the cephalic vein insertion into the subclavian vein. Occasionally, overlying muscle may give the appearance of a stenosis at the insertion of the cephalic vein into the subclavian vein. Placing the patient's arm by his/her side (rather than in an abducted position) may alleviate an apparent cephalic vein stenosis.

If the cephalic vein is not adequate, the basilic vein in the forearm is assessed. If the basilic vein is not adequate, the volar surface of the forearm, followed by the dorsal surface of the forearm is assessed for a suitable vein. If no vein is sufficient in the forearm, a frequent finding in the end-stage renal patient, the same protocol should be followed in the dominant forearm.

UPPER ARM ASSESSMENT

If a forearm fistula is not possible, the upper arm should be assessed for anatomy suitable for fistula placement. A tourniquet is placed at the axilla. The brachial artery is measured above its bifurcation into the radial and ulnar arteries. Satisfactory internal diameter should be 2 mm or greater (Figure 16-5).

The cephalic vein diameter is then measured at the antecubital fossa. For a brachiocephalic fistula, it should measure at least 2.5 mm and extend approximately 2 cm below the antecubital fossa. Several centimeters of vein are needed

to make the anastomosis with the brachial artery near the antecubital fossa. Alternatively, the surgeons may use a median cubital branch of the cephalic vein as it travels close to the brachial artery; therefore, this branch can also be evaluated, depending on the surgeon's preference.

If an adequate cephalic vein is not found (Figure 16-6), the basilic vein (Figure 16-7) is evaluated. A basilic vein suitable for a basilic vein transposition must extend at least 4 cm caudal to the antecubital fossa to provide a suitable length to loop around and connect with the brachial artery. If the basilic vein does not extend 4 cm into the forearm, it may still be of adequate diameter for a graft (4 mm).

If a suitable vein is found, its continuity with the deep venous system must be confirmed. To this end, the vein is followed cephalad to ensure that it is continuous and of adequate size along its entire course, until it empties into the deep venous system. The diameter of the deep vein is also evaluated to the point at which it empties

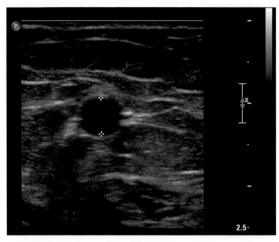

FIGURE 16-7 Normal basilic vein in upper arm. Transverse gray-scale image shows a normal basilic vein diameter measuring 4.4 mm *(cursors)*. The vein depth is not considered, since the vein will be surgically isolated and superficially tunneled within the upper arm to the brachial artery for anastomosis.

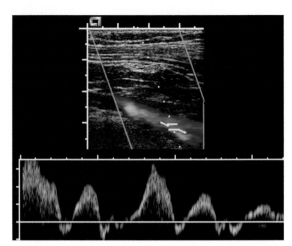

FIGURE 16-8 Normal subclavian vein. Longitudinal duplex Doppler image demonstrates color Doppler flow signals filling the vein and a normal spectral waveform with phasic temporary reversal of flow during atrial contraction.

into the subclavian vein. If no anatomy suitable for an AVF, forearm loop, or upper arm straight graft is found, the axillary vein and axillary artery diameters are measured for a possible upper arm loop graft.

SUBCLAVIAN, INTERNAL JUGULAR, AND CENTRAL VEIN ASSESSMENT

The subclavian and internal jugular (IJ) veins are then evaluated for the presence of stenotic lesions, occlusions, or thrombus. It is easiest to perform this portion of the study in the supine position, to increase venous filling. Spectral waveforms should be assessed in the medial portion of the subclavian vein and the caudal portion of the IJ for respiratory phasicity and transmitted cardiac pulsatility (Figure 16-8). If normal flow features are absent (monophasic flow is demonstrated), central venous stenosis or obstruction is inferred. The contralateral subclavian and IJ should then be examined. If the flow abnormality is unilateral, brachiocephalic vein stenosis or occlusion is likely. If bilateral, a superior vena cava (SVC) stenosis or occlusion is likely. Figure 16-9 shows abnormal unilateral respiratory phasicity and transmitted cardiac pulsatility in the left subclavian vein, consistent with a brachiocephalic vein stenosis or occlusion. Occasionally, the brachiocephalic veins and SVC can be directly visualized with ultrasound. In such cases, they are best seen with a small-footprint transducer placed above the medial clavicle or in the sternal notch, using

central angulation. Assessment of the brachiocephalic veins and SVC, if visible, should be performed both with gray scale and with color and spectral Doppler.

KEY ADDITIONAL POINTS REGARDING PREOPERATIVE MAPPING

1. It may be possible to create a forearm cephalic vein AVF, even if the cephalic vein in the upper arm is small or occluded by thrombus. The cephalic vein in the forearm should then drain into the brachial or basilic veins via an adequately sized median cubital or other branch vein.

2. It is important to carefully assess vein branch points, because areas of focal stenosis can occur at accessory vein takeoffs. These stenoses may significantly limit blood flow in a subsequently created access.

3. The cephalic vein may meet diameter criteria for AVF creation yet lie too deep to access easily. Therefore, the depth of the cephalic vein from the skin surface should be measured during the ultrasound mapping procedure. If the vein is greater than 0.5 cm in depth, it will likely be difficult to palpate the vein with sufficient confidence to permit the insertion of a 15-gauge needle into it for hemodialysis.[11] Detection of a vein that is too deep but otherwise suitable for an AVF allows the surgeon to inform the patient preoperatively about the potential need for a second procedure to

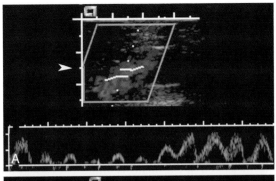

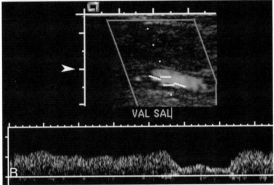

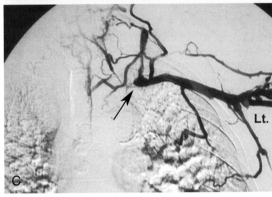

FIGURE 16-9 Abnormal subclavian vein waveform. **A,** Longitudinal duplex Doppler shows normal phasic flow within the right subclavian vein. **B,** Duplex Doppler of the left subclavian vein depicts abnormal monophasic venous waveforms. **C,** Subsequent venogram confirms occlusion of the left brachiocephalic vein *(arrow).*

"superficialize" the vein in the subcutaneous tissues. This discussion allows the patient to decide whether to accept the possibility of multiple surgical procedures needed to create a mature AVF.

4. Normally, the radial artery originates from the brachial artery near the elbow. A high radial artery takeoff from the brachial or even axillary artery is a common anatomic variant. This variant is likely when two arteries with accompanying paired veins are seen in the upper arm. Both arteries should be followed into the forearm, as they become respectively the radial and ulnar arteries. Hemodialysis access surgeons are reluctant to place a forearm graft or upper arm straight graft in a patient with a high radial artery takeoff because the chance for arterial steal is increased. Infrequently, a prominent arterial branch that courses posteriorly toward the elbow can mimic a high radial artery takeoff. Following the course of the artery more distally allows differentiation between the two possibilities.

5. It is important to analyze the Doppler spectral waveform of the brachial and radial arteries to detect either proximal or distal arterial obstruction. With proximal obstruction, the waveforms are monophasic and dampened, with a tardus-parvus pattern (low resistance flow). With distal obstruction, the waveforms have a normal triphasic pattern, but the velocity may be reduced because of diminished outflow (high resistance flow). Malovrh[12] noted a higher success rate in forearm fistulas in patients who converted from triphasic to monophasic flow after release of a clenched fist. In his series, no radial artery diameter threshold was applied. In our experience, neither arterial peak systolic velocity (PSV) or change in resistive index following a clenched-fist maneuver are predictive of subsequent AVF maturation.[13] We do not recommend the use of arterial PSV or resistive index criteria if the artery has a diameter of 2 mm or more.[13]

AVF MATURITY ASSESSMENT

GENERAL PRINCIPLES

Definitions of a mature AVF in the United States include a fistula that is usable for hemodialysis at a flow of 300 to 350 mL/min at six to eight dialysis sessions in 1 month.[5,14] Practitioners in other countries, particularly in Europe, accept lower AVF flows with subsequently longer dialysis times.[1,2] A mature AVF can be identified clinically as one that has a large, easily palpable vein that can provide access for two 15-gauge needles.[15] Experienced dialysis nurses were found to have an 80% accuracy rate in determining whether an AVF was mature enough to successfully undergo hemodialysis.[11] For the obviously mature AVF, clinical examination by an experienced nephrologist or dialysis nurse is sufficient. If there is doubt, an ultrasound examination is useful for assessing adequacy of the AVF. Ultrasound findings can also serve a triage function, directing the patient to either the interventional radiologist or surgeon.[6] Sonographic evaluation can address multiple anatomic features of the AVF, including the presence of stenosis, minimum vein diameter, and the maximum vein depth from the skin surface.

SONOGRAPHIC EVALUATION OF AVF MATURITY

The ultrasound protocol for assessing AVF for maturity has been previously described,[11] as well as associated diagnostic pitfalls.[16] The evaluation of the AVF is a more focused sonographic examination than vascular mapping before hemodialysis access placement. A tourniquet is not used during the routine AVF examination. A high-resolution (9 MHz or higher) linear ultrasound probe is used to evaluate the AVF feeding artery and draining vein or veins. Gray-scale imaging in the transverse plane is used to identify and evaluate vessel diameter, wall thickness, and compressibility. Color Doppler images and Doppler spectral waveforms are acquired in the longitudinal plane, at the feeding artery, the draining vein, and any visualized stenosis.

The arm is placed in a comfortable position on towels on a procedure stand or phlebotomy chair. Minimal pressure and abundant ultrasound gel are used while evaluating the feeding artery, arteriovenous anastomosis, and draining vein. The diameter of the draining vein is measured routinely in the caudal, mid, and cranial portions of the forearm, and similarly in the upper arm when an upper arm AVF is evaluated. The entire draining vein should be scanned, and the minimum diameter should be measured, even if it occurs at a location not routinely measured. The distance from the anterior wall of the efferent vein of the AVF to the skin surface is measured in the forearm or upper arm depending on the type of AVF. If the depth of the vein is greater than 0.5 cm, it will likely be too deep for easy access with a 15-gauge needle[11] (Figure 16-10).

The AVF feeding artery, anastomosis, and draining vein are evaluated. Peak systolic velocities are measured at the anastomosis and 2 cm cephalad to the anastomosis in the feeding artery. A PSV ratio is then calculated by dividing the PSV at the anastomosis by the PSV obtained 2 cm cranial to the anastomosis (Figure 16-11). We generally begin to be concerned about stenosis at the arteriovenous anastomosis when the PSV ratio is 3.0 or greater.[16] Visual confirmation of a stenosis at the arteriovenous anastomosis is useful, because the PSV in the draining vein may be significantly elevated merely because of the acute angulation of the draining vein at the anastomosis.

If the draining vein is visibly narrowed, PSVs are measured at the stenosis and 2 cm caudal to the stenosis. A PSV ratio is calculated by dividing the PSV at the stenosis by the PSV obtained 2 cm caudal to the stenosis. If the PSV ratio is 2 or more, it is classified as a stenosis of greater than or equal to 50% diameter reduction. Both arteriovenous and draining vein stenoses may be treated with angioplasty or surgical revision. The most frequent location of AVF stenosis is juxtaanastomotic.[17]

Blood flow is measured in the midportion of the AVF in milliliters per minute, using the volume flow measurement function on the ultrasound scanner. It is important to use careful technique while measuring blood flow in the fistula, as there are many potential pitfalls in volume flow measurement. The blood flow should be measured approximately 10 cm from the anastomosis, in a straight nontapering segment of the draining vein. The highest-frequency transducer available

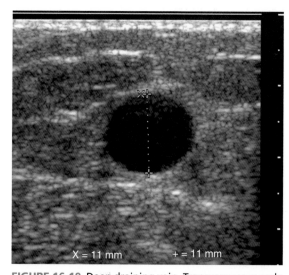

FIGURE 16-10 Deep draining vein. Transverse gray-scale image of draining cephalic vein *(cursors)* of an upper arm brachiocephalic fistula shows normal diameter of a mature fistula measuring 11 mm. However, the depth of the vein, 11 mm, may limit palpation and cannulation with dialysis needles.

that gives optimal lumen definition should be used, with the focal zone centered at the vessel. Abundant gel, beam steering, and potential heel-toe angulation of the transducer should be used to achieve an angle of 60 degrees or less between the Doppler signal and the back wall of the AVF. The Doppler sample volume (gate) is adjusted to encompass the entire vessel width, not extending significantly past the wall. The velocity scale should be adjusted so that the spectral waveform occupies approximately 75% of the spectral window with the baseline adjusted to avoid aliasing. At least three cardiac cycles should be used to estimate the time-averaged mean velocity. The internal diameter measurement should be placed perpendicular to the back wall of the vessel. The scanner then calculates the volume blood flow as the time-averaged velocity multiplied by the vessel cross-sectional area.[18]

If the blood flow equals or exceeds 500 mL/min, the likelihood of fistula adequacy is nearly twice as great as with lower flow rates. We find that combining venous diameter and volume flow measurement increases our ability to predict fistula adequacy. A venous diameter of 4 mm or greater and flow volume equaling or exceeding 500 mL/min confirms AVF maturity in 95% of cases, versus a maturity rate of only 33% when neither criterion is met.[11]

KEY ADDITIONAL POINTS REGARDING AVF EVALUATION

1. Look for the presence of large vein branches involving the first 10 cm of the draining vein (Figure 16-12). These accessory branches can divert a significant amount of flow from the primary draining vein with resultant decrease in AVF blood flow to below functional levels. Such diversion of blood flow is a frequent reason for AVF immaturity.[17] These branches can be surgically ligated, thereby increasing the likelihood that the AVF will mature.[6]

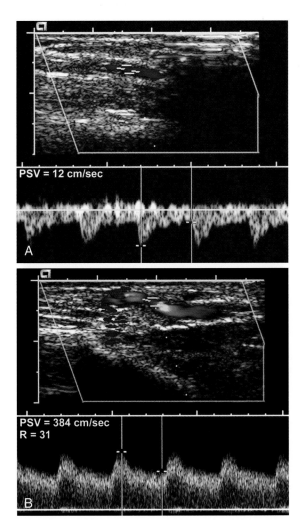

FIGURE 16-11 Anastomotic stenosis of arteriovenous fistula. **A,** Longitudinal color and spectral Doppler of the feeding artery 2 cm upstream from the arteriovenous anastomosis shows normal arterial waveform with peak systolic velocity (PSV) of 12 cm/sec. **B,** Color and spectral Doppler at the anastomosis shows elevated PSV of 384 cm/sec yielding a ratio much greater than 3.1, consistent with arteriovenous fistula (AVF) stenosis.

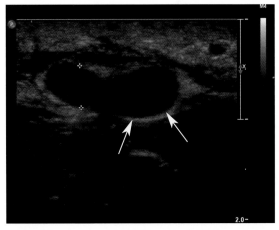

FIGURE 16-12 Large draining vein branch at 10 cm from the anastomotic region. Transverse gray-scale image shows a large venous branch *(cursors)* measuring 4.2 mm, which is similar in size to the draining cephalic vein *(arrows)*. A large draining vein branch may divert blood flow away from the draining vein and hinder fistula maturation.

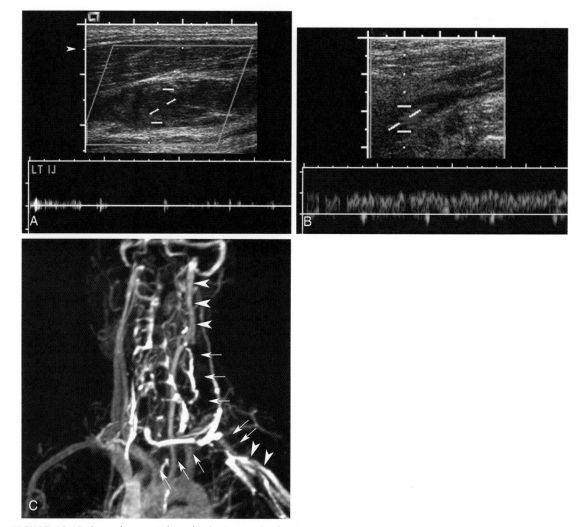

FIGURE 16-13 Central venous thrombosis. **A,** Longitudinal color Doppler of left internal jugular vein demonstrates heterogeneous clot within the vessel, which has no visible flow. **B,** Monophasic flow in the left lateral aspect of the sub-clavian vein on spectral Doppler suggests thrombosis or stenosis of the brachiocephalic vein. Note that normal venous waveforms in the right internal jugular and subclavian veins (not shown) excluded superior vena cava location of the obstruction. **C,** Magnetic resonance venography of the chest and neck shows flow within the cranial left internal jugu-lar vein and lateral subclavian vein *(arrowheads)*. There is no flow in the expected course of the left brachiocephalic vein, caudal internal jugular vein, and medial subclavian vein *(arrows)*.

2. Occasionally a patient with an AVF may pres-ent for evaluation of arm swelling. Respi-ratory phasicity and transmitted cardiac pulsatility should be evaluated in the subcla-vian and IJ veins to assess for the possibil-ity of a central venous obstruction (Figure 16-13). There may be high blood flow rates in an AVF despite central stenosis or occlu-sion severe enough to cause arm swelling. If no etiology for significant arm swelling is found, magnetic resonance imaging (MRI) may be useful to evaluate the central veins. The brachial veins should also be evaluated with ultrasound for the presence of deep venous thrombosis.

3. Infrequently a patient will have symptoms of arterial steal with an AVF, such as hand pain and numbness, particularly during dialysis. Direction of blood flow in the distal radial artery is then evaluated with color Doppler imaging and Doppler spectral waveforms. Arterial steal is diagnosed when the direction of blood flow in the radial artery is reversed.[16] It is important to recognize that an asymp-tomatic arterial steal can be present in AVFs and not be clinically significant.

GRAFT EVALUATION

GENERAL PRINCIPLES

Compared with AVFs, grafts are generally considered a less-desirable method for permanent hemodialysis access because of their higher rates of stenosis, infection, and pseudoaneurysm formation.[1,2] Graft stenosis occurs because of intimal hyperplasia, most commonly located at the venous anastomosis.[19] Many surveillance methods for the detection of graft stenosis have been proposed, including physical examination, various laboratory measurements, static and dynamic pressure measurements performed during hemodialysis, duplex ultrasound, and ultrasound dye dilution.[1,2] Although it is widely agreed that surveillance may increase secondary graft patency rates, no definite consensus has been established regarding the best surveillance method at the time of this writing.

The clinically symptomatic graft should be referred to angiography for diagnosis, and should be treated with angioplasty with possible stent placement if any stenosis is found. Ultrasound graft assessment is reserved for patients with a palpable focal mass in the vicinity of the graft and those in whom there is an intermediate likelihood of graft stenosis. Color Doppler imaging is useful for the evaluation of a focal mass, differentiating a hematoma from a pseudoaneurysm. An area of graft with a relatively larger diameter because of graft degeneration is another potential cause of a palpable mass. Additional indications for graft ultrasound include the evaluation of clinically significant arterial steal,[16] resulting in arterial insufficiency to the hand.

SONOGRAPHIC EVALUATION OF GRAFTS

The protocol for evaluation of dialysis access grafts for stenosis and perigraft findings has been previously described,[20] as well as a discussion of diagnostic pitfalls.[16] A tourniquet is not used during a graft examination. A high-resolution linear ultrasound probe, generally 9 MHz or greater, is used to evaluate the artery feeding the graft, the arterial anastomosis, the graft body, the venous anastomosis, and the draining vein or veins. Gray-scale evaluation in the transverse plane is used to identify graft anatomy and to evaluate graft and vessel diameters. Color Doppler imaging and Doppler spectral waveforms are performed in the longitudinal plane of the anastomoses, within the graft, and at any visualized stenosis.

The arm is placed in a comfortable position on towels on a procedure stand. The feeding artery, graft, arterial and venous graft anastomoses, and draining vein are evaluated in both the transverse and longitudinal planes, using gentle pressure with the transducer. Most current graft material is readily identified sonographically by the presence of two echogenic parallel lines representing the polytetrafluoroethylene (PTFE) graft wall. An initial sonographic survey is used to familiarize oneself with the patient's particular graft anatomy before attempting analysis for the presence or absence of stenosis. For example, identification of the direction of blood flow in a loop graft is useful, allowing identification and labeling of the arterial limb (the side of the loop graft closest to the arterial anastomosis) and the venous limb (the side of the loop graft closest to the venous anastomosis).

PSVs are assessed 2 cm cranial to the arterial anastomosis (within the feeding artery), 2 cm caudal to the venous anastomosis (within the graft), at the arterial and venous anastomoses, and midgraft. A PSV ratio is calculated at the anastomoses (as described previously for AVFs) and at any visible stenosis. A venous anastomotic or draining vein stenosis with a PSV ratio of 2.0 or greater is classified as equaling or exceeding 50% diameter reduction. A stenosis with a PSV ratio of 3.0 or greater indicates a stenosis of 75% or greater.[20] We use a PSV equaling or exceeding 3.0 and visual confirmation of a stenosis on direct imaging for the arterial anastomosis since the abrupt angulation typically seen there causes an increase in PSV. Figure 16-14 shows a significant stenosis at the graft venous anastomosis, with angiographic confirmation and treatment. When the PSV is close to 2.0, a significant stenosis is likely.

KEY ADDITIONAL POINTS REGARDING GRAFT EVALUATION

1. The IJ and subclavian veins should be evaluated routinely for respiratory phasicity and transmitted cardiac pulsatility. However, particularly in the presence of an upper arm graft, monophasic blood flow may be seen in the subclavian vein in the absence of a central stenosis. This is related to the high-volume of blood flow and low-resistance pattern of flow in the graft.

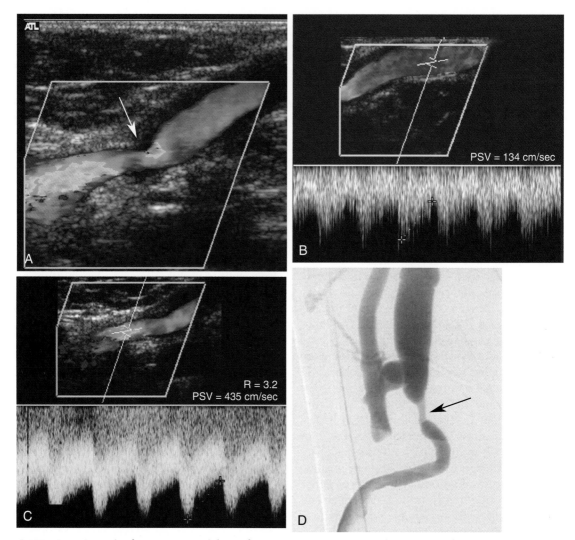

FIGURE 16-14 Stenosis of upper arm straight graft venous anastomosis. **A,** Color Doppler of the venous anastomosis *(arrow)* shows color aliasing at the stenosis. **B,** Duplex Doppler within the graft 2 cm upstream from the venous anastomosis has normal flow, with peak systolic velocity (PSV) of 134 cm/sec. **C,** Spectral Doppler at the venous anastomosis shows turbulent flow with PSV of 435 cm/sec, which yields a PSV ratio of 3.2, consistent with stenosis. **D,** Angiography of the graft demonstrates a focal venous anastomotic stenosis with greater than 50% narrowing *(arrow)*. The stenosis was successfully treated with balloon angioplasty (not shown).

2. An arterial steal distal to the arterial anastomosis occurs when the venous outflow from the graft exceeds the capacity of the inflow artery. This causes the graft to "steal" blood from more caudal portions of the extremity, which can cause symptoms of arterial insufficiency, particularly during dialysis. To assess for arterial steal, a Doppler spectral waveform is obtained in the radial artery distal (caudal) to the graft insertion, usually at the wrist. If the direction of flow is reversed caudal to the graft, the diagnosis of a complete arterial steal can be made. If the spectral waveform is biphasic, a partial steal is present. Gentle, brief compression of the graft returns the abnormally reversed arterial flow direction to normal, confirming the existence of the steal phenomenon. Asymptomatic steal is relatively common and of no clinical significance. However, severely symptomatic patients may require graft ligation to correct the steal.

Acknowledgments. We acknowledge the invaluable time and dedication of the sonographers at the University of Alabama at Birmingham (UAB) hospital and The Kirklin Clinic (particularly Michael Clements, BS, RDMS, RVT) and the UAB hemodialysis access program physicians and personnel. We also thank Trish Thurman and Tonya Braddy for their assistance with manuscript preparation.

REFERENCES

1. Allon M, Robbin ML: Increasing arteriovenous fistulas in hemodialysis patients: Problems and solutions, *Kidney Int* 62:1109–1124, 2002.
2. National Kidney Foundation: K/DOQI clinical practice guidelines for vascular access, 2006, *Am J Kid Dis* 48(Suppl 1):S176–S247, 2006.
3. Robbin ML, et al: US vascular mapping before hemodialysis access placement, *Radiology* 217:83–88, 2000.
4. Allon M, et al: Effect of preoperative sonographic mapping on vascular access outcomes in hemodialysis patients, *Kidney Int* 60:2013–2020, 2001.
5. Dember LM, et al: Effect of clopidogrel on early failure of arteriovenous fistulas for hemodialysis: A randomized controlled trial, *JAMA* 299:2164–2171, 2008.
6. Singh P, et al: Clinically immature arteriovenous hemodialysis fistulas: Effect of US on salvage, *Radiology* 246:299–305, 2008.
7. Miller CD, et al: Comparison of arteriovenous grafts in the thigh and upper extremities in hemodialysis patients, *J Am Soc Nephrol* 14:2942–2947, 2003.
8. Moss AH, et al: Use of a silicone dual-lumen catheter with a Dacron cuff as a long-term vascular access for hemodialysis patients, *Am J Kidney Dis* 16:211–215, 1990.
9. Fan PY, Schwab SJ: Vascular access: concepts for the 1990s, *J Am Soc Nephrol* 3:1–11, 1992.
10. Silva MB Jr, et al: A strategy for increasing use of autogenous hemodialysis access procedures: impact of preoperative noninvasive evaluation, *J Vasc Surg* 27:302–308, 1998.
11. Robbin ML, et al: Hemodialysis arteriovenous fistula maturity: US evaluation, *Radiology* 225:59–64, 2002.
12. Malovrh M: Non-invasive evaluation of vessels by duplex sonography prior to construction of arteriovenous fistulas for haemodialysis, *Nephrol Dial Transplant* 13(1):125–129, 1998.
13. Lockhart ME, et al: Preoperative sonographic radial artery evaluation and correlation with subsequent radiocephalic fistula outcome, *J Ultrasound Med* 23:161–168, 2004. quiz 169–171.
14. Miller PE, et al: Predictors of adequacy of arteriovenous fistulas in hemodialysis patients, *Kidney Int* 56:275–280, 1999.
15. Beathard GA: Physical examination of the dialysis vascular access, *Semin Dial* 11:231–236, 1998.
16. Lockhart ME, Robbin ML: Hemodialysis access ultrasound, *Ultrasound Q* 17:157–167, 2001.
17. Beathard GA, et al: Aggressive treatment of early fistula failure, *Kidney Int* 64:1487–1494, 2003.
18. Hoyt K, et al: Accuracy of volumetric flow rate measurements: an in vitro study using modern ultrasound scanners, *J Ultrasound Med* 28:1511–1518, 2009.
19. Swedberg SH, et al: Intimal fibromuscular hyperplasia at the venous anastomosis of PTFE grafts in hemodialysis patients. Clinical, immunocytochemical, light and electron microscopic assessment, *Circulation* 80:1726–1736, 1989.
20. Robbin ML, et al: Hemodialysis access graft stenosis: US detection, *Radiology* 208:655–661, 1998.

ULTRASOUND ASSESSMENT OF LOWER EXTREMITY ARTERIES

17

R. EUGENE ZIERLER, MD

The purpose of noninvasive testing for lower extremity arterial disease is to provide objective information that can be combined with the clinical history and physical examination to serve as the basis for decisions regarding further evaluation and treatment. One of the most critical decisions relates to whether a patient requires therapeutic intervention and should undergo additional imaging studies. Catheter contrast arteriography has generally been regarded as the definitive examination for lower extremity arterial disease, but this approach is invasive, expensive, and poorly suited for screening or long-term follow-up testing. In addition, arteriography provides anatomic rather than physiologic information, and it is subject to significant variability at the time of interpretation.[1,2] Magnetic resonance angiography (MRA) and computed tomographic angiography (CTA) can also provide an accurate anatomic assessment of lower extremity arterial disease without some of the risks associated with catheter arteriography.[3-5] There is evidence that the application of these less-invasive approaches to arterial imaging has decreased the utilization of diagnostic catheter arteriography.[6] The most valid physiologic method for detecting hemodynamically significant lesions is direct, intra-arterial pressure measurement, but this method is impractical in many clinical situations.

As discussed in Chapter 14, the nonimaging or indirect physiologic tests for lower extremity arterial disease, such as measurement of ankle systolic blood pressure and segmental limb pressures, provide valuable physiologic information, but they give relatively little anatomic detail.[7] Duplex scanning extends the capabilities of indirect testing by obtaining anatomic and physiologic information directly from sites of arterial disease. The initial application of duplex scanning concentrated on the clinically important problem of extracranial carotid artery disease.

The focal nature of carotid atherosclerosis and the relatively superficial location of the carotid bifurcation contributed to the success of these early studies.[8] Ongoing clinical experience and advances in technology, particularly the availability of lower-frequency duplex transducers, have made it possible to obtain image and flow information from the deeply located vessels in the abdomen and lower extremities. This chapter reviews the current status of duplex scanning for the initial evaluation of lower extremity arterial disease. The more specialized applications of intraoperative assessment and follow-up after arterial interventions are covered in Chapter 18.

INSTRUMENTATION

A standard duplex ultrasound system with high-resolution B-mode imaging, pulsed Doppler spectral waveform analysis, and color flow Doppler imaging is adequate for scanning of the lower extremity arteries. A variety of transducers is often needed for a complete lower extremity arterial duplex examination. Low-frequency (2 MHz or 3 MHz) transducers are best for evaluating the aorta and iliac arteries, whereas a higher-frequency (5 MHz or 7.5 MHz) transducer is adequate in most patients for the infrainguinal vessels. In general, the highest-frequency transducer that provides adequate depth penetration should be used. The color flow image helps to identify vessels and the flow abnormalities caused by arterial lesions (Figures 17-1 and 17-2). The ability to visualize flow throughout a vessel improves the precision of pulsed Doppler sample volume placement for obtaining spectral waveforms. Thus, color flow imaging reduces examination time and improves overall accuracy. Power Doppler is an alternative method for displaying flow information that is particularly sensitive to low flow rates. The power Doppler display is also less dependent on the direction of flow and the

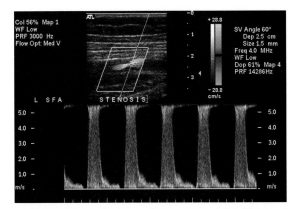

FIGURE 17-1 Duplex scan of a severe superficial femoral artery stenosis. Color flow image shows a localized, high-velocity jet. Spectral waveforms obtained from the site of stenosis indicate peak velocities over 500 cm/sec.

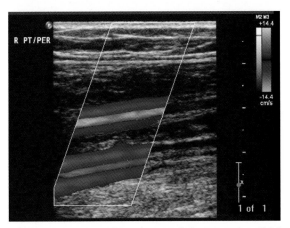

FIGURE 17-2 Color flow image of the posterior tibial and peroneal arteries and veins. The posterior tibial vessels are located more superficially (toward the top of the image). The single arteries and paired veins are identified by their flow direction (color).

angle of the ultrasound beam than color Doppler, and it tends to produce a more "arteriogram-like" vessel image.

Duplex instruments are equipped with presets or combinations of ultrasound parameters for gray-scale and Doppler imaging that can be selected by the examiner for a particular application. These presets can be helpful, especially during the learning process, but these parameters may not be adequate for all patient examinations. A complete understanding of the ultrasound parameters that are under the examiner's control (i.e., color gain, color velocity scale, wall filter) is essential for optimizing arterial duplex scans.

DUPLEX ULTRASOUND TECHNIQUE

Similar to other arterial applications of duplex scanning, the lower extremity assessment relies on high quality B-mode imaging to identify the artery of interest and facilitate precise placement of the pulsed Doppler sample volume for spectral waveform analysis.[9] Both color flow and power Doppler imaging provide important flow information to guide spectral Doppler interrogation. These imaging modalities are also valuable for recognizing anatomic variations and for identifying arterial disease by showing plaque or calcification. However, it should be emphasized that color flow Doppler and power Doppler imaging are not replacements for spectral waveform analysis, the primary method for classifying the severity of arterial disease.[10]

When examining an arterial segment, it is essential that the ultrasound probe be sequentially displaced in small intervals along the artery in order to evaluate blood flow patterns in an overlapping pattern. This is necessary because the flow disturbances produced by arterial lesions are propagated along the vessel for a relatively short distance. Experimental work has shown that the high-velocity jets and turbulence associated with arterial stenoses are damped out over a distance of only a few vessel diameters.[11] Consequently, failure to identify localized flow abnormalities could lead to underestimation of disease severity. Because local flow disturbances are usually apparent with color flow imaging (see Figure 17-1), pulsed Doppler flow samples may be obtained at more widely spaced intervals when color flow Doppler is used. Nonetheless, it is advisable to assess the flow characteristics with spectral waveform analysis at frequent intervals, especially in patients with diffuse arterial disease. Lengths of occluded arterial segments can be measured with a combination of B-mode, color flow, and power Doppler imaging by visualizing the point of occlusion proximally and the distal site where flow reconstitutes through collateral vessels. Because flow velocities distal to an occluded segment may be low, it is important to adjust the Doppler imaging parameters of the instrument to detect low flow rates.

For ultrasound examination of the aorta and iliac arteries, patients should be fasting for about 12 hours to reduce interference by bowel gas. Satisfactory aortoiliac Doppler signals can be obtained from approximately 90% of individuals that are prepared in this way. It is usually convenient to examine patients early in the morning

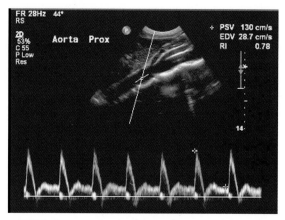

FIGURE 17-3 Longitudinal B-mode image of the proximal abdominal aorta. The origins of the celiac and superior mesenteric arteries are well visualized. Spectral waveforms obtained just proximal to the origin of the celiac artery show a normal aortic flow pattern.

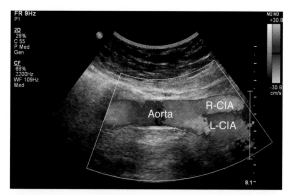

FIGURE 17-4 Color flow image of a normal aortic bifurcation obtained from an oblique approach at the level of the umbilicus. The changes in color are the result of different flow directions with respect to the transducer. R-CIA, right common iliac artery; L-CIA, left common iliac artery.

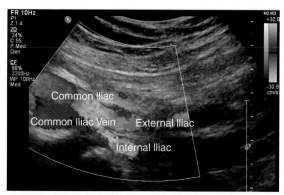

FIGURE 17-5 Color flow image of a normal right common iliac artery bifurcation obtained at the level of the iliac crest. The color change in the common iliac segment is related to different flow directions with respect to the transducer. A portion of the common iliac vein is visualized deep to the common iliac artery.

after an overnight fast. The patient is initially positioned supine with the hips rotated externally. A left lateral decubitus position may also be advantageous for the abdominal portion of the examination. An electric blanket placed over the patient prevents vasoconstriction caused by low room temperatures.

For a complete lower extremity arterial evaluation, scanning begins with the upper portion of the abdominal aorta. An anterior midline approach to the aorta is used, with the transducer placed just below the xyphoid process. Both ultrasound images and Doppler signals are best obtained in the longitudinal plane of the aorta, but transverse views are useful to define anatomic relationships, assess branch vessels, and determine the cross-sectional lumen (Figure 17-3). If specifically indicated, the mesenteric and renal vessels can be examined at this time, although these do not need to be examined routinely when evaluating the lower extremity arteries. The aorta is followed distally to its bifurcation, which is visualized by placing the transducer at the level of the umbilicus and using an oblique approach (Figure 17-4). The iliac arteries are then examined separately to the level of the groin with the transducer placed at the level of the iliac crest to evaluate the middle to distal common iliac and proximal external iliac arteries (Figure 17-5). This may require applying considerable pressure with the transducer to displace overlying bowel loops. The origin of the internal iliac artery is used as a landmark to separate the common iliac from the external iliac artery.

Each lower extremity is examined in turn, beginning with the common femoral artery and working distally. After the common femoral and the proximal deep femoral arteries are studied, the superficial femoral artery is followed as it courses down the thigh. At the distal thigh, it is often helpful to turn the patient into the prone position to examine the popliteal artery. However, some examiners prefer to image the popliteal segment with the patient supine and the leg externally rotated and flexed at the knee. As the popliteal artery is scanned in a longitudinal view, the first branch encountered below the knee joint is usually the anterior tibial artery. The tibial and peroneal arteries distal to the tibioperoneal trunk can be difficult to examine completely, but they can usually be imaged with color flow or power Doppler. Identification of these vessels

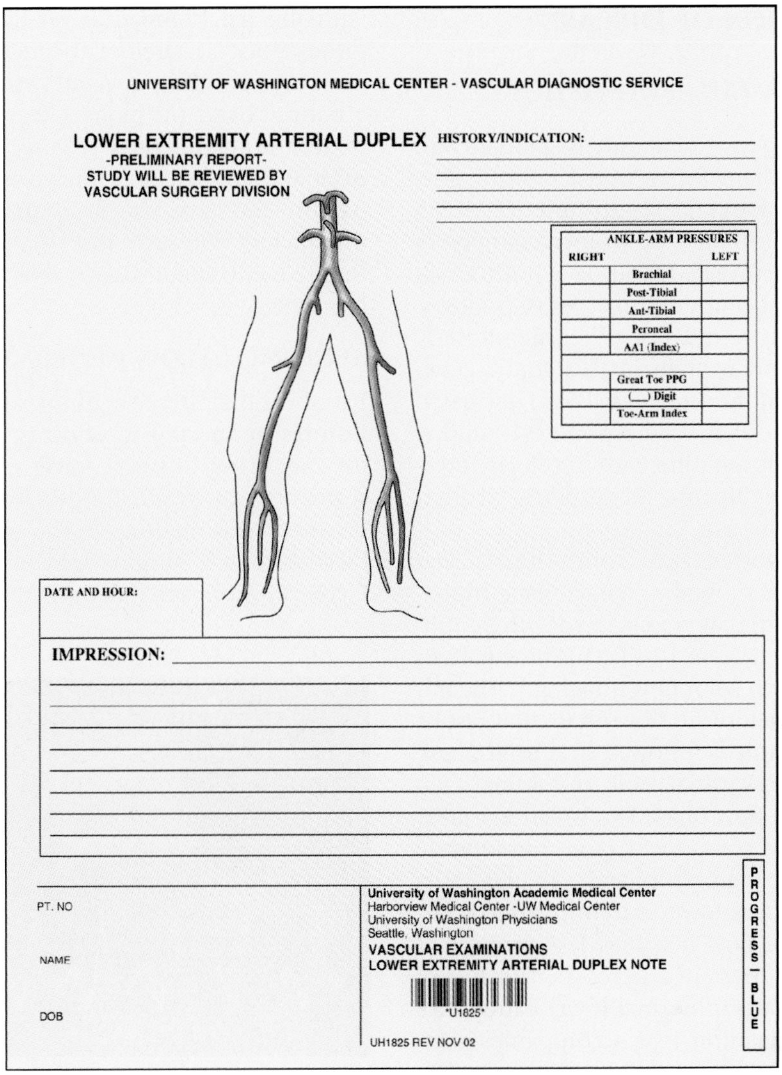

UNIVERSITY OF WASHINGTON MEDICAL CENTER - VASCULAR DIAGNOSTIC SERVICE

LOWER EXTREMITY ARTERIAL DUPLEX
-PRELIMINARY REPORT-
STUDY WILL BE REVIEWED BY
VASCULAR SURGERY DIVISION

HISTORY/INDICATION: _____

ANKLE-ARM PRESSURES		
RIGHT		LEFT
	Brachial	
	Post-Tibial	
	Ant-Tibial	
	Peroneal	
	AA1 (Index)	
	Great Toe PPG	
	(__) Digit	
	Toe-Arm Index	

DATE AND HOUR:

IMPRESSION: _____

PT. NO

NAME

DOB

University of Washington Academic Medical Center
Harborview Medical Center -UW Medical Center
University of Washington Physicians
Seattle. Washington
VASCULAR EXAMINATIONS
LOWER EXTREMITY ARTERIAL DUPLEX NOTE

U1825

PROGRESS - BLUE

UH1825 REV NOV 02

FIGURE 17-6 Example of a vascular laboratory worksheet used for lower extremity arterial assessment.

is facilitated by visualization of the adjacent paired veins (see Figure 17-2). These vessels are best evaluated by identifying their origins from the distal popliteal artery and scanning distally or by finding the arteries at the ankle and working proximally. Several large branches can often be seen originating from the distal superficial femoral and popliteal segments. These are readily visualized with color flow or power Doppler imaging and represent the geniculate and sural arteries.

Pulsed Doppler spectral waveforms are recorded from any areas in which increased velocities or other flow disturbances are noted. Recordings should also be made at the following standard locations: (1) the proximal and distal abdominal aorta; (2) the common, internal, and external iliac arteries; (3) the common femoral and proximal deep femoral arteries; (4) the proximal, middle, and distal superficial femoral artery; (5) the popliteal artery; and (6) the tibial/peroneal arteries at their origins and at the level of the ankle. As with other applications of arterial duplex scanning, Doppler angle correction is required for accurate velocity measurements. Although an angle of 60 degrees is usually obtainable, angles below 60 degrees can be utilized to provide clinically useful information.

A complete examination of the aortoiliac system and the arteries in both lower extremities may require 1 to 2 hours, but a single leg can usually be evaluated in less than 1 hour. An example of a vascular laboratory worksheet for lower extremity arterial duplex scanning is shown in Figure 17-6.

CLASSIFICATION OF DISEASE

NORMAL FLOW CHARACTERISTICS

Jager and colleagues[12] determined standard values for arterial diameter and peak systolic flow velocity in the lower extremity arteries of 55 healthy subjects (30 men, 25 women) ranging in age from 20 to 80 years (Table 17-1). Although women had smaller arteries than men, peak systolic flow velocities did not differ significantly between men and women in this study. However, the peak systolic velocities (PSVs) decreased steadily from the iliac to the popliteal arteries. There is no significant difference in velocity measurements among the three tibial/peroneal arteries in normal subjects.

Spectral waveforms taken from normal lower extremity arteries show the characteristic triphasic velocity pattern that is associated with peripheral arterial flow (Figure 17-7). This flow pattern is also apparent on color flow imaging.[13] The initial high-velocity, forward flow phase that results from cardiac systole is followed by a brief phase of reverse flow in early diastole and a final low-velocity, forward flow phase late in late diastole. The reverse flow component is a consequence of the relatively high peripheral vascular resistance in the normal lower extremity arterial circulation. Reverse flow becomes less prominent when peripheral resistance decreases. This loss of flow reversal occurs in normal lower extremities with the vasodilatation that accompanies exercise, reactive hyperemia, or limb warming. The reverse flow component is also absent distal to severe occlusive lesions. A similar triphasic flow pattern is seen in the peripheral arteries of the upper extremities (see Chapter 15).

The flow pattern in the center stream of normal lower extremity arteries is relatively uniform, with the red blood cells all having nearly the same velocity. Therefore, the flow is laminar, and the corresponding spectral waveform contains a narrow band of frequencies with a clear area under the systolic peak (Figures 17-7 and 17-8). Arterial lesions disrupt this normal laminar flow pattern and give rise to characteristic changes that include increases in PSV and a widening of the frequency band that is referred to as *spectral broadening*.

ABNORMAL FLOW PATTERNS

Based on the established normal and abnormal features of spectral waveforms, a set of criteria for classifying diseased lower extremity arterial segments was originally developed at the University of Washington.[9,12] The current version of these criteria is summarized in Table 17-2 and Figure 17-8. Minimal disease (1%-19% diameter

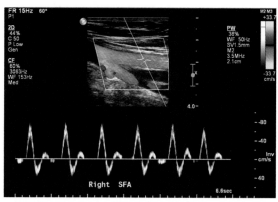

FIGURE 17-7 Spectral waveforms obtained from a normal proximal superficial femoral artery. The waveforms show a triphasic velocity pattern and contain a narrow band of frequencies with a clear area under the systolic peak. Peak systolic velocities are approximately 80 cm/sec. The color flow image shows the common femoral artery bifurcation and the location of the pulsed Doppler sample volume.

TABLE 17-1 Mean Arterial Diameters and Peak Systolic Flow Velocities*		
Artery	**Diameter ± SD (cm)**	**Velocity ± SD (cm/sec)**
External iliac	0.79 ± 0.13	119.3 ± 21.7
Common femoral	0.82 ± 0.14	114.1 ± 24.9
Superficial femoral (proximal)	0.60 ± 0.12	90.8 ± 13.6
Superficial femoral (distal)	0.54 ± 0.11	93.6 ± 14.1
Popliteal	0.52 ± 0.11	68.8 ± 13.5

Data from Jager KA, Ricketts HJ, Strandness DE Jr: Duplex scanning for the evaluation of lower limb arterial disease. In Bernstein EF, editor: *Noninvasive diagnostic techniques in vascular disease*, St. Louis, 1985, Mosby, pp 619–631.
*Measurements by duplex scanning in 55 healthy subjects.
SD, standard deviation.

reduction) is indicated by a slight increase in spectral width (spectral broadening), without a significant increase in PSV (<30% increase in PSV compared to the adjacent proximal segment). This minimal spectral broadening is usually found in late systole and early diastole. Moderate stenosis (20%-49% diameter reduction) is characterized by more prominent spectral broadening and by an increase in PSVs up to 100% compared to the adjacent proximal segment. High-grade stenosis (50%-99% diameter reduction) produces the most severe flow disturbance, with markedly increased PSVs (>100% compared to the adjacent proximal segment), extensive spectral broadening, and loss of the reverse flow component. Occlusion of an arterial segment is documented when no Doppler flow signals can

be detected in the lumen of a clearly imaged vessel. Spectral waveforms obtained distal to a high-grade stenosis or occlusion are generally monophasic, with reduced systolic velocities (Figure 17-9). The features of spectral waveforms taken proximal to a stenotic lesion are variable and depend primarily on the status of the intervening collateral circulation. Immediately proximal to an arterial occlusion, the spectral waveforms typically show extremely low PSVs and little or no flow in diastole.

The PSV ratio, dividing the maximum velocity within a stenosis by the peak velocity in a normal arterial segment just proximal to the stenosis, is also a useful approach to grading the severity of arterial lesions. The PSV ratio is relatively independent of changes in blood pressure,

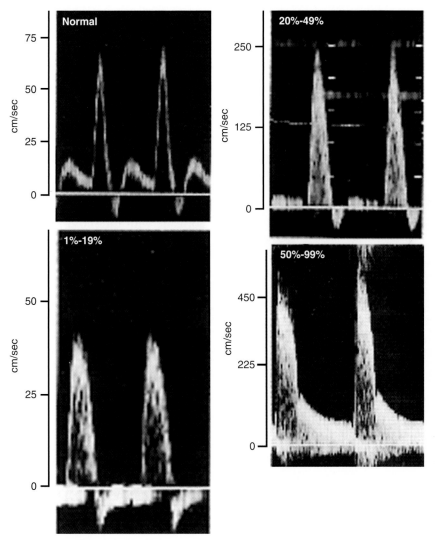

FIGURE 17-8 Lower extremity artery spectral waveforms. These are typical waveforms for each of the stenosis categories described in Table 17-2.

TABLE 17-2 University of Washington Duplex Criteria for Classification of Lower Extremity Arterial Stenosis	
Disease Severity	**Spectral Waveform Features**
Normal	Triphasic waveform No spectral broadening
1%-19% diameter reduction	Triphasic waveform with minimal spectral broadening Peak systolic velocities increased <30% relative to the adjacent proximal segment Proximal and distal waveforms remain normal
20%-49% diameter reduction	Triphasic waveform usually maintained (although reverse flow component may be diminished) Spectral broadening is prominent, with filling in of the clear area under the systolic peak Peak systolic velocity is increased 30%-100% relative to the adjacent proximal segment Proximal and distal waveforms remain normal
50%-99% diameter reduction	Monophasic waveform with loss of the reverse flow component and forward flow throughout the cardiac cycle Extensive spectral broadening Peak systolic velocity is increased >100% relative to the adjacent proximal segment Distal waveform is monophasic with reduced systolic velocity
Occlusion	No flow detected within the imaged arterial segment Preocclusive "thump" may be heard just proximal to the site of occlusion Distal (collateral) waveforms are monophasic with reduced systolic velocities

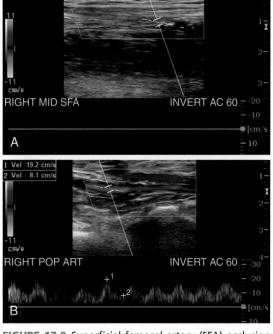

FIGURE 17-9 Superficial femoral artery (SFA) occlusion with abnormal distal flow. **A,** Color and pulsed Doppler image reveals no flow in SFA. **B,** Flow in reconstituted popliteal artery (POP ART) demonstrates low-velocity, low-resistance monophasic (tardus-parvus) waveforms consistent with proximal obstruction to flow.

cardiac output, and vascular compliance. Grading stenoses using the PSV ratio has been found to be highly reproducible.[14,15] Hemodynamically significant stenoses in lower extremity arteries correlate with threshold PSV ratios from 1.4 to 3.0.[9,16-18] A PSV ratio of 2.0 or greater is a reasonable compromise and is used by many vascular laboratories as a threshold for a peripheral artery stenosis of 50% or greater diameter reduction.

An important difference between spectral waveform analysis and color flow imaging is that spectral waveforms display the entire frequency and amplitude content of the pulsed Doppler signal at a specific site, whereas the color flow image provides a single estimate of the Doppler shift frequency or flow velocity for each site within the B-mode image. Consequently, spectral waveform analysis provides considerably more flow information from each individual site than color flow imaging. The main advantage of the color flow display is that it presents flow information throughout the B-mode image, although the actual amount of data for each site is reduced. Color Doppler displays flow abnormalities as focal areas of aliasing or color bruit artifacts that enable the sonographer to place the sample volume in the region of flow disturbance and obtain spectral information. Spectral waveforms contain a range of frequencies and amplitudes that allow determination of flow direction and parameters such as mean, mode, and peak frequency or velocity. In contrast, color assignments are based on flow direction and a single mean or average frequency estimate. Therefore, the peak or maximum Doppler frequency shifts found with spectral waveforms are generally higher than those indicated by the color flow image.

VALIDATION STUDIES

Although the criteria listed in Table 17-2 include several categories for lesions of less than 50% diameter reduction, the distinction between these categories is often subjective and rarely of clinical importance. The most useful classification for clinical purposes recognizes those lesions of less than 50% diameter reduction, 50% to 99% diameter reduction, and occlusion. Leng and colleagues[15] did not find further classification of diameter reduction within the 50% to 99% stenosis category to be reliable based on commonly used spectral waveform and color flow parameters. Jager and associates[9] used duplex scanning to evaluate 338 arterial segments in 54 lower extremities of 30 patients and compared the severity of stenosis as classified by spectral waveform analysis to the results of independently interpreted catheter contrast arteriograms. For all segments, duplex scanning differentiated between normal and diseased arteries with a sensitivity of 96% and a specificity of 81%. Duplex scanning distinguished between stenoses of greater or less than 50% diameter reduction with a sensitivity of 77% and a specificity of 98%. This study was performed before the addition of color Doppler imaging to the duplex scanner. These results compare favorably with the variability found when two different radiologists interpreted the same lower extremity arteriograms as either normal or diseased (sensitivity, 98%; specificity, 68%), or as greater or less than 50% diameter reduction (sensitivity, 87%; specificity, 94%).[2]

A second validation study was reported by Kohler and co-workers,[19] who evaluated 393 lower extremity arterial segments in 32 patients by both duplex scanning and arteriography. This study was also conducted before color Doppler imaging was available. By correctly identifying stenoses that had a significant (measured) pressure gradient or those lesions with diameter reduction more than 50%, duplex scanning had a sensitivity of 82%, a specificity of 92%, a positive predictive value of 80%, and a negative predictive value of 93%. The results were especially good for lesions in the iliac arteries (sensitivity, 89%; specificity, 90%). Lesions distal to very high grade stenoses or complete occlusions were difficult to detect because of the low flow velocities in these segments. This limitation was also observed by Allard and colleagues,[20] who found that the presence of 50% to 99% stenoses in adjacent arterial segments decreased both the sensitivity and specificity of lower extremity duplex scanning.

Moneta and associates[18] documented the accuracy of lower extremity duplex scanning in 286 limbs of 150 patients undergoing preoperative arteriography. Ninety-nine percent of arterial segments from the common iliac to the popliteal level were successfully visualized by duplex scanning, whereas 95% of the anterior and posterior tibial arteries and 83% of the peroneal arteries were adequately imaged. For arterial segments proximal to the tibial level, duplex scanning was evaluated for its ability to identify stenoses of greater than 50% diameter reduction and for its ability to distinguish between stenosis and occlusion. In the tibial and peroneal arteries, the ability of duplex scanning to predict continuous patency from the popliteal to ankle level was assessed. In the proximal arterial segments, the overall sensitivities for detecting a greater than 50% stenosis ranged from 67% in the popliteal to 89% in the iliac arteries; corresponding specificities ranged from 97% to 99%. Stenosis was successfully distinguished from occlusion in 98% of proximal arterial lesions. For the more distal arteries, overall sensitivities for predicting continuous patency ranged from 93% to 97%. Contrary to other reported experience,[20] the accuracy of lower extremity duplex scanning was not significantly affected by the presence of multiple-level disease.

CLINICAL APPLICATIONS

The clinical role of noninvasive vascular testing can be considered in three general categories: *screening, definitive diagnosis,* and *follow-up.* Because the purpose of screening is to detect disease in a patient population in which the prevalence of disease is presumed to be relatively low, a screening test should be low in cost and must not expose the patient to any significant risk. Screening also requires that the test have a high sensitivity or low false-negative rate to minimize the possibility of failing to detect disease. False-positive test results tend to be less problematic, because the results of screening are generally confirmed by further diagnostic tests before intervention. Appropriate patient selection can improve the yield of screening by increasing the pretest probability of detecting a disease.

Testing performed for definitive diagnosis is meant to provide the precise anatomic or physiologic information required for planning treatment. Ever since it was first described in 1927, contrast arteriography has served as the "gold standard" for the anatomic diagnosis of arterial disease.[21,22] However, the high cost and invasive nature of arteriography make it unsuitable for many clinical applications, such as screening or follow-up testing. Continued improvements in the accuracy of duplex scanning, together with a mandate to reduce the risks and cost of health care, have prompted many vascular surgeons to consider performing surgical procedures based on the results of noninvasive tests alone. This trend is particularly evident in the assessment of carotid artery disease, and the planning of carotid endarterectomy based on duplex scanning alone has become a standard of practice in selected patients.[23,24] A similar trend can be seen for patients undergoing lower extremity arterial bypass procedures.[25,26]

The purpose of follow-up testing is to detect progressive or recurrent disease at a previously diagnosed or treated site. Although this is similar to screening, it typically requires serial studies over time, and the terms *follow-up* and *surveillance* are often used interchangeably. Examples of surveillance include serial duplex scanning of infrainguinal vein grafts and repeat evaluation of patients following peripheral angioplasty and stent procedures. These applications are discussed in Chapter 18.

SCREENING

It should be emphasized that it is not necessary to obtain a complete duplex scan on every patient who requires a noninvasive lower extremity arterial evaluation. In most clinical situations, the history, physical examination, and indirect physiologic tests are sufficient to assess the presence and severity of arterial occlusive disease. Initial therapeutic plans can often be based on

this information alone. If intervention is not warranted, then more sophisticated testing is usually not necessary. However, if more detailed anatomic information is needed for clinical decision making, duplex scanning is a reasonable next step. Experience has shown that duplex scanning is superior to segmental pressure measurement for localization and classification of lower extremity arterial lesions.[27]

Lower extremity duplex scanning is generally helpful for those patients being considered for direct intervention—either a catheter-based intervention or open surgical repair. The goal in this setting is to determine the location and extent of arterial lesions so that decisions can be made regarding the need for additional imaging studies and the most appropriate therapeutic approach. For example, duplex scanning is valuable for the preoperative assessment and follow-up evaluation of the iliac artery after stent placement (Figure 17-10). Whether a particular arterial segment is suitable for an endovascular procedure or open surgical reconstruction depends on the specific features of the lesion. For example, focal stenoses or short occlusions in the iliac or superficial femoral arteries are often suitable for percutaneous transluminal angioplasty and stenting, whereas arterial segments with long, irregular stenotic lesions or extensive occlusions may be better treated by a surgical bypass graft. The anatomic features that are important in making this determination are the site, severity, and length of the lesion. In addition, it is essential to assess the status of the arterial inflow and the quality of the

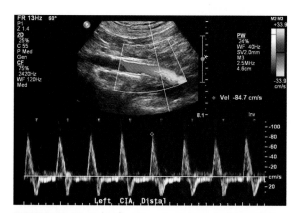

FIGURE 17-10 Color flow image and spectral waveforms obtained from a stented left common iliac artery (CIA). The stent is visualized on the left side of the color Doppler image. The spectral waveforms from the distal common iliac artery show a normal flow pattern with a peak velocity of 85 cm/sec.

distal runoff vessels. Duplex scanning provides a practical means for obtaining this information without resorting to catheter contrast arteriography or other anatomic imaging techniques such as MRA or CTA.

Edwards and co-workers[28] reported on 110 patients who underwent lower extremity duplex scanning before catheter contrast arteriography. Based on the duplex scan findings, 50 lesions were considered suitable for percutaneous transluminal angioplasty. Of these, the procedure was actually performed in 47 (94%). In the remaining three cases, lesions were present as predicted by the duplex scan, but angioplasty was not performed for various technical reasons. No angioplasties were performed in patients who were found not to be candidates by duplex scanning. The characterization of lesions before catheter contrast arteriography and angioplasty facilitates the intervention by directing attention to the appropriate arterial segment and indicating the optimal puncture site for catheter access to the target lesion.[28,29] Thus, with a preintervention duplex scan, it should not be necessary to perform separate diagnostic and therapeutic catheter procedures. It is often valuable to screen older adult or debilitated patients with duplex scanning. The goal in such patients is to identify lesions that can be treated by percutaneous techniques. If such lesions are not found and if open surgery is contraindicated, then further evaluation with catheter contrast arteriography is not necessary.

DEFINITIVE DIAGNOSIS AND PLANNING OF TREATMENT

The high accuracy of duplex scanning compared with catheter contrast arteriography has raised the issue of whether duplex scanning might replace arteriography in the preoperative evaluation of lower extremity arterial disease. Kohler and associates[30] performed a study to determine if vascular surgeons would choose different therapeutic procedures when provided with basic clinical information and the results of either lower extremity duplex scanning or arteriography. Relatively little disparity was found when decisions based on the two tests were compared for each individual surgeon. However, significant disagreement was noted among the clinical decisions made by various surgeons, even when the duplex scan and arteriogram reports agreed. These data suggest that most of the observed

variability in patient management was caused by diversity in the clinical approach to particular patterns of disease rather than actual differences in the results of the two diagnostic tests.

The most important considerations in planning a surgical lower extremity revascularization procedure are the location and severity of arterial lesions, adequacy of inflow to the femoral level, and the identification of a distal target vessel for a bypass graft. Ligush and co-workers[25] compared the types of operations predicted by duplex scanning or conventional arteriography with the actual operations performed in 36 patients undergoing 40 infrainguinal bypass grafts for critical limb ischemia. A hemodynamically significant stenosis was defined by a twofold increase in the PSV at the site of the lesion relative to a normal segment immediately proximal to the stenosis (PSV ratio of 2.0 or greater). The mean time required for duplex scanning was 30 minutes (range, 20-55 minutes). Of the actual operations performed, 83% were correctly predicted by duplex scanning, and 90% were correctly predicted by arteriography. There was no significant difference in the ability of the two preoperative imaging methods to predict operative strategy. A similar study was reported by Wain and associates,[26] who evaluated 41 patients having infrainguinal bypass grafts. The same velocity criterion was used for a hemodynamically significant stenosis, and the typical duplex scanning time was approximately 60 minutes. Duplex scanning correctly predicted whether a femoropopliteal or infrapopliteal bypass graft was required in 90% of the cases. Both anastomotic sites were correctly predicted in 90% of femoropopliteal grafts (18 of 20 patients) but only 24% of infrapopliteal grafts (5 of 21 patients). These authors concluded that duplex scanning was a reliable predictor of the distal anastomotic site for femoropopliteal bypass grafts but not for bypass grafts to the tibial or peroneal arteries.

A study by Grassbaugh and colleagues[31] evaluated whether preoperative duplex scanning could take the place of catheter contrast arteriography in selecting the target vessel for distal anastomosis in patients undergoing bypass grafts to the tibial or peroneal arteries. Forty lower extremities in 38 patients were examined by both duplex scanning and arteriography, and observers blinded to the actual operation performed reviewed either the ultrasound or arteriographic results and selected the optimal target vessel. The target vessel actually used was correctly predicted by duplex scanning in 88% of patients and by contrast arteriography in 93% of patients, a difference that was not statistically significant ($P = .59$). The distal arteries used for bypass grafting had significantly higher PSVs (mean 35 cm/sec vs 25 cm/sec; $P = .04$) and end-diastolic velocities (mean 15 cm/sec vs 9 cm/sec; $P = .005$) compared with those not selected as target vessels. These authors noted occasional difficulty in visualizing the peroneal artery, but they concluded that duplex scanning and contrast arteriography usually agree when selecting the distal target vessel for a tibial or peroneal artery bypass graft.

The experience summarized above suggests that duplex scanning alone is adequate for the preoperative evaluation of selected patients who require infrainguinal bypass grafting. However, it may be necessary to combine preoperative duplex scanning with intraoperative, prebypass contrast arteriography to clearly define the target vessel and anastomotic site, particularly when the distal anastomosis is to the tibial or peroneal arteries. Some investigators have found the predictive value of duplex scanning to be limited when bypass to a tibial or peroneal artery is required and multiple patent target vessels are identified.[26,32] Intraoperative, prebypass contrast arteriography is a simple and rapid method for identifying the most suitable target vessel while avoiding the cost and risk of a formal preoperative arteriogram.

Preoperative arteriography is still advisable for patients who are found on duplex scanning to have significant aortoiliac occlusive disease, who do not appear to have an adequate distal target vessel for bypass, and in whom the ultrasound evaluation is limited by obesity, vessel calcification, or open wounds. This should avoid the distressing problem of taking a patient to the operating room for a bypass graft and being unable to complete the procedure. Mapping and marking of superficial veins by duplex ultrasound is also valuable to ensure that a satisfactory venous conduit is available.

EVALUATION OF LOWER EXTREMITY TRAUMA

Vascular injuries in the lower extremities can produce acute arterial insufficiency or exsanguinating hemorrhage that require rapid diagnosis and treatment. In these situations, the conventional history, physical examination, and diagnostic tests are often impractical. Patients with lower extremity vascular trauma can present in two ways. Some have clear evidence of a vascular injury with obvious distal limb ischemia or massive hemorrhage. These patients generally undergo immediate operative exploration and repair. A second and more common presentation is when a patient has sustained blunt or penetrating trauma to an extremity but does not have specific signs or symptoms of a vascular problem. In this setting, the mechanism of trauma or location of a wound raises the clinical suspicion of an occult vascular injury.

Routine surgical exploration of vessels in proximity to traumatic wounds has been practiced but has a relatively low diagnostic yield. On the other extreme, the sensitivity of the physical examination alone may not be high enough to serve as a basis for treatment.[33] For many years, catheter contrast arteriography was the standard method for definitive diagnosis of acute arterial trauma. In a series of 100 extremity injuries published in 1991, catheter contrast arteriography took a mean of 2.4 hours to perform.[34] This represents an unacceptable delay in patients with major vascular injuries or multiple-system trauma who require ongoing resuscitation and immediate treatment. The use of catheter contrast arteriography for screening stable patients with suspected occult arterial injuries is more feasible but is associated with considerable cost and some increased risk. Furthermore, experience has shown that many posttraumatic arteriographic lesions, such as intimal flaps, pseudoaneurysms, and arteriovenous fistulas, follow a benign course and heal over time.[33] In many centers, CTA has replaced catheter contrast arteriography for the urgent assessment of extremity vascular trauma.[35,36]

Both indirect measurement of limb systolic blood pressure and duplex scanning have been used in patients with extremity trauma to avoid unnecessary arteriography and determine the need for surgical exploration. Lynch and Johansen[34] obtained Doppler pressure measurements in 100 injured limbs of 93 trauma victims who also had catheter contrast arteriography. An arterial pressure index (systolic pressure distal to the site of injury/brachial systolic pressure in an uninvolved arm) of greater than 0.90 was considered normal. Compared with the arteriographic findings, the arterial pressure index had a sensitivity of 87%, specificity of 97%, and overall accuracy of 95% for detecting arterial injuries. When the results of two false-positive arteriograms were excluded, the sensitivity, specificity, and accuracy increased to 95%, 98%, and 97%, respectively. The selection of trauma patients with possible occult vascular injuries for arteriography based on an arterial pressure index of less than 0.90 was prospectively evaluated in 100 limbs of 96 patients.[37] Among the 17 limbs with a decreased arterial pressure index, 16 had an abnormal arteriogram and 7 underwent arterial repair. For the 83 limbs with a normal arterial pressure index, follow-up revealed 6 minor lesions but no major injuries.

Although the arterial pressure index is a simple, rapid, and clinically valuable screening test, it has several important limitations. This approach cannot be used in cases where extensive wounds prevent placement of a pneumatic cuff on the injured extremity. In addition, it will not differentiate between an intrinsic arterial lesion, extrinsic compression, and vasospasm. Finally, distal limb pressure measurement will not detect non–flow-limiting lesions or injuries to nonaxial arteries, such as the deep femoral artery.

Duplex scanning has been applied to the diagnosis of arterial trauma in the cervicothoracic region and the extremities.[38-41] Panetta and associates[42] reported an experimental study of duplex scanning and arteriography in a canine model of arterial injury (occlusion, laceration, intimal flap, hematoma, and arteriovenous fistula). Although duplex scanning and arteriography had equivalent overall accuracy in detecting arterial injuries, duplex scanning was significantly more sensitive (90% vs 80%) and was more accurate than arteriography in identifying arterial lacerations. This high sensitivity makes duplex scanning particularly useful as a screening test in patients with suspected arterial injuries.

Meissner and co-workers[39] used duplex scanning as a screening test to evaluate 89 patients with suspected arterial trauma. Among 60 scans performed for wound proximity to adjacent vascular structures, only 4 (7%) were positive. Of the 19 scans done for specific clinical signs of arterial injury, 13 (68%) were positive (Figure 17-11). Clinical follow-up or catheter contrast arteriography confirmed that no major arterial injuries were missed. A similar experience was reported by Bynoe and colleagues,[40] who prospectively evaluated 319 potential vascular injuries in 198 patients. Duplex scanning showed a sensitivity of 95%, specificity of 99%, and overall accuracy of 98% for identifying arterial injuries.

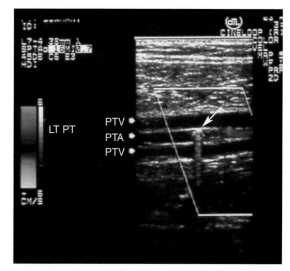

FIGURE 17-11 Color flow image from a patient with a lower extremity gunshot wound showing a bullet fragment *(arrow)* in the posterior tibial artery (PTA). The color flow stream stops at the bullet, where marked acoustic shadowing is present. Two posterior tibial veins (PTV) are also visualized. *(From Zierler RE, Zierler BK: Duplex sonography of lower extremity arteries,* Semin Ultrasound CT MR *18:39–56, 1997.)*

Although most of the experience with duplex scanning for lower extremity vascular injuries has been limited to a small number of trauma centers, it is clearly effective in this clinical setting. It is particularly important to follow patients with initially negative duplex scans when there is ongoing suspicion of an arterial injury, since lesions may become apparent on later examinations.[38,43,44]

CONCLUSIONS

In well-trained hands, duplex ultrasound with color flow and Doppler waveform evaluation of the lower extremity arteries is a useful adjunct to the indirect physiologic assessment of arterial disease. It can be used selectively as a substitute for more sophisticated imaging techniques such as MRA, CTA, and contrast arteriography.

REFERENCES

1. Slot HB, Strijbosch L, Greep JM: Interobserver variability in single-plane aortography, *Surgery* 90:497–503, 1981.
2. Thiele BL, Strandness DE Jr: Accuracy of angiographic quantification of peripheral atherosclerosis, *Prog Cardiovasc Dis* 26:223–236, 1983.
3. Bui TD, et al: Comparison of CT and catheter arteriography for evaluation of peripheral arterial disease, *Vasc Endovasc Surg* 39:481–490, 2005.

4. Met R, et al: Diagnostic performance of computed tomography angiography in peripheral arterial disease: a systematic review and meta-analysis, *JAMA* 301:415–424, 2009.

5. Collins R, et al: A systematic review of duplex ultrasound, magnetic resonance angiography and computed tomography angiography for the diagnosis and assessment of symptomatic, lower limb peripheral arterial disease, *Health Technol Assess* 20:iii-iv, xi-xiii,1–184, 2007.

6. Levin DC, et al: The effect of the introduction of MR and CT angiography in the utilization of catheter angiography for peripheral arterial disease, *J Am Coll Radiol* 4:457–460, 2007.

7. Zierler RE, Strandness DE Jr: Doppler techniques for lower extremity arterial diagnosis. In Zwiebel WJ, editor: *Introduction to Vascular Ultrasonography*, ed 2, Orlando, FL, 1986, Grune & Stratton, pp 305–331.

8. Zierler RE: Carotid artery evaluation by duplex scanning, *Semin Vasc Surg* 1:9–16, 1988.

9. Jager KA: Noninvasive mapping of lower limb arterial lesions, *Ultrasound Med Biol* 11:515–521, 1985.

10. Hatsukami TS, et al: Color Doppler imaging of infrainguinal arterial occlusive disease, *J Vasc Surg* 16:527–533, 1992.

11. Thiele BL, et al: Pulsed Doppler waveform patterns produced by smooth stenosis in the dog thoracic aorta. In Taylor DEM, Stevens AL, editors: *Blood Flow Theory and Practice*, San Diego, CA, 1983, Academic Press, pp 85–104.

12. Jager KA, Ricketts HJ, Strandness DE Jr: Duplex scanning for the evaluation of lower limb arterial disease. In Bernstein EF, editor: *Noninvasive Diagnostic Techniques in Vascular Disease*, St. Louis, 1985, Mosby, pp 619–631.

13. Hatsukami TS, et al: Color Doppler characteristics in normal lower extremity arteries, *Ultrasound Med Biol* 18:167–171, 1992.

14. Whyman MR, et al: Accuracy and reproducibility of duplex ultrasound imaging in a phantom model of femoral artery stenosis, *J Vasc Surg* 17:524–530, 1993.

15. Leng GC, et al: Accuracy and reproducibility of duplex ultrasonography in grading femoropopliteal stenoses, *J Vasc Surg* 17:510–517, 1993.

16. Sacks D, et al: Peripheral arterial Doppler ultrasonography: Diagnostic criteria, *J Ultrasound Med* 11:95–103, 1992.

17. de Smet AA, Ermers EJ, Kitslaar PJ: Duplex velocity characteristics of aortoiliac stenoses, *J Vasc Surg* 23:628–636, 1996.

18. Moneta GL, et al: Accuracy of lower extremity arterial duplex mapping, *J Vasc Surg* 15:275–284, 1992.

19. Kohler TR, et al: Duplex scanning for diagnosis of aortoiliac and femoropopliteal disease: A prospective study, *Circulation* 76:1074–1080, 1987.

20. Allard L, et al: Limitations of ultrasonic duplex scanning for diagnosing of lower limb arterial stenoses in the presence of adjacent segment disease, *J Vasc Surg* 19:650–657, 1994.

21. Moniz E: L'encephalographie arterielle: Son importance dans la localisation des tumeurs cerebrales, *Rev Neurol* 2:72–90, 1927.

22. Dos Santos R, Lamas A, Pereira CJ: L'arteriographie des membres de l'aorte et ses branches abdominales, *Bull Soc Natl Chir* 55:587–601, 1929.

23. Dawson DL, et al: The role of duplex scanning and arteriography before carotid endarterectomy: A prospective study, *J Vasc Surg* 18:673–683, 1993.

24. Zwolak RM: Carotid endarterectomy without angiography: Are we ready? *Vasc Surg* 31:1–9, 1997.

25. Ligush J, et al: Duplex ultrasound scanning defines operative strategies for patients with limb-threatening ischemia, *J Vasc Surg* 28:482–491, 1998.

26. Wain RA, et al: Can duplex arterial mapping replace contrast arteriography as the test of choice before infrainguinal revascularization? *J Vasc Surg* 29:100–109, 1999.

27. Moneta GL, et al: Noninvasive localization of arterial occlusive disease: A comparison of segmental Doppler pressures and arterial duplex mapping, *J Vasc Surg* 17:578–582, 1993.

28. Edwards JM, et al: The role of duplex scanning in the selection of patients for transluminal angioplasty, *J Vasc Surg* 13:69–74, 1991.

29. Van Der Heijden FHWM, et al: Value of duplex scanning in the selection of patients for percutaneous transluminal angioplasty, *Eur J Vasc Surg* 7:71–76, 1993.

30. Kohler T, et al: Can duplex scanning replace arteriography for lower extremity arterial disease? *Ann Vasc Surg* 4:280–287, 1990.

31. Grassbaugh JA, et al: Blinded comparison of preoperative duplex ultrasound scanning and contrast arteriography for planning revascularization at the level of the tibia, *J Vasc Surg* 37:1186–1190, 2003.

32. Hingorani AP, et al: Limitations of and lessons learned from the clinical experience of 1,020 duplex arteriography, *Vascular* 16:147–153, 2008.

33. Johansen K: Evaluation of vascular trauma. In Bernstein EF, editor: *Vascular Diagnosis*, ed 4, St. Louis, 1993, Mosby, pp 575–578.

34. Lynch K, Johansen K: Can Doppler pressure measurement replace "exclusion" arteriography in the diagnosis of occult extremity arterial trauma? *Ann Surg* 241:737–741, 1991.

35. Peng PD, et al: CT angiography effectively evaluates extremity vascular trauma, *Am Surg* 74:103–107, 2008.

36. Fleiter TR, Mervis S: The role of 3D-CTA in the assessment of peripheral vascular lesions in trauma patients, *Eur J Radiol* 64:92–102, 2007.

37. Johansen K, et al: Non-invasive vascular tests reliably exclude occult arterial trauma in injured extremities, *J Trauma* 31:515–519, 1991.

38. Fry WR, et al: Duplex scanning replaces arteriography and operative exploration in the diagnosis of potential cervical vascular injury, *Am J Surg* 168:693–695, 1994.

39. Meissner M, Paun M, Johansen K: Duplex scanning for arterial trauma, *Am J Surg* 161:552–555, 1991.

40. Bynoe RP, et al: Non-invasive diagnosis of vascular trauma by duplex ultrasonography, *J Vasc Surg* 14:346–352, 1991.

41. Fry WR, et al: The success of duplex ultrasonography scanning in diagnosis of extremity vascular proximity trauma, *Arch Surg* 128:1368–1372, 1993.

42. Panetta TF, et al: Duplex sonography versus arteriography in the diagnosis of arterial injury: An experimental study, *J Trauma* 33:627–635, 1992.

43. Sorrell K, Demasi R: Delayed vascular injury: The value of follow-up color flow duplex ultrasonography, *J Vasc Technol* 20:93–98, 1996.

44. Bergstein JM, et al: Pitfalls in the use of color flow duplex ultrasound for screening of suspected arterial injuries in penetrated extremities, *J Trauma* 33:395–402, 1992.

ULTRASOUND ASSESSMENT DURING AND AFTER CAROTID AND PERIPHERAL INTERVENTION

18

KELLEY HODGKISS-HARLOW, MD, and DENNIS F. BANDYK, MD

The application of vascular laboratory testing after peripheral arterial intervention can improve procedural and patient outcomes.[1-6] Clinical efficacy requires use of appropriate testing methods and interpretation criteria. Duplex ultrasound imaging alone or in conjunction with extremity systolic blood pressure measurements provides accurate diagnostics to identify both technical problems and occlusive lesions that can occur following open surgical bypass or endovascular therapy. Duplex testing is portable and thus suitable for intraprocedural assessment with the goal of testing to improve the technical precision of the arterial intervention. Repair site abnormalities (stenosis, kinks, dissection, thrombus, low-volume flow) interfere with normal functional patency and contribute to early failure.[3-8] Routine duplex testing has demonstrated residual stenosis is a common finding following percutaneous transluminal angioplasty (PTA; 5%-25%) as well as infrainguinal vein bypass (10%-15%).[1,7-10] When these duplex-detected lesions are identified and promptly revised, the incidence of arterial repair failure is low (1%-2%), which contributes to cost-effective patient care.

In the outpatient setting, duplex testing is the cornerstone of a vascular laboratory–based surveillance program.[3,4] Serial testing is performed; initially to confirm that the repair simulates "normal" arterial blood flow, and thereafter to detect developing stenosis caused by myointimal hyperplasia (a common mode of arterial repair failure) or to identify atherosclerotic disease progression. Repeat intervention based on threshold duplex velocity spectra criteria has been shown to increase long-term patency compared to a clinical follow-up regimen that relies on a recurrence of symptoms or signs of peripheral arterial occlusive disease.[5]

INTRAPROCEDURAL DUPLEX ULTRASOUND ASSESSMENT

Assessment of an arterial intervention by inspection, pulse palpation, and continuous-wave, handheld Doppler signal analysis is safe and easy to perform but lacks diagnostic sensitivity to identify moderate to severe stenosis or intraluminal defects (dissection, intimal flaps, and thrombus). Although fluoroscopic digital subtraction angiography (DSA) is considered a "gold standard" for arterial repair assessment, the technique is invasive, requiring arterial puncture, radiation exposure, and contrast-induced toxicity. Study interpretation even with multiple imaging runs is prone to false-negative errors.[11-13] Duplex testing has emerged as a preferred intraprocedural diagnostic technique since it provides real-time, high-resolution vessel imaging coupled with physiologic information using pulsed-Doppler velocity spectra analysis. Essentially all open and endovascular extremity procedures capable of being insonated with a transducer (either placed directly over the repair or transcutaneous) can be evaluated for technical adequacy using similar interpretation criteria (Table 18-1). Endovascular interventions of the extracranial carotid, subclavian, renal, or mesenteric arteries should be assessed using either DSA alone, with catheter pullback systolic pressure measurement to verify a gradient of less than 10 mm Hg, or intravascular ultrasound. For open arterial surgical repairs, (carotid endarterectomy [CEA], renal/visceral artery bypass or endarterectomy, extremity arterial bypass), intraoperative duplex scanning is easy to perform and interpret using imaging and velocity spectra criteria associated with high diagnostic accuracy (sensitivity and negative predictive value rates of >90%). Procedural

TABLE 18-1 Diagnostic Methods and "Normal" Threshold Criteria for Commonly Used for Intraprocedural Assessments of Surgical and Endovascular Peripheral Arterial Reconstructions

Procedure	Angiogram*	Measurement of Systolic Arterial Pressure Gradient†	Duplex Ultrasound‡
"Open" Surgical Repair			
Carotid endarterectomy	Yes, <20% DR	Not used	Yes, PSV <150 cm/sec
Renal bypass	Not used	Not used	Yes, PSV <180 cm/sec
Mesenteric bypass	Not used	Not used	Yes, PSV <180 cm/sec
Infrainguinal bypass	Yes, <30% DR	Not used	Yes, PSV <180 cm/sec
Endovascular Intervention-Angioplasty (PTA)			
Carotid stent-angioplasty	Yes, <20% DR	Not used	Yes, PSV<150 cm/sec
Renal PTA	Yes, <30% DR	Yes, <10 mm Hg	Not used
Mesenteric PTA	Yes, <30% DR	Yes, <10 mm Hg	Not used
Iliac PTA	Yes, <30% DR	Yes, <10 mm Hg	Yes, PSV <180 cm/sec
Infrainguinal PTA	Yes, <30% DR	Not used	Yes, PSV <180 cm/sec
Vein bypass balloon PTA	Yes, <30% DR	Not used	Yes, PSV <180 cm/sec

DR, diameter reduction; PSV, peak systolic velocity; PTA, percutaneous transluminal angioplasty.
*Criteria for acceptable residual stenosis, expressed as diameter reduction.
†Catheter measurement of pressure gradient during systole across angioplasty site.
‡Peak systolic velocity threshold for revision of residual stenosis, used in conjunction with B-mode imaging criteria of stenosis and peak systolic velocity ratio of >2.0 at site of abnormality.

duplex imaging can be completed within 5 to 10 minutes and is more convenient than completion arteriography.[1,2,14]

The type of repair site abnormality varies with procedure type, but stenosis caused by residual disease, plaque dissection, or improper suturing is the most common irregularity identified using either duplex scanning or DSA. When a duplex-detected abnormality has velocity spectra indicative of a severe stenosis, the blood flow turbulence produced reduces volume flow and downstream pressure and alters blood coagulability; these conditions can result in platelet-thrombus formation and repair site thrombosis. Failure to identify the "abnormal" repair increases the likelihood of procedure failure—an outcome that requires a secondary salvage procedure and has associated increased morbidity and health care costs.

It is recommended that a vascular technologist participate in duplex ultrasound evaluations performed in the operating room or angiography suite. The technologist assists in instrument setup to optimize image resolution and color Doppler settings that are essential for quality, interpretable studies. For intraoperative assessment, a 10- to 15-MHz linear array transducer with a small footprint should be used to afford high-resolution imaging and placement within the surgical wound, directly on the repair. For transcutaneous imaging of bypass grafts or extremity angioplasty/atherectomy procedures, 5- to 7-MHz linear array transducers are necessary to image the deeper-positioned vessels. By placing the transducer within a sterile plastic sleeve containing acoustic gel together with sterile gel on the prepped operative field or saline in the wound, acoustic coupling necessary for duplex imaging is achieved.

Reluctance to adopt routine intraprocedural duplex assessment is based on the false belief that testing is difficult to perform and interpret, whereas clinical assessment and arteriography provide equivalent diagnostic accuracy. Intraoperative duplex assessment of infrainguinal vein bypass doubles the immediate revision rate compared to completion DSA, and early (30-day) thrombosis/revision rate is halved. The recommended velocity criteria threshold for repair of a duplex-detected stenosis varies, but a peak systolic velocity (PSV) greater than 150 to 180 cm/sec associated with a velocity ratio (Vr) greater than 2 across the imaged stenosis has been shown to predict both lower extremity bypass and PTA failure. Revision rates based on duplex testing are higher with infrainguinal bypass to an infrageniculate artery (17%), when arm (27%) versus saphenous (15%) vein conduit is used, and when PTA is performed by atherectomy (20%) versus balloon (15%) or stent-angioplasty (5%).[15,16]

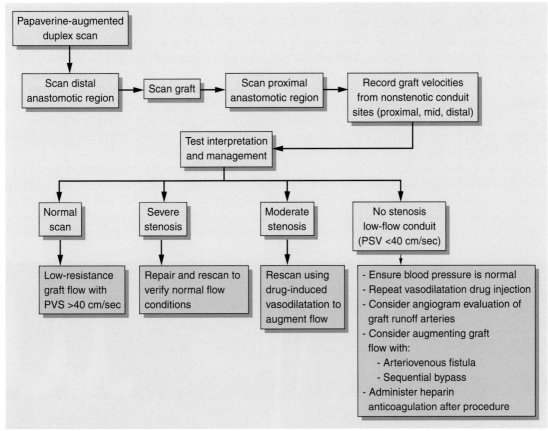

FIGURE 18-1 Algorithm for intraoperative duplex scanning of an infrainguinal vein bypass. Following duplex assessment, the study is classified into one of four categories—normal, severe stenosis identified, moderate stenosis identified, or no stenosis identified but hemodynamic assessment of graft flow demonstrates low flow velocity (peak systolic velocity [PSV] <40 cm/sec). BP, blood pressure.

INFRAINGUINAL BYPASS ASSESSMENT

The intraoperative scanning algorithm relies on real-time color Doppler imaging to identify lumen stenosis and sites of disturbed, turbulent flow.[10,17] The entire bypass should be imaged to the extent possible beginning at the distal anastomotic region and then proceeding proximally (Figure 18-1). Before duplex scanning, papaverine hydrochloride (30-60 mg) is administered (via a 27-gauge needle into the conduit) to vasodilate the runoff arterial bed and augment graft blood flow. This technique, termed *papaverine-augmented duplex scanning*, improves diagnostic sensitivity for the detection and grading of residual stenosis severity. Use of a vasodilator drug is also useful to confirm the presence of low resistance flow pattern in distal bypass graft and runoff arteries (Figure 18-2)—a hemodynamic characteristic associated with successful lower limb bypass grafting. Pulsed Doppler velocity spectra are recorded using a Doppler angle of 60 degrees relative to the vessel wall and the sample volume placed in the center stream of flow.

Based on the duplex scan findings, the repair is classified as normal (no stenosis, low resistance graft flow with PSV >40 cm/sec), residual stenosis (moderate, severe), or a low-flow condition is present (Table 18-2). The duplex criteria for a greater than 50% stenosis include color Doppler imaging of an anatomic defect with disturbed color flow pattern and a PSV greater than 180 cm/sec. The PSV ratio across the stenosis should be greater than or equal to 2.5—a level of hemodynamic abnormality that is clinically significant and warrants correction, or at the very least additional evaluation by DSA. An elevated PSV in the range of 125 to 180 cm/sec may be recorded from small-diameter (<3 mm) vessels and should not be considered abnormal if Vr is less than 2.

A high-resistance waveform (antegrade flow only during systole) in the distal bypass graft is abnormal and when associated with a low systolic flow velocity (PSV ≤40 cm/sec) indicates a "low-flow conduit" and is predictive of early graft failure. In these instances, a careful evaluation for residual proximal or distal occlusive disease should be undertaken. Depending on angiographic and repeat papaverine-augmented duplex scan findings, procedures to augment graft flow, such as construction of a distal arteriovenous fistula or bypass to a second outflow artery, can be considered.

The entire infrainguinal bypass should be imaged for anatomic and flow abnormalities, especially if the bypass technique utilized the in situ saphenous vein with valvulotome vein

leaflet lysis. A vein valve site with velocity spectra indicating stenosis (PSV >180 cm/sec; Vr >2.5) should be revised by repeat valve lysis (Figure 18-3). Duplex scanning can also be used to locate patent vein side-branches for ligation. In general, the duplex assessment of prosthetic bypass grafts is limited to imaging of anastomotic sites, since ultrasound insonation of grafts constructed of polytetrafluoroethylene (PTFE) is attenuated by air in the graft wall.

Intragraft platelet thrombus formation is an abnormality that develops in 3% of bypass grafting procedures and has the duplex features of high-grade stenosis (PSV >300 cm/sec) with mobile lumen thrombus seen on real-time

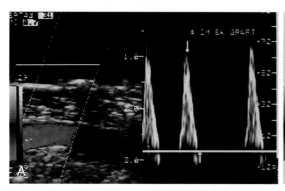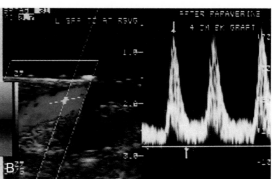

FIGURE 18-2 Velocity spectra recorded from the below-knee (BK) graft segment of an infrainguinal saphenous vein bypass before **(A)** and following **(B)** the administration of an intragraft injection of papaverine HCl (30 mg) to produce vasodilatation of the graft runoff. Velocity spectra contour changes from high peripheral vascular resistance, with flow only during systole, to a low peripheral vascular resistance contour, with antegrade flow during the entire pulse cycle, indicating an increase in graft volume flow. Note that peak systolic velocity does not change appreciably.

TABLE 18-2 Interpretation and Recommended Management Based on Intraoperative Duplex Ultrasound Assessment of Infrainguinal Vein Bypasses			
Duplex Scan Category	Graft Flow Velocity (cm/sec)	Peripheral Vascular Resistance	Interpretation and Perioperative (24-hr) Management
Normal	>40	Low	No stenosis identified and graft PSV is normal. Administer dextran-40 (25 mL/hr, 500 mL) and oral ASA (325 mg/d).
Severe stenosis: PSV >180 cm/sec; Vr >2.5	<40	Low	Correct lesion and rescan graft. If no residual stenosis identified but graft PSV is low (<40 cm/sec), administer low-molecular-weight heparin (1 mg/kg SC bid), dextran-40 (25 mL/hr), and oral ASA (325 mg/d).
Moderate stenosis: PSV <125-200 cm/sec; Vr 1.5-2.5	>40	Low	Rescan after 10 min to confirm no progression. Administer low- molecular-weight heparin (1 mg/kg SC bid), dextran-40 (25 mL/hr), and oral ASA (325 mg/d).
Low flow, no graft stenosis	<40	High	Consider an adjunctive procedure to increase graft flow (distal arteriovenous fistula, jump/sequential graft to another outflow artery); if not possible, treat as low-flow graft with antithrombotic regimen of heparin anticoagulation, dextran-40, and ASA (325 mg/d).

ASA, acetylsalicylic acid (aspirin); bid, twice a day; PSV, peak systolic velocity; SC, subcutaneously; Vr, velocity ratio.

B-mode imaging. This lesion is best treated by replacement of the involved vein graft segment, perfusion of the distal graft, and runoff with a thrombolytic agent, followed by reimaging the entire repair for residual flow abnormality as well as the adequacy of graft flow velocity (GFV).

Graft or anastomotic sites with velocity spectra of a moderate stenosis (PSV 125-200 cm/sec; Vr 1.5-2.5) should be carefully imaged (Figure 18-4) for any lumen defects (thrombus, stricture, valve cusp) and rescanned after drug-induced vasodilatation to verify PSV at the site remains less than 180 cm/sec. When elevated velocity spectra (PSV >180 cm/sec) are recorded in an outflow tibial artery but the Vr is less than 2.5 compared to the distal anastomosis PSV, spasm or hyperemic flow is likely the cause and revision is not required. Whenever a low-PSV graft velocity or moderate stenosis is confirmed on the intraoperative study but left unrepaired, a predischarge duplex scan is recommended to verify presence of normal graft hemodynamics versus a persistent residual stenosis or low-flow condition.

A study of 626 consecutive infrainguinal vein bypasses found intraoperative duplex findings predicted outcome (Table 18-3).[10] A study interpreted as "normal" had a bypass graft failure rate of 1% at 30 days and 1.5% from 30 to 90 days. If moderate stenosis was identified and not repaired, the incidence of graft thrombosis was 8% at 30 days and the 90-day graft revision rate was 30%. The finding of low graft flow (PSV <40 cm/sec) with no identified graft abnormality was present in only 2% of all bypasses studied, but 5 (38%) of 13 bypasses failed within 90 days. These data indicate that residual duplex-identified defects and low graft flow are risk factors for thrombosis as well as the development of graft stenosis. Intraoperative duplex assessment produced similar primary patency rates at 90 days relative to saphenous vein grafting technique: in situ bypass (94%), nonreversed translocated bypass (94%), and reversed saphenous vein bypass (89%); but lower for arm vein bypasses (82.5%, P <0.01). The application of both intraoperative and predischarge duplex

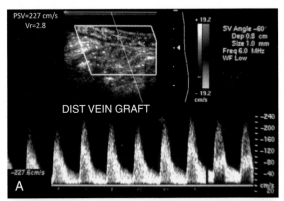

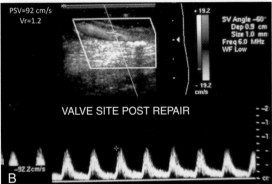

FIGURE 18-3 Intraoperative duplex scan of distal vein graft demonstrating abnormal velocity spectra **(A)**, with peak systolic velocity (PSV) of 227 cm/sec and lumen narrowing. Normal velocity spectra are recorded (PSV = 92 cm/sec) following valve lysis **(B)**.

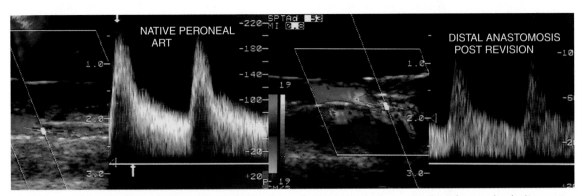

FIGURE 18-4 Intraoperative duplex scan of distal vein graft anastomosis demonstrating abnormal velocity spectra *(left image)*, with peak systolic velocity (PSV) of 220 cm/sec and lumen narrowing. Following revision *(right image)*, normal velocity spectra are recorded (PSV = 100 cm/sec).

TABLE 18-3 **Results of Intraoperative Duplex Assessment of Infrainguinal Vein Bypass**	
Incidence of Graft Revision	**Percent Revised**
Outflow Artery	
Above-knee popliteal	13
Below-knee popliteal	16
Anterior tibial	20
Posterior tibial	12
Peroneal	15
Pedal	17
Bypass Grafting Technique	
In situ saphenous vein bypass	16
Reversed saphenous vein bypass	10
Nonreversed, translocated saphenous vein bypass	13
Arm vein bypass	27
Site of Graft Problem Repaired	
	Percent of Total Lesions Repaired
Inflow artery	8
Proximal anastomotic region	7
Venous conduit	59
Distal anastomotic region	26

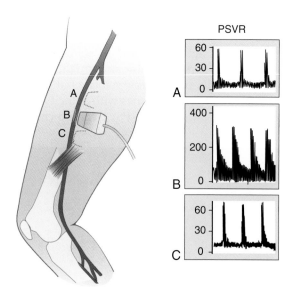

FIGURE 18-5 Transcutaneous use of duplex ultrasound to assess velocity spectra proximal to **(A)**, at an occlusive lesion **(B)**, and distal to a stenosis in the superficial femoral artery **(C)**. PSVR, peak systolic velocity ratio.

assessment with subsequent revision as necessary resulted in a secondary graft patency of 99.4% at 30 days and 98.8% at 90 days. The observed 15% intraoperative revision rate and a low (2.5%) 90-day failure/revision rate provide the rationale for routine duplex assessment to enhance early outcomes after infrainguinal vein bypass.

DUPLEX-MONITORED PERIPHERAL ANGIOPLASTY

The use of duplex ultrasound to perform and assess an endovascular procedure is a novel but proven application. Angiographic criteria for grading angioplasty site stenosis using diameter-reduction (DR) criteria are inaccurate due to presence of plaque dissection, and the absence of multiplanar image interpretation. Duplex testing is more precise in detection of PTA site stenosis. Successful endovascular therapy of femoropopliteal occlusive disease by balloon PTA (i.e., <30% residual angiogram stenosis) had duplex findings of greater than 50% stenosis (PSV >180 cm/sec; Vr >2) in 20% of limbs.[6,14] By life-table analysis, a greater than 50% duplex-detected PTA stenosis was associated with only a 15% 1-year clinical success rate compared to 84% stenosis-free patency when the postprocedural scan was normal.

Duplex scanning has been used as the sole imaging technique to perform peripheral endovascular procedures (lower limb, dialysis access). The occlusive lesion to be treated is scanned before PTA to verify its severity (PSV, velocity ratio across the stenosis) and to confirm that the site can be interrogated by duplex ultrasound (Figure 18-5). Duplex ultrasound is used to guide arterial puncture, monitor guidewire passage across the lesion, and visualize balloon angioplasty or stent deployment. The goal of duplex-monitored angioplasty is to not terminate the endovascular intervention until normal hemodynamics is verified. Pre-PTA velocity values typically indicate high-grade, pressure-reducing stenosis, with PSV of more than 300 cm/sec and end-diastolic velocity of more than 40 cm/sec. Following successful angioplasty, the PSV at the angioplasty site should be less than 180 cm/sec with Vr in the treated segment less than 2. If abnormal velocity spectra are recorded, reintervention is performed at the same procedure. Treatment options may include atherectomy, dilatation with a larger balloon, stent placement, or prolonged balloon inflation. When a lesion is judged to be maximally dilated (e.g., for PTA of vein graft stenosis) and a persistent stenosis is identified by duplex scanning, operative intervention or frequent duplex surveillance after the procedure is recommended, depending on the

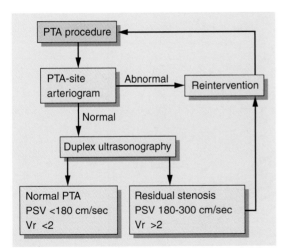

FIGURE 18-6 Algorithm of duplex-monitored angioplasty based on arteriography and duplex ultrasound findings. PSV, peak systolic velocity; PTA, percutaneous transluminal angioplasty; Vr, velocity ratio.

severity of the residual stenosis (Figure 18-6). A persistent duplex-detected stenosis at the angioplasty site has been correlated with early failure, as indicated by progression of stenosis to a velocity level similar to the primary lesion or progression to occlusion (Figure 18-7). Our experience in using duplex-monitored PTA of femoropopliteal-tibial stenosis or infrainguinal vein bypass graft stenosis resulted in reintervention for residual duplex-detected stenosis in approximately 20% of cases (balloon angioplasty, 15%; stent-angioplasty, 5%; vein graft stenosis, 20%). Additional intervention resulted in further decrease in PSV at the lesion site and resulted in more than 95% of angioplasty sites having velocity values indicating stenosis of less than 50% on initial postprocedural duplex surveillance testing.

SURVEILLANCE AFTER INTERVENTION

Failure of a peripheral arterial intervention within the first year is commonly the result of the development of myointimal hyperplasia, with failure beyond 1 year more likely caused by atherosclerotic disease progression. Myointimal hyperplasia consists of smooth muscle cell proliferation and matrix formation, producing occlusive lesions at anastomotic, vein valve, angioplasty, or endarterectomy sites that, when progressive, reduce flow and distal perfusion pressure. The development and progression of myointimal and atherosclerotic stenotic lesions can be monitored using serial duplex testing. Identification of a

progressive stenosis permits elective intervention, usually with endovascular therapy since the lesion is focal (i.e., involving a short vessel segment). Duplex ultrasound surveillance has been shown to yield superior assisted patency rates after infrainguinal vein bypass, peripheral angioplasty, and carotid intervention (endarterectomy, stent-angioplasty) compared to clinical assessment alone.[5,15-19] Surveillance is associated with a greater number of secondary procedures to repair identified high-grade (>70%-80%), typically asymptomatic stenosis. The efficacy of surveillance has been best demonstrated following infrainguinal vein bypass (78% versus 53% assisted primary patency) with lesser levels of benefit documented after prosthetic lower limb bypass grafting, dialysis access placement, or carotid intervention.[20-25] Infrainguinal prosthetic bypass graft surveillance is also recommended based on the observation of a higher diagnostic accuracy of duplex scanning (81%) compared to clinical evaluation with ankle-brachial systolic pressure index (ABI) measurement (24%) in identification of graft stenosis that warranted repair.[26] The accuracy of predicting graft failure or the need for revision was higher for femorotibial than for femoropopliteal grafts.

Timing of the initial vascular laboratory surveillance study varies with procedure type and whether an intraprocedural ultrasound study was performed and its interpretation. If the intraprocedural or predischarge ultrasound assessment was normal, surveillance should be initiated within 1 month after infrainguinal bypass or peripheral endovascular intervention, and 2 to 3 months after CEA or stent-angioplasty. Procedures with residual stenosis by arteriography or ultrasound assessment should be evaluated earlier, especially if the predischarge duplex scan identified a moderate stenosis. In general, duplex surveillance at 6-month intervals is sufficient to detect developing stenosis. Beyond 1 year, the incidence of failure due to myointimal hyperplasia decreases and surveillance intervals can be lengthened to 9 to 12 months for the detection of atherosclerotic disease progression or aneurysm formation.

INFRAINGUINAL BYPASS GRAFT SURVEILLANCE

Duplex surveillance is used to confirm graft patency, identify stenotic lesions, assess their risk for producing graft thrombosis, and, if not

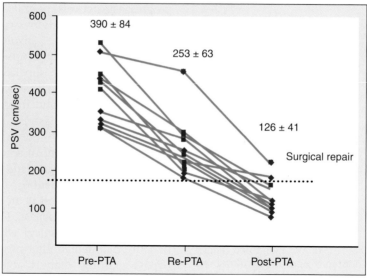

FIGURE 18-7 Peak systolic velocity (PSV) changes before reintervention, at the time of reintervention, and following balloon percutaneous transluminal angioplasty (PTA) of 11 vein graft stenoses with abnormal duplex scan despite an angiogram showing less than 30%-diameter-reducing stenosis. Reintervention resulted in PSV of less than 180 cm/sec in all but two procedures. Surgical repair was performed on one graft lesion with PSV of 235 cm/sec after balloon angioplasty.

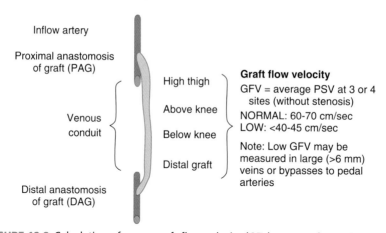

FIGURE 18-8 Calculation of mean graft flow velocity (GFV). PSV, peak systolic velocity.

repaired, monitor stenosis progression.[17] The surveillance protocol begins with questioning the patient for symptoms of recurrent limb ischemia, performing a pulse (femoral, pedal) evaluation, and measuring the ABI. Color Doppler imaging of the entire bypass, including adjacent inflow and outflow arteries, is performed, and the hemodynamics of graft flow is characterized by measurement of graft PSV along the length of the bypass. Mean systolic GFV, calculated as the average PSV recorded from three or four nonstenotic graft sites, correlates with volume flow, and if low (<40-45 cm/sec), indicates a graft at increased risk

for thrombosis (Figure 18-8). GFV may be below 40 cm/sec in large-caliber (>6-mm diameter) grafts or bypasses to a pedal or isolated tibial artery. If color Doppler imaging identifies a stenosis, measurements of PSV and Vr are obtained, as well as measurements of the lesion length and the graft/vessel diameter (Figure 18-9). Lesions with duplex-derived velocity spectra of a high-grade stenosis (PSV >300 cm/sec; end-diastolic velocity >20 cm/sec; Vr stenosis/prestenosis >3.5) correlate with greater than 70% angiogram-measured DR stenosis and should be repaired. In a prospective study, the application of these threshold

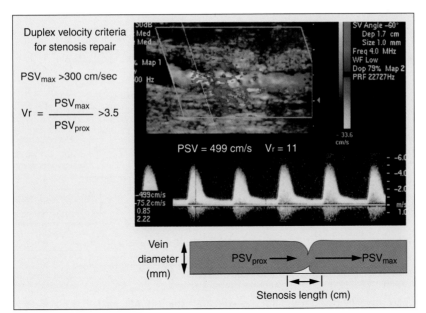

FIGURE 18-9 Measurements recorded at site(s) of color Doppler–detected vein graft stenosis. A peak systolic velocity (PSV) of more than 300 cm/sec in conjunction with a velocity ratio (Vr) of more than 3.5 are the duplex criteria for repair.

TABLE 18-4 Risk Stratification for Graft Thrombosis Based on Surveillance Data

Category*	High-Velocity Criteria		Low-Velocity Criteria		ABI Change
I (highest risk)	PSV >300 cm/sec and Vr >3.5	*and*	GFV <45 cm/sec	*and*	>0.15
II (high risk)	PSV >300 cm/sec or Vr >3.5	*and*	GFV <45 cm/sec	*or*	>0.15
III (intermediate risk)	180 < PSV <300 cm/sec or Vr >2	*and*	GFV >45 cm/sec	*and*	<0.15
IV (low risk)	PSV <180 cm/sec and Vr <2.0	*and*	GFV >45 cm/sec	*and*	<0.15

ABI, Doppler-derived ankle-brachial systolic pressure index; GFV, graft flow velocity (global or distal); PSV, duplex-derived peak systolic velocity at site of flow disturbance; Vr, PSV ratio at maximum stenosis compared to proximal graft segment without disease.
*Category I: Prompt repair of lesion is recommended—patients are hospitalized and anticoagulated before repair. Category II: Lesions are repaired electively (within 2 weeks). Category III: Lesions are observed with serial duplex examination at 4- to 6-week intervals and repaired if they progress. Category IV: Lesions are at low risk for producing graft thrombosis—follow-up every 6 months; few (<3%/yr) failures observed in this group.

criteria identified all grafts at risk for thrombosis, and only one lesion with these high-velocity criteria regressed.[27] Multiple investigators have observed an approximate 25% incidence of graft thrombosis in stenotic bypasses when a policy of no intervention was followed.[3-5,8,22]

The risk for graft thrombosis is predicted by using the combination of high- and low-velocity duplex criteria discussed previously and the ABI values (Table 18-4). In the highest-risk group (Category I), the development of a pressure-reducing stenosis has produced low flow velocity levels in the graft, which, if the level decreases below the "thrombotic threshold velocity," will result in graft thrombosis. Prompt repair of Category I lesions is recommended, while Category

II lesions (>70% stenosis but mean graft velocity >40 cm/sec) can be scheduled for elective repair within 1 to 2 weeks. A Category III moderate stenosis (PSV, 180-300 cm/sec; Vr <3.5) is not pressure or flow reducing in the resting limb. Serial scans at 4- to 6-week intervals are recommended to determine the hemodynamic course of these lesions (Figure 18-10). Among graft stenoses detected within the first 3 months of surgery, spontaneous regression of the lesion occurs in less than one-third of cases, whereas 40% either remain stable or progress (40%-50% likelihood) to high-grade stenosis. In general, serial duplex scans will determine if a lesion will progress and become "graft threatening" within 4 to 6 months of identification.[8,9,28] Important features of the

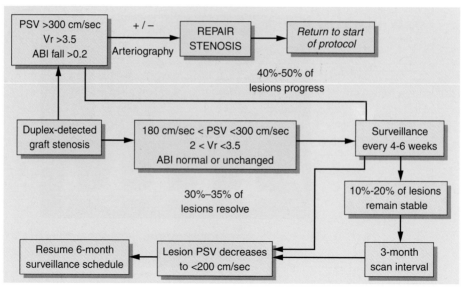

FIGURE 18-10 Duplex surveillance algorithm for detected graft stenosis. ABI, ankle-brachial index; PSV, peak systolic velocity; Vr, velocity ratio.

"graft-threatening" stenosis are its propensity to progress in severity, reduce graft flow, and form surface thrombus, events that ultimately will precipitate thrombosis. Using serial duplex testing, the one-half of Category III stenoses that do not progress can be distinguished from the progressive lesion needing repair. The majority (approximately 80%) of lower limb bypass grafts during duplex surveillance will have no abnormality identified (i.e., Category IV interpretation). Testing at 6-month intervals is generally recommended, except when the GFV is less than 40 cm/sec, signifying a "low-flow" bypass. These bypasses require a diligent search for additional inflow or outflow occlusive lesions. If none are detected, oral anticoagulation (sodium warfarin) is prescribed to maintain the prothrombin time at an international normalized ratio (INR) of 1.6 to 2.0; aspirin (325 mg/day) is also prescribed. This anticoagulation regimen is also prescribed following femoral-distal PTFE bypass grafting when a peak velocity of less than 60 cm/sec is measured in the graft by duplex scanning before discharge. The rationale for this practice is based on the concept of the "thrombotic threshold velocity," which is lower in autologous vein grafts than in prosthetic bypasses.

When duplex surveillance is performed, approximately 20% of infrainguinal vein bypasses will have a Category I or II stenosis identified within the first year after grafting. The likelihood of graft stenosis is influenced by a number of factors,

including small (<3 mm) vein caliber, a prior graft revision procedure, use of an arm vein conduit, and an initial "abnormal" duplex scan. When the early duplex scan is abnormal (i.e., identification of a moderate stenosis [PSV ≥180 cm/sec; Vr ≥2]), the clinical outcome was inferior compared with bypasses with normal duplex scans—such grafts require more frequent graft revision (51% versus 24%), require earlier revision (7 versus 11 months), and have a lower 3-year assisted primary patency (68% versus 87%).[12] Multivariate analysis confirmed a significant association between graft revision and an abnormal first postoperative duplex scan (P <.001, odds ratio >3.2). The primary patency of bypasses with "abnormal" first duplex scans is less (P <.0001) than those with no stenosis and a mean GFV less than 45 cm/sec (28% versus 61% at 3 years). Despite surveillance and reintervention for duplex-detected stenosis, this high-risk graft cohort had a lower 3-year assisted primary patency (65% versus 84%; P<.001) than bypasses with normal first duplex scans.[29]

Two-thirds of duplex-detected graft stenoses are focal (<2 cm in length) and can be treated by balloon angioplasty, including cutting balloon or cryoangioplasty. More extensive graft stenosis or early (<3months) appearing lesions are best treated by surgical repair. Stenosis-free patency at 2 years was identical for surgical (63%) and endovascular intervention (63%), and overall assisted graft patency by life-table analysis was

91% at 1 year and 80% at 3 years. Following endovascular or open surgical repair, the subsequent graft surveillance schedule is the same as after the primary grafting procedure—1 month, 4 months, then every 6 months thereafter for bypasses with Category I scans.

Based on the costs of graft surveillance, the salvage of 7% to 8% of bypasses would be cost-effective. Many vascular groups believe duplex surveillance should be "part of the service" after infrainguinal vein bypass grafting. It should be emphasized that the benefit of surveillance is highly dependent on the durability and morbidity of the procedures used to repair graft stenoses. Most series have reported a mortality of less than 0.5%, early failure rate of less than 1%, and late failure rate of less than 15% with graft revision procedures.[6]

In summary, routine duplex ultrasound surveillance of lower limb bypass grafts is recommended. Because the majority of graft abnormalities identified may be asymptomatic, appropriate criteria to recommend repair by either balloon angioplasty or open surgical repair should be used. The likelihood of graft revision varies with the vein bypass type and is increased when a graft stenosis is identified on a predischarge or early (<4 weeks) duplex scan. With time, the incidence of vein graft stenosis decreases, but because of atherosclerotic disease progression in native arteries and aneurysm formation in the vein conduit, lifelong surveillance (yearly after 3 years) is recommended.[17,30]

PERIPHERAL ANGIOPLASTY/STENT SURVEILLANCE

Late failure (>3 months) of peripheral angioplasty or stent placement can result from restenosis caused by myointimal hyperplasia within the treated segment or progression of atherosclerosis at or remote from the PTA site. On occasion, both disease processes can occur and produce recurrent limb ischemia. Identification of a hemodynamically failing PTA site or stented arterial segment does not preclude and can often precipitate endovascular reintervention, which can be potentially cost-effective in the long-term (i.e., delaying graft failure). Since angioplasty and stent failures are expensive, efforts to improve the technical success or durability of these procedures are worthwhile. Repeat PTA is generally associated with a patency prognosis identical to a primary procedure.

Timing of initial assessment following peripheral angioplasty depends on the indications for the PTA or stent procedure. For patients with claudication and palpable pulses after the angioplasty, lower limb duplex scanning and measurement of ABI within 2 weeks of the procedure is sufficient. For critical limb ischemia, duplex testing before discharge is recommended to verify DR of less than 50% at the PTA site (PSV< 180 cm/sec) and to document an increase in the ABI greater than 0.2, compared with the pre-PTA level. The duplex criteria for grading lower limb PTA site stenosis from two vascular groups indicate substantial agreement on PSV and Vr thresholds for greater than 50% DR (Table 18-5). Criteria for recurrent stent stenosis are less well studied. The University of Pittsburgh reported positive predictive values of greater than 95% for greater than 50% or greater than 80% in-stent stenosis after femoropopliteal angioplasty for Transatlantic Inter-Society Consensus (TASC) B and C lesions.[30]

Subsequent surveillance of "normal" PTA sites (i.e., less than 50% stenosis) is recommended at 3 months and then every 6 months thereafter. If the post-PTA duplex scan identifies a stenosis with a DR of 50% to 70% (PSV 180-300 cm/sec), but the ABI has increased appropriately (i.e., >0.2), a repeat scan in 1 month should be performed to assess for improvement or deterioration in functional patency. A progressing PTA site stenosis with a PSV of more than 300 cm/sec and a Vr of more than 3.5 should be considered for repeat endovascular therapy, depending on the anatomic characteristics and the arterial segment involved.

After iliac angioplasty or stent placement, surveillance should include both indirect (clinical status, ABIs, toe pressures in diabetics, and femoral artery waveform analysis) and direct (aortoiliac duplex scanning) evaluation of the treated iliac system (Figure 18-11). If the Doppler velocity waveform of the common femoral artery distal to the treated iliac segment is normal, duplex imaging of the iliac angioplasty is not necessary, as no significant hemodynamic lesion is present. The normal waveform is triphasic, or in the case of an occluded superficial femoral artery, the waveform is monophasic but the acceleration time is less than 200 msec. When the femoral pulse is abnormal or a damped, monophasic femoral artery waveform is identified, direct aortoiliac duplex imaging should be performed.

TABLE 18-5 University of South Florida Published Duplex Velocity Criteria for Classification of Angioplasty-Site Stenosis

Stenosis Category	Peak Systolic Velocity (cm/sec)	Velocity Ratio	End-Diastolic Velocity (cm/sec)	Distal Artery Waveform
<50% DR	<180	<2	NA	Normal
>50% DR; moderate	180-300	2-3.5	>0	Monophasic
>70% DR; severe	>300	>3.5	>45	Damped, monophasic, low velocity
Occluded		No flow detected		Damped, monophasic, low velocity

From Armstrong PA, Bandyk DF: Surveillance after peripheral artery transluminal angioplasty. In Zierler RE, Meissner MH, editors: *Strandness—duplex scanning in vascular disorders,* Philadelphia, 2009, Lippincott Williams & Wilkins, pp 302-327.

TABLE 18-6 University of Pittsburgh Criteria for Classification of Superficial Femoral Artery Stent Stenosis

Stenosis Category	Peak Systolic Velocity (cm/sec)	Velocity Ratio
<50% DR	<190	<1.5
>50% DR	190-275	1.5-3.5
>80% DR	>275	>3.5
Occluded	No flow detected	

Baril DT, Marone LK, Kim J, et al: Outcomes of endovascular interventions for TASC II B and C femoropopliteal lesions, *J Vasc Surg* 48:627-633, 2008.
DR, diameter reduction.

A linear array (L4-7 MHz) transducer is used to map the external iliac artery, with deeper imaging of the common iliac and aorta in obese individuals performed using a curvilinear array (3-MHz) probe. Color Doppler imaging is performed in the infrarenal aorta, along the treated and native iliac segments, and through the common femoral artery as well as the proximal deep and superficial femoral arteries. Velocity spectra of center stream flow are recorded at multiple sites using a Doppler-correction angle of 60 degrees or less. PSVs within the iliac angioplasty segments are compared with velocities in the adjacent native iliac artery, and the peak Vr is calculated at sites of stenosis. Detection of an iliac lesion by duplex scanning with a PSV of more than 300 cm/sec and a Vr of more than 2.0 indicates a hemodynamically failing iliac intervention site, and the patient should be recommended for arteriography and possible secondary endovascular intervention. Reports of duplex surveillance after iliac angioplasty have demonstrated a 20% incidence of PTA stenosis within 2 years. In a prospective study, duplex surveillance resulted in reintervention in 10% of iliac PTAs and was associated with

a secondary patency of 95% at 2 years, with 4% of the treated iliac segments thrombosed.[31] Criteria for iliac stent reintervention are less well documented but, in essence, are similar to those for primary angioplasty.

Serial clinical evaluation, measurement of limb pressures, and Doppler waveform analysis at 6-month intervals can reliably identify failing iliac artery intervention sites. Progression to occlusion is uncommon, and most recurrent lesions are amenable to endovascular therapy. If limb pressures and segmental Doppler waveforms are normal or unchanged, routine duplex scanning is avoided, which reduces overall costs. The clinical usefulness of a surveillance algorithm is predicated not only upon the ability to detect intervention sites at risk for failure but also on the success of reintervention and the overall rate of secondary patency. Failure of the treated iliac system may threaten patency of a downstream lower limb bypass graft and substantially increase the risk for limb loss. Angioplasty failure is more common in patients with multilevel atherosclerosis, and, thus, this cohort should be considered high risk and offered routine duplex ultrasound surveillance. The utility of surveillance in patients with claudication is less clear, since patency rates after PTA are better in this group than in patients with multilevel disease, and the ischemic sequelae of treatment site failure may be less significant clinically.

SURVEILLANCE AFTER CAROTID INTERVENTION

Based on prospective randomized clinical trials (Asymptomatic Carotid Atherosclerosis Study [ACAS], North American Symptomatic Carotid Endarterectomy Trial [NASCET], and Carotid Revascularization Endarterectomy versus Stenting Trial [CREST]), carotid intervention has been

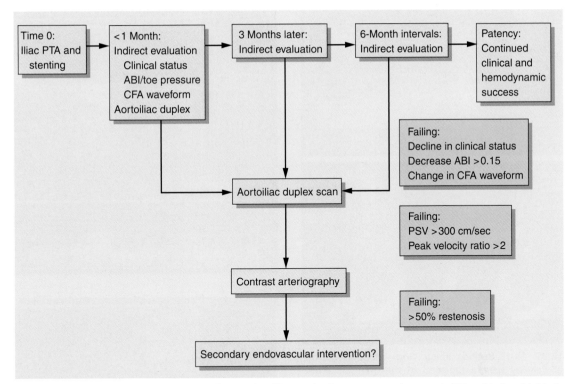

FIGURE 18-11 Algorithm for duplex surveillance after iliac angioplasty or stent placement. ABI, ankle-brachial index; CFA, common femoral artery; PSV, peak systolic velocity; PTA, percutaneous transluminal angioplasty.

shown to be more effective than medical therapy in prevention of stroke. The efficacy of CEA and carotid artery stenting (CAS) is highly dependent on completing the procedure with a low perioperative morbidity rate (<5%) and producing a durable repair with a low incidence of recurrent disease or occlusion. Multiple reports have documented a low (<1%/yr) stroke rate in patients undergoing routine duplex surveillance to identify high-grade (>70%) recurrent carotid stenosis or progression of unoperated internal carotid artery (ICA) stenosis. Duplex testing after CEA and CAS procedures has shown a varied (4%-22%) incidence of greater than 50% DR residual or recurrent stenosis.[31] In the clinical trials early restenosis (>60% DR) was identified in 7% to 11% of cases, whereas late restenosis occurred in 2% to 5% of cases. When intraoperative duplex assessment of carotid surgery is applied to ensure a precise anatomic and hemodynamic result, the rate of restenosis can be decreased further (<5% early and late combined).

Carotid repair (CEA, CAS) imaging with B-mode ultrasound has characteristic features. Following the endarterectomy, the normal intimal-media stripe is absent within the repair site and

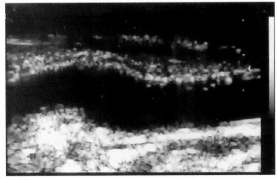

FIGURE 18-12 B-mode image of carotid endarterectomy site showing absence of intimal-media stripe in the internal and distal common carotid artery, compared with the proximal common carotid artery *(far right)*. Sutures used for artery closure are seen in anterior wall of common carotid artery closure as focal, bright reflections.

arteriotomy closure sutures appear as bright reflectors in the anterior wall (Figure 18-12). As wall remodeling occurs (weeks to months), wall thickening (neointima) develops (Figure 18-13), but its clinical importance is minimal unless associated with lumen reduction and an increase in PSV. Recurrent stenoses at the site of primary closure of the carotid artery are often easily corrected by placement of a synthetic or vein patch

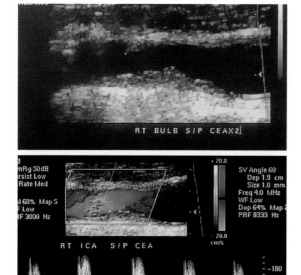

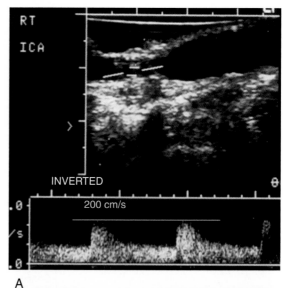

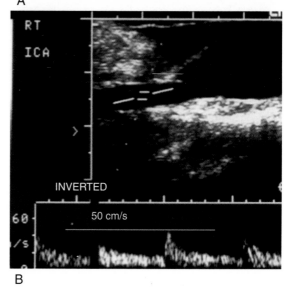

FIGURE 18-13 B-mode image *(top)* and pulsed Doppler velocity spectra *(bottom)* of the internal carotid artery (ICA) with recurrent stenosis caused by myointimal hyperplasia. A peak systolic velocity of 218 cm/sec indicates a 50% to 79% diameter-reducing stenosis. CEA, carotid endarterectomy.

(Figure 18-14). After CAS, the stent is easily seen with ultrasound (Figure 18-15). Slight lumen narrowing may persist at the ends of the stent, but these anatomic changes should not result in significant velocity elevation. Typically, blood flow is laminar or only slightly disturbed within both CEA and CAS sites. However, increased PSVs are very common at the site of stent placement despite the absence of any measurable lesion.[32]

Abnormal postendarterectomy findings include flow disturbances (usually caused by an intimal flap or retained plaque), stenosis, and occlusion. Intimal flaps and retained plaque are immediately apparent postoperatively and should not be encountered on a follow-up basis if intraoperative sonography was performed. Typically, intimal flaps occur at the distal end of the endarterectomy, where the cut edge of the intima is subject to dislodgement by the flow stream moving cephalad. This elevated intima can cause tremendous flow disturbance and may ultimately lead to restenosis or thrombosis. Myointimal hyperplasia (see Figure 18-13) is a delayed complication that develops over a period of months after CEA or CAS (usually within the first 2 years). This process can result in

FIGURE 18-14 **A,** Duplex examination shows a recurrent stenosis following endarterectomy. **B,** The stenosis and associated blood flow abnormality are corrected following placement of a patch closure.

either focal or diffuse narrowing at the endarterectomy/angioplasty site, and is associated with elevation of flow velocity and poststenotic flow disturbance. Velocity criteria for stenosis grading are presented below. Additional abnormal duplex findings may be encountered post-CAS, including malposition of the stent and separation of the stent from the vessel wall, which can be seen immediately following stent deployment.

The natural history of recurrent internal carotid stenosis caused by myointimal hyperplasia (smooth muscle and fibrous overgrowth of

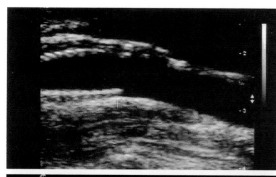

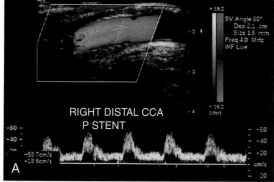

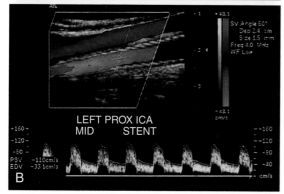

FIGURE 18-15 **A** and **B,** Duplex scan following carotid stent angioplasty. Stents are easily visualized. Note the close apposition of the stent to the artery wall. Velocity spectra indicate nondisturbed (laminar) flow conditions and normal carotid systolic velocity. CCA, common carotid artery; ICA, internal carotid artery.

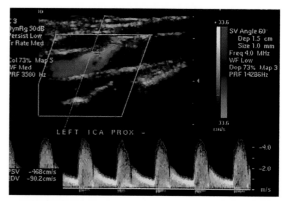

FIGURE 18-16 Duplex scan of the proximal internal carotid artery (ICA) showing a high-grade (>75%) recurrent carotid stenosis caused by myointimal hyperplasia. Peak systolic velocity, 468 cm/sec; end-diastolic velocity, 90 cm/sec.

the tissue layer that replaces the intima following carotid intervention) is thought to be associated with a lower risk for stroke or occlusion, as compared to atherosclerosis, and some early postoperative lesions (10%) have demonstrated regression on serial duplex scans. These lesions occur within the first 3 years; lesions identified after this time frame are more apt to resemble atherosclerotic plaque, with abundant collagen, foam cells, and calcium deposits. High-grade ICA restenosis (>75% DR; PSV >300 cm/sec, and end-diastolic velocity >125-140 cm/sec),

whether from recurrent myointimal hyperplasia or primary atherosclerosis, is associated with an increased risk for ICA thrombosis and late stroke (Figure 18-16). Considering the potential for recurrence of carotid stenosis, duplex surveillance after CEA or CAS is highly recommended (Figure 18-17). Testing intervals of 1 year for less than 50% DR stenosis and every 6 months for greater than 50% DR stenosis appear to be sufficient to detect development of restenosis and follow its progression. In the majority of patients, however, the main reason for duplex surveillance is to identify progression of contralateral ICA stenosis of more than 50%, rather than to detect restenosis of the CEA or CAS site. An early duplex scan of the CEA or CAS site (other than intraoperative) at 1 to 3 months is useful to exclude residual stenosis. High-grade ICA stenosis (PSV >300 cm/sec; diastolic velocity >125 cm/sec; ICA/common carotid artery ratio >4) should prompt consideration for reintervention, especially if the stenosis is rapidly progressing, is longer than 1 cm, or occurs following CAS. The majority of patients demonstrate no stenosis after CEA/CAS, and if less than 50% DR contralateral ICA stenosis is present, duplex surveillance every 1 to 2 years is adequate (see Figure 18-17). Surveillance every 6 months is indicated in patients with residual or recurrent ipsilateral stenosis and contralateral ICA occlusion. The yield (i.e., intervention rate for severe stenosis) of duplex surveillance after CEA (5%-7%) is less than after CAS (10%) or infrainguinal vein bypass (15%-20%).[33] Progression of contralateral disease, however, is five times more common.

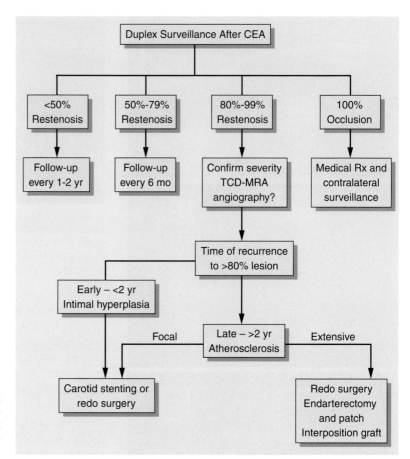

FIGURE 18-17 Algorithm for duplex surveillance after carotid endarterectomy (CEA). MRA, magnetic resonance angiography; TCD, transcranial Doppler.

A policy of duplex ultrasound surveillance and reintervention for high-grade stenosis is associated with a low (<1%/yr) incidence of ipsilateral hemispheric, disabling stroke. The development of hemispheric symptoms in the presence of ICA stenosis with a DR of more than 50%, or asymptomatic disease progression to a high-grade stenosis (>75%-80% DR; end-diastolic velocity >125-140 cm/sec) should prompt a recommendation of intervention in appropriate patients.

CONCLUSIONS

The outcome of arterial intervention can be improved by the application of duplex ultrasound assessment. When used at the time of the procedure, testing can identify residual stenosis, lumen thrombus, or other conditions that increase the likelihood of procedure failure. With recognition, immediate correction by surgery or endovascular intervention is possible, or additional imaging (i.e., arteriography) can be performed to further define and treat the abnormality. The criteria for reintervention vary with the procedure type, but Doppler velocity criteria indicating arterial stenosis of more than 70% are generally used to select lesions to be corrected. The majority of arterial repairs are followed by normal duplex studies, and these patients, who have a clinically predictable higher success rate, can be restudied less frequently than when testing indicates an abnormality. Lesions that reduce flow increase the likelihood for repair failure and have Doppler velocity findings of severe stenosis—high PSV (>300 cm/sec), turbulent flow, and damped distal velocity waveform. Interventions to correct these lesions should also be evaluated using duplex ultrasound, since clinical assessment and arteriography are imperfect measures of technical adequacy. All patients undergoing peripheral interventions should be enrolled in a surveillance program that includes duplex ultrasound. These surveillance programs are cost-effective by decreasing the number of failures, despite the expense of serial examinations at 3- to 6-month intervals and the performing of secondary procedures to repair progressive, severe duplex-detected stenosis.

REFERENCES

1. Bandyk DF, et al: Intraoperative duplex scanning of arterial reconstructions: Fate of repaired and unrepaired defects, *J Vasc Surg* 20:426–433, 1994.
2. Bandyk DF, et al: Nature and management of duplex abnormalities encountered during infrainguinal vein bypass grafting, *J Vasc Surg* 24:430–438, 1996.
3. Bandyk DF, et al: Monitoring functional patency of in situ saphenous vein bypasses: The impact of a surveillance protocol and elective revision, *J Vasc Surg* 9:284–296, 1989.
4. Armstrong PA, Bandyk DF: Surveillance after peripheral artery transluminal angioplasty. In Zierler RE, Meissner MH, editors: *Strandness's Duplex Scanning in Vascular Disorders*, Philadelphia, PA, 2009, Lippincott Williams & Wilkins, pp 302–327.
5. Tinder CN, et al: Duplex surveillance after infrainguinal vein bypass may be enhanced by identification of characteristics predictive of graft stenosis development, *J Vasc Surg* 48:613–618, 2008.
6. Idu MM, et al: Impact of a color flow duplex surveillance program on infrainguinal graft patency: A five-year experience, *J Vasc Surg* 17:42–53, 1993.
7. Kundell A, et al: Femoropopliteal graft patency is improved by an intensive surveillance program: A prospective-randomized study, *J Vasc Surg* 21:26–34, 1995.
8. Wixon CL, et al: An economic appraisal of lower extremity bypass graft maintenance, *J Vasc Surg* 32:89–95, 2000.
9. Spijkerboer AM, et al: Iliac artery stenoses after percutaneous transluminal angioplasty: Follow-up with duplex ultrasonography, *J Vasc Surg* 23:691–697, 1996.
10. Johnson BL, et al: Intraoperative duplex monitoring of infrainguinal vein bypass procedures, *J Vasc Surg* 31:678–690, 2000.
11. Mills JL, Fujitani RM, Taylor SM: The contribution of routine intraoperative completion arteriography to early graft patency, *Am J Surg* 164:506–511, 1992.
12. Miller A, et al: Comparison of angioscopy and angiography for monitoring infrainguinal vein bypass grafts: Results of prospective randomized trial, *J Vasc Surg* 17:382–398, 1993.
13. Dalman RL, Harris EJ, Zarins CK: Is completion arteriography mandatory after reversed-vein bypass grafting? *J Vasc Surg* 23:637–644, 1996.
14. Mewissen MW, et al: The role of duplex scanning versus angiography in predicting outcome after balloon angioplasty in the femoropopliteal artery, *J Vasc Surg* 15:860–864, 1992.
15. Johnson BL, Avino AJ, Bandyk DF: Duplex-monitored angioplasty of peripheral artery and infrainguinal vein graft stenosis. In Whittemore AD, editor: *Advances in Vascular Surgery*, Vol 8, St. Louis, 2000, Mosby, pp 83–95.
16. Gupta AK, et al: Natural history of infrainguinal vein graft stenosis relative to bypass grafting technique, *J Vasc Surg* 25:211–225, 1997.
17. Mills JL, et al: The origin of infrainguinal vein graft stenosis: A prospective study based on duplex surveillance, *J Vasc Surg* 21:16–25, 1995.
18. Bandyk DF: Infrainguinal vein bypass graft surveillance. How to do it, when to intervene, and is it cost-effective? *J Am Coll Surg* 194:S40–S52, 2002.
19. Moody AP, Gould DA, Harris PL: Vein graft surveillance improves patency in femoropopliteal bypass, *Eur J Vasc Surg* 4:117–120, 1990.
20. Mills JL, et al: The importance of routine surveillance of distal bypass grafts with duplex scanning: A study of 379 reversed vein grafts, *J Vasc Surg* 12:379–389, 1990.
21. Spijkerboer AM, et al: Evaluation of femoropopliteal arteries with duplex ultrasound after angioplasty. Can we predict results at one year? *Eur J Vasc Endovasc Surg* 12:418–423, 1996.
22. Tielbeek AV, et al: The value of duplex surveillance after endovascular intervention for femoropopliteal obstructive disease, *Eur J Vasc Endovasc Surg* 12:145–150, 1996.
23. Bandyk DF, Chauvapun JP: Duplex surveillance can be worthwhile after arterial intervention, *Perspect Vasc Surg Endovasc Ther* 19:354–359, 2007.
24. Cluley SR, et al: Transcutaneous ultrasonography can be used to guide and monitor balloon angioplasty, *J Vasc Surg* 17:23–31, 1993.
25. Ramaswami G, et al: Duplex controlled angioplasty, *Eur J Vasc Surg* 8:457–463, 1994.
26. Calligaro KD, et al: Duplex ultrasonography to diagnose failing arterial prosthetic grafts, *Surgery* 120:455–459, 1996.
27. Westerband A, et al: Prospective validation of threshold criteria for intervention in infrainguinal vein grafts undergoing duplex surveillance, *Ann Vasc Surg* 11:44–48, 1997.
28. Caps T, et al: Vein graft lesions: Time of onset and rate of progression, *J Vasc Surg* 22:466–475, 1995.
29. Erickson CA, et al: Ongoing vascular laboratory surveillance is essential to maximize long-term in situ saphenous vein bypass patency, *J Vasc Surg* 23:18–24, 1996.
30. Baril DT, et al: Outcomes of endovascular interventions for TASC II B and C femoropopliteal lesions, *J Vasc Surg* 48:627–633, 2008.
31. Back MR, et al: Utility of duplex surveillance following iliac artery angioplasty and primary stenting, *J Endovasc Ther* 8:629–637, 2001.
32. Lal BK, et al: Duplex ultrasound velocity criteria for the stented carotid artery, *J Vasc Surg* 47:63–73, 2008.
33. Roth SM, et al: A rational algorithm for duplex surveillance following carotid endarterectomy, *J Vasc Surg* 30:453–460, 1999.

ULTRASOUND IN THE ASSESSMENT AND MANAGEMENT OF ARTERIAL EMERGENCIES

19

BRIAN J. BURKE, MD, RVT

Vascular emergencies require a prompt diagnosis, as timely intervention is often critically important. Delays of minutes or hours in management may mean the difference between life and death, or limb preservation or loss. Ultrasound plays an important role in the diagnosis and management of many vascular emergencies.

Since vascular emergencies often are managed nonoperatively, an accurate diagnosis is critical to appropriate patient triage. Several diagnostic modalities can be applied in such cases. In addition to duplex ultrasound, other modalities include computed tomographic angiography, magnetic resonance angiography, digital subtraction angiography, and intravascular ultrasound. The advantages of ultrasound for emergencies include ready availability, portability, speed, and high temporal and spatial resolution. A relative disadvantage is the acoustic barrier presented by bone; air in lung, soft tissue, or bowel; and tissue edema; these limit the use of ultrasound at the skull base, in the chest, deep pelvis, and injured extremities with extensive tissue disruption. Depiction of regional arterial supply through collateral pathways associated with an injured vessel is also less complete with ultrasound than with angiography. The choice of ultrasound as a diagnostic modality reflects these factors as well as the clinical information needed to direct management.

RUPTURED ABDOMINAL AORTIC ANEURYSM

An aneurysm is a localized dilatation of an artery, with an increase in diameter of greater than 50% of the normal size. Abdominal aortic aneurysms (AAAs) are most commonly encountered in the infrarenal region. In general, AAAs occur when the maximal anteroposterior diameter is greater than 3 cm. As the population ages, the incidence of AAAs is increasing. Approximately 1.5 million

Americans have AAAs, and 200,000 are diagnosed each year.[1] Most AAAs are asymptomatic and are detected during routine physical examinations or radiologic procedures for other problems. Elective repair is reserved for subjects with AAAs of at least 5 cm in diameter, and postoperative survival is approximately 95%. Symptomatic aneurysms may result in abdominal, flank, or back pain, distal embolization, thrombosis, or rupture. The latter complication is usually fatal if untreated; surgical repair carries a 30% to 65% survival rate. Success is highly dependent on rapid diagnosis and transport to the operating room.[2]

Ultrasonography is often used as the initial procedure for diagnosis of AAAs. It is also used for screening and serial measurement of AAA size. When aneurysms rupture, only 50% of patients present with the "classic" triad of abdominal or back pain, hypotension, and pulsatile abdominal mass. The clinical diagnosis may, therefore, pose a challenge, particularly in patients without a known history of AAA. An accurate imaging diagnosis of retroperitoneal hematoma in the presence of AAA enables prompt initiation of surgical treatment.

Although noncontrast computed tomography (CT) is also useful for this purpose, ultrasound is more expeditious in these potentially unstable patients. Ultrasound diagnosis of an abdominal aneurysm has a sensitivity of 98% and specificity of 95% in the setting of abdominal pain and hemodynamic instability.[3] Although active extravasation is never brisk enough to demonstrate by Doppler ultrasound, the resultant hematoma provides evidence of rupture (Figure 19-1). Initially, intramural hemorrhage may be visible as an echogenic crescent within the aneurysmal wall. Following rupture, blood initially accumulates in the para-aortic space, extending toward the flanks via the pararenal space. Hemorrhage may track along the course of the iliac arteries to the extraperitoneal spaces of the pelvis (Figure 19-2).

324

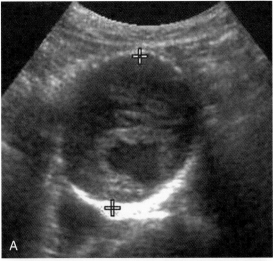

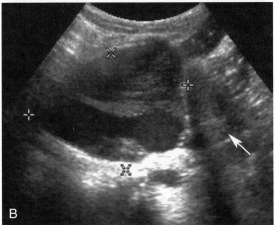

FIGURE 19-1 Ruptured aortic aneurysm. Transverse **(A)** and oblique **(B)** views of aortic aneurysm *(cursors)* with abundant mural thrombus and a small periaortic hematoma *(arrow)*.

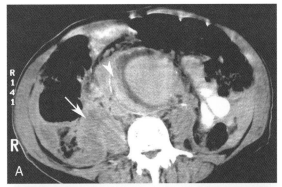

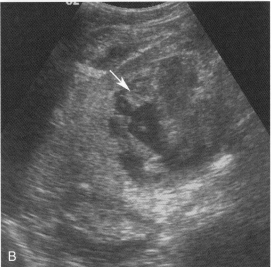

FIGURE 19-2 Retroperitoneal hematoma. **A,** Computed tomographic image shows a large abdominal aortic aneurysm with intramural *(arrowhead)* and retroperitoneal *(arrow)* hemorrhage. **B,** Ultrasound shows a large retroperitoneal hematoma in the left flank, infiltrating the psoas muscle *(arrow)* and distorting tissue planes.

Anterior extension may transgress the posterior peritoneum, resulting in hemoperitoneum.

When the patient presents with abdominal pain, the operator may be reluctant to use probe pressure to visualize the aorta for fear of provoking or exacerbating rupture. Although this is rarely a practical concern, the use of a coronal approach from the left flank avoids trapping the aneurysm between the transducer and the spine. In addition, this approach frequently provides improved visualization of the aorta by circumventing overlying bowel gas.

Nonetheless, conventional sonography has some limitations in imaging patients with a ruptured aneurysm because retroperitoneal hematoma is not always readily apparent, and the rupture itself is not directly visualized. In the

appropriate clinical setting, contrast-enhanced sonography can be performed in less time than is required for contrast-enhanced CT. Findings associated with aneurysm rupture in these studies include delayed or protracted aortic lumen opacification, contrast leakage through luminal thrombus or around the aneurysm, and dependent contrast pooling around the aneurysm.[4] There are no large studies evaluating the diagnostic accuracy of ultrasound in patients with suspected acute rupture of an AAA.

Aortic dissection may be encountered as an alternative diagnosis in patients with a clinical presentation suggesting aneurysm rupture. Although ultrasound is not a primary diagnostic modality, since it cannot reveal the full extent of dissection in the thorax, the characteristic intimal flap and altered blood flow pattern are readily visible on

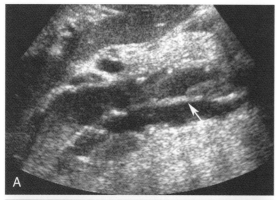

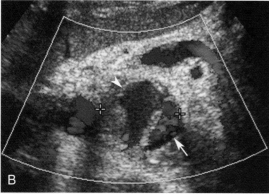

FIGURE 19-3 Aortic dissection. Sagittal **(A)** image of the abdominal aorta shows an echogenic intimal flap *(arrow)*. Transverse color view **(B)** clearly distinguished the patent true lumen *(arrow)* from the thrombosed false lumen *(arrowhead)*.

abdominal sonography and can lead to appropriate workup and treatment (Figure 19-3).[5] In a recent study, the use of contrast-enhanced sonography increased the sensitivity for abdominal aortic dissection to 97%, from 68% for combined gray scale and duplex sonography.[6] Additional details about aortic aneurysm and dissection are presented in Chapter 27.

CAROTID ARTERY STENOSIS

Symptomatic carotid artery stenosis is manifested by transient ischemic attacks (TIAs) or stroke (cerebrovascular accident, CVA). Neurologically unstable patients in whom there is no evidence of intracranial hemorrhage are potential candidates for emergency carotid endarterectomy. These cases include patients presenting with crescendo TIAs, stroke in evolution, fluctuating or fixed neurologic deficits caused by acute carotid artery thrombosis, and free-floating thrombus. In these cases, rapid sonographic evaluation of the

carotid bifurcation can result in timely intervention to prevent stroke or death.

Sonographic detection and quantification of carotid stenosis in the emergency setting (i.e., progressive neurologic deficit) is similar to the nonacute setting and is described in Chapter 9. It is important to distinguish acute carotid thrombosis from stable (chronic) carotid occlusion. Whereas revascularization of a chronic occlusion is generally contraindicated, timely intervention may avoid or limit neurologic sequelae in cases of acute thrombosis.

Acute thrombosis may occur as a complication of endarterectomy or stenting, or it may represent acute progression of carotid stenosis. The thrombus is usually heterogeneously echogenic (Figure 19-4). The vessel lumen is of normal caliber or slightly expanded, as opposed to chronic occlusion, which may result in luminal narrowing or obliteration.[7] Pulsations may be observed in the vessel wall, which retains its normal compliance. Swirling, sludgelike flow may be observed in the carotid bulb at the interface of the thrombosed and patent lumen. Spectral waveforms assume a high-impedance, hammerlike, or to-and-fro configuration proximal to the thrombus. Internalization of the external carotid artery waveform is uncommonly seen with acute thrombosis due to insufficient time to develop collateral pathways.

If the thrombus is nonocclusive, its free edge may oscillate back and forth in the bloodstream; the "free-floating" thrombus has a characteristic appearance at real-time examination (Figure 19-5).[8] The risk for embolization is related to the extent of attachment of the base of the thrombus to the vessel wall; this can be depicted with the aid of color Doppler or B-flow imaging.[9]

When patients with acute carotid thrombosis undergo thrombectomy or revascularization, intraoperative ultrasound is a useful adjunctive technique. Scanning directly over the vessel in the exposed surgical field yields superb resolution of the vessel wall. It is possible to visualize small intimal flaps, ulcerative plaques, or retained thrombi, leading to immediate surgical revision, which favorably impacts patency rates.[10]

CAROTID ARTERY DISSECTION

There are two types of carotid artery dissection. The "primary" dissection is in the cervical internal carotid resulting from hemorrhage into the

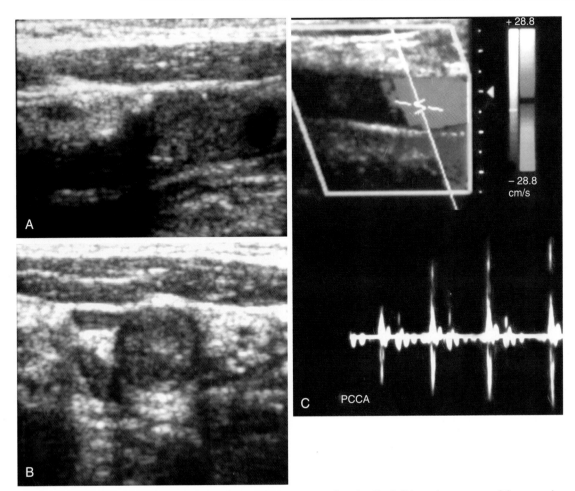

FIGURE 19-4 Carotid thrombosis. Shortly after endarterectomy, longitudinal **(A)** and transverse **(B)** scans show hypoechoic thrombus filling the common carotid artery. Duplex scan **(C)** shows "water-hammer" waveforms at the interface of the patent lumen and acute thrombus. PCCA, proximal common carotid artery.

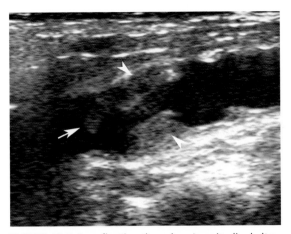

FIGURE 19-5 Free-floating thrombus. Longitudinal ultrasound in the distal common carotid artery shows nonocclusive thrombi *(arrowheads)* with a nonadherent tail *(arrow)* seen to move back and forth in the bloodstream on real-time examination.

wall of the carotid artery and extending distally to the carotid canal in the petrous portion of the temporal bone. The second type of carotid dissection usually extends into the common carotid artery from a type A dissection of the aortic arch.

We will be discussing the primary type of internal carotid artery dissection where the media is the most common location for hemorrhage, with extension into the subintimal or subadventitial layers. The former may result in thrombosis of the vessel; aneurysms may occur from the latter. Spontaneous dissections may be associated with type IV Ehler-Danlos syndrome, Marfan syndrome, fibromuscular dysplasia, and cystic medial necrosis; however, most spontaneous dissections are idiopathic. They often happen in previously healthy individuals younger than 40 years.[11] Most traumatic carotid dissections result from motor vehicle accidents in which the neck is hyperextended, compressing the carotid artery against the atlas or second cervical vertebra. Blunt trauma, penetrating injuries, and catheter injuries during arteriography also cause traumatic dissections.[12]

In the United States, the annual incidence of symptomatic carotid artery dissection is 2.6 per 100,000. The actual incidence may be higher, since many episodes may be asymptomatic or cause only minor transient symptoms, thereby remaining undiagnosed. Morbidity from carotid artery dissection varies in severity from transient neurologic deficit to permanent deficit and death. Dissection of the intracranial portion of the internal carotid artery, although rare, is associated with a 75% mortality rate. The male-to-female ratio of carotid dissection is 1.5:1. The mean age for extracranial internal carotid artery dissection is 40 years; intracranial dissections are more common in patients 20 to 30 years old. Approximately 20% of strokes in young patients are caused by carotid artery and vertebral artery dissections in the neck, compared with 2.5% in older patients.

Patients with carotid dissection often complain of neck pain, headache, tinnitus, or a focal neurologic deficit. Horner syndrome, transient monocular blindness, neck swelling, and cranial nerve palsy may also result. The onset of symptoms may be hours to days after the dissection occurs.[13]

Duplex scanning of patients with suspected carotid dissection can be performed quickly in the emergency department to make this diagnosis. Typical findings with duplex scanning include a patent carotid bifurcation with tapering of the internal carotid artery, leading to a distal stenosis or occlusion (Figure 19-6). Intimal flaps or membranes may be seen (Figure 19-7), and spectral analysis reveals high-resistance waveforms with reduced flow velocity in the internal carotid artery.[14] Ultrasound demonstrates a sensitivity of 70% for the diagnosis of spontaneous dissection in the cervical carotid artery, and 75% to 86% in the vertebral artery.[15] Follow-up scanning can be useful to monitor vessel recanalization and to determine the duration of anticoagulation therapy.

The false lumen may be thrombosed or patent. If acutely thrombosed, the intimal flap may bulge in convex fashion toward the true lumen. A patent false lumen usually exhibits flow characteristics differing from the true lumen, unless a second intimal tear downstream reestablishes continuity between the true and false lumen.

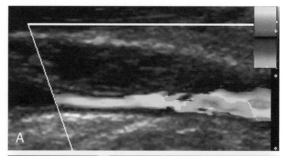
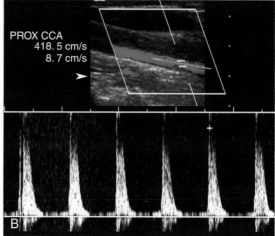

PROX CCA
418.5 cm/s
8.7 cm/s

FIGURE 19-6 Common carotid artery (CCA) dissection. **A,** The true lumen tapers distally, compressed by the thrombosed false lumen. **B,** High-velocity, high-impedance flow reflects the degree of stenosis caused by the displaced intimal flap.

More commonly, the false lumen demonstrates low peak velocity with reversal of flow during diastole (to-and-fro pattern).

If the site of dissection is near the skull base, it may not be visible with ultrasound. In such cases, altered hemodynamics in the internal carotid artery proximal to the dissection (reduced peak velocity, increased impedance) constitute indirect evidence for the diagnosis in a patient with a compatible clinical presentation. Magnetic resonance imaging will typically show the presence of acute thrombus as a zone of increased T1 signals in the wall of the internal carotid artery. Magnetic resonance or CT angiography can confirm the presence of luminal narrowing and establish the extent of dissection.

ACUTE LOWER EXTREMITY ISCHEMIA

Acute ischemia of the lower extremity is caused by an embolism from the heart or a more proximal arterial location, or from acute thrombosis of the affected artery. Approximately 80% of

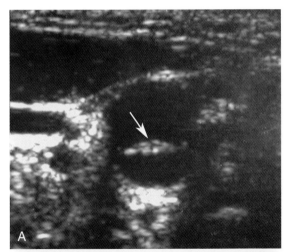

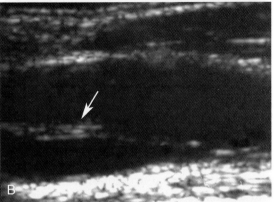

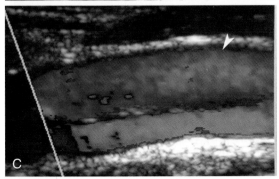

FIGURE 19-7 Carotid dissection. Transverse **(A)** and longitudinal **(B)** images demonstrate an echogenic intimal flap *(arrows)*. Color image **(C)** shows retrograde diastolic flow in the patent false lumen *(arrowhead)*.

peripheral arterial emboli originate in the heart, often secondary to myocardial infarction, endocarditis, or arrhythmia. An embolism can also originate from any artery outside the heart, and the abdominal aorta is the most common source of artery-to-artery emboli. Atherosclerotic plaques and small aneurysms of the aorta or iliac arteries account for approximately 70% of these emboli. More distal lower extremity arteries

(e.g., popliteal) account for most of the other cases of emboli of arterial origin. Duplex imaging of infrainguinal arterial occlusive disease has become popular in elective revascularization cases, leading some practitioners to abandon angiography.[16] The same arguments supporting preferential use of ultrasonography in acute situations will undoubtedly lead to its use in cases of acute arterial thrombosis.

Detection of lower extremity aneurysms that may be the source of emboli is readily accomplished with ultrasound. The upper limit of the normal arterial diameter is 10 mm in the common femoral artery, 8 mm in the superficial femoral artery, and 5 to 6 mm in the popliteal artery. Fusiform enlargement is often accompanied by vessel tortuosity and may be multifocal. Popliteal aneurysms are associated with AAA in 30% to 35% of cases. Intraluminal plaque and thrombus with an irregular luminal contour and heterogeneous echogenicity may be of higher risk for embolization than smooth, homogeneous plaque without thrombus (Figure 19-8).[17] Acute limb-threatening ischemia may be the initial presentation of popliteal aneurysms; although the diagnosis may be missed by contrast angiography, the aneurysm is readily detected with duplex sonography.[18]

In acute arterial thrombosis, nonduplex physiologic testing (i.e., segmental arterial pressure measurement and volume plethysmography) is useful to confirm the presence of a flow-limiting lesion, and this test can often indicate the involved vascular segment (Figure 19-9). Duplex scanning can then be directed to the area of suspicion, and the site of embolization can be identified (Figure 19-10). For example, when segmental pressure measurements demonstrate a pressure gradient across the knee, duplex scanning should begin above this level, in the mid–superficial femoral artery. The examination should proceed distally to the point of obstruction. Color Doppler is essential for surveying long segments of vessel for the presence of flow and to identify the disturbed color pattern and collateral branches at the site of occlusion. Sampling of the Doppler spectral waveforms at intervals along the vessel may demonstrate characteristic changes in the arterial waveform. Proximal to the occlusion, the waveform shows increased impedance and may convert from triphasic to biphasic flow, with flow reversal in end diastole. Downstream from the occlusion, waveforms are typically

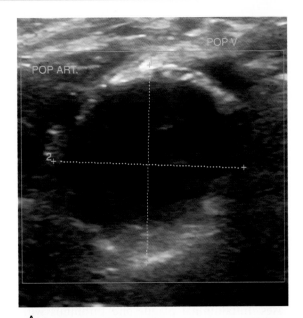

A

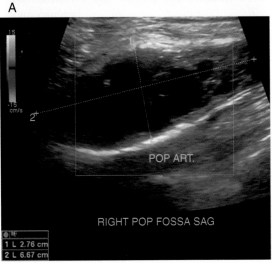

B

FIGURE 19-8 Popliteal aneurysm. Transverse **(A)** and longitudinal **(B)** images of 2.8-cm aneurysm with irregular intimal plaque and thrombus.

monophasic and often low resistance, with diminished peak velocities. Caution is necessary with such waveform analysis in patients with significant atherosclerosis, as serial-segment or long-segment stenosis upstream and downstream from the occlusion may exert unpredictable effects on regional hemodynamics.

After an acute embolic occlusion, the artery may undergo retrograde thrombosis to the nearest proximal branch that provides a collateral pathway around the obstruction. It is seldom feasible to track the entire course of the small, tortuous collateral vessels, but when following the thrombosed arterial trunk with color Doppler, one can often detect the point at which arterial patency is reconstituted. Tracking the thrombosed artery is complicated by the lack of color signal within its lumen, but the accompanying vein (or in the calf, paired veins) provides a useful landmark. Small vessel size, as well as extensive atheromatous disease and collaterals in patients with chronic ischemia, limit the use of duplex scanning in the infrapopliteal arteries. However, the distal anterior and posterior tibial arteries are readily accessible to duplex sampling due to their constant superficial location.[19,20]

Patients with failed infrainguinal bypass grafts may present acutely with lower extremity ischemia. The cause of graft failure usually relates to stenosis within or adjacent to the graft, impairing blood flow and ultimately leading to thrombosis. The usual causes of graft failure are related to the age of the graft. In the early postoperative period (<1 month), technical problems with vein selection or anastomosis construction are often implicated. At graft maturity (1 month to 2 years), the development of fibrointimal hyperplasia at vein valves and anastomoses leads to stenoses. In the later period (>2 years), graft failure is usually due to progression of atherosclerotic disease as well as fibrointimal hyperplasia in the adjacent native circulation. A program of duplex graft surveillance is beneficial in improving graft patency by detecting asymptomatic lesions before graft thrombosis. In one study of 101 infrainguinal vein grafts, no grafts with normal duplex examinations progressed to occlusion, while 54% of grafts with abnormal duplex examinations proceeded to failure.[21] Correction of asymptomatic lesions before graft failure improves secondary patency rates.[22]

When patients present with acute ischemia, duplex scanning often reveals graft thrombosis with absence of flow (Figure 19-11). When flow is present within the graft, average peak velocity of less than 45 cm/sec and interval decrease (compared with prior examinations) in ankle-brachial index of more than 0.15 are signs of impending graft failure (Figure 19-12). Other graft complications detectable by duplex scanning include arterial-venous shunting through unligated vein branches, anastomotic pseudoaneurysm, and perigraft abscess.

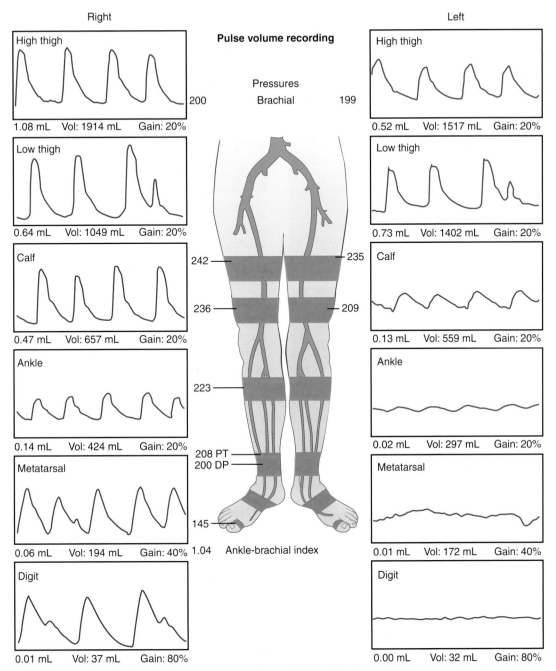

FIGURE 19-9 Atheroembolic occlusion. Lower extremity arterial physiologic examination on a patient presenting with cold left foot. The ankle-brachial index is unobtainable due to inaudible pulses in the left foot. Pulse volume recordings show progressively diminishing amplitude and pulsatility below the left knee. DP, dorsalis pedis; PT, posterior tibial.

FEMORAL PSEUDOANEURYSM

Thousands of diagnostic coronary and peripheral arterial catheterization procedures are performed daily in the United States. The most common entry route is the femoral artery. Femoral pseudoaneurysms occur in up to 0.2% of diagnostic and 8% of interventional procedures.[23] A pseudoaneurysm, or false aneurysm, is a confined collection of thrombus and blood associated with disruption of all three layers of an artery wall. This occurs at the puncture site as a complication of percutaneous arterial catheterization.

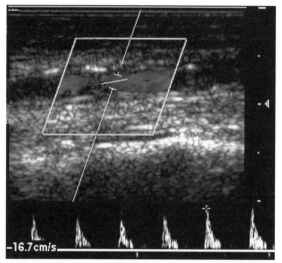

A

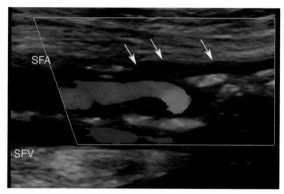

FIGURE 19-11 Bypass graft failure. Color flow is seen in the proximal superficial femoral artery (SFA), but echogenic thrombus occludes the proximal segment of this autologous vein graft (arrows). SFV, superficial femoral vein.

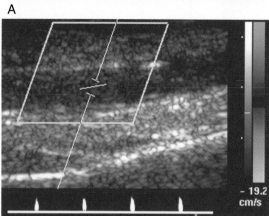

B

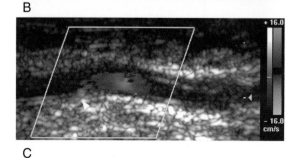

C

FIGURE 19-10 Atheroembolic occlusion. High-impedance, low-velocity flow is present in the posterior tibial artery (A) proximal to an occlusive thrombus (B). A small collateral vessel (arrowhead) is seen just above the thrombus (C).

Pseudoaneurysms differ from true aneurysms in that the latter contain all three histologic layers of the arterial wall, whereas pseudoaneurysms contain none of these layers.

Modern duplex imaging makes the diagnosis of femoral artery pseudoaneurysm routine.[24] The pseudoaneurysm usually arises from the superficial aspect of the artery at the site of puncture. This occurs most often at the level of the common femoral artery, but occasionally puncture occurs above the inguinal ligament in the external iliac artery or below the bifurcation in the superficial or deep femoral artery. The pseudoaneurysm lumen is connected to the underlying artery by a cylindrical neck—variable in length and diameter—which takes the course of the needle tract. Color Doppler is useful for detection of the pseudoaneurysm and its neck. A Doppler spectral waveform showing bidirectional to-and-fro flow within the neck is diagnostic (Figure 19-13).

The pseudoaneurysm lumen is often 1 to 3 cm in diameter, although large pseudoaneurysms can exceed 5 cm, and the presence of a string or series of pseudoaneurysms can be seen (Figure 19-14). Sometimes flow within a needle tract is detectable by color Doppler imaging without an associated lumen.[25] A swirling pattern of blood flow in the lumen often appears on color Doppler imaging as a characteristic "yin-yang" sign (Figure 19-15). The lumen may be partially thrombosed at the time of diagnosis.

Because of the potential risk for expansion, pseudoaneurysms are usually treated at the time of diagnosis. Since initial description of the technique in 1992, ultrasound-guided compression repair has been efficacious and safe.[26] Approximately 75% of femoral pseudoaneurysms are successfully thrombosed with this method; success rate is diminished in anticoagulated patients. Prolonged compression (up to or exceeding 1 hour) may be necessary and is tedious for the operator and painful for the patient.

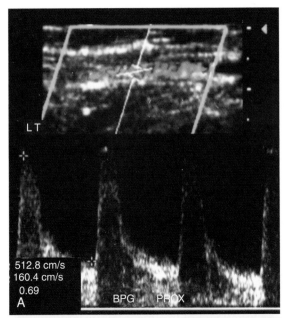

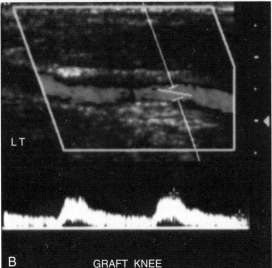

FIGURE 19-12 Impending graft failure. **A,** Disturbed color flow and high peak velocity (512.8 cm/sec) are demonstrated by duplex study at a high-grade stenosis just beyond the proximal graft anastomosis. **B,** Low-velocity flow (<45 cm/sec) downstream from the stenosis portends impending graft failure.

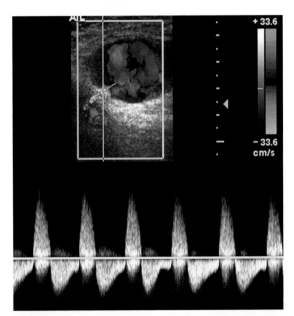

FIGURE 19-13 Femoral artery pseudoaneurysm. Duplex sampling in the pseudoaneurysm neck demonstrates characteristic to-and-fro flow.

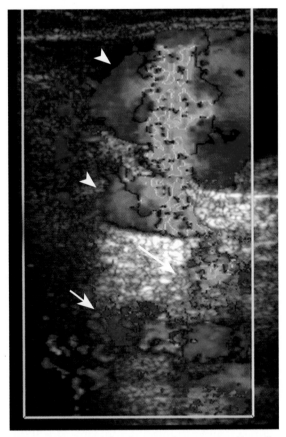

FIGURE 19-14 Multilocular pseudoaneurysm. Two distinct lumens *(arrowheads)* communicate with the common femoral artery *(short arrow)* via a single neck *(long arrow)*.

Ultrasound-guided thrombin injection is the current treatment of choice for femoral pseudoaneurysms and can be used in elective or emergency situations.[27] A review of 19 studies of more than 400 patients undergoing thrombin injection of femoral pseudoaneurysms revealed an initial success rate of 99%.[28] In most cases, pseudoaneurysm thrombosis occurred within seconds of the initial injection. Few cases required more than 15 minutes

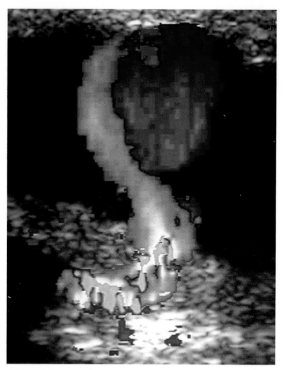

FIGURE 19-15 Femoral artery pseudoaneurysm. The lumen shows the distinctive "yin-yang" appearance.

to complete. The complication rate with this technique was strikingly low, although potential risks include pseudoaneurysm expansion and inadvertent arterial or venous thrombin injection. No cases of limb-threatening ischemia were reported following thrombin injection of pseudoaneurysms. The following technique is employed.

Either a linear or curved array transducer is used for scanning and guidance for thrombin injection, depending on the depth of the underlying artery. The pseudoaneurysm is identified and characterized with color Doppler imaging. Spectral Doppler waveform analysis is performed to demonstrate characteristic blood flow pattern in the neck of the pseudoaneurysm. A 22-gauge spinal needle is advanced into the false aneurysm under direct ultrasound visualization. Color Doppler is turned off during placement of the needle into the lumen to improve visualization of the needle tip. Color Doppler imaging is then used to assess thrombosis during thrombin injection. Once the needle tip is seen within the lumen, a 1-mL syringe is used to inject 0.5 to 1 mL of a 1000-IU/mL solution of thrombin. The majority of cases require only 0.5 mL or less of thrombin to accomplish pseudoaneurysm thrombosis

(Figure 19-16). The needle tip is directed away from the pseudoaneurysm neck to avoid injection into the femoral artery. Color Doppler imaging is performed after injection to assess the degree of thrombosis and to check patency of the femoral artery and vein. Distal pulses should be assessed before and after treatment. After successful aneurysm thrombosis, patients are maintained at bed rest for several hours. A follow-up duplex scan is obtained to assess for pseudoaneurysm recurrence before discharge.

Occasionally blood flow will persist within the neck after luminal thrombosis. Although this finding often resolves spontaneously, it may be associated with a higher rate of recurrence. Although reinjection of the neck is technically challenging and potentially risky, ultrasound-guided compression may succeed in eliminating any residual flow.

Overall rate of treatment failure and/or recurrence is estimated at up to 9%. Many of these cases are due to an elongated laceration in the arterial wall at the site of arteriotomy. Some, but not all, of these pseudoaneurysms are associated with a short, wide neck (Figure 19-17). Other risk factors include multilocularity and combined arteriovenous (AV) fistula. Factors that are not associated with failure include volume of pseudoaneurysm lumen, blood flow velocity within the neck, and use of systemic anticoagulation therapy.[29] Repeat thrombin injection can be performed, although human thrombin is preferred in these cases due to the risk for IgE-mediated anaphylaxis following repeated exposure to bovine thrombin.[30]

TRAUMATIC ARTERIOVENOUS FISTULA

AV fistulas of the peripheral vascular system can occur following penetrating trauma. In the ultrasound laboratory, these are most often encountered from iatrogenic injury to the femoral vessels. In a large prospective series, 0.6% of patients undergoing cardiac catheterization developed a femoral AV fistula.[31] These can occur in isolation or combined with a pseudoaneurysm. Small AV fistulas are often asymptomatic, but high-flow lesions may cause distal ischemia or high-output heart failure. Up to one-third ultimately close spontaneously, but symptomatic fistulas may require surgery or covered stent placement.[32]

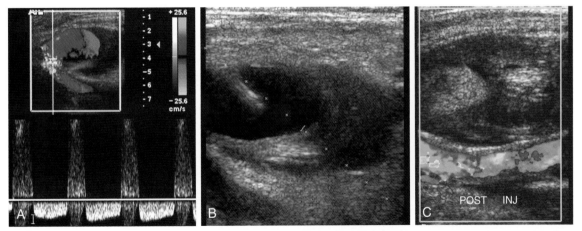

FIGURE 19-16 Pseudoaneurysm thrombin injection. **A,** Unilocular pseudoaneurysm with a long, broad neck. **B,** A 22-gauge needle is placed in the pseudoaneurysm lumen under direct ultrasound guidance. Note that the lumen has undergone partial spontaneous thrombosis. **C,** Complete thrombosis immediately following thrombin injection.

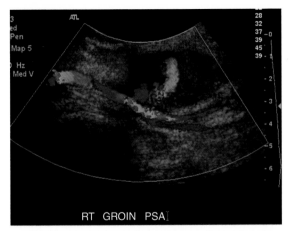

FIGURE 19-17 Common femoral artery laceration. Partially thrombosed pseudoaneurysm shows recurrent intraluminal blood flow 24 hours following thrombin injection. Note absence of a true neck between the lumen and the underlying artery. A transmural laceration was discovered at subsequent surgical repair.

On color Doppler imaging, the fistulous tract is not always visualized, especially when the involved artery and vein are immediately apposed to each other. A color bruit surrounding the vessels corresponds to an overlying palpable thrill and represents soft tissue motion induced by turbulent blood flow through the fistula (Figure 19-18). Markedly increased blood flow velocities necessitate increasing the color Doppler pulse repetition frequency (PRF) to reduce color aliasing. Increasing the color Doppler wall filter reduces the bruit artifact. Pulsed Doppler sampling demonstrates high-velocity, pulsatile venous flow downstream from the AV connection. Low-flow

AV fistulas may not alter the hemodynamics within the feeding femoral artery, but in larger fistulas, the normal triphasic arterial waveform is replaced by one of lower impedance manifesting antegrade flow throughout diastole.[33] AV fistulas manifesting with arterial waveform abnormalities are more often symptomatic and less likely to undergo spontaneous closure.

PENETRATING ARTERIAL TRAUMA

Penetrating trauma is the most common cause of noniatrogenic injury to blood vessels. The anatomic distribution of penetrating vascular injuries depends on the mechanism of injury. Nonfatal gunshot wounds usually involve abdominal vessels, followed by the lower extremities.[34] Shotgun wounds are more likely to involve extremity blood vessels, and truncal shotgun wounds are more often fatal. Stab wounds are most common in the neck, arms, and trunk.

Some patients with extremity trauma have clear evidence on examination of significant vascular injury and undergo surgical exploration without imaging. In some cases, however, a vascular injury is suspected without hemodynamic compromise, based on the location or nature of the injury. Most of these patients undergo arteriography or CT angiography, but some centers have investigated the diagnostic utility of duplex ultrasound for intimal injury to the artery wall, arterial thrombosis, traumatic pseudoaneurysms, and AV fistulas (Figure 19-19). In an experimental study comparing duplex sonography and arteriography in a canine model of arterial injury, duplex

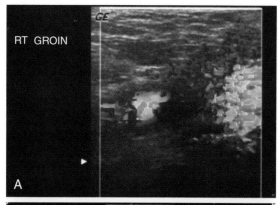

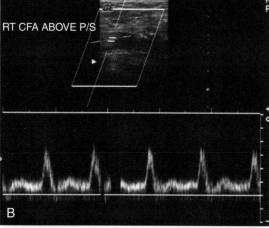

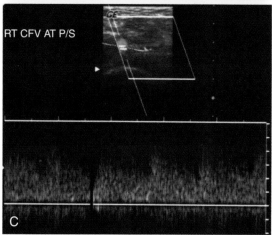

FIGURE 19-18 Iatrogenic arteriovenous (AV) fistula. **A,** Color bruit surrounds the affected segment of the common femoral vein. **B,** Low impedance waveform from the common femoral artery feeding the fistula. **C,** High-velocity, pulsatile flow in the common femoral vein immediately distal to the AV fistula.

scanning was significantly more accurate than angiography in identifying arterial lacerations.[35]

An extremity/brachial pressure index in the affected limb of less than 0.90 has been used as a threshold to prompt duplex evaluation. Bynoe and colleagues[36] used duplex scanning in 198 patients; they achieved a sensitivity of 95%, a specificity of 99%, and an overall accuracy of 98% for identifying arterial injuries. However, most physicians consider a negative arterial pressure index as a poor indicator of some potentially unstable injuries, such as arterial dissections, disruptions, and pseudoaneurysms. In a study by Lynch and Johansen[37] use of an arterial pressure index threshold of 0.9 had a sensitivity of only 80% for the presence of arterial disruption.

Patients undergoing duplex evaluation to assess for occult vascular injury from penetrating trauma in proximity to the vascular bundle are by definition hemodynamically stable; thus, the examination does not have to be performed immediately on admission to the trauma room. However, it should be done expeditiously to facilitate management, especially in multitrauma victims. Since the site of vessel injury is difficult to predict based on the location of entry and exit wound, the study should extend to the joints above and below the level of injury. For shotgun wounds, where the injury is often more diffuse, the examiner should be especially careful to evaluate the entire affected area. Evaluation should include veins as well as arteries to assess for traumatic AV fistulas, as well as isolated injuries.

Several factors can complicate performance of the duplex examination in the trauma setting. Uncooperative or combative patients may require sedation to limit motion of the extremity. Acoustic access may be limited by the presence of wound dressings, orthopedic immobilizing devices, and air or metallic foreign bodies in the soft tissues. Soft tissue hematomas increase the depth of sound penetration needed to visualize the vessels. Repositioning of the transducer may provide an alternative window to overcome some of these obstacles. Scanning through an open wound requires the use of a sterile probe cover and sterile gel to minimize risk of infection.

Color Doppler survey of the regional arteries and veins facilitates rapid assessment of the affected area. Sites of disturbed or absent color flow signals or extravascular flow should prompt close inspection. Gray-scale imaging should be performed to evaluate for intimal irregularity, flap formation, and the presence of intraluminal thrombus. Because it does not overwrite the vessel wall like color flow Doppler, B-flow imaging can be especially useful in visualizing a vessel wall abnormality in relation to the local flow

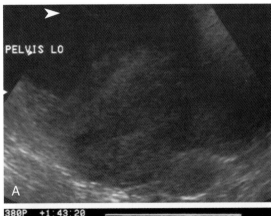

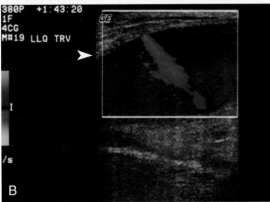

FIGURE 19-20 Active arterial hemorrhage. **A,** Swirling internal echoes were seen within this pelvic hematoma at gray-scale sonography. **B,** Color jet shows active extravasation from the inferior epigastric artery.

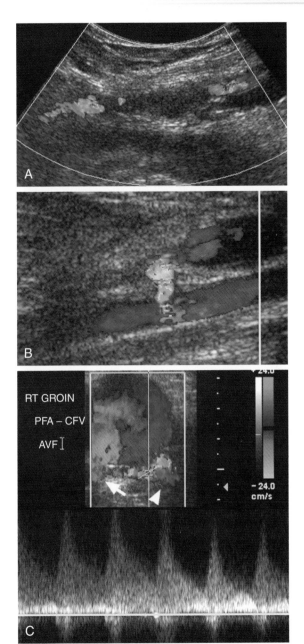

FIGURE 19-19 Peripheral arterial trauma. **A,** Segmental thrombosis of the common femoral artery after blunt trauma. **B,** Brachial artery extravasation due to penetrating injury. **C,** Combined pseudoaneurysm and arteriovenous (AV) fistula formation following deep femoral artery laceration. Spectral tracing shows high-velocity low-resistance shunt flow in the AV fistula. *Arrow,* deep femoral artery; *arrowhead,* common femoral vein.

disturbance. Assessment of the degree of narrowing incurred at the site of injury requires the evaluation of Doppler spectral waveforms.

Arterial injuries from penetrating trauma detectable by duplex scanning include arterial stenosis or occlusion (from intramural hematoma or transmural laceration), intimal dissection, pseudoaneurysm, and AV fistula. Venous injuries include thrombosis, extrinsic compression (from hematoma or soft tissue swelling), and fistula. Diagnostic criteria for these entities are similar to those that apply in the nontrauma setting.

Soft tissue hematoma results from blunt or penetrating injury causing vascular disruption. The hematoma may be discrete if constrained within muscle or may be diffuse if it tracks along fascial planes. Large hematomas may cause extrinsic compression and narrowing of adjacent vessels. Gray-scale sonographic findings vary depending on the age of the hematoma. Recent hemorrhage tends to appear solid and heterogeneously echogenic, whereas with time and liquefaction the hematoma may resemble a complex cyst.

Serial sonographic measurements of the hematoma may be useful to assess for ongoing or recurrent hemorrhage. Active bleeding is seldom visible sonographically, although brisk hemorrhage may be detectable with color Doppler (Figure 19-20). Some centers have explored the potential use of contrast-enhanced sonography for identification of the site of extremity or solid visceral hemorrhage.[38]

CONCLUSIONS

Algorithms for the diagnosis of arterial pathology are evolving with the rapidly advancing capabilities of cross-sectional imaging. The expanding therapeutic role associated with catheter angiography has made this traditional mainstay of vascular diagnosis and intervention even more valuable. In this perspective, the ultimate role of duplex sonography in the workup of arterial emergencies is unsettled. Its strengths are most clearly displayed in the acute care setting, where rapid resolution of a focused clinical question results in timely intervention in a critically ill patient. This role has led to increasing use of portable ultrasound devices in the operating room, emergency department, and intensive care unit settings, as well as in out-of-hospital environments (i.e., combat fields). If it can be shown that high rates of diagnostic accuracy achieved by experienced sonographers using high-end equipment can be achieved in these alternative settings, ultrasound will have a definite role in the management of these challenging problems.

REFERENCES

1. Powell JT, Brown LC: The natural history of abdominal aortic aneurysms and their risk of rupture, *Adv Surg* 35:173–185, 2001.
2. Sebesta P, et al: Ruptured abdominal aortic aneurysm: role of initial delay on survival, *J Mal Vasc* 23:361–367, 1998.
3. Shuman WP, et al: Suspected leaking abdominal aortic aneurysm: Use of sonography in the emergency room, *Radiology* 168:117–119, 1988.
4. Catalano O, et al: Contrast-enhanced sonography for diagnosis of ruptured abdominal aortic aneurysm, *Am J Radiol* 184:423–427, 2005.
5. Thomas EA, Dubbins PA: Duplex ultrasound of the abdominal aorta – a neglected tool in aortic dissection, *Clin Radiol* 42:330–334, 1991.
6. Clevert DA, et al: Contrast-enhanced ultrasound versus conventional ultrasound and MS-CT in the diagnosis of abdominal aortic dissection, *Clin Hemorheol Microcirc* 43:129–139, 2009.
7. Kimura K, et al: Duplex carotid sonography in distinguishing acute unilateral atherothrombotic from cardioembolic carotid artery occlusion, *Am J Neuroradiol* 18:1447–1452, 1997.
8. Kimura K, et al: Oscillating thromboemboli within the extracranial internal carotid artery demonstrated by ultrasonography in patients with acute cardioembolic stroke, *Ultrasound Med Biol* 24:1121–1124, 1999.

9. Kemany V, Jung DK, Devuyst G: Ultrasound characteristics of adherent thrombi in the common carotid artery, *Circulation* 104:E24–E25, 2001.
10. Padayachee TS, et al: Value of intraoperative duplex imaging during supervised carotid endarterectomy, *Br J Surg* 88:389–392, 2001.
11. Schievink WI, Mokri B, Piepgras DG: Spontaneous dissections of the cervicocephalic arteries in childhood and adolescence, *Neurology* 44:1607–1612, 1994.
12. Sanzone AG, Torres H, Doundoulakis SH: Blunt trauma to the carotid arteries, *Am J Emerg Med* 13:327–330, 1995.
13. Siblert PL, Mokri B, Schievink WI: Headache and neck pain in spontaneous internal carotid and vertebral artery dissections, *Neurology* 45:1517–1522, 1995.
14. Sturzenegger M, Mattle H, Rivoir A: Ultrasound findings in carotid artery dissection: Analysis of 43 patients, *Neurology* 45:691–698, 1995.
15. Benninger DH, Baumgartner RW: Ultrasound diagnosis of cervical artery dissection, *Front Neurol Neurosci* 21:70–84, 2006.
16. Grassbaugh JA, et al: Blinded comparison of preoperative duplex ultrasound scanning and contrast arteriography for planning revascularization at the level of the tibia. *J Vasc Surg* 37:1186–1190, 2003.
17. MacGowan SW, et al: Ultrasound examination in the diagnosis of popliteal artery aneurysms, *Br J Surg* 72:528–529, 1985.
18. Kallakuri S, et al: Impact of duplex arteriography in the evaluation of acute lower limb ischemia from thrombosed popliteal aneurysms, *Vasc Endovascular Surg* 40(1):23–25, 2006.
19. Ascher E, et al: Acute lower limb ischemia: the value of duplex ultrasound arterial mapping (DUAM) as the sole preoperative imaging technique, *Ann Vasc Surg* 17(3):284–289, 2003.
20. Lafberg AM, et al: The role of duplex scanning in the selection of patients with critical lower-limb ischemia for infrainguinal percutaneous transluminal angioplasty, *Cardiovasc Intervent Radiol* 24(4):229–232, 2001.
21. Westerband A, et al: Prospective validation of threshold criteria for intervention in infrainguinal vein grafts undergoing duplex surveillance, *Ann Vasc Surg* 11:44–48, 1997.
22. Mofidi R, et al: Significance of the early postoperative duplex result in infrainguinal vein bypass surveillance, *Eur J Vasc Endovasc Surg* 34(3):327–332, 2007.
23. Ahmad F, et al: Iatrogenic femoral artery pseudoaneurysms – a review of current methods of diagnosis and treatment, *Clin Radiol* 63(12):1310–1316, 2008.
24. Middleton WD, Dasyam A, Teefey SA: Diagnosis and treatment of iatrogenic femoral artery pseudoaneurysms, *Ultrasound Q* 21(1):3–17, 2005.
25. O'Malley C Jr, et al: Color Doppler sonographic appearance of patent needle tracts after femoral arterial catheterization, *Radiology* 197:163–165, 1995.
26. Feld R, et al: Treatment of iatrogenic femoral artery injuries with ultrasound-guided compression, *J Vasc Surg* 16:832–840, 1992.
27. Paulson EK, et al: Treatment of iatrogenic femoral artery pseudoaneurysms: Comparison of US-guided thrombin injection with compression repair, *Radiology* 215:403–408, 2000.

28. Friedman SG, et al: Ultrasound-guided thrombin injection is the treatment of choice for femoral pseudoaneurysms, *Arch Surg* 137:462–464, 2002.

29. Sheiman RG, Mastromattreo M: Iatrogenic femoral pseudoaneurysms that are unresponsive to percutaneous thrombin injection: potential causes, *Am J Roentgenol* 181(5):1301–1304, 2003.

30. Vazquez V, et al: Human thrombin for treatment of pseudoaneurysms: comparison of bovine and human thrombin sonogram-guided injection, *Am J Roentgenol* 184(5):1665–1671, 2005.

31. Ohlow MA, Secknus MA, von Korn H: Incidence and outcome of femoral vascular complications among 18,165 patients undergoing cardiac catheterization, *Int J Cardiol* 135(1):66–71, 2009.

32. Gonzalez SB, et al: Imaging arteriovenous fistulas, *Vasc Intervent Radiol* 193(5):1425–1433, 2009.

33. Igidbashian VN, et al: Iatrogenic femoral arteriovenous fistula: diagnosis with color Doppler imaging, *Radiology* 170(3):749–752, 1989.

34. Mattox KL, et al: Five thousand seven hundred sixty cardiovascular injuries in 4459 patients: Epidemiologic evolution 1958 to 1987, *Ann Surg* 209:698–705, 1989.

35. Panetta TF, et al: Natural history, duplex characteristics, and histopathologic correlation of arterial injuries in a canine model, *J Vasc Surg* 16:867–874, 1993.

36. Bynoe RP, et al: Noninvasive diagnosis of vascular trauma by duplex ultrasonography, *J Vasc Surg* 14:346–352, 1991.

37. Lynch K, Johansen K: Can Doppler pressure measurement replace "exclusion" arteriography in the diagnosis of occult extremity arterial trauma? *Ann Surg* 214(6):737–741, 1991.

38. Catalano O, et al: Real-time, contrast-enhanced sonography: a new tool for detecting active bleeding, *J Trauma* 59(4):933–939, 2005.

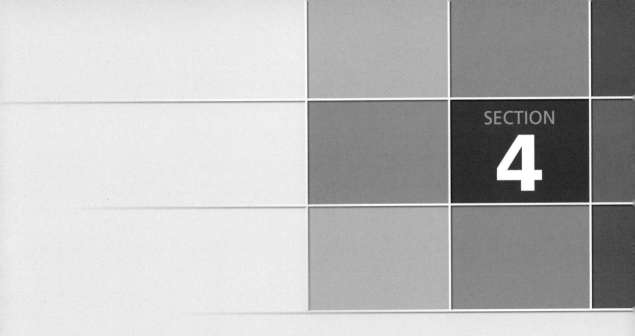

Extremity Veins

RISK FACTORS AND THE ROLE OF ULTRASOUND IN THE MANAGEMENT OF EXTREMITY VENOUS DISEASE

20

JOSEPH F. POLAK, MD, MPH, and JOHN S. PELLERITO, MD, FACR, FSRU, FAIUM

Duplex sonography can effectively diagnose the presence of acute or chronic venous thrombosis in the extremity veins. Most commonly, duplex sonography is used when acute deep venous thrombosis (DVT) is suspected, but it is also a reliable method of determining the extent of chronic venous disease and the accompanying physiologic alterations in venous hemodynamics.

ACUTE VENOUS THROMBOEMBOLIC DISEASE

Suspected venous thromboembolic disease (VTE) is the most common reason for the clinical evaluation of the extremity veins. While a comprehensive review of VTE is beyond the scope of this chapter, a brief review of risk factors and conditions fostering the development of VTE is in order. *VTE refers to DVT and pulmonary embolism (PE)*, related aspects of the same disease process. The annual incidence of VTE in the United States is estimated at over 2.5 million cases.[1] Roughly 25% of untreated patients with DVT will sustain a nonfatal PE. Moreover, without treatment, PE is associated with a mortality rate of approximately 30%.[2] The population at risk represents a myriad of clinical conditions that predispose to venous thrombosis. This susceptibility to develop venous thrombosis was first described in 1865 as Virchow's triad: venous stasis, endothelial damage, and hypercoagulability.

Thrombogenesis occurs through the activation of enzymatic reactions in the intrinsic and tissue factor pathways, leading to the ultimate formation of thrombin via the prothrombin enzyme complex. The thrombomodulin–protein C system primarily limits coagulation, while the fibrinolytic system further limits fibrin deposition. This homeostatic system is continuously active and balances activation and inhibition of coagulation and fibrinolysis. The predisposition to thrombus formation results either from inherited (nonreversible) or acquired(reversible) prothrombotic conditions.

Inherited prothrombotic disease states have been described with increasing frequency over the past 20 years. This category of venous thrombosis is considered nonreversible and as such, the patient keeps his/her increased risk for developing venous thromboembolic disease throughout life.

Antithrombin III deficiency was the first reported congenital thrombotic condition.[3] It is transmitted in an autosomal dominant pattern with a prevalence of 1:5000. Isolated spontaneous thrombosis has been described with this condition. Precipitating circumstances, such as trauma, pregnancy, and surgical procedures, seem to lower the threshold for the development of DVT.

Protein C and protein S are vitamin K–dependent cofactors that facilitate degradation of activated factor V. Deficiencies, therefore, predispose to thrombosis. Congenital deficiencies of these factors are well described.[4] Since these proteins are synthesized in the liver, acquired deficiencies also may occur from variations in liver function as well as with dietary changes. Protein C or S deficiency confers a roughly sevenfold increased risk for developing venous thrombosis. *Resistance to activated protein C* is also known as factor V Leiden. This disorder results from a point mutation in the factor V gene, rendering activated factor V resistant to degradation by activated protein C. It is present in 12% to 33% of patients with spontaneous VTE,[5] thereby making it the most common inherited hypercoagulable condition.

Factor II (prothrombin) G20210A is a mutation seen in 2% to 3% of individuals, predominantly those of European descent. In a recent study, it was observed to confer a 2.8-fold increase in relative risk for VTE.[6]

Primary hyperhomocysteinemia increases risk for VTE, along with the development of premature atherosclerosis. Serum elevation of *coagulation factors*

TABLE 20-1	Acquired Risk Factors for VTE

Immobilization
Surgery within 3 mo
Stroke, paralysis of extremities
History of VTE
Malignancy
Obesity
Cigarette smoking
Hypertension
Oral contraception, hormone replacement therapy
Pregnancy and puerperium
Secondary hyperhomocysteinemia
Antiphospholipid syndrome
Congestive heart failure
Myeloproliferative disorders
Nephrotic syndrome
Inflammatory bowel disease
Sickle cell anemia
Marked leukocytosis in acute leukemia
Prior VTE

VTE, venous thromboembolic disease.

VIII, IX, and XI have been shown to confer elevated risk for venous thrombosis in the Leiden thrombophilia study.[7] Factor IX and XI levels greater than the 90th percentile confer a 2.5-fold and 2.2-fold increased risk for VTE, respectively. *Dysfibrogenemias and hypofibrinolysis* impair the steps involved in the generation, cross-linkage, and breakdown of fibrin. Bleeding diathesis, as well as VTE, has been described with this condition.

Acquired prothrombotic states are more numerous than inherited states. Table 20-1, modified from the Prospective Investigation of Pulmonary Embolism Diagnosis (PIOPED) study,[8] shows clinical conditions that predispose to VTE. Several of these conditions are briefly considered. *Pregnancy* and the postpartum period confer a higher risk for developing VTE than the nonpregnant state. PE is a leading cause of maternal death after childbirth, with 1 fatal PE per 100,000 births.[9,10] *Oral contraceptives* and *hormone replacement therapy* can increase the risk for VTE in premenopausal and postmenopausal women. Lidegaard and colleagues reported a prevalence of VTE in women receiving oral contraceptives of 1 to 3 in 10,000.[11] Women receiving hormone replacement therapy have a twofold increased risk for VTE with rates depending on the type of contraceptive and decreasing with duration of use.[11] *Antiphospholipid antibody*

syndrome refers to the presence of either the lupus anticoagulant antibody or anticardiolipin antibodies. Overall, the syndrome can be identified in 1% to 5% of the population. Among those with positive titers for the lupus anticoagulant, the risk for developing VTE is 6% to 8%. Patients with anticardiolipin antibody titers greater than the 95th percentile have a 5.3-fold increased risk for developing VTE.[12]

An important consideration for the triage of patients is the application of the Well's score (see Chapter 23). This clinical instrument is a useful guide in determining the need to perform a diagnostic imaging test, most often venous ultrasound, given an a priori likelihood that the patient has VTE.[13]

ANTICOAGULATION AND THROMBOLYSIS IN THE MANAGEMENT OF VENOUS THROMBOEMBOLIC DISEASE

Heparin anticoagulation is standard for initial management of VTE. Heparin potentiates the action of antithrombin III, thereby preventing additional thrombus formation and permitting endogenous fibrinolysis.

In the absence of contraindication to anticoagulation, prompt institution of heparin therapy is indicated for patients with either confirmed VTE (through imaging techniques) or among patients in whom a moderate or high clinical suspicion of VTE exists. Either unfractionated or low-molecular-weight heparin is effective. Oral warfarin therapy is instituted once therapeutic heparin anticoagulation has been achieved. Warfarin dosing is guided by measuring the international normalized ratio (INR), a reflection of the inhibition of vitamin K–dependent cofactors. While the target INR will vary, depending on the clinical circumstance, it is important to understand that early elevations in the INR (1 to 3 days after institution of warfarin therapy [with an INR target of 2 to 3]) usually result from inhibition of factor VII because of its short half-life. Effective anticoagulation depends on the depletion of factor II (thrombin) and typically requires about 3 to 4 days of warfarin therapy[14] to achieve a stable INR. Therapy with oral warfarin in the absence of heparin anticoagulation should be avoided, as days will pass before anticoagulation is adequate, leaving the patient unprotected against PE. Moreover, warfarin therapy in the absence of heparin anticoagulation may paradoxically intensify hypercoagulability and predispose to recurrent VTE.

The necessary duration for anticoagulation varies with the clinical scenario. In general, for initial cases of uncomplicated DVT, 3 months of anticoagulation is recommended. PE, inherited and acquired procoagulant states, and cases of recurrent VTE usually require longer anticoagulation therapy, typically 6 months. In some cases of recurrent VTE and irreversible risk factors, lifelong anticoagulation is recommended.

Thrombolysis is not commonly used among patients with VTE, but there are situations in which it should be considered. Thrombolysis can be lifesaving for patients in whom massive PE causes hemodynamic instability, but this situation is rare. More commonly, thrombolysis may be useful for patients with extensive iliofemoral venous thrombosis, where the risk for development of the postthrombotic syndrome is high. The prevalence and severity of the postthrombotic syndrome are believed to be decreased if rapid thrombolysis is achieved.[15] However, the substantial proportion of patients with contraindications to thrombolysis and the associated increase in major bleeding severely limit the use of thrombolytic therapy.

NEW THERAPEUTIC AGENTS

Oral agents not based on suppression of vitamin K–dependent coagulation factors are increasingly available. For example, a factor Xa inhibitor is showing much promise as the equivalent of vitamin K antagonists for the treatment of DVT.[16]

ACUTE DEEP VENOUS THROMBOSIS OF SPECIFIC EXTREMITY VEINS

CALF VEIN THROMBOSIS

Most lower extremity DVTs originate in the deep veins of the calf,[17,18] although acute thrombus can form anywhere in the venous system. The soleal sinuses of the calf are thought to be the most common site of origin of DVT.[19] Untreated calf vein thrombus can progress into the popliteal and femoral veins in up to 30% of cases,[20] whereas this risk is drastically reduced by anticoagulation.[21] Once the thrombus propagates into the popliteal or femoral vein, therapeutic anticoagulation is needed to decrease the likelihood of pulmonary embolism.

In cases where there is a contraindication to anticoagulation, inferior vena cava placement may be required to prevent PE. However, the clinical importance of isolated calf DVT remains uncertain. Abundant literature has been published, but much of it is contradictory. Although there is no strong consensus over the prevalence of isolated calf DVT, current clinical practice guidelines favor treatment of calf DVT due to its propensity to progress, the underlying risk for PE, and the likelihood of the postthrombotic syndrome.[20,22]

The prevalence of isolated calf DVT in specific patient groups is difficult to establish, because many studies include mixed patient populations and a variety of diagnostic techniques. For example, a study by Atri and colleagues[23] attempted to better separate patient populations by examining an asymptomatic postoperative high-risk group and a symptomatic ambulatory group. In the asymptomatic postoperative group, 20% of patients were found to have isolated calf DVT; in the symptomatic ambulatory group, the prevalence was 30%. These studies indicate that although it is difficult to establish precisely, isolated calf DVT is not uncommon.

Since most DVTs arise in calf veins, calf DVT can obviously propagate to the popliteal vein and more proximally. More important, do *all* calf DVTs propagate, and can those that do so be identified? The reported frequency of calf DVT propagation varies markedly. In postoperative patients, the reported rate of propagation varies from 6% to 34%.[24-26] Unfortunately, it is not possible to identify thrombi that are likely to propagate and distinguish them from those that are not.

Some authors argue that few, if any, significant pulmonary emboli arise from isolated calf DVT[27-29] and therefore that anticoagulation is unnecessary in the absence of demonstrable propagation. Other investigators have reported that patients with PE have calf-only thrombi about 5% of the time.[30] These studies are limited by the fact that they are not prospective. Meta-analysis of the importance of calf vein thrombosis provides indeterminate results.[31]

There is no general agreement on the management of isolated calf DVT since no well-controlled, prospective, randomized trial of treatment of patients with isolated calf DVT has been published. The closest studies by design show an advantage to treatment.[20,32,33]

Recent American College of Chest Physicians' guidelines recommend anticoagulation for isolated calf vein DVT. The current recommended length of anticoagulation for calf vein DVT is 3 months, although prior guidelines had recommended 6 weeks.[22]

FEMOROPOPLITEAL VEIN THROMBOSIS

DVT proximal to the calf is a more serious clinical problem than isolated calf DVT. The risk for PE is greater, thus absolutely requiring therapeutic anticoagulation. For patients in whom anticoagulation is contraindicated, vena cava filter placement is the therapeutic alternate. The clinical presentation of DVT may change appreciably as thrombus propagates more proximally. The calf is usually painful when the lower femoral vein or upper popliteal vein is involved. Swelling and warmth are typically evident on physical examination. With thrombus extension into the common femoral or iliac vein, the leg becomes painful and the patient will complain that it "feels tight." Swelling may extend to the inguinal ligament, and the patient may be tender over the course of the veins, particularly in the inguinal region.

Duplex sonography is now accepted as the definitive diagnostic test in patients suspected of having femoropopliteal DVT. Duplex sonography easily permits visualization of occlusive as well as partially occlusive thrombi. The presence of very proximal party occlusive thrombi is thought by some to indicate an increased risk for embolization, although there are no large studies confirming this concern.

While duplex sonography is a useful technique for distinguishing acute from chronic thrombus, it can be difficult to distinguish acute from subacute thrombus. Although the degree of spontaneous lysis of thrombosed venous segments can be monitored, the value of such a strategy is unproven.

ILIAC VEIN THROMBOSIS

The clinical presentation and therapeutic implications of iliac vein thrombosis are generally similar to those of femoropopliteal vein thrombosis, and the diagnostic approach is identical. The difference in the diagnostic approach is the decreased reliability of duplex sonography to directly visualize the length of the iliac veins.

If iliac vein thrombi are visualized, the diagnosis of DVT is established. However, despite a convincing clinical scenario, the only evidence of proximal DVT may come from Doppler waveform alterations distal to the thrombus.

Indirect Doppler evidence of proximal thrombosis includes the loss of respiratory phasicity on the spectral Doppler venous waveforms obtained below the level of the thrombus and the inability to augment the Doppler signal with calf or distal thigh compression. It is important to recognize that these signs may be absent in the presence of partially occlusive thrombi. Partially occlusive common or external iliac vein thrombi, or thrombi isolated to the internal iliac vein, are likely to be missed by duplex sonography. Therefore, when needed, further evaluation of the deep venous system could be obtained with venography but is more commonly achieved with either magnetic resonance venography or computed tomographic venography.

EXTREMITY VEIN DUPLEX SCANNING TO DIAGNOSE PULMONARY EMBOLISM

Because duplex ultrasound has become the diagnostic test of choice in DVT evaluation and because the majority of pulmonary emboli originate in lower extremity veins, some clinicians now utilize lower extremity duplex ultrasound as the first diagnostic study in the evaluation for possible PE. This approach is based on the noninvasive nature of the study, the portability of the machine, and the rapidity with which results may be obtained in institutions where technical support is readily available. The merit to this approach is supported when the diagnosis of extremity DVT is confirmed, because the diagnosis of PE may then be safely assumed in the appropriate clinical setting and therapy begun.

The two major limitations are (1) the yield of positive lower extremity duplex sonography is low and (2) a negative venous ultrasound test does not exclude pulmonary embolism.

Beecham and colleagues[34] reviewed 225 patients who underwent both ventilation perfusion $(\dot{V}/\dot{Q})$ scans and lower extremity duplex sonography in the evaluation of suspected PE. Of 56 patients with high-probability $\dot{V}/\dot{Q}$ scans, only 36% demonstrated duplex evidence of DVT. Furthermore, of 22 patients without evidence of DVT by duplex scanning, 25% were found to have suffered PE detected by angiography. Killewich and co-workers[35] similarly documented the absence of duplex-diagnosed DVT in 60% of patients with PE confirmed by pulmonary angiography. Eze and associates[36] demonstrated the usefulness of stratifying patients with suspected PE based on unilateral leg symptoms. In their series of 336 patients with clinically suspected PE, 7% demonstrated proximal DVT by duplex sonography. However, in the 25 patients with unilateral leg swelling, 40% were found to have DVT by duplex scanning, whereas DVT was evident in only 5% of patients in the absence of leg swelling. This group further confirmed that most patients with high-probability $\dot{V}/\dot{Q}$ scans had no DVT visualized by duplex sonography. Other studies have reaffirmed the overall low yield of venous duplex examination in the evaluation of PE and the finding that the majority of patients with confirmed PE do not demonstrate DVT,[37,38] although the yield is higher if the patient has a swollen leg.

In summary, it appears that the lower extremity venous duplex examination may be useful in the patient who is suspected of having suffered PE and has unilateral lower extremity swelling. In the absence of leg swelling, computed tomographic angiography or $\dot{V}/\dot{Q}$ scanning are the first tests of choice. Furthermore, in a patient with suspected pulmonary embolism, a negative venous duplex study must be followed by $\dot{V}/\dot{Q}$ imaging or by computed tomographic pulmonary angiography since up to half of the patients who have suffered a pulmonary embolism do not have evidence of DVT by ultrasound.

SUPERFICIAL VENOUS THROMBOSIS

Superficial venous thrombosis has traditionally been considered a relatively benign disease. It is now recognized as an important marker of coexistent DVT and hypercoagulability.[39,40]

The diagnosis of superficial venous thrombosis has typically been made clinically. Physical findings include a painful superficial cord with surrounding erythema in the course of the vein. Treatment of patients with superficial venous thrombosis used to be symptomatic and included ambulation, heat application, compression, and nonsteroidal antiinflammatory drug therapy. The new treatment guidelines recommend treatment with low-molecular-weight heparin for 4 weeks.[22]

Duplex evaluation of superficial venous thrombosis, especially occurring in the great (large) saphenous vein, is important for two reasons. First, although the clinical examination is useful

in establishing the diagnosis, it is not reliable in identifying the extent of the thrombus. Thrombus often extends beyond the apparent area of involvement particularly into the common femoral vein.[41] Duplex sonography documents the proximal extent and can be used to monitor progression. Although data are limited, it appears that a small proportion (approximately 10%) of patients with isolated superficial venous thrombosis of the great saphenous vein progress to DVT if untreated. Of that group, those with superficial venous thrombosis in the thigh are at highest risk, with 70% of untreated patients progressing to thrombosis of the femoral vein. Most clinicians either disconnect the saphenofemoral junction surgically or institute systemic anticoagulation if proximal saphenous thrombosis progresses to the saphenofemoral junction.

Duplex sonography of the extremity with superficial venous thrombosis is also useful to identify concomitant but clinically silent involvement of the deep system. Some series have demonstrated the presence of unapparent DVT in 20% to 40% of patients with superficial venous thrombosis.[40-42] Confirmation of concurrent deep vein involvement leads to long-term anticoagulation for at least 3 months. Occasionally an apparent superficial phlebitis is, in fact, a soft tissue infection or hematoma. These conditions can easily be distinguished from superficial venous thrombosis with duplex scanning but may be more difficult to differentiate clinically.

AXILLARY-SUBCLAVIAN VENOUS THROMBOSIS

DVT of the upper extremities can be divided into two categories based on whether or not there is an indwelling venous catheter. The incidence of axillary-subclavian DVT is increasing, paralleling the increased use of central venous catheters.[43,44] In the absence of central catheters, axillary-subclavian DVT may be seen among patients affected by certain cancers (especially mediastinal lymphomas), trauma, surgery, and radiation therapy. However, spontaneous effort thrombosis, also known as the *Paget-Schroetter syndrome*, is the most common presentation of axillary-subclavian DVT in the ambulatory population.[45] This condition may be associated with demonstrable anatomic abnormalities of the thoracic inlet (e.g., cervical rib). Men are affected more often than women, and the incidence is higher in the veins of the dominant arm. The clinical presentation of an upper extremity DVT can be dramatic. The acute onset of marked arm swelling and of prominent superficial veins leaves little doubt of the clinical diagnosis, and the role of duplex sonography is a confirmatory one. Sometimes the presentation is subtle. The patient may complain of vague discomfort, with minimal swelling; in these cases, duplex sonography is an effective way of evaluating the status of the deep venous system. The proximal upper extremities are drained by a rich collateral venous network around the neck and shoulder, confirming the need for direct visualization of the veins with duplex sonography. Duplex ultrasound is, however, limited by the bony structures in the neck and shoulder, impeding imaging of the medial portion of the subclavian vein. Blood flow characteristics of the proximal subclavian and brachiocephalic veins may offer indirect evidence of central vein patency, by showing preservation of cardiac phasicity.[46]

Initial treatment of axillary-subclavian thrombosis follows standard guidelines for VTE. If there is no obvious underlying cause for DVT, a thrombophilia workup, including antithrombin III, factor V Leiden, antiphospholipid antibodies, and protein C and S levels, should be performed. Prompt heparin anticoagulation is undertaken to protect from pulmonary emboli, reported to occur in up to 36% of patients.[43,44] For thromboses caused by catheters, anticoagulation, along with removal of the catheter, if possible, appears to be sufficient. However, anticoagulation alone among young, healthy patients may lead to an unacceptably high rate of postthrombotic disability, caused by incomplete recanalization of the axillary-subclavian system. Increased arterial flow with use of the arm can lead to venous hypertension from outflow obstruction. In the most severe cases, venous claudication, a bursting sensation in the arm, may develop, leading to significant disability. Local thrombolysis is reserved for low risk patients who are very symptomatic.[22]

The most common extrinsic cause of axillary-subclavian thrombosis is compression of the vein between the clavicle and the first rib. Additional causes of extrinsic compression include hypertrophic scalene or subclavius muscles, the costoclavicular ligament, or the head of the clavicle. Congenital or acquired intrinsic venous lesions also may cause venous stenosis, leading to thrombosis. Extrinsic causes are usually treated by thoracic inlet

decompression, typically including first rib resection and resection of the anterior scalene muscle. A combination of thrombolysis, surgical decompression, and endovascular intervention is often used to treat these patients.[47,48] The order of the interventions varies with local practice patterns. After thoracic inlet decompression, intrinsic venous lesions can be treated, either concurrently, with open surgical reconstruction, or through endovascular techniques performed 1 to 2 days postoperatively. The timing of decompression after thrombolysis varies with the surgeon's preference. Some prefer to wait 1 to 3 months after lysis while anticoagulating the patient to reduce thrombogenesis of the local venous endothelium. Others advocate decompression 1 to 2 days after lysis to minimize the probability of rethrombosis.[47] Nevertheless, utilizing this general approach, Machleder[48] reported reduced upper extremity disability from 60% to 12%, compared with anticoagulation alone.

SEQUELAE OF DEEP VENOUS THROMBOSIS

The sequelae of DVT result from proximal chronic venous obstruction, acquired incompetence of the valves of the deep venous system following recanalization, or both. In most patients who have suffered from DVT, the thrombosed vein recanalizes over a period of months, allowing adequate restoration of flow to the central circulation. Despite recanalization, the vein wall and valves are permanently damaged in at least 60% of cases,[15,49] leaving the valve leaflets immobile and fixed to the vein wall. Failure of the venous valve mechanism causes venous reflux and prolonged residence time of deoxygenated blood in the lower extremity, especially in the standing position. In some individuals, the thrombosed veins do not recanalize, resulting in chronic obstruction to venous return. Venous obstruction, venous reflux, or both in combination manifest clinically as chronic leg swelling, ankle pigmentation, and, ultimately, ankle ulceration in the "gaiter zone," just above the ankle. Collectively, this is known as the *postthrombotic syndrome* (Figure 20-1).

The pathophysiology underlying the swelling and discoloration is straightforward. Increased hydrostatic pressure in the deep venous system causes extravasation of protein-rich tissue fluid, presenting clinically as interstitial edema. If venous

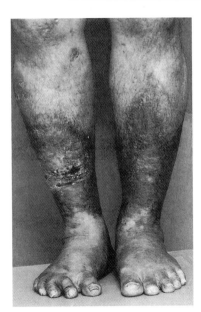

FIGURE 20-1 The *gaiter zone* is located in the lower calf and ankle. In this region, the ambulatory superficial venous pressures are the highest, leading to edema, pigmentation, and ultimately, ulceration. The skin, after years of edema, is difficult to examine for incompetent perforators (both clinically and with duplex sonography) because of extensive fibrosis.

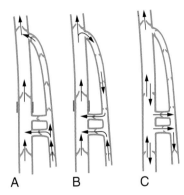

FIGURE 20-2 With incompetent deep veins and perforating veins, venous hypertension below the fascia of the leg is transmitted to the superficial system. **A,** Normal. **B,** Greater saphenous incompetence. **C,** Deep and perforator vein incompetence.

hypertension persists, acquired incompetence of the valves of the perforating veins results in secondary varicose veins (Figure 20-2). Red blood cells are deposited in the subcutaneous tissue surrounding the perforators. Metabolic breakdown of the hemoglobin is responsible for the characteristic brown skin pigmentation seen in the postphlebitic syndrome. Eventually, ulceration can develop, either spontaneously or as the result of minor trauma. Although the pathophysiology of the ulceration is not clear, it appears to be related to an inflammatory reaction in the tissue, fibrin cuffing, and eventual lipodermatosclerosis. Whatever the cause, ulceration is undoubtedly related to persistent chronic elevations in venous pressures.

Duplex ultrasound assessment of the postthrombotic extremity is useful for both diagnosis and therapy. First, indirect confirmation of the diagnosis of venous hypertension can be made with duplex ultrasound by direct observation of deep vein valve incompetence or documentation of chronic deep vein obstruction. The perforating veins and the superficial venous system can be similarly assessed. This information assists in planning therapy; for example, if the deep venous system is widely incompetent, valve repair

or transplantation may be required. However, if the deep venous system is competent, perforator interruption or stripping of the superficial venous system may suffice.

VARICOSE VEINS

Primary varicose veins are abnormally dilated and tortuous components of the superficial venous system, *in the absence of coexisting deep venous disease.* Varicose veins are classified as *secondary* when they are associated with obstruction or incompetence of the deep venous system and *recurrent* if they reappear after ablation. For most patients, the medical history and physical examination provide sufficient information to distinguish between primary and secondary varicose veins.

In the patient with primary varicose veins, a history of DVT is rare. Physical signs of the postthrombotic syndrome, such as brown skin coloration in the lower ankle (gaiter zone) and venous stasis ulcers, are uncommon. However, in the occasional patient, it can be difficult to rule out involvement of the deep venous system by the medical history and physical examination. In this instance, duplex sonography can be especially helpful. Exclusion of pathology of the deep venous system confirms the diagnosis of primary varicose veins and predicts a high likelihood of cure with complete excision of the varicosities or endovascular ablation of the superficial veins.

A careful assessment of the great saphenous vein is critical before considering treatment of varicose veins. If the saphenous vein is competent, treatment can be confined to the clinically evident varicosities. Conversely, if the great

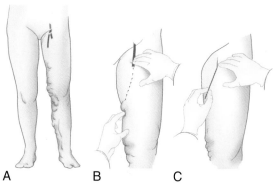

A   B   C

FIGURE 20-3 Varicose veins in the calf may be isolated to the superficial calf veins, or they may be associated with incompetence of the entire saphenous vein (**A**). Physical examination (**B** and **C**) and duplex sonography can determine the extent of superficial venous involvement.

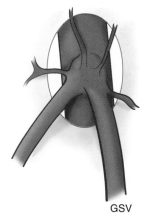

GSV

FIGURE 20-4 The great (long) saphenous vein (GSV) enters the femoral vein through the fossa ovalis. There are several large superficial branches that enter the saphenous vein at the saphenous bulb. These veins, as well as the greater saphenous vein, must be ligated to prevent recurrence of varicose veins.

saphenous is incompetent, the vein should be ablated to reduce the probability of recurrence, even if it is not clinically apparent that it is varicose. A careful evaluation of the saphenofemoral junction is needed. Valvular incompetence at the saphenofemoral junction occurs in most cases of primary varicose veins. Nevertheless, the varicosities may be clinically apparent in only the calf or distal thigh (Figure 20-3). If the saphenofemoral valve is incompetent, the saphenous vein must be either ligated at the saphenofemoral junction and stripped or endovascular ablation must extend to a few centimeters below the saphenofemoral junction.

Perforator incompetence may also cause or accompany varicose veins in the absence of deep venous incompetence. Occasionally an incompetent perforator causes primary varicose veins, even though the deep venous system is intact. Ligation of the incompetent perforator and ablation of the varicosities are the key to successful management of the problem. Incompetent perforator veins are easily localized with duplex sonography.

Recurrence of primary varicose veins is caused either by inadequate initial treatment or by development of new primary varicose veins. Initial treatment unwittingly directed at secondary varicose veins uniformly results in recurrence. The most easily identified and managed cause of recurrent primary varicose veins is inadequate high ligation of the greater saphenous vein at the saphenofemoral junction with persistence of an incompetent valve (Figure 20-4) or recanalization of a vein treated with laser or radiofrequency

ablation. Failure to ligate the great saphenous vein flush with the common femoral vein preserves the incompetent valve, allowing reflux into the subcutaneous branches at the saphenous bulb. This condition may be identified, either by physical examination or by duplex scanning, as a cluster of veins in the inguinal region. When incompetence and reflux are identified in these veins, flush ligation is curative.

A variety of other causes of recurrent primary varicosities are known, including incomplete ligation of incompetent perforators, a duplicated saphenous system, and failure to differentiate great from small saphenous vein incompetence. As usual, careful physical examination, complemented with duplex sonography, determines the cause of recurrent varicosities. The importance of evaluation of the deep venous system cannot be overstated because secondary varicose veins resulting from deep venous incompetence are a common cause of recurrence.

MAPPING FOR BYPASS SURGERY

Evaluation of the presence, location, and adequacy of a proposed bypass conduit before harvest for bypass surgery is helpful especially in individuals with a history of thrombophlebitis or prior harvesting of the superficial veins. This is accurately done with duplex sonography. In the obese patient, for example, the course of the vein may be hidden by subcutaneous tissue. Duplex scanning can confirm the patency and location of the veins, avoiding the undesirable consequence of raising large skin flaps.

Similarly, in the patient who has suffered previous saphenous vein thrombosis, duplex scanning can identify chronic occlusion or valvular insufficiency, conditions that obviate vein use as a bypass graft. In those patients who have undergone venous surgery or prior vein harvesting, the great saphenous vein may be absent. A diligent search using the duplex scanner can facilitate identification of alternative bypass conduits for the planned procedure. In our experience, the great and small saphenous, cephalic, and basilic veins are all potentially useful as bypass conduits and are easily evaluated and mapped with duplex sonography.

REFERENCES

1. White RH: The epidemiology of venous thromboembolism, *Circulation* 107:I4–8, 2003.
2. Kroegel C, Reissig A: Principle mechanisms underlying venous thromboembolism: epidemiology, risk factors, pathophysiology and pathogenesis, *Respiration* 70:7–30, 2003.
3. Egeberg O: Inherited antithrombin deficiency causing thrombophilia, *Thromb Diath Haemorrh* 13:516–530, 1965.
4. Miletich J, Sherman L, Broze G Jr: Absence of thrombosis in subjects with heterozygous protein-C deficiency, *N Engl J Med* 317:991–996, 1987.
5. Svensson PJ, Dahlback B: Resistance to activated protein C as a basis for venous thrombosis, *N Engl J Med* 330:517–522, 1994.
6. Anderson FA Jr, Spencer FA: Risk factors for venous thromboembolism, *Circulation* 107:I9–16, 2003.
7. van Hylckama Vlieg A, et al: High levels of factor IX increase the risk of venous thrombosis, *Blood* 95:3678–3682, 2000.
8. PIOPED: Value of the ventilation/perfusion scan in acute pulmonary embolism. Results of the Prospective Investigation of Pulmonary Embolism Diagnosis (PIOPED). The PIOPED investigators, *JAMA* 263:2753–2759, 1990.
9. Hogberg U: Maternal deaths in Sweden, 1971-1980, *Acta Obstet Gynecol Scand* 65:161–167, 1986.
10. Nijkeuter M, Ginsberg JS, Huisman MV: Diagnosis of deep vein thrombosis and pulmonary embolism in pregnancy: a systematic review, *J Thromb Haemost* 4:496–500, 2006.
11. Lidegaard O, et al: Hormonal contraception and risk of venous thromboembolism: National follow-up study, *BMJ* 339, 2009. b2890.
12. Ginsburg KS, et al: Anticardiolipin antibodies and the risk for ischemic stroke and venous thrombosis, *Ann Intern Med* 117:997–1002, 1992.
13. Wells PS, et al: Use of a clinical model for safe management of patients with suspected pulmonary embolism, *Ann Intern Med* 129:997–1005, 1998.
14. Bates SM, Ginsberg JS: Clinical practice. Treatment of deep-vein thrombosis, *N Engl J Med* 351:268–277, 2004.
15. Meissner MH, et al: Determinants of chronic venous disease after acute deep venous thrombosis, *J Vasc Surg* 28:826–833, 1998.
16. EINSTEIN Investigators, et al: Oral rivaroxaban for symptomatic venous thromboembolism, *N Engl J Med* 363:2499–2510, 2010.
17. Nicolaides AN, Kakkar VV, Renney JT: The soleal sinuses: Origin of deep-vein thrombosis, *Br J Surg* 57:860, 1970.
18. Rollins DL, et al: Origin of deep vein thrombi in an ambulatory population, *Am J Surg* 156:122–125, 1988.
19. Sevitt S, Gallagher N: Venous thrombosis and pulmonary embolism. A clinico-pathological study in injured and burned patients, *Br J Surg* 48:475–489, 1961.
20. Lautz TB, et al: Isolated gastrocnemius and soleal vein thrombosis: Should these patients receive therapeutic anticoagulation? *Ann Surg* 251:735–742, 2009.
21. Galanaud J-P, et al: Comparison of the clinical history of symptomatic isolated muscular calf vein thrombosis versus deep calf vein thrombosis, *J Vasc Surg* 52:932–938, 2010.
22. Kearon C, et al: Antithrombotic therapy for venous thromboembolic disease: American college of chest physicians evidence-based clinical practice guidelines, ed 8, *Chest* 133:454S–545S, 2008.
23. Atri M, et al: Accuracy of sonography in the evaluation of calf deep vein thrombosis in both postoperative surveillance and symptomatic patients, *AJR Am J Roentgenol* 166:1361–1367, 1996.
24. Doouss TW: The clinical significance of venous thrombosis of the calf, *Br J Surg* 63:377–378, 1976.
25. Kakkar VV, et al: Natural history of postoperative deep-vein thrombosis, *Lancet* 2:230–232, 1969.
26. Thomas ML, McAllister V: The radiological progression of deep venous thrombus, *Radiology* 99:37–40, 1971.
27. Dorfman GS, et al: Occult pulmonary embolism: A common occurrence in deep venous thrombosis, *AJR Am J Roentgenol* 148:263–266, 1987.
28. Moser KM, LeMoine JR: Is embolic risk conditioned by location of deep venous thrombosis? *Ann Intern Med* 94:439–444, 1981.
29. Solis MM, et al: Is anticoagulation indicated for asymptomatic postoperative calf vein thrombosis? *J Vasc Surg* 16:414–418, 1992.
30. Haas SB, et al: The significance of calf thrombi after total knee arthroplasty, *J Bone Joint Surg Br.* 74:799–802, 1992.
31. Righini M, et al: Clinical relevance of distal deep vein thrombosis. Review of literature data, *Thromb Haemost* 95:56–64, 2006.
32. Gillet J-L, Perrin MR, Allaert FA: Short-term and mid-term outcome of isolated symptomatic muscular calf vein thrombosis, *J Vasc Surg* 46:513–519, 2007.
33. Galanaud J-P, et al: Comparative study on risk factors and early outcome of symptomatic distal versus proximal deep vein thrombosis: results from the OPTIMEV study, *Thromb Haemost* 102:493–500, 2009.
34. Beecham RP, et al: Is bilateral lower extremity compression sonography useful and cost-effective in the evaluation of suspected pulmonary embolism? *AJR Am J Roentgenol* 161:1289–1292, 1993.
35. Killewich LA, Nunnelee JD, Auer AI: Value of lower extremity venous duplex examination in the diagnosis of pulmonary embolism, *J Vasc Surg* 17:934–938, 1993.

36. Eze AR, et al: Is venous duplex imaging an appropriate initial screening test for patients with suspected pulmonary embolism? *Ann Vasc Surg* 10:220–223, 1996.

37. Matteson B, et al: Role of venous duplex scanning in patients with suspected pulmonary embolism, *J Vasc Surg* 24:768–773, 1996.

38. Daniel KR, Jackson RE, Kline JA: Utility of lower extremity venous ultrasound scanning in the diagnosis and exclusion of pulmonary embolism in outpatients, *Ann Emerg Med* 35:547–554, 2000.

39. Ascher E, et al: Lesser saphenous vein thrombophlebitis: Its natural history and implications for management, *Vasc Endovasc Surg* 37:421–427, 2003.

40. Decousus H, et al: Superficial venous thrombosis and venous thromboembolism: a large, prospective epidemiologic study.[summary for patients in Ann Intern Med. 2010;152(4):I-48;], *Ann Intern Med* 152:218–224, 2010.

41. Pulliam CW, Barr SL, Ewing AB: Venous duplex scanning in the diagnosis and treatment of progressive superficial thrombophlebitis, *Ann Vasc Surg* 5:190–195, 1991.

42. Jorgensen JO, et al: The incidence of deep venous thrombosis in patients with superficial thrombophlebitis of the lower limbs, *J Vasc Surg* 18:70–73, 1993.

43. Prandoni P, et al: The long term clinical course of acute deep vein thrombosis of the arm: Prospective cohort study, *BMJ* 329:484–485, 2004.

44. Prandoni P, et al: Upper-extremity deep vein thrombosis. Risk factors, diagnosis, and complications, *Arch Intern Med* 157:57–62, 1997.

45. Brandao LR, et al: Exercise-induced deep vein thrombosis of the upper extremity. I. Literature review, *Acta Haematol* 115:214–220, 2006.

46. Patel MC, et al: Subclavian and internal jugular veins at Doppler US: Abnormal cardiac pulsatility and respiratory phasicity as a predictor of complete central occlusion, *Radiology* 211:579–583, 1999.

47. Angle N, et al: Safety and efficacy of early surgical decompression of the thoracic outlet for Paget-Schroetter syndrome, *Ann Vasc Surg* 15:37–42, 2001.

48. Machleder HI: Evaluation of a new treatment strategy for Paget-Schroetter syndrome: Spontaneous thrombosis of the axillary-subclavian vein, *J Vasc Surg* 17:305–315, 1993.

49. Meissner MH, et al: Deep venous insufficiency: The relationship between lysis and subsequent reflux, *J Vasc Surg* 18:596–605, 1993.

EXTREMITY VENOUS ANATOMY AND TECHNIQUE FOR ULTRASOUND EXAMINATION

21

STEVEN R. TALBOT, RVT, FSVU, and JOHN S. PELLERITO, MD, FACR, FSRU, FAIUM

Veins are not arteries. They *are* cylindrical structures that transport blood like their thicker-walled counterparts. However, they are dissimilar in many other ways. Veins are multitaskers. Their job description includes transporting blood back to the heart, helping to regulate body temperature and cardiac output, and providing a storage reservoir for blood. While being stored, blood can stagnate, making the formation of life-threatening blood clots more likely.

When imaging the veins, the examiner must work from a different mindset than when imaging arteries. When imaging the arteries, the most important thing is to determine how narrowed or obstructed a given vessel is. When imaging the veins, the most important thing is to detect the presence or absence of thrombus and determine, if possible, how well attached the thrombus is to the vein wall. A nonobstructive thrombus, for example, may pose a larger risk for breaking loose and traveling to the lungs than a totally obstructive clot because it may be more poorly attached to the vein wall. Fortunately, duplex imaging is a perfect tool for identifying and evaluating these clots, thus allowing physicians to take actions to minimize the risks of clot embolization and pulmonary embolism.

The three main goals in diagnosing venous thrombosis are to determine the following:
1. The presence or absence of thrombus
2. The relative risk for the thrombus dislodging and traveling to the lungs
3. The competence of the venous valves

Venous duplex is uniquely suited for each of these tasks.

In order to perform venous duplex ultrasound of the veins, the examiner must understand the venous anatomy[1-4] and be fully acquainted with the examination protocols for imaging the veins. In this chapter we will review the venous anatomy and the examination protocols.

ANATOMY OF THE LOWER EXTREMITY

There are three kinds of veins that will be examined by duplex imaging:
1. Deep veins
2. Superficial veins
3. Perforator veins

DEEP VEINS

The deep veins are accompanied by an artery and are, by definition, surrounded by muscle. Their job is to act as the main conduits that transport blood back to the heart. Clots within the deep veins are more likely to produce a clinically significant pulmonary embolism because these clots are usually larger than those in the superficial system. Also, because they are surrounded by muscle, the chance of the clot being dislodged during muscle contraction is higher than for a clot in the superficial veins. For these reasons, the main focus in a lower extremity venous duplex examination is on the deep system.

SUPERFICIAL VEINS

The superficial veins are, by definition, located near the skin, superficial to the muscle. The main superficial veins usually travel without an accompanying artery within the border that separates the fascia from the muscle. Their job is not to be the primary source for returning blood to the heart, but rather to get blood close to the skin surface so the veins can help to regulate body temperature. They constrict if the environment is cold to help preserve body heat. When the body needs to cool down, they enlarge to shunt large amounts of warm blood to the skin so that heat escapes the body.

There is a mistaken idea that clots within the superficial veins pose no threat of producing a pulmonary embolism. Clots can and do break loose from superficial veins and travel to the pulmonary arteries. These clots in the superficial system are less likely to cause major, clinically significant pulmonary embolism because they are usually smaller than clots found in the deep veins, and they are less likely to be dislodged because they are not surrounded by muscle. Examination of the superficial veins is still an important part of a complete evaluation of the lower extremity because superficial clots may become large (as the normally small superficial vein is expanded by the contained thrombus) and cause considerable discomfort. There is also potential danger that a superficial vein clot can extend into the deep system.

PERFORATORS

Perforator veins are veins that connect the deep veins with the superficial veins. Their job is to keep blood moving from the superficial system into the deep system. When they are working properly, they keep blood from pooling at the level of the skin. When they do not function, blood can pool at the skin level and chronic stasis changes and even ulcers may result. While a full examination of the lower extremity need not include detailed evaluation of perforators, more attention is paid to them when the question of chronic swelling or venous stasis is being evaluated.

VENOUS DUPLEX IMAGING EXAMINATION TECHNIQUE AND PROTOCOL

The biggest disadvantage to venous duplex imaging is its operator-dependent nature. The quality of venous imaging studies varies tremendously from institution to institution and between individual sonographers. This is true because of the lack of standardized training and standardized protocols. Following the protocol described in this chapter will increase your likelihood of performing accurate, reliable venous duplex examinations.

There are three factors that will dramatically influence the quality of venous duplex imaging studies:

1. Equipment selection
2. Proper patient positioning
3. Proper education and examination techniques

EQUIPMENT SELECTION

The quality of imaging equipment varies widely. Attempting to do venous duplex imaging with inadequate equipment is frustrating and potentially dangerous. The equipment needed for venous imaging will have excellent gray-scale image quality, with the ability to image from the skin line to a depth of about 6 cm. This may require the use of several transducers: a high-frequency linear probe (10-18 MHz) with a small footprint for superficial veins like the saphenous, distal tibial veins, and most of the arm veins; a midrange linear probe (5-9 MHz) for most of the deep veins of the legs and deeper veins of the arm; and a lower-frequency probe (2-5 MHz) for the iliac veins and inferior vena cava and also to see leg veins in heavy patients.

PATIENT POSITIONING FOR THE LOWER EXTREMITY

When imaging the lower extremity, the bed should be tilted to allow blood to dilate the leg veins so they can be imaged clearly. Omitting this seemingly insignificant step is one of the most common reasons for missing small clots, especially in the calf. The bed should be placed in a reversed Trendelenburg's position (head elevated) at about 20 degrees (Figure 21-1, *A*). Another technique to distend the calf veins is to allow the patient to sit up during calf evaluation (Figure 21-1, *B*). This is extremely effective but is clumsy and can make the veins difficult to compress. In this situation, veins filled with stagnant flow may be mistaken for thrombus-filled veins.

After the bed is tilted, the patient must be positioned properly. For the lower extremity, this means having the knee slightly bent and the hip externally rotated (Figure 21-2). This allows full access to the medial portion of the thigh and calf and also allows access to the popliteal fossa. Trying to image the leg without proper positioning will lead to inadequate views and errors in diagnosis.

PATIENT POSITIONING FOR THE UPPER EXTREMITY

The upper extremity veins are examined with the bed flat and the patient in the supine position. It is especially important that the bed be flat while the jugular and subclavian veins are examined because they will collapse if the head of the bed is up. Once these vessels are imaged, the bed can be raised to allow for imaging of the arm veins. The arm is positioned at the patient's side for examination of the neck veins and the subclavian vein. When examining the axillary veins, the

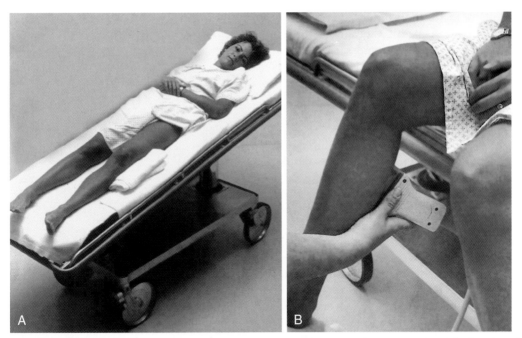

FIGURE 21-1 Patient positions for lower extremity venous examination. **A,** Supine, reverse Trendelenburg's position. **B,** Upright position. *(Modified from Zwiebel WJ, Priest DL: Color duplex sonography of extremity veins,* Semin Ultrasound CT MR *11:136-167, 1990.)*

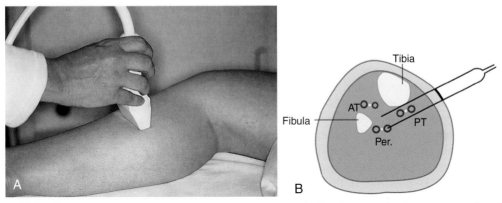

FIGURE 21-2 **A,** Posteromedial position for viewing the posterior tibial and peroneal veins. **B,** Image plane for the posterior tibial and peroneal veins.

arm is repositioned with the arm raised to allow access to the axilla. It is repositioned again in a slightly lower position with the arm externally rotated to allow access to the medial portion of the upper and lower arm.

PROPER TECHNIQUE AND DIAGNOSTIC CRITERIA

Before the 1980s, venograms were the only method available for looking inside the veins of the extremities. It was thought that ultrasound would not be useful in imaging the *veins* because clots were thought to be invisible to ultrasound

(this was the so-called wisdom of the experts of the day). Despite this false assumption, attempts to image the veins with ultrasound began in the early 1980s. In attempting to find diagnostic criteria for identifying clots, investigators discovered not only that you actually *could* see clot on ultrasound, but also that normal veins are so easily compressed with light probe pressure that vein compression could be used to unequivocally determine the absence of thrombus in that vein.[5] Defining compression of the vein as the primary criterion for duplex imaging for deep venous thrombosis (DVT) was the major factor in its universal acceptance. Using compression in this way allows for the examination to quickly progress in a transverse plane to evaluate the extensive venous anatomy.[6-10]

IMAGING NORMAL, THROMBUS-FREE VEINS

Most of the imaging performed during the venous duplex examination is done in a transverse plane. The vein and its accompanying artery (if a deep vessel) are identified alongside each other. The artery is thicker walled but usually the smaller of the two (if the limb being examined is positioned below the heart). Light probe pressure is exerted directly over the vessels. The thicker-walled artery will resist compression (it is also under higher pressure). The vein should compress easily. If there is any confusion about which vessel is the artery or vein, the examiner should use Doppler and color to completely and accurately separate the two structures before proceeding.

If the vein is thrombus-free, it will compress completely so that the inner vein walls actually touch each other. When the vein collapses completely with light probe pressure, it can be determined to be unequivocally thrombus-free at that location (Figure 21-3). This is the key to venous duplex imaging of the veins. The pressure on the vein is released, and the vein will reopen. The examiner then moves the probe along the length of the vessel, compressing every centimeter or so, until the entire vein has been imaged in this way. It is important to ensure that these compression maneuvers are as close together as possible. If the "cuts" are too far apart, a major section of vein containing thrombus can be missed. As a rule, the smaller the cuts, the less chance there is of missing a thrombus.

After the entire segment of vein has been evaluated in the transverse plane, the examiner can rotate the probe and rescan the segment in the longitudinal plane and add color and pulsed Doppler (Figure 21-4). These views provide additional information regarding blood flow through the venous system. These longitudinal views, however, are only an addition to the information already gathered by the transverse compression views and cannot substitute for them. Substituting longitudinal views with color Doppler for the transverse compression views will result in missing partially obstructive thrombus.

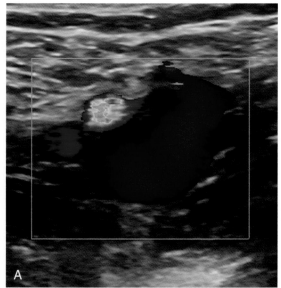

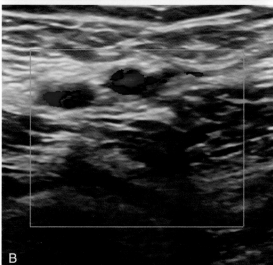

FIGURE 21-3 A split-screen image. Transverse view demonstrating proper compression of a vein. **A,** In this example, the arteries and vein are seen side by side. **B,** Only the arteries are seen because the vein is being collapsed by light probe pressure being exerted over the vessels. Note that the vein is completely collapsed. This is the key maneuver in diagnostic venous imaging. When the vein compresses as shown in this example, the vein can be said to be thrombus-free at this given position. In this example, color is used to show the location of the vessels. However, in practice, transverse compression views are often obtained with the color turned off so that color does not obscure the vessel walls.

COLOR AND DOPPLER INFORMATION ADDED TO TRANSVERSE COMPRESSION VIEWS

Present accreditation protocols require transverse compression views and longitudinal views with color and pulsed Doppler information to

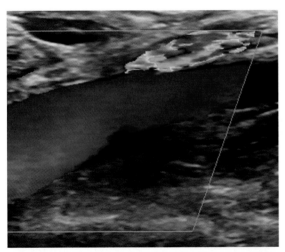

FIGURE 21-4 Longitudinal view of an artery and vein positioned side by side. The blue vessel in this example is the femoral vein.

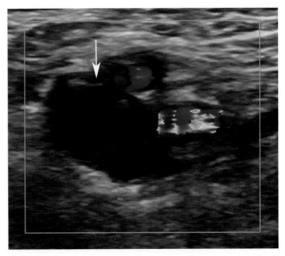

FIGURE 21-6 Transverse view of thrombus in the femoral vein. Note the slightly echogenic material *(arrow)* within the vein.

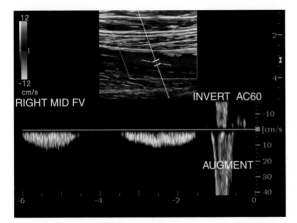

FIGURE 21-5 Longitudinal view of the femoral vein. Note the Doppler spectral waveform that shows normal phasicity of flow. Then note the spike in the Doppler signal as the examiner squeezes the calf (AUGMENT).

be performed at specific levels. Doppler signals in the normal leg vein will be phasic (suggesting an absence of *obstruction* of the major veins above the level of the probe). The flow in the vein should stop completely as the patient takes a breath in and should resume spontaneously as the patient exhales. Squeezing of the leg distal to the level of the transducer should produce an augmentation of flow during this maneuver (Figure 21-5). This indicates the lack of an *obstruction* of the major veins from the level of the squeeze to the level of the transducer. The examiner must understand the limitations of information gathered by pulsed or color Doppler; a partially obstructive thrombus may be missed using these methods—thus the need for the transverse compressions.

DETERMINING THE PRESENCE OF THROMBUS

Thrombus is present within the vein when echogenic material is identified within the lumen of the vein (Figure 21-6) *and* when full compression of the vein is impeded. It is crucial to note that both of these things must occur together to definitively make the diagnosis of thrombus in the vein (Figure 21-7). Too many institutions simply look for noncompressibility of the vein (some institutions refer to duplex venous imaging as "compression ultrasound"). Failure to link these two will result in false-positive results in cases where the veins are difficult to compress—not because of the presence of thrombus—but because of a myriad of other factors. For example, proximal compression of the vein causing stagnation and increased echogenicity of blood flow may simulate intraluminal thrombus. Complete compression of the vein lumen excludes thrombus (Figure 21-8). Other pitfalls include incomplete compression from a patient bearing down in response to painful probe compressions (Figure 21-9), compression being limited by a nearby bone, and other factors. In the case where the vein is not compressing but thrombus cannot be seen directly (poor views or views of very small or deep structures), an additional maneuver is essential to determine whether the noncompressibility is due to the presence of thrombus or some other factor. This additional maneuver may involve compressing harder until the artery next to the vein starts to compress. If the artery next to the vein compresses and the vein does not, thrombus is likely to be present

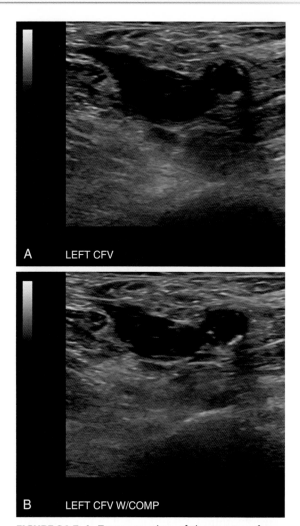

FIGURE 21-7 A, Transverse view of the common femoral vein (CFV) with faintly echogenic material within it. **B,** Probe pressure is being exerted over the vein, and the thrombus is preventing the compression of the vein. This is the key to positively identifying the presence of thrombus within the vein.

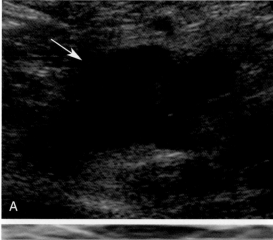

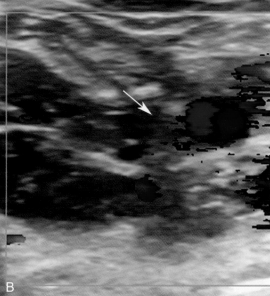

FIGURE 21-8 A, Transverse view of echogenic material seen within the vein *(arrow)* that appears to be thrombus. **B,** Transverse view of the same vein with probe compression. Note how the vein compresses completely *(arrow),* indicating the material previously visualized was only stagnant blood, not a thrombus.

within the vein despite the fact that the clot is relatively anechoic or is not directly visualized. Augmentation of flow through the noncompressible segment may also demonstrate patency, although this maneuver may not exclude a partially occlusive clot. If there is uncertainty regarding the presence of DVT, a correlative study with magnetic resonance venography or computed tomographic scanning may be required for further evaluation.

CHARACTERIZATION OF THROMBUS

Once thrombus has been identified, the next step is to try to gain some information about how fixed or poorly attached the clot is and the likelihood of embolization. Generally speaking, the newer the clot, the more likely it is to embolize. This, as you might imagine, is a very difficult task and not an exact science. However, there are clues to the age and stability of a given thrombus. Characteristics usually associated with *acute clot* are the following:

1. Faintly echogenic (hypoechoic) thrombus
2. Poorly attached thrombus
3. Spongy-texture thrombus
4. Dilated vein (when totally obstructed)

Characteristics usually associated with *chronic clot* are the following:

1. Brightly echogenic (hyperechoic) thrombus
2. Well-attached thrombus

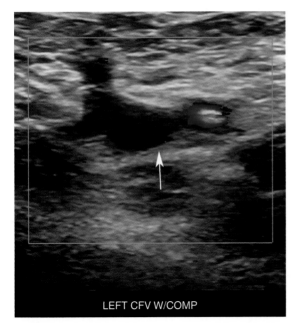

LEFT CFV W/COMP

FIGURE 21-9 Compression of the vein *(arrow)* is being attempted. It is uncertain whether there is echogenic material seen within the vein. However, the vein does not fully compress. This might suggest the presence of thrombus that is lightly echogenic. In this case, the lack of compressibility of the vein is occurring because the patient is bearing down in response to the painful compression, thus not allowing the vein to collapse completely. This is a common cause of a false-positive venous duplex. For this reason, whenever echogenic material is not directly visualized but the vein does not compress fully, the examiner must either equivocate, try another position for compression, perform the augmentation maneuver with color Doppler, or compress harder over the vessels so that the artery compresses. These techniques improve the detection of thrombus within the vein.

3. Rigid texture of thrombus
4. Contracted vein (if totally obstructed)
5. Large collaterals
6. Thickened vein walls

ACUTE THROMBUS

When a thrombus has just formed, it is very faintly echogenic—almost invisible. When the clot is acute, it may be detected by limiting the compression of the vein and by the presence of a faintly visible edge to the thrombus (Figure 21-10). The experienced examiner will spot faint echoes within the vein and note the difficulty in compression (Figure 21-11). Thrombi at this stage are extremely spongy in texture, so the vein will deform with probe compression (but still not allow complete collapse of the vein). Thrombi at this stage of formation may be attached to the vein wall over only a small

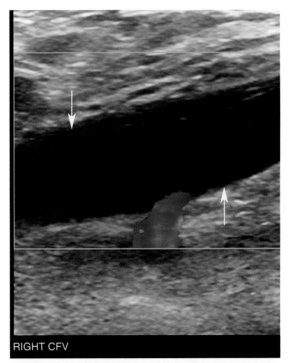

RIGHT CFV

FIGURE 21-10 Longitudinal view of a vein containing a fresh thrombus. Note that the only indication of the contained thrombus is the presence of faint white lines *(arrows)* that actually are the reflection from the thrombin net that has recently captured the blood components to form a thrombus.

area with the remainder of the clot looking like a snake that sways back and forth in the flow stream ("free-floating" DVT) (Figure 21-12). The fact that these poorly attached clots might be more likely to break loose seems logical, although this seemingly obvious conclusion is not universally accepted.

When a new clot fully obstructs a vein, it may continue to enlarge as the compliant vein struggles to stay patent (because veins have the ability to enlarge several times because they serve as a storage area for blood). Eventually the vein loses the battle, and the contained thrombus stretches the vein to its maximum size. This makes a newer obstructive clot stand out in the transverse plane on the venous duplex examination (Figure 21-13).

CHRONIC THROMBUS

Complete dissolution of thrombus may occur naturally over time. However, most of the time, clinically significant thrombi will, as they age, become more solid (as the thrombin net squeezes the fluid components out of the thrombi, leaving the more solid components). Thus, older

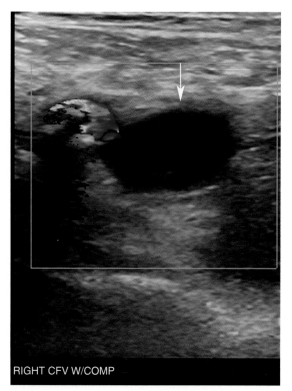

RIGHT CFV W/COMP

FIGURE 21-11 Transverse view of a fresh thrombus *(arrow)*. The thrombus is only faintly echogenic along the periphery but anechoic in the center. Note that the vein shows minimal compression.

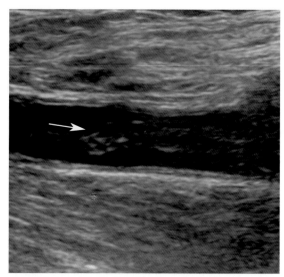

FIGURE 21-12 Longitudinal view of the femoral vein demonstrates a long "tail" of thrombus in the lumen *(arrow)*. Note that no attachment point is seen for the thrombus. This view is of a free-floating thrombus that is attached to the vein at a level below this view.

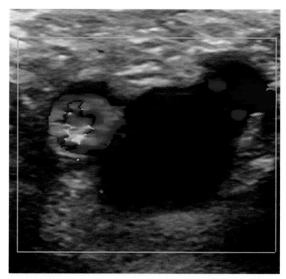

FIGURE 21-13 Transverse view of the common femoral vein, distended with clot. This thrombus is so fresh that the stagnated flow around the contained thrombus is more echogenic than the thrombus itself. Note the flow in the great saphenous vein and common femoral artery.

clots will be firm (they will not deform with probe pressure as newer clots do). They will also be more echogenic (Figure 21-14). The longer the thrombus is present without new clot formation, the better attached it will become to the vein wall (Figure 21-15) and therefore pose less of a threat of embolization into the pulmonary system.

A clot that causes complete venous obstruction will usually produce venous distension, but as the clot ages, it contracts, along with the vein wall. With healing, the vein gets smaller and smaller with time. Thus, a clot that has been present for years will become so small and contracted that it will be difficult to detect. As the clot gets older, it becomes more echogenic and may blend in with the surrounding tissue. These chronic stable clots are no longer at risk for breaking loose.

If a clot does not fully obstruct the vein, it will attach to part of the vein wall while flow moves through the residual channel (Figure 21-16). The contained thrombus will shrink as it ages to fill less and less of the vein (recanalization). Eventually it will appear on ultrasound as a brightly echogenic scar along the vein wall or within the vein lumen (Figure 21-17). Its borders may become irregular (Figure 21-18). Often, the residual clot will look (from a longitudinal view) like a string or cord residing within the vein lumen (Figure 21-19).

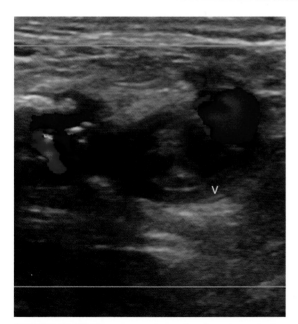

FIGURE 21-14 Transverse view of a chronic occlusive deep venous thrombosis. Note that the clot is more echogenic and that the lumen is less distended than the acute examples previously presented.

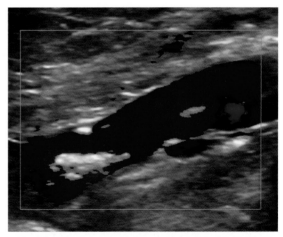

FIGURE 21-16 Longitudinal view of blood flowing around chronic echogenic clot that is partly occlusive.

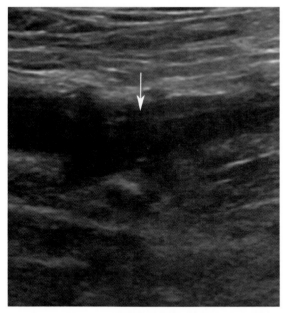

FIGURE 21-15 Longitudinal view of chronic clot adherent to the vein wall *(arrow)*. Note the smooth margins and echogenic border due to recanalization and remodeling.

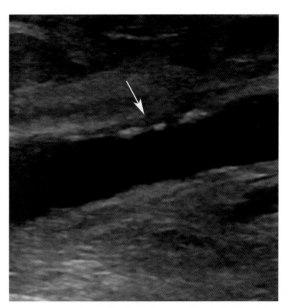

FIGURE 21-17 Longitudinal view of old, brightly echogenic scar or calcification *(arrow)* within the vein wall.

Another observation that can be made, as a clot ages, is the presence of large collaterals. Collaterals develop when a main drainage channel is obstructed and a smaller vein has to enlarge to reroute the flow. When large collaterals are seen, it is a reliable indicator of a chronic problem.

The sonographer who adds these observations to his/her report will provide the physician with valuable information that will often, especially when combined with clinical information, drive the appropriate treatment of the patient.

VALVES AND REFLUX

In addition to checking for thrombus, a full examination of the veins includes checking for reflux in the deep and superficial veins. There may be several different protocols added to a regular venous duplex examination that involve investigating the veins for reflux. Please see Chapter 24 for a full discussion of venous insufficiency, including

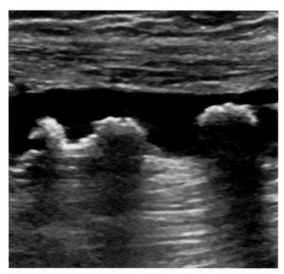

FIGURE 21-18 Longitudinal view of chronic, brightly echogenic deep venous thrombosis with irregular borders.

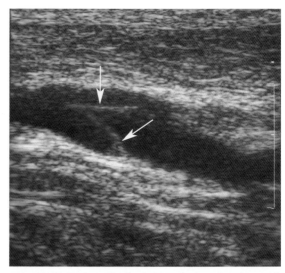

FIGURE 21-20 Longitudinal view of vein valves *(arrows)*. Color and pulsed Doppler should be utilized to check for venous reflux.

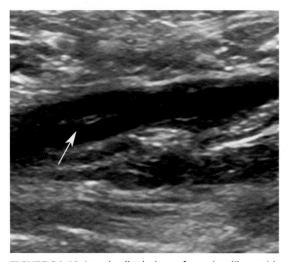

FIGURE 21-19 Longitudinal view of a string-like residual clot. Note the thickening of the vein walls and central stranding consistent with chronic deep venous thrombosis or scarring.

scanning techniques and criteria for diagnosis. A check for venous reflux in the femoral and great saphenous vein may be appropriate in a routine venous duplex examination. The sonographer may perform a more detailed examination if reflux seems to be a major factor for leg swelling. A much more detailed examination will be needed to plan an intervention such as a venous ablation.

There are essentially four ways to check for reflux:

1. Direct visualization of valve closure
2. Doppler waveform evaluation
3. Color flow evaluation
4. Gray-scale evaluation

The least reliable way to check for reflux is to directly visualize the vein valve and watch its function (Figure 21-20). You would think that this would be reliable; however, the valve may appear to be functioning on visual inspection, but when the examiner turns on color Doppler, reflux is discovered.

Color Doppler evaluation is accurate for severe and moderate reflux (Figure 21-21) but will miss mild or minimal reflux. Doppler waveform evaluation is accurate for detecting severe, moderate, and even mild reflux but may miss minimal reflux (Figure 21-22).

The most accurate technique for detecting the most minimal reflux is using the gray scale to actually watch the blood flow directly. This is not always possible but should be tried if one wants to make sure minimal reflux is not being missed.

THE VENOUS ANATOMY AND EXAMINATION PROTOCOL

START AT THE GROIN CREASE

The examination of the lower extremity veins usually begins at the groin crease (Figure 21-23). Just above the crease the main venous trunk is called the external iliac. As it crosses the groin crease, it becomes the common femoral (Figures 21-24 and 21-25).

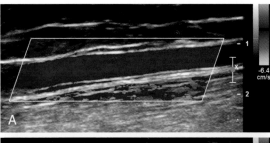
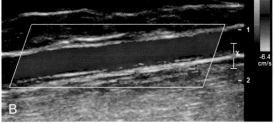

FIGURE 21-21 Using color Doppler, the examiner views the blood flow in the vein moving away from the transducer (back toward the heart), displayed as blue **(A)**. During the Valsalva maneuver, the direction of blood flow reverses to red, suggesting the presence of venous reflux **(B)**. If the valves were competent, no flow would be seen during the Valsalva maneuver.

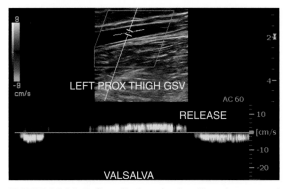

FIGURE 21-22 Reflux displayed using Doppler spectral analysis. Note how flow is below the base line at rest and switches to above the line with Valsalva. If the valves were competent, no flow would be seen during the Valsalva maneuver.

COMMON FEMORAL AND LARGE SAPHENOUS VEINS

The common femoral vein gives off a superficial branch just below the inguinal ligament (Figure 21-26). This is the large saphenous (great saphenous) vein (Figure 21-27). This vein has traditionally been called the greater saphenous vein but has recently been renamed the great saphenous. The great saphenous (Figure 21-28) travels (close to the skin line) down the medial aspect of the thigh (Figure 21-29) and eventually continues in the anterior medial calf all the way into the foot (Figure 21-30).

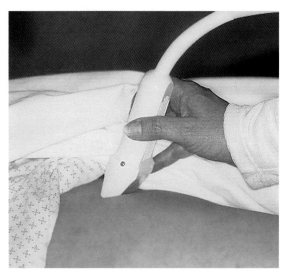

FIGURE 21-23 Short-axis femoral vein examination. Transducer position, upper thigh.

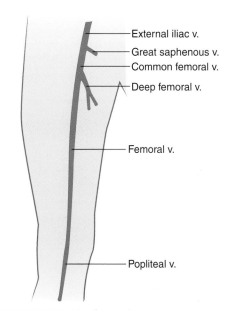

FIGURE 21-24 The femoral venous system. v., vein.

After the great saphenous vein unites with the deep system, the common femoral continues as a single trunk accompanied by the common femoral artery until it bifurcates to form the femoral (superficial femoral) and deep femoral (profunda femoris) veins (Figure 21-31; see Figure 21-24).

FEMORAL VEIN (SUPERFICIAL FEMORAL) AND DEEP FEMORAL (PROFUNDA FEMORIS)

The names of these veins (femoral and deep femoral) continue to create confusion. The vein previously called the superficial femoral has recently

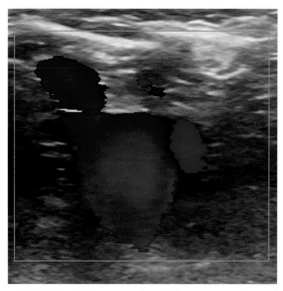

FIGURE 21-25 Transverse view of the common femoral artery and vein at the groin crease. The common femoral artery is the red circle at the right, while the common femoral vein is at the center and appears blue on color Doppler imaging . Note that blood flow in the long (great) saphenous vein is displayed as blue when it empties into the common femoral vein.

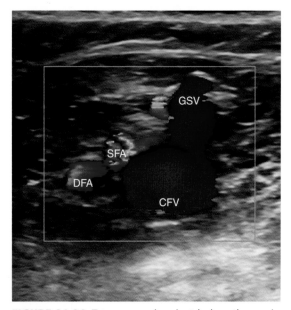

FIGURE 21-26 Transverse view just below the groin crease. The great saphenous vein (GSV) empties into the common femoral vein (CFV). The veins are coded in blue. The superficial femoral artery (SFA) and deep femoral artery (DFA) are identified on the left, color coded in red.

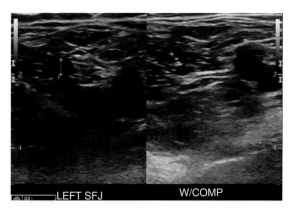

FIGURE 21-27 A view of the great saphenous (GSV) vein (measured) emptying into the common femoral vein just below the level of the groin crease. Note there is complete compression (W/COMP) of the GSV and CFV.

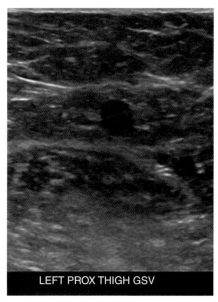

FIGURE 21-28 Transverse view of the great saphenous vein (GSV) traveling within the fascial border in the midthigh.

been renamed the femoral vein. This was done because many people would hear the term *superficial* femoral and get it confused with the great saphenous vein. The vein previously called the profunda femoris is now called the deep femoral. However, it seems that the renaming of these vessels has only made things more confusing. In this text, we will use the updated names: the superficial femoral vein will be called the femoral vein, while the profunda will be called the deep femoral vein. Just remember, the femoral vein is the main deep vein through the thigh.

The femoral vein courses down the thigh alongside the femoral artery (Figures 21-32 and 21-33) with the deep femoral vein on a parallel course deeper in the thigh (see Figure 21-24). The femoral vein is bifid or duplicated in about 25% of patients (Figure 21-34). It continues

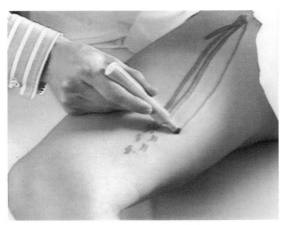

FIGURE 21-29 The medial thigh with the common femoral, femoral (superficial femoral), deep femoral, and great saphenous (greater saphenous) veins being drawn to illustrate their location in the thigh. The marker is pointing out the course of the great saphenous vein.

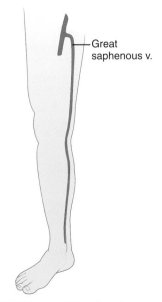

Great saphenous v.

FIGURE 21-30 The great (long) saphenous vein. v., vein.

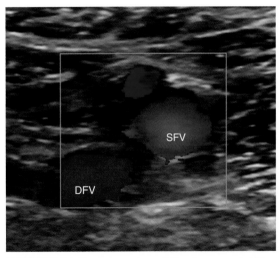

FIGURE 21-31 Transverse view of the deep vessels bifurcating just below the groin crease high in the medial thigh. The superficial femoral artery (in red) is located at the mid-left portion of the image with the femoral vein (labeled SFV for superficial femoral vein) just below it. The next circle below it represents the deep femoral vein (DFV).

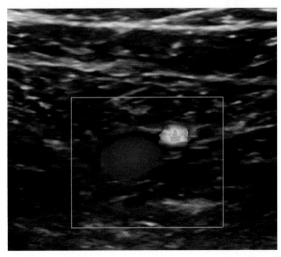

FIGURE 21-32 Transverse view of the superficial femoral artery (red) and femoral vein (blue) at midthigh level.

down the thigh, serving as the primary route of venous drainage until, at the proximal end of the adductor canal, it dives deep and becomes the popliteal vein.

POPLITEAL VEIN

After passing though the adductor canal, this main trunk (the femoral vein) becomes the popliteal vein (Figure 21-35; see Figure 21-24). The popliteal vein is the main drainage conduit for blood flow leaving the calf (Figure 21-36). In the popliteal fossa, the popliteal vein is accompanied

by the popliteal artery (Figure 21-37). Sometimes, (approximately 25% of the time) the popliteal will be, or appear to be, bifid. Usually, however, this is the result of an unusually high junction of the posterior tibial and peroneal trunks.

ANTERIOR TIBIAL VEIN

The anterior tibial vein will leave the popliteal vein high in the popliteal fossa (see Figure 21-36) but is not easily visualized on duplex. It leaves the popliteal vein as a single trunk (the common anterior tibial trunk) and quickly bifurcates

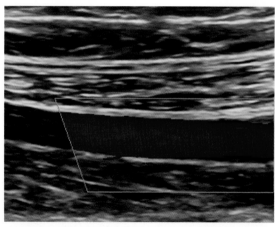

FIGURE 21-33 Longitudinal view of the femoral vein at midthigh level.

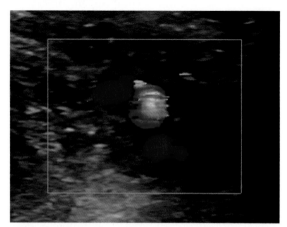

FIGURE 21-34 Transverse view of a bifid femoral vein. Note how the veins (blue) are on either side of the accompanying superficial femoral artery (red). A typical paired femoral vein commonly originates as a single vein, bifurcates into two vessels as seen here, and then eventually rejoins as a single trunk.

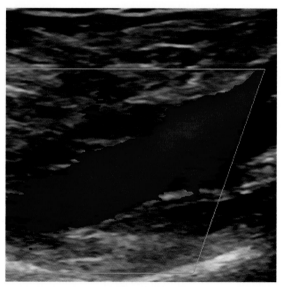

FIGURE 21-35 Longitudinal view of the popliteal vein in the upper portion of the popliteal fossa.

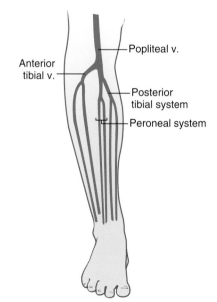

FIGURE 21-36 The popliteal vein and the calf veins. v., vein.

to form the two anterior tibial veins (accompanied by the anterior tibial artery). Although its trunk origin is hard to image, the remainder of the anterior tibial vein is easily imaged from the anterior-lateral projection (Figure 21-38) when performing duplex imaging (Figure 21-39). Unlike the posterior tibial and peroneal veins, the anterior tibial veins do not communicate directly with the soleal sinus veins in the calf. For this reason, the anterior tibial veins almost never develop venous thrombosis (with few exceptions, of course). That is why imaging of the anterior tibial veins is commonly omitted from the basic protocols of most laboratories. Examination of the anterior tibial veins may be added to standard protocols whenever there is injury

to the lateral calf or in instances where pain is reported in the area of the anterior tibial veins.

GASTROCNEMIUS VEINS

As the popliteal continues its course through the popliteal fossa, it joins with branches called the gastrocnemius veins. Each "gastroc" will branch from the popliteal vein as a single trunk that quickly bifurcates into two veins accompanied by a small artery (Figure 21-40). There

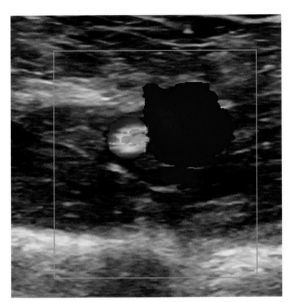

FIGURE 21-37 Transverse view of the popliteal artery (red) and vein (blue) high in the popliteal fossa.

will be several branches that serve to drain each gastrocnemius muscle (Figure 21-41). The gastrocnemius veins are contained in the gastrocnemius muscle and eventually disappear at the distal end of the muscle. This is one way the examiner can make sure he/she is in the gastroc as opposed to one of the tibial veins; the gastroc veins cannot be followed to the foot as the tibials can.

SMALL SAPHENOUS (LESSER SAPHENOUS) VEIN

The vein traditionally called the lesser saphenous has not escaped the name changes that affected the superficial femoral and greater saphenous veins. The lesser saphenous, now called the small saphenous, empties into the popliteal vein (Figure 21-42) at about the same level as the gastrocnemius veins. Sometimes the small saphenous vein will actually share a common trunk with the gastrocs for a time. The small saphenous then passes down the posterior calf (Figure 21-43) and passes behind the lateral malleolus and eventually merges over the top of the foot with the great saphenous vein. There are some variations where the small saphenous (a superficial vein) rejoins the deep system. Sometimes the small saphenous will run the usual course in the calf but not connect with the popliteal vein; rather it will continue up into the thigh, where it may eventually join the deep system (the femoral) or remain superficial and join the great saphenous vein.

TIBIOPERONEAL TRUNK

As the popliteal continues below the level where the anterior tibial and gastrocnemius veins merge, it is called the tibioperoneal trunk. Some still continue to call this short segment of deep vein the popliteal vein. Either is acceptable. In this text, we will refer to this segment as the tibioperoneal trunk.

COMMON TIBIAL AND COMMON PERONEAL TRUNKS

Lower in the popliteal fossa, the tibioperoneal trunk will bifurcate into the common tibial and common peroneal trunks (Figure 21-44). This bifurcation is sometimes mistaken for a bifid popliteal. These trunks will bifurcate again, one trunk to form the paired posterior tibial veins and the other trunk to form the paired peroneal veins (see Figure 21-36).

POSTERIOR TIBIAL VEINS

The posterior tibial veins (paired) will take a course near the tibia (Figure 21-45) on either side of the posterior tibial artery that will eventually end up passing between the medial malleolus and the Achilles tendon at the ankle (see Figure 21-36).

PERONEAL VEINS

The peroneal veins (paired) will follow a deep course near the fibula on either side of the peroneal artery (Figure 21-46; see Figure 21-36). Throughout the calf, the paired posterior tibial and peroneal veins can be viewed side by side from a medial projection (Figures 21-47 and 21-48).

SOLEAL SINUS VEINS

Embedded deep within the soleal muscle in the calf are the extensive network of soleal sinus veins (Figure 21-49). These veins are a major storage area for blood that will empty into either the posterior tibial or peroneal veins (see Figure 21-41). These veins may appear insignificant, but actually they are some of *the* most important veins in the leg for one reason: clots form in these veins because of stagnation of blood when the calf muscle is not active (Figure 21-50). Most blood clots that extend into the larger deep veins like the popliteal originate in these soleal sinus veins. Evaluation of this area is essential to a comprehensive venous imaging study.

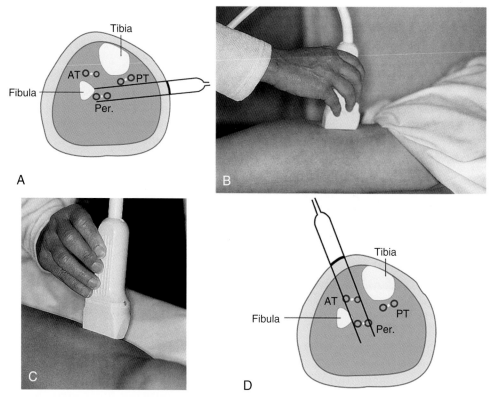

FIGURE 21-38 Calf vein transducer positions. **A,** Posterior tibial (PT) and peroneal (Per.) vein image planes. **B,** "Stocking seam" transducer approach to the peroneal veins. **C,** Anterolateral transducer position for viewing the anterior tibial veins. **D,** Anterior tibial (AT) vein image plane.

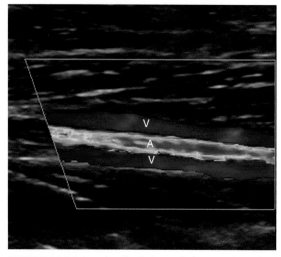

FIGURE 21-39 Longitudinal view of the anterior tibial artery (A) and veins (V).

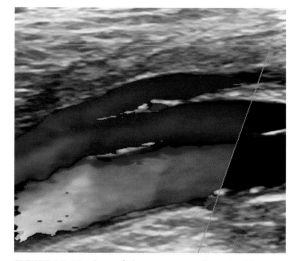

FIGURE 21-40 View of the gastrocnemius vein. The gastrocnemius vein empties into the popliteal vein. The popliteal artery (in red) is seen below the popliteal vein (in blue).

IMAGING THE ILIAC VEINS

Imaging the veins above the inguinal ligament is not routinely done in most institutions. Instead, Doppler waveforms of the common femoral vein are obtained. If good phasic flow is detected, the iliac veins are assumed to be patent. This, of course, will not detect a partially obstructive thrombus, so extension of the venous duplex examination into the pelvis is occasionally appropriate. Imaging the iliac veins is difficult because

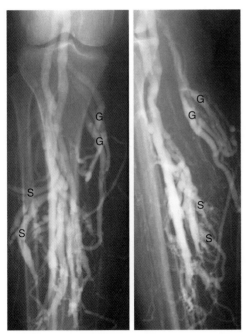

FIGURE 21-41 The gastrocnemius (G) and soleal (S) veins are shown on anteroposterior *(left)* and lateral *(right)* contrast venography images.

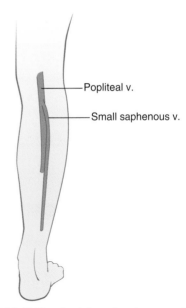

FIGURE 21-43 The short (lesser) saphenous vein. v., vein.

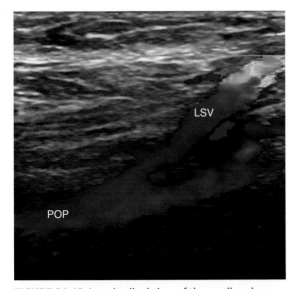

FIGURE 21-42 Longitudinal view of the small saphenous (lesser saphenous) vein (LSV) as it enters the popliteal vein (POP) at the midportion of the popliteal fossa.

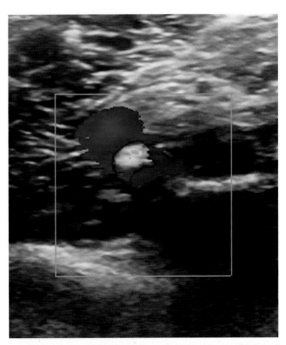

FIGURE 21-44 Transverse view of the common tibial and common peroneal trunks (blue) low in the popliteal fossa. Note how this could easily be mistaken for a bifid popliteal vein. The popliteal artery is central, color coded in red.

of their depth and the presence of bowel gas. Also, compression of the iliac veins is usually not possible, so the diagnostic criteria used in the leg must be altered, relying on gray-scale image and color Doppler flow to identify a thrombus. This significantly reduces the reliability of imaging in this area.

As the common femoral vein is followed superiorly at the inguinal ligament, the vein will quickly dive deeply as it becomes the external iliac vein. At the level of the sacroiliac joints, the external iliac vein becomes the common iliac vein as it is followed upward. This transition occurs as the internal iliac vein joins the external iliac vein. The

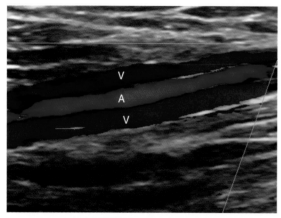

FIGURE 21-45 Longitudinal view of the posterior tibial artery (A) and two veins (V). All of the main-line deep veins of the calf will look similar to this—one artery accompanied by two veins. Sometimes, especially in the distal portion of the calf, there may be three veins for each artery.

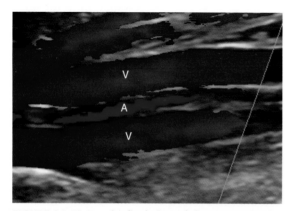

FIGURE 21-46 Longitudinal view of the peroneal veins (V) in the calf. They are located deeper than the posterior tibial veins, so getting them to fill with color flow signals can sometimes be difficult. They are commonly larger than the posterior tibial veins, so once the examiner is used to knowing where to look for them, they are fairly easy to see. A, artery.

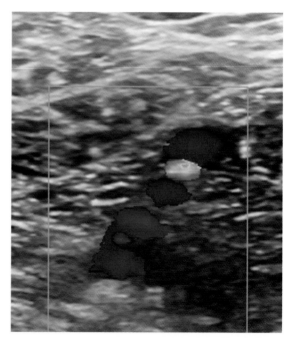

FIGURE 21-47 Transverse view of the upper midportion of the calf from a medial projection. The posterior tibial veins are located anterior to the peroneal veins. Both veins (blue) are paired and flank the artery (red) of the same name. The two sets of vessels parallel each other throughout the calf, so once they are identified at this location they can be easily followed throughout the calf.

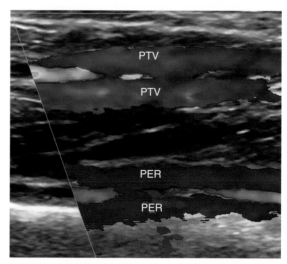

FIGURE 21-48 Longitudinal view of the posterior tibial (PTV) and peroneal (PER) veins at the midportion of the calf. The distal calf is being squeezed to improve the visualization of color flow in both sets of vessels.

internal iliac vein may be difficult to identify, so it may be hard to know when this transition has occurred. Eventually the common iliac will be joined by the common iliac vein from the other leg to form the inferior vena cava (Figure 21-51).

ANATOMY OF THE UPPER EXTREMITY

There are two major differences to be aware of when considering venous thrombosis of the upper extremity versus venous thrombosis of the lower extremity, as follow:

1. Most clots in the upper extremity are the result of injury to the vein wall (usually needle punctures) as opposed to stasis as

seen in the lower extremity. The reason for this is that the upper extremities have no soleal sinuses. Without these sinuses, clots in the arm are less common unless the patient had a recent needle stick or an indwelling venous catheter. The exceptions

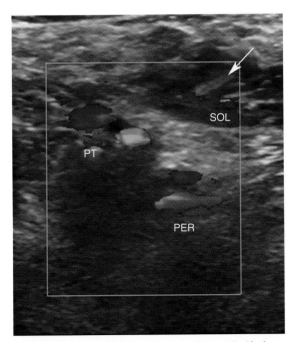

FIGURE 21-49 Transverse view at the midcalf from a medial projection showing a soleal sinus vein (SOL) *(arrow)*. Note its close proximity to the posterior tibial (PT) and peroneal (PER) veins in this view. Soleal sinus veins will be located in the soleal muscle deep in the calf and will connect to either the posterior tibial or peroneal veins.

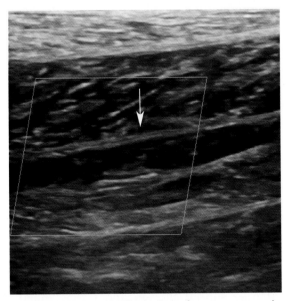

FIGURE 21-50 Longitudinal view of an acute, nonobstructive thrombus residing within a soleal sinus vein *(arrow)*. The thrombus is hypoechoic with stranding (thrombin net) seen within the clot.

to this rule include clots caused by chronic injury to the subclavian vein as the result of thoracic outlet obstruction, underlying coagulopathy, obstruction to blood flow, compression by a mass, and other factors.

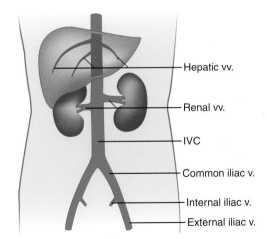

FIGURE 21-51 The inferior vena cava (IVC) and the iliac veins. v., vein; vv., veins.

2. There is much more variation in the anatomy in the upper extremity. Most of this variation involves the median cubital veins and their connection with the basilic and cephalic veins.

UPPER EXTREMITY EXAMINATION PROTOCOL

JUGULAR VEIN

The complete examination of the upper extremity always includes the internal and external jugular veins in the neck. The internal jugular is followed in the lateral neck alongside the carotid artery (Figure 21-52). The external jugular vein lies superficial and posterior to the internal jugular (Figure 21-53) and joins the internal jugular low in the neck to form the subclavian and brachiocephalic veins.

BRACHIOCEPHALIC VEIN

Following the brachiocephalic (innominate) vein is usually difficult because of the sternum and air-filled lungs that block ultrasound transmission. Small footprint probes that operate at lower frequencies can improve visualization of this region. Doppler signals in this area may assist in determining patency of areas that are poorly visualized (Figure 21-54).

SUBCLAVIAN VEIN

The subclavian vein moves from its junction with the jugular and brachiocephalic veins toward the arm. It passes under the clavicle, and shortly thereafter a superficial branch empties into the subclavian vein, the cephalic vein. The subclavian vein

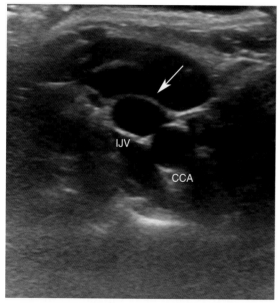

FIGURE 21-52 Transverse view of the internal jugular vein (IJV) *(arrow)* alongside the common carotid artery (CCA).

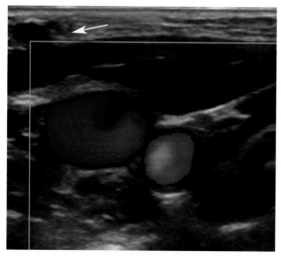

FIGURE 21-53 Transverse view of the external jugular vein located at the top left portion of the frame *(arrow)*. The external jugular vein is located by first finding the internal jugular vein (coded in blue) and then moving a little posterior. Care must be taken to use little or no probe pressure because the external jugular vein is very easily compressed. A large amount of gel to create a standoff is often required to ensure that no pressure is being exerted to inadvertently compress this vein.

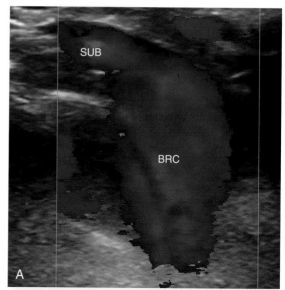

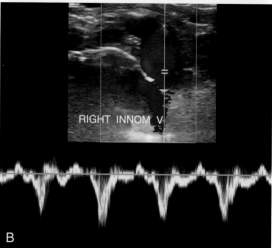

FIGURE 21-54 **A,** The subclavian vein (SUB) emptying into the brachiocephalic vein (BRC). **B,** A pulsed Doppler tracing from the brachiocephalic vein (INNOM V) with marked pulsatility from atrial contractions.

is a large deep vein that runs alongside the subclavian artery (Figures 21-55 and 21-56). Because of its position beneath the clavicle, it is difficult to perform compression maneuvers to check the patency of this vein. To check for collapsibility of the vein, the examiner has the patient take a quick breath in with pursed lips, which allows the vein to collapse.

CEPHALIC VEIN

The cephalic is a superficial vein that empties into the subclavian vein and travels superficially (without an accompanying artery) (Figure 21-57) across the shoulder and down the anterior-lateral border of the biceps muscle. At the level of the anticubital fossa, there is a branch (median cubital vein) that will connect the cephalic to the basilic vein that travels in the medial portion of the arm (Figures 21-58 and 21-59). After communicating with the median

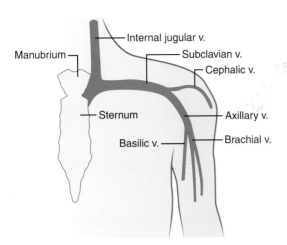

FIGURE 21-55 The subclavian vein and its tributaries. v., vein.

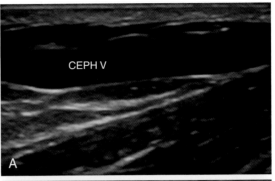

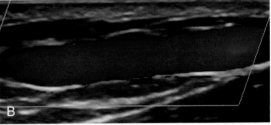

FIGURE 21-57 **A,** Gray-scale longitudinal view of the cephalic vein (CEPH V) in the upper arm, proximal to emptying into the subclavian vein. **B,** Longitudinal view of the cephalic vein with color Doppler.

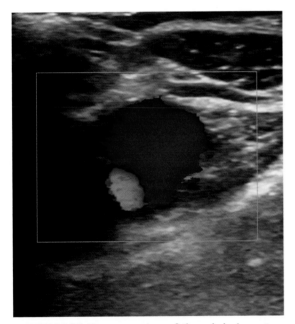

FIGURE 21-56 Transverse view of the subclavian artery (red) and vein (blue). This image is taken below the clavicle just before the level where the cephalic vein leaves the subclavian vein.

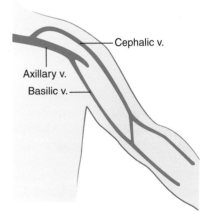

FIGURE 21-58 The superficial veins of the upper extremity. v., vein.

cubital vein, the cephalic vein continues into the forearm. There are commonly two branches of the cephalic vein in the forearm. One will travel down the volar (palmar) aspect of the forearm to the wrist, while the other will roll onto the dorsal aspect of the forearm as it approaches the wrist.

MEDIAN CUBITAL VEIN

As mentioned earlier, the median cubital vein is a superficial vein that connects the cephalic and basilic veins. This usually occurs in the anticubital

fossa where the median cubital vein crosses over the brachial artery and vein (see Figure 21-59). However, this connection is quite variable from person to person.

AXILLARY VEIN

Below the level where the subclavian receives the cephalic vein, the subclavian becomes the axillary vein (Figure 21-60). The axillary vein travels through the axilla (Figures 21-61 and 21-62). In most parts of the body the deep vein will travel directly alongside the artery of the same name;

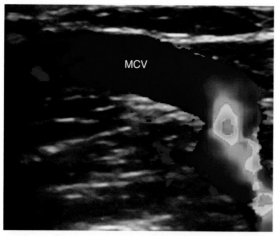

FIGURE 21-59 The median cubital vein (MCV) crosses the antecubital fossa and connects the cephalic and basilic veins. Following the median cubital toward the inside of the arm will lead the examiner to the basilic vein. Following the median cubital in the other direction (toward the outside of the arm) will lead the examiner to the cephalic vein. This proves to be a useful landmark where many examiners choose to begin their examination of the arm.

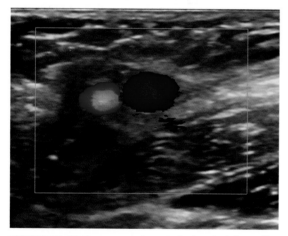

FIGURE 21-60 Transverse view at the level of the axilla. The axillary artery (red) is on the left of the frame with the axillary vein on the right.

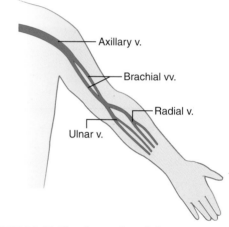

FIGURE 21-61 Longitudinal view of the axillary vein.

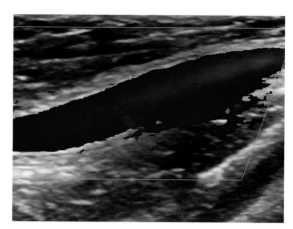

FIGURE 21-62 The deep veins of the upper extremity. v., vein; vv., veins.

however, the armpit is one area where the artery and its accompanying vein have some distance between them for a short while.

At a point usually about halfway down the upper arm, a vein will empty into the axillary vein from the superficial tissues. This vein is called the basilic vein (Figure 21-63). It is usually fairly large and will travel along the medial border of the biceps muscle without an artery (Figure 21-64), taking a parallel course with the brachial vein.

The level where the basilic vein joins the axillary vein is extremely variable. Sometimes it occurs high in the upper arm, but often it occurs in the mid to lower third of the forearm.

BRACHIAL VEIN

The brachial vein continues down the arm as two small paired veins on either side of the brachial artery (Figure 21-65). These deep veins may become very small compared to the superficial veins. The brachial veins continue to follow the artery of the same name until just below the bend in the elbow. At this level, the brachial veins split into a pair of radial and a pair of ulnar veins that accompany the artery of the same name.

RADIAL VEINS

The radial veins course along the volar aspect of the forearm on the radial side towards the thumb (Figure 21-66). They are two very small veins that accompany the artery all the way into the hand near the thumb.

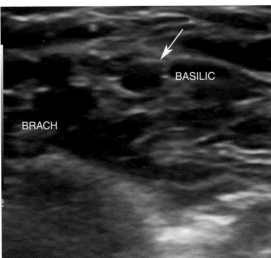

FIGURE 21-63 A transverse view in the mid upper arm from a medial projection. To the left of the frame, the brachial vessels (BRACH) are seen. In the middle of the frame, the basilic vein *(arrow)* is seen traveling without an artery.

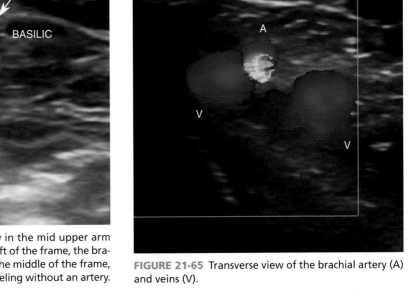

FIGURE 21-65 Transverse view of the brachial artery (A) and veins (V).

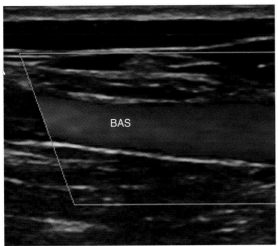

FIGURE 21-64 Longitudinal color flow image of the basilic vein (BAS) traveling without an artery.

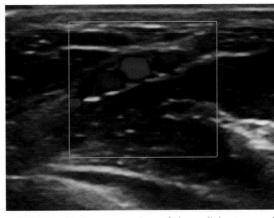

FIGURE 21-66 Transverse view of the radial artery and two veins in the forearm.

ULNAR VEINS

From the level of the brachial vein, the ulnar veins travel along the volar aspect of the forearm and enter the hand at the wrist on the ulnar side (Figure 21-67).

BASILIC VEIN

To examine the basilic vein, we go back to the midportion of the upper arm and find its distal end from the axillary vein. The basilic (a superficial vein) will travel without an artery along the medial forearm and will, for a time, parallel the

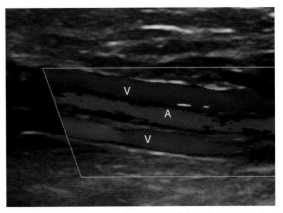

FIGURE 21-67 Longitudinal view of the ulnar artery (A) and two veins (V) in the forearm.

brachial veins. At a point near the anticubital fossa, the basilic vein joins with the median cubital vein, which crosses over the top of the brachial artery and vein like a freeway overpass to eventually connect to the cephalic vein (see Figure 21-59). This vein is a great landmark that many examiners use as a starting point during the venous examination of the upper arm because it is superficial, easy to find, and communicates medially with the basilic vein and laterally with the cephalic vein. After examining these veins, the examiner returns to the overpass portion of the median cubital vein to identify the brachial vessels and evaluate the deep system. The examiner may also continue down the forearm and follow the basilic vein to the wrist. There are commonly two branches of the basilic vein at the distal forearm level; one will run mostly on the volar (palmar) aspect of the forearm, while the other will eventually roll onto the dorsal aspect.

REFERENCES

1. Hollinshead WH: *Textbook of anatomy*, ed 3, New York, 1974, Harper and Row, p 75.
2. Kadir S: *Diagnostic angiography*, Philadelphia, 1986, WB Saunders, p 541.
3. DeWeese JA, Rogoff SM, Tobin CE: *Radiographic anatomy of major veins of the limb*, Rochester, NY, Eastman Kodak.
4. Blackburn DR: Venous anatomy, *J Vasc Technol* 12:78–82, 1988.
5. Talbot SR: Use of real-time imaging in identifying deep venous obstruction: a preliminary report, *Bruit* Vol VI(41), 1982.
6. Cronan JS: History of venous ultrasound, *J Ultrasound Med* 22(11):1144–1145, 2003.
7. Talbot SR: B-mode evaluation of peripheral veins, *Semin Ultrasound CT MR* 9:295–319, 1988.
8. Sullivan ED, Peters BS, Cranley JJ: Real-time B-mode venous ultrasound, *J Vasc Surgery* 1:465–471, 1984.
9. Oliver MA: Duplex scanning in venous disease, *Bruit* 9:206–209, 1985.
10. Talbot SR, Oliver MA: *Techniques of venous imaging*, 1992, Pasadena Calif, Appleton Davies, pp 37–133.

ULTRASOUND DIAGNOSIS OF LOWER EXTREMITY VENOUS THROMBOSIS

22

LESLIE M. SCOUTT, MD; JOSHUA CRUZ, RVT; and ULRIKE M. HAMPER, MD, MBA

Deep venous thrombosis (DVT) is an extremely common medical problem worldwide. The incidence of DVT is estimated to be close to 120 per 100,000 person years,[1-3] and recent modeling data suggest that over 900,000 cases of venous thromboembolism occur in the United States per year.[3,4] Sequelae of lower extremity DVT include recurrence, postthrombophlebitic syndrome, and chronic venous insufficiency. However, pulmonary embolism (PE) is the most serious consequence of DVT. Fifteen percent of all in-hospital related deaths and up to 20% to 30% of deaths related to pregnancy and delivery are caused by PE with an average case fatality rate estimated to be close to 11%.[5] It is estimated that at least 80% of PEs originate from DVT in the lower extremity.[6]

Lower extremity DVT most commonly originates in the calf veins at the valve leaflets and may extend proximally into the calf and the thigh. The pathophysiology of DVT is best described by the constellation of findings in Virchow's triad, namely endothelial damage, venous stasis, and hypercoagulable state. Risk factors are listed in Table 22-1 and can be divided into hereditary and acquired causes. The incidence is higher among women than men, higher among African Americans than whites, and lower in Asian and Native Americans.[3] The incidence of DVT also increases with age. The most common risk factors include immobilization, pregnancy, major surgery, birth control pills, and hormonal replacement therapies. Because both the age of the population and obesity are increasing in the United States, the incidence of DVT is expected to increase as well.[7]

The most common signs and symptoms of DVT are lower extremity swelling and pain, particularly if the swelling is unilateral. Bilateral lower extremity swelling is more likely cardiovascular in origin and secondary right to heart failure. A positive Homans' sign, or pain on forced dorsiflexion of the foot, is considered an unreliable diagnostic criterion. A palpable cord is also an unreliable sign of DVT but is often found in patients with superficial rather than deep venous thrombosis. However, pain and swelling are nonspecific findings, and many patients with DVT are asymptomatic. Therefore, the accuracy of the clinical diagnosis of DVT is extremely poor and estimated at 50%. Compression ultrasound (US) is considered the imaging modality of choice for the diagnosis of DVT. US examination is extremely accurate for the diagnosis of lower extremity DVT in the thigh with reported sensitivities ranging from 88% to 100%, and specificities ranging from 92% to 100%.[8-11] Furthermore, US is readily available, inexpensive, noninvasive, and without contraindication or risk. However, US examination is less accurate in detecting calf DVT, where sensitivity is reported to be only 60% to 80%.[8,12,13]

In many institutions, patients with a high clinical suspicion of DVT or even asymptomatic patients with significant risk factors (prolonged bed rest, major surgery, or malignancy) are immediately evaluated with US examination since it is reliable, safe, and relatively inexpensive. However, despite the efficacy and safety of US for making the diagnosis of DVT, the American Academy of Family Physicians and the American College of Physicians recently published a joint statement recommending that a pretest probability of DVT be estimated before obtaining an US examination.[14] The most common means of establishing pretest probability of DVT is with the Wells score (Table 22-2)[15] and the D-dimer assay.[16-19] The Wells score is based on clinical risk factors. A Wells score less than or equal to 0 is considered low probability; a score of 1 to 2 is consistent with intermediate probability; and a score greater than or equal to 3 is considered high probability for DVT.[15] The D-dimer assay measures fibrin degradation products that accumulate in the blood when thrombus forms. If a high resolution D-dimer assay is negative, DVT is

TABLE 22-1 Risk Factors for Deep Venous Thrombosis

Hereditary Factors	Acquired Factors
Antithrombin deficiencies	
(Protein C and S)	Age
Factor V Leiden mutation	Malignancy (advanced)
Plasminogen deficiency	Surgery (orthopedic, neurologic)
Non-O blood group	Trauma
Elevated levels of clotting factors	Immobilization
(II, VII, VIII, IX, X, and XI)	Pregnancy and postpartum state
Elevated plasminogen activator	Obesity
Inhibitor–I	Oral contraceptive use
Hyperhomocysteinemia	Hormonal replacement therapy
	Hyperviscosity syndromes
Antiphospholipid antibody syndrome	
	Chemotherapy
	Heparin-induced thrombocytopenia
	Myelodysplasia
	Polycythemia vera

TABLE 22-2 Wells Scoring for Estimating Pretest Probability of Deep Venous Thrombosis

+1 Point for Each:

Active malignancy (within 6 months or palliative)

Paralysis, paresis, or recent plaster immobilization of lower limb

Recently bedridden >3 days

Major surgery/trauma within past 4 weeks

Localized tenderness along distribution of lower extremity veins

Swelling of entire lower limb

Calf swelling >3 cm compared with asymptomatic leg

Pitting edema of symptomatic leg

Collateral superficial veins or symptomatic leg

–2 Points for:

Alternative diagnosis at least as likely as deep vein thrombosis

Probability

High ≥3 points

Intermediate 1-2 points

Low ≤0 points

very unlikely. Studies have shown that if there is a low pretest probability and a negative D-dimer assay, no treatment or ultrasound examination is necessary.[7] However, in patients with a high pretest probability for PE or DVT, the D-dimer assay should not be obtained since the negative predictive value of the assay is low in this clinical situation.[5] There are many causes of false positive D-dimer assays, and, therefore, patients should not be treated on the basis of a positive D-dimer assay alone. If the D-dimer assay is positive, an US examination should be performed to evaluate for the presence of DVT. In general, the D-dimer assay is not considered to be helpful or discriminatory in patients who are over 80 years of age, hospitalized, pregnant, or who have cancer since there is frequently a nonspecific elevation of D-dimer levels in these patient subgroups.[5,16-19]

TECHNIQUE AND NORMAL ANATOMY

The deep venous system of the lower extremity begins with the three paired calf veins (Figure 22-1). The posterior tibial veins (PTVs) arise posterior to the medial malleolus and ascend posterior to the tibia in the posterior calf muscles. The peroneal veins (PEVs) course laterally in the calf medial and posterior to the fibula. The PTVs and PEVs join in the upper calf to form the tibioperoneal trunk (TPT). The anterior tibial veins (ATVs) drain the anterior compartment of the calf, travel up the calf between the tibia and fibula, and lie anterior to the interosseous membrane. The ATVs join the TPT after crossing the interosseous membrane in the upper calf. The PTVs, PEVs and ATVs are always found adjacent to their corresponding artery and, barring very rare congenital variants, are always paired. Occasionally one or both of the paired veins may be duplicated. Muscular branches within the calf include the gastrocnemius and soleus branches. The soleal branches join either the peroneal or the posterior tibial veins. The gastrocnemius branches join the popliteal above the knee and are typically duplicated and accompanied by gastrocnemius artery.

The TPT and ATVs combine to form the popliteal vein (PV) (see Figure 22-1). The PV courses superficial to the popliteal artery in the popliteal fossa. When the PV enters the adductor canal, it becomes the femoral vein (FV), which travels medial and deep to the superficial femoral artery in the thigh. In the upper thigh, the FV is joined by the deep femoral or profunda femoris vein

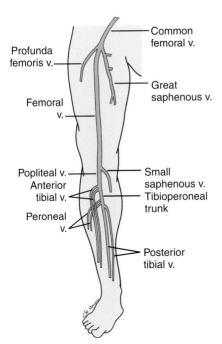

FIGURE 22-1 Schematic drawing demonstrating the anatomy of the deep veins of the lower extremity. v., vein. *(Courtesy of Ms. Geri Mancini.)*

(PFV) and is then called the common femoral vein (CFV). The CFV runs medial and slightly posterior to the common femoral artery. The external iliac vein (EIV) is the continuation of the CFV above the inguinal ligament. The deep veins of the thigh are duplicated in up to 25% of patients.[20] Duplication may be segmental or unilateral. It is advisable to describe duplicated segments in dictated reports so that thrombosis of one of the duplicated veins is not missed on follow-up studies. Unless duplicated, the deep veins of the thigh are generally larger than the accompanying artery and in all cases should run parallel and immediately adjacent to the accompanying artery. The term *femoral vein* should be used instead of *superficial femoral vein* in order to avoid confusion in distinguishing the deep from the superficial venous systems. The great saphenous vein (GSV), a superficial vein, joins the CFV medially just above its bifurcation into the FV and PFV.

Venous Doppler US examination of the lower extremities is optimally performed with a high-resolution 5- to 7.5-MHz linear array transducer. However, if the patient is large and if the vessels are deep to the skin surface, a lower-frequency 2- to 5-MHz curved array transducer may be required to ensure adequate depth of penetration. Gain

settings are optimized to avoid creating artifactual echoes that may be mistaken for thrombus. Color Doppler parameters should be optimized for detection of low-velocity, low volume.

At a minimum, the deep venous system should be examined from the level of the inguinal ligament (CFV) to the tibioperoneal trunk. The CFV and FV are examined with the patient supine and the leg slightly externally rotated. The PV is best evaluated with the knee flexed 20 to 30 degrees and externally rotated (frog's-leg position) or in the decubitus position. Examination of the proximal GSV, the saphenofemoral junction (SFJ), and the origin of the PFV should also be included according to the practice guidelines recommended by the American College of Radiology (Figure 22-2).[21] If desired, the examination may be extended to include the lower EIVs and the calf veins (see later). The CFV, FV, and PV, as well as the origins of the GSV and PFV, should be examined in the transverse plane with and without compression every 2 to 3 cm. With compression, the normal vein wall should completely coapt with obliteration of the vessel lumen (Figure 22-3; see Figure 22-2, C). How much compression is adequate or necessary? In general, if the degree of compression is enough to deform the adjacent artery, it should be adequate to coapt the walls of a normal vein. Compression of the deep veins of the lower extremity may be difficult in the obese or edematous patient, particularly in the adductor canal. In the adductor canal, a two-handed technique may be necessary to demonstrate complete compression of the femoral vein. The examiner places his/her free hand behind the patient's leg in the adductor canal and pushes the soft tissue toward the transducer until complete venous compression is visualized and documented. Although compression US examination is the key to identification of DVT, some authors advocate avoiding compression in the setting of clearly visualized acute thrombus, particularly if nonadherent or free floating, because of the theoretic risk for embolization (Figure 22-4). However, despite concern for potential embolization of a partially occlusive or free-floating clot, one must be certain that luminal echoes represent DVT and not slow-flowing, echogenic blood. In this case, a single compression event may be sufficient for clarification.

Compression maneuvers should be performed with gray-scale imaging, and it is completely adequate to perform the examination of the venous

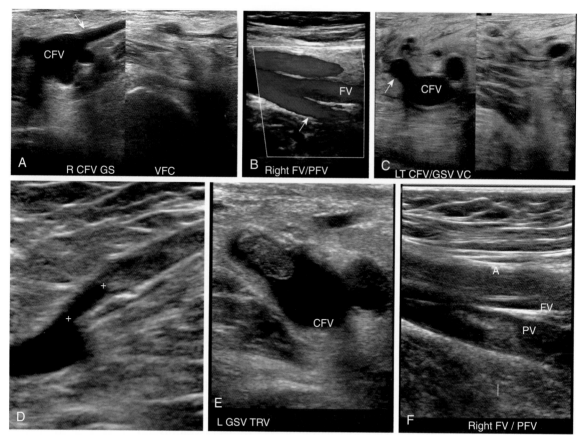

FIGURE 22-2 Origins of the great saphenous (GSV) and profunda femoris (PFV) veins. The origins of the GSV and PFV should be examined longitudinally with color and gray scale as well as in the transverse plane with compression as part of the routine protocol for ultrasound examination of the lower extremities. **A,** Oblique gray-scale split-screen image of the saphenofemoral junction (SFJ) showing the GSV *(arrow)* and common femoral vein (CFV). On the compression image *(right)* the CFV and GSV completely compress. **B,** Color Doppler image of the origin of the profunda femoris vein *(arrow).* FV, femoral vein. **C,** Gray-scale split-screen transverse image of the SFJ demonstrating complete compression of the GSV *(arrow)* and CFV on the compression (VC; *right*) image. **D,** Thrombus in the GSV. Note echogenic thrombus in the proximal GSV. If thrombus is noted in the GSV, the distance from the edge of the thrombus to the SFJ should be measured *(calipers)* since some clinicians will anticoagulate patients with thrombus extending to within 0.5 to 1 cm of the SFJ. **E,** In another patient with thrombus in the left GSV, a transverse gray-scale image demonstrates that the clot extends just into the CFV. This would, therefore, be considered deep venous thrombosis, and the patient would be treated with anticoagulation. **F,** Note echogenic intraluminal echoes indicative of thrombus at the origin of the profunda femoris vein (PV). Isolated thrombus in the PFV can occasionally be observed. However, more commonly thrombus in the PFV is seen in conjunction with thrombus elsewhere in the deep system, usually in the femoral vein. A, superficial femoral artery; FV, femoral vein.

system to exclude DVT with gray-scale imaging alone. However, color or power Doppler imaging, particularly in the longitudinal plane, may be useful to quickly identify the absence of flow due to an occlusive thrombus or a color void due to partially occlusive thrombus. In addition, color flow imaging may be helpful in examining the obese patient to identify venous structures and demonstrate blood flow signals following the augmentation maneuver when spontaneous flow cannot be demonstrated because of problems with depth penetration and resolution.

Consensus regarding the necessity for evaluation of the calf veins and optimal imaging protocol has not been reached. In 2007, the American College of Chest Physicians' published guidelines recommended treatment of DVT regardless of location,[22] and in accordance that same year, the Intersocietal Commission for the Accreditation of Vascular Laboratories changed their standard to require evaluation of the calf veins.[23] While the American Institute of Ultrasound in Medicine (AIUM)/ American College of Radiology (ACR) DVT practice guideline does not require routine calf vein

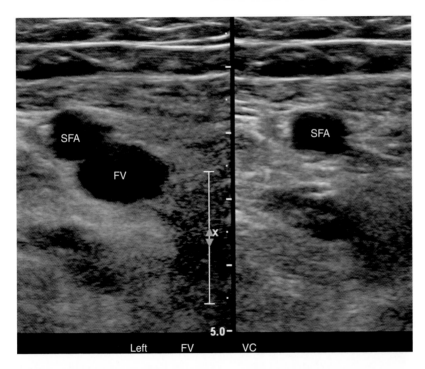

FIGURE 22-3 Normal venous compression. Split-screen grayscale image demonstrating normal compression of the femoral vein (FV) posterior to the superficial femoral artery (SFA) on the right-hand image. The venous lumen is completely obliterated, and the venous walls cannot be seen. VC, venous compression.

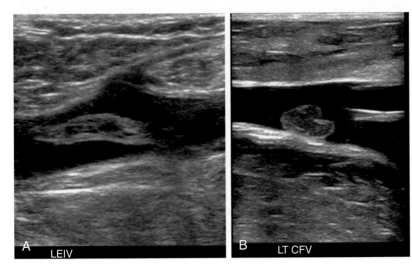

FIGURE 22-4 Free-floating clot. Sagittal **(A)** and transverse **(B)** gray-scale images demonstrating echogenic free-floating intraluminal clot in two different patients. When thrombus is incompletely adherent to the vessel wall and surrounded by flowing blood (anechoic lumen), compression maneuvers pose an increased risk for embolization and should be avoided.

evaluation, AIUM/ACR does require evaluation of the veins of the calf in the patient with calf pain.[21] Rationales for calf vein evaluation and treatment include calf DVT, prevention of thrombus progression and PE, reduction in the risk of recurrent DVT, prevention of venous insufficiency, and the making of a specific diagnosis, thus excluding other causes of pain/swelling. In addition, there is increasing recognition that bilateral calf vein DVT may not be a self-limited disease process in comparison to unilateral calf DVT, with substantially increased risk of PE, cancer, recurrence, and chronic venous insufficiency and lower 2-year survival.[24]

Most calf vein protocols require evaluation of the PTVs and PEVs. If these veins cannot be followed inferiorly from the bifurcation of the TPT, one can identify the PTVs posterior to the medial malleolus and the peroneal veins in the lateral calf above the ankle and attempt to follow these paired veins superiorly. The calf veins are typically duplicated and accompany the named artery that serves as a landmark (Figure 22-5). It may be difficult to identify the calf veins with US due to their small size and slow flow. Color and power Doppler imaging as well as distal augmentation can facilitate visualization of these small veins.

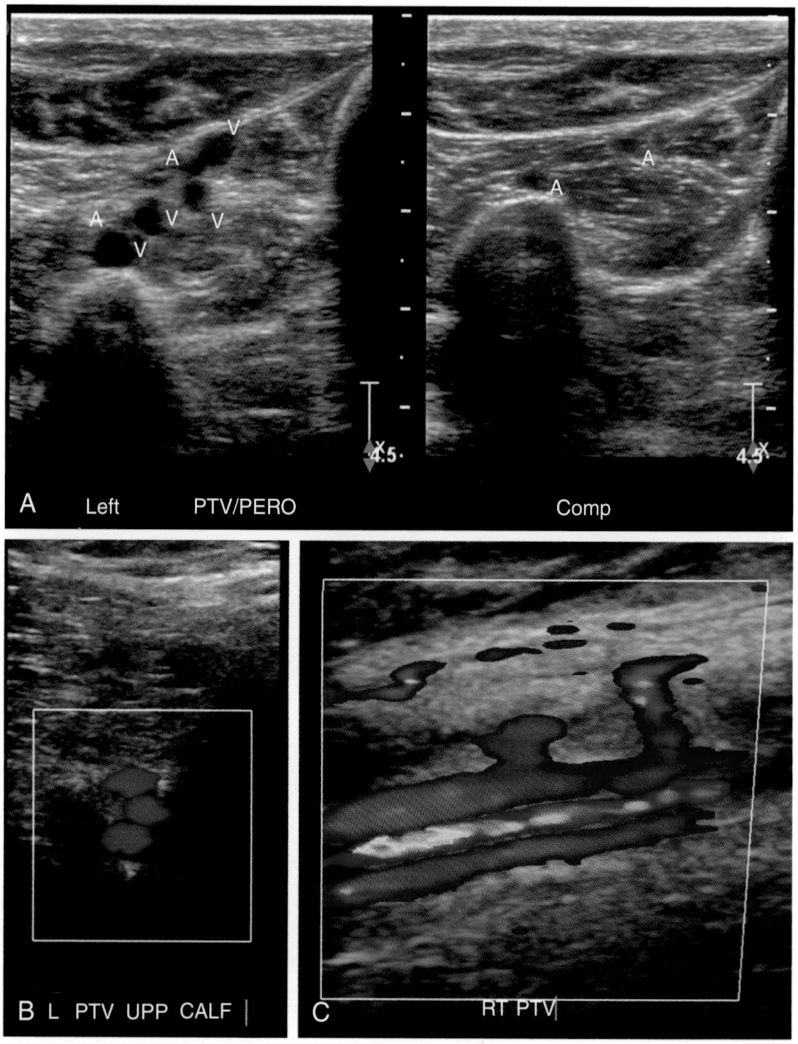

FIGURE 22-5 Normal calf veins. **A,** Split-screen transverse gray-scale image demonstrates the paired posterior tibial (anterior) and peroneal (posterior) veins (V) adjacent to the named arteries (A). Whether the posterior tibial veins (PTVs) are anterior or posterior relative to the peroneal veins (PEVs) depends upon the angle of interrogation. The PTVs run medially in the calf, and the PEVs run laterally near the fibula and do not cross the ankle joint. Note complete compression of these normal four veins on the compression (Comp) image *(right)*. Transverse **(B)** and sagittal **(C)** color Doppler images of the paired PTVs (blue) on either side of the posterior tibial artery (red).

In addition, dangling the lower leg over the edge of the bed, scanning in the reverse Trendelenburg position, or even gentle placement of a tourniquet near the knee can distend the calf veins, making them easier to visualize. Since isolated thrombus occurs infrequently in the ATVs and examination of the normal ATVs is difficult, visualization of these veins is not required for most protocols. The ATVs can be most easily found branching anteriorly from the popliteal artery below the knee or on the dorsum of the foot at the level of the dorsalis pedis arteries.

In addition to gray-scale compression and color Doppler evaluation, spectral Doppler waveforms should be obtained bilaterally from the EIVs or CFVs to assess for respiratory phasicity (Figure 22-6) and from the PVs to assess for augmentation (Figure 22-7).[21,23] It may be useful to assess for respiratory phasicity below and augmentation above

any nonvisualized venous segment in the thigh. Augmentation is a useful maneuver to demonstrate venous flow in the calf, thigh, and pelvic veins and to exclude occlusive thrombus in a nonvisualized venous segment. However, augmentation maneuvers should not be performed if free-floating or partially occlusive thrombus is visualized in order to avoid the theoretic possibility of dislodging and embolizing the thrombus. A recent report suggests that evaluation of augmentation in the lower extremities adds little to the sensitivity or accuracy of the Doppler examination and therefore can be safely eliminated from the venous DVT protocol.[25]

A unilateral examination is acceptable in a patient with unilateral symptoms, although spectral Doppler waveforms are required, according to recommended protocols, from both CFVs or EIVs.[21] However, in a patient with bilateral leg symptoms or central cardiac and/or pulmonary

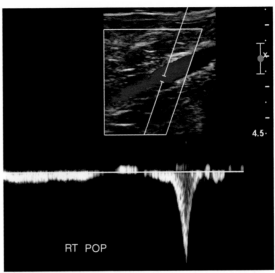

FIGURE 22-7 Normal augmentation. Spectral Doppler waveform from the right popliteal (RT POP) vein demonstrates venous augmentation following compression of the calf. If the caudal veins are patent, compression from below will create a spike of high-velocity blood flowing toward the heart. This provides indirect evidence that the caudal veins are patent. This maneuver can be useful in the thigh if part of the femoral vein is obscured by overlying bandages or surgical hardware. However, augmentation is less useful in the popliteal vein as there are three paired veins below this level. Calf augmentation will only be absent if all six veins are thrombosed and may still be observed if only one or two veins below the knee are patent.

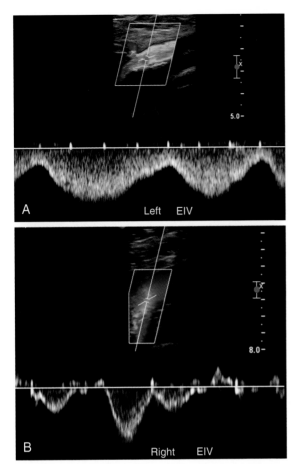

FIGURE 22-6 Normal respiratory variation. **A,** Spectral Doppler waveform of the lower left external iliac vein (EIV) demonstrating decreased flow velocity in inspiration due to increased intra-abdominal pressure. On expiration venous velocity increases. **B,** Mild cardiac pulsatility indicative of changes in right heart pressure during the cardiac cycle also can be transmitted to the iliac and femoral veins in normal patients as noted on this spectral Doppler waveform of the lower right EIV.

symptoms (i.e., PE, shortness of breath or tachycardia), a bilateral examination is necessary. Although examinations limited to the CFV and PV have been proposed to decrease examination time with acceptable accuracy in detection of DVT, this approach has not been generally accepted[8,20] unless a repeat examination is performed in all cases with a negative study, typically 5 to 7 days after the first study. These controversial topics are addressed in greater detail in Chapter 23.

NORMAL FINDINGS

The walls of the normal veins are thin and practically imperceptible and will completely coapt, obliterating the vein lumen, with slight pressure from the transducer (see Figures 22-2, *C*, and 22-3). The lumen of the vein should be anechoic, without internal echoes. Color flow imaging should demonstrate spontaneous flow with no evidence of a color void. Spectral Doppler interrogation should demonstrate respiratory variation in the EIV or CFV (see Figure 22-6, *A*). Transmitted cardiac pulsatility may also be noted in the EIV or CFV (see Figure 22-6, *B*). Tricuspid regurgitation and/or right heart failure will increase the pulsatility of the Doppler waveform of the EIV or CFV (Figure 22-8). Compression of the calf veins will produce augmentation and increased blood flow signals toward the heart in the above-the-knee veins (see Figure 22-7).

ULTRASOUND FINDINGS OF VENOUS THROMBOSIS

The primary criterion for the diagnosis of venous thrombosis is lack of coaptation of the vein walls with compression (Figure 22-9). Intraluminal echoes may be noted on gray-scale imaging

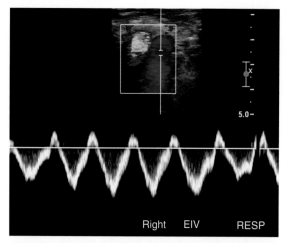

FIGURE 22-8 Tricuspid regurgitation. Spectral Doppler waveform from the right external iliac vein (EIV) demonstrating tricuspid regurgitation. The sawtooth pattern of the spectral Doppler waveform of the right external vein indicates severe increased right-sided venous pressure and can be seen in patients with tricuspid regurgitation, pulmonary hypertension, or severe right heart failure.

(Figure 22-10). However, slow-flowing blood may also demonstrate luminal echoes, although compression US will be normal (Figure 22-11). Lack of spontaneous flow (Figure 22-12) is a suggestive but not a specific finding of DVT as slow flow may not be detectable on Doppler interrogation and, therefore, may mimic DVT. Color Doppler interrogation will demonstrate no flow if the thrombosis is occlusive and a color void in the setting of partially occlusive thrombus (Figure 22-13). Extensive thrombus in the calves may blunt augmentation of blood flow signals in the popliteal veins. Thrombus in the iliac veins or inferior vena cava (IVC) will flatten the Doppler tracing in the distal (caudal) veins and eliminate respiratory variation and cardiac pulsatility in the EIV, CFV, and below.[26] External compression by pelvic or inguinal masses and/or a large volume of ascites will also eliminate or reduce respiratory variation in the veins below the inguinal ligament (Figures 22-14 and 22-15).[26]

COMMON PITFALLS

The most common pitfall in the use of US to diagnose DVT is inability to see the veins due to large body habitus, overlying bandages or hardware, or slow blood flow. Use of a curved array transducer may improve penetration, and the reversed Trendelenburg position or dangling the leg over the side of the bed may dilate the veins,

making them easier to visualize. If the veins cannot be seen on gray-scale imaging alone, use of color or power Doppler following distal augmentation may be helpful to demonstrate preserved blood flow. If blood flow can be documented, occlusive thrombus can be excluded, but partially occlusive thrombus may still be present. If a vein segment cannot be seen, the examination is indeterminate in this region and DVT cannot be excluded. Follow-up sonography to exclude propagation or referral for magnetic resonance imaging can be recommended. On occasion, the veins can be seen but are not compressible due to pain, obesity, and/or edema. In this situation, color Doppler can be used to exclude occlusive thrombus but partially occlusive thrombus cannot be ruled out.

Color Doppler facilitates the performance of the US examination, by affording rapid identification of the veins and showing a color void in cases of partially occlusive DVT. Unfortunately, color blooming can overwrite or obscure visualization of partially occlusive thrombus, thereby giving a false-negative diagnosis (Figure 22-16). Compression US should demonstrate the partially occlusive clot. Color blooming is more likely to occur when flow is increased, for example, following augmentation or coughing. Thrombus in only one limb of a duplicated deep venous segment has also been reported as a cause of a false-negative US examination for DVT (Figures 22-17 and 22-18),[20] as the unwary may consider the single patent vein to be normal and miss the thrombosed vein, which may be more echogenic and fade into the surrounding soft tissues. A vein diameter that is less than the diameter of the adjacent artery should raise the possibility of a duplicated vein or scarring and fibrosis from a prior DVT.

ACUTE VERSUS CHRONIC DVT

Following an episode of acute DVT, complete resolution occurs in approximately 20% of patients. In others, no or partial recanalization and/or collateralization may occur.[8] Differentiation of acute superimposed on chronic DVT may be difficult. Acute thrombus tends to be hypoechoic and expand the vein diameter (larger than the adjacent artery). Chronic thrombus usually appears irregular, eccentric, and echogenic with the vein often contracted and smaller than the adjacent artery. However, there is overlap in the US appearance.

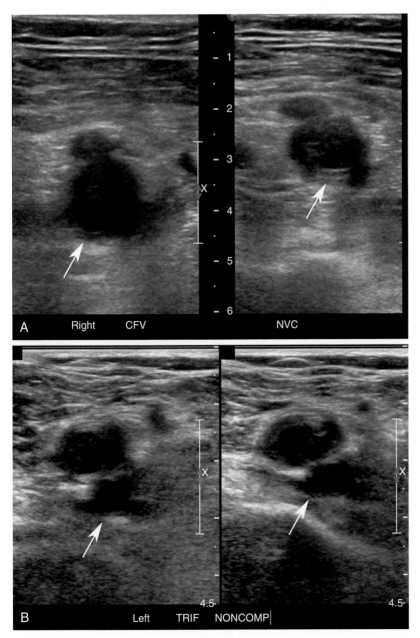

FIGURE 22-9 Ultrasound findings of deep venous thrombosis (DVT): Lack of compression. **A,** Split-screen gray-scale image demonstrating lack of compression on the right hand image (NVC) of the right common femoral vein (CFV; *arrow*) posterior to the common femoral artery, which also does not compress. **B,** Note lack of compression on right-hand image in a second patient with acute DVT in the left tibioperoneal trunk superficial to the popliteal artery. The artery *(arrow)* has a thicker, more echogenic wall than the normal vein.

Thickening of the vein wall, calcification, echogenic webs or synechiae within the vessel lumen, and serpiginous collateral vessels suggest chronic thrombus, although collateral channels may develop relatively quickly (Figure 22-19). Since any episode of DVT increases the risk for recurrent DVT, such patients may develop acute superimposed on chronic DVT, making differentiation extremely difficult. Fortunately, this clinical scenario is rare. It is helpful to obtain a baseline study upon completion of anticoagulation therapy as the identification of thrombus in a new location is the single best indicator that acute DVT is present in a patient with recurrent symptoms. In addition, several recent studies have suggested that documentation of residual or persistent DVT might be extremely helpful in patient management. A study reported by Siragusa and colleagues[27] suggests that if a repeat US examination at 3 months documents no residual DVT, anticoagulation may be safely stopped with a very low risk for recurrence. Conversely, Prandoni and associates[28] reported that extending the duration of anticoagulation therapy in patients with evidence of persistent DVT on follow-up US examination after 3 months of therapy reduced the rate of recurrent DVT.

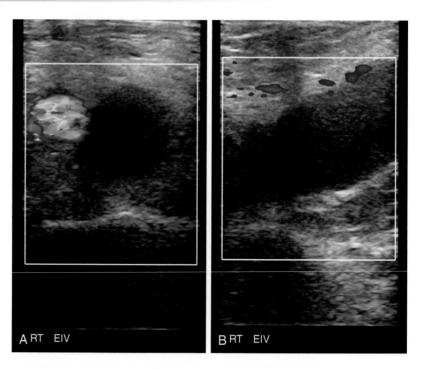

FIGURE 22-10 Ultrasound findings of deep venous thrombosis (DVT): Intraluminal echoes. Transverse **(A)** and sagittal **(B)** color Doppler images of the right external iliac vein (RT EIV) demonstrate intraluminal echoes filling the vein lumen. Color signal fills the lumen of the adjacent external iliac artery in **A.** The echoes are hypoechoic and expand the venous diameter. There is no peripheral blood flow. These findings are indicative of occlusive acute DVT.

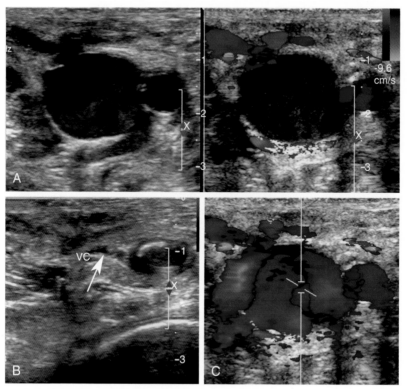

FIGURE 22-11 Slow flow mimicking deep venous thrombosis (DVT). **A,** Split-screen gray-scale *(left)* and color *(right)* images of the common femoral vein reveal internal echoes and a color flow void suggestive of DVT. However, the internal echoes were noted to swirl on real time, suggesting slow flow rather than DVT. **B,** On gray-scale transverse compression image, there is complete coaptation of the vessel wall (VC, *arrow*), confirming that these echoes merely represent swirling of aggregates of red blood cells (rouleaux formation) in the setting of slow flow. **C,** Color Doppler image following augmentation demonstrates fill-in of the vessel lumen with color. However, this is not a reliable finding to exclude DVT, as color bleeding may bloom and overwrite partially occlusive thrombus.

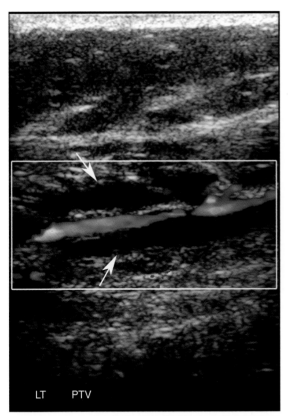

FIGURE 22-12 Ultrasound findings of deep venous thrombosis (DVT): Lack of spontaneous flow. Sagittal color Doppler image of the left posterior tibial veins (LT PTV) reveals lack of spontaneous flow *(arrows)* in distended veins. The vessel lumen appears anechoic at these gain settings without intraluminal echoes. These findings are suggestive of acute DVT but are not diagnostic as slow flow may not be detected on color Doppler interrogation. Augmentation from below may be attempted to demonstrated fill-in of the vessel lumen with color signal. However, color blooming from the augmented blood flow may obscure partially occlusive thrombus. Therefore, compressive ultrasound maneuvers must be performed to confirm vessel patency. Posterior tibial artery (red) is patent.

INCIDENTAL FINDINGS/ALTERNATIVE DIAGNOSES

Leg pain and swelling are the most common clinical presentations of acute DVT but are nonspecific. In most institutions, DVT will be diagnosed in only approximately 10% to 25% of patients referred for venous duplex Doppler examinations of the lower extremities. This means that nearly 7 out of 10 patients referred for evaluation of leg pain and swelling will have a cause other than DVT.[29,30] Studies have shown that careful ultrasound examination will identify the cause of

symptoms in over 10% of patients.[29,31] One of the most common causes of calf pain and swelling other than DVT is a ruptured popliteal or Baker's cyst. The presence of a cystic mass in the popliteal fossa connecting to the joint space or coursing between the medial head of the gastrocnemius muscle and the semimembranous tendon is diagnostic of a Baker's cyst[32,33] (Figure 22-20). A Baker's cyst develops secondary to distension of the semimembranous gastrocnemius bursa usually secondary to degenerative changes. However, Baker's cysts are also associated with inflammatory arthritis (especially rheumatoid arthritis), trauma, infection, and pigmented villonodular synovitis. Baker's cysts have been reported as incidental findings in over 3% of patients.[34] On US, a ruptured Baker's cyst will have an irregular elongated or tear-shaped configuration, often dissecting in the subcutaneous tissues superficial to the gastrocnemius muscle (Figure 22-21). Internal echoes may indicate internal debris, hemorrhage, or infection.[32,33] Other causes of calf pain and swelling that may be diagnosed on US examination include arterial thrombosis (Figure 22-22), popliteal artery aneurysms, hematomas, soft tissue abscesses, muscle tears (Figure 22-23), tendon tears, and muscle or soft tissue masses (Figure 22-24) including lymphadenopathy, cellulitis, joint effusions, and thrombosed superficial varicosities (Figure 22-25).[29,31-33] Please see Chapter 25 for other nonvascular pathologies encountered during venous sonography.

CONCLUSIONS

The compression ultrasound examination has become the gold standard for the evaluation of DVT. The primary diagnostic criterion for the diagnosis of DVT is lack of venous compression or complete coaptation of the vein walls. Other diagnostic criteria include intraluminal echoes, a color void, lack of spontaneous flow, and absence of respiratory variation (suggestive of clot within or external compression of the veins above the level of examination). While US is highly accurate in the diagnosis of DVT in the thigh, the sensitivity of Doppler US for the detection of calf thrombus is much lower, perhaps only 60% to 80%. As clinicians increasingly recommend treatment of calf DVT, examination of calf veins has become part of the routine protocol for sonographic venous evaluation of the lower extremity in many centers. Sensitivity and

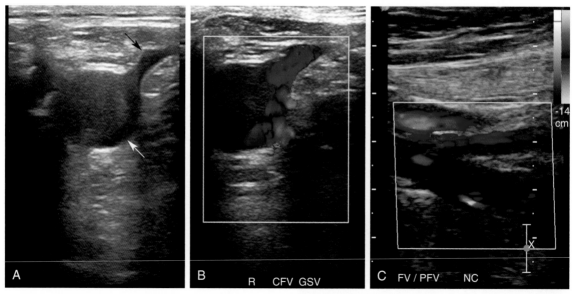

FIGURE 22-13 Ultrasound findings of deep venous thrombosis (DVT): Color void. **A,** Transverse gray-scale image of the common femoral vein (CFV) near the saphenofemoral junction (SFJ) demonstrates an enlarged vein containing intraluminal echoes. The great saphenous vein is indicated by the black arrow. Peripherally the lumen is more anechoic *(white arrow),* suggesting that the vessel is partially patent, a finding that is confirmed by the presence of color flow on the transverse color Doppler image **(B). C,** Longitudinal color Doppler image from another patient demonstrates peripheral flow and a central flow void consistent with partially occlusive thrombus in the femoral vein (FV) and profunda femoris vein (PFV).

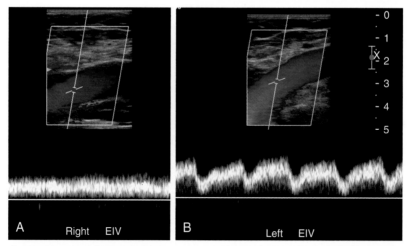

FIGURE 22-14 Indirect Ultrasound findings of deep venous thrombosis (DVT): Asymmetric respiratory variation. Spectral Doppler waveform in the right external iliac vein (EIV, **A**) is flat in comparison to the spectral Doppler waveform in the left EIV **(B).** The flat waveform was due to compression of the upper right EIV and common iliac vein in the pelvis by a large, pedunculated uterine leiomyoma.

accuracy of US examination for the diagnosis of DVT is limited by obesity, pain on compression, immobility, and overlying bandages or surgical hardware. US examination of the lower extremity in the symptomatic patient can be extremely useful in identifying alternative causes of leg pain and swelling, including musculoskeletal etiologies such as Baker's cysts and muscle tears as well as arterial causes such as arterial thrombosis or popliteal artery aneurysms.

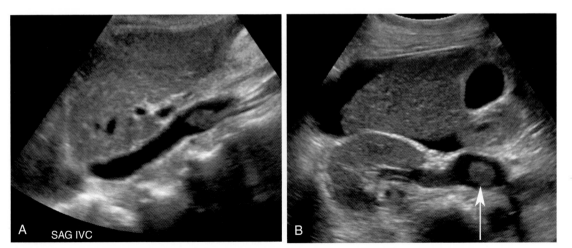

FIGURE 22-15 Inferior vena cava (IVC) thrombus. Sagittal (SAG; **A**) and transverse **(B)** gray-scale images demonstrate thrombus *(arrow)* in the IVC. IVC thrombus can cause flattening of the waveforms in the external iliac veins (EIVs) and common femoral veins (CFVs) bilaterally. If thrombus is noted in the EIV, the examination protocol should be extended to include the pelvic veins and IVC to identify the superior extent of the thrombus. In addition, the contralateral EIV and CFV should be examined as the presence of contralateral clot may affect potential venous access if direct clot lysis is to be considered as a therapeutic option.

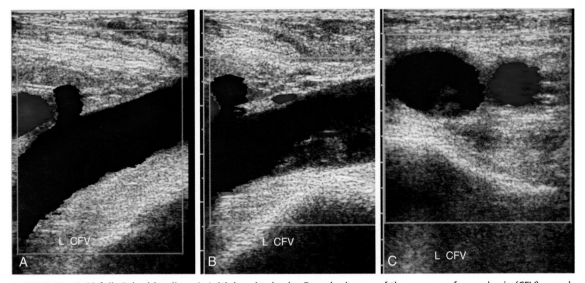

FIGURE 22-16 Pitfall: Color bleeding. **A,** Initial sagittal color Doppler image of the common femoral vein (CFV) reveals complete fill-in with color (i.e., no evidence of deep venous thrombosis [DVT]). However, sagittal **(B)** and transverse **(C)** color Doppler images reveal a color void consistent with DVT. In the first image the color Doppler signal blooms or covers up the intraluminal echoes from the partially occlusive DVT, giving a false-negative color Doppler examination. Color blooming is more prominent following augmentation and is more likely to occur if a low color-velocity scale or low-frequency transducer is used. Increasing the velocity scale or examining the patient in subsequent deep inspiration can reduce color-blooming artifact.

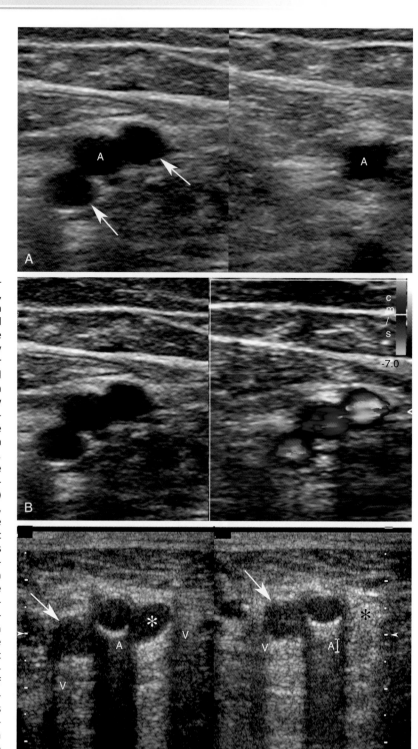

FIGURE 22-17 Pitfall: Duplication of the femoral vein. **A,** Transverse gray-scale split-screen image demonstrates two femoral veins (FVs; *arrows*) on either side of the superficial femoral artery (A). Note that each FV is smaller than the adjacent superficial femoral artery (SFA). When a single FV is present, it is normally larger than the SFA. Note normal compression of both of the duplicated segments of the FV on the compression image *(right)*. **B,** Split-screen transverse image with color Doppler *(right)* revealing duplication of the FVs (blue) adjacent to the SFA (red). **C,** Split-screen transverse gray-scale image from a second patient with a duplicated FV (V) reveals lack of compression of one segment *(arrow)* consistent with deep venous thrombosis. The second segment (*) is fully compressible and normal. A, superficial femoral artery. Visualization of normal compressibility of one limb of a duplicated FV without realizing that a duplicated segment is thrombosed is a cause of false-negative ultrasound examinations. A clue to this diagnosis is the recognition that the visualized patent vein is smaller than the accompanying artery. If the vein is smaller in diameter than the adjacent artery, a careful search for a thrombosed duplicated segment should be made.

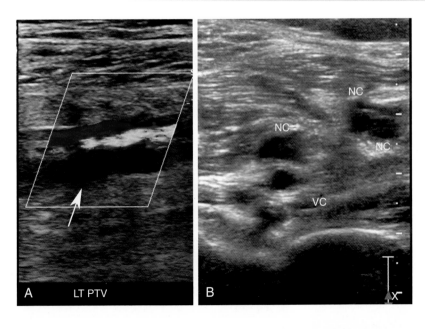

FIGURE 22-18 Deep venous thrombosis (DVT) in one posterior tibial vein (PTV). **A,** Sagittal color Doppler image demonstrating internal echoes and lack of spontaneous flow in the more posterior of the two PTVs *(arrow).* The more anterior PTV is patent (blue). Posterior tibial artery (red) is in between the two veins. **B,** Transverse gray-scale image with compression demonstrates lack of compression of one of the PTVs and both peroneal veins (NC). VC, venous compression.

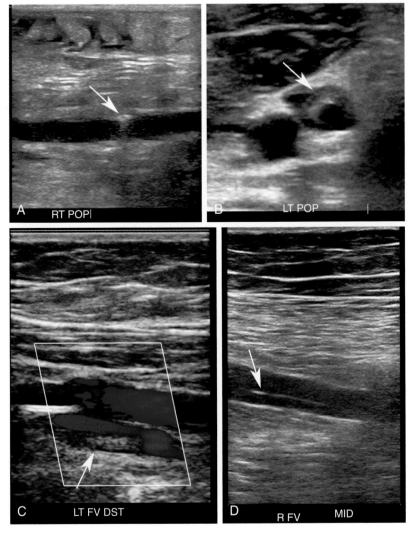

FIGURE 22-19 Chronic deep venous thrombosis (DVT). **A,** Sagittal gray-scale image demonstrating an echogenic plaque-like area *(arrow)* in the wall of the right popliteal vein (RT POP), most likely due to scarring of the venous wall from a prior episode of DVT. **B,** Transverse gray-scale image of the left popliteal vein (LT POP) in another patient demonstrates retractile, echogenic thrombus *(arrow)* that appears adherent to the vessel wall. **C,** Sagittal color Doppler image from a third patient demonstrates a long segment of echogenic mural thrombus in the distal (DST) left femoral vein (FV; blue) consistent with partially occlusive chronic DVT. Superficial femoral artery is color coded in red. On transverse imaging, chronic thrombus such as this often appears as echogenic thickening of the vein wall. **D,** Sagittal gray-scale image of the mid right FV from a fourth patient demonstrates a linear intraluminal echogenic focus *(arrow),* likely representing fibrin stranding or scarring, which may be seen following resolution of acute DVT.

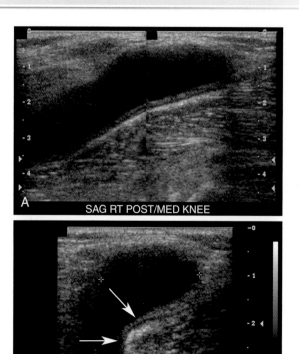

SAG RT POST/MED KNEE

2.14cm

TRV RT POST/MED KNEE

FIGURE 22-20 Baker's cyst. **A,** Sagittal gray-scale image demonstrates an anechoic cystic mass medial in the popliteal fossa anterior to the striated gastrocnemius muscle. **B,** The diagnosis of a Baker's cyst is confirmed by the transverse image demonstrating that the fluid collection wraps around the medial head of the gastrocnemius muscle *(arrows)*. *(Reprinted with permission from Hamper UM, DeJong MR, Scoutt LM: Ultrasound evaluation of the lower extremity veins,* Radiol Clin North Am *45:525–547, 2007.)*

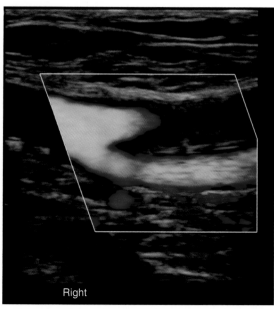

Right

FIGURE 22-22 Arterial occlusion. Longitudinal power Doppler image demonstrates complete occlusion of the superficial femoral artery just beyond the bifurcation of the common femoral artery in a patient who presented with acute onset of right leg pain. The profunda femoris artery is patent.

FIGURE 22-21 Ruptured Baker's cyst. Extended field of view ultrasound image demonstrates a large complex cystic mass *(calipers)* anterior to the striated gastrocnemius muscle extending inferiorly in the subcutaneous tissues of the calf. *(Reprinted with permission from Hamper UM, DeJong MR, Scoutt LM: Ultrasound evaluation of the lower extremity veins,* Radiol Clin North Am *45:525–547, 2007.)*

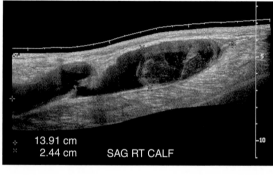

13.91 cm
2.44 cm   SAG RT CALF

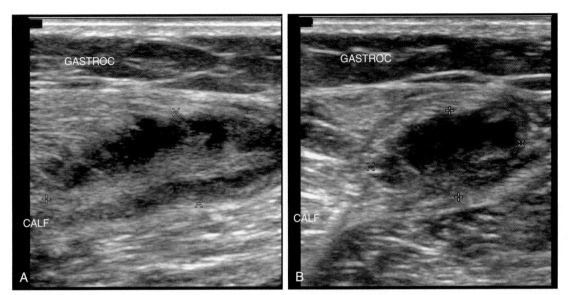

FIGURE 22-23 Muscle tear. Gray-scale longitudinal **(A)** and transverse **(B)** images demonstrate a hypoechoic area *(calipers)* within the gastrocnemius muscle (GASTROC), consistent with a tear or hematoma.

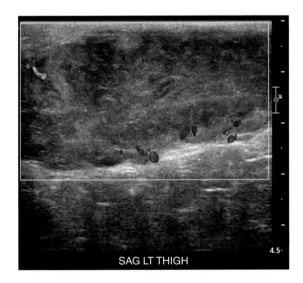

FIGURE 22-24 Soft tissue metastasis. This patient with stage IV lung cancer presented with left thigh pain, and an ultrasound examination was ordered to rule out deep venous thrombosis (DVT). Sagittal color Doppler image reveals a vascular subcutaneous soft tissue mass in the region of the patient's pain. Biopsy confirmed lung cancer metastasis.

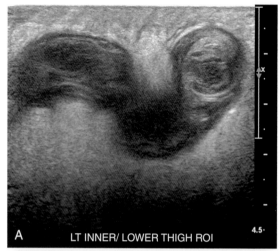

A LT INNER/ LOWER THIGH ROI   4.5·

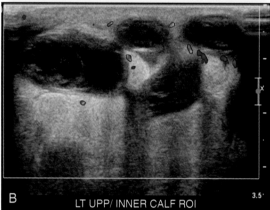

B LT UPP/ INNER CALF ROI   3.5·

FIGURE 22-25 Thrombosed superficial varicosities. This patient presented with a palpable cord. Gray-scale image of the thigh **(A)** and color Doppler image **(B)** of the inner calf demonstrate serpiginous tubular structures with internal echoes consistent with thrombosed varicose veins arising from posteromedial branches of the great saphenous vein.

REFERENCES

1. Silverstein M, et al: Trends in the incidence of deep vein thrombosis and pulmonary embolism: a 25 year population-based cohort study, *Arch Intern Med* 158:585–593, 1998.
2. Heit J, et al: Trends in incidence of deep vein thrombosis and pulmonary embolism: a 35 year population-based study, *Blood* 108(430a), 2006.
3. Heit JA: The epidemiology of venous thromboembolism in the community, *Arterioscler Thromb Vasc Biol* 28:370–372, 2008.
4. Heit J, Cohen A, Anderson FJ: Estimated annual number of incident and recurrent, non-fatal and fatal venous thromboembolism (VTE) events in the US, *Blood* 106:267A, 2005.
5. Konstantinides S: Acute pulmonary embolism, *N Engl J Med* 359:2804–2813, 2008.
6. Tapson VF: Acute pulmonary embolism, *N Engl J Med* 358:1037–1050, 2008.
7. Needleman L: Ultrasound in the diagnosis of lower extremity venous diseases: 2009 Update, *ARRS Categorical Course Syllabus* 85–91, 2009.
8. Cronan JJ: Venous thromboembolic disease: the role of ultrasound, *Radiology* 186:619–650, 1993.
9. Cornuz J, Pearson SD, Polak JF: Deep venous thrombosis: complete lower extremity venous US evaluation in patients without known risk factors – outcome study, *Radiology* 211:637–641, 1999.
10. Heijboer H, et al: A comparison of real-time compression ultrasonography with impedance plethysmography for the diagnosis of DVT in symptomatic outpatients, *N Engl J Med* 329:1365–1369, 1993.
11. White Rh, et al: Diagnosis of deep-vein thrombosis using duplex ultrasound, *Ann Intern Med* 111:297–304, 1989.
12. Yucel EK, et al: Isolated calf venous thrombosis: diagnosis with compression US, *Radiology* 179:443–446, 1991.
13. Rose SC, et al: Symptomatic lower extremity deep venous thrombosis: accuracy, limitations and the role of color duplex imaging in diagnosis.
14. Snow V, et al: Management of venous thromboembolism: a clinical practice guideline from the American College of Physicians and the American Academy of Family Physicians, *Ann Intern Med* 146:204–210, 2007.
15. Wells PS, et al: Value of assessment of pretest probability of deep-vein thrombosis of the lower limbs: an epidemiological study, *J Thromb Haemost* 3:1362–1367, 2005.
16. American College of Radiology: *ACR practice guideline for the performance of peripheral venous ultrasound examination, 2006.* American College of Radiology Website. www.acr.org/SecondaryMainMenuCategories/quality_safety/guidelines/us/us_periphera_l venous.aspx. Accessed December 15, 2008.
17. Righini M, et al: D-dimer for venous thromboembolism diagnosis: 20 years later, *J Thromb Haemost* 6:1059–1071, 2008.
18. Hargett CW, Tapson VFR: Clinical probability and D-dimer testing: How should we use them in clinical practice? *Semin Respir Crit Care Med* 29:15–24, 2008.
19. Wells PS, et al: Evaluation of D-dimer in the diagnosis of suspected deep vein thrombosis, *N Engl J Med* 349:1227–1235, 2003.
20. Hamper UM, DeJong MR, Scoutt LM: Ultrasound evaluation of the lower extremity veins, *Radiol Clin North Am* 45:525–547, 2007.
21. American College of Radiology: *ACR practice guideline for the performance of peripheral venous ultrasound examination, 2006.* American College of Radiology Website. www.acr.org/SecondaryMainMenuCategories/quality_safety/guidelines/us/us_periphera_l venous.aspx Accessed December 15, 2008.
22. Hirsch J, et al: American College of Chest Physicians evidence-based clinical practice guidelines, ed 8, *Chest* 133(suppl):71S–109S, 2008.
23. *ICAVL Standards for accreditation in noninvasive vascular testing. Part 2. Vascular laboratory operations: peripheral venous testing, 2006:*Intersocietal Commission for the Accreditation of Vascular Laboratories Website. www.icavl.org/icavl/pdfs/venous2007.pdf:Accessed January 15, 2009.
24. Seinturier C, et al: Site and clinical outcome of deep vein thrombosis of the lower limbs: an epidemiological study, *J Thromb Haemost* 3:1362–1367, 2005.

25. Lockhart ME, Sheldon HI, Robbin ML: Augmentation in lower extremity sonography for the detection of deep venous thrombosis, *AJR Am J Roentgenol* 184:419–422, 2005.

26. Lin EP, Bhatt S, Rubens D: The importance of monophasic Doppler waveforms in the common femoral vein, *J Ultrasound Med* 26:885–891, 2007.

27. Siragusa S, et al: Residual vein thrombosis to establish duration of anticoagulation after a first episode of deep vein thrombosis: the duration of anticoagulation based on compression ultrasonography (DACUS) study, *Blood* 112:511–515, 2008.

28. Prandoni P, et al: Residual thrombosis on ultrasonography to guide the duration of anticoagulation in patients with deep venous thrombosis, *Ann Intern Med* 150:577–585, 2009.

29. Borgestede JP, Clagett GE: Types, frequency, and significance of alternative diagnoses found during duplex Doppler venous examinations of the lower extremities, *J Ultrasound Med* 11:85–89, 1992.

30. Kahn SR: The clinical diagnosis of deep venous thrombosis: integrating incidence, risk factors, and symptoms and signs, *Arch Intern Med* 158:2315–2323, 1998.

31. Sutter ME, et al: Venous ultrasound testing for suspected thrombosis: incidence of significant non-thrombotic findings, *J Emerg Med* 36:55–59, 2009.

32. Useche JN, et al: Use of US in the evaluation of patients with symptoms of deep venous thrombosis of the lower extremities, *Radiographics* 28:1785–1797, 2008.

33. Jamadar DA, et al: Sonography of the painful calf: differential considerations, *AJR Am J Roentgenol* 179:709–716, 2002.

34. Langsfeld M, et al: Baker's cysts mimicking the symptoms of deep vein thrombosis: diagnosis with venous duplex scanning, *J Vasc Surg* 25:658–662, 1997.

CONTROVERSIES IN VENOUS ULTRASOUND

23

JOHN J. CRONAN, MD

Venous ultrasound has become the diagnostic tool of choice in assessing extremity veins for deep venous thrombosis (DVT). In less than 20 years, this technique has replaced venography in clinical practice. Although compression ultrasound was embraced by radiologists, it has been adopted as a replacement for impedance plethysmography and phleborheography by all other specialties, including vascular surgery, emergency medicine, and vascular medicine.

Many questions regarding the performance and interpretation of venous ultrasound remain. In this chapter we will review several issues that continue to cause controversy in the employment of compression ultrasound for assessment of venous clot.

HOW MUCH IS ENOUGH?

The venous ultrasound technique is primarily dependent on compression of the vein lumen as the signature of normality. Assessment with color flow Doppler imaging and Doppler spectral waveforms add little value except in the few cases of proximal (iliac or vena cava) venous obstruction. What remains unanswered is, how much of the venous system needs to be interrogated? The minimalists advocate "two-point compression," while the more compulsive examiners demand that every centimeter of the vein from the groin to the ankle be evaluated. Succinctly stated, there is no agreement regarding the extent of a lower venous ultrasound examination. Adding complexity to the imaging evaluation is the use of serum D-dimer[1] tests, with their poor specificity and high false-positive rates. In addition, there is an increasing interest in incorporating clinical prediction tools for DVT such as the 10 items assessed by the Wells score for DVT (Table 23-1).[2]

THE ROLE OF THE UNILATERAL VENOUS ULTRASOUND EXAMINATION IN THE PATIENT WITH UNILATERAL SYMPTOMS

In the era of venography, when the radiologist was requested to evaluate a patient for acute DVT, only the symptomatic leg was studied.[3] Because of the risk for reactions to intravenous contrast material and the invasiveness of venography, the asymptomatic leg was not studied. Historically, noninvasive vascular laboratories employing impedance plethysmography or phleborheography routinely evaluated both the symptomatic leg and the asymptomatic leg. These laboratories, which are usually directed by surgeons, not radiologists, utilized the physiologic information obtained from the asymptomatic leg as a frame of reference to help diagnose any thrombus that might be present in the symptomatic leg. Following the introduction of venous ultrasound, some sonographers continued to evaluate only the symptomatic leg, while many vascular laboratories, which had developed a pattern of noninvasively evaluating both the symptomatic leg and the asymptomatic leg, continued to evaluate both legs.

Until 1995, a Correct Procedural Terminology (CPT) code existed only to evaluate bilateral lower extremities. In 1995, a code for a unilateral or limited examination of the leg was introduced (CPT 93971). Also in 1995, the Intersocietal Commission for the Accreditation of Vascular Laboratories (ICAVL) acknowledged the need for limited unilateral studies with the publication of their revised guidelines. Up until that time, ICAVL had indicated that an examination of a symptomatic extremity also required a study of the asymptomatic leg.

Controversy had existed regarding the importance and frequency of finding thrombus in the

TABLE 23-1 The Wells Score for DVT

Clinical Characteristics	Points
Active cancer (patient receiving treatment for cancer within the previous 6 months or currently receiving palliative treatment)	+1
Paralysis, paresis, or recent plaster immobilization of the lower extremities	+1
Recently bedridden for 3 days or more or major surgery within the previous 12 weeks requiring general or regional anesthesia	+1
Localized tenderness along the distribution of the deep venous system	+1
Entire leg is swollen	+1
Calf swelling at least 3 cm larger than that on the asymptomatic side (measured 10 cm below tibial tuberosity)	+1
Pitting edema confined to the symptomatic leg	+1
Collateral superficial veins (nonvaricose)	+1
Previously documented DVT	+1
Alternative diagnosis at least as likely as DVT	-2

Total Score	Clinical Probability	Prevalence of DVT
<2 points	DVT unlikely	5.5% (95% CI, 3.8%-7.6%)
≥2 points	DVT likely	27.9% (95% CI, 23.9%-31.8%)

CI, confidence interval; DVT, deep venous thrombosis.

asymptomatic leg.[4,5] Historically, the literature indicated that the asymptomatic leg did not harbor thrombus. Articles were then published suggesting that thrombus could be found in the asymptomatic leg, but the frequency of this finding in a patient with a negative evaluation of the symptomatic leg was less than 1%.[3,6-8] Certainly, finding thrombus in the asymptomatic leg of a patient with thrombus in the symptomatic leg would not have altered treatment. The likelihood of finding thrombus solely in the asymptomatic leg was estimated to be between 0% and 1% if the patient did not have any risk factors such as a malignancy.

This low frequency of thrombus does not justify a routine evaluation of the asymptomatic leg in a patient presenting with symptoms limited to one extremity. However, this applies to outpatients without contralateral symptoms and without a risk factor such as a malignancy.

BILATERAL SYMPTOMS: THE ROLE OF THE BILATERAL VENOUS EXAMINATION

As discussed previously, the situation of a patient presenting with bilateral lower leg swelling or bilateral leg pain would have been triaged in

the era of venography with reevaluation of the patient or, more likely, with a contrast venogram of only one extremity. It has been suggested that most of these patients have cardiac disease or peripheral vascular disease as the dominant cause of their bilateral swelling.[8] However, an alternative should be considered: a significant percentage of these patients harbor lower extremity venous thrombus.[7]

Certainly, the important factor to consider in the subgroup of patients with bilateral leg swelling would be the presence of risk factors.[3] If the Wells score for DVT (see Table 23-1) indicates DVT is unlikely, then the bilateral ultrasound examination will, in my experience and that of others, always be negative. If a patient has a significant underlying risk for DVT, such as malignancy, then the bilateral examination should be performed. If there are no risk factors for DVT, the first assumption should be that the patient has heart disease or underlying peripheral vascular disease as the cause of the bilateral leg swelling. The probability of finding thrombus in the leg is related to the presence of risk factors for DVT. In the absence of any risk factors for DVT, it is unusual to find extremity thrombus. It has been stated that the majority of patients with DVT have one or more risk factors.[9]

THE EXTENT OF THE ULTRASOUND EXAMINATION: HOW MUCH NEEDS TO BE STUDIED?

Proper technique for ultrasound evaluation of the vein, as stated both in the American College of Radiology standards in 1993 (revised in 2006) and by the ICAVL, indicates that a patient with a symptomatic extremity should be evaluated from the level of the inguinal ligament to the popliteal fossa in as continuous a manner as possible (Figure 23-1).[10] Evaluation of the calf veins is also done in most vascular laboratories.

Symptomatic patients tend to have lengthy thrombi involving one or more venous segments.[11,12] Symptomatic thrombus may involve multiple venous segments and is biologically different from thrombus that develops in the asymptomatic high-risk patients, where thrombus preferentially involves valve cusps in the calf.[13] This observation was demonstrated on retrospective review of venograms and has been confirmed in our ultrasound laboratory. We demonstrated that in approximately 99% of symptomatic cases, evaluation of the femoral or popliteal vein, employing the two-point compression technique, would detect thrombus that extends above the knee. This two-point evaluation requires examination of only the common femoral and popliteal venous areas (Figure 23-2).[14]

This very abbreviated study detects a high percentage of cases with DVT. The overall decrease in the examination time is slightly in excess of 50%. The potential of the two-point technique has been confirmed by others who have demonstrated that approximately 90% to 95.4% of thrombus would be detected using a two-point compression technique.[15] Obviously, there is some degree of compromise with the two-point technique, balancing simplicity versus accuracy. This limited-compression technique is not the accepted standard within the medical community in North America but may have utility in the emergency department and for evaluating the patient with extremely restricted mobility. As an alternative to evaluating the entire leg, this two-point technique provides an equivalent degree of certainty when combined with serial ultrasound examinations in patients with a negative ultrasound examination at baseline (Figure 23-3).[16] From the point of view of outcomes, two two-point examinations separated by 7 days, in combination with a D-dimer test,

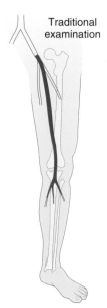

FIGURE 23-1 Topographic delineation of the lower extremity venous system as examined in routine evaluation.

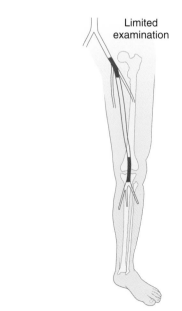

FIGURE 23-2 Proposed two-point lower extremity venous evaluation.

are equivalent to a full-length examination of the lower extremity veins.[17]

SIGNIFICANCE OF A NEGATIVE ULTRASOUND EXAMINATION

Evidence exists that a negative compression ultrasound study of a symptomatic lower extremity, employing complete evaluation of both the femoral and popliteal veins, provides sufficient

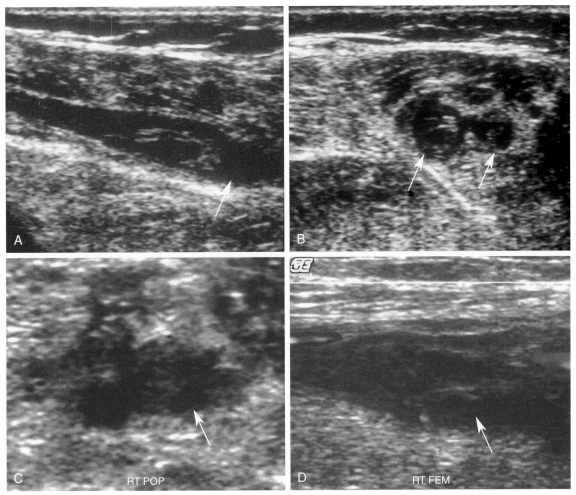

FIGURE 23-3 Propagation of calf vein thrombus. Long-axis **(A)** and short-axis **(B)** views of a distended, thrombus-filled gastrocnemius vein (*arrows*). The popliteal and femoral veins were normal. **C,** Compression of the popliteal (POP) vein (*arrow*) 12 days later demonstrates the presence of acute thrombus. **D,** The femoral (FEM) vein (*arrow*) now is also filled with thrombus, which has propagated upward from the calf.

validation to withhold anticoagulation.[6,18] The need for any follow-up studies in these cases is somewhat less well defined, but the evidence suggests that if the patient remains symptomatic, a repeat study of the lower extremity should be performed 3 to 5 days after the initial examination. An alternative proven technique to end the workup is to demonstrate a normal study of the proximal veins combined with a negative D-dimer. Such a negative combination obviates the need to reassess the leg.[19] In 1% to 2% of cases,[19] small focal calf thrombi might propagate upward into the popliteal vein and cause symptoms. As will be mentioned in the next section, the direct evaluation of the calf veins needs to be considered as a more direct approach to immediate diagnosis.

CALF VEIN THROMBOSIS

The clinical acceptance of venous ultrasound as a diagnostic technique in the evaluation of the symptomatic patient occurred based on clinical series that did not attempt direct evaluation of calf veins. The initial reports and literature were based only on evaluation of the femoral and popliteal veins. It was with this examination format that the compression ultrasound examination was acknowledged as clinically useful.[20] Although isolated calf thrombi are common, they often arise in the hospitalized postoperative or immobile bed-bound patient and, in this context, rarely cause acute clinical problems or clinical symptoms. The outpatient with localized calf symptoms and calf DVT may represent a more aggressive manifestation of thromboembolic disease.

Eighty-eight percent of calf thrombus occurs in the asymptomatic patient, and this accounts for 50% of thrombi in the asymptomatic population. Similarly, the presence of calf thrombus is unlikely to lead to clinically significant pulmonary embolus (PE).[21] As pointed out by Moser and LeMoine,[22] patients with calf thrombus are unlikely to have signs or symptoms of PE. PE that originates from the calf is usually asymptomatic because of the small clot load. Alternatively, patients with above-knee thrombus have PE in more than 50% of cases, despite the fact that they may not have any signs or symptoms of this phenomenon and evidence of PE is detected only on ventilation/perfusion scans, computed tomographic pulmonary arteriography (CTPA), or pulmonary arteriograms.[23-25]

Our knowledge of calf vein clot and its clinical impact remains in flux. However, there are two distinct points of view regarding treatment of calf DVT. If thrombus is isolated to the calf veins, it appears to have little or no impact in the *acute* setting. Calf clot usually does not cause clinically significant DVT/PE. The 3-month outcome when calf veins are evaluated and clot treated is equivalent to that when the calf veins are not interrogated.[1,17,26] The risk of anticoagulation is significant and in many circles is deemed to outweigh the value of treating acute calf clot.[27]

In the long-term, *chronic* setting, the issue now swings toward treatment since data suggest a lower recurrence rate and decreased percentage of chronic venous insufficiency when treatment of the initial clot occurs. The impetus for acute treatment stems from the recommendation by the American College of Chest Physicians.[28] Hence, the reason for evaluating the calf in the acute setting allows for a specific diagnosis of calf DVT. If no clot is seen, no further study is necessary. However, if the calf is not evaluated acutely, one needs to reevaluate the proximal veins within a week or confirm negative D-dimer test results at the time of the initial study. This algorithm detects calf clot migration into the proximal veins.[27]

Therapeutic management of patients with documented calf thrombus is debatable. Some suggest that observation of the thrombus with serial ultrasound studies is all that is necessary. A second examination, performed at 3 to 5 days from the baseline study, detects proximal propagation of thrombus into the popliteal system, and if this

occurs, treatment ensues. However, there is now convincing evidence that calf thrombus does contribute to subclinical pulmonary embolism.[22-25]

Another issue that strongly endorses the evaluation of the calf veins and treatment of calf thrombus relates to the development of chronic venous insufficiency. Most venous valves are located below the knee. If thrombus develops in the calf area, this could lead to destruction of the valves and initiate chronic venous insufficiency. Therefore, logic strongly endorses direct evaluation of the calf veins to search for thrombus. Detection of thrombus permits treatment to be initiated so that the extent of valve destruction in the calf veins is minimized.

This belief that calf thrombus does embolize and produces valve destruction is a forceful argument to support early diagnosis and treatment of thrombus isolated to calf veins.[29-32] The argument for direct calf evaluation, however, is countered with the risk of anticoagulation and the data showing that 3-month outcomes are the same with or without evaluation of the distal veins.

If a patient has signs or symptoms of calf thrombus, venous ultrasound of the calf should be performed.[33] The presence of calf signs or symptoms necessitates a look at the calves because other disorders such as calf hematoma, muscle rupture, or popliteal cyst may be the cause of symptoms.

MUSCULAR VEINS IN THE CALF

Improved resolution of lower extremity venous ultrasound has permitted the visualization of calf muscular veins such as the gastrocnemius, soleus, and conduit veins and the detection of thrombus within them. Approximately 2% of symptomatic patients were found to have isolated muscular vein thrombus.[34] Unfortunately, the implications of finding such thrombus are not clear. No treatment guidelines are available for this variant of DVT. There is no definitive proof that this thrombus should be treated in view of the risks of anticoagulation.[34,35] These muscle veins drain into the deep veins of the lower extremity. The soleal veins drain into the peroneal and posterior tibial veins, and the gastrocnemial veins drain into the popliteal veins. A recent series demonstrated 16% of clots in the muscular veins extended into the tibial peroneal system. Only 3% of isolated muscle vein clots extended into the popliteal vein, and this occurred within 15 days.[34] A short course of anticoagulation may be all that is necessary. One may also consider withholding anticoagulation and reevaluate in 7 to 10 days to confirm the absence of migration.[26]

COMPRESSION ULTRASOUND CAUSING PULMONARY EMBOLUS

Compression ultrasound has always had the potential to break off thrombus in the femoral vein and lead to pulmonary embolization. While this has been a theoretic consideration, there exists a paucity of reports that patients who had diagnostic compression ultrasound were subsequently found to have developed PE.[36,37] The temporal relationship of the ultrasound examination to the actual occurrence of PE is somewhat uncertain. This is particularly noteworthy given the fact that patients with above-knee DVT have clinically unsuspected PE in greater than 50% of cases.[18] It should be noted that the risks of compression ultrasound are quite small if one takes care to avoid excessive venous compression and manipulation of the vein beyond that which is necessary for diagnosis. When concerns are raised about the risk for causing PE, the scenario typically involves free-floating thrombus in the upper femoral vein (Figure 23-4), which is at greater risk for embolization. Obviously, compression should be minimized in this scenario.

DVT IN OCCULT MALIGNANCY

Trousseau's sign concerns hypercoagulability associated with cancer and is based on the finding of spontaneous venous thrombosis in patients with underlying malignancy.[38-41] When patients present with DVT and have no known risk factors, there is an underlying concern that they may indeed have an occult malignancy. Several published series have looked at this issue and observed a 10% to 34% incidence of cancer developing in patients who lack any apparent cause for thrombosis.[38-41] The controversy regarding the actual percentage of patients with underlying malignancy is less important. The real issue is that all sources support a causal relationship. DVT associated with malignancy tends to be much more extensive and aggressive than DVT in the nonmalignant setting.[42] The clinical examination demonstrates an extremity that is very swollen and painful (Figure 23-5).

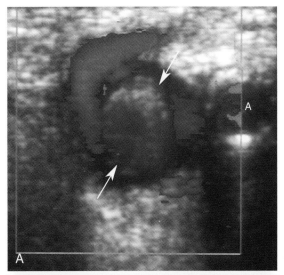
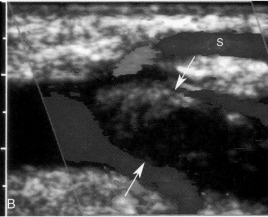

FIGURE 23-4 Short-axis **(A)** and long-axis **(B)** views showing free-floating thrombus (*arrows*) in the femoral vein at the level of the saphenous vein inflow (S). Caution should be exercised when applying compression to the veins. A, femoral artery.

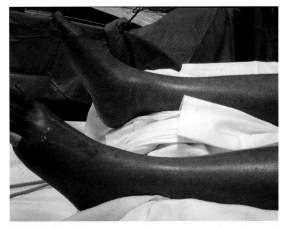

FIGURE 23-5 Malignancy-induced venous thrombosis is often associated with extreme leg swelling and a tense appearance.

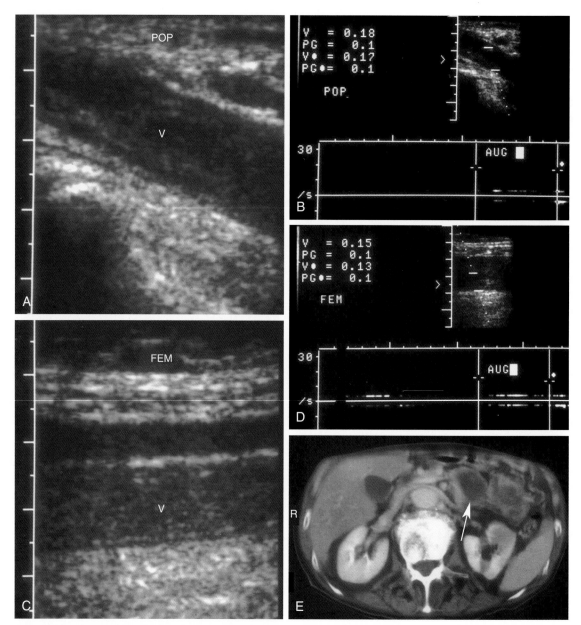

FIGURE 23-6 A patient without a known history of malignancy presents with a tensely swollen extremity, which demonstrates occlusion of all the veins. **A,** The popliteal (POP) vein (V) is markedly distended with occlusive thrombus. **B,** Pulsed Doppler indicates absence of flow in the popliteal vein. **C** and **D,** Likewise, the entire femoral (FEM) vein (V) is occluded by thrombus. **E,** Computed tomography image obtained several days after the venous examination demonstrates a 5-cm pancreatic tail mass (*arrow*). This was biopsied and yielded adenocarcinoma of the pancreas.

Controversy also exists regarding whether a diagnostic workup should be initiated following documentation of DVT in a patient without risk factors (Figure 23-6). There is evidence to indicate that a workup searching for occult malignancy is not cost-effective and that the cancers are already metastatic.[43] Alternatively, there is an opinion that an aggressive workup is warranted in these situations.[44,45] Patients with DVT related to Trousseau's syndrome usually clinically manifest the cancer within 1 to 2 years. Malignancies associated with venous thrombosis typically arise in the breast, the gastrointestinal or genitourinary tracts, the lung, and the brain. Of note, if a patient presents with recurrent episodes of DVT and has no known risk factors, the risk of an underlying malignancy is markedly increased.[44]

ULTRASOUND FOR THE ASSESSMENT OF PULMONARY EMBOLUS

CTPA has become the standard technique to assess for pulmonary embolism. Of note, the recent concern regarding radiation risks has tempered the exuberance for CTPA.[46-48] Because the majority of PEs are felt to originate from the lower extremity, a teleologic assessment employing noninvasive venous imaging to clarify an indeterminate lung scan or to confirm a clinical impression of PE has been utilized.[49] By establishing the presence of thrombus in the lower extremity, adequate therapy could be initiated, as the treatment for DVT and PE is essentially the same (i.e., anticoagulation). However, it has been observed for several decades that even when bilateral venography is employed, nearly a third of patients who have documented PE will not demonstrate any thrombus in the lower extremities.[18] A recent review indicated that compression ultrasound detects proximal vein thrombosis in 20% of patents with pulmonary embolism, and the rate is twice as high when the distal veins are included; no pertinent reference was quoted however.[50] Hence, *a negative lower extremity venous ultrasound study cannot exclude PE.* The explanation for the absence of lower extremity thrombus in the setting of proven PE remains a conjecture. A big bang theory, that all the lower extremity clot embolized in toto, is most likely. This is an important concept to convey to the clinician, as he/she should not terminate consideration of PE based on a negative noninvasive study if there is a strong clinical suspicion for PE. Similarly, the value of employing lower extremity venous ultrasound in the absence of leg symptoms, to diagnose PE, is questionable.[51-53]

A recent proposal has been to employ CTPA in the workup of PE and to complement CT with compression ultrasound (Figure 23-7).[54,55] The suggestion has been made that if a patient presents *with symptoms of both DVT and PE,* ultrasound of the lower extremities should be obtained first. If the test is positive for thrombus, treatment for venous thromboembolic disease should be initiated. A negative venous ultrasound study would be followed by CTPA to exclude PE via direct visualization of the pulmonary arteries. Either a multidetector CT scan demonstrating pulmonary artery thrombus or compression ultrasound demonstrating lower extremity DVT would permit treatment to be started. Negative studies would permit anticoagulation to be withheld.[56]

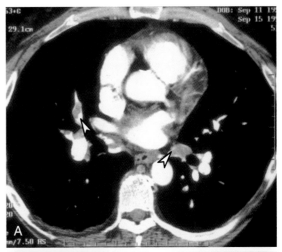

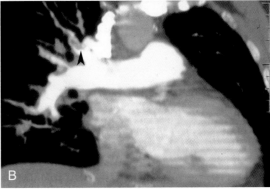

FIGURE 23-7 Pulmonary thromboembolus. A middle-age man presented with leg pain and swelling. Ultrasound (not shown) demonstrated acute thrombus in the right femoral vein. **A,** The onset of chest pain the same day led to computed tomographic pulmonary angiography, which confirmed pulmonary embolization (*arrowheads*). **B,** This reformatted coronal computed tomography image shows acute thrombus in the right pulmonary artery (*arrowhead*).

CONFUSING TERMINOLOGY

Proper anatomic terminology in the venous system is important because many primary care physicians have often misinterpreted reports generated by sonographers. The common interpretation that the deep veins distal to the common femoral are the "deep femoral vein" and the "superficial femoral vein" is confusing.[57] This confusion comes from the use of the term *superficial femoral vein* to describe a *component of the deep venous system.* A thrombus in this location requires treatment. When this venous segment is labeled as "superficial," a clinician unfamiliar with the terminology might assume that it is not an important vein (because it is a superficial

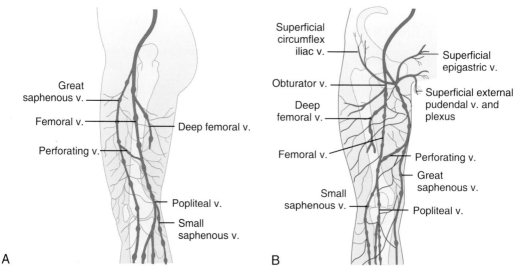

FIGURE 23-8 Correct terminology. Avoid reference to the femoral vein as "superficial." Lateral **(A)** and anterior **(B)** lower extremity views illustrating preferred terminology. v., vein.

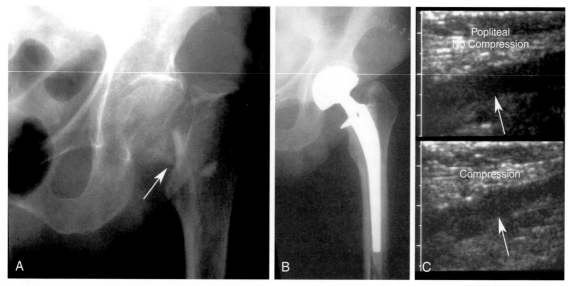

FIGURE 23-9 Acute hip fracture and immobilization as risk factors for deep venous thrombosis (DVT). This 69-year-old woman developed acute DVT 1 week after falling (risk = trauma) and surgery (risk = immobilization + trauma). **A,** Hip film demonstrating acute left hip fracture (*arrow*). **B,** Hemiarthroplasty was performed. **C,** One week later, the popliteal vein (*arrows*) is occluded by acute thrombus.

vein) and decide not to initiate treatment The correct anatomic term is the *femoral vein* and not the "superficial" femoral vein (Figure 23-8).[57]

RISK FACTORS FOR DEEP VENOUS THROMBOSIS

Our knowledge regarding the causation of DVT is expanding, revealing our initial ignorance regarding the etiology of venous thrombosis. A recognizable cause for DVT is evident in nearly 70% of cases.[58] Our knowledge gap is manifested in the 30% of patients in whom no known risk factor is apparent.

Most sonographers are familiar with the established causes of DVT: immobilization, trauma, pregnancy, and childbirth, as well as malignancy (Figure 23-9).[59,60] The relationship between estrogen and DVT has been established for 25 years.[61] In the past decade, mutations and conditions associated with thrombophilia have been defined—antithrombin, protein C or protein S deficiency, factor V Leiden, prothrombin G20210A mutation, hyperhomocysteinuria, and lupus anti-coagulants.[62,63]

More recently, a link between DVT and atherosclerosis has been established.[58] The actual etiologic relationship is uncertain, but a diffuse underlying inflammation involving both the arterial and venous systems is possible. There is confirmation of a relationship between asymptomatic atherosclerotic lesions and spontaneous venous thrombosis of the legs.

Presently, it is important that the clinician be aware of the many causes and realize that unless they are corrected, repeat episodes of DVT will occur.

A FOLLOW-UP STUDY TO DETERMINE RISK FOR RECURRENT DVT

In nearly 50% of initial lower extremity DVT, the vein lumen remains abnormal with residual vein thrombosis (RVT). Initially the RVT was deemed a potential masquerader for acute DVT.[64] Over time, chronic thrombus adheres to the vein wall and causes a diffuse thickening.[65] The ability of the vein to collapse normally, as well as the restoration of a normal-sized lumen, are very helpful in excluding the presence of chronic thrombus. If the findings remain perplexing, a repeat study in 24 to 72 hours will confirm stability or demonstrate progression.

RVT may be a marker of increased risk for recurrent DVT. Patients without RVT can be treated with only 3 months of anticoagulation. RVT may be a marker of a prothrombotic state, and individuals with RVT might be prone to recurrent episodes of DVT.[66,67]

CONCLUSIONS

This chapter has presented several issues that are in evolution and remain somewhat controversial. However, it is important to realize that this is by no means an all-inclusive list of controversial topics, and many other issues could be discussed. However, in spite of these controversies, ultrasound for evaluation of the venous system, particularly in the acute situation, remains the dominant diagnostic technique.

REFERENCES

1. Buller HR, et al: Safely ruling out deep venous thrombosis in primary care, *Ann Intern Med* 150:229–235, 2009.
2. Wells PS, Anderson DR: Value of assessment of pretest probability of deep-vein thrombosis in clinical management, *Lancet* 350:1795–1798, 1997.
3. Cronan JJ: Deep venous thrombosis: One leg or both legs? *Radiology* 200:323–324, 1996.
4. Sheiman RG, McArdle CR: Bilateral lower extremity US in the patient with unilateral symptoms of deep venous thrombosis: Assessment of need, *Radiology* 194:171–173, 1995.
5. Strotham G, et al: Contralateral duplex scanning for deep venous thrombosis is unnecessary in patients with symptoms, *J Vasc Surg* 22:543–547, 1995.
6. Cronan JJ: Controversies in venous ultrasound, *Semin Ultrasound CT MR* 18:33–38, 1997.
7. Naidich JB, et al: Suspected deep venous thrombosis: Is US of both legs necessary? *Radiology* 200:429–431, 1996.
8. Sheiman RG, Weintrub JL, McArdle CR: Bilateral lower extremity US in the patient with bilateral symptoms of deep venous thrombosis: Assessment of need, *Radiology* 196:379–381, 1995.
9. Anderson FA, Wheeler HB: Physician priorities in the management of venous thromboembolism: A community wide survey, *J Vasc Surg* 15:707–714, 1992.
10. ACR Standards for the performance of peripheral venous ultrasound examination (revised 2001), *ACR Standards* 579–581, 2002–2003.
11. Cogo A, et al: Distribution of thrombosis in patients with symptomatic deep vein thrombosis, *Arch Intern Med* 153:2777–2780, 1993.
12. Markel A, et al: Patterns and distribution of thrombi in acute venous thrombosis, *Arch Surg* 127:305–309, 1992.
13. Rose SC, Zwiebel WJ, Miller FJ: Distribution of acute lower extremity deep venous thrombosis in symptomatic and asymptomatic patients: Imaging implications, *J Ultra Med* 13:243–250, 1994.
14. Pezzullo JA, Perkins AB, Cronan JJ: Symptomatic deep vein thrombosis: Diagnosis with limited compression US, *Radiology* 198:67–70, 1996.
15. Frederick MG, et al: Can the US examination for lower extremity deep venous thrombosis be abbreviated? A prospective study of 755 examinations, *Radiology* 199:45–47, 1996.
16. Jacoby J, et al: Can emergency medicine residents detect acute deep venous thrombosis with a limited, two-site ultrasound examination? *J Emerg Med* 32:197–200, 2007.
17. Bernardi E, et al: Serial 2-point ultrasonography plus D-dimer vs whole-leg color-coded Doppler ultrasonography for diagnosing suspected symptomatic deep vein thrombosis, *JAMA* 300:1653–1659, 2008.
18. Cronan JJ: Venous thromboembolic disease: The role of US, *Radiology* 186:619–630, 1993.
19. Kearon C, et al: A randomized trial of diagnostic strategies after normal proximal vein ultrasonography for suspected deep venous thrombosis: D-dimer testing compared with repeated ultrasonography, *Ann Intern Med* 142:490–496, 2005.
20. Vaccaro JP, Cronan JJ, Dorfman GS: Outcome analysis of patients with normal compression US examinations, *Radiology* 175:645–649, 1990.
21. Huisman MV, et al: Serial impedance plethysmography for suspected deep venous thrombosis in outpatients, *N Engl J Med* 314:823–828, 1986.
22. Moser KM, LeMoine JR: Is embolic risk conditioned by location of deep venous thrombosis? *Ann Intern Med* 94:439–444, 1981.

23. Huisman MV, et al: Unexpected high prevalence of silent pulmonary embolism in patients with deep venous thrombosis, *Chest* 95:498–502, 1989.

24. Philbrick JT, Becker DM: Calf deep vein thrombosis: A wolf in sheep's clothing? *Arch Intern Med* 148:2131–2138, 1988.

25. Lohr JM, et al: Lower extremity calf thrombosis: To treat or not to treat? *J Vasc Surg* 14:618–623, 1991.

26. Righini M, Bounameux H: Clinical relevance of distal deep vein thrombosis, *Curr Opin Pulm Med* 14:408–413, 2008.

27. Landefeld CS: Noninvasive diagnosis of deep vein thrombosis, *JAMA* 300:1696–1697, 2008.

28. Kearon C, et al: Antithrombotic therapy for venous thromboembolic disease: American College of Chest Physicians Evidence-Based Clinical Practice Guidelines (8th Edition), *Chest* 133:454S–545S, 2008.

29. Kakkar VV, et al: Natural history of postoperative deep venous thrombosis, *Lancet* 2:230–232, 1969.

30. Langerstedt CL, et al: Need for long-term anticoagulant treatment in symptomatic calf vein thrombosis, *Lancet* 2:515–518, 1985.

31. Cornuz J, Pearson SD, Polak JF: Deep venous thrombosis: Complete lower extremity venous US examination in patients without known risk factors—outcome study, *Radiology* 211:637–641, 1999.

32. Atri M, et al: Accuracy of sonography in the evaluation of calf deep vein thrombosis in both postoperative surveillance and symptomatic patients, *AJR Am J Roentgenol* 166:1361–1367, 1996.

33. Gottlieb RH, et al: Randomized prospective study comparing routine versus selective use of sonography of the complete calf in patients with suspected deep venous thrombosis, *AJR Am J Roentgenol* 180:241–245, 2003.

34. MacDonald PS, et al: Short-term natural history of isolated gastrocnemius and soleal vein thrombosis, *J Vasc Surg* 37:523–527, 2003.

35. Schwartz T, et al: Therapy of isolated calf muscle vein thrombosis with low-molecular-weight heparin, *Blood Coagul Fibrinolysis* 12:597–599, 2001.

36. Perlin SJ: Pulmonary embolism during compression US of the lower extremity, *Radiology* 184:165–166, 1992.

37. Schroder WB, Bealer JF: Venous duplex ultrasonography causing acute pulmonary embolism: A brief report, *J Vasc Surg* 15:1082–1083, 1992.

38. Silverstein RL, Nachman RL: Cancer and clotting—Trousseau's warning, *N Engl J Med* 327:1163–1164, 1992.

39. Goldberg RJ, et al: Occult malignant neoplasm in patients with deep venous thrombosis, *Arch Intern Med* 147:251–253, 1987.

40. Aderka D, et al: Idiopathic deep vein thrombosis in an apparently healthy patient as a premonitory sign of occult cancer, *Cancer* 57:1846–1849, 1986.

41. Monreal M, et al: Occult cancer in patients with deep venous thrombosis, *Cancer* 67:541–545, 1991.

42. Schulman S, Lindmarker P: Incidence of cancer after prophylaxis with warfarin against recurrent venous thromboembolism, *N Engl J Med* 342:1953–1958, 2000.

43. Sorenson HT, et al: Prognosis of cancers associated with venous thromboembolism, *N Engl J Med* 343:1846–1850, 2000.

44. Prandoni P, et al: Deep-vein thrombosis and the incidence of subsequent symptomatic cancer, *N Engl J Med* 327:1128–1133, 1992.

45. Prins MH, Lensing AWA, Hirsh J: Idiopathic deep vein thrombosis. Is a search for malignant disease justified? *Arch Intern Med* 154:1310–1312, 1994.

46. Brenner DJ, Hall EJ: Computed tomography – an increasing source of radiation exposure, *N Engl J Med* 357:2277–2284, 2007.

47. Einstein AJ, Henzlova MJ, Rajagopalan S: Estimating risk of cancer associated with radiation exposure from 64-slice computed tomography coronary angiography, *JAMA* 298:317–323, 2007.

48. Killewich LA, Nunnelee JD, Auer AI: Value of lower extremity venous duplex examination in the diagnosis of pulmonary embolism, *J Vasc Surg* 17:934–939, 1993.

49. Smith LL, Iber C, Sirr S: Pulmonary embolism: Confirmation with venous duplex US as adjunct to lung scanning, *Radiology* 191:143–147, 1994.

50. Konstantinides S: Acute pulmonary embolism, *N Engl J Med* 359:2804–2813, 2008.

51. Turkstra F, et al: Diagnostic utility of ultrasonography of leg veins in patients suspected of having pulmonary embolism, *Ann Intern Med* 126:775–781, 1997.

52. Sheiman RG, McArdle CR: Clinically suspected pulmonary embolism: Use of bilateral lower extremity US as the initial examination—a prospective study, *Radiology* 212:75–78, 1999.

53. MacGilavry MR, et al: Compression ultrasonography of the leg veins in patients with clinically suspected pulmonary embolism. Is a more extensive assessment of compressibility useful? *Thromb Haemost* 84:973–976, 2000.

54. Rosen MP, et al: Compression sonography in patients with indeterminate or low-probability lung scans: Lack of usefulness in the absence of both symptoms of deep vein thrombosis and thromboembolic risk factors, *AJR Am J Roentgenol* 166:285–289, 1996.

55. Hull RD, et al: Pulmonary angiography, ventilation lung scanning, and venography for clinically suspected pulmonary embolism with abnormal perfusion lung scan, *Ann Intern Med* 98:891–899, 1983.

56. Goodman LR, Lipchik RJ: Diagnosis of acute pulmonary embolism: Time for a new approach, *Radiology* 199:25–27, 1996.

57. Bundens WP, et al: The superficial femoral vein: A potentially lethal misnomer, *JAMA* 274:1296–1298, 1995.

58. Prandoni P, et al: An association between atherosclerosis and venous thrombosis, *N Engl J Med* 348:1435–1441, 2003.

59. Geerts WH, et al: A prospective study of venous thromboembolism after major trauma, *N Engl J Med* 331:1601–1606, 1994.

60. Toglia MR, Weg JG: Venous thromboembolism during pregnancy, *N Engl J Med* 335:108–114, 1996.

61. Vandenbroucke JP, et al: Oral contraceptives and the risk of venous thrombosis, *N Engl J Med* 344:1527–1535, 2001.

62. Seligsohn U, Lubetsky A: Genetic susceptibility to venous thrombosis, *N Engl J Med* 344:1222–1231, 2001.

63. Den Heijer M, et al: Hyperhomocysteinemia as a risk factor for deep-vein thrombosis, *N Engl J Med* 334:759–762, 1996.

64. Cronan JJ, Leen V: Recurrent deep venous thrombosis, *Radiology* 170:739–742, 1989.

65. Prandoni P, et al: Residual venous thrombosis as a predictive factor of recurrent venous thromboembolism, *Ann Intern Med* 137:955–960, 2002.

66. Prandoni P, et al: Residual thrombosis on ultrasonography to guide the duration of anticoagulation in patients with deep venous thrombosis, *Ann Intern Med* 150: 577–585, 2009.

67. Siragusa S, et al: Residual vein thrombosis to establish duration of anticoagulation after a first episode of deep vein thrombosis: the Duration of Anticoagulation based on Compression UltraSonography (DACUS) study, *Blood* 112:511–515, 2008.

ULTRASOUND DIAGNOSIS OF VENOUS INSUFFICIENCY

24

MARSHA M. NEUMYER, BS, RVT, FSDMS, FSVU, FAIUM

The term *chronic venous insufficiency* is associated with a form of venous dysfunction that has been widely researched and yet is poorly understood. Most often, the term refers to venous valvular incompetence in the superficial, deep, and/or perforating veins. Incompetence of the vein valves permits reversal of flow and promotes venous hypertension in distal segments. This form of venous dysfunction may be the result of recanalization of thrombosed venous segments, pathologic dilatation of the vein, or the congenital absence of competent valves. It is important to understand that venous valvular incompetence may occur alone or in association with venous obstruction. Venous insufficiency is associated with physical findings that are characteristic, yet these findings are nonspecific with respect to cause. They do not differentiate between obstruction and valvular incompetence, nor do they define the location or extent of valvular dysfunction.

Historically, chronic venous insufficiency was evaluated using methods that were inaccurate, nonspecific for incompetence or obstruction, or invasive and associated with patient discomfort and poor acceptance. For these reasons, investigators have pursued a variety of noninvasive vascular procedures that have defined lower extremity venous flow dynamics globally or segmentally. As a pathway to understanding these laboratory procedures, it is important to review the mechanism of venous valvular incompetence.

PATHOPHYSIOLOGY OF VENOUS INSUFFICIENCY

Normal venous anatomy and physiology were described in Chapters 20 and 21. It is necessary to appreciate that venous valves are present throughout the lower extremity venous system in the deep, superficial, and perforating veins. The concentration of valves is higher in the calf veins than in the deep veins of the thigh.

Ambulation results in activation of the calf muscle pump. With calf muscle contraction, venous blood is propelled, or augmented, toward the heart. The valves distal to the contracting muscles, and those in the perforating veins, close to prevent reflux. This reduces venous pressure in the foot from the pressure of a standing column of blood, approximately 90 mm Hg while standing at rest, to 20 to 30 mm Hg during walking. During muscle relaxation, there is slow filling of the venous system from arterial inflow, but venous pressure remains low if the valves are competent. In the limb with chronic venous insufficiency, incompetent valves allow blood to move from the deep to the superficial system during muscle contraction. During relaxation, incompetent valves in the deep, superficial, and perforating veins allow blood to flow back toward the foot. This results in an uninterrupted column of blood with gravity and hydrostatic pressure causing persistently elevated venous pressure, both at rest and during exercise. Venous hypertension may lead to leakage of protein-rich fluid and blood cells through the capillary walls into the intercellular space. The immediate result is soft tissue edema, but the long-term result is skin thickening and hyperpigmentation, and, ultimately, skin ulceration. The pathogenesis of stasis-related ulceration is not well understood, but the chronic debilitating effects of ulceration are easily appreciated.

Chronic venous insufficiency may affect only the superficial veins, or it may be related to deep venous thrombosis. The valves below the knee are most often implicated in the clinical sequelae of venous thrombosis. Patients who develop ulceration following an episode of deep venous thrombosis quite often exhibit both deep venous incompetence and incompetence of the great and small saphenous veins. It is of interest to note that patients without significant incompetence of the deep veins below the knee may not suffer from ulceration if there is normal valvular function in the superficial veins.

CLINICAL SIGNS AND SYMPTOMS

Patients with chronic venous insufficiency typically present with symptoms of leg pain and clinical signs of edema, dilated veins, and skin changes in the region of the ankle. Patients with incompetent venous valves involving the superficial, perforating, and deep venous systems may demonstrate the full spectrum of signs and symptoms, whereas those with only segmental incompetence of the superficial veins may experience lesser degrees of disability.

Mild swelling in the region of the ankle is usually the first sign seen in patients with valvular dysfunction. The edema usually resolves with bed rest or with elevation of the limb. In patients with severe venous insufficiency, the swelling may involve the lower limb to the midcalf level and may or may not be associated with pitting in response to moderate pressure applied to the skin.

The increased venous pressure that results from incompetence of the superficial vein valves causes dilatation of the superficial veins in the distal extremity (Figure 24-1). This is generally noted first on the medial aspect of the lower calf and around the ankle. With progressively worsening dysfunction, the veins become enlarged and tortuous.

Patients with valvular dysfunction frequently complain of a feeling of heaviness and aching in the legs after prolonged standing or sitting with the legs dependent. In patients with valvular incompetence in the absence of venous obstruction, the feeling may subside with walking or with elevation of the limb, actions that relieve venous congestion. In contrast, if the deep veins are obstructed, exercise results in venous claudication, consisting of severe cramping, burning pain that persists as long as the veins remain congested. Several investigators have shown that venous claudication is caused by a rapid increase in pressure in both the superficial and deep venous systems.[1,2] This is usually the result of obstruction of the iliofemoral venous segment with inadequate collateral compensatory flow.

The goals of the noninvasive evaluation of patients with symptoms of venous insufficiency are to define which venous systems are involved (superficial and/or deep), the anatomic level of dysfunction, and whether the pathologic process includes both incompetence and obstruction.

VASCULAR LABORATORY TEST PROCEDURES

Historically, investigators relied on the invasive procedures (namely, ascending and descending venography and ambulatory venous pressure measurements) to evaluate chronic venous insufficiency. Venography was considered to be the gold standard for visualization of anatomy, confirmation of the presence of venous obstruction and collateralization, and definition of the location and extent of valvular reflux. Ambulatory venous pressure measurements were used as a hemodynamic complement to the anatomic information obtained from venography.[3] Pressures could be measured with the patient at rest in a supine position, while standing, and during exercise. This procedure had value as a means for recording venous pressure recovery time, which has been used as the basis for more recent plethysmographic studies.

The modern vascular laboratory evaluation of venous insufficiency has evolved steadily from continuous-wave Doppler velocimetry to indirect, plethysmographic procedures and finally, to

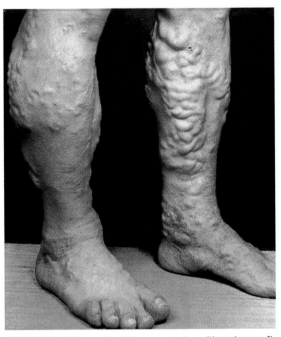

FIGURE 24-1 Lower limb demonstrating dilated superficial veins and varicosities on the medial aspect of the calf and around the ankle.

quantification of venous reflux using duplex ultrasound imaging. Although duplex sonography is currently the most accurate method for assessing venous incompetence, continuous-wave Doppler remains in use as a convenient, "low-tech" method for diagnosing venous reflux. This technique is therefore included in this chapter. Plethysmographic methods also remain in clinical use as a means of assessing venous hemodynamics, and for that reason, they too are discussed.

BIDIRECTIONAL CONTINUOUS-WAVE DOPPLER

Equipment

Bidirectional, continuous-wave Doppler uses separate transmitting and receiving crystals that operate continuously to detect flow at all depths along the emitted sound beam (Figure 24-2). Because of this, the signal that is received may contain echoes from more than one vessel lying within the beam path. The depth of penetration of a sound beam is inversely proportional to the carrier Doppler frequency. For this reason, lower-frequency transducers (3-5 MHz) are required when studying the deeper veins of the thigh, whereas higher frequencies (8-10 MHz) may be used for evaluating the superficial and calf veins of patients with a normal body habitus.

Quadrature phase separation is used to detect the direction of flow. The analog waveform of the Doppler signal is displayed using a frequency-to-voltage converter and a zero-crossing detector. The voltage output is proportional to the number of zero crossings (Figure 24-3). This display method is highly dependent on the signal-to-noise ratio and on the amplitude of the return signal.[4,5]

Patient Positioning

Patients are examined in a warm room while lying supine in reverse Trendelenburg's (10-15 degrees, feet down) position or standing to promote venous filling. In the supine reverse Trendelenburg's position, the patient's head is slightly elevated and the legs are externally rotated at the hip with the knees comfortably flexed. In the upright position, the patient should initially face the examiner with the body weight supported mainly on the contralateral leg. The limb must remain immobile throughout the examination to prevent muscle contraction and inadvertent augmentation of venous flow. The examination is facilitated if the patient stands on a platform that is approximately 2 feet high with a support railing on three sides.

Examination Technique and Diagnostic Criteria

The examination is initiated with the continuous-wave Doppler probe placed over the femoral vein pointing toward the head (cephalad) at an angle approximating 45 degrees to the skin. The identification of the vein is confirmed by first insonating the common femoral artery (noting the pulsatile, multiphasic, caudad flow signal) and then moving the probe in a medial direction to locate the common femoral vein. Care must be taken to avoid pressure on the probe, because the veins are quite easily compressed.

Normal venous blood flow is spontaneous and phasic during respiration, yielding a wind-like audible Doppler signal. Manual compression of the limb below the probe should augment

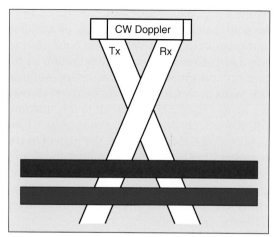

FIGURE 24-2 Diagram of a continuous-wave (CW) Doppler demonstrating transmitting and receiving crystals with the ultrasound beam intersecting both an artery *(red)* and a vein *(blue)*. Rx, receiving crystal, Tx, transmitting crystal.

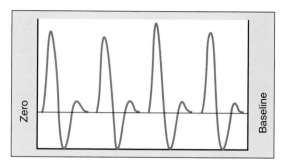

FIGURE 24-3 Analog waveform from a continuous-wave Doppler using a zero-crossing detector and quadrature phase separation to show direction of flow. *(Modified from Scissons R: Physiological testing techniques and interpretation, North Kingstown, RI, 2003, Unetixs Educational Publishing.)*

forward flow, with resultant increased amplitude of the audible Doppler signal. When the limb is compressed above the probe, the Doppler signal will normally cease, because competent valves restrict retrograde venous flow. When compression above the probe is released, an augmented, forward flow signal should be noted. Blood flow signals will also decrease when the patient coughs or performs a Valsalva maneuver. Both actions cause an increase in intra-abdominal pressure, which restricts escape of blood from the lower limb. The same compression and/or respiration procedure is repeated over the femoral, popliteal, and posterior tibial veins and in the regions of the saphenofemoral and saphenopopliteal junctions. Spontaneous Doppler signals are most often present in the larger-diameter thigh and popliteal veins. If the patient is examined in a cool room, however, vasoconstriction may reduce extremity blood flow, and augmentation of flow signals may be required to confirm patency of the small-diameter tibial veins.

If the valve immediately *distal* to the site of probe placement is incompetent, reversed blood flow signals will be noted with compression of the limb *above* the probe. Given this, a retrograde Doppler flow signal over the common femoral vein following an appropriately performed Valsalva maneuver should suggest an incompetent valve immediately *distal* to that site. Moreover, the presence of a single competent valve at any site proximal to the probe will prevent reflux and may lead to a false-negative result.

The anatomic location of valvular incompetence can be inferred by simple compression maneuvers that exclude the superficial venous system during the examination. The continuous-wave Doppler probe is placed over the region of the saphenofemoral junction, and the presence of retrograde flow is confirmed with release of compression of the limb *below* the level of the probe. A tourniquet is placed around the limb approximately 10 cm distal to the expected location of the saphenofemoral junction and tightened sufficiently to compress the great saphenous vein (Figure 24-4). Compression of the limb below the level of the probe is repeated. The continued presence of reversed blood flow signals suggests incompetence of the common femoral and/or proximal femoral vein(s). If retrograde blood flow is abolished by tourniquet application, incompetence of the great saphenous vein is suggested. The saphenopopliteal junction should be examined in a similar manner to distinguish

popliteal/gastrocnemius reflux from incompetency of the small saphenous vein.

Absence of a Doppler signal along the anatomic course of a vein suggests occlusion of the vessel. Remembering that the major arteries and veins course together through the lower extremity, a venous signal found at a distance of more than 1 cm from the corresponding artery suggests the presence of a large collateral and occlusion of the primary vein. Low-amplitude Doppler signals may imply partial thrombosis, a collateralized venous occlusion, or a recanalized vein.

Advantages

In the hands of experienced examiners, bidirectional, continuous-wave Doppler velocimetry has been shown to have excellent sensitivity (92%) with acceptable specificity (73%) for the assessment of venous incompetence.[6] While some applaud this method as a valuable portable tool for detection of valvular incompetence or obstruction of the deep and superficial veins,[7-9] others note that the continuous-wave Doppler test is extremely operator dependent and subjective.[10]

Limitations

It is important to be aware of the considerable limitations associated with continuous-wave Doppler examination of the extremity veins. Because this

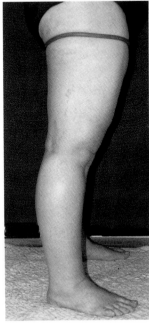

FIGURE 24-4 Lateral view of a lower extremity showing placement of an upper-thigh tourniquet used to compress and stop blood flow through the great saphenous vein.

is a nonimaging modality, there is no way to be certain which veins are being insonated. Duplication of the deep and superficial veins is common, and a Doppler signal may be elicited from a patent vein that lies adjacent to a thrombosed venous segment or from a large collateral vein. It is often quite difficult to differentiate reflux in the deep venous system from reflux in a superficial vein or major tributary at the saphenofemoral and saphenopopliteal junctions. Similarly, incompetence of large perforating veins may be confused with reflux in the saphenous or deep veins. Finally, standardization of the testing protocol is not possible because of the variability associated with tourniquet application. There is no assurance that the superficial veins are adequately compressed or that the compression does not obliterate flow in the deep venous system or perforating veins.

PHOTOPLETHYSMOGRAPHY

Equipment

Photoplethysmography is a relatively simple tool used to screen for valvular incompetence. This technique employs an infrared light-emitting diode, with a second diode used to sense light reflected from subdermal venous flow. The photoplethysmographic probe is most commonly affixed to the skin in the supramalleolar region, using double-stick tape (Figure 24-5). The plethysmograph is coupled to a direct current recorder (DC mode) to track the average changes in reflected light that occur over time in association with alterations in blood flow volume. In the normal limb, the volume of blood in the skin decreases in response to manual compression of the calf or dorsiflexion of the foot and ankle. In the absence of obstruction to arterial inflow, the venous microcirculation refills slowly. If venous valves are incompetent, however, reflux occurs and the microcirculation refills rapidly. The quality of venous emptying with calf muscle compression can be assessed subjectively, and the length of time required for venous refill can be calculated from the calibrations on the strip chart recording.

Patient Positioning

The patient is seated forward on a bed or examination table with the legs unsupported. The photoplethysmographic sensors are affixed to the medial aspect of the leg above the malleolus. Care is taken to avoid positioning the sensor over regions of inflammation or ulceration.

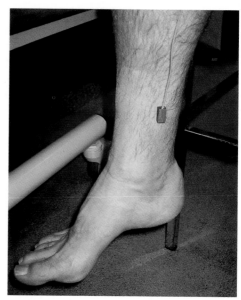

FIGURE 24-5 Medial view of the lower calf demonstrating correct placement of a photoplethysmographic sensor used for the evaluation of venous refill time.

Examination Technique and Diagnostic Criteria

The patient is initially requested to relax the limb while a baseline tracing is recorded on the plethysmographic strip chart recorder. The stylus for the recorder is positioned near the top of the tracing.

The patient is then requested to dorsiflex the foot four or five times. This causes the calf muscles to contract, simulating ambulation, and empties the calf veins in normal individuals. Manual calf compression can be used for patients who are unable to achieve adequate emptying of the venous pool with dorsiflexion. When the leg is relaxed and immobile, the calf veins refill. The venous refilling time is defined as the number of seconds required for the photoplethysmographic tracing to reach a stable endpoint for at least 5 seconds. The refill time is measured from the time exercise ceases to the stable endpoint (Figure 24-6, *A*). As noted previously, normally there is a rapid reduction of venous volume (and venous pressure) with limb exercise. Capillary refilling is primarily a function of arterial inflow when vein valves are competent and venous refilling is relatively slow. In patients with competent deep and superficial veins, the venous refill time is lengthened and usually exceeds 20 seconds.

A venous refill time less than 20 seconds suggests venous insufficiency (Figure 24-6, *B*).

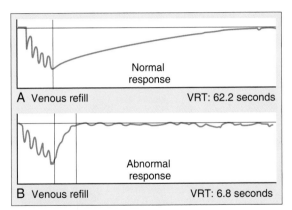

FIGURE 24-6 Strip chart recordings of photoplethysmographic measurement venous refill time (VRT). Note the placement of calipers at completion of exercise and at a stable endpoint. **A,** Normal venous refill time, exceeding 20 seconds. **B,** Abnormal response consistent with venous reflux. Venous refill time is only 6.8 seconds. *(From Scissons R: Physiological testing techniques and interpretation, North Kingstown, RI, 2003, Unetixs Educational Publishing.)*

Superficial venous reflux can be differentiated from deep venous reflux by application of tourniquets to compress the great and small saphenous veins. A tourniquet (latex tubing or blood pressure cuff inflated to 45 mm Hg) is initially placed above the knee. The test is repeated as described previously. If the venous refill time normalizes to longer than 20 seconds, the superficial venous system is implicated as the source of incompetence. If the refill time improves but does not normalize, the data imply that both the deep and superficial systems are incompetent. The tourniquet is then moved below the knee. If the refill time normalizes, this is diagnostic of superficial venous incompetence alone. If the refill time remains less than 20 seconds with tourniquet compression of the superficial veins, this suggests deep venous insufficiency.

Advantages

Photoplethysmographic determination of venous refill time correlates with ambulatory venous pressure measurements.[11] The application is technically simple, and the equipment is inexpensive and portable. This modality serves as a useful screening tool for evaluation of patients in whom venous insufficiency is suspected on the basis of history or physical findings.

Limitations

While attractive as a screening tool because of its technical simplicity, photoplethysmographic assessment of venous refill time has significant limitations. Most notable is the fact that it is a subjective and nonquantitative modality. It also is not capable of anatomically localizing the site of incompetence. As with bidirectional continuous-wave Doppler, the technique cannot be standardized because of variability in sensor placement and tourniquet pressure. The sensor may be placed over incompetent perforators or a region of localized inflammation or ischemia. There is no assurance that the superficial veins are compressed or that the deep veins remain patent with tourniquet application. In addition, it must be recognized that the results of photoplethysmographic studies may be influenced by body temperature, with alterations of blood flow and filling time occurring in response to vasodilatation and/or vasoconstriction.

AIR PLETHYSMOGRAPHY

Air plethysmography (APG) was first introduced in the 1960s to study lower extremity volume changes that occur in response to alterations in posture and muscular exercise. Once it became possible to calibrate the system, interest was renewed in this noninvasive modality that could replace the older diagnostic devices such as strain gauge, segmental volume, and water plethysmographs. Christopoulos and colleagues[12] introduced APG as a diagnostic tool in 1987 to detect global limb volume changes that occur with exercise and gravity.

With respect to venous incompetence, APG measures the following: (1) calf venous volume, (2) the rate at which calf venous volume is restored normally or as a result of reflux, (3) the effectiveness of the calf muscle pump, and (4) ambulatory venous pressure (indirectly).

Equipment

APG uses an air-filled, polyvinyl cuff, which surrounds the calf and functions as a sensing device to detect calf volume changes. The cuff is connected to an air-calibrated pressure transducer, amplifier, and recorder (Figure 24-7).

Patient Positioning

The patient initially reclines in the supine position with the heel slightly elevated on a support and the limb externally rotated and flexed to allow application of the cuff. Volume changes in the limb are recorded during limb elevation (which empties the veins), venous refilling, and a series of maneuvers with the patient upright, as shown in Figure 24-8 and described in the following section.

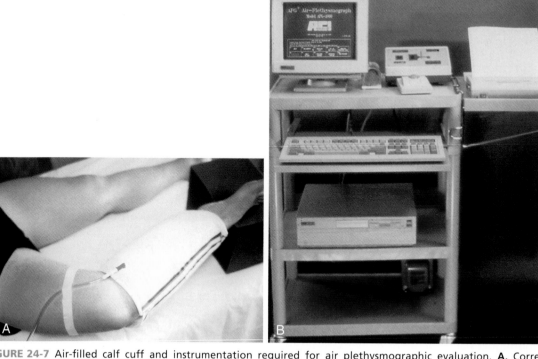

FIGURE 24-7 Air-filled calf cuff and instrumentation required for air plethysmographic evaluation. **A,** Correct placement of the air-filled cuff on the patient's calf. **B,** Air-calibrated pressure transducer, amplifier, recorder, and display system.

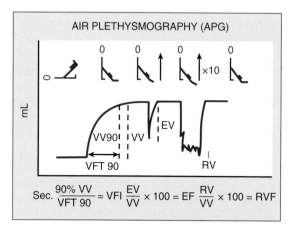

FIGURE 24-8 *Top row:* Typical positions of the lower limb during an air plethysmographic study. Upward arrows indicate transient elevation of the leg. *Bottom row:* Resulting air plethysmographic tracings and measurement of the venous filling index (VFI), ejection fraction (EF), and residual volume fraction (RVF). EV, ejection volume; RV, residual volume; VFT, venous filling time; VV, venous volume. *(From Christopoulos DG, Nicolaides AN, Szendro G, et al: Air plethysmography and the effects of elastic compression on venous hemodynamics of the leg, J Vasc Surg 5:148-159, 1987.)*

Examination Technique and Diagnostic Criteria

With the patient's heel supported and the limb properly positioned, the air-filled cuff is adjusted over the calf so that it encloses the calf from the knee to the ankle. The patient's limb is elevated 45 degrees to empty the calf veins (see Figure 24-8). Maximal venous emptying is indicated when the baseline recording stabilizes. The patient is then quickly brought to a standing position with the weight supported on the opposite limb. Filling of the calf veins is recorded continuously until a steady baseline is again obtained. This indicates that functional *venous volume* (VV) has been reached. Venous filling should result in an increase in leg VV of 100 to 150 mL in limbs with competent vein valves and 100 to 350 mL in limbs with venous insufficiency.

The *venous filling index* (VFI) is the ratio of 90% of the VV divided by the time required to achieve 90% venous filling (*venous filling time,* or VFT90%). The VFI, which evaluates overall valvular competence, is calculated from the equation

VFI = 90% VV/VFT90%. This measurement of average filling rate is expressed in milliliters per second. A VFI of 2 mL/sec or less indicates normal valvular function, while a VFI greater than 7 mL/sec is consistent with deep and/or superficial incompetence and is associated clinically with symptoms of chronic venous insufficiency. Application of a narrow below-knee tourniquet to occlude the small and great saphenous veins may reduce the VFI to less than 5 mL/sec in limbs with incompetent common femoral vein valves but competent popliteal valves.[13] Christopoulos and associates[12] found that a VFI between 2 and 30 mL/sec was associated with superficial venous incompetence, while patients with a VFI between 7 and 28 mL/sec had evidence of deep venous insufficiency.

After the measurements cited previously are obtained, the patient is asked to rise up once on the toes and return to normal position. This maneuver activates the calf muscle pump, which decreases venous volume. The *ejection volume* (EV) measures the decrease in VV achieved with one heel raise exercise and represents the volume of blood expelled by the calf with a single calf muscle contraction. The *ejection fraction* (EF) represents the emptying power of a single calf contraction and normally exceeds 60% of the baseline VV. The ejection volume and ejection fraction can be calculated from the equation $EF = (EV/VV) \times 100$.

The patient then performs 10 heel raises to completely empty the calf veins and returns to the resting position. The *residual venous volume* (RV) is recorded at the end of the exercise. The *residual venous volume fraction* (RVF) is calculated as $RV/VV \times 100$ to determine the percentage of total calf blood volume that remains following this level of exercise. Normally this value is less than 35% and represents overall calf muscle pump function. While some investigators believe that this value correlates with ambulatory venous pressure,[12] others have challenged this opinion.[14,15]

Advantages

APG has value as a tool for studying calf muscle pump function and global lower limb venous hemodynamics. As such, it can be used to select patients who will benefit from surgical intervention to correct venous valvular dysfunction and to evaluate the effect of noninvasive therapeutic measures such as limb compression.

Limitations

While APG has shown value as a noninvasive means for assessing global venous hemodynamics in the lower extremity, specific incompetent valve sites cannot be identified. Although the technique has merit for quantification of venous reflux and outflow obstruction, it is difficult for many patients to move from the supine to upright position rapidly and to perform the heel-raise maneuvers. A small number of patients cannot undergo testing because of extensive limb swelling and discomfort or their inability to perform the exercise routine.

DUPLEX ULTRASONOGRAPHY

Duplex ultrasound, the combination of B-mode (gray-scale) imaging and pulsed Doppler velocity spectral analysis, has become the primary diagnostic procedure for identification of deep venous thrombosis and superficial thrombophlebitis. This technique, complemented with color flow imaging, provides an excellent tool for demonstration of venous obstruction and reflux. The B-mode image allows definition of the vein lumen, vein valve leaflets, and vein wall morphology, as well as compressibility of the vein, and assessment of the acoustic properties of thrombus. Pulsed Doppler velocity spectral analysis is used to ensure accurate differentiation of venous and arterial blood flow, to document venous flow patterns and flow direction, and for timing the duration of venous reflux through incompetent valves. Color flow imaging is used to differentiate venous occlusion from partial thrombosis of the vein, to distinguish reflux in the deep veins from reflux in the superficial system at the saphenofemoral and saphenopopliteal junctions, to identify incompetent perforating veins, and to demonstrate recanalization and collateralization of chronically thrombosed venous segments.

Equipment

Accurate assessment of lower extremity venous morphology and hemodynamics requires a high-resolution ultrasound system equipped with pulsed Doppler transducers with frequency ranges from 2 to 10 MHz. This frequency range allows interrogation of the inferior vena cava, deep pelvic veins, and the veins of the thigh and calf. Excellent spatial resolution is necessary to ensure identification of acute, acoustically homogeneous thrombus. In addition, Doppler spectral and color wall filters must be independently controlled to ensure detection of low-amplitude, low-velocity flow associated with partially occlusive thrombus, recanalized venous segments, and venous collaterals.

Patient Positioning

The patient is placed in the supine position with the head slightly elevated and the examination table in the reverse Trendelenburg's position (feet 10-15 degrees below the level of the heart) to maximize venous pooling in the lower limbs. The patient's hips are externally rotated, and the knees are slightly flexed. This position permits easy access to the common femoral, femoral, deep femoral, posterior tibial, peroneal, and great saphenous veins. Moving the patient to the lateral decubitus position facilitates examination of the common iliac, external iliac, popliteal, and small saphenous veins. The popliteal and small saphenous veins may also be interrogated with the patient lying prone with the feet elevated slightly on a rolled towel or pillow. Elevation in this manner prevents hyperextension of the knee and resulting extrinsic compression of the popliteal vein and the saphenopopliteal junction. The inferior vena cava may be evaluated with the patient lying in the supine position, or a coronal image plane can be used with the patient in a left lateral decubitus position.

Examination Technique and Diagnostic Criteria

The examination is initiated with a longitudinal B-mode image of the common femoral vein. Confirmation of venous flow is established by placing the Doppler sample volume within the vein lumen. Normal venous blood flow signals are spontaneous and show phasicity with respiration (Figure 24-9). As described in the discussion of bidirectional continuous-wave Doppler, forward (cephalad) flow occurs when the limb is compressed *distal* to the probe. There should be no evidence of retrograde flow with release of distal compression, with a Valsalva maneuver, or with limb compression *proximal* to the probe.

The venous competency examination may be complemented with color flow imaging to facilitate recognition of blood flow direction, the identification of anatomic landmarks and blood flow patterns, and the detection of morphologic and hemodynamic abnormalities (Figure 24-10). Color flow imaging parameters

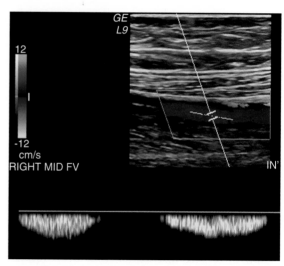

FIGURE 24-9 Color flow image of the femoral vein (FV) demonstrating appropriate flow direction and spontaneous respiratory phasicity. Note that the spectral display is inverted; blood flow toward the probe is displayed below the baseline. *(Courtesy of John Pellerito, Vascular Laboratory at North Shore University Hospital, Manhasset, NY.)*

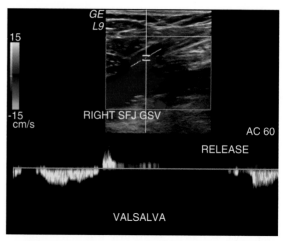

FIGURE 24-10 Color flow image of the saphenofemoral junction with reflux identified on the spectral tracing with the Valsalva maneuver. SFJ, saphenofemoral junction; GSV, great saphenous vein. *(Courtesy of John Pellerito, Vascular Laboratory at North Shore University Hospital, Manhasset, NY.)*

must be optimized for detection of low-velocity blood flow by decreasing the color velocity scale and wall filters and taking care to use an appropriately angled, narrow color box. Doppler spectral waveforms should confirm normal blood flow direction at rest and the absence of retrograde flow with application of proximal limb compression or release of distal compression. Abnormal blood flow direction can also be confirmed with color flow imaging.

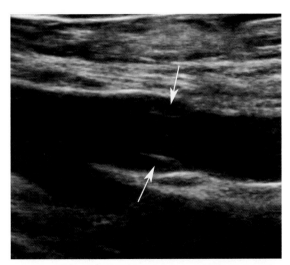

FIGURE 24-11 B-mode image of a valve sinus demonstrating the thin, echogenic valve leaflets *(arrows)*. *(Courtesy of Michael Aboulafia, Zwanger-Pesiri Radiology, Long Island, NY.)*

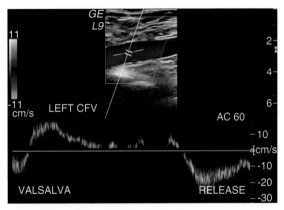

FIGURE 24-12 Color flow image and Doppler spectral waveform demonstrating significant reflux through an incompetent valve in the common femoral vein (CFV). *(Courtesy of John Pellerito, Vascular Laboratory at North Shore University Hospital, Manhasset, NY.)*

The B-mode examination of the femoral area is continued by moving the transducer slightly distally or proximally to identify the saphenofemoral junction. The common femoral vein and the saphenofemoral junction are interrogated carefully for evidence of intraluminal echoes that suggest the presence of thrombus. Care should be taken to identify valve sinuses in the common femoral and proximal great saphenous veins. The sinuses most commonly have an elliptical configuration. By imaging perpendicular to the anterior wall of the vein, the thin, mobile valve leaflets can be visualized (Figure 24-11). Compression of the limb proximal to the probe, a Valsalva maneuver, or release of distal compression will normally elicit no evidence of retrograde venous flow (Figure 24-12). The scan is continued throughout the common femoral to its bifurcation into the profunda femoris and femoral veins. The profunda femoris vein is examined as far along its course as possible with careful attention to ensure the absence of thrombus and reflux. The femoral vein is examined throughout its length in a similar manner to evaluate the valve sinuses, to confirm the absence of intraluminal echoes, and to ensure valvular competency. B-mode image resolution may be compromised in the distal thigh because of the depth of the vein. To overcome this obstacle, the transducer is placed in the popliteal fossa to image the popliteal vein longitudinally. Counterpressure is applied to the patient's knee while the

scan is continued in a cephalad direction into the distal femoral vein.

The transducer is returned to the popliteal fossa to insonate the popliteal vein throughout its length, ensuring the absence of thrombus and confirming the competence of this important valve site. The scan is continued distally to identify the anterior tibial and tibioperoneal trunks. In a manner identical to that used for examination of the proximal veins, posterior tibial and peroneal veins are interrogated throughout their length. The anterior tibial veins may be interrogated only proximally or throughout their length, as clinically indicated. Color flow imaging may facilitate identification of the tibial veins, duplicated venous segments, and the absence of reflux.

Following the longitudinal examination of the deep veins, the transducer is returned to the level of the common femoral vein and a transverse image of the vein is obtained at the saphenofemoral junction. Compressibility of the vein is then confirmed by applying pressure with the ultrasound transducer on the venous segment proximal and distal to the saphenofemoral junction. Vein walls normally coapt easily with pressure in the absence of thrombosis or abnormal venous pressure resulting from extrinsic compression of the vein proximal to the image site. Compressibility is then assessed sequentially throughout all venous segments from the common femoral vein distally to the tibial veins at ankle level.

When assessment of the deep veins is complete, the great and small saphenous veins are insonated in an identical manner. Longitudinal and transverse B-mode imaging is used to ensure

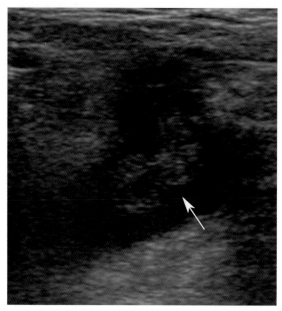

FIGURE 24-13 Cross-sectional image of the common femoral vein demonstrating partially occlusive, organized thrombus *(arrow)*. *(Courtesy of John Pellerito, Vascular Laboratory at North Shore University Hospital, Manhasset, NY.)*

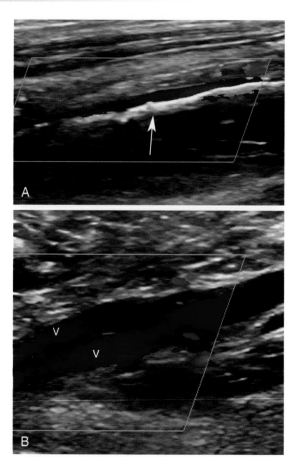

FIGURE 24-14 Color flow images of recanalized venous segments. **A,** Note the narrowed lumen and calcified wall *(arrow)*. **B,** Note the small parallel channels that reconstitute the previously thrombosed segment. V, venous channels. *(Courtesy of John Pellerito, Vascular Laboratory at North Shore University Hospital, Manhasset, NY.)*

the absence of thrombus, evaluate valve sites, and assess venous compressibility.

Intraluminal echogenicity suggests venous thrombosis, and affected venous segments are noncompressible or partially compressible (Figure 24-13). As described in Chapter 22, acute thrombus most often appears lightly echogenic with a spongy texture and may be poorly attached to the vein wall. As the thrombus organizes in the subacute and chronic phases, it becomes more echogenic, because of the increased collagen content, and it becomes more rigid. It is then well attached to the vein wall, and as it continues to organize, it contracts, pulling the walls of the vein inward. The vein may appear to be small in diameter with thickened, irregular walls. Over time, recanalization may occur or collateral veins may develop (Figure 24-14).

Doppler spectral waveforms become continuous and nonphasic when venous outflow is obstructed by thrombus or extrinsic compression. Augmentation of flow with distal limb compression also is diminished, as compared to flow at the same level in a normal contralateral limb. Color flow imaging is useful in differentiating a totally thrombosed vein from one that is partially obstructed (Figure 24-15). Careful imaging is necessary to ensure that blood flow characteristics are recorded from the primary superficial and deep veins rather than from large venous collaterals.

Quite often, deep venous thrombosis damages the vein valves, causing them to thicken and scar. As a result, the valve leaflets cannot function properly, leading to reflux of blood through incompetent sites. Improperly functioning valve leaflets can be identified with B-mode imaging, and reversed blood flow through such valves is demonstrated with spectral and color Doppler (Figure 24-16).

Incompetent perforating veins can be identified with duplex sonography complemented with color flow imaging (Figure 24-17). Perforating veins connect the superficial and deep systems and have one-way valves that normally allow blood flow *only* from the superficial to the deep veins. Large perforating veins are commonly found in the distal calf and in the proximal and mid thigh. In the thigh, identification of

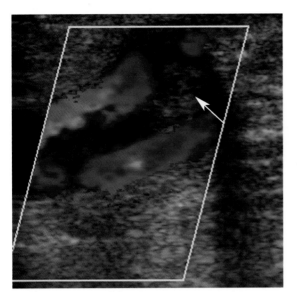

FIGURE 24-15 Color flow image of a femoral vein demonstrating partially occluding thrombus *(arrow). (Courtesy of John Pellerito, Vascular Laboratory at North Shore University Hospital, Manhasset, NY.)*

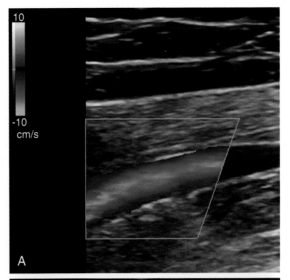

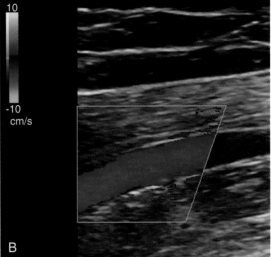

FIGURE 24-16 Color flow images demonstrating valvular incompetence. **A,** Venous flow is antegrade through an incompetent valve when manual compression is applied distal to the valve. **B,** Blood flow direction is retrograde (reflux) through the incompetent valve when manual compression is released. (Color assignment is red for flow toward the transducer and blue for flow away from the transducer.) *(Courtesy of John Pellerito, Vascular Laboratory at North Shore University Hospital, Manhasset, NY.)*

the medial perforating veins is best accomplished with transverse B-mode imaging beginning at the level of the common femoral vein. The perforating veins penetrate the deep fascia and connect the great saphenous vein to the deep veins of the thigh.[16-18] When a perforating vein is identified, manual compression of the limb above and below the transducer can be used to detect abnormal retrograde flow toward the skin.[17,19] Color flow imaging can also identify retrograde blood flow toward the transducer, consistent with valvular incompetence. Incompetent perforating veins are usually larger than competent ones. Phillips and associates[20] noted that all perforating veins larger than 4 mm in diameter were incompetent, while those smaller than 3 mm were competent.

In the calf, there are major groups of medial perforating veins that are rather constant in their anatomic location. They are typically located 6, 12, 18, 24, and 28 to 32 cm above the heel. The first three groups are referred to as the Cockett's perforators and the highest (anteromedial) perforating vein is called the Boyd perforator.[21] Identification of these medial perforating veins should be included in the scanning protocol for venous insufficiency because they account for approximately 40% of incompetent perforating veins.[18]

Lateral calf perforating veins vary in location. Imaging in the transverse plane with color Doppler, beginning at the level of the proximal small saphenous and peroneal veins, facilitates localization of the major lateral perforators. In the proximal calf, two perforating veins connect the small saphenous vein to the gastrocnemius veins.[18] In the distal calf, there are usually two lateral perforating veins located approximately 5 and 12 cm above the ankle.

When venous insufficiency is suggested during the recumbent sonographic examination,

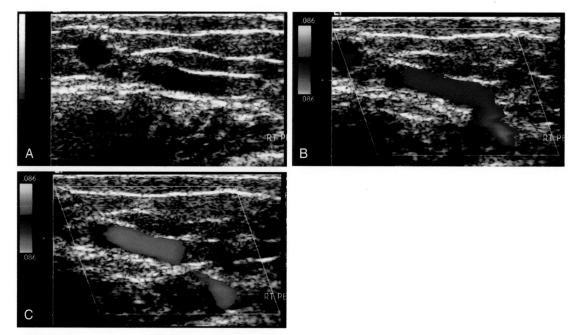

FIGURE 24-17 B-mode and color flow images of an incompetent perforating vein. **A,** B-mode image of a Cockett's perforator in the distal calf. **B,** Color flow image of the same perforator with manual compression of the limb distal to the vein. Blood flow through the perforator is normal and directed toward the skin. **C,** Color flow image demonstrating abnormal blood flow and reflux (blood flow from the deep veins to the skin) through the perforator after release of compression. *(Courtesy of the Ultrasound Department, Memorial Hospital of Sweetwater County, Rock Springs, WY.)*

confirmation is obtained by moving the patient to the standing position to impose the usual circumstances of valve function. The examination is facilitated by use of a platform as described previously in the section on continuous-wave Doppler. Color flow imaging is repeated in the longitudinal plane over the saphenofemoral and saphenopopliteal junctions and along the deep and superficial venous segments where valvular incompetence was previously suggested. If the patient is able to perform an adequate Valsalva maneuver, this method may be used to produce reflux. Otherwise, manual limb compression proximal and distal to the suspect valve sites is employed.

With the Doppler sample volume placed center stream in the vein distal to a valve site that appears to be incompetent on color flow examination, Doppler spectral waveforms are recorded during normal respiration and with manual limb compression or the Valsalva maneuver. The duration of retrograde venous flow is determined. Welch and colleagues[22] have termed this the valve closure time. The University of Washington vascular laboratory team[23,24] has shown that the normal valve closure time is less than 0.5 second (Figure 24-18).

Venous valves close when reversal of the normal transvalvular pressure gradient results in sufficient retrograde flow velocity to force the valve leaflets to coapt. Van Bemmelen and associates[25] noted that valve closure was achieved when the reverse velocities exceeded 30 cm/sec. During sonographic examination, the velocity of retrograde flow is related to the external pressure on the vein. Reflux can be demonstrated only when a significant transvalvular pressure gradient is present. It must be noted that sufficient pressure is not uniformly achieved with either the Valsalva maneuver or manual compression, particularly in the more distal veins. This can result in failure to detect venous incompetence.

Advantages

Duplex ultrasound, complemented with color flow imaging, has been validated as a sensitive and specific modality for identification of superficial and deep venous thrombosis.[26-28] Valvular incompetence can be confirmed with spectral and color Doppler, and, unlike photoplethysmography and APG, venous insufficiency can be localized to specific valve sites in the deep and superficial veins. Incompetent perforators

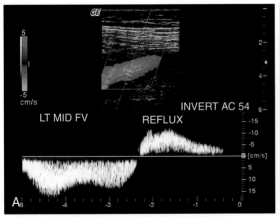
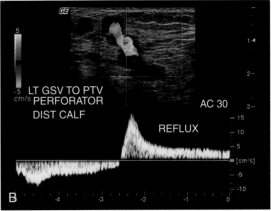
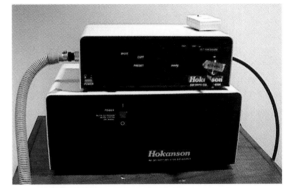

FIGURE 24-18 Color flow images and Doppler waveforms demonstrating clinically significant reflux (duration longer than 0.5 second) in a femoral vein **(A)** and in a calf perforating vein **(B;** blood flow from the great saphenous vein[GSV] to the posterior tibial vein [PTV]). The duration of reflux is determined using the timing monitor on the bottom of the image display. *(Courtesy of the Hershey Vascular Laboratory, the Penn State Vascular Institute, Hershey, PA.)*

can similarly be identified and mapped before any intervention.

Limitations

Accuracy of the technique is entirely dependent upon the experience of the sonographer and physician interpreter. In parallel with continuous-wave Doppler and photoplethysmography, the intensity of the Valsalva maneuver or manual compression cannot be standardized and may be insufficient to produce reflux. This was shown by van Bemmelen and colleagues[25] to be a significant problem, particularly in the distal veins. Because of the inability to ensure adequate venous pressure to produce reflux with Valsalva or manual compression, the severity of venous insufficiency cannot be quantitated.

QUANTITATIVE MEASUREMENT OF VENOUS INCOMPETENCE

Given the inability to standardize duplex ultrasound identification of reflux using the Valsalva maneuver or manual compression, investigators sought a method that would remove the variability of the procedure and permit quantification of valvular incompetence. In 1989 the vascular laboratory teams in Seattle at the University of Washington and at St. Mary's Hospital in London published reports using cuff-deflation techniques.[23,29] The method proposed by van Bemmelen and colleagues has been adopted by many laboratories as a reliable, reproducible procedure for identification and quantification of segmental venous reflux.

FIGURE 24-19 Shown in this picture is a device capable of rapid cuff inflation and deflation.

Equipment

Quantitative measurement of venous insufficiency requires a high-resolution ultrasound system and range of pulsed Doppler transducers identical to those used for duplex scanning. Although not required for accurate testing, color flow imaging facilitates venous identification and recognition of retrograde flow.

A rapid cuff inflator and air source are required to ensure inflation of large (24-cm) thigh cuffs within 0.3 second (Figure 24-19). In addition, a 12-cm cuff is applied to the patient's calf, and a 7-cm cuff is wrapped around the foot.

Patient Positioning

For duplex ultrasound examination of the common femoral and proximal femoral veins and the saphenofemoral junction, the patient stands on a platform, facing the examiner, with the body weight shifted to the leg opposite that being investigated. For evaluation of the popliteal vein and proximal small saphenous vein, the patient faces away from the examiner, again standing in a non–weight-bearing position. The knee is flexed slightly to prevent extrinsic compression of the popliteal vein. This position also may be used for examination of the midsegment of the great saphenous vein, the anterolateral and accessory posterior branches of the great saphenous vein, and the posterior tibial and peroneal veins.

Technique and Diagnostic Criteria

A large (24-cm) blood pressure cuff is placed around the patient's thigh. This is connected to the air source with the automatic cuff inflator and is intermittently inflated to 80 mm Hg pressure during the course of the examination.

Step 1. The examination begins with identification of the common femoral vein in the longitudinal plane using B-mode imaging (Figure 24-20). Color flow imaging may be used to facilitate identification of the vein and the recognition of flow direction. The Doppler sample volume is placed center stream in the common femoral vein, and spectral waveforms are obtained during normal respiration. The thigh cuff is then inflated for 3 seconds and then rapidly deflated while Doppler spectral waveforms are continuously recorded. Careful attention should be given to the direction of flow during cuff deflation and, if present, the length of time during which retrograde venous flow persists. Calipers associated with the ultrasound calculation software can be used to determine the duration of reflux. Reflux that persists for longer than 0.5 second is considered to be clinically significant.[25]

Step 2. The saphenofemoral junction is identified, and the inflation and deflation procedure is repeated in a manner identical to that used for evaluation of the common femoral vein. Doppler spectral waveforms are recorded continuously throughout inflation and deflation of the cuff. This procedure is next repeated with Doppler spectral waveform recordings from the proximal femoral vein (Figure 24-21).

Step 3. The patient is now turned to face away from the examiner, and the 12-cm blood pressure cuff is placed around the

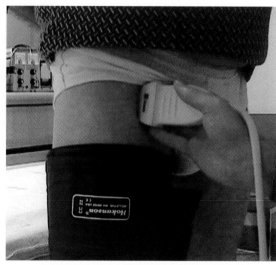

FIGURE 24-20 Appropriate positioning of the patient, thigh cuff, and transducer for obtaining Doppler spectral recordings from the common femoral, proximal femoral, and proximal great saphenous veins.

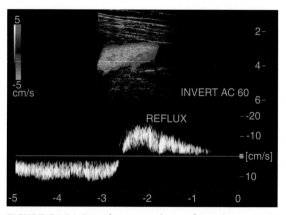

FIGURE 24-21 Doppler spectral waveform demonstrating significant reflux in the proximal femoral vein. The color Doppler image is acquired during augmentation (blood flow away from the transducer), whereas the Doppler waveform shows the time course of blood flow during (away from the probe) and following augmentation (toward the probe). *(Courtesy of the Hershey Vascular Laboratory, the Penn State Vascular Institute, Hershey, PA.)*

calf (Figure 24-22). The popliteal vein is imaged in the longitudinal plane, and Doppler spectral waveforms are obtained during normal respiration. The cuff is then inflated to 100 mm Hg pressure for 3 seconds and then rapidly deflated. Spectral waveforms are recorded continuously during inflation and deflation.

Step 4. Following completion of the popliteal recording, the midsegment and distal segment of the femoral vein, and the major

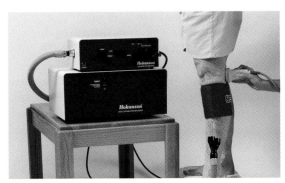

FIGURE 24-22 Appropriate positioning of the patient, calf cuff, and transducer for recording Doppler spectral tracings from the popliteal, distal femoral, and thigh perforating veins. *(Courtesy of D.E. Hokanson, Inc, Bellevue, WA.)*

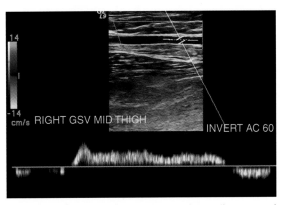

FIGURE 24-23 Color flow image and Doppler spectral waveforms demonstrating significant reflux in the great saphenous vein (GSV). *(Courtesy of John Pellerito, Vascular Laboratory at North Shore University Hospital, Manhasset, NY.)*

perforating veins along the medial side of the thigh are tested in an identical manner.

Step 5. The confluence of the small saphenous vein with the popliteal vein is identified and imaged in the longitudinal plane. Doppler spectral waveforms are recorded during normal respiration and during cuff inflation to 100 mm Hg pressure and rapid deflation. Careful attention is given to flow direction and, if present, to the duration of retrograde venous flow.

Step 6. The midsegment of the great saphenous vein is identified on the medial aspect of the knee and imaged in its longitudinal plane. Using a cuff inflation pressure of 100 mm Hg, the presence of reflux is confirmed in a manner similar to that used for the deep veins of the thigh. Next, the anterolateral branch of the great saphenous vein is located on the lateral aspect of the knee and evaluated in the longitudinal plane in an identical fashion (Figure 24-23).

Step 7. The blood pressure cuff is moved to the level of the ankle. The posterior tibial and peroneal veins are identified using B-mode and/or color flow imaging. Doppler spectral waveforms are recorded from the posterior tibial veins during normal respiration and with the cuff inflated to 100 mm Hg. Waveforms are continuously recorded during rapid cuff deflation. The test is repeated in an identical manner for evaluation of the peroneal veins.

Step 8. The posterior arch vein and the midsegment of the small saphenous vein should be examined using a cuff inflation pressure of 100 mm Hg, with the cuff at ankle level.

Step 9. A 7-cm-wide blood pressure cuff is wrapped around the foot. Color flow imaging is used to locate the posterior tibial veins in long axis just anterior to the medial malleolus. The blood pressure cuff is inflated to 120 mm Hg pressure. Doppler spectral waveforms are recorded during cuff inflation and deflation. The peroneal veins and the distal segment of the great saphenous vein are interrogated for reflux in an identical fashion.

Step 10. Large perforating veins associated with the posterior arch vein that were identified in the distal calf during the initial duplex evaluation of the limb may be tested using the 7-cm metatarsal cuff and an inflation pressure of 120 mm Hg.

As noted previously, reflux that persists for longer than 0.5 second at any level is considered to be clinically significant. In addition, O'Donnell[18] has shown that a sum of the venous closure times from the femoral and popliteal veins exceeding 4 seconds is accurate in predicting severe venous reflux.

Advantages

The standing cuff inflation-deflation technique, combined with duplex sonography, provides a quantitative estimate of valve closure time in specific segments of the deep and superficial venous systems. All venous segments, including major perforating veins, can be studied using this method, which mimics venous valvular physiology. The deficiencies of the Valsalva maneuver and manual compression techniques, cited previously, are overcome by use of distal limb cuff compression to ensure adequate extrinsic venous pressure and transvalvular pressure gradients. The accuracy of the cuff inflation-deflation technique does not depend on the presence of incompetent valves proximal to the venous segment being studied, as does the Valsalva maneuver.

Limitations

Although they are relatively inexpensive items, an automatic cuff inflator and an air source capable of rapid cuff inflation are not common to all noninvasive vascular laboratories. Some laboratories find it helpful to have one sonographer perform the imaging component of the study while a second member of the staff assists with the cuff inflation and deflation procedures. Other laboratories employ a foot pedal to activate the inflation-deflation sequence, which obviates the need for assistance from a second sonographer. In addition, sonographer and patient comfort is best achieved if the patient is examined while standing on a platform that is 18 to 24 inches in height surrounded on three sides by a support railing. This places the patient's lower limb at a level approximating the ultrasound system controls and allows the sonographer to assume an ergonomically correct position throughout the procedure. Such platforms are not universally available and may need to be specially constructed to meet individual laboratory designs.

Care must be taken to observe the patient throughout the examination, as a small percentage of patients with impaired venous function and venous dilatation may experience dizziness, as noted by Ballard and associates.[30] This is most likely the result of decreased venous return during the cuff inflation procedure.

SEGMENTAL VENOUS INCOMPETENCE

It is not uncommon to find segmental valvular dysfunction in both the deep and superficial veins. Patients with venous ulceration most often have three or four incompetent segments, involving either the deep or superficial systems.[31] Incompetence of the superficial veins is present in at least 92% of cases with ulceration, whereas incompetence of the deep veins at ankle level is less common.[12]

Van Bemmelen and Bergan[31] have described the distribution of incompetent segments of the great saphenous vein in patients with superficial venous insufficiency. The great saphenous vein was incompetent at knee level in 61% of limbs, at calf level in 49%, and in the proximal thigh in 32% of limbs. This finding emphasizes the prevalence of distal superficial vein incompetence, while the more proximal valves of the great saphenous vein remain functional. In patients with incompetence of the great saphenous vein at knee level, van Bemmelen and Bergan noted that less than 50% had multisegmental incompetence from the saphenofemoral confluence to the level of the knee. A total of 34% of patients with great saphenous incompetence at knee level and functional proximal superficial venous segments demonstrated deep venous reflux in the femoral and popliteal veins. In these cases, an incompetent perforating vein was identified at the upper end of the incompetent segment of the great saphenous vein.

Small saphenous venous reflux is often found to occur segmentally. Incompetency of the proximal segment of the small saphenous vein has been reported in 36% of lower limbs, while 31% of limbs demonstrated reflux in the calf segments.[31] If the valves in the distal segments remain competent, flow from incompetent proximal valves is diverted to superficial branches.

THE ROLE OF SONOGRAPHY IN THE TREATMENT OF CHRONIC VENOUS INSUFFICIENCY

Historically, severe chronic venous insufficiency has been treated conservatively with application of compression stockings to promote appropriate valve function, by chemical sclerosis of incompetent vein segments, use of transilluminated powered phlebectomy, surgical saphenectomy, or vein avulsion. Most recently, clinicians have used endovenous therapy for treatment of chronic venous valvular incompetence. With this nonsurgical procedure, incompetent vein segments can be ablated by applying either radiofrequency (RF) energy to the vein wall or treating the incompetent vein with endovenous laser energy. When compared to surgical methods for treating superficial venous valvular incompetence, endovenous therapy has several distinct advantages. The procedure is performed using local anesthetic and is minimally invasive. Therefore, there is reduced risk for postoperative scarring or infection. The treatment time required for endovenous ablation of incompetent veins and the amount of postoperative discomfort experienced by patients are significantly less than associated with surgical stripping or avulsion of the saphenous vein. Most often, patients can resume normal activities within days following endovenous therapy. Excellent clinical and aesthetic results have been reported with both RF and laser treatment methods.

Duplex sonography has shown value in the assessment of patients before, during, and following endovenous treatment of chronic venous insufficiency. Using a combination of B-mode, color, power, and spectral Doppler, sonography is used to define incompetent valve sites, determine the diameter of veins, guide placement of catheters and tumescent anesthetic (local anesthetic diluted in saline), and to confirm successful ablation of superficial veins and perforators.

Equipment

The ultrasound system requirements for sonographic evaluation of patients presented for endovenous treatment of chronic venous insufficiency parallel those described previously. The instrument should be equipped with pulsed Doppler linear array transducers ranging in frequency from 5 to 10 MHz to allow interrogation of the superficial veins. Examination of small, superficial veins, and some perforating veins, may be facilitated by use of a linear, "hockey-stick" style of transducer with a frequency range of 5 to 12 MHz.

Patient Positioning

The initial assessment begins with the patient standing on a platform, facing the examiner, so that the limb can be examined for evidence of telangiectasias, reticular veins, and varicose veins. For the purposes of this initial screening examination, a handheld continuous-wave Doppler device can be used for detection of superficial venous reflux while a vein light (cold light transillumination) facilitates identification of reticular veins.[32]

The detailed diagnostic sonographic examination, which confirms and localizes sites of valvular incompetence, is also performed with the patient in the standing position to maximize dilatation of the limb veins and to optimize vein valve function.[33]

TECHNIQUE: BEFORE ENDOVENOUS THERAPY

To rule out deep venous thrombosis and valvular incompetence, a complete and thorough examination of the deep venous system, as described previously in this chapter, is performed before mapping the superficial and perforating veins for evidence of valvular incompetence. The great saphenous vein is then imaged in longitudinal and transverse planes from the saphenofemoral junction to the foot. Care should be taken to identify the accessory saphenous veins, including the anterior lateral vein in the upper thigh; the posterior medial vein, which connects the great and small saphenous veins; the superior epigastric vein; the superior circumflex vein; and the superior external pudendal vein. The location of the confluence of the superior epigastric vein with the great saphenous may be marked on the skin with indelible ink. This site, typically within 2 cm of the terminal valve in the great saphenous vein, serves as a landmark for positioning the ablation catheter during endovenous therapy. During the procedure, the ablation catheter will be advanced to a position that is 1 cm distal to this confluence.

The locations of duplicated saphenous vein segments and the takeoff of venous tributaries (major branches above the deep fascia) and perforating veins are noted. These sites are either marked on the skin with indelible ink or entered on a diagram that can be referred to during the ablation procedure. The diameters of the femoral vein and the saphenofemoral junction are measured to determine suitability for RF closure and/or endovenous laser ablation.[34-36] In addition to measuring the diameter of the great saphenous at the saphenofemoral junction, it is also important to measure the diameter of the great saphenous vein in the mid and distal thigh. Care should be taken to note the depth of the vein above, at, and just below the knee as this will be the region of access for ablation catheters.[34,37]

Venous patency and the presence and location of venous reflux are assessed using compression maneuvers as previously described. The evaluation can be facilitated and standardized by use of rapid inflation-deflation cuffs.[17,24,38] Valvular reflux that persists for longer than 0.5 second, in any segment of the superficial venous system, is considered to be clinically significant.[29,33] As noted, these criteria are identical to those used for diagnosis of significant valvular incompetence involving the deep venous system.

The diameters of the popliteal vein, the saphenopopliteal junction, and the small saphenous vein are measured, and the location of intersaphenous veins is defined. Because the small saphenous

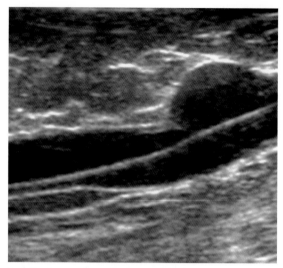

FIGURE 24-24 B-mode image illustrating a linear, hyperechoic laser fiber within the lumen of a great saphenous vein during endovenous therapy. *(Courtesy of Robert Scissons, Jobst Vascular Institute, Toledo, OH.)*

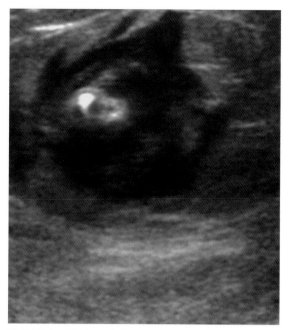

FIGURE 24-25 B-mode image demonstrating tumescent anesthetic (local anesthetic diluted in saline) surrounding a great saphenous vein. The echogenic tip of a laser catheter can be seen within the vein lumen. *(Courtesy of Robert Scissons, Jobst Vascular Institute, Toledo, OH.)*

vein may terminate in the popliteal, femoral, or great saphenous vein, it is important to note the site of termination of this vein carefully.

The preprocedure evaluation should also include assessment of perforating veins and mapping of their exit and reentry locations along the course of the saphenous veins.[39] Labropoulos and Leon[40] have shown that sensitivity for detection of perforating vein reflux is enhanced when the limb is compressed distal to the perforator site. Clinically significant incompetence is present when augmented blood flow through the perforator to the superficial system exceeds 350 msec.[40]

TECHNIQUE: DURING ENDOVENOUS THERAPY

To initiate the procedure, a nontortuous segment of the supragenicular saphenous vein is cannulated and a catheter sheath is advanced, using ultrasound guidance, to a position 1 cm distal to the confluence of the superior epigastric and great saphenous veins. The laser fiber or a 6 or 8 Fr RF catheter is introduced and positioned for ablation. The sheathed fiber or catheter can readily be visualized sonographically as a linear hyperechoic structure within the lumen of the saphenous vein (Figure 24-24). Sonographic imaging is used to guide and monitor placement of tumescent anesthetic into the saphenous compartment (Figure 24-25). The perivenous anesthetic is used to reduce heat conduction during the endovenous procedure.

Venous ablation occurs when RF or laser energy is applied to the endothelial surface of vein walls.[41] The energy causes heating and vaporization of blood within the vein lumen, resulting in carbonization and thermal destruction of the vein wall. The sonographic image may initially reveal evidence of venous spasm and contraction followed by formation of thrombus (Figure 24-26). Coagulation is most often visualized within 10 to 20 seconds following application of RF or laser energy.

TECHNIQUE: FOLLOWING THE ENDOVENOUS PROCEDURE

Immediately following the procedure, the saphenofemoral junction and the length of the ablated saphenous vein are scanned thoroughly. Spectral Doppler and color flow imaging should confirm continued patency of the common femoral and proximal femoral veins. Flow may be noted at the saphenofemoral confluence, but there should be no evidence of thrombus proximal to the terminal valve of the great saphenous or extending into the deep veins. Successful ablation will reveal a contracted saphenous vein with a diameter less than 2 mm and acoustically heterogeneous echoes throughout its lumen. Because inflammation of

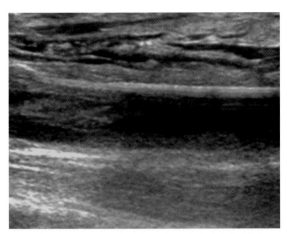

FIGURE 24-26 B-mode image demonstrating saphenous vein thrombus following ablation with endovenous laser therapy. *(Courtesy of Robert Scissons, Jobst Vascular Institute, Toledo, OH.)*

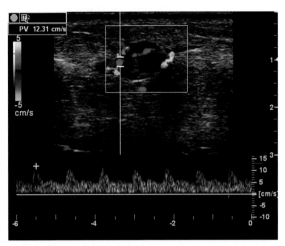

FIGURE 24-27 Color flow image and Doppler spectral waveforms illustrating low-resistance arterial blood flow in a vein wall following ablation of an incompetent venous segment. *(Courtesy of Robert Scissons, Jobst Vascular Institute, Toledo, OH.)*

the vein walls is normally noted in the early post-treatment period, Doppler interrogation of the ablated segments may demonstrate arterialized spectral waveforms (Figure 24-27).

Within 7 to 10 days following the procedure, the sonographic examination should demonstrate a contracted, noncompressible vein with thickened walls and an echogenic, cord-like appearance. There should be no evidence of flow in any ablated venous segment.

CONCLUSIONS

The vascular laboratory approach to diagnosis of venous insufficiency is dependent on the clinical questions that are to be answered. The question of whether the patient has venous insufficiency can be answered with a thorough medical history, physical examination, and determination of photoplethysmographic refill time. APG is reserved for patients whose global limb venous hemodynamics and the effectiveness of the calf muscle pump must be determined to define therapeutic options. To accurately assess the deep, superficial, and perforating venous systems for valvular incompetence and to exclude residual venous obstruction, a complete venous duplex sonographic examination should be performed, complemented by color flow imaging. To ensure the most accurate, site-specific definition of clinically significant valvular incompetence, segmental quantitative measurement of reflux using the standing cuff inflation-deflation technique is recommended.

The value of sonography has extended beyond diagnosis of venous insufficiency into the realm of treatment, where it has increased the accuracy and reliability of endovenous therapies. Before endovenous treatment, sonographic imaging is used to localize incompetent valves in the superficial and perforating veins and to confirm clinically significant valvular reflux. Sonographic guidance enhances placement of sheaths and/or catheters and tumescent anesthetic and is used to monitor the coagulation process during the ablation procedure. Following treatment for venous insufficiency, confirmation of successful ablation is facilitated by sonographic imaging.

As with all areas of diagnostic sonography, accurate patient evaluations depend on the knowledge, experience, and expertise of the sonographer and the physician interpreter. High-quality patient care is best achieved when the studies are performed and interpreted by credentialed sonographers and physicians in accredited vascular facilities.

REFERENCES

1. Negus D, Cockett FB: Femoral vein pressures in postphlebitic iliac vein obstruction, *Br J Surg* 54:522, 1967.
2. Killewich LA, Martin R, Cramer M: Pathophysiology of venous claudication, *J Vasc Surg* 1:502, 1984.
3. Nicolaides AN, Zukowski AJ: The value of dynamic venous pressure measurements, *World J Surg* 10:919–924, 1986.
4. Johnston KW, Maruzzo BC, Cobbold RSC: Inaccuracies of a zero-crossing detector for recording Doppler signals, *Surg Forum* 28:201–203, 1977.

5. Strandness DE Jr: Doppler ultrasonic techniques in vascular disease. In Bernstein EF, editor: *Noninvasive Diagnostic Techniques in Vascular Disease*, 3rd edition, St. Louis, 1985, CV Mosby, pp 13–18.

6. Raju S, Fredericks R: Evaluation of methods for detecting venous reflux. Perspectives in venous insufficiency, *Arch Surg* 125:1463–1467, 1990.

7. Barnes RW: Noninvasive tests for chronic venous insufficiency. In Bergan JJ, Yao JST, editors: *Surgery of the Veins*, Orlando, FL, 1985, Grune & Stratton, pp 99–109.

8. Sigel B, et al: Doppler ultrasound method for diagnosing lower extremity venous disease, *Surg Gynecol Obstet* 127:339–350, 1968.

9. Miller SS, Foote AV: The ultrasonic detection of incompetent perforating veins, *Br J Surg* 61:653–656, 1974.

10. O'Donnell TF, et al: Doppler examination versus clinical and phlebographic detection of the location of incompetent perforating veins, *Arch Surg* 112:31–35, 1977.

11. Abramowitz HB, et al: The use of photoplethysmography in the assessment of venous insufficiency: A comparison to venous pressure measurements, *Surgery* 86:434–441, 1979.

12. Christopoulos DG, et al: Air plethysmography and the effects of elastic compression on venous hemodynamics of the leg, *J Vasc Surg* 5:148–159, 1987.

13. Herman RJ, et al: Descending venography: a method of evaluating lower extremity valvular function, *Radiology* 137:63–69, 1980.

14. Payne S, et al: Venous assessment using air plethysmography: a comparison with clinical examination, ambulatory venous pressure measurement, and duplex scanning, *Br J Surg* 80:967–970, 1993.

15. Lees TA, Lambert D: A comparative study of air plethysmography and Doppler colour flow imaging with ambulatory venous pressure measurements in the diagnosis of venous reflux in the lower limb. In Raymond-Martinbeau R, Prescott RM, Zummo M, editors: *Phlebologie 92*, Paris, 1992, John Libbey Eurotext, pp 594–596.

16. Oliver MA: Anatomy and physiology. In Talbot SR, Oliver MA, editors: *Techniques of Venous Imaging*, Pasadena, CA, 1992, Appleton Davies, pp 11–20.

17. Masuda EM, Kistner RL, Eklof B: Prospective study of duplex scanning for venous reflux: comparison of Valsalva and pneumatic cuff techniques in the reverse Trendelenburg and standing position, *J Vasc Surg* 20:711–719, 1994.

18. O'Donnell TF: Surgical treatment of incompetent communicating veins. In Bergan JJ, Kistner RL, editors: *Atlas of Venous Surgery*, Philadelphia, 1992, Saunders, pp 111–124.

19. Lees TA, Lambert D: Patterns of venous reflux in limbs with skin changes associated with chronic venous insufficiency, *Br J Surg* 6:725–728, 1993.

20. Phillips GWL, Paige J, Molan MP: A comparison of colour duplex ultrasound with venography and varicography in the assessment of varicose veins, *Clin Radiol* 50:20–25, 1995.

21. Mozes G, et al: Surgical anatomy for endoscopic subfascial division of perforating veins, *J Vasc Surg* 23:800–808, 1996.

22. Welch HJ, et al: Comparison of descending phlebography with quantitative photoplethysmography, air plethysmography, and duplex quantitative valve closure time in assessing deep venous reflux, *J Vasc Surg* 16:913–919, 1993.

23. van Bemmelen PS, et al: Quantitative segmental evaluation of venous valvular reflux with duplex ultrasound scanning, *J Vasc Surg* 10:425–431, 1989.

24. Markel A, et al: A comparison of the cuff deflation method with Valsalva's maneuver and limb compression in detecting venous valvular reflux, *Arch Surg* 129:701–705, 1994.

25. van Bemmelen PS, et al: The mechanism of venous valve closure, *Arch Surg* 125:617–619, 1990.

26. Talbot SR: Use of real time imaging in identifying deep venous obstruction: A preliminary report, *Bruit* 6:41–44, 1984.

27. Mattos MA, et al: Color flow duplex scanning for the surveillance and diagnosis of acute deep venous thrombosis, *J Vasc Surg* 15:366–376, 1992.

28. Kerr TM, et al: Analysis of 1084 consecutive lower extremities involved with acute venous thrombosis diagnosed by duplex scanning, *Surgery* 108:520–527, 1990.

29. Vasdekis SN, Clarke GH, Nicolaides AN: Quantification of venous reflux by means of duplex scanning, *J Vasc Surg* 10:670–677, 1989.

30. Ballard JL, Bergan JJ, DeLange M: Venous imaging for reflux using duplex ultrasonography. In AbuRahma AF, Bergan JJ, editors: *Noninvasive Vascular Diagnosis*, London, 2000, Springer-Verlag, pp 329–334.

31. van Bemmelen PS, Bergan JJ: Segmental duplex reflux examination and color flow imaging. *Medical Intelligence Unit: Quantitative Measurement of Venous Incompetence*, Austin, TX, 1992, RG Landes Company, pp 51–66.

32. Mekenas L, Bergan J: Venous reflux examination: Technique using miniaturized ultrasound scanning, *J Vasc Technol* 2(26):139–146, 2002.

33. Labropoulos N, et al: Definition of venous reflux in lower extremity veins, *J Vasc Surg* 38(4):793–798, 2003.

34. Sadick NS: Advances in the treatment of varicose veins: Ambulatory phlebectomy, foam sclerotherapy, endovascular laser, and radiofrequency closure, *Dermatol Clin* 23(3):443–455, 2005.

35. Pichot O, et al: Role of duplex imaging in endovenous obliteration for primary venous insufficiency, *J Endovasc Ther* 7(6):451–459, 2000.

36. Min RJ, Khilnani N, Zimmet SE: Endovenous laser treatment of saphenous vein reflux: long-term results, *J Vasc Intervent Radiol* 14(8):991–996, 2003.

37. Puggioni A, et al: Endovenous laser therapy and radiofrequency ablation of the great saphenous vein: analysis of early efficacy and complications, *J Vasc Surg* 42(3):488–493, 2005.

38. Delis KT, et al: Enhancing venous outflow in the lower limb with intermittent pneumatic compression. A comparative haemodynamic analysis of the effect of foot vs calf vs foot and calf compression, *Eur J Vasc Endovasc Surg* 19(3):250–260, 2000.

39. Delis KT, et al: In situ hemodynamics of perforating veins in chronic venous insufficiency, *J Vasc Surg* 33(4):773–782, 2001.

40. Labropoulos N, Leon LR Jr: Duplex evaluation of venous insufficiency, *Semin Vasc Surg* 18(1):5–9, 2005.

41. Weiss RA: Comparison of endovenous radiofrequency versus 810 nm diode laser occlusion of large veins in an animal model, *Dermatol Surg* 28(1):56–61, 2002.

NONVASCULAR PATHOLOGY ENCOUNTERED DURING VENOUS SONOGRAPHY

25

JOHN S. PELLERITO, MD, FACR, FSRU, FAIUM

Numerous findings may be encountered during the course of a venous examination. These findings may indicate the cause of extremity pain or swelling apart from venous disease. Recognition of the sonographic features associated with these pathologies is critical for accurate diagnosis.[1-12] Many of these diagnoses are common, such as edema, hematoma, lymph nodes, or popliteal (Baker's) cysts. Other findings are less common, but no less important, including abscess, joint effusion, adenopathy, benign or malignant tumor, and metastatic disease.

Soft Tissue Edema

Lower extremity edema is a common cause of limb swelling and is associated with elevated venous pressures. Causes of increased hydrostatic pressure within the venous system include congestive heart failure (CHF; venous congestion), fluid overload, deep vein thrombosis (DVT), venous compression, and other causes of venous obstruction. These problems result in leg swelling and soft tissue edema.

There is a change in venous flow patterns associated with CHF. Normally, phasic, nonpulsatile waveforms are seen in the lower extremity veins. In the setting of CHF, the waveforms are usually more pulsatile and typically bidirectional, with components seen above and below the baseline[2] (Figure 25-1). As noted in Chapter 1, causes of increased venous pressure such as CHF or tricuspid insufficiency lead to increased transmission of cardiac phasic changes in pressure and blood flow to the peripheral veins of the upper and lower limbs. These changes result in increased pulsatility in the peripheral vein waveforms. Pulsatility in the venous system may resemble arterial pulsations because of the bidirectional pattern of blood flow. Comparison of the arterial and venous flow patterns is key to distinguishing pulsatile venous signals from arterial flow. On close

inspection, one will note that the phases of the venous pattern are less periodic than the typical triphasic waveforms found in the arterial system. Other clues to the nature of the flow abnormality are the direction of flow and the communications with the superficial veins. Changes in venous flow will also be seen with the Valsalva maneuver.

Pulsatile venous waveforms from venous congestion are frequently mistaken for signals associated with arteriovenous fistula (AVF). Although flow patterns seen with both venous congestion and AVF will demonstrate increased pulsatility, there are major differences. The waveforms identified from both the arterial and venous sides of an AVF will show an arterialized pattern with a low-resistance (high-diastolic) component. Flow in the fistula will only be in one direction on one side of the baseline (toward the venous or lower-pressure side) without reversal of flow. This is very different from the typical biphasic (above and below the baseline) pattern seen with venous congestion.

Gray-scale imaging may show a marbled, reticulated pattern when edema collects in the subcutaneous fat. Small collections of fluid may be seen when edema collects in the superficial tissues (Figure 25-2). This can be associated with significant soft tissue swelling and attenuation of sound that can restrict visualization of deep tissues and underlying vascular structures. A "sound" approach to this problem is to switch transducers to allow lower-frequency imaging. Changing from the usual 5- to 7-MHz linear array probe to a 2- to 5-MHz curved array transducer should allow deeper penetration of sound and visualization of the area of interest.

Bilateral leg swelling is a typical presentation for patients with venous congestion. It is also a common indication for venous sonography. Studies have shown that the likelihood of identifying DVT in patients with bilateral leg swelling and no significant risk factors is low (≤5%).[3] Naidich and associates[4] showed that 23% of patients

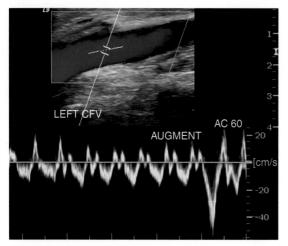

FIGURE 25-1 Pulsatile venous flow. Common femoral vein (CFV) flow signals are markedly pulsatile in this patient with leg swelling due to right heart failure.

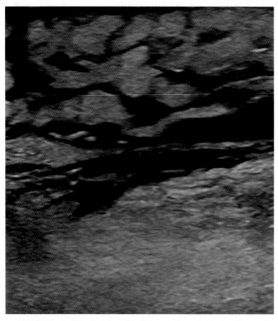

FIGURE 25-2 Marked soft tissue edema gives the subcutaneous fat a marbled appearance in this patient with renal failure and fluid overload.

with bilateral symptoms and risk factors had underlying DVT. In this group, 78% of patients had risk factors for DVT.[5] DVT cannot be reliably diagnosed or excluded on clinical grounds alone.

LYMPHEDEMA

Lymphedema is also associated with leg swelling and mimics DVT.[5] Obstruction of the lymphatics due to malignancy, trauma, or surgery will cause extremity swelling and pain. Patients will typically present with unilateral or bilateral leg swelling. The appearance of lymphedema is indistinguishable from soft tissue edema associated with venous congestion. There may or may not be lymph node enlargement to suggest the etiology of the leg swelling.

HEMATOMA

Another common cause of leg swelling and pain is soft tissue hematoma. These patients may have focal or diffuse swelling of the extremity. There is usually a history of trauma, vigorous exercise, or prior surgery or intervention. There may also be a history of anticoagulation, which suggests the correct diagnosis.

Sonographic examination of a focal mass will reveal a cystic, complex, or solid lesion, which is typically found in the superficial tissues. The mass may initially have irregular borders and demonstrate areas of fluid and solid tissue depending on the amount of clot in the hematoma (Figure 25-3). Over time, the mass will retract and become better defined and ovoid. Hematoma may also be spread through fascial or muscle planes and seen as hypoechoic or isoechoic tissue. This may be very difficult to identify as there is no significant difference in echogenicity from adjacent structures. Leg swelling may be the only clue to the soft tissue infiltration with hematoma. Magnetic resonance imaging (MRI) provides superior soft tissue contrast and displays the extent of soft tissue hematoma.

Color and duplex Doppler will demonstrate no flow within hematoma. This is very helpful to distinguish a hematoma from other soft tissue masses such as lymph nodes or tumors. Although hematoma may compress or displace adjacent vascular structures, demonstration of patent veins will allow exclusion of DVT. With significant compression by large hematomas, adjacent veins may be difficult to identify. Low-velocity blood flow below the level of compression may also be difficult to detect.

MUSCLE INJURY

Muscle injury may result from a blow (contusion), from a penetrating injury, or from a "muscle pull," which is a tearing of muscle bundles in response to vigorous exercise or abrupt straining. Tearing of the muscle is accompanied

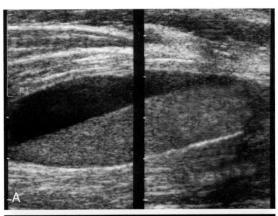

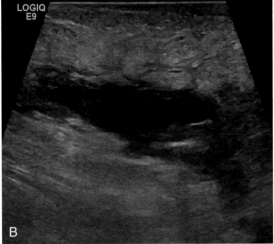

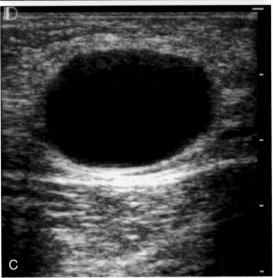

FIGURE 25-3 Various appearances of soft tissue hematomas. **A,** Composite image of an acute (hours-old) arm hematoma related to poorly controlled warfarin (Coumadin) therapy. Note the fluid/fluid level resulting from settling of nonclotted blood cells. **B,** A subacute hematoma in the calf. This hematoma is fairly hypoechoic with irregular borders. **C,** Two-month-old asymptomatic hematoma at a saphenous vein harvest site. The well-defined collection is anechoic because the clot has lysed and the collection resembles a simple cyst.

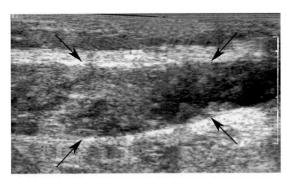

FIGURE 25-4 Muscle injury. A fusiform, heterogeneous region *(arrows)* is seen within the calf musculature at a site of pain and tenderness. The symptoms began 1 day earlier, after the patient helped push a stalled automobile.

initially by varying degrees of bleeding and, subsequently, by inflammation. Kim and colleagues[8] reported that injured muscle initially is hyperechoic and either homogeneous or heterogeneous. By about 7 days after injury, the affected muscle is intermediate to low in echogenicity and heterogeneous. These findings persist for at least 3 weeks after injury (Figure 25-4). Long-term follow-up information is not available. With a muscle pull, the area of injury may be quite focal and possibly fusiform in shape. Larger areas of abnormality may be seen with contusion.

LYMPH NODES

Lymph nodes are commonly seen in the groin, neck, and axillary regions. They may also be seen adjacent to the aorta, inferior vena cava, and iliac vessels. In general, lymph nodes have a characteristic appearance with a hypoechoic mantle of peripheral tissue surrounding an echogenic hilum containing fat and feeding vessels (Figure 25-5).

Lymph nodes are typically less than 1 cm in diameter but can attain large sizes with inflammatory or malignant infiltration. They may be seen as discrete almond-shaped nodules or large

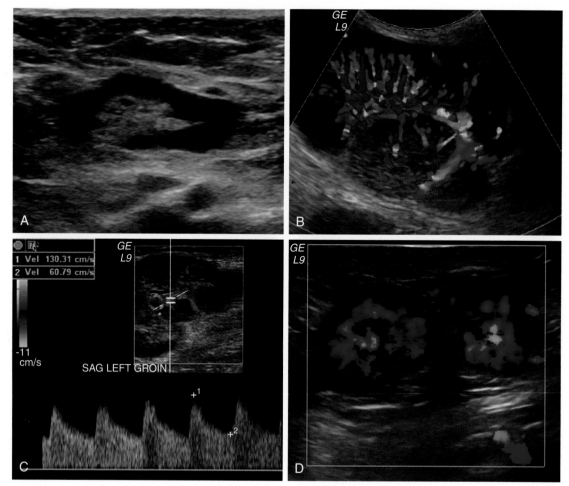

FIGURE 25-5 Lymph nodes. **A,** A normal lymph node with ovoid appearance and echogenic fatty hilum. **B,** Arterial and venous branches are identified coursing through the hilum of the node. **C,** Pulsed Doppler sample of the hilum demonstrates low-resistance arterial flow. **D,** Power Doppler image reveals disorganized vascularity in these rounded nodes due to lymphomatous infiltration.

irregular solid masses. Enlarged lymph nodes (adenopathy) may cause swelling when associated with lymphatic or venous obstruction. Inflamed lymph nodes are commonly tender on examination and indicate the cause of leg pain during Doppler study.

Color Doppler evaluation reveals arterial flow in the hilum or central portion of the lymph node. Arterial branching is seen from the center to the periphery of the node. Pulsed Doppler interrogation usually demonstrates low-resistance arterial signals with continuous forward flow in systole and diastole.

Differentiation of inflammatory from malignant lymph nodes may be difficult. Benign lymph nodes tend to maintain an ovoid shape with the short-axis diameter not exceeding half of the length of the node. Malignant nodes are

typically rounder and less ovoid than inflamed nodes. They can lose the normal architecture and are more uniform in echotexture than inflammatory nodes. They may lose the central echogenic hilum because of tumor infiltration. Doppler may also demonstrate irregular branching, peripheral vascular invasion, or disordered vascularity within the node, suggesting malignant infiltration.[9-11]

POPLITEAL (BAKER'S) CYSTS

Popliteal cysts are focal fluid collections that are found behind the knee, typically posterior and medial to the knee joint.[12,13] They are seen posterior to the medial femoral condyle between the tendons of the gastrocnemius and semimembranosus muscles. These cysts result from fluid collections in the gastrocnemius-semimem-branosus bursa, an extension of the knee joint, usually related to inflammation or irritation. Multiple conditions are associated with popliteal cysts, including arthritides such as degenerative joint disease and rheumatoid arthritis, trauma, infection, dialysis, and hemophilia.

As these cysts enlarge, they may dissect through the tissue planes and extend down into the calf musculature. They are also prone to spontaneous rupture. They can produce pain, tenderness, and swelling and mimic symptoms of DVT.

Popliteal cysts are usually discovered on ultrasound examinations performed to identify DVT. The classic Baker's cyst is seen along the posterior medial aspect of the joint, adjacent to the medial head of the gastrocnemius muscle. It usually demonstrates the typical characteristics of a simple cyst with no internal echoes, well-defined walls, and posterior sound enhancement (Figure 25-6, *A*). Rupture of the cyst is usually associated with irregular cyst margins, heterogeneous cyst contents or echogenic debris, and extension into the calf (Figure 25-6, *B*). Differential considerations include hematoma, abscess, tumor, and soft tissue edema. Unlike tumor, complex or ruptured popliteal cysts, abscesses, and hematoma demonstrate no internal blood flow on Doppler examination. A popliteal artery aneurysm may also be seen in this location. The aneurysm may be patent, or occluded and continuity with the popliteal or femoral artery should be easy to establish.

JOINT EFFUSION

Like popliteal cysts, joint effusion usually results from an inflammatory, infectious, or traumatic insult to the joint with distension of the joint capsule with fluid. The fluid may be simple or complex on ultrasound evaluation (Figure 25-7). Joint effusion is another cause of leg pain and swelling and can be diagnosed with ultrasound during an investigation for DVT. As indicated, ultrasound may also be used to sample or drain fluid from the joint for diagnostic or therapeutic reasons.[14]

INFECTION

Infectious processes in the soft tissues may be difficult to identify sonographically. Patient tenderness and erythema are clues to the underlying pathology. Skin thickening, edema, and swelling

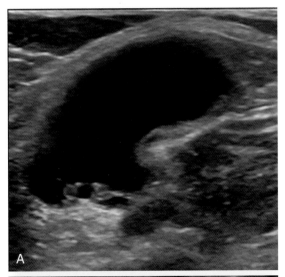
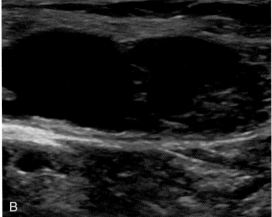

FIGURE 25-6 Baker's cyst. **A,** Longitudinal view of a simple Baker's cyst. **B,** Thickened septation is present in a complicated popliteal cyst, which may contain hemorrhage or fibrinoid material.

of the subcutaneous tissues may be identified during ultrasound examination. Cellulitis is a diffuse soft tissue inflammation of the skin and subcutaneous tissues usually caused by bacterial infection. This usually results from a break in the skin from trauma, surgery, or bite. Cellulitis is often a clinical diagnosis but often requires the exclusion of DVT from the differential diagnosis.

Abscesses are seen as well-circumscribed fluid collections within the soft tissues. An abscess demonstrates a well-defined peripheral wall and contains simple or complex fluid (Figure 25-8, *A*). Posterior sound enhancement is usually seen. Gas bubbles, seen as bright reflectors with posterior shadowing, may be identified within the collection (Figure 25-8, *B*). There may be increased vascularity in the wall of the abscess.

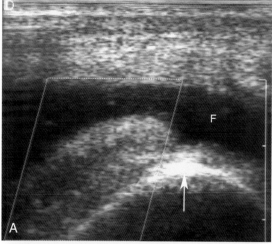

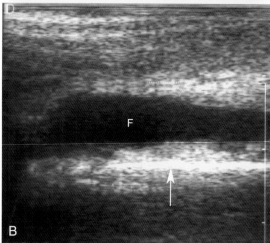

FIGURE 25-7 Knee joint effusion. Images obtained along the medial **(A)** and lateral **(B)** borders of the patella show joint fluid (F), which would not be visible in a normal knee. Note that the bony structure of the knee *(arrows)* is quite close to the fluid.

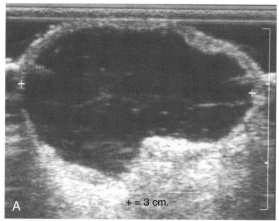

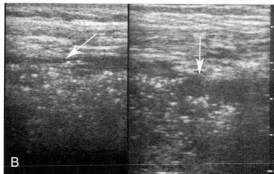

FIGURE 25-8 Various appearances of soft tissue abscesses. **A,** This is an incisional abscess that developed after arterial bypass graft. Note the thick, irregular walls and low-level internal echoes. Enhanced through-transmission of ultrasound is present, as the contents are watery and produce little attenuation. **B,** Composite image of an extensive, poorly defined medial arm abscess in a diabetic patient. This abscess is much different than that shown in **A.** The borders of the abscess are not visualized at all. The presence of infection is indicated only by heterogeneous material *(arrows)* containing myriad tiny air bubbles that produce tiny bright reflections. Enhanced through-transmission is absent due to the echogenic, attenuating nature of the abscess contents. Magnetic resonance imaging was needed to demonstrate the full extent of the abscess, which was not encapsulated.

The diagnosis is suggested by the typical sonographic appearance of the mass, tenderness on examination, and history of sepsis.

SOFT TISSUE TUMORS

Soft tissue tumors are unlikely causes of leg swelling and tenderness. Solid masses identified in the tissue must be distinguished from superficial or deep vein phlebitis. Large masses in the tissues may be benign or malignant. Benign soft tissue tumors include lipoma, fibroma, leiomyoma, desmoid tumor, neurofibromatosis, and hemangioma.[15-18] Lipomas are the most common benign lesions and are usually isoechoic or hyperechoic on ultrasound with scant internal vascularity. Soft tissue hemangiomas have a homogeneous or complex appearance with variable vascularity. Phleboliths may be present with acoustic shadowing. Most solid benign tumors are not specific on ultrasound and require further characterization with computed tomography (CT) or MRI. Malignant masses may be due to primary or metastatic disease. Primary tumors include sarcoma and lymphoma. These masses may be quite large and heterogeneous, requiring cross-sectional imaging with CT or MRI to determine the origin of the lesion and

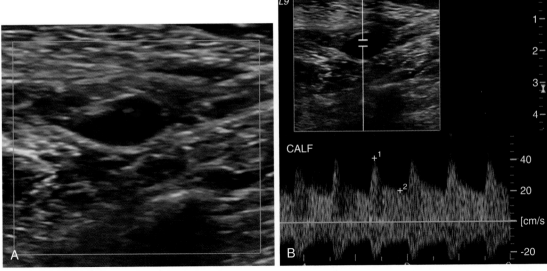

FIGURE 25-9 Soft tissue tumor. **A,** A solid hypoechoic mass is seen in the soft tissues of the calf. Color flow demonstrates internal vascularity within the lesion. This is a lung carcinoma metastasis. **B,** Pulsed Doppler demonstrates low-resistance arterial flow consistent with malignant vascularity.

the full extent of tumor invasion. Metastatic disease to the extremity is uncommon and may be related to lymphoma, leukemia, or other primary tumors. Malignant masses may have a solid or complex appearance, depending on the degree of necrosis (Figure 25-9). Color and pulsed Doppler demonstrates arterial flow within solid areas of the tumor with a high-velocity, low-resistance flow pattern. A review of the clinical history usually provides insight into this process.

REFERENCES

1. Borgstede JP, Clagett BS: Types, frequency and significance of alternative diagnoses found during duplex Doppler venous examination of the lower extremities, *J Ultrasound Med* 11:85–89, 1992.
2. Abu-Yousef MM, Kakish ME, Mufid M: Pulsatile venous Doppler flow in lower limbs: highly indicative of elevated right atrium pressure, *AJR Am J Roentgenol* 167:977–980, 1996.
3. Sheiman RG, Weintraub JL, McArdle CR: Bilateral lower extremity US in the patient with bilateral symptoms of deep venous thrombosis: assessment of need, *Radiology* 196:379–381, 1995.
4. Naidich JB, et al: Suspected Deep Venous Thrombosis: Is US of Both Legs Necessary? *Radiology* 200:429–431, 1996.
5. Drinman KJ, et al: Duplex imaging in lymphedema, *J Vasc Technol* 17:23–26, 1993.
6. Goldhaber SZ: Pulmonary embolism, *N Engl J Med* 339:93–104, 1998.
7. Weinman EE, Salzman EW: Deep-vein thrombosis, *N Engl J Med* 331:1630–1641, 1994.
8. Kim HJ, et al: Correlation between sonographic and pathologic findings in muscle injury: experimental study in the rabbit, *J Ultrasound Med* 21:1113–1119, 2002.
9. Ott G, et al: Lymphadenopathy: Differentiation of benign from malignant disease—color Doppler US assessment of intranodal angioarchitecture, *Radiology* 208:117–123, 1998.
10. Ying M, et al: Power Doppler sonography of normal cervical lymph nodes, *J Ultrasound Med* 19:511–517, 2000.
11. Tschammler A, et al: Pathological angioarchitecture in lymph nodes: Underlying histopathologic findings, *Ultrasound Med Biol* 26:1089–1097, 2000.
12. Ward EE, et al: Sonographic detection of Baker's cysts: comparison with MR imaging, *AJR Am J Roentgenol* 176:373–380, 2001.
13. Langsfeld M, et al: Baker's cysts mimicking the symptoms of deep vein thrombosis: diagnosis with venous duplex scanning, *J Vasc Surg* 25:658–662, 1997.
14. Fessell DP, et al: Using sonography to reveal and aspirate joint effusions, *AJR Am J Roentgenol* 174:1353–1362, 2000.
15. Inampudi P, et al: Soft-Tissue Lipomas: accuracy of Sonography in Diagnosis with Pathologic Correlation, *Radiology* 233:763–767, 2004.
16. Belli P, et al: Role of color Doppler sonography in the assessment of musculoskeletal soft tissue masses, *J Ultrasound Med* 19:823–830, 2000.
17. Needleman L, Nack TL: Vascular and nonvascular masses, *J Vasc Technol* 18:299–306, 1994.
18. Mitchell DG, et al: Superficial masses with color flow Doppler imaging, *J Clin Ultrasound* 19:555–560, 1991.

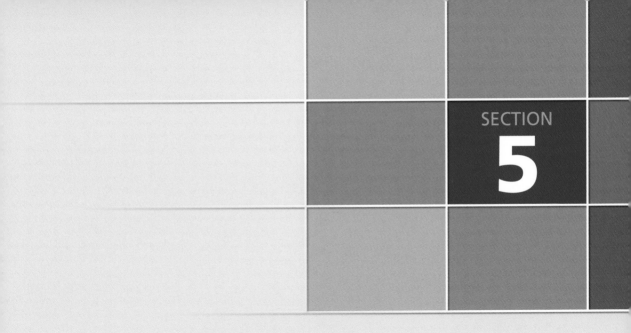

Abdomen and Pelvis

ANATOMY AND NORMAL DOPPLER SIGNATURES OF ABDOMINAL VESSELS

26

JOHN S. PELLERITO, MD, FACR, FSRU, FAIUM

Recognition of normal vascular anatomy is essential for any investigation into abdominal vascular problems. Doppler studies of the abdominal vessels demand an understanding of normal and abnormal blood flow patterns. The recognition of changes in abdominal blood flow allows accurate diagnosis of arterial and venous abnormalities, including stenosis, occlusion, and thrombosis. This chapter will review the normal flow patterns seen in abdominal arteries and veins that will be encountered in our Doppler examinations.

ABDOMINAL AORTA

It is important to recognize that all abdominal arterial branches identified during our Doppler studies receive blood supply via the abdominal aorta. The abdominal aorta leaves its vascular "imprint" on all its branches. Therefore, changes in aortic blood flow related to stenosis (high-velocity flow) or aneurysmal dilatation (low-velocity flow) will be transmitted to its branches. All of our examinations of the mesenteric and renal arteries always begin with an evaluation of the abdominal aorta for plaque, stenosis, aneurysm, dissection, or occlusion. Waveforms are obtained from the abdominal aorta at the level of the branch vessel of interest and compared to the vessel to assess for changes in flow. It is good practice to look at the aorta for all abdominal studies to detect aneurysm or significant atherosclerotic disease. The presence of significant atherosclerotic plaque in the abdominal aorta certainly increases your suspicion of underlying branch disease, particularly at the origin of the vessels.

Doppler waveforms obtained from the proximal abdominal aorta near the origins of the celiac and renal arteries usually have a low-resistance flow pattern, reflecting the need for continuous forward diastolic flow by the liver, spleen, and kidneys. Remember that, like the brain, the highly metabolic parenchymal organs of the abdomen (liver, spleen, kidneys) demand forward flow in systole and diastole (low-resistance flow). The arteries that feed these organs will generate waveforms that look like the internal carotid artery waveforms.

Waveforms obtained from the distal abdominal aorta near the iliac bifurcation usually have a higher-resistance flow pattern, reflecting the peripheral resistance of the lower extremity arteries. Waveforms obtained from the peripheral arteries demonstrate a triphasic character in the resting state with reversal of flow during diastole. This is due to branching into smaller arteries and capillary beds. The average velocity range for the abdominal aorta is 60 to 100 cm/sec.

CELIAC ARTERY

The celiac artery, also called the *celiac trunk* or *celiac axis*, is the first major visceral branch of the abdominal aorta. It arises from the anterior aortic surface, between the diaphragmatic crura (Figure 26-1). It then bifurcates about 1 to 3 cm from its origin into the common hepatic and splenic arteries, which are readily visualized with ultrasound. The celiac artery also gives rise to the left gastric artery, which is generally not visible sonographically. The branching pattern of the celiac artery is quite constant, occurring in approximately 93% of individuals. In the most common variations, one or more of the celiac branches arises separately from the aorta or from the superior mesenteric artery (SMA). In less than 1% of individuals, the celiac artery and the SMA arise from the aorta as a common trunk. In such cases, the common trunk splits into the celiac artery and the SMA within 1 or 2 cm from the aorta.[1,2]

Ultrasound examination of the celiac artery usually begins with a transverse sweep of the proximal abdominal aorta. The transverse approach allows visualization of the bifurcation of the

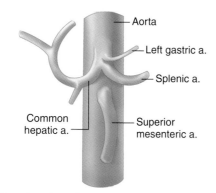

FIGURE 26-1 The celiac artery and its branches. a., artery.

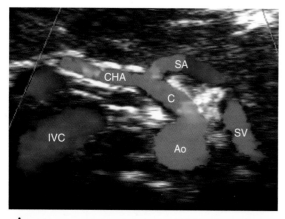

A

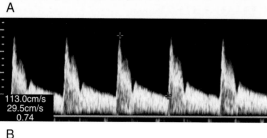

B

FIGURE 26-2 Celiac artery. **A,** Transverse sonogram of the celiac axis (C) as it divides into the common hepatic artery (CHA) and splenic artery (SA). Ao, aorta; IVC, inferior vena cava; SV, a segment of the splenic vein. **B,** Normal, low-resistance Doppler signal in the celiac artery. Peak systolic velocity is 113 cm/sec, and end-diastolic velocity is 30 cm/sec.

hepatic and splenic branches, usually resembling a T or "seagull" (Figure 26-2, *A*). The longitudinal approach is preferred for evaluation of the celiac artery origin. We also utilize the longitudinal view for Doppler interrogation of the celiac artery. Consistent angle correction of greater than or equal to 60 degrees is obtained in this projection. This view also permits evaluation of the SMA, which is found just inferior to the celiac artery.

The characteristic Doppler waveform is a low-resistance arterial waveform (Figure 26-2, *B*). As mentioned above, continuous forward flow throughout diastole is required for adequate perfusion of the liver and spleen. The hepatic and splenic branches will also demonstrate the low-resistance pattern.[3]

The mesenteric circulation is notable for extensive arterial anastomoses and rich collateral network. This network allows for continuous circulation to the splanchnic vessels in the event of stenosis or occlusion of mesenteric branches, avoiding significant ischemic insult. With occlusion of the celiac artery, there is collateralization through the pancreaticoduodenal arterial arcade, a network of small vessels surrounding the pancreas and duodenum. These vessels enlarge and feed into the gastroduodenal artery. When the celiac is occluded, there is retrograde flow through the gastroduodenal artery to supply blood to the common hepatic artery. Thus, blood supply to the liver and spleen can be maintained.[4]

SPLENIC ARTERY

The splenic artery (limb of the celiac T toward patient's left) follows a tortuous course along the posterosuperior margin of the pancreatic body and tail (Figure 26-3, *A*) and terminates by splitting into a number of branches in the hilum of the spleen. Along the way, the splenic artery gives rise to several pancreatic branches, short gastric branches, and the left gastroepiploic artery. These vessels are usually not seen with ultrasound. Transverse scans from a midline approach usually reveal the proximal portion of the splenic artery (see Figure 26-2, *A*). The distal portion of the splenic artery is best seen through the splenic hilum from a left lateral approach. Because of the tortuous course of the splenic artery, flow in this vessel is typically turbulent, (Figure 26-3, *B*).

HEPATIC ARTERY

The common hepatic artery (Figure 26-4) is the limb of the celiac T that heads toward the patient's right. After running a short distance along the superior border of the pancreatic head, the common hepatic artery gives rise to the gastroduodenal artery, which can often be seen with ultrasound at the anterosuperior border of the pancreatic head. Beyond the gastroduodenal artery origin, the *common* hepatic artery becomes

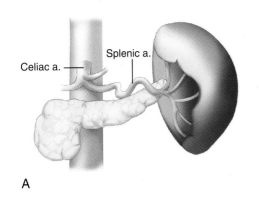

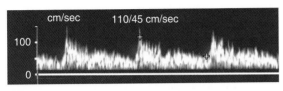

FIGURE 26-3 A, Splenic artery anatomy. a., artery. **B,** Normal, low-pulsatility Doppler signal from the splenic artery. Peak systolic velocity is 110 cm/sec, and end-diastolic velocity is 45 cm/sec.

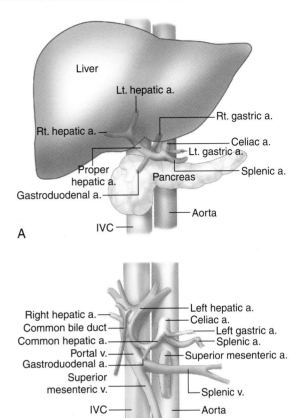

FIGURE 26-4 A, The hepatic artery and its branches. **B,** Anatomic relationships among the hepatic artery, the portal vein, and the extrahepatic bile ducts. a., artery; IVC, inferior vena cava; Lt., left; Rt., right; v., vein.

the *proper* hepatic artery, which follows the portal vein to the porta hepatis. At this point, it divides into the left and right hepatic arteries, which penetrate into the hepatic substance. The anatomic relationships among the hepatic artery, the portal vein, and the extrahepatic bile ducts are shown in Figure 26-4, *B*.

The classic hepatic artery configuration just described is seen in 72% of individuals.[5] A number of alternative patterns may occur, the most noteworthy of which are the following: (1) the common (4%) or right (11%) hepatic artery may arise from the SMA, and (2) the left hepatic artery may arise from a shared trunk with the left gastric artery (10%).[2]

The hepatic arteries are usually well visualized sonographically from an anterior abdominal approach. The common hepatic artery is most easily identified at its origin from the celiac artery (see Figure 26-2, *A*). The proper hepatic artery is seen on ultrasound images near the porta hepatis, anterior to the portal vein, in short- or long-axis views, as can be seen in Figure 26-5. The right and left hepatic artery branches can be followed into the substance of the liver to a variable distance from the porta hepatis. As noted previously, the hepatic arterial system has low-resistance flow characteristics, with continuous forward flow throughout diastole. It is interesting to note that

blood flow in the proper hepatic artery and portal vein are both hepatopetal, delivering blood flow toward the liver.

SUPERIOR AND INFERIOR MESENTERIC ARTERIES

The SMA arises from the anterior surface of the aorta, immediately distal to the origin of the celiac artery (Figure 26-6). The SMA generally consists of a short, anteriorly directed segment and a much longer inferiorly directed segment that ends in the vicinity of the ileocecal valve. SMA branches supply the jejunum, ileum, cecum, and ascending colon, as well as the proximal two-thirds of the transverse colon and portions of the duodenum and pancreatic head. As noted previously, the SMA may also give rise to an aberrant right hepatic artery (11%) or common hepatic artery (4%).[1] The SMA communicates with the celiac artery via the pancreaticoduodenal arcade.

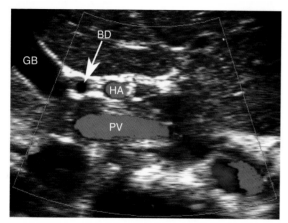

FIGURE 26-5 Ultrasonography of the hepatic artery. At the porta hepatis, the hepatic artery (HA) can be differentiated from the bile duct (BD), because blood flow is present in the former and not in the latter. Blood flow is also seen in the portal vein (PV). GB, gallbladder.

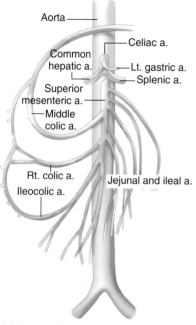

FIGURE 26-6 Superior mesenteric artery anatomy. a., artery; Lt., left; Rt., right.

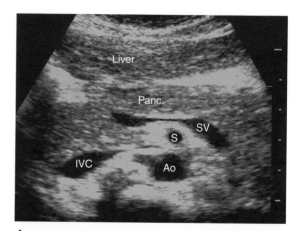

A

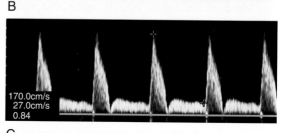

B

C

D

FIGURE 26-7 Ultrasound of the superior mesenteric artery (SMA). **A,** Anatomic relationships of the SMA (S). Note that the SMA is surrounded by a distinctive layer of echogenic fat. The pancreas (Panc.) is anterior to the SMA. The aorta (Ao) is posterior to the SMA. IVC, inferior vena cava; SV, splenic vein. **B,** A long-axis view shows the origin of the celiac artery and the SMA from the aorta (Ao). **C,** Normal, high-resistance Doppler signal in the SMA of a fasting patient. **D,** Normal high-resistance fasting waveform in the inferior mesenteric artery.

The SMA is easily identified on longitudinal or transverse ultrasound images (Figure 26-7). The SMA serves as an important landmark for identifying upper abdominal structures that are well seen on transverse ultrasound images. The SMA lies to the right of the superior mesenteric vein. The pancreas and the splenic vein lie anterior to the SMA. In contrast, the left renal vein (discussed later) lies posterior to the SMA (between the SMA and the aorta). These anatomic features are very distinctive, making the SMA an excellent point of orientation for abdominal scanning.

The inferior mesenteric artery (IMA) arises from the abdominal aorta below the renal arteries, above the iliac bifurcation. It originates at the left anterolateral aspect of the aorta and proceeds inferiorly and to the left. The IMA provides blood supply to the distal colon and proximal rectum. There are multiple collateral circuits between the SMA and the IMA, including the arc of Riolan and the marginal artery of Drummond.

The IMA is seen in the majority of patients studied for mesenteric vascular integrity. The best approach is a transverse view, sliding down the abdominal aorta below the renal arteries. The IMA is visualized arising from the anterolateral aorta on the left.

SMA and IMA blood flow is best evaluated with longitudinal ultrasound images, because a lengthy segment of the vessel is visualized from a single perspective. Doppler waveforms are usually obtained from this longitudinal view at the level of the origin and proximal segments.

The SMA and IMA Doppler waveforms show mild turbulence near the arterial origin; however, as one moves distally, flow becomes more uniform. In a fasting patient, a high-resistance flow pattern is seen in the SMA and IMA (see Figure 26-7, *C* and *D*), with sharp systolic peaks and little diastolic flow. Within 30 to 90 minutes after eating, however, the SMA and IMA waveforms may assume a low-resistance pattern, with broad systolic peaks and continuous diastolic flow.[3]

PORTAL VENOUS SYSTEM

The portal venous system transports blood from the bowel and spleen to the liver. The portal vein (Figure 26-8) originates at the junction of the splenic and superior mesenteric veins, which converge immediately posterior to the pancreatic neck. The portal vein courses obliquely toward the right to terminate at the porta hepatis, where it divides into right and left portal branches. Each branch enters the corresponding lobe of the liver.

The splenic vein lies immediately posterior to the pancreas and follows a straight course (unlike the tortuous splenic artery) to the hilum of the spleen. The body and tail of the pancreas are seen anterior to the splenic vein; hence, the pancreas is a good landmark for finding the splenic vein.

The superior mesenteric vein proceeds inferiorly from the portal vein junction and parallels

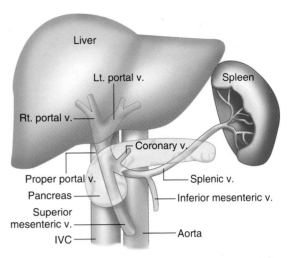

FIGURE 26-8 Portal venous system anatomy. IVC, inferior vena cava; Lt., left; Rt., right; v, vein.

the course of the SMA, which lies to its left. The superior mesenteric vein is best seen with ultrasound in longitudinal views.

Other tributaries of the portal venous system include the coronary vein and the inferior mesenteric vein, which are illustrated in Figure 26-8. The inferior mesenteric vein empties into the splenic vein in 38% of individuals. Alternatively, it may terminate at the splenic–superior mesenteric vein junction (32%) or into the superior mesenteric vein itself (25%).[2] The coronary vein runs along the posterior aspect of the stomach toward the gastroesophageal junction. This vein usually enters the superior aspect of the portal vein near the portosplenic junction,[2] where it can be seen with ultrasound. The coronary vein may enlarge and shunt blood from the portal to the systemic circulation in cases of portal hypertension (see Chapter 30).

Doppler assessment of portal vein flow is usually conducted along the long axis of the portal vein, as shown in Figure 26-9. Flow in the portal vein and its tributaries is normally *toward* the liver (hepatopetal). Portal vein Doppler waveforms exhibit subtle phasic variations caused by respiration-related changes in pressure and cardiac contractility. The phasic pattern generates a "windstorm" sound in the audible Doppler signal, which is quite distinct from the pulsatile sound of the hepatic artery and other arterial branches. Flow is unidirectional toward the liver and similar in appearance to the lower extremity veins. With right heart failure and fluid overload, right atrial pulsations may be transmitted

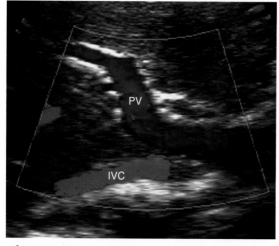

A

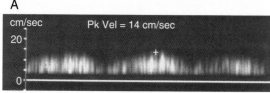

B

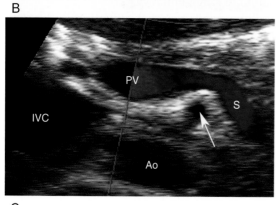

C

FIGURE 26-9 Ultrasound of the portal vein and its tributaries. **A,** Long-axis view of the portal vein (PV). IVC, inferior vena cava. **B,** Normal phasic Doppler spectrum in the portal vein. Peak velocity (Pk Vel) is 14 cm/sec. **C,** The splenic vein (S) is seen at its junction with the portal vein (PV). Arrow represents the superior mesenteric artery. Ao, aorta; IVC, inferior vena cava.

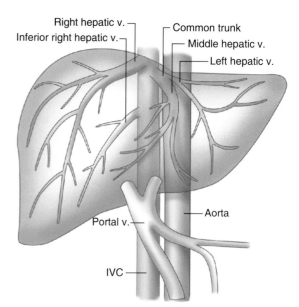

FIGURE 26-10 Hepatic vein anatomy. IVC, inferior vena cava; v, vein.

veins, which normally increase 50% to 100% in diameter from quiet respiration to deep inspiration.[7,8] With portal hypertension, the portal vein may dilate and respiratory variation in the portal and splenic/superior mesenteric veins may be obliterated.

HEPATIC VEINS

There are three major hepatic veins (Figure 26-10), which converge on the inferior vena cava (IVC) at the diaphragm. The right hepatic vein runs in a coronal plane between the anterior and posterior segments of the right hepatic lobe. The middle hepatic vein lies between the right and left hepatic lobes and may be seen prominently on sagittal or parasagittal images of the liver. The left hepatic vein runs between the medial and lateral segments of the left hepatic lobe. In 96% of individuals, the middle and left hepatic veins join to form a common trunk before entering the IVC.[9] The caudate lobe has its own venous drainage, directly into the IVC. The hepatic veins and other anatomic structures are important landmarks that define hepatic lobar anatomy, as listed in Table 26-1 and illustrated in Figure 26-11.

The left hepatic vein frequently is duplicated, and a number of other variations of hepatic vein anatomy may occur.[9] Accessory hepatic veins, which enter the IVC in locations other than at the diaphragm (see Figure 26-10), occur commonly, although they are rarely identified

through the liver to the portal vein, which then exhibits pulsatile Doppler waveforms. These waveforms may be bidirectional and appear "arterialized," but they do not follow cardiac systole.

The normal portal vein measures up to 13 mm in diameter during quiet respiration in a supine patient.[6] The caliber of the portal vein and its tributaries normally increases substantially during sustained deep inspiration. This is best seen in the splenic and superior mesenteric

TABLE 26-1 Structures Defining Hepatic Lobar Anatomy

Structure	Location
Right hepatic vein	Separates anterior and posterior segments, right lobe
Middle hepatic vein	Separates right and left lobes
Gallbladder fossa	Separates right and left lobes
Ascending branch, left portal vein	Separates lateral and medial segments, left lobe
Falciform ligament	Separates lateral and medial segments, left lobe

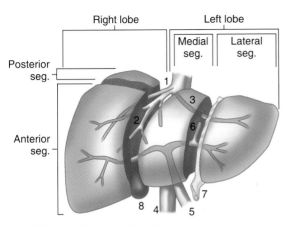

1. Right hepatic v.
2. Middle hepatic v.
3. Left hepatic v.
4. Inferior vena cava
5. Portal v.
6. Ascending left portal v.
7. Falciform lig.
8. Gallbladder

FIGURE 26-11 Anatomic landmarks that define the major hepatic lobes and segments (seg). lig., ligament; v., vein.

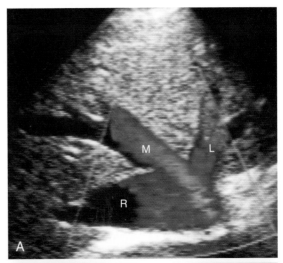

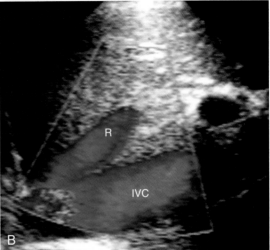

FIGURE 26-12 Hepatic vein sonography. **A,** Transverse view of the three main hepatic vein trunks as they enter the inferior vena cava. L, left hepatic vein; M, middle hepatic vein; R, right hepatic vein. **B,** Coronal view showing the right hepatic vein (R) at its junction with the inferior vena cava (IVC).

sonographically.[10] Occasionally, one of the three major hepatic veins is absent, typically, the right hepatic vein (6%), or less commonly, the middle or left hepatic veins.

The hepatic veins are best visualized with ultrasound using a transverse subxiphoid approach, which yields an image of the three main hepatic trunks converging on the IVC, such as is seen in Figure 26-12, A. From this perspective, however, blood flow often cannot be visualized in the right hepatic vein with color Doppler, because the axis of this vein is perpendicular to the ultrasound beam. The right hepatic vein is seen to better advantage using a longitudinal scan plane and an intercostal transducer position (Figure 26-12, B).

Pulsed Doppler waveforms obtained from the hepatic veins differ from those of the portal veins. The hepatic veins demonstrate a pulsatile flow pattern with a W configuration. This pattern demonstrates blood flow that is predominately away from the liver toward the heart (hepatofugal). The pulsatility is related to atrial contraction and reversal of blood flow back toward the liver (Figure 26-13).

Hepatic veins may be differentiated from portal veins by the following sonographic features:
1. Course: Hepatic veins are more or less longitudinally oriented, whereas portal veins run in transverse planes.
2. Convergence: The hepatic veins converge on the IVC at the diaphragm, whereas the portal veins converge on the porta hepatis.

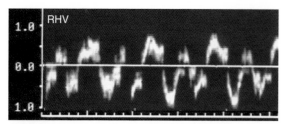

FIGURE 26-13 Normal hepatic vein Doppler signals. Note that these pulsatile signals are quite different from normal portal vein Doppler signals.

3. Changes in size: The hepatic veins enlarge progressively toward the diaphragm, whereas the portal veins become larger as they approach the porta hepatis.
4. Margins: Hepatic veins have "naked" margins, whereas the portal veins are surrounded by a heavy sheath of echogenic fibrous tissue.
5. Waveform pattern: Hepatic vein Doppler signals are pulsatile and bidirectional, whereas portal vein waveforms are monophasic and unidirectional.

INFERIOR VENA CAVA

The normal IVC is situated anterior to the spine and to the right of the aorta. The IVC begins at the junction of the common iliac veins and terminates in the right atrium (Figure 26-14). The upper abdominal portion of the IVC is easily visualized sonographically,[11-13] using the liver as an acoustic window (see Chapter 30). The inferior portion of the IVC may also be visualized, depending on the body habitus of the patient and the amount of overlying bowel gas. The size of the IVC varies markedly with respiration and throughout the cardiac cycle, but the IVC seldom exceeds 2.5 cm in diameter.[13] Deep inspiration limits venous return to the chest, markedly dilating the IVC. Expiration has the opposite effect. The IVC diameter is also dependent on patient size and right atrial pressure. The IVC and the hepatic veins become enlarged with fluid overload and heart failure.

Doppler flow signals in the IVC are pulsatile near the heart because of reflected right atrial pulsations with reversal of flow during atrial systole. The pattern is similar to the hepatic veins with the characteristic W appearance (see description of hepatic vein flow earlier). The flow pattern becomes less phasic near the iliac vein bifurcation and is similar to the pattern seen in extremity veins.

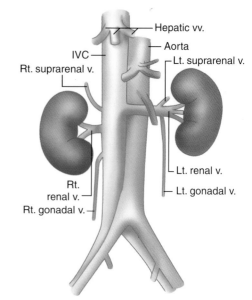

FIGURE 26-14 The inferior vena cava (IVC) and its tributaries. Lt., left; Rt., right; v, vein; vv., veins.

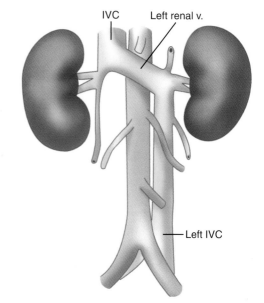

FIGURE 26-15 Anomalous, left-sided inferior vena cava (IVC). v., vein.

Most anomalies of the IVC occur at and below the level of the renal veins.[10] Of these, the most common are duplication (0.2%-3.0%) and transposition (0.2%-0.5%). In both of these anomalies, the left-sided IVC usually joins the left renal vein and crosses over to join the normal right-sided IVC (Figure 26-15). Interruption of the IVC with azygos or hemiazygos continuation (0.6%) results from failure of the intrahepatic segment of the IVC to form. Flow is diverted to the heart

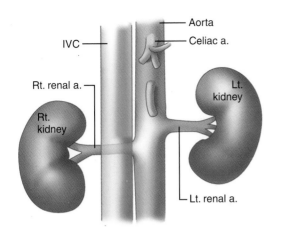

FIGURE 26-16 Renal artery anatomy. a., artery; Lt., left; Rt., right; IVC, inferior vena cava.

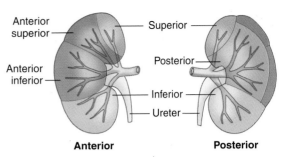

FIGURE 26-17 Distal arborization of the renal arteries.

via the azygos and hemiazygos veins, and the hepatic veins drain directly into the right atrium.

RENAL ARTERIES

The renal arteries (Figure 26-16) arise from the aorta, slightly below the origin of the SMA. The origin of the right renal artery is usually slightly superior to the left, but this relationship is not constant. The right renal artery arises from the anterolateral aspect of the aorta and then passes *posterior* to the IVC as it courses toward the right renal hilum. The left renal artery arises from the lateral or posterolateral aspect of the aorta and follows a posterolateral course to the left renal hilum.

Almost one-third of kidneys are supplied by two or more arteries arising from the aorta.[14] In some cases, the main renal artery is duplicated. In other instances, small accessory renal arteries arise from the aorta superior or inferior to the main renal artery and may enter the kidneys either at the renal hilum or at the poles of the kidney. Extrahilar duplicated or accessory renal arteries also may arise from the ipsilateral renal artery, the ipsilateral iliac artery, the aorta, or, occasionally, from other arteries in the retroperitoneum.

The branching pattern of the renal arteries is illustrated in Figure 26-17. The renal arteries typically divide into anterior and posterior divisions that lie, respectively, anterior and posterior to the renal pelvis. The anterior division branches into four segmental arteries, whereas the posterior division supplies only a single renal segment. The segmental arteries branch farther within the

renal sinus, forming interlobar arteries that penetrate the renal parenchyma. These terminate in arcuate arteries that curve around the corticomedullary junction, giving rise to cortical or interlobular branches.[14]

During Doppler examination, the renal artery origins (Figure 26-18, *A* to *C*) are usually visualized by scanning either transversely from a midline anterior approach or in the coronal plane in the decubitus position, depending on body habitus and degree of bowel gas. In the decubitus position with a posterolateral transducer approach, the kidney is used as an acoustic window to visualize the renal artery. This is the approach preferred by my sonographers as the window is almost universally available and the renal artery may be seen in its entirety on this single view, as noted on Figure 26-18. In many cases, a combination of both approaches allows complete visualization of the renal arteries.

Renal artery Doppler signals have a low-resistance flow pattern with a rapid systolic upstroke, as seen in Figure 26-18, *D*. Continuous forward flow is present in diastole because of low resistance in the renal vascular bed. This flow pattern is evident at all locations in the renal arteries, including the intrarenal branches.[5]

RENAL VEINS

Each renal vein is formed from tributaries that coalesce in the renal hilum. As illustrated in Figure 26-14, the left renal vein usually receives the left suprarenal (adrenal) vein from above and the left gonadal (ovarian or testicular) vein from below. The left renal vein then passes anterior to the aorta and posterior to the SMA, to enter the left side of the IVC. The right renal vein, which is shorter than the left renal vein, extends directly to the IVC from the right renal hilum and usually receives no tributaries.

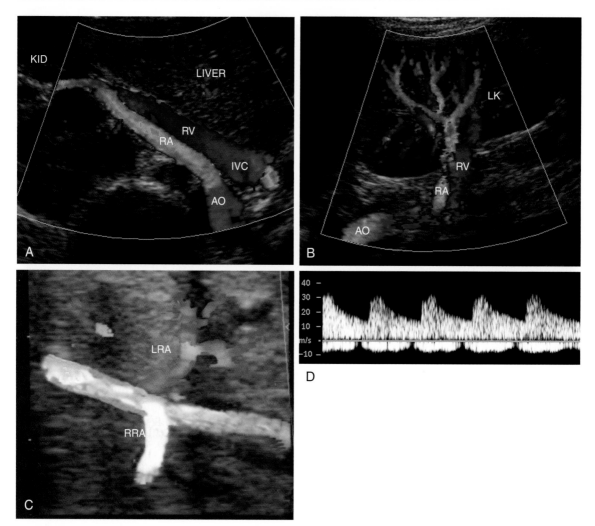

FIGURE 26-18 Sonographic appearance of the renal arteries and veins. **A,** Transverse image of the right renal artery (RA) and right renal vein (RV). Note that the artery lies posterior to the inferior vena cava (IVC) and the renal vein. AO, aorta; KID, right kidney. **B,** Coronal decubitus view of the left renal artery (RA) and the left renal vein (RV). AO, aorta, LK, left kidney. **C,** Coronal view of the left (LRA) and right (RRA) renal arteries in a premature infant (head to left). **D,** Pulsed Doppler demonstrates normal, low-pulsatility renal artery waveforms above the baseline and normal phasic renal vein waveforms below the baseline.

The left renal vein may be circumaortic (1.5%-8.7%), with separate veins passing anterior and posterior to the aorta. The left renal vein may also be retroaortic in location (1.8%-2.4%), with a single branch passing posterior to the aorta, rather than anterior. Accessory renal veins are commonly present on the right side, draining directly into the IVC.[11,14]

The renal veins are visualized with ultrasound (see Figure 26-18, *A* and *B*) on transverse scans from an anterior approach and coronally from a posterolateral approach. Sonographers should be mindful that the left renal vein crosses the midline *between* the aorta and the SMA. This differentiates

the left renal vein and the nearby splenic vein, which lies anterior to the SMA. Doppler signals in the renal veins (see Figure 26-18, *D*) show phasic flow variations. Transmitted cardiac pulsations may be evident in the renal veins near the IVC.

REFERENCES

1. Ruzika FF Jr, Rossi P: Normal vascular anatomy of the abdominal viscera, *Radiol Clin North Am* 8:3–29, 1970.
2. Michels NA: *Blood Supply and Anatomy of the Upper Abdominal Organs*, Philadelphia, 1955, JB Lippincott.
3. Lewis BD, James EM: Current applications of duplex and color Doppler ultrasound imaging: abdomen, *Mayo Clin Proc* 64:1158–1169, 1989.

4. Geelkerken RH, et al: Pitfalls in the diagnosis of origin stenosis of the coeliac and superior mesenteric arteries with transabdominal color duplex instrumentation, *Ultrasound Med Biol* 22:695–700, 1996.

5. Taylor KJW, et al: Blood flow in deep abdominal and pelvic vessels: ultrasonic pulsed Doppler analysis, *Radiology* 154:487–493, 1985.

6. Weinreb J, et al: Portal vein measurements by real-time sonography, *AJR Am J Roentgenol* 139:497–499, 1982.

7. Bolondi L, et al: Ultrasonography in the diagnosis of portal hypertension: diminished response of the portal vessels to respiration, *Radiology* 142:167–172, 1982.

8. Bellamy EA, Bossi MC, Cosgrove DO: Ultrasound demonstration of changes in the normal portal venous system following a meal, *Br J Radiol* 57:147–149, 1984.

9. Cosgrove DO, Arger PH, Coleman BG: Ultrasonic anatomy of hepatic veins, *J Clin Ultrasound* 15:231–235, 1987.

10. Makuuchi M, et al: The inferior right hepatic vein: Ultrasonic demonstration, *Radiology* 148:213–217, 1983.

11. Kellman GH, et al: Computed tomography of vena caval anomalies with embryologic correlation, *Radiographics* 8:533–556, 1988.

12. Needleman L, Rifkin MD: Vascular ultrasonography: Abdominal applications, *Radiol Clin North Am* 24:461–484, 1986.

13. Mintz GS, et al: Real-time inferior vena caval ultrasonography: normal and abnormal findings and its use in assessing right-heart function, *Circulation* 64:1018–1024, 1981.

14. Hollinshead WH: *Textbook of Anatomy*, ed 3, Hagerstown, MD, 1974, Harper & Row, pp 649-650.

ULTRASOUND ASSESSMENT OF THE ABDOMINAL AORTA

JOSEPH F. POLAK, MD, MPH

The abdominal aorta is the major conduit artery distributing blood to the abdominal organs and then to the lower extremities. Pathologic processes that can affect it are, in order of incidence rates, atherosclerosis, abdominal aortic aneurysm formation, various vasculitides, genetically based degenerative disease of the aortic wall, and the extension of proximal dissections of the aorta.

ANATOMY

The abdominal aorta extends from the level of the diaphragm to the iliac artery bifurcation. It is an elastic artery in which elastin and collagen provide mechanical strength. Alterations in collagen levels, due to exposure to the stresses of the pulse pressure over time (cystic medial degeneration) or because of an inherent congenital defect in the quality of the collagen (Marfan's or Ehlers-Danlos syndromes), cause the media to be susceptible to dissection. Blood supply to the artery wall is a dual one because the small arterioles (vasa vasorum) in the adventitia and the arterial lumen are the source of oxygen to the deeper layers of the wall. A region of relatively poor perfusion, at the junction of the middle and external third of the media, causes cystic medial degeneration to develop. The abdominal aortic wall is less prone to cystic medial degeneration (necrosis) than the thoracic aorta. Cystic medial degeneration predisposes to aortic wall dissection and development of intramural hematoma in the media.

The major branches of the aorta include the celiac axis, the superior mesenteric artery, the renal arteries, the inferior mesenteric artery, and the lumbar arteries.

The celiac axis has an anterior origin, most often near the midline at approximately the level of the twelfth thoracic vertebral body and the first lumbar vertebral artery. The superior mesenteric artery originates at approximately the level of the first and second lumbar vertebral bodies and slightly to the left. The renal arteries have their origins just inferior to the superior mesenteric artery and are located to the side of the aorta. The inferior mesenteric artery has its origin just above the level of the aortic bifurcation and oriented slightly to the left of the midline. The lumbar arteries are located on both sides, on the posterior aspect of the aorta. There are normally four pairs of lumbar branches, the lower one possibly arising from iliac artery branches.

NORMAL SIZES

The abdominal aorta gradually tapers as it courses through the abdomen. The average diameter of the aorta is smaller in women than in men. Normal values vary with age, progressively increasing from childhood into adulthood. By adulthood, the average diameter of the abdominal aorta is approximately 27 mm at the diaphragm, tapering to approximately 21 mm at the iliac bifurcation.[1] For women, diameters are smaller by approximately 3 to 5 mm.

NORMAL DOPPLER VELOCITY PROFILES

Peak systolic velocities in the abdominal aorta average 110 cm/sec in the population with an average age of 12 years.[2] With aging, the average velocity decreases, ranging from 70 to 100 cm/sec. Proximally, the waveforms are triphasic but with noticeable forward blood flow during diastole (Figure 27-1, A). This diastolic component is a reflection of the low impedance of vascular beds located slightly lower in the abdominal aorta: the liver, the spleen, and the kidneys. These organs have low-resistance blood flow patterns, in essence monophasic. Below the renal arteries, the aortic Doppler tracings will show a typical "peripheral" waveform (Figure 27-1, B) with a relative decrease in forward diastolic blood flow and

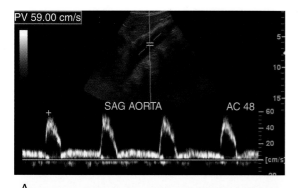

A

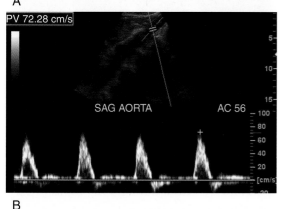

B

FIGURE 27-1 A, Proximal abdominal aortic waveform showing a low-resistance component during diastole. **B,** More distal aortic Doppler waveform showing a typical "peripheral" triphasic waveform.

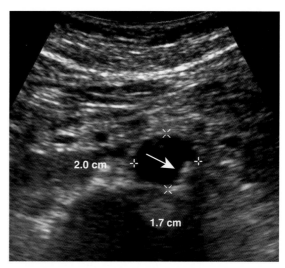

FIGURE 27-2 Plaque formation in the posterolateral aortic *(arrow)* wall of a 55-year-old adult.

more prominent flow reversal in early diastole. In summary, the aortic blood flow profiles are triphasic[3] and the diastolic component decreases with distance from the diaphragm. Blood flow patterns through the abdominal aorta will therefore be affected, to a certain extent, by the state of the renal arteries and of the celiac axis. There have not been any systematic studies of the variations of adult abdominal Doppler tracings linked to pathologic changes in these organs. For example, no specific studies have looked at the Doppler aortic waveforms in the presence of chronic renal failure.

PATHOLOGIC STATES

ATHEROSCLEROSIS AND OCCLUSIVE ARTERIAL DISEASE

The atherosclerotic process affects the aortic wall relatively early in life and is prevalent by the late 50s in men (Figure 27-2) and later, by approximately 10 years, in women. Most autopsy studies of the distribution of arterial disease show that the abdominal aorta is one of the first affected vessels with the thoracic aorta possibly showing some of the earliest changes.[4,5] Isolated high-grade stenoses and full occlusions of the abdominal aorta are uncommon in the spectrum of peripheral arterial disease.[6,7] Isolated aortic lesions that become symptomatic can be seen in younger patients (less than 55 years) and more often in women. Clinically, the development of high-grade lesions tends to be slow and progressive with the concurrent development of collateral blood flow channels. Acute aortic occlusions can occur very rapidly and compromise blood supply to the lower extremities and even the mesenteric and renal arteries. More commonly, progressive aortic occlusive narrowing is accompanied by slowly increasing lower extremity symptoms. Symptoms can be very restrictive, and the patients adapt by decreasing the distances and frequency over which they walk, progressing to rest pain and then impotence in men; the syndrome is referred to as Leriche's syndrome. Full occlusions of the abdominal aorta tend to occur in the lower portion of the aorta with thrombus spreading upward (cephalad). Normally the occlusive process and the associated thrombus formation will extend to the level of the renal arteries. The renal arteries tend to stay patent and rarely occlude. The superior mesenteric artery is rarely affected and serves as a source of collateral blood flow to the lower extremities via colonic collaterals to the inferior mesenteric artery branches and then into the internal iliac arteries.

Doppler imaging at the level of the common femoral arteries can suggest the diagnosis of either

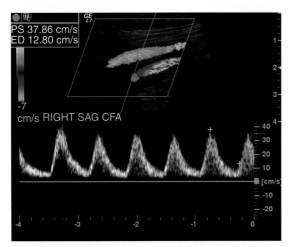

FIGURE 27-3 Doppler waveform obtained distal to a proximal aortoiliac occlusion. Note the tardus-parvus waveform and low peak systolic velocity. CFA, common femoral artery.

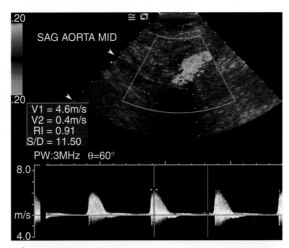

A

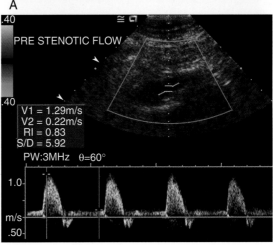

B

FIGURE 27-4 A, Doppler velocity waveform obtained at site of a midaortic stenosis. The peak systolic velocity is markedly elevated at 460 cm/sec. **B,** Doppler velocities obtained just above the site of velocity elevation. Comparing the stenotic peak of 460 cm/sec to 129 cm/sec gives a ratio of 3.6, corresponding to a stenosis in the 50% to 75% diameter stenosis range.

occlusion or severe stenosis of the abdominal aorta (Figure 27-3). This indirect approach will of course fail to fully document the extent of aortic involvement. Doppler tracings will typically show a monophasic pattern common to any severe proximal arterial occlusion with peak velocities of 45 cm/sec or less.[8-10] With acute occlusions, the relative magnitude of the diastolic velocities compared to the systolic velocities may not be as well developed. The monophasic waveform and the extent of diastolic flow reflect the ability of the peripheral circulation to recruit collateral blood flow and to vasodilate.

Doppler ultrasound can be used to confirm the diagnosis of an aortic occlusion by verifying the absence of blood flow in the involved aortic segment. No large series has evaluated the accuracy of this approach. Grading of stenosis severity in the aorta by Doppler criteria has also not been extensively studied because of the rarity of isolated aortic stenoses and occlusions. Implicitly, the diagnostic criteria used to grade stenosis severity are adapted from the criteria used for the lower extremity arteries, and a peak systolic velocity ratio is used (Figure 27-4). As discussed in Chapter 17, the Doppler peak systolic velocity ratio is determined by performing a Doppler velocity measurement at the site of maximal blood flow velocity and then dividing this peak systolic velocity by a " normal" aortic peak systolic velocity. This "normal" value is measured in a contiguous segment of the aorta located above the site of stenosis. In cases of diffuse disease or absence

of a good acoustic window, distal peak systolic velocities can be used to calculate this ratio when "disturbed flow" seen distal to a stenosis becomes normal again. As in the lower extremity, a velocity ratio of 2 or greater is used to indicate the presence of a 50% or greater diameter stenosis.[11]

ABDOMINAL AORTIC ANEURYSM

TYPES OF ANEURYSMS

A general overview of aneurysm disease is shown in Figure 27-5. A summary of the different types of abdominal aortic aneurysms is shown in

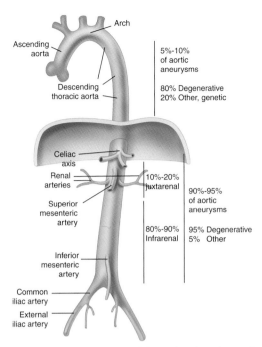

FIGURE 27-5 Diagram summarizing the location of aneurysms. Most aneurysms are infrarenal.

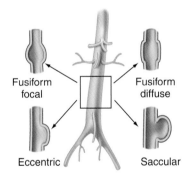

FIGURE 27-6 Diagram summarizing the types of aortic aneurysms: fusiform, eccentric, and saccular. Eccentric aneurysms are a form of fusiform aneurysms because all three layers of the arterial wall are intact.

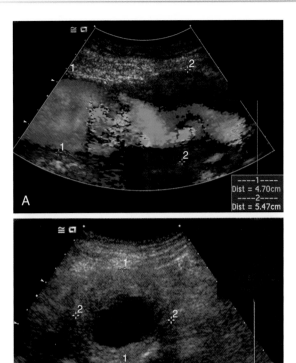

FIGURE 27-7 **A,** This long fusiform aneurysm has a proximal component without thrombus (left of image) and a distal component with mural thrombus (right of image). **B,** Transverse view at the level of the distal component shows the symmetric deposition of mural thrombus.

Figure 27-6. It is generally accepted that there are two types of aneurysms: fusiform (Figure 27-7; see Videos 27-1 and 27-2) and saccular (Figure 27-8). By far, the most common form of aneurysm is the fusiform type. Fusiform describes a concentric enlargement of the aorta but also includes cases where there can be extensive eccentric enlargement. By definition, all three layers of the abdominal aorta are intact in a fusiform aneurysm. Saccular aneurysms are, by their nature, eccentric because the artery wall has a dissection, and they are much less common than fusiform aneurysms, making up less than 1% of

all aortic aneurysms. This number is a bit misleading because most saccular aneurysms occur in the thoracic aorta and are very rare in the abdominal aorta.

There are various possible etiologies for aneurysm formation: traumatic, infectious, vasculitides, and those associated with spontaneous dissections into the aortic wall. Although traumatic pseudoaneurysms typically rupture through all three layers of the aortic wall, they can sometimes lead to saccular aneurysms. By far, the most common location is the thoracic aorta.[12] Prior instrumentation, such as placement of cannulas in the aortic wall, can be the source of saccular aneurysm formation. A second type of saccular aneurysm has typically been termed a *mycotic aneurysm*. Mycotic aneurysms develop because of an acute infection in the layers of the aortic wall, typically by bacteria such as nontyphoid *Salmonella* species, *Streptococcus pneumoniae*, and *Staphylococcus* species, although any organism can potentially be a source. Interestingly, the term

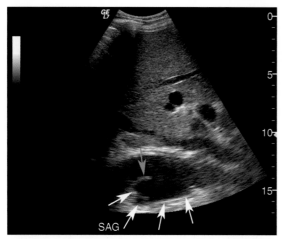

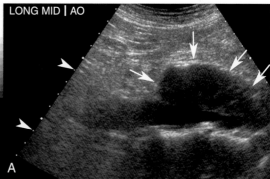

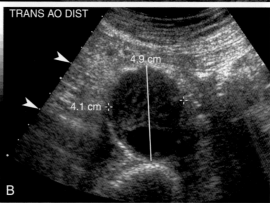

FIGURE 27-8 Saccular aneurysm *(white arrows)* at the level of the diaphragm. The integrity of the aortic wall has been compromised as shown by the presence of a dissection flap *(green arrow).*

FIGURE 27-9 **A,** Eccentric aneurysm containing thrombus. The very eccentric nature of the aneurysm may mimic the appearance of a saccular aneurysm. However, all three layers of the aortic wall are intact. **B,** Transverse scan of the aneurysm shown above. The eccentric component is again shown to be thrombus filled.

mycotic implies that a fungal source would be the cause of the infection, though this is uncommon. *Candida* is the most common fungal organism seen in mycotic aneurysms. The distinction between saccular and mycotic aneurysm can only be made by means of cultures for the suspected organisms and the patient's clinical presentation. The third type of saccular aneurysm is associated with a vasculitis. The inflammatory process affects the vasa vasorum of the adventitia, then spreads to cause fibrosis and degeneration of the media. The aortic wall ruptures into the media, causing a saccular aneurysm. This is typical of Behçet's syndrome. The fourth type of saccular aneurysm occurs when a penetrating ulcer ruptures into the media of the aorta.[13] This leads to a contained leak into the wall with eccentric pressure effects that promote the formation of the aneurysm. The saccular aneurysm is therefore associated with a compromise of the aortic wall. The major difference with a pseudoaneurysm is the fact that the adventitia and very commonly a part of the media remain intact in a saccular aneurysm. All three layers are ruptured in the case of a pseudoaneurysm.

Confusion can arise when a very eccentric fusiform aneurysm is imaged (Figure 27-9). The eccentricity does not represent a saccular aneurysm because all three layers of the abdominal aorta are intact. The edges of the eccentric aneurysm appear smooth, whereas a defect is seen in the aortic wall at the beginning of a saccular aneurysm.

In summary, the majority of abdominal aneurysms that are seen during a sonographic examination is fusiform. If a saccular aneurysm is seen or suspected, then the patient should be referred to a surgeon as soon as possible. Confusion can arise when distinguishing a saccular aneurysm from an eccentric aneurysm.

ANEURYSM FORMATION

The magic number for abdominal aortic intervention is 5.5 cm. The use of diagnostic ultrasound is based on detecting aneurysms below this threshold because the most serious complication of abdominal aortic aneurysm is rupture into the retroperitoneum. Although patients can present with symptoms (Table 27-1), the use of ultrasound has significantly increased the detection of smaller asymptomatic aneurysms. Rupture of an abdominal aortic aneurysm is a catastrophic event with low survival rates. The risk for rupture increases so rapidly for diameters above 5.5 cm that surgical or endovascular intervention

TABLE 27-1 Complications of Abdominal Aortic Aneurysms

Complication	Mechanism	Comment
Rupture	Increases as size increases	Lags by 10 years in women
Pain (back pain or lower abdominal)	More likely in adults 50 years or less	Possibly due to inflammatory component
Hydronephrosis	Compression of the ureters	Large aneurysms
Distal embolization	Associated with mural thrombus	Uncommon
Acute thrombosis	Associated with athero-sclerosis	Rare

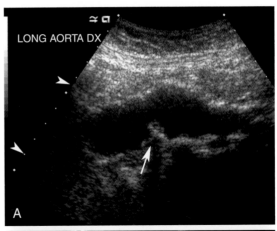

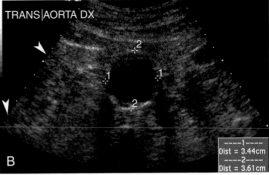

FIGURE 27-10 A, This longitudinal image of the aorta shows coexistence of a large calcified plaque *(arrow)* in a small fusiform aortic aneurysm. **B,** Transverse diameter measurements confirm that the aorta is enlarged above 3.0 cm.

is recommended in almost all instances once the diameter reaches 5.5 cm.

The pathologic processes that lead to the formation of abdominal aortic aneurysm are not fully understood. It is clear that elevated blood pressure, cigarette smoking, and a genetic predisposition are the major factors contributing to aneurysm formation. Aneurysms are also much more common in men than in women, with a ratio estimated from 4 to 13:1.[14]

The common belief that aneurysm formation is an atherosclerotic process needs to be placed in context (Figure 27-10). Elevated blood pressure and cigarette smoking are risk factors that are causally linked to the development of atherosclerosis. In the aorta, these risk factors will promote the formation of early atherosclerotic plaque and continue to promote growth and remodeling of these lesions. Continued exposure to cigarette smoke and elevated blood pressure can act directly on the constituents of the aortic wall and degrade the elastin in the artery wall. For example, cigarette smoke is associated with increased activity of elastase. Elastase will enzymatically break down the elastin in the aortic wall and compromise the mechanical integrity of the wall. Elevated blood pressure, especially pulse pressure, will cause repetitive mechanical stress on the wall of the aorta. This repeated stress leads to mechanical fatigue of the elastin, as well as the other elements of the wall, and ultimately to fragmentation and local mechanical disruption of fibers within the wall. In addition, the proportion of collagen in the aortic wall increases (types I and III). This process, occurring over time, weakens the wall of the aorta and leads to aneurysm formation.

There are genetic factors that have been associated with aneurysm formation. The most common is simple inheritance of a familial risk for developing aneurysms with a male predominance. Some groups had lower amounts of type III collagen in the aortic media, suggesting that abnormalities in type III collagen may be one of the genetic factors. Another type of genetic inheritance is that of disease states in which collagen constituents in the aortic wall are abnormal due to an inherited defect in the structure of collagen, such as Marfan's and Ehlers-Danlos syndromes.

ULTRASOUND EXAMINATION

PREPARATION

The most common reason for a failed examination of the abdominal aorta is the presence of bowel gas. Fasting after midnight and abstinence from actions that lead to air swallowing, such as smoking or chewing gum, are recommended.

In some instances, a bowel preparation can be used to guarantee a better-quality examination.

The examination will typically include an evaluation of the full length of the aorta from the diaphragm to the iliac artery bifurcation. The common iliac artery bifurcation should be evaluated for the following reasons: extension of an abdominal aortic aneurysm into the common iliac artery, the primary formation of common iliac artery aneurysms, or the presence of iliac artery stenoses.

A gray-scale frequency of 3 to 4 MHz or greater is normally used, and a curved array transducer offers the most flexibility. A sector transducer or a linear array transducer can be used if needed. We prefer to use one to two focal points in order to keep a high frame rate during the examination. The basic images stored are a transverse image of the proximal, mid, and distal abdominal aorta with the associated wall measurements. Measurements are made outer wall to outer wall, perpendicular to the long axis of the aorta. The tendency of the abdominal aortic aneurysm to rupture is linked to the stress on the outer wall and not on the lumen of the artery. Typically, both anteroposterior and transverse diameter measurements are made. Anteroposterior measurements are more reliable since they are based on the reflection of the ultrasound beam from the aortic wall interfaces. These are best seen when the ultrasound beam is perpendicular to the wall. The lateral wall can be difficult to measure. We also include a transverse image of each common iliac artery, including the respective diameter measurements. The sagittal images also allow detection of aortic ectasia, a relative enlargement of the aortic diameter of 20% or more but less than 50%, and better define the extent of thrombus deposition (Figure 27-11).

The reported 95% confidence intervals for replicate measurements of the abdominal aorta are 4.0 mm. Based on these numbers, serial changes of less than 4.0 mm should be considered to be within the measurement error of the technique. This measurement error estimate includes the error linked to repositioning the ultrasound probe and replicating the site of measurement.[15]

The following protocol, as shown in Table 27-2, should be considered:

1. Always measure an aneurysm the way a surgeon does in the operating room, from the outer surface of the artery (outer to outer).

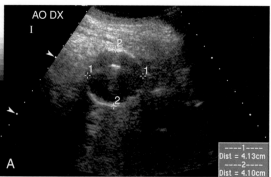

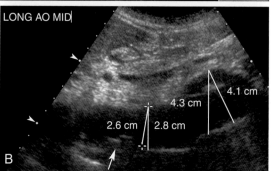

FIGURE 27-11 A, Transverse image taken of a low abdominal aortic aneurysm showing typical measurements. The anteroposterior measurement (outer wall to outer wall) is the most reliable because the probe is perpendicular to the aorta. **B,** Longitudinal image can be used to confirm the measurement made in **A.** The arrow points to an atherosclerotic plaque that obscures a reliable diameter measurement. The next measurement to the right, at 2.6 cm, falls short to the interfaces. The next measurement is a correct estimate of the aortic diameter at 2.8 cm. After this is an angled measurement where the size of the aneurysm is overestimated at 4.3 cm. The last measurement of 4.1 cm on the right is taken perpendicular to the aorta lumen and confirms the measurement made in **A.**

2. Sagittal and coronal planes are recommended for aneurysm measurement, as well as the transverse plane. The use of these planes shows the point of maximum dilatation clearly in a way that is reproducible from one examination to the next. It also avoids error resulting from oblique transverse measurements.
3. Coronal views are generally easier to obtain from the left side of the aorta than from the right side.
4. The maximum interobserver variability for aortic measurement is approximately 4 mm.[15] Therefore, an increase in size of less than 4 mm from one examination to another may not be significant. Gradual size increase on serial examination is important.

TABLE 27-2 Examination Protocol for Aortic and Iliac Aneurysms

1. Longitudinal

Examine aorta, diaphragm to bifurcation using gray-scale and color Doppler imaging to identify dissection, if present.

Determine location and longitudinal extent of any aortic aneurysm.

Measure aortic aneurysm anteroposterior diameter, outer diameter to outer diameter.

Examine iliac arteries to iliac bifurcation. Use color Doppler, at least briefly, to detect flow disturbances associated with iliac artery stenosis. Document severity of stenosis, if present, as per Chapter 17.

Measure iliac artery aneurysm(s), if present, outer diameter to outer diameter.

2. Transverse

Document the maximum diameter of the aorta at the diaphragm, superior mesenteric artery, and distally near the aortic bifurcation.

Measure aortic diameters in anteroposterior and transverse planes, outer diameter to outer diameter.

Visualize the iliac arteries, and ensure iliac artery diameter; measure aneurysm(s) size, if present, outer diameter to outer diameter.

3. Coronal (difficult to perform)

Measure aortic aneurysm, transverse dimension, outer diameter to outer diameter.

Examine iliac arteries, and measure aneurysm(s), if present.

4. Color Doppler examination

Measure distance from renal arteries to aneurysm neck.

Alternatively, measure distance from superior mesenteric artery to aneurysm neck.

5. Kidneys: longitudinal and transverse views

Document kidney length and normal features.

Document hydronephrosis, if present.

---

5. Remember, aneurysms do not decrease in size! To avoid looking foolish, be aware of the measurements reported previously before giving current measurements.

6. If possible, determine whether an aneurysm extends to, or above, the renal arteries. This is done best by directly visualizing the renal artery origins and measuring the distance from these vessels to the origin of the aneurysm. Time constraints often do not permit direct visualization of the renal arteries, but their location may be quickly inferred by measuring the distance from the superior mesenteric artery to the aneurysm. The renal arteries arise no more than 2 cm below the superior mesenteric artery; therefore, the renal arteries should be unaffected if the aneurysm begins 2 cm or more below the superior mesenteric artery.

7. The entire abdominal aorta must be examined to ensure that suprarenal aneurysms are not overlooked.

8. An aneurysm at the bifurcation of the iliac arteries can easily be overlooked, because this area is difficult to visualize. A transducer position lateral to the rectus muscles aids iliac artery visualization.

9. Color Doppler imaging should always be used at some point in the aortic examination to exclude aortic dissection and to identify iliac artery stenosis.

DEFINITION OF AN ANEURYSM: SIZE THRESHOLDS

Aneurysm formation should not be viewed as an all-or-none phenomenon with a fixed diameter value defining the presence of an aneurysm. The major reason for this is the fact that the aortic diameter increases with age and is a function of body size.[16] The latter is the main reason why aortic diameters are smaller in women than in men.

Specific cut-points of 3 cm or 4 cm have been used for defining an aortic aneurysm. However, there are various criteria that can be used to define the presence of an aneurysm.[14] A relative increase in the diameter of an aortic segment by 50% or at least 1.5 times greater than the adjacent unaffected segment is considered to be an aneurysm, irrespective of the absolute size.[14,17]

However, longitudinal scans will often show areas of ectasia (Figure 27-12) where local diameter increases and causes a small bulge in the aortic wall. It is not clear at what point these areas of ectasia will lead to aneurysm formation. We define these as increases in the aortic diameter of approximately 20% or more in aortas smaller than 3.0 cm.[18] Recent reviews of the natural history of aneurysm formation show that even aortic bulges with diameters of 2.5 cm to 3.0 cm can go on to form aneurysms.[19] These small zones of ectasia likely represent the earliest manifestation of aneurysmal disease of the aorta.

Data recently reported in a large cohort of patients followed for 10 years[20] showed that after 5 years, 2.4% of aortas measuring 2.6 to 2.9 cm reached a threshold of 5.5 cm or received surgery, whereas 5% of aneurysms between 3.0 and 3.4 cm

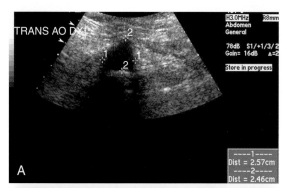

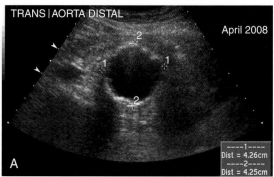

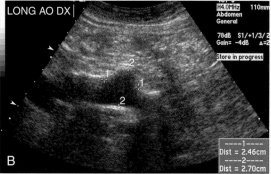

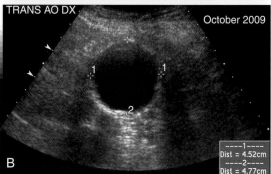

FIGURE 27-12 A, Transverse scan of the distal abdominal aorta showing a small zone of ectasia that is less than 3.0 cm. **B,** The longitudinal image confirms that this represents a significant bulge as compared to the normal-caliber aorta.

FIGURE 27-13 A, Baseline diameter obtained in April 2008 shows a fusiform aneurysm, without thrombus, measuring 4.25 cm in anteroposterior diameter. **B,** Follow-up examination in October 2009 shows a diameter of 4.77 cm. The aneurysm growth rate is at the upper range of expected growth. Closer follow-up at 3-6 months should now be performed.

had surgery or reached 5.5 cm within 3 years. Of the aneurysms measuring 3.5 to 3.9 cm in size, 1.2 % expanded to 5.5 cm at 1 year, whereas 10.5% reached 5.5 cm or required surgery by 2 years (an additional 1.4% presenting with acute rupture).

In summary, classification of aneurysm disease of the aorta includes frank aneurysms of 3 cm or more and should also include a broad category of localized aortic bulges referred to as aortic ectasia. An absolute cut-point of 3.0 cm is not a gold-standard definition of an aortic aneurysm.

GROWTH RATE OF ANEURYSMS

Most of the literature on growth rates was adapted from studies combining both thoracic and abdominal aneurysms. The common factor is that growth rate seems to be proportional to aneurysm size: basically the larger the aneurysm, the faster the growth rate. Typically growth rates of aneurysms are 1 to 2 mm/yr in aneurysms measuring 3 to 4 cm and then increase to rates of 4 to 5 mm/yr or even more (Figure 27-13). There is a belief that the growth rate increase represents a transition point where the stresses have lead to a mechanical

compromise of the wall and that the wall of the aorta is starting to fail mechanically. This also corresponds to the increasing likelihood for aortic rupture. What is interesting is that not all patients with large aneurysms have accelerated growth rates. If this were true, the rupture rate of 25% over 5 years for aneurysms 5.5 cm or more would be greater. There is therefore some variability in the growth rate and likelihood of aortic rupture that depends on individual patient characteristics.

Aneurysms tend to develop mural thrombus over time. It is not clear how this affects the growth rate of the aneurysm. Some authors believe that the thrombus cushions the aortic wall from the mechanical stresses of blood pressure. However, analysis of the content of the thrombus shows that this is not a passive accumulation of fibrin, but a metabolically active mesh. Enzymes produced within the thrombus can contribute to the mechanical breakdown of the aneurysm wall. At least one report has suggested that eccentric thrombus is associated with increased expansion rates in aneurysms sized 4.0 to 4.9 cm.[21]

TABLE 27-3 Proposed Screening Intervals for Abdominal Aortic Aneurysms	
Size of Aorta	Interval Between Visits*
Ectatic aorta (local bulges >20%)	2 to 3 years
3 to 4 cm	Every year
4 to 4.5 cm	Every 6 months
4.5 to 5.0 cm	Every 3 to 6 months
5.0 to 5.5 cm	Every 3 months

*These estimated time intervals are based on estimated rates of expansion and not based on a cost-effectiveness evaluation.

If a patient experiences a diameter change of 4 mm/year or more during yearly follow-up, the next follow-up should be at 3 months. A decision is then made to do either 3- or 6-month follow-up depending on the findings at that time.

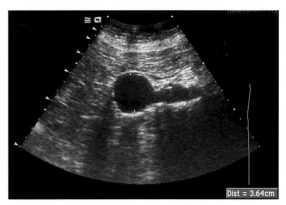

FIGURE 27-14 Transverse view of the common iliac artery bifurcations showing a markedly enlarged right common iliac artery (3.64-cm diameter) as compared to the left common iliac artery (1.5-cm diameter).

Expected growth rates in one series are 0.9 mm/yr for aortas measuring 2.6 to 2.9 cm, increasing to 1.6 mm/yr for aortic diameters of 3.0 to 3.4 cm, and finally 3.2 mm/yr for aneurysms 3.5 to 3.9 cm in size.[20] It is not clear from this review whether the expansion rates for aortic sizes of 2.6 to 2.9 cm apply to ectatic aortas or simply large aortas. A study of ectatic aortas less than 3.0 cm showed that the expansion rates average 0.65 mm/yr, but a subset of 9.5% of this group had expansion rates of 3 mm/yr, while 30 of the 116 ectatic aortas did not show any expansion.[18] Table 27-3 summarizes proposed time intervals for the follow-up of aortic aneurysms. Some authors recommend that a 3-month visit take place after the original diagnosis to protect against the possibility of a rapidly expanding aneurysm.

It appears that traditional cardiovascular risk factors are not associated with expansion rates of abdominal aortic aneurysms once they have formed.[22,23] In addition, lowering blood pressure with beta-blockers does not seem to affect the expansion rates of aneurysms,[24] whereas antiinflammatory agents and statins reduce the expansion rates.[23,24] These data apply to well-established aneurysms and not to smaller aneurysms or even ectatic aortas.

COMMON ILIAC ARTERY ANEURYSMS

Common iliac arteries are normally 0.8 to 1.2 cm in diameter. At somewhere between 1.3 and 1.4 cm they are considered ectatic. A practical definition of an iliac artery aneurysm can therefore be taken as a diameter of 1.5 cm or more (Figure 27-14). The presence of a focal region of dilatation, as

discussed for the aorta, should be considered as a potential precursor to the development of an aneurysm. Although common iliac artery aneurysms are commonly present in patients with aortic aneurysms, they can be isolated. The prevalence of iliac artery aneurysms is low, about 2% of that of abdominal aortic aneurysms.[25] An association between common iliac artery diameter and the diameter of the aortic aneurysm has been reported.[26]

A cut-point of 3.5 cm has been recommended as the threshold for intervention. Growth rates are equivalent to those of the abdominal aorta and increase with aneurysm size.[27] Typically the expansion rate remains close to 1.0 mm/yr or less until the aneurysm reaches 3.0 cm. At that point, the expansion rates are double or more.[27]

ANEURYSM COMPLICATIONS

The most common complication of aortic aneurysm disease is rupture of the aneurysm with acute retroperitoneal or intraperitoneal hemorrhage. The probability of this occurrence increases with the size of the aneurysm. It is generally accepted that once the size reaches 5.0 cm or more, this risk starts to increase.[28-30] Above 5.5 cm, this risk is even larger and can reach 10% per year and increases even more for larger aneurysms (Figure 27-15).

Another complication is the development of peripheral embolization. This is normally associated with the presence of thrombus in the aneurysm (also called aneurysm sac). There have not been any studies correlating this risk with the amount of thrombus present in the aneurysm sac, but it seems logical that this risk should increase in larger aneurysms that also have a large amount of thrombus.

A rare complication is that of a contained rupture into the wall of the aorta. This can be suggested by the presence of different echogenic zones within the aneurysm sac. This is uncommon and is usually inferred by the sonographic appearance unless serial measurements were performed on that same patient. This intrathrombus rupture can cause a rapid expansion of the aneurysm diameter and is more clearly shown by computed tomography (CT).[31] Although this can be hard to document, a zone with low echogenicity may represent an acute rupture into the mural thrombus (Figure 27-16).

VARIED PATHOLOGIES

VASCULITIS

Aortitis is a generic classification used to describe an inflammatory process affecting the wall of the aorta. This typically extends from the outer layers of the aorta inward, adventitia to the media. Abdominal aortic involvement with vasculitis has been described in patients with Takayasu's arteritis, giant cell arteritis, polychondritis, and various bacterial organisms.[32] Wall thickening can be seen on CT and sonographic scans, although ultrasound findings may be difficult to document in the aorta (Figure 27-17, *A*), whereas involvement of the common carotid arteries is often seen (Figure 27-17, *B*).

An entity called nonspecific aortitis has been described in individuals who present with

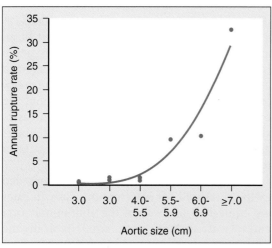

FIGURE 27-15 Diagram summarizing the risk for abdominal aneurysm rupture as a function of size. A sharp inflection is seen at around 5.5 cm. The data shown are a combination of separate studies that evaluated the risk for abdominal aneurysm rupture.[28-30]

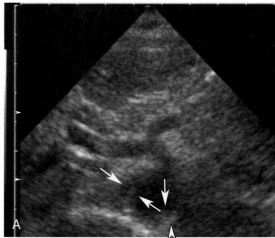

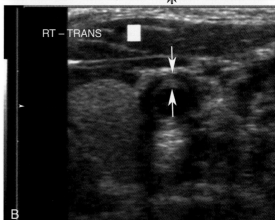

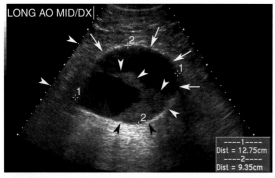

FIGURE 27-16 Aneurysm containing zones of different echogenicity, suggesting that the outer layer of thrombus (less echogenic; *arrows*) may be due to a dissection into the original inner layer of thrombus (echogenic; *arrowheads*).

FIGURE 27-17 A, Transverse image of the proximal aorta at the level of the celiac axis showing diffuse wall thickening *(arrows)*. **B,** Diffuse thickening of the common carotid wall is more easily documented in this same patient *(arrows)*.

localized pain to a very specific portion of the abdomen and are subsequently shown to have an area of abnormal aortic wall thickening. However, this diagnosis is most often made by CT or magnetic resonance imaging rather than by ultrasound.

The presence of vasculitis is a risk factor for the subsequent development of aneurysms, possibly saccular as described in the cases of Behçet's disease.[33]

DISSECTIONS

The most common instance of aortic dissection is the extension of the dissecting flap of a proximal thoracic aortic dissection. Localized dissections in the abdominal aorta have been reported but they are very rare[34] and are most often associated with penetrating ulcers in the aortic wall.

The classic ultrasound finding is that of two lumens separated by a membrane representing the intimal flap of the aortic wall (Figure 27-18).[35] The false lumen tends to be larger than the smaller true lumen. However, this can vary from individual to individual. Color Doppler ultrasound and B-flow ultrasound have been reported to have a high accuracy for this diagnosis.[36] The flap can be difficult to visualize when parallel to the ultrasound beam. However, in such cases, a blood flow disturbance should be seen on color Doppler imaging (see Video 27-3). It can be difficult to distinguish between patent true and false lumens, although absence of blood flow usually signifies thrombosis of the false lumen.[37]

POSTOPERATIVE ASSESSMENT

The traditional method of aortic aneurysm repair is surgical bypass grafting using synthetic graft material. Endovascular aneurysm repair (EVAR) has gained much popularity in the last few years and is covered in Chapter 28.

It is important that sonographers be familiar with the surgical repair method, because a great number of patients remain alive who have had surgical repair and a significant number continue to have surgical repair when stent grafting is not possible.

Three types of surgical graft procedures have commonly been used for aortic aneurysm repair (Figure 27-19): (1) simple tube grafts for aneurysms limited to the aorta (see Figure 27-19, *A*); (2) end-to-end aortoiliac grafts (see Figure 27-19, *B*); and (3) end-to-side aortobiiliac or aortobifemoral grafts (see Figure 27-19, *C*). With simple tube grafts the aortic aneurysm is opened longitudinally, the graft is placed inside, and the native aorta is wrapped around the graft (see Figure 27-19, *D*). This is done to isolate the graft and the duodenum, lessening the chance of graft infection. The wrapping procedure creates a potential space that normally contains fluid during the immediate postoperative period.[38,39] However,

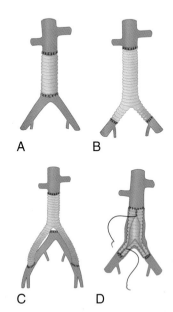

FIGURE 27-19 Types of aortic grafts. **A,** Tube graft with end-to-end proximal and distal anastomoses. **B,** Aorto-bifemoral graft with end-to-end distal anastomoses. **C,** Aortobifemoral graft with end-to-side distal anastomoses. **D,** The native aorta is wrapped around the graft and sewn closed.

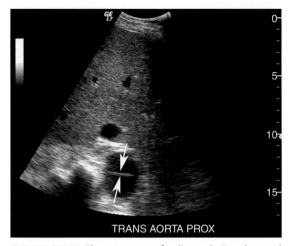

TRANS AORTA PROX

FIGURE 27-18 The presence of a linear lesion *(arrows)* in this transverse view of the aorta is consistent with a dissection.

during and after this time period, the postoperative site can be indistinguishable from a normal aorta by ultrasound imaging.

Tube grafts are normally placed as an end-to-end procedure, but occasionally an end-to-side anastomosis is used (end of graft to side of aorta). Aortoiliac and aortofemoral grafts have two components: the body, which is attached to the aorta, and two limbs, which are attached to the common iliac, external iliac, or common femoral arteries. The distal anastomosis can be end-to-end or end-to-side for aorto–common iliac grafts, likely end-to-side for aorto–external iliac grafts, and almost exclusively end-to-side for aortofemoral grafts. A femoral attachment is used when atherosclerosis or iliac aneurysm precludes attachment of the graft limbs to the iliac arteries. The end-to-side configuration permits retrograde blood flow from the external iliac artery into the internal iliac branches.

TECHNIQUE AND NORMAL APPEARANCE OF GRAFTS

The objectives of postoperative ultrasound examination are to detect pathologic fluid collections and pseudoaneurysm formation at the anastomotic sites, to examine the full length of the graft, and to use Doppler ultrasound for evaluating the graft and the anastomoses for stenosis. The ultrasound graft examination generally is fairly quick and easy. The sonographer begins at the proximal end and follows the graft to the distal end (or vice versa) using color Doppler imaging. Blood flow disturbances indicating stenosis in the graft are uncommon. The sonographer should document the appearance of the proximal and distal anastomoses, as well as the diameter of the graft body and limbs, and document Doppler waveforms and velocities in the runoff vessels, just beyond the distal anastomoses.

The graft material used for aortic bypass grafts is Dacron or polytetrafluoroethylene (PTFE). Dacron grafts generally have a textured, or tramtrack, appearance and are fairly echogenic (Figure 27-20); therefore, this type graft can usually be identified easily. The exception to this rule is an old graft (e.g., >8 years) that is invested with fibrous tissue or atherosclerotic plaque. These grafts can be difficult to identify. Slight puckering of the graft and the native artery is seen normally at the suture lines, causing visible thickening of the artery wall at the anastomosis. A small layer of fluid can be present around the graft during the postoperative period. This fluid may be focal or diffuse and

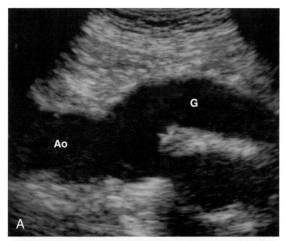

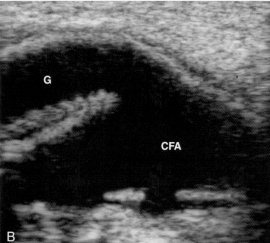

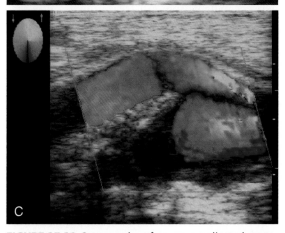

FIGURE 27-20 Sonography of an uncomplicated aorto-bifemoral graft. **A,** Proximal end-to-end anastomosis of the mildly dilated aorta (Ao) and the smaller-diameter graft (G). **B,** End-to-side anastomosis of the left graft limb (G) with the common femoral artery (CFA). Note that the weave of the graft is visible. **C,** Color flow image, same as **B.**

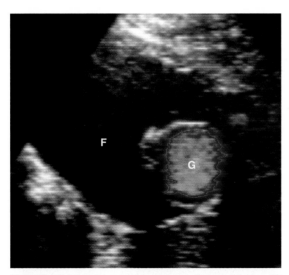

FIGURE 27-21 A large postoperative fluid collection (F) is present between the aneurysm sac and the body of this graft (G).

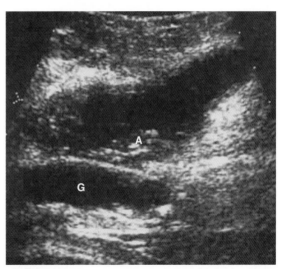

FIGURE 27-22 An abscess (A) is present in a groin incision. Unfortunately, the abscess extends to the graft (G), implying that the graft is infected as well.

may persist for more than a week. Large fluid collections may be present postoperatively around the body of an aortic graft if the native aorta is wrapped around it (Figure 27-21), and this fluid may persist for months. The important thing about postoperative fluid is that it should decrease in volume with time and ultimately disappear. Increasing fluid volume suggests graft infection. PTFE grafts can be more difficult to identify and are normally used as tube grafts. Reinforced PTFE is used when aortoiliac and aortofemoral grafts are inserted.

COMPLICATIONS

Complications of aortic graft surgery may be divided into early and late periods. In the early period (weeks/months), surgery-related hematomas and seromas, as well as infection, are the principal problems. Hematomas are collections of blood, and seromas are collections of tissue fluid or serum. Either type of fluid is normally present adjacent to the graft in the days following surgery, and these fluid collections occasionally may be large focally or may be located somewhat distant from the graft within the retroperitoneum. The sonographic appearance is that of any fluid collection: anechoic or mildly echogenic; homogeneous or heterogeneous. Although they cannot be differentiated from abscesses, postoperative hematomas and seromas should recede within weeks of surgery, as mentioned previously. Furthermore, they are not associated with

leukocytosis or other clinical signs of infection. These inconsequential fluid collections do not increase in size, and if they do, abscess should be considered. Abscess can be diagnosed in two ways: (1) by aspirating fluid from the sonographically identified collection and subsequently demonstrating the presence of bacteria via culture or Gram stain, or (2) by a combination of sonographic and clinical findings (e.g., perigraft fluid, leukocytosis, and fever). When abscess is diagnosed, it is important to determine whether the collection is immediately adjacent to the graft or remote from it. A remote abscess (e.g., in a surgical incision) may be drained percutaneously without significant clinical consequences, whereas a perigraft abscess necessitates graft removal (Figure 27-22) and insertion of a new bypass. Finally, it should be noted that graft infection may not be accompanied by sonographic abnormalities if the infection is indolent. In such cases, infection may be accompanied only by perigraft inflammation that is not visible sonographically. Chronic infection is generally diagnosed by a combination of laboratory findings, clinical symptomatology, and CT findings.

In most patients, aortic bypass grafting is a durable procedure, and the graft may be expected to function without complications for 10 years or more.[40] Late graft failure may occur, however, from a variety of causes. With time, the graft material may weaken due to fatigue imposed by the repeated stress of arterial pulsation. Fatigue

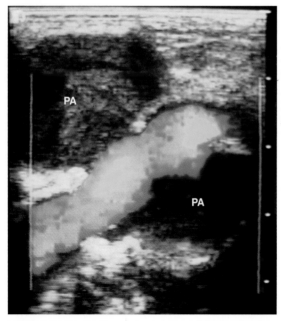

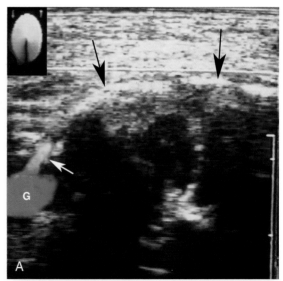

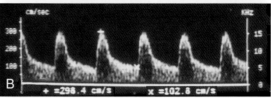

FIGURE 27-23 Graft pseudoaneurysm. A large pseudoaneurysm (PA) extends both superficial and deep to the distal anastomosis of an aortoexternal iliac bypass graft.

FIGURE 27-24 Graft aneurysm and stenosis (68-year-old man with claudication, 8 years after aortobifemoral graft). **A,** A large aneurysm *(black arrows)* is present at the right femoral anastomosis of an aortofemoral graft (G). Only the near surface of the aneurysm is visible because extensive calcification of the aneurysm obscures deeper structures. A tiny residual lumen is present along the near surface of the aneurysm *(white arrow).* **B,** Doppler investigation of the stenotic segment shows a peak systolic velocity of 298 cm/sec and an end-diastolic velocity of 103 cm/sec, consistent with severe narrowing.

may cause the graft to stretch and dilate, like an old sock, or it may lead to localized failure and the development of a leak accompanied by a pseudoaneurysm.[41] These modes of failure are uncommon, however. The majority of long-term complications occur instead at the distal anastomoses, which tend to stretch and/or break down with time (Figures 27-23 and 27-24). Stretching causes a true aneurysm to form at the anastomosis, involving both the graft and the native artery. More commonly breakdown of the sutured graft-artery interface leads to pseudoaneurysm formation. Although these complications may occur at any anastomosis, they are usually seen at the distal anastomosis and are particularly common at aortofemoral anastomoses. The fact that most graft complications occur at the anastomoses is the reason for emphasizing the identification of the proximal and distal anastomoses in the course of every sonographic graft examination.

Aortic grafts are also subject to the development of stenosis and occlusion. Again, these are usually late problems and almost invariably occur at the distal anastomosis or in the runoff vessel. Stenoses usually occur not in the graft, but in the runoff vessel at or beyond the distal anastomosis. Occasionally, however, stenosis develops in a graft limb. Regardless of location, severe stenosis may cause stagnation of flow and thrombus formation

in a graft limb, leading to occlusion. On ultrasound examination, stenosis is indicated by focal high velocity and disturbed flow that is readily detected with color flow sonography. Stenosis severity is judged with Doppler velocity measurements, as discussed in Chapters 17 and 18. Occlusion is diagnosed by the absence of flow and the presence of echogenic material in the graft lumen.

CONCLUSIONS

Ultrasound imaging has demonstrated strong diagnostic performance for the detection and follow-up of abdominal aortic aneurysms. It can also be used to detect the presence of hemodynamically significant stenoses, although this is a relatively uncommon entity. The role of ultrasound in other pathologies such as aortic dissections and aortitis is limited.

REFERENCES

1. Grimshaw GM, Thompson JM: Changes in diameter of the abdominal aorta with age: an epidemiological study, *J Clin Ultrasound* 25:7–13, 1997.
2. Wilson N, et al: Normal intracardiac and great artery blood velocity measurements by pulsed Doppler echocardiography, *Br Heart J* 53:451–458, 1985.
3. Fraser KH, et al: Characterization of an abdominal aortic velocity waveform in patients with abdominal aortic aneurysm, *Ultrasound Med Biol.* 34:73–80, 2008.
4. Holman RL, et al: The natural history of atherosclerosis: the early aortic lesions as seen in New Orleans in the middle of the 20th century, *Am J Pathol* 34:209–235, 1958.
5. Strong JP, et al: Prevalence and extent of atherosclerosis in adolescents and young adults: implications for prevention from the pathobiological determinants of atherosclerosis in youth study, *JAMA* 281:727–735, 1999.
6. Staple TW: The solitary aortoiliac lesion, *Surgery* 64: 569–576, 1968.
7. Cronenwett JL, et al: Aortoiliac occlusive disease in women, *Surgery* 88:775–784, 1980.
8. Audet P, et al: Infrarenal aortic stenosis: long-term clinical and hemodynamic results of percutaneous transluminal angioplasty, *Radiology* 209:357–363, 1998.
9. Sensier Y, Bell PR, London NJ: The ability of qualitative assessment of the common femoral Doppler waveform to screen for significant aortoiliac disease, *Eur J Vasc Endovasc Surg* 15:357–364, 1998.
10. Shaalan WE, et al: Reliability of common femoral artery hemodynamics in assessing the severity of aortoiliac inflow disease, *J Vasc Surg* 37:960–969, 2003.
11. Polak JF, et al: Determination of the extent of lower-extremity peripheral arterial disease with color-assisted duplex sonography: comparison with angiography, *AJR Am J Roentgenol* 155:1085–1089, 1990.
12. Taylor BV, Kalman PG: Saccular aortic aneurysms, *Ann Vasc Surg* 13:555–559, 1999.
13. Minor ME, Menzoian JO, Raffetto JD: Noninfectious saccular abdominal aortic aneurysm–a report of two cases, *Vasc Endovascular Surg* 37:353–358, 2003.
14. Wanhainen A, et al: Influence of diagnostic criteria on the prevalence of abdominal aortic aneurysm, *J Vasc Surg* 34:229–235, 2001.
15. Singh K, et al: Intra- and interobserver variability in ultrasound measurements of abdominal aortic diameter. The Tromso study, *Eur J Vasc Endovasc Surg* 15:497–504, 1998.
16. Sonesson B, et al: Infrarenal aortic diameter in the healthy person, *Eur J Vasc Surg* 8:89–95, 1994.
17. Johnston KW, et al: Suggested standards for reporting on arterial aneurysms. Subcommittee on Reporting Standards for Arterial Aneurysms, Ad Hoc Committee on Reporting Standards, Society for Vascular Surgery and North American Chapter, International Society for Cardiovascular Surgery, *J Vasc Surg* 13:452–458, 1991.
18. Basnyat PS, et al: Natural history of the ectatic aorta, *Cardiovasc Surg* 11:273–276, 2003.
19. Biancari F, et al: Ten-year outcome of patients with very small abdominal aortic aneurysm, *Am J Surg* 183:53–55, 2002.
20. McCarthy RJ, et al: Recommendations for screening intervals for small aortic aneurysms, *Br J Surg* 90:821–826, 2003.
21. Vega de Ceniga M, et al: Analysis of expansion patterns in 4-4.9 cm abdominal aortic aneurysms, *Ann Vasc Surg* 22:37–44, 2008.
22. Vega de Ceniga M, et al: Growth rate and associated factors in small abdominal aortic aneurysms, *Eur J Vasc Endovasc Surg* 31:231–236, 2006.
23. Schlosser FJV, et al: Growth predictors and prognosis of small abdominal aortic aneurysms, *J Vasc Surg* 47:1127–1133, 2008.
24. Guessous I, et al: The efficacy of pharmacotherapy for decreasing the expansion rate of abdominal aortic aneurysms: A systematic review and meta-analysis, *PLoS ONE* 3:e1895, 2008.
25. Huang Y, et al: Common iliac artery aneurysm: expansion rate and results of open surgical and endovascular repair, *J Vasc Surg* 47:1203–1210, 2008. discussion 1201-1210.
26. Richards T, et al: Natural history of the common iliac artery in the presence of an abdominal aortic aneurysm, *J Vasc Surg* 49:881–885, 2009.
27. Santilli SM, Wernsing SE, Lee ES: Expansion rates and outcomes for iliac artery aneurysms, *J Vasc Surg* 31:114–121, 2000.
28. Anonymous. Mortality results for randomised controlled trial of early elective surgery or ultrasonographic surveillance for small abdominal aortic aneurysms. The UK small aneurysm trial participants, *Lancet* 352:1649–1655, 1998.
29. Lederle FA, et al: Rupture rate of large abdominal aortic aneurysms in patients refusing or unfit for elective repair, *JAMA* 287:2968–2972, 2002.
30. Vardulaki KA, et al: Growth rates and risk of rupture of abdominal aortic aneurysms, *Br J Surg* 85:1674–1680, 1998.
31. Roy J, et al: Bleeding into the intraluminal thrombus in abdominal aortic aneurysms is associated with rupture, *J Vasc Surg* 48:1108–1113, 2008.
32. Marie I, et al: Long-term follow-up of aortic involvement in giant cell arteritis: a series of 48 patients, *Medicine* 88: 182–192, 2009.
33. Matsumoto T, Uekusa T, Fukuda Y: Vasculo-Behçet's disease: a pathologic study of eight cases, *Hum Pathol* 22: 45–51, 1991.
34. Farber A, et al: Isolated dissection of the abdominal aorta: clinical presentation and therapeutic options, *J Vasc Surg* 36:205–210, 2002.
35. Bresnihan ER, Keates PG: Ultrasound and dissection of the abdominal aorta, *Clin Radiol* 31:105–108, 1980.
36. Clevert DA, et al: Improved diagnosis of vascular dissection by ultrasound B-flow: a comparison with color-coded Doppler and power Doppler sonography, *Eur Radiol* 15:342–347, 2005.
37. Risse JH, et al: [Color-coded duplex ultrasound in chronic dissecting abdominal aortic aneurysm. Differentiation between true and false aortic lumen with reference to the blood supply to larger abdominal arteries], *Radiologe* 35:759–766, 1995.
38. Hilton S, et al: Computed tomography of the postoperative abdominal aorta, *Radiology* 145:403–407, 1982.
39. Mark A, et al: CT evaluation of complications of abdominal aortic surgery, *Radiology* 145:409–414, 1982.
40. Liapis C, et al: Changes of the infrarenal aortic segment after conventional abdominal aortic aneurysm repair, *Eur J Vasc Endovasc Surg* 19:643–647, 2000.
41. Polak JF, et al: Pulsatile masses surrounding vascular prostheses: real-time US color flow imaging, *Radiology* 170:363–366, 1989.

ULTRASOUND IMAGING ASSESSMENT FOLLOWING ENDOVASCULAR AORTIC ANEURYSM REPAIR

28

GEORGE L. BERDEJO, BA, RVT, and EVAN C. LIPSITZ, MD

Frequent assessment and objective follow-up are critical following endovascular aneurysm repair. Endografts, sometimes referred to as endovascular grafts, stent-grafts or transluminally placed endovascular grafts, continue to evolve and change in their design. Patients undergoing endovascular abdominal aortic aneurysm (AAA) repair require routine, lifelong follow-up and imaging surveillance.

Color Doppler ultrasound has been used for aortic endovascular graft evaluation and has the advantage of being noninvasive, inexpensive, rapid, safe, nontoxic, easily repeatable, and well tolerated by patients. This technique has already become an important tool in both the planning and the postoperative evaluation of endovascular grafts placed for a variety of vascular lesions and complications.[1-9] Color Doppler imaging combines many of the ideal features of both angiography and spiral computed tomography (CT). It allows the examiner to make both quantitative and qualitative assessments of blood flow through the endovascular graft, and via a combination of pulsed-wave and color flow Doppler, can easily demonstrate normal blood flow patterns or abnormal flow patterns associated with specific pathologies. Because color Doppler is relatively inexpensive, easily repeatable, and without known risks, it has become a primary means of surveillance for endovascular interventions.[2,4,5,7,10] The *primary* objectives of the color Doppler examination following endovascular AAA repair are to:

1. Determine whether there is any persistent perigraft flow in the aneurysm sac (endoleak)
2. Characterize the type of endoleak, if present
3. Measure maximal residual aneurysm sac diameter.
4. Assess flow through the graft, including the identification of any kinking, stenosis, or thrombosis

It is important to determine the origin of any blood flow signals identified within the aneurysm sac (endoleak source, Table 28-1) because the source of the blood flow signals and their characteristics may determine subsequent treatment.

Cross-sectional diameter measurements are recorded at each visit to determine maximum aneurysm size. When an aneurysm sac is excluded from the circulation, an aneurysm should remain stable or decrease in size over time.[10,11] Any increase in size suggests that there is preserved blood flow into the aneurysm sac (endoleak) and because of the associated increase in blood pressure, a continued risk for rupture.[11,12] However, increases in size have been reported without CT, angiographic, or color Doppler evidence of endoleak (endotension) and proven by direct pressure measurements in the aneurysm sac.[13-15]

It is also important to determine that the distal arterial circulation has been preserved by ensuring that there are no graft-threatening abnormalities within the body of the endovascular graft, the graft limb(s) or in the inflow and outflow arteries. We previously described a protocol for evaluation of endovascular grafts placed at the aortoiliac level.[2]

If abnormalities are detected by color Doppler imaging, contrast arteriography and spiral CT may then be used to further characterize the abnormality when an intervention is being considered. This chapter describes a protocol for assessing endovascular grafts performed for the repair of isolated aneurysms of the abdominal aorta as well as aortoiliac aneurysms.

ENDOVASCULAR GRAFTS: OVERVIEW AND GENERAL CONSIDERATIONS

The endoluminal placement of stent-grafts, at sites remote from where the graft is introduced, allows for repair of a variety of complex lesions while reducing the relatively high morbidity

TABLE 28-1	Endoleak Types
Type 1a, 1b	Endoleak whose origin is at the proximal (1a) or distal (1b) stent attachment site.
Type 2	Endoleak originating from a branch vessel. Possible sources include patent lumbar (posterior to the endovascular graft sonographically), inferior mesenteric (anterolateral to the endovascular graft sonographically), accessory renal or hypogastric arteries, or other patent branches of the abdominal aorta. These are best seen in the transverse orientation.
Type 3	Endoleak that originates at the junctions between components of modular devices or from fabric tears within the graft.
Type 4	Transgraft flow or flow that fills the aneurysm sac because of porosity of the graft.
Endotension	Increase in aneurysm size in the absence of endoleak.

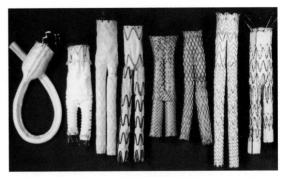

FIGURE 28-1 Commercially available endografts.

TABLE 28-2 Food and Drug Administration–Approved Grafts for Endovascular Abdominal Aortic Aneurysm Repair

- AneuRx Stent Graft System (Medtronic Vascular, Santa Rosa, CA)
- Zenith AAA Endovascular Graft and H&L-B One-Shot Introduction System (Cook Incorporated, Bloomington, IN)
- EXCLUDER AAA Endoprosthesis Bifurcated Endoprosthesis (W.L. Gore & Associates, Inc., Flagstaff, AZ)
- Endologix PowerLink System (Endologix, Inc., Irvine, CA).
- Talent Abdominal Stent Graft System (Medtronic Vascular, Santa Rosa, CA)
- Endurant (Medtronic Vascular, Santa Rosa, CA)

and mortality associated with traditional open operative repair. The first series of transluminally placed endovascular grafts for the repair of abdominal aortic aneurysms in high-risk patients was reported in 1991.[16] Since that time, significant advances in the design of endovascular stents and grafts have facilitated their deployment in aortic and aortoiliac aneurysms, permitting a greater number of patients to be treated with these devices.[17-20] We have extensive experience with the Montefiore Endovascular Graft System (MEGS), which has now expanded to include a number of commercially available endografts (Figure 28-1).

Currently several devices (Table 28-2) have been granted U.S. Food and Drug Administration approval for the treatment of aortoiliac aneurysms and are available for widespread use in the United States. Many other devices are undergoing clinical trials in the United States and abroad.[21-23]

Endovascular grafts are a combination of intravascular metallic stents and prosthetic graft materials. The stent functions as the fixation component of the endovascular graft, anchoring it to normal portions of the aorta and iliac arteries in lieu of standard suture anastomotic techniques. Fixation of the graft can be based on the column strength of the device, the net radial force that pushes outward onto the neck of the

aneurysm, or the suprarenal stent components. The stent can be made of nitinol, stainless steel, or a cobalt-chromium alloy. Gore-Tex (polytetrafluoroethylene [PTFE]) and Dacron are the fabrics most commonly used as the prosthetic graft material component of the endograft. Once the endovascular graft is fixed into position, blood should flow only through the endovascular graft, thereby excluding the aneurysm sac from the effects of blood pressure and blood flow. Endovascular grafts come in many types and configurations (Figure 28-2). It is not uncommon for endovascular aortic aneurysm repair to be supplemented by other ancillary procedures such as femorofemoral artery bypass, intra-arterial coil vessel occlusion, or other vessel occlusion procedures (Figure 28-3). Newer endovascular grafts can treat a variety of complex arterial pathologies, and their surveillance becomes more complex. Examples include grafts with hypogastric branches and endografts with incorporated proximal fenestrations and branches.

Since most aortic aneurysms are infrarenal, the proximal component of the endovascular

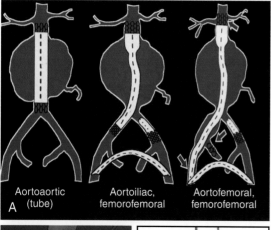

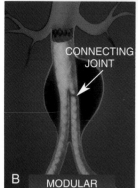

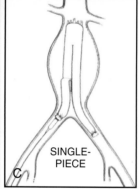

A Aortoaortic (tube)   Aortoiliac, femorofemoral   Aortofemoral, femorofemoral

B MODULAR — CONNECTING JOINT

C SINGLE-PIECE

FIGURE 28-2 Examples of the various configurations of endovascular grafts that may be encountered. **A,** On the left is a simple tube graft with stent attachments at the proximal and distal aneurysm necks. In the center is an aortoiliac endovascular graft, and on the right, an aortofemoral endovascular graft (used for complex aortoiliac aneurysm repair), with the *top blue arrow* indicating use of an occluding device and the *bottom blue arrow* an anastomotic site to a femoro-femoral by pass graft. Note the use of occluder devices and coils in the grafts in the center and right of the figure (also see Figure 28-3). The proximal stent crosses the renal arteries in the figure on the far right *(top blue arrow)*. **B,** A bifurcated modular device with a connecting joint. **C,** A single-piece, aorto-bi-iliac design.

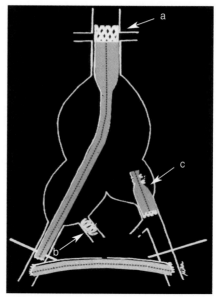

FIGURE 28-3 Multiple interventions performed in conjunction with aortounifemoral, femorofemoral endovascular graft. The proximal fixation site is located at the level of the renal arteries, and the stent crosses the renal arteries *(a)*. Coils have been deployed in the right internal iliac artery *(b)*, and an occluder device is deployed in the contralateral common iliac artery *(c)*, both to prevent backflow into the aneurysm sac. An endoluminal anastomosis is performed at the distal end of the endovascular graft in the right femoral artery. Outflow to the extremities is via the ipsilateral (right) common femoral artery and through a right-to-left femorofemoral graft. Retrograde flow in the left external iliac artery perfuses the pelvis.

TABLE 28-3 Advantages of Endovascular Graft Exclusion of Abdominal Aortic Aneurysms
• Procedure is performed from a remote site and avoids laparotomy.
• Small incisions (femoral, brachial, or carotid artery cutdown for access).
• No prolonged aortic clamping.
• Decreased or no stay in intensive care unit.
• Decreased length of stay (1-2 days for endovascular vs 6-8 days for open repair).
• Decreased recovery time (to resumption of normal activity level).

graft is deployed immediately below the lowest renal artery and extends distally as close as possible to the common iliac bifurcation. The device has an uncovered metal component when there is need for suprarenal fixation. The uncovered part of the stent crosses the orifices of the renal arteries. This design is thought to provide better fixation of the graft to the surrounding arterial wall, thereby reducing the potential for proximal graft migration and providing for a better proximal seal (Figure 28-4).

While the endovascular repair of AAAs offers many benefits (Table 28-3), there are several potential complications specific to this technique. The most significant of these complications are endoleaks[24,25] and graft migration. These two complications have been seen in all of the endovascular graft designs that have been used for endovascular AAA repair.

An endoleak is defined as blood flow outside of the endovascular graft into the aortic aneurysm sac. This leak pressurizes the aneurysm sac

Types of Grafts

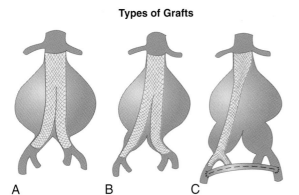

A   B   C

FIGURE 28-4 Various configurations seen in patients with coexisting aortic and iliac artery aneurysms. In type 2A, there is no distal iliac involvement, and an aorto-bi-iliac bifurcated endovascular graft to the proximal common iliac artery is used. In type 2B, there is common iliac artery involvement, and the bifurcated graft is extended to the distal common iliac artery bifurcation. In type 2C, there is extensive iliac artery involvement, and the endovascular graft configuration described in Figure 28-3 is used.

TABLE 28-4 Complications Associated With Endovascular Repair of Abdominal Aortic Aneurysms
Aneurysm growth
Embolization
Endoleak*
Fabric tears
Graft infection
Graft migration*
Limb thrombosis
Limb separation
Stent and/or attachment site fracture

*Common to all endovascular grafts used to date.

and leads to continued risk for aneurysm enlargement and rupture. The presence of an endoleak, therefore, negates the primary goal of the endovascular procedure and results in an aneurysm that remains inadequately treated.[11,24-30] Considerable progress in patient selection and surgical technique has reduced the overall rate of all types of complications seen after endovascular AAA repair (Table 28-4). Traditionally the optimal method for postendovascular graft screening and the most reliable method for detecting complications is a contrast CT scan. However, this method is invasive, expensive, and involves radiation exposure to the patient and risk for possible contrast nephrotoxicity. Color Doppler ultrasound has been increasingly and successfully used to follow patients after endograft placement. It can be used to identify patients who may require further intervention with or without the need for additional preprocedural imaging.[31,32]

COLOR DOPPLER ULTRASOUND TECHNIQUE

We generally allocate 60 to 90 minutes and up to 2 hours per study depending on the complexity of the intervention and the patient's body habitus. This allows enough time to prepare the patient and room, perform the imaging component of the examination, and provide a preliminary report for the interpreting physician after the scan is completed.

PATIENT PREPARATION

As with all abdominal scanning, the quality of the examination may be degraded in the obese or gaseous patient, and preprocedural patient preparation may be necessary. The patient may be required to fast overnight or for at least 8 hours before the study to decrease intestinal gas and avoid nonvisualization of the graft and attachment sites. Usually, no other patient preparation is necessary.

TECHNOLOGIST PREPARATION

Before ultrasound evaluation, the technologist/sonographer performs a brief history for symptoms of claudication (hip, buttock, or lower extremity) and impotence (as applicable), and a physical examination that includes palpation of the aortic and femoral pulses. An ankle-brachial index and/or pulse volume recording can be obtained bilaterally and compared to the preoperative measurement, where available, to ensure that baseline blood flow to the extremities has been maintained.

To perform a thorough and optimal examination of the endovascular graft, the examiner must have considerable knowledge of the endovascular technique and of the various endovascular graft designs and configurations that are available and must be familiar with the details of the surgical procedure.

To this end, a review of all previous imaging studies is mandatory. This includes any preoperative or postoperative CT scans, color Doppler scans, or angiograms, as well as any intraoperative imaging studies that have been performed. This review is important because the examiner must be familiar with the configuration and specific anatomy of the endovascular graft,[17,33,34] including the locations of the proximal and distal

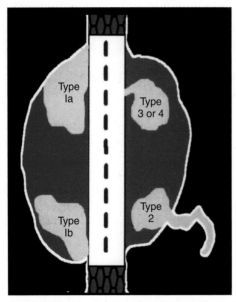

FIGURE 28-5 Potential endoleak sites. Types 1a and 1b: Leakage occurs at the proximal or distal stent attachment sites, as shown in yellow in the left panel. Type 2: Backflow enters the aneurysm sac from patent aortic branches (yellow, bottom right), or from back-bleeding through the iliac arteries. Type 3 or 4: Flow through the graft body itself (yellow, top right).

attachment sites. This information is used to document endovascular graft migration (if it occurs) and to identify all possible endoleak sources in advance of the color Doppler examination (Figure 28-5). In addition, review of the operative report or discussion with the operating surgeon is recommended to determine if the following apply: (1) coil embolization of branch vessels or use of other vessel occlusion devices, (2) supplemental proximal or distal arterial reconstructive procedures, and (3) other vessels have been treated with stents, either within the endovascular graft to support a portion of the graft or in the native artery to treat occlusive disease. The sonographic examination includes not only the aortic/iliac stent graft but also all other related arterial occlusion/reconstruction procedures.

ULTRASOUND EQUIPMENT

The examination is performed using a high-resolution, state-of-the-art, duplex scanner that provides color flow capability. A low-frequency (2.5-4 MHz) sector or curved array transducer is necessary to visualize these deep structures. A variety of differently configured (linear) and/or higher-frequency transducers may be needed to accomplish a complete study. The equipment selected must allow enough penetration to permit adequate insonation of the deep structures in the abdomen and pelvis with color flow sensitivity that allows the detection of slow flow velocities seen in endoleak, at reasonable frame rates.

The addition of color Doppler flow imaging is essential to the examination and allows for quick identification and evaluation of blood flow within the endovascular graft and aneurysm sac. The pulse repetition frequency (PRF) must be adjusted to allow for slow flow velocities in deep structures, and a narrow color box will maximize frame rate. Special attention must be directed to the color flow gain so as to not overgain and risk a false-positive result of endoleak based on the presence of color within the aneurysm sac. Conversely, undergaining may fail to detect the presence of a true endoleak. By convention we overgain the color flow image and then slowly decrease the gain to eliminate noise and color speckling within the image.

All studies are digitally recorded or videotaped for review by an interpreting physician, review by the sonographer/technologist before follow-up studies, and for archiving purposes.

GENERAL CONSIDERATIONS

Patients are generally scanned in the supine position initially using a midline approach; however, a left lateral decubitus position will facilitate visualization of the entirety of the aneurysm sac. Occasionally a right lateral decubitus approach may be necessary. These technically challenging studies will require multiple views to detect abnormalities that may not be appreciated in any one projection. Any examination that does not achieve visualization of the entire aneurysm sac may be considered of limited diagnostic value, and the examination can be repeated to correct the limitation, as deemed necessary by the interpreting physician.

TECHNICAL PROTOCOL[4,5]

Ultrasound assessment begins with identification of the intra-aneurysm sac portion of the endovascular graft in a transverse plane (Figure 28-6). The endovascular graft is then followed proximally to the superior attachment site, where the endovascular graft–artery interface is seen. This site is typically at, or immediately distal to, the level of the renal arteries, which are visible in the

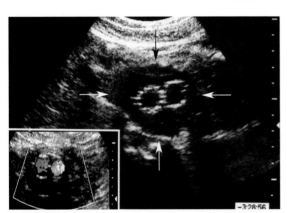

FIGURE 28-6 Transverse image of an abdominal aortic aneurysm treated with a bifurcated endovascular graft. The arrows mark the outer dimensions of the aortic sac. An encapsulated color flow image is seen in the lower left of the figure.

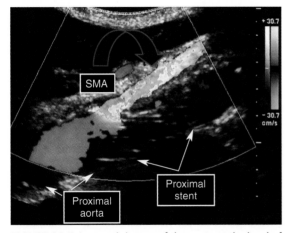

FIGURE 28-7 Long axis image of the aorta at the level of the superior mesenteric artery (SMA; *curved arrow*) origin. The proximal stent has been deployed distal to the SMA origin. The renal arteries, crossed by the proximal stent, are not seen in this projection.

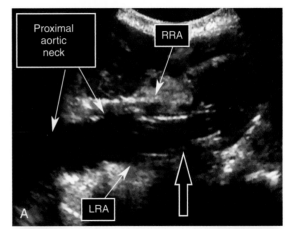

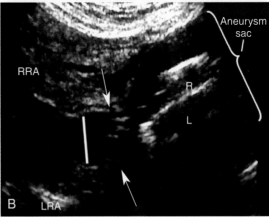

FIGURE 28-8 A, Long-axis image of the neck of an abdominal aortic aneurysm. The uncovered part of the stent has been deployed across the renal arteries in this patient. The large open arrow identifies the proximal stent. **B,** Long-axis image of an endovascular graft at the level of the proximal fixation site. On the left side of the image is the aortic neck. The diameter of the proximal neck is measured using electronic calipers *(solid white line)*. The arrows mark the stent. The right (R) and left (L) limbs of the endovascular graft are seen to the right of the image. LRA, left renal artery; RRA, right renal artery.

transverse plane. The renal arteries are important landmarks in the evaluation of endovascular AAA repair.

When the superior end of the endovascular graft is identified, the transducer is turned longitudinally to view the long axis of the aorta. Alternatively, longitudinal assessment of the aorta begins immediately inferior to the xiphoid process in the midline or slightly to the left.[35] After identification of the origins of the celiac or superior mesenteric arteries (Figure 28-7), scanning distally permits visualization of the stent or fixation component of the endovascular graft, which may cross the orifices of both renal arteries or may be deployed

immediately below the takeoff of the *lowest* renal artery (Figure 28-8).

The endovascular graft should be closely apposed to the arterial wall at the proximal end of the prosthesis. The aortic diameter at this site (proximal neck of the aneurysm) is measured and compared on follow-up examinations to assess for dilatation of the aneurysm neck, as this can result in endovascular graft migration and/or endoleak (see Figure 28-8). Occasionally the endovascular graft takes a sharp turn immediately distal to the proximal attachment site. This occurs because the endovascular graft follows the tortuous course of the aorta caused by the surrounding aneurysm.

After the proximal fixation site is identified and evaluated, the transducer is moved proximally and the suprarenal aorta is visualized and examined for defects, such as dissection and intimal flaps that may have resulted from the introduction and manipulation of devices used during endovascular graft deployment (e.g., catheters, guide wires, sheaths). Blood flow velocity is recorded immediately proximal to the endovascular graft device. The body of the endovascular graft is then scanned along its entire length in the color Doppler mode, and a search is made for sites of color flow signals and associated intraluminal defects. Flow velocities and waveforms are recorded in the intra-aneurysm portion of the graft body with particular attention to any sites of kinking and/or twisting that may result in stenosis and decreased distal flow.

For aortoiliac or aortofemoral endovascular grafts, the iliofemoral segment of the endovascular graft (and the femorofemoral crossover graft when present) is next examined for any abnormalities. Flow velocity and waveforms are obtained at the distal endovascular graft termination and in the outflow artery distal to the graft. For these and all other velocity measurements, typical procedures are followed: the Doppler angle is maintained at 60 degrees (or less if necessary), and the angle cursor is aligned so that it is parallel to the vessel/graft wall. The distal end of the endovascular graft is usually attached to the surrounding artery wall by the supporting stent of the endovascular graft but otherwise may be sutured endoluminally in the setting of a non-supported endovascular graft.[36]

To this point, the ultrasound examination has focused principally on the endovascular graft. The focus is then turned to the surrounding aneurysm sac. Special attention is directed to the detection of any flow outside the endovascular graft (endoleak), to measuring the size of the aneurysm sac (outer wall to outer wall of the original aneurysm), and to assessing for the presence and evolution of clot formation within the aneurysm sac.

Finally, a worksheet with a diagram detailing the anatomy of the endovascular graft, adjacent vessels, flow velocities and waveforms, and the site(s) of any abnormalities that are detected is created as a reference for follow-up studies. Ideally, the same examiner performs the follow-up studies; however, a detailed worksheet can avoid the problems of interexaminer or intraexaminer variability when serial studies are performed.

ENDOLEAK DETECTION

CT is considered by many to be the gold standard for the detection of endoleak following endovascular AAA repair. In skilled hands, however, color Doppler ultrasound is an accurate, cost-effective, noninvasive method to evaluate and follow endovascular grafts. It is a valuable adjunct to CT scanning and in some instances can be superior to CT. Because of its obvious advantages, color Doppler is now being advocated by many as the test of choice to screen for endoleaks and to follow aneurysm size serially.[31,32]

CT is fundamentally a static imaging system that requires precision in the timing of contrast injection and the acquisition of multiple image sets to obtain optimum diagnostic results. More than one CT scan is typically performed at the same imaging session. A typical study consists of scans taken without contrast, during the early venous phase and following a variable time delay. Several studies have demonstrated the superiority of color Doppler ultrasound over CT for identifying small, low-flow, type 2 side branch leaks, and for documenting the source of an endoleak.[3,6,8,9,10] These studies conclude that side branch endoleak is more readily detected with color Doppler because it is a real-time imaging modality (i.e., there is no dilution of contrast material and no need to obtain delayed images). Special care, however, must be taken to adjust the PRF/velocity range and color flow gain of the ultrasound equipment to allow for detection of the very low flow rates that exist in the aneurysm sac and are associated with type 2 endoleak.

Both CT and color Doppler confirm the diagnosis of endoleak by identifying the presence of active blood flow into the aneurysm sac. CT does this by documenting accumulation of contrast in the aneurysm sac, whereas color flow looks for flow signals within the aneurysm sac (Figure 28-9). Side branch endoleaks fill the aneurysm sac in a retrograde manner via patent collaterals and may fill the aneurysm sac slowly, which is a problem for CT, since a short time delay after contrast injection may fail to detect these leaks. This is not a problem for color Doppler imaging because it visualizes the leak directly, without the need for a contrast agent. In

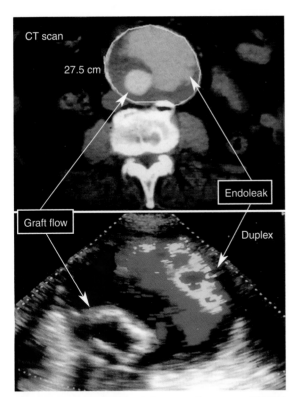

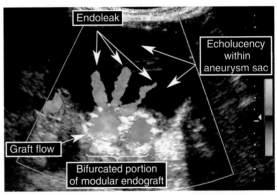

FIGURE 28-10 A type 3 endoleak. The flow in the aneurysm sac results from a defect at the junction of two limbs of a modular endovascular graft. Although thrombus has started to form, there are significant areas of echolucency within the aneurysm sac, suggesting the presence of endoleak confirmed by the color flow image.

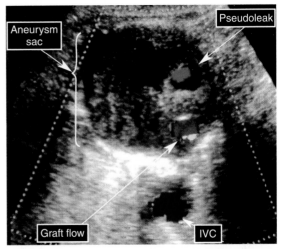

FIGURE 28-11 Cross-sectional color Doppler image of a pseudoleak. There is an area of color within a focal fluid collection (pseudoleak) within the aneurysm sac that results from transmitted pulsations from the nearby endovascular graft. Thrombus has filled the remainder of the sac. No endoleak source was identified, and the Doppler signal at the area of color was atypical and not consistently reproducible. This patient had a computed tomographic scan that was endoleak negative. IVC, inferior vena cava.

FIGURE 28-9 *Upper panel:* Computed tomographic (CT) scan with contrast that shows a large type Ia endoleak that arises from the proximal attachment site. Contrast is seen both in the endovascular graft (graft flow) and within the aneurysm sac. *Lower panel:* Duplex scan image of the same patient. The indwelling endovascular graft is seen in the lower left of the aneurysm sac (graft flow). Color is seen both within the endovascular graft and the aneurysm sac. Note how closely the duplex image resembles the CT scan.

an increasing number of laboratories, the use of color Doppler flow imaging is used to confirm or exclude the presence of an endoleak.

When an aneurysm is successfully treated, the blood within its sac tends to clot. These areas of thrombus are generally easy to visualize on the B-mode image. The examiner, therefore, must be suspicious for the presence of endoleak when echolucent areas are present within the aneurysm sac (Figure 28-10). These lucent areas within the sac must be fully interrogated with Doppler, as they may represent islands of non-clotted blood that still communicate with the arterial circulation (endoleak). In the early post-operative period, the movement of nonclotted blood within the aneurysm sac, caused by the pulsatile wall motion of the adjacent endovascular graft, may create color artifacts that mimic a true endoleak. We refer to this phenomenon

as a pseudoleak (Figure 28-11). Therefore, one must avoid the temptation to report an endoleak based solely on the presence of color flow within the aneurysm sac.

True endoleaks typically produce a uniform color Doppler appearance and should be easily reproducible. In order to reduce false-positive findings, the technologist must take special care to correctly readjust the PRF and color flow gain settings during the ultrasound examination. The use of spectral Doppler also can be helpful in this situation. Endoleaks should produce Doppler waveforms that are reproducible, similar to the flow patterns seen within the peripheral circulation, and synchronous with the patient's cardiac cycle.

Spectral Doppler may also play a role in distinguishing the endoleaks that may thrombose from those that might persist. A study by Carter and associates[37] revealed that endoleaks with very attenuated, monophasic, or bidirectional (to and fro) Doppler waveforms in the source vessel tended to occlude spontaneously, whereas the presence of normal, biphasic peripheral flow waveforms in the source vessel portended endoleak persistence. The number of patients in this study was small, however, and these preliminary results have not yet correlated with our experience.

As noted earlier, a thorough examination to determine the presence of endoleak not only includes visualization of the endovascular graft attachment sites and the graft body, but also visualization and interrogation of the *entire* AAA sac, in both the long and short axis. Thorough assessment also requires color Doppler interrogation of all potential leak sites suggested by the preoperative, intraoperative, and postoperative imaging studies. It is critical, therefore, that the vascular technologist be cognizant of the results of any preoperative imaging studies, the sites for potential endoleaks, and the details of the surgical procedure, including any problems that occurred preoperatively, intraoperatively, or during any postoperative supplemental procedures.

In our opinion, definitive identification of a distinct site of abnormal Doppler signals is the most important step needed to confirm a true endoleak. It is important to examine the entire aneurysm sac, identify patent side branches, and document the direction of flow within these side branches in an attempt to identify the source of any endoleak. In addition, this must be done in multiple approaches, because endoleak can be positional in nature. For example, some endoleaks can occur when the patient is standing and be absent when the patient is supine.

Endoleak flow can originate from proximal or distal endovascular graft attachment sites (type 1) (Figure 28-12), through the endovascular graft itself (types 3 or 4), or from patent aortic branches (side branch or type 2 endoleaks) (Figures 28-13 and 28-14). Potential arterial

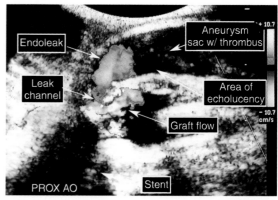

FIGURE 28-12 Type 1a endoleak. Long-axis image at the level of the proximal aortic attachment site (PROX AO). Flow is entering the aneurysm sac through a channel at the proximal attachment site (endoleak). Note the area of echolucency near the endoleak flow.

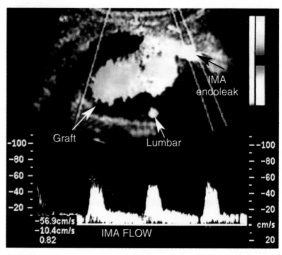

FIGURE 28-13 Type 2 endoleak. In this patient with a bifurcated endovascular graft, the inferior mesenteric artery (IMA) is seen in the upper right of the ultrasound image and is the channel for outflow, and a lumbar artery posteriorly is the afferent tract. The sample volume placed within the lumen of the IMA yields a negative Doppler shift, confirming the IMA to be the outflow tract.

sources for type 2 endoleaks include the lumbar arteries, the inferior mesenteric artery (IMA), the hypogastric arteries, the right gonadal artery, and accessory renal arteries that communicate with the aneurysm.[24] The IMA is typically found sonographically anterior and to the left of the aneurysm sac. The lumbar arteries are located posterior to the aneurysm sac, and the right gonadal artery inferior to the renal artery. The accessory renal arteries may be seen at any location (Figures 28-12 to 28-15).

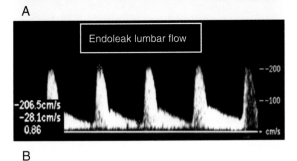

A

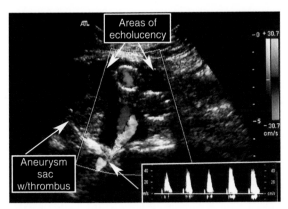

B

FIGURE 28-14 Combination endoleak. **A,** This patient has inflow from a proximal attachment site defect (type 1a) not seen in this projection and outflow via multiple patent lumbar arteries (type 2). **B,** Because of the direct aortic inflow, velocity in the lumbar artery is in excess of 200 cm/sec.

FIGURE 28-15 Type 2 endoleak with a single lumbar artery acting as both the outflow and inflow tracts. The corresponding spectral waveform is on the bottom right of the image. The spectral waveform captured in the lumbar artery in systole yields a positive Doppler shift.

Even in the absence of detectable flow within the sac, Doppler flow signals seen in the IMA or in the lumbar arteries adjacent to the aneurysm sac indicate the presence of an endoleak, because these vessels should occlude after deployment of

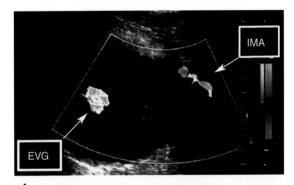

A

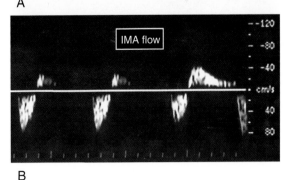

B

FIGURE 28-16 A cross-sectional image of an abdominal aortic aneurysm after endovascular graft repair with a type 2 endoleak. **A,** The endovascular graft (EVG) is seen as an area of color flow within the aneurysm sac. The inferior mesenteric artery (IMA) is clearly patent and perfusing the aneurysm sac (although in this image the flow within the sac is not seen). In this case, the IMA acts as both inflow and outflow channel. **B,** This phenomenon is reflected in the spectral waveform (to-and-fro flow similar to a pseudoaneurysm tract) but is strikingly different (velocity and morphology) from the spectral waveform seen in Figure 28-15. The prognostic value of the waveform information is yet to be determined.

the endovascular graft. If these vessels are patent, the flow direction must be assessed to determine whether the vessels are afferent or efferent channels, relative to the aneurysm sac (Figure 28-16).

In cases where no endoleak is identified yet the aneurysm sac continues to grow, special care must be taken to evaluate the aneurysm sac from multiple projections and with the patient in various positions, including supine, upright, and right and left lateral decubitus. Endoleaks can be positional in nature and seen in one but not other imaging windows or patient positions.

ANEURYSM SIZE

After endovascular AAA repair, aneurysms that have been totally excluded from the circulation usually decrease in size or remain stable (Figure 28-17).

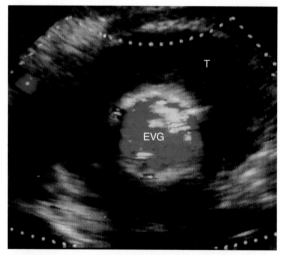

FIGURE 28-17 This cross-sectional color Doppler image shows complete exclusion after endovascular graft repair. There is color flow seen only with the indwelling endovascular graft (EVG). The *T* seen above the endovascular graft indicates thrombus that has completely filled the residual aneurysm sac.

Conversely, AAAs with a documented endoleak often increase in size. It is therefore critical to measure AAA sac size at every examination. A transverse sweep of the aneurysm sac is performed to determine the site of its maximal diameter. With the scan plane aligned with the short axis of the vessel, the outer-to-outer diameter of the aneurysm sac is measured in the anteroposterior and transverse planes, and an image is obtained with recorded measurements (Figure 28-18). The image plane is then oriented with the long axis of the aneurysm, and the maximum anteroposterior dimension is again measured and recorded. Review of previous imaging studies is recommended to ensure that the location of the current measurements corresponds with those obtained previously. Comparison of CT and ultrasound measurements taken at different times is not recommended.[38] Any patient with a significant increase in aneurysm size (>0.5 cm) detected with ultrasound during the follow-up period should be suspected of having an endoleak, even if no leak can be shown, and further imaging with CT or contrast arteriography should be performed as indicated.

ENDOVASCULAR GRAFT DEFORMITY AND NATIVE ARTERY COMPLICATIONS

Late postoperative kinking of the endovascular graft body within the aneurysm sac can develop despite having been absent in the perioperative

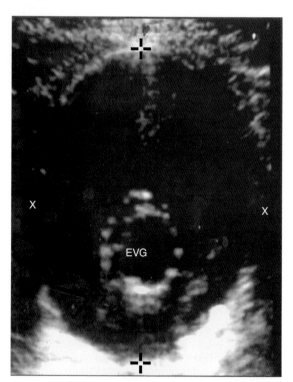

FIGURE 28-18 Transverse image of a large (7.16 cm anteroposterior × 7.47 cm transverse) abdominal aortic aneurysm with an indwelling endovascular graft (EVG). Note the cursors on the anteroposterior and lateral walls of the aneurysm. Aortic aneurysm size should be measured at the level of maximal aneurysm size and/or at the proximal and mid aorta.

or early postoperative period. The cause of such kinking is likely due to continued increase in the diameter or length of the aneurysm sac, leading to buckling of the aorta. Morphologic alterations of this sort can lead to significant conformational changes of the sac and the indwelling endovascular graft. Ultimately this can lead to disassociation or kinking of the endovascular graft limb(s). Possible consequences include lower extremity ischemia, due to kinking and decreased flow, or endoleak, due to disassociation of the endograft limbs. When the aorta is effectively excluded and shrinks in diameter or length, this subjects the endovascular graft to stress, especially at limb junctions and at the proximal and/or distal attachment sites. The consequence, once again, may be a late-onset endoleak.

Endovascular graft deformation, in the form of extrinsic graft compression, twisting (torsion), or kinking can lead to stenosis or thrombosis of the distal endovascular graft limb(s), potentially causing lower extremity ischemia. The superiority of ultrasound for demonstrating these problems has been documented in several studies[2,39] and is largely due to the dynamic, real-time capabilities of ultrasound, as opposed to the limited temporal sampling of CT.

Extrinsic endovascular graft compression is sometimes caused by atherosclerotic plaque in the wall of the artery that surrounds the endovascular graft but is usually due to tortuosity of the endovascular graft. Because these atherosclerotic stenotic lesions have been excluded from the arterial circulation, they may not progress. They are followed, however, per our endovascular graft surveillance protocol, in the setting of aortoiliac arterial occlusive disease.[2] Hemodynamically significant atherosclerotic plaques cause focal increases in flow velocity along the iliofemoral limb of the endovascular graft. When deemed to be flow limiting on the basis of spectral Doppler findings (see Chapter 17), they are treated with balloon angioplasty, with or without stenting. Kinks and twists are often due to severe vessel tortuosity or graft redundancy (excessive graft length) and can cause hemodynamically significant flow reduction.

Another consideration during endograft follow-up is iatrogenic trauma to the distal vessels secondary to arterial manipulations performed through tortuous and diseased vessels during endovascular graft deployment. Such trauma may cause various complications, including dissection, intramural or extramural hematoma, pseudoaneurysm, arteriovenous fistula, and emboli to the lower extremities. The ultrasound findings associated with these complications are described elsewhere in this text.

Personal Commentary

Color Doppler endovascular graft evaluation is a technically challenging endeavor that should be reserved for senior-level technologists. These individuals must be facile with ultrasound technique, have accrued the considerable skills required to scan the deep structures of the abdomen, and have extensive knowledge of the endovascular exclusion of AAAs and its associated complications. In addition, there must be a commitment to endovascular graft evaluation on the part of the technologist, the interpreting physician, and the institution. The major weaknesses of the majority of the negative literature reports concerning color Doppler endovascular graft assessment can be attributed to a lack of commitment to the education of the technologist, a lack of appropriate time allocation for performing

the examinations, and opposition to investment of funds for the high-end, state-of-the-art equipment necessary to adequately image aortic endovascular grafts. Those facilities that have made these commitments have had excellent results using color Doppler in this setting.

Another important factor standing in the way of the color Doppler technique is a lack of standardization of the endovascular graft examination protocol, such as we see in other areas of vascular ultrasound (e.g., lower extremity venous and cerebrovascular testing) where color Doppler is proven to be extremely accurate and has been widely accepted as the gold standard. With the increasing prevalence of the endovascular technique, and continued sharing of common experiences among vascular laboratories around the country, we feel that this weakness can be overcome. In addition, the Society for Vascular Ultrasound has published examination guidelines that should further decrease the variability seen in the performance of this examination.[40]

Finally, the addition of ultrasound contrast agents to the color Doppler examination has been shown to increase the sensitivity of ultrasound to the detection of endoleak (see Chapter 4).[3,41] Although not currently approved for widespread use in the United States, this adjunctive procedure, in addition to advances in ultrasound technology such as tissue harmonic imaging, promises to add to the utility of color Doppler ultrasound for the detection of endoleak.

Sac Pressure Measurement

Some authors have recommended sac pressure monitoring[42-45] as an alternative to image-based follow-up. The pressure measurements obtained with an implantable sensor have been shown to correlate well with the pressure measurements obtained through a catheter in the sac, and low sac pressures predict aneurysm shrinkage. One potential role for monitoring sac pressure is for cases of known type 2 endoleak. Currently, aneurysm dilatation is the primary indication for reintervention. At this time, the use of wireless pressure sensors is not widespread.

Conclusions

This chapter reviews the complications associated with endovascular AAA repair and demonstrates the effectiveness of color Doppler sonography for their evaluation. As with the entire field of endovascular surgery, imaging techniques and recommendations regarding endovascular graft use are evolving rapidly. Although contrast arteriography and spiral CT are important methods for endovascular graft evaluation, we feel that a combination of examinations is superior to any single test. In centers of excellence, color Doppler is an important adjunctive study and can decrease the required frequency for more expensive studies, such as CT, thus allowing color Doppler to be the principal screening modality in the postoperative period for endoleak detection and surveillance after endovascular exclusion of AAAs. Finally, because of its noninvasive nature, patient compliance and satisfaction may also be improved by the use of ultrasound.

REFERENCES

1. Berdejo GL, et al: Value of color Doppler ultrasonography in the planning and assessment of endovascular stented grafts for traumatic arterial injuries, *J Vasc Technol* 20(3):178, 1996. (Abstract).
2. Berdejo GL, et al: Color Doppler ultrasonography for the evaluation of endovascular PTFE stented grafts for occlusive disease, *J Vasc Technol* 21(1):11–15, 1997.
3. Heilberger P, et al: Postoperative color flow duplex scanning in aortic endografting, *J Endovasc Surg* 4:262–271, 1997.
4. Johnson BL, et al: Color duplex evaluation of endoluminal aortic stent grafts, *J Vasc Technol* 22(2):97–104, 1998.
5. Berdejo GL, et al: Color duplex ultrasound evaluation of transluminally placed endovascular grafts for aneurysm repair, *J Vasc Technol* 22(4):201–207, 1998.
6. Sato DT, et al: Endoleak after aortic stent graft repair: Diagnosis by color duplex ultrasound vs. CT scan, *J Vasc Surg* 28(4):657–663, 1998.
7. Lyon RT, Berdejo GL, Veith FJ: Ultrasound imaging techniques for evaluation of endovascular stented grafts. In Parodi JC, Veith FJ, Marin ML, editors: *Endovascular Grafting Techniques*, Media, PA, 1999, Williams & Wilkins.
8. Wolf YG, et al: Duplex ultrasonography vs. CT angiography for postoperative evaluation of endovascular abdominal aortic aneurysms repair, *J Vasc Surg* 32(6):1142–1148, 2000.
9. Zannetti S, et al: Role of duplex scan in endoleak detection after endoluminal aortic repair, *Eur J Vasc Endovasc Surg* 19:531–535, 2000.
10. Parent FN, et al: The incidence and natural history of type 1 and 2 endoleak: A 5 year follow-up assessment with color duplex ultrasound scan, *J Vasc Surg* 35(3):474–481, 2002.
11. Matsumura JS, Moore WS: Clinical consequences of periprosthetic leak after endovascular repair of abdominal aortic aneurysm, *J Vasc Surg* 27:606–613, 1998.
12. Matsumura JS, et al: Reduction in aortic aneurysm size: Early Results after endovascular graft placement, *J Vasc Surg* 25(1):113–123, 1997.
13. Gilling-Smith G, et al: Endotension after endovascular aneurysm repair: definition, classification and strategies for surveillance and intervention, *J Endovasc Surg* 6(4):305–307, 1999.
14. White GH, May J: How should endotension be defined? History of a concept and evolution of a new term, *J Endovasc Ther* 7(6):435–438, 2000. discussion 439-440.
15. Gilling-Smith G, et al: Freedom from endoleak after endovascular aneurysm repair does not equal treatment success, *Eur J Vasc Endovasc Surg* 19(4):421–425, 2000.
16. Parodi JC, Palmaz JC, Barone HD: Transfemoral intraluminal graft implantation for abdominal aortic aneurysms, *Ann Vasc Surg* 5:491–499, 1991.
17. Veith FJ, et al: Guidelines for development and use of transluminally placed endovascular prosthetic grafts in the arterial system, *J Vasc Surg* 21:67–685, 1995.
18. Marin ML, et al: Transfemoral endovascular stented graft treatment of aorto-iliac and femoropopliteal occlusive disease for limb salvage, *Am J Surg* 168:156–162, 1994.
19. Panetta TF, Marin ML, Veith FJ: Endovascular stent grafts in the management of vascular trauma. In Veith FJ, editor: *Current Critical Problems in Vascular Surgery*, Vol 6, St. Louis, MO, 1994, Quality Medical Publishing, Inc.
20. Lipsitz EC, Ohki T, Veith FJ: Overview of techniques and devices for endovascular abdominal aortic aneurysm repair, *Semin Interv Cardiol* 5(1):21–28, 2000.
21. Zarins CK, et al: The AneuRx stent graft: Four year results and worldwide experience 2000, *J Vasc Surg* 33(2 Suppl):S135–S145, 2001.
22. Moore WS, Rutherford RB: Transfemoral endovascular repair of abdominal aortic aneurysms: Results of the North American EVT Phase 1 Trial, *J Vasc Surg* 23:543–553, 1996.
23. Greenberg R: Zenith investigators. The zenith AAA endovascular graft for abdominal aortic aneurysms: clinical update, *Semin Vasc Surg* 16(2):151–157, 2003.
24. Wain RA, et al: Endoleaks after endovascular graft treatment of aortic aneurysms: classification, risk factors and outcome, *J Vasc Surg* 27:69–80, 1998.
25. White GH, Yu W, May J: Endoleak—a proposed new terminology to describe incomplete aneurysm exclusion by an endoluminal graft, *J Endovasc Surg* 3:124–125, 1996.
26. Zarins CK, White RA, Fogarty TJ: Aneurysm rupture after endovascular repair using AneuRx stent graft, *J Vasc Surg* 31:960–970, 2000.
27. Chuter TA, et al: Clinical experience with a bifurcated endovascular graft for abdominal aortic aneurysm repair, *J Vasc Surg* 24:655–666, 1996.
28. White GH, Yu W, May J: Endoleak following endoluminal repair of AAA: Diagnosis, significance and management, *J Endovasc Surg* 3:339–340, 1996. (abstract).
29. Zarins CK, White RA, Fogarty TJ: Aneurysm rupture after endovascular repair using the AneuRx stent graft, *J Vasc Surg* 31(5):960–970, 2000.
30. Lumsden AB, Allen RC, Chaikoff EL: Delayed rupture of aortic aneurysms following endovascular stent grafting, *Am J Surg* 170:174–178, 1995.
31. Chaer RA, et al: Duplex ultrasound as the sole long-term surveillance method post-endovascular aneurysm repair: a safe alternative for stable aneurysms, *J Vasc Surg* 49(4):845–849, 2009. discussion 849-50.
32. Beeman BR, et al: Duplex ultrasound factors predicting persistent type 2 endoleak and increasing AAA sac diameter after EVAR, *J Vasc Surg* 52(5):1147–1152, 2010.
33. Chuter T, DeWeese JA: Treatment of abdominal aortic aneurysm by endovascular grafting. In Ernst CB, Stanley JC. (eds): *Current Therapy in Vascular Surgery*, ed 3, St. Louis, MO: Mosby-Yearbook Inc., pp 265–270.

34. May J, White GH, Harris JP: Devices for aortic aneurysm repair, *Surg Clin North Am* Vol. 79:507–527, June 1999. No 3.

35. Cramer MM: Color flow duplex examination of the abdominal aorta: atherosclerosis, aneurysm and dissection, *J Vasc Technol* 19(5-6):249–260, 1995.

36. Wain RA, et al: Alternative techniques for management of distal anastomoses of aortofemoral and iliofemoral endovascular grafts, *J Vasc Surg* 32(2):307–314, 2000.

37. Carter KA, et al: Doppler Waveform Assessment of Endoleak Following Repair of Abdominal Aortic Aneurysm: Predictors of endoleak thrombosis, *J Vasc Technol* 24(2):119–122, 2000.

38. Sprouse RL, et al: Comparison of abdominal aortic aneurysm diameter measurements obtained with ultrasound and computed tomography: Is there a difference? *J Vasc Surg* 38:466–472, 2003.

39. Lyon RT, et al: *Utility of operative intravascular ultrasound for the assessment of endovascular procedures*, Boston, MA, 1997 June 1-4, Proceedings of the Joint Annual Meeting of the Society for Vascular Surgery / North American Chapter, International Society for Cardiovascular Surgery.

40. *"Members Only" Section of the Society for Vascular Ultrasound website*, www.svunet.org.

41. Napoli V, et al: Abdominal aortic aneurysm: Contrast enhanced US for missed endoleaks after endoluminal repair, *Radiology* 233:217–225, 2004.

42. Ellozy SH, et al: First experience in human beings with a permanently implantable intrasac pressure transducer for monitoring endovascular repair of abdominal aortic aneurysms, *J Vasc Surg* 40:405–412, 2004.

43. Ohki T, et al: Initial results of wireless pressure sensing for endovascular aneurysm repair: the APEX Trial—Acute Pressure Measurement to Confirm Aneurysm Sac EXclusion, *J Vasc Surg* 45:236–242, 2007.

44. Hoppe H, et al: Aortic aneurysm sac pressure measurements after endovascular repair using an implantable remote sensor: initial experience and short-term follow-up, *Eur Radiol* 18:957–965, 2008.

45. Hinnen JW, et al: Aneurysm sac pressure monitoring: Does the direction of pressure measurement matter in fibrinous thrombus? *J Vasc Surg* 245:812–816, 2007.

ULTRASOUND ASSESSMENT OF THE SPLANCHNIC (MESENTERIC) ARTERIES

29

MARGARITA V. REVZIN, MS, MD, and JOHN S. PELLERITO, MD, FACR, FSRU, FAIUM

Color and pulsed Doppler evaluation of the splanchnic arteries is performed to evaluate for possible compromise of intestinal blood flow in patients presenting with abdominal pain. This examination is frequently requested for patients with abdominal pain that is unexplained, chronic, and atypical. The concern is that decreased blood flow to the bowel could be the cause of the patient's symptoms. This examination includes the evaluation of the abdominal aorta, celiac, superior mesenteric (SMA), and inferior mesenteric (IMA) arteries. Doppler ultrasonography can assess vessel patency, degree of vessel lumen stenosis, and the number of arteries affected, factors that are critical for patient management. Similar to the examination of the renal arteries, these studies are technically challenging and rely on operator experience and expertise. This chapter provides a review of general concepts, technical factors, diagnostic criteria, and insights that allow for the successful evaluation of the splanchnic arteries:

ANATOMY, PHYSIOLOGY, AND NATURAL HISTORY OF BOWEL ISCHEMIA

ANATOMY

Understanding the mesenteric circulation provides a foundation for the interpretation of the sonographic examination. The splanchnic, or mesenteric, arteries comprise the celiac, superior mesenteric, and inferior mesenteric arteries (Figure 29-1). All three vessels arise from the abdominal aorta. The celiac artery is the first major branch of the abdominal aorta. The SMA is located just inferiorly to the celiac artery. On occasion, the celiac and SMA may share a common origin or trunk. The renal arteries are the next major branches of the abdominal aorta and arise laterally, toward the kidneys. The IMA

is identified just below the renal arteries and originates at the left anterolateral aspect of the abdominal aorta. The IMA can be identified in the majority of patients studied for mesenteric insufficiency.

The celiac artery supplies blood to the solid visceral organs (liver, pancreas, and spleen) and the stomach and proximal small bowel. The SMA supplies the bowel from the duodenum to the splenic flexure. The IMA supplies the descending and rectosigmoid colon. A rich collateral network exists between the different mesenteric vessels through the mesenteric arcades and marginal artery. Additional vascular protection is obtained from direct communication between the three mesenteric arteries. Communication between the celiac artery and the SMA occurs by way of the gastroduodenal artery (also known as the pancreatoduodenal arcade; Figure 29-2, A). The superior and inferior mesenteric arteries are connected by the arc of Riolan and the marginal artery of Drummond. The arc of Riolan, also known as the "meandering mesenteric artery" connects the middle colic artery with the left colic artery, and the marginal artery of Drummond connects the ileocolic, right colic, and middle colic branches of the SMA with the left colic and sigmoid branches of the IMA (Figure 29-2, B). In addition, communication also exists between the IMA and branches of the internal iliac arteries. Given this extensive collateral circulation, patients may remain asymptomatic despite the presence of severe mesenteric vascular disease.[1-4] In general, severe compromise (>70% stenosis or occlusion) of at least two of the three mesenteric arteries is required for symptoms of mesenteric ischemia to be present. Mesenteric stenosis or occlusion of a single vessel does not usually produce symptoms in light of a patent collateral network. The "two-vessel rule" holds in most patients and is utilized clinically for the diagnosis of chronic mesenteric ischemia.[5]

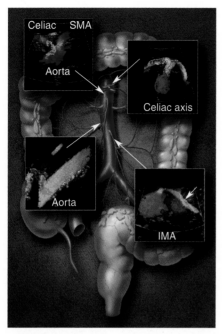

FIGURE 29-1 Montage with normal color flow images of the aorta, celiac artery, superior mesenteric artery (SMA), and inferior mesenteric artery (IMA).

PHYSIOLOGY

Normal flow patterns differ between the celiac artery and the mesenteric arteries (Figure 29-3). The celiac artery supplies blood to the low-resistance vascular beds of the liver, spleen, and stomach via the hepatic, splenic, and left gastric branches. Pulsed Doppler demonstrates low-resistance flow in the celiac artery, with high end-diastolic velocities (Figure 29-4, *A*). This low-resistance flow pattern relates to the need for continuous forward flow in both systole and diastole to supply the high oxygen demands of the liver and spleen throughout the cardiac cycle. This flow pattern is similar to the low-resistance signals seen in the renal and internal carotid arteries. The celiac artery low-resistance flow pattern is not dependent on food intake. In other words, there is no significant change in peak systolic or end-diastolic velocities obtained from the celiac artery after a meal.[6-9]

The superior and inferior mesenteric arteries supply the high-resistance vascular beds of the small intestine and colon. Pulsed Doppler examination reveals high impedance flow with low diastolic velocities in the fasting state (Figure 29-4, *B*). This is due to the relative vasoconstriction of the splanchnic branch vessels before a meal, when the bowel is empty and quiescent. After a meal, there is an increase in mesenteric arterial blood

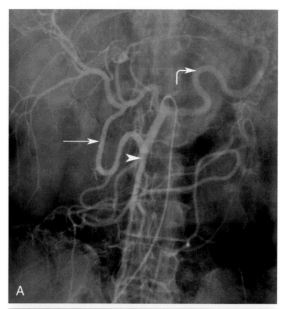

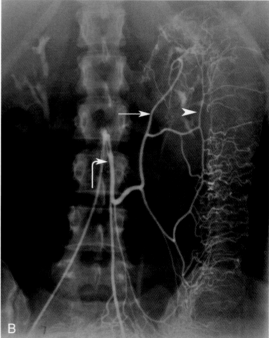

FIGURE 29-2 A, Selective superior mesenteric artery (SMA) arteriogram demonstrating gastroduodenal artery *(straight arrow)* serving as a collateral between the celiac artery and SMA *(arrowhead)*. Note splenic artery *(curved arrow)*. **B,** Selective inferior mesenteric artery (IMA) arteriogram demonstrating IMA *(curved arrow)*, portions of the arc of Riolan *(straight arrow)* and marginal artery of Drummond *(arrowhead)*.

flow to assist digestion. Vasodilatation of the mesenteric branches allows increased blood flow to the intestines. Moneta and colleagues[10] showed that both peak systolic and end-diastolic velocities increase after a meal. The authors described at

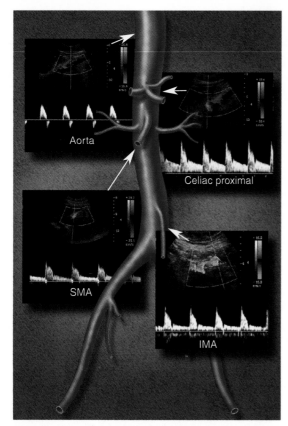

FIGURE 29-3 Montage of normal Doppler waveforms. IMA, inferior mesenteric artery; SMA, superior mesenteric artery.

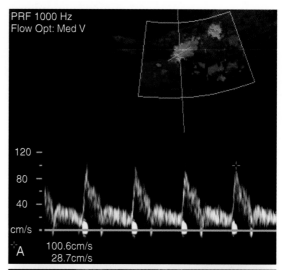

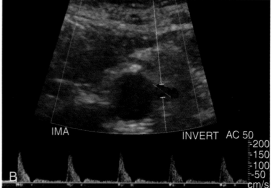

FIGURE 29-4 **A,** Pulsed Doppler waveforms of the celiac artery with low-resistance flow with high-diastolic velocity. **B,** Pulsed Doppler waveforms from the inferior mesenteric artery (IMA) with a high-resistance flow pattern.

least doubling of the end-diastolic velocity (EDV) in the SMA after eating. They found the greatest increase in flow after a meal that includes fat, carbohydrate, and protein, and they concluded that this provocative test provides a mechanism for evaluating the reactivity of the splanchnic circulation. The presence of increased flow velocities after a meal was used to infer the adequacy of the splanchnic blood supply in their studies.

Although duplex ultrasound examinations of the mesenteric arteries can be performed before and after a meal to identify physiologic changes in blood flow, there appears to be significant variability in the response to food. Healy and associates[11] found that postprandial duplex studies were not dependable and did not improve diagnostic accuracy in their series of patients. We no longer routinely perform preprandial and postprandial duplex examinations of the mesenteric vessels because we found these examinations to be less reliable for the diagnosis of stenosis, as compared with other direct measurements.

NATURAL HISTORY OF BOWEL ISCHEMIA

Mesenteric ischemia can be classified into four major subcategories according to the cause of vascular compromise. Acute arterial occlusive disease is caused by embolus, thrombosis, or external compression of the vessel. Doppler sonography is generally not useful in this situation because of the rapid time course of the disease and necessity for emergent intervention. Nonobstructive mesenteric arterial insufficiency is the second subcategory and is attributable to hypotensive shock, blood loss, or sepsis that leads to insufficient blood supply to the bowel. Treatment of the underlying condition is key to the management of this type of bowel ischemia. The third category of bowel ischemia is related to venoocclusive disease. Unfortunately, Doppler sonography plays a lesser role in the investigation of this type of bowel ischemia because of the limited ability to detect

slow venous blood flow in the main mesenteric and portal veins and their branches. Contrast-enhanced computed tomography (CT) or magnetic resonance imaging (MRI) are more valuable to assess venous patency. The fourth type is chronic mesenteric ischemia (CMI), which in 95% of cases is attributable to atherosclerotic disease causing arterial stenosis or occlusion in the main mesenteric arteries.[12] This condition typically occurs in older adult patients with stenosis or occlusion of at least two of the three principal mesenteric vessels (celiac, SMA, and IMA).[13] Doppler sonography can play a major role in screening patients with suspected chronic mesenteric ischemia.[14-16]

Patients with suspected *chronic* mesenteric ischemia classically present with abdominal pain apparently related to recent ingestion of a meal. Patients typically complain of postprandial pain, bloating, weight loss, and diarrhea. They may describe a "fear of food," as they experience pain after meals. They may change their diet or eating habits to more frequent, smaller meals to avoid discomfort. In some cases, this change of eating habits is not recognized by the patient, who notes only weight loss. Other patients have a confusing clinical picture with vague symptoms of pain that may or may not be related to meals.[17] CMI should be considered in older adult patients with unexplained abdominal pain and weight loss.

Evaluation of the mesenteric arteries is helpful to work through the differential diagnosis in this group of patients with an unclear etiology for their clinical symptoms. Until recently, visceral angiography was the primary diagnostic modality used in the assessment of patients with suspected CMI. With advances in technology, Doppler ultrasound, MR and CT angiography have proven to be accurate noninvasive alternatives to conventional arteriography for the evaluation of mesenteric arteries.[18-20] Advantages of Doppler ultrasonography include direct evaluation of all three mesenteric vessels, assessment of the hemodynamics of blood flow, and determination of the significance of lesions involving the visceral vessels. It is an inexpensive, noninvasive method that requires no radiation or contrast material, can be performed portably, and does not have any of the inherent risks associated with other angiographic studies.[14] Doppler ultrasound determines the hemodynamic significance of stenotic lesions by demonstrating prestenotic and poststenotic waveform changes. These findings can influence the decision to intervene in the appropriate clinical setting.

TECHNIQUE

The duplex and color Doppler examination of the mesenteric arteries usually includes the evaluation of the proximal abdominal aorta as well as the ostia and proximal portions of the celiac, SMA, and IMA. The distal segments of the mesenteric arteries cannot be seen with ultrasound. Most atherosclerotic lesions typically occur at the ostia of these vessels, and this is the main focus of investigation.

In preparation for our abdominal Doppler studies, we ask our patients to fast for at least 12 hours. This reduces the amount of scatter and attenuation from intra-abdominal bowel gas. Fasting also avoids the elevated velocities noted in the postprandial state, which can be confused with stenotic flow. We give no medication before the examination. Mesenteric Doppler studies should be performed on modern ultrasound instruments with high-quality color and power Doppler imaging and with sensitive pulsed Doppler capability. Given that mesenteric vessels are situated deep in the abdomen, a Doppler scanner with a low-frequency 2- to 5-MHz convex (curvilinear) transducer is used. This allows for adequate visualization and resolution over a large field of view.

Patients are examined most often in the supine position by way of an anterior approach. If visualization of the vessels is limited because of overlying bowel gas, patients may be turned to the decubitus or oblique positions for better visualization of the vessels of interest, occasionally using the liver as an acoustic window. During the study, the patient is asked to breath-hold or breathe quietly to obtain adequate Doppler spectral samples.

The aorta is evaluated by an anterior approach by placing the transducer just below the xiphoid process of the sternum. Transverse and sagittal planes are used for evaluation of aortic diameter and velocity. The aorta lies anterior to the spine and slightly to the left of midline throughout its course. The evaluation of the abdominal aorta is included in the mesenteric examination to assess for aortic aneurysm, dissection, and significant atherosclerotic disease.

Visualization of the celiac artery origin is initially performed in the sagittal plane. On the transverse view, the branches of the celiac artery have a distinctive appearance with a T-shaped bifurcation ("seagull sign"; Figure 29-5, *A*). The

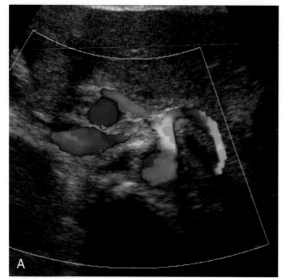

A

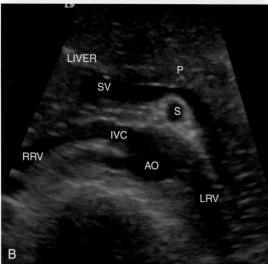

LIVER

SV

P

S

IVC

RRV

AO

LRV

B

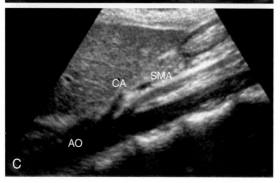

CA

SMA

AO

C

FIGURE 29-5 A, Transverse color Doppler image reveals a T-shaped bifurcation, the characteristic landmark of the celiac artery. **B,** Anatomic relationships of the superior mesenteric artery (SMA; S). Transverse gray-scale image shows the SMA surrounded by a layer of echogenic fat. Anterior to the SMA is the pancreas (P), posterior to the SMA is the aorta (AO), to the left is the left renal vein (LRV), and to the right is the right renal vein (RRV) and inferior vena cava (IVC). Splenic vein (SV) is situated between the pancreas and SMA. **C,** Sagittal gray-scale image shows the abdominal aorta (AO), celiac artery (CA), and SMA.

by a prominent ring of retroperitoneal fat that separates the SMA from the pancreas. In patients with normal bowel rotation, the SMA lies to the right of the superior mesenteric vein (SMV). The splenic vein and pancreas lie anterior to the SMA, whereas the left renal vein is situated posteriorly. (Figure 29-5, *B* and *C*). Visualization of these anatomic structures helps to avoid possible misinterpretation and errors in diagnosis in patients with variant vascular anatomy. One of the most common vascular variants is a separate origin of one of the celiac artery branches arising directly from the aorta or from the SMA. The IMA can be found on the transverse view arising from the anterolateral aspect of the aorta just below the renal arteries.

Several techniques are utilized to optimize assessment of the mesenteric vessels. Harmonic imaging is routinely employed to improve resolution and decrease noise in the image. It has been noted in the literature that studies performed by experienced vascular technologists, sonographers, or sonologists provide the best results.[21] Indeed, we have noted that our finest abdominal vascular studies are performed by sonographers and physicians with at least 1 year of experience with abdominal Doppler examinations and a working knowledge of Doppler physics. The learning curve for these examinations depends on the technical ability, motivation, and patience of the examiner. It is clear that a steady volume of abdominal Doppler studies is required to gain proficiency with these examinations. It is also clear that experience with these studies allows the examiner to determine, in short order, whether a successful study will be obtained in any given patient. It should be obvious in most cases whether excessive bowel gas, shortness of breath, large body size, or severe

SMA is seen on the sagittal view arising from the anterior aspect of the aorta, just below the origin of the celiac artery. The SMA serves as a landmark for identification of other major mesenteric vessels because of its unique anatomic location. On the transverse view, it is surrounded

atherosclerotic disease will preclude a complete study. This is usually determined within the first 10 minutes of examination.

The experienced examiner employs a number of techniques to improve visualization of the abdominal vessels and the detection of significant lesions. Optimization of gray-scale and color Doppler parameters assists in the visualization of vessel walls, the detection of atherosclerotic plaque, and assessment of the residual lumen. The color Doppler gain, pulse repetition frequency, and wall filter are adjusted such that laminar flow in the normal segment of the aorta and branch vessel has a homogeneous color flow pattern (Figure 29-6). These adjustments should be tailored to each patient, because mesenteric arterial velocities vary widely. Proper adjustment of the color Doppler parameters aids in the observation of vessel patency and visualization of normal flow in the vessel. Equally important, correct instrument adjustment permits the examiner to screen the vessel quickly for flow abnormalities and to detect color aliasing and color bruit artifacts that occur with significant flow disturbance (Figure 29-7). Demonstration of these color flow changes increases the sensitivity for stenosis detection and decreases the time of examination.

Pulsed Doppler waveforms are obtained with a small sample volume (1.5 to 3 mm) to ensure that velocity information is derived from the vessel of interest and not from adjacent structures. Angle correction is always performed for correct Doppler analysis. Most studies are performed at a Doppler angle of insonation of 60 degrees or less to provide accurate velocity estimation. The angle of insonation used in evaluating the mesenteric arteries should not exceed 60 degrees because higher Doppler angles tend to overestimate the measured velocity in the region of interest. Rizzo and co-workers[22] showed that varying the angle of insonation from 0 to 80 degrees produces marked increases in SMA peak systolic velocity (PSV) in normal volunteers. They found that for the SMA, 70-degree and 80-degree angles produced 16% and 120% increases, respectively, in PSV. Because estimation of PSV is inversely proportional to the cosine of the angle of insonation, accurate measurement is dependent on precise Doppler angle correction. Errors in angle correction will result in changes in velocity calculation, particularly at higher angles. This phenomenon, they noted, also occurs in other arterial systems, including the carotid arteries.

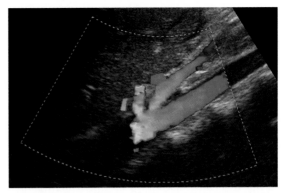

FIGURE 29-6 Color Doppler image of the aorta, celiac origin, and superior mesenteric artery demonstrates normal homogeneous color flow pattern.

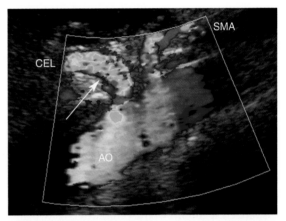

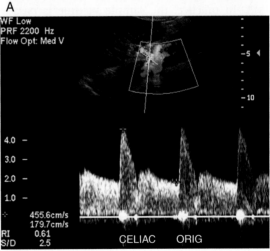

FIGURE 29-7 A, Color Doppler image demonstrates aliasing artifact *(arrow)* in the proximal celiac artery (CEL) consistent with stenosis. Note the normal color flow patterns in the aorta (AO) and superior mesenteric artery (SMA). **B,** Pulsed Doppler evaluation at the site of aliasing in the celiac artery demonstrates high-velocity (456 cm/sec) flow, confirming the presence of a high-grade stenosis.

Although many examiners prefer to obtain Doppler velocity measurements at 60 degrees (similar to carotid artery studies), a 60-degree angle of insonation may be difficult to obtain in the celiac artery, since the artery projects toward the probe at a 0- to 30-degree angle. In these cases, a lower Doppler angle is used for celiac artery velocity measurement. This should be noted in the report or patient's chart so that the same angle can be used on follow-up evaluations. Most spectral samples are obtained from a sagittal projection of the aorta and mesenteric vessels. The direction of blood flow in the celiac and SMA is more easily established in the sagittal plane. An oblique plane is used for Doppler evaluation of the IMA along the direction of blood flow.

EXAMINATION PROTOCOL

Our protocol includes the initial evaluation of the abdominal aorta with gray-scale and color Doppler to assess for the presence or absence of plaque, luminal narrowing, and aneurysm. Pulsed Doppler samples are obtained from the abdominal aorta at the level of the mesenteric arteries (Figure 29-8). This measurement provides a baseline velocity for comparison with the mesenteric artery PSVs. Peak velocity measurements are also obtained from the origin and visualized segments of the celiac artery, SMA, and IMA. In practice, the sample volume is passed slowly from the abdominal aorta into the ostium and proximal segment of each artery, in search of the highest PSV and signs of poststenotic turbulence and bruit (Figure 29-9). Remember, the highest velocity measurement will be obtained within the stenosis.

DIAGNOSTIC CRITERIA

The range of normal blood flow velocity in the celiac artery is quite small: from 98 to 105 cm/sec.[23] Much wider normal ranges are reported in the SMA (97 to 142 cm/sec) and in the IMA (93 to 189 cm/sec).[23]

A review of the literature reveals that many different criteria have been proposed for the diagnosis of splanchnic artery stenosis and no consensus has been reached regarding the optimal Doppler criteria for the diagnosis of significant mesenteric artery stenosis. The most popular and widely accepted criteria are based on PSV measurements of the mesenteric arteries, as reported by Moneta

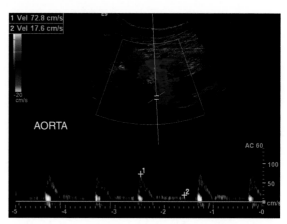

FIGURE 29-8 Pulsed Doppler evaluation of the abdominal aorta at the level of the celiac and superior mesenteric artery demonstrates forward flow in systole with continuous low-velocity forward flow in diastole.

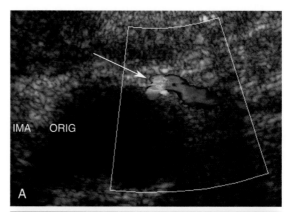

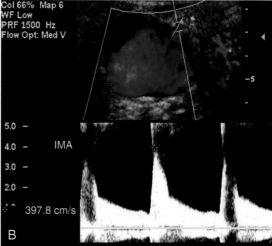

FIGURE 29-9 A, Color Doppler image demonstrates focal color aliasing *(arrow)* at the origin of the inferior mesenteric artery (IMA). **B,** Pulsed Doppler sampling of the origin of the IMA reveals markedly elevated peak systolic velocity (398 cm/sec) consistent with severe stenosis.

and colleagues.[24] In a retrospective review of mesenteric duplex examinations and arteriograms in 34 patients, these authors showed that a PSV greater than or equal to 200 cm/sec in the celiac artery and a PSV greater than or equal to 275 cm/sec in the SMA were predictive of stenosis of 70% or more. Sensitivity, specificity, and positive predictive values for the SMA were 89%, 92%, and 80%, respectively; and 75%, 89%, and 85% for the celiac artery. These parameters were not obtained for the IMA, which was not assessed in that study. Moneta and associates found that end-diastolic velocities and velocity ratios did not offer any advantage over arterial PSV measurements. A follow-up prospective study of 100 patients by Moneta and colleagues[25] supported the authors' initial results and suggested that duplex evaluation may be clinically useful as a screening examination to detect celiac and SMA stenosis. In a study of 82 patients, Lim and associates[26] confirmed the value of the Moneta criteria for the detection of mesenteric stenosis with an overall sensitivity of 100% and specificity of 87% for the celiac artery and 100% sensitivity and specificity for the SMA.

Bowersox and co-workers[27] concluded that an EDV greater than 45 cm/sec was the best indicator of hemodynamically significant SMA stenosis (considered ≥50% diameter reduction). In this series, elevated PSV was less sensitive but more specific for severe SMA stenosis. Other investigators have also indicated that the EDV was the more accurate parameter for the detection of significant mesenteric stenosis. Zwolak and colleagues[28] published a series of 243 mesenteric scans with 46 correlative angiograms. Perko and associates[29] studied 39 patients with duplex ultrasonography and arteriography. Both investigators concluded that the EDV was the superior threshold value for identification of SMA and celiac artery stenosis. They also considered a stenosis with diameter reduction greater than or equal to 50% as clinically significant.

It is interesting to note that the studies discussed previously did not include the IMA in their investigations. This is pertinent in light of the fact that most clinicians follow the "two-vessel rule" in the diagnosis of chronic mesenteric ischemia. A complete study requires identification and Doppler analysis of all three mesenteric arteries. We believe it is imperative to visualize the IMA to exclude mesenteric insufficiency when a significant stenosis or occlusion is identified in the celiac artery or SMA.

Recent studies have shown that the IMA is readily visible in most patients, and adequate Doppler waveforms can be obtained that allow calculation of the PSV, EDV, and resistivity index. Mirk and co-workers[30] visualized the IMA in 88.8% of studies in 116 patients. Denys and associates[31] were successful in demonstrating the IMA in 92% of cases in their study of 100 consecutive fasting adults. PSV and resistivity index measurements differed among the studies. The PSV of the IMA ranged from 93 to 189 cm/sec in normal patients. Erden and colleagues[32] showed that the PSV varies with the degree of collateral flow through the IMA when there is occlusive disease of the abdominal aorta and other mesenteric vessels. Increases in IMA PSV up to 190 cm/sec were seen in patients with occlusion of the celiac, SMA, and common iliac arteries. In our recent retrospective review of 205 studies, Pellerito and colleagues were successful in visualization of the IMA in 86% of cases.[33] The ranges of PSVs, EDV, and mesenteric artery–aortic velocity ratio (MAR) in the nonstenotic IMA were 70 to 200 cm/sec, 0 to 33 cm/sec, and 0.7 to 3.7, respectively.

The ranges of the PSV, EDV, and MAR in IMA stenosis were 200 to 485 cm/sec, 0 to 177 cm/sec, and 0.69 to 8.1, respectively. The threshold values for hemodynamically significant IMA stenosis were as follows: PSV, greater than 200 cm/sec; EDV, greater than 25 cm/sec; and MAR, greater than 2.5, with sensitivities of 90%, 40%, and 80%; specificities of 97%, 91%, and 88%; positive predictive values (PPVs) of 90%, 57%, and 67%; negative predictive values (NPVs) of 97%, 83%, and 93%; and accuracy of 95%, 79%, and 86%, respectively. We found that a PSV of greater than 200 cm/sec was the best criterion for the diagnosis of IMA stenosis. The sensitivity, specificity, PPV, NPV, and accuracy for the PSV were 93%, 97%, 93%, 97%, and 95%, respectively.[33]

It may be valuable to include the velocity ratio in the evaluation for significant mesenteric artery stenosis. This is similar to the calculation of the renal-aortic ratio (RAR) used to diagnose renal artery stenosis. The velocity ratio is calculated by dividing the PSV at the site of the stenosis in the mesenteric artery by the PSV in the abdominal aorta. The normal MAR is usually slightly greater than 1.0. In general, the MAR associated with hemodynamically significant stenosis is greater than 3.0. We find this ratio particularly useful in patients with abnormally high or low velocities in the aorta and branch vessels. Low-velocity flow is seen in patients with poor cardiac function and diffuse atherosclerotic disease. Significant stenosis may be present with lower velocities, sometimes less than 200 cm/sec. An MAR greater than 3.0 suggests severe stenosis, even when PSVs at the site of stenosis are lower than the established threshold for a high-grade lesion. Conversely, elevated velocities may occur in patients without underlying stenosis. This is seen especially in young adults and children with high cardiac output or increased metabolic state. Although elevated velocities are detected in these patients, there is no focal elevation of velocity or significant increase in the MAR to suspect significant disease. Validation of the MAR is based on our experience and a recent retrospective review of more than 1000 abdominal Doppler studies performed at our institution. The MAR greater than or equal to 3.5 demonstrated a specificity of 87% and NPV of 81% for the detection of significant mesenteric artery stenosis.[33]

ROLE OF DUPLEX ULTRASOUND IN SURVEILLANCE FOLLOWING MESENTERIC REVASCULARIZATION (STENT ANGIOPLASTY AND BYPASS GRAFT ASSESSMENT)

At the present time, surgical revascularization remains the treatment of choice for most patients presenting with clinical symptoms and angiographic evidence of CMI. The entire spectrum of vascular reconstructive techniques, including bypass, endarterectomy, reimplantation, and angioplasty, has been used to improve blood flow in the mesenteric vessels. The preferred technique is not yet established, and the choice of operation depends on clinical circumstances and judgment of the operating surgeon. The results of the various revascularization techniques are generally satisfactory and quite comparable. Despite strong institutional preferences, no prospective randomized clinical trial has clearly documented superiority of any single revascularization technique.[34-38]

Duplex testing is implemented to evaluate functional patency following visceral bypass grafting procedures or angioplasty with endovascular stent placement. The focus of duplex surveillance after visceral artery intervention is to identify recurrent stenosis, which can develop and cause symptoms of bowel ischemia. In-stent restenosis, which develops in 20% to 40% of patients after SMA or celiac angioplasty, is caused by myointimal hyperplasia.[39] In his practice, Armstrong[39] uses the following criteria for detection of significant stenosis of the bypass graft or stent-angioplasty site: PSV greater than 300 cm/sec with EDVs greater than 50 to 70 cm/sec, presence of poststenotic turbulence, or a graft PSV less than 40 cm/sec. Criteria for an occluded angioplasty site or bypass graft include a clearly visualized vessel and no detection of color Doppler flow or spectral flow signals within the occluded angioplasty site or bypass graft. In addition, waveforms from the mid-SMA and distal SMA are evaluated for flow velocity damping due to proximal occlusive disease and inadequate collateral artery flow. Following a positive duplex scan for restenosis, further evaluation with angiography to confirm lesion severity and potential intervention should be considered. Bypass grafts are imaged along their length for luminal narrowing or color flow abnormality with particular attention to proximal and distal anastomotic sites. Recording of a midgraft spectral waveform and volume measurement facilitate the diagnosis of graft stenosis and disease progression when complete graft imaging is difficult. In his vascular laboratory, Armstrong found that an interpretable study can be obtained in 80% of patients, with the major limitation being the presence of excessive bowel gas. He states that an increase in PSV greater than 150 cm/sec on serial testing has been associated with the development of either clinical symptoms or an angiographic stenosis. Although surveillance guidelines have been validated for carotid and lower limb interventions, similar criteria for prediction of stenosis following mesenteric revascularization continue to evolve. Among reported series of mesenteric revascularizations, clinical follow-up alone inaccurately predicted graft occlusion and was associated with a sensitivity as low as 33%.[39] For this reason, duplex testing should be utilized to follow up mesenteric bypass grafts and stents to improve patency rates and prevent graft/stent thrombosis.

KEYS TO SUCCESSFUL EXAMINATION

The keys to a successful abdominal Doppler examination include adequate patient preparation, modern ultrasound equipment, examiner experience, proven diagnostic criteria, and correlation with confirmatory studies, when available. We schedule the majority of our patients for morning ultrasound evaluation, following an overnight fast. Abdominal Doppler studies are usually performed by our more experienced sonographers. They choose to perform these examinations on our best Doppler units. Our junior sonographers and trainees observe and perform these studies with supervision by the more experienced senior technologists.

We utilize a practical approach to the interpretation of abdominal Doppler studies. Similar to other Doppler examinations, significant arterial occlusive disease is usually associated with gray-scale, color, and pulsed Doppler abnormalities. Gray-scale evaluation should disclose atherosclerotic plaque or thrombus at the site of stenosis or occlusion (Figure 29-10). The absence of plaque, wall thickening, or thrombus reduces the likelihood of a stenotic lesion in the visualized segment of the vessel.

Color Doppler is extremely useful in the diagnosis of stenosis and occlusion. Luminal narrowing, color flow aliasing, color bruit artifacts and the presence of collateral vessels are important color Doppler findings in arterial stenosis (Figure 29-11). A search for these findings ("Doppler clues") with color and power Doppler imaging facilitates the diagnosis of stenosis. The absence of color flow in the vessel leads to the diagnosis of arterial occlusion. This is confirmed by the absence of arterial signals during pulsed Doppler interrogation. Reversal of flow in the mesenteric arteries is an additional sign of significant disease of the mesenteric circulation. Reversal of flow in the hepatic and gastroduodenal arteries is seen with celiac artery occlusion. Similarly, reversal of flow in the SMA is seen with occlusion at the origin of this vessel. The presence of a color bruit increases suspicion for significant stenosis (Figure 29-12). Bruit artifacts are also associated with arteriovenous fistula and pseudoaneurysms. Color bruit artifacts are produced by low-level frequency shifts. These frequency shifts occur when high-velocity jets induce vibrations in the tissues surrounding the stenotic lesion. Pulsed Doppler sampling at the site of the bruit usually demonstrates elevated PSVs.

Pulsed Doppler is essential in the identification and characterization of stenosis and occlusion. Pulsed Doppler demonstrates elevated velocities and poststenotic turbulence, diagnostic of a hemodynamically significant lesion (Figure 29-13). In most patients, PSVs greater than 200 cm/sec are associated with stenosis. In addition to sampling the site of stenosis, it is important to sample the poststenotic region. A poststenotic signal confirms

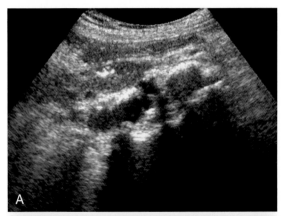

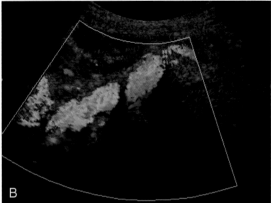

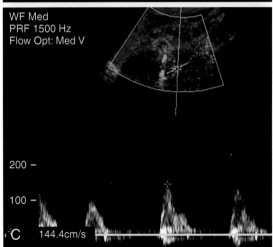

WF Med
PRF 1500 Hz
Flow Opt: Med V

200 –

100 –

C 144.4cm/s

FIGURE 29-10 A, Sagittal gray-scale image of the abdominal aorta reveals marked calcified plaque with luminal irregularity. **B,** Color Doppler image of the abdominal aorta demonstrates color aliasing suspicious for stenosis. **C,** Pulsed Doppler interrogation of the abdominal aorta at the site of flow disturbance reveals increased velocities consistent with moderate stenosis.

the presence of a pressure-reducing lesion. In the poststenotic zone, the systolic jet dissipates into eddy currents, with red blood cells moving in different directions at different velocities. This is termed *poststenotic turbulence* and is recognized as

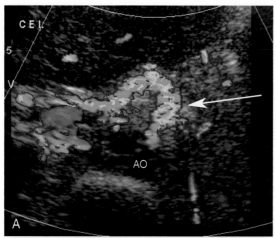

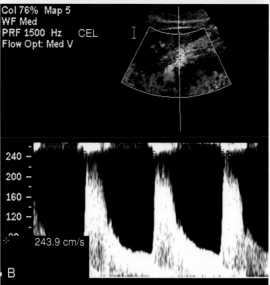

FIGURE 29-11 **A,** Color flow aliasing *(arrow)* allows rapid identification of stenosis in the proximal celiac (CEL) artery. AO, aorta. **B,** Pulsed Doppler evaluation of the proximal celiac artery demonstrates increased velocities consistent with stenosis.

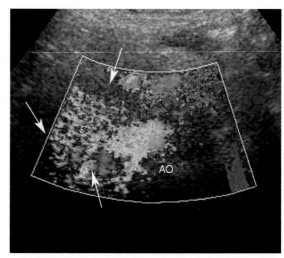

FIGURE 29-12 Marked color bruit artifact *(arrows)* is noted in the region of the celiac artery origin consistent with severe stenosis. AO, aorta.

on pulsed Doppler are typical of a high-grade lesion. Further investigation is warranted when there is discordance between gray-scale, color, and pulsed Doppler findings. We recommend other noninvasive tests, including CT or MR angiography for the difficult cases in which the study is indeterminate and intervention is not immediately indicated.

PITFALLS

Several pitfalls should be considered in the evaluation of the mesenteric arteries. As was stated previously, there are normal variants in vascular anatomy that investigators should recognize. These variants include a replaced right hepatic artery that originates not from the celiac trunk, but from the SMA, anomalous origin of the common hepatic artery from the SMA or aorta, and a common celiac-SMA trunk. The low-resistance hepatic artery waveform could be misinterpreted as increased diastolic flow associated with SMA stenosis. This pitfall is avoided by following the course of these arterial branches.

A potential pitfall for celiac artery stenosis is the **median arcuate ligament syndrome (MALS).** The median arcuate ligament (MAL) is a fibrous arch that units the diaphragmatic crura on either side of the aortic hiatus. The MAL usually passes just superior to the celiac artery. In some people, the MAL passes anteriorly to the celiac artery and may cause celiac artery compression during expiration secondary to upward motion of the diaphragm.

a lower-velocity waveform with irregular borders, usually with a simultaneous bidirectional pattern (see Figure 29-13). This "shaggy" waveform is seen within 1 to 2 cm distal to the stenosis and dissipates with increasing distance from the stenosis. Poststenotic waveforms usually also show a delay to peak systole that is called the tardus-parvus pattern. A rounded, low-velocity waveform, characteristic of tardus-parvus flow, is a marker of a proximal stenosis or occlusion (Figure 29-14).

To summarize, findings of plaque on gray-scale imaging, narrowing, aliasing and bruit artifacts on color Doppler, and elevated peak systolic velocities and ratios with poststenotic turbulence

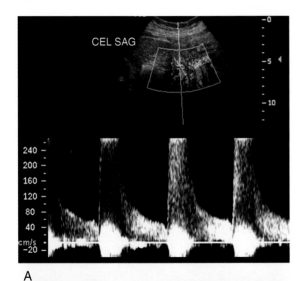

A

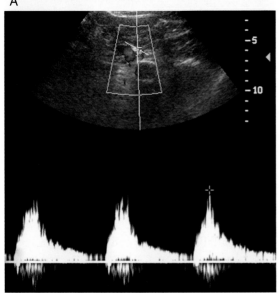

B

FIGURE 29-13 A, Spectral analysis of the region of flow disturbance in the celiac (CEL) artery demonstrates markedly elevated peak systolic velocities consistent with significant stenosis. SAG, sagittal. **B,** Pulsed Doppler sampling of the poststenotic region reveals lower-velocity flow with irregular borders, slow systolic rise, and a bidirectional flow pattern.

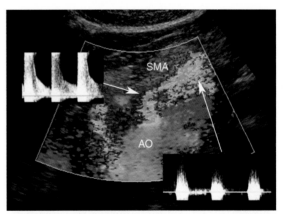

FIGURE 29-14 This montage of waveforms shows high-velocity continuous flow at the site of superior mesenteric artery (SMA) stenosis *(short arrow)* and low-velocity, rounded (tardus-parvus) waveforms *(long arrow)* in the poststenotic zone. Note the abnormal turbulent color flow pattern in the SMA. AO, aorta.

stenosis of the celiac artery with elevated PSV that persists with inspiration.

Doppler insonation of the mesenteric vessels, especially the celiac artery, can be challenging due to vessel tortuosity. It may not be possible to maintain a constant angle of insonation in these vessels. Increasing Doppler angles can produce spuriously increased velocity measurements. It should also be remembered that there is a wide range of normal velocities in the splanchnic vessels.[22]

Low flow velocities in the mesenteric arteries may be due to aneurysmal dilatation of the abdominal aorta. This is one reason that the evaluation of the mesenteric arteries should include the abdominal aorta (Figure 29-16). Elevated PSVs occur with marked narrowing of the abdominal aorta. These high-velocity signals may be transmitted to the mesenteric arteries suggesting mesenteric arterial stenoses. Incorporating the MAR is helpful in this situation since the ratio will not be elevated. Variable flow velocities may be seen in patients who have cardiac arrhythmias, caused by disproportionately high cardiac output during postectopic heartbeats.(Figure 29-17). Color and pulsed Doppler can also detect aneurysmal dilatation of the mesenteric vessels (Figure 29-18).

In the presence of significant stenotic disease of one of the mesenteric vessels, an increase in flow velocity in another mesenteric vessel may occur, caused by compensatory blood flow to the intestines.[40] It is believed that the compensatory increase in blood flow allows perfusion of collateral channels (i.e., pancreaticoduodenal

With pulsed Doppler, mechanical compression of the celiac artery by the MAL is detected as increased PSV during expiration. On inspiration, however, the celiac artery is in its noncompressed (neutral) caudad position, and a normal PSV is observed. When MALS is suspected, inspiratory and expiratory velocity measurements therefore should be obtained (Figure 29-15). Chronic compression of the celiac artery by the MAL may produce a fixed

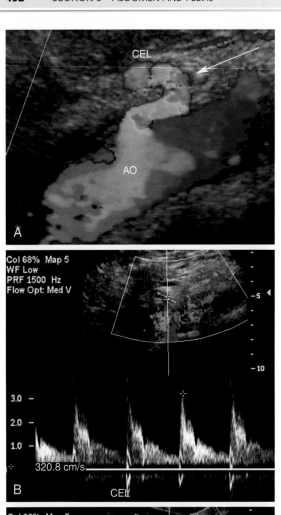

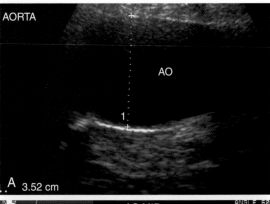

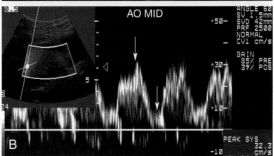

FIGURE 29-16 **A,** Gray-scale image demonstrates an abdominal aortic aneurysm measuring 3.5 cm. AO, aorta. **B,** Color and pulsed Doppler evaluation of the aneurysm reveals low-velocity flow, with peak systolic velocity measuring 32 cm/sec.

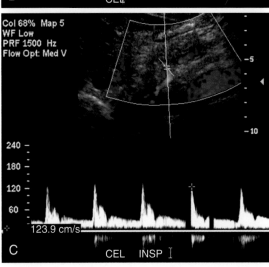

FIGURE 29-15 **A,** Median arcuate ligament syndrome. Color Doppler image reveals a "fishhook" appearance *(arrow)* of the celiac (CEL) artery in expiration. AO, aorta. **B,** Pulsed Doppler sample of the celiac artery in expiration reveals elevated velocities due to compression from the median arcuate ligament. **C,** There is a marked decrease in peak systolic velocity in the celiac artery in inspiration.

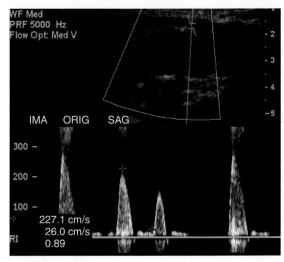

FIGURE 29-17 Pulsed Doppler evaluation of the inferior mesenteric artery (IMA) demonstrates variable peak systolic velocities due to cardiac arrhythmia. No secondary signs of stenosis are identified.

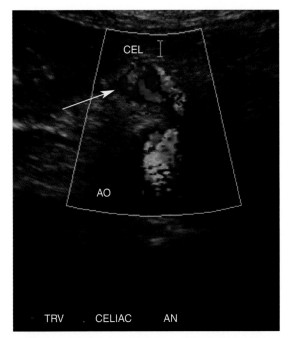

FIGURE 29-18 Celiac (CEL) artery aneurysm. The lumen of the celiac artery is dilated *(arrow)* and demonstrates disturbed flow on the color Doppler image. AO, aorta.

artery) that exist between the celiac artery and SMA. Elevated velocities will be detected *throughout* the nonstenotic vessel, unlike the *focal* increased velocity seen in a stenotic vessel. In this situation, the absence of secondary signs of stenosis such as color flow aliasing, bruit artifact, and tardus-parvus waveforms may be helpful. As noted previously, low mesenteric arterial velocities may be seen in older adult patients and patients with poor cardiac output, even with significant mesenteric disease.[41] Conversely, elevated velocities are commonly seen in younger patients in the absence of significant mesenteric stenosis. Velocity ratios tend to work better than PSV criteria in these patients who have baseline velocities outside the normal range. Elevated velocities may also be noted in vessels serving as major collateral channels. Finally, careful history of fasting or recent meal is necessary to avoid misinterpretation of elevated PSVs on the basis of a postprandial increase in intestinal blood flow.[10,42]

CONCLUSIONS

Doppler ultrasound has proven value in the detection of mesenteric artery stenosis and occlusion. Proper patient preparation and the use of sensitive Doppler equipment are necessary to start the investigation. Operator experience and knowledge of technical shortcuts increase accuracy and decrease the time of the examination. Finally, the use of proven diagnostic criteria and correlation with confirmatory studies are also keys to diagnostic success.

Acknowledgments. I would like to thank Saiedeh "Nanaz" Maghool for her excellent images and James Cooper for his wonderful illustrations.

REFERENCES

1. Ruzika FF Jr, Rossi P: Normal vascular anatomy of the abdominal viscera, *Radiol Clin North Am* 8:3–29, 1970.
2. Michels NA: *Blood supply and anatomy of the upper abdominal organs*, Philadelphia, 1955, JB Lippincott.
3. Kornblith PL, Boley SJ, Whitehouse BS: Anatomy of the splanchnic circulation, *Surg Clin North Am* 72:1–30, 1992.
4. Lin PH, Chaikof EL: Embryology, anatomy and surgical exposure of the great abdominal vessels, *Surg Clin North Am* 80:417–433, 2000.
5. Baxter BT, Pearce H: Diagnosis and surgical management of chronic mesenteric ischemia. In Strandness DE, Van Brida A, editors: *Vascular Diseases Surgical and Interventional Therapy*, New York, 1994, Churchill Livingstone Publishers, pp 795–802.
6. Van Bel F, et al: Superior mesenteric artery blood flow velocity and estimated volume flow: duplex Doppler US study of preterm and term neonates, *Radiology* 174:165–169, 1990.
7. Perry MA, et al: Physiology of splanchnic circulation. In Kveitys PR, Barrowman JA, Granger DN, editors: *Pathophysiology of the Splanchnic Circulation*, Vol. 1, Boca Raton, Fla, 1987, CRC, pp 1–56.
8. Granger DN, et al: Intestinal blood flow, *Gastroenterology* 78:837–863, 1980.
9. Lewis BD, James EM: Current applications of duplex and color Doppler ultrasound imaging: Abdomen, *Mayo Clin Proc* 64:1158–1169, 1989.
10. Moneta GL, et al: Duplex ultrasound measurement of postprandial intestinal blood flow: Effect of meal composition, *Gastroenterology* 95:1294–1301, 1988.
11. Healy DA, et al: Evaluation of celiac and mesenteric vascular disease with duplex ultrasonography, *J Ultrasound Med* 11:481–485, 1992.
12. Cunningham CG, Reilly LM, Stoney R: Chronic visceral ischemia, *Surg Clin North Am* 72:231–244, 1992.
13. Mikkelson WP: Intestinal angina: its surgical significance, *Am J Surg* 94:262–269, 1957.
14. Zwolak RM: Can duplex ultrasound replace arteriography in screening for mesenteric ischemia? *Semin Vasc Surg* 12:252–260, 1999.
15. Harward TR, Smith S, Seeger JM: Detection of celiac axis and superior mesenteric artery occlusive disease with use of abdominal duplex scanning, *J Vasc Surg.* 17(4):738–745, 1993.
16. Moneta GL: Screening for mesenteric vascular insufficiency and follow-up of mesenteric artery bypass procedures, *Semin Vasc Surg.* 14(3):186–192, 2001.

17. Moawad J, Gewertz BL: Chronic mesenteric ischemia. Clinical presentation and diagnosis, *Surg Clin North Am* 77:357–369, 1997.

18. Meany JF, Prince MR, Nostrand TT: Gadolinium-enhanced magnetic resonance angiography in patients with suspected chronic mesenteric ischaemia, *J Magn Reson Imaging* 7:171–176, 1997.

19. Carlos RC, et al: Interobserver variability in the evaluation of chronic mesenteric ischemia with gadolinium enhanced MR angiography, *Acad Radiol* 8(9):879–887, 2001.

20. Savastano S, et al: Multislice CT angiography of the celiac and superior mesenteric arteries: Comparison with arteriographic findings, *Radiol Med* 103(5-6):456–463, 2002.

21. Nicoloff AD, et al: Duplex ultrasonography in evaluation of splanchnic artery stenosis, *Surg Clin North Am* 77:339–355, 1997.

22. Rizzo RJ, et al: Mesenteric flow velocity variations as a function of angle of insonation, *J Vasc Surg* 11:688–694, 1990.

23. Jager K, et al: Measurement of mesenteric blood flow by duplex scan, *J Vasc Surg* 3:462–469, 1986.

24. Moneta GL, et al: Duplex ultrasound criteria for diagnosis of splanchnic artery stenosis or occlusion, *J Vasc Surg* 14:511–520, 1991.

25. Moneta GL, et al: Mesenteric duplex scanning: A blinded prospective study, *J Vasc Surg* 17:79–86, 1993.

26. Lim HK, et al: Splanchnic arterial stenosis or occlusion: Diagnosis at Doppler US, *Radiology* 211:405–410, 1999.

27. Bowersox JC, et al: Duplex ultrasonography in the diagnosis of celiac and mesenteric artery occlusive disease, *J Vasc Surg* 14:780–788, 1991.

28. Zwolak RM, et al: Mesenteric and celiac duplex scanning: A validation study, *J Vasc Surg* 27:1078–1088, 1998.

29. Perko MJ, Just S, Schroeder TV: Importance of diastolic velocities in the detection of celiac and mesenteric artery disease by duplex ultrasound, *J Vasc Surg* 26:288–293, 1997.

30. Mirk P, et al: Sonographic and Doppler assessment of the inferior mesenteric artery: Normal morphologic and hemodynamic features, *Abdom Imaging* 23:364–369, 1998.

31. Denys AL, et al: Doppler sonography of the inferior mesenteric artery: A preliminary study, *J Ultrasound Med* 14:435–439, 1995.

32. Erden A, Yurdakul M, Cumhur T: Doppler waveforms of the normal and collateralized inferior mesenteric artery, *Am J Roentgenol* 171:619–627, 1998.

33. Pellerito JS, et al: Doppler sonographic criteria for the diagnosis of inferior mesenteric artery stenosis, *J Ultrasound Med* 28:641–650, 2009.

34. Patel B, Widdowson J, Smith RC: Superior mesenteric artery bypass for chronic mesenteric ischaemia: a DGH experience, *J R Coll Surg Edinb* 45:285–287, 2000.

35. Baur GM, et al: Treatment of chronic visceral ischaemia, *Am J Surg* 148:138–144, 1984.

36. Johnston KW, et al: Mesenteric artery bypass graft: early and late results and suggested surgical approach for chronic and acute mesenteric ischaemia, *Surgery* 118:1–7, 1995.

37. Rapp JH, et al: Durability of endarterectomy and antegrade graft in the treatment of chronic visceral ischaemia, *J Vasc Surg* 3:799–806, 1986.

38. Kieny R, Battellier J, Kertz JG: Aortic reimplantation of the superior mesenteric artery for atherosclerotic lesion of the visceral arteries: sixty cases, *Ann Vasc Surg* 4:122–125, 1990.

39. Armstrong PA: Visceral duplex scanning: Evaluation before and after artery intervention for chronic mesenteric ischemia, *Perspect Vasc Surg Endovasc Ther* Vol. 19(No. 4):386–392, 2007.

40. Healy DA, et al: Evaluation of celiac and mesenteric vascular disease with duplex ultrasonography, *J Ultrasound Med* 11:481–485, 1992.

41. Perko MJ, et al: Changes in superior mesenteric artery Doppler waveform during reduction of cardiac stroke volume and hypotension, *Ultrasound Med Biol* 22(1):11–18, 1996.

42. Gentile AT, et al: Usefulness of fasting and postprandial duplex ultrasound examination for predicting high grade superior mesenteric artery stenosis, *Am J Surg* 169:476–479, 1995.

ULTRASOUND ASSESSMENT OF THE HEPATIC VASCULATURE

30

WILLIAM D. MIDDLETON, MD, FACR, and KATHRYN A. ROBINSON, MD

Because chronic liver disease is the tenth most common cause of death in the United States, evaluation of the liver and its vasculature is a very common indication for abdominal Doppler assessment.[1,2] The liver vessels are effectively imaged with ultrasound in a high percentage of patients. Therefore, Doppler sonography is frequently the first modality used to evaluate patients with suspected hepatic vascular disorders. This chapter reviews the normal hemodynamics of the liver and the sonographic assessment of portal hypertension, portal vein obstruction, hepatic vein obstruction, and intrahepatic portosystemic shunts.

TECHNIQUE AND NORMAL HEMODYNAMICS

HEPATIC VEINS

The Doppler signal from the left hepatic vein is usually best optimized with the transducer in a subxyphoid approach. The right hepatic vein is best seen from a lateral intercostal approach near the mid axillary line. Optimization of the middle hepatic vein signal is more variable, ranging from subxyphoid to intercostal near the anterior axillary line to subcostal. In all of these locations, the transducer is generally positioned so that forward flow in the hepatic veins (i.e., out of the liver, toward the inferior vena cava [IVC] and the heart) is away from the probe and is displayed below the baseline, while reversed flow (away from the heart and into the liver) is above the baseline.

With that in mind, it is easiest to understand the morphology of the hepatic vein waveform by relating it to activity in the right atrium. When the right atrium contracts, forward flow from the hepatic veins into the IVC and right atrium slows and eventually reverses. The reversal of flow produces a short period of flow above the baseline. As the right atrium relaxes, there is relatively rapidly accelerating flow from the liver into the atrium. This is reflected in the waveform as a rapid downslope below the baseline. With progressive atrial filling, the velocity of flow from the hepatic veins into the atrium starts to slow and the Doppler signal starts to approach the baseline. This deceleration of hepatic vein outflow continues until the tricuspid valve opens. At this point there is a short period of passive atrial emptying into the ventricle, which produces a second phase of accelerating hepatic vein flow into the atrium and another downslope below the baseline. The right atrium then starts to contract, and the hepatic vein flow toward the atrium slows and eventually reverses (Figure 30-1).[3]

It is important to recognize that deep inspiration can blunt the normal hepatic vein pulsatility and should be avoided when possible. To improve demonstration of the normal waveform morphology, it is best to obtain the waveform at the end of a normal breath out. Specific instructions to the patient that tend to work well are "take a *normal* breath in, take a *normal* breath out, stop breathing," and then obtain a waveform.

Predictably, right heart failure and alterations in right atrial filling and emptying cause changes in the hepatic vein waveform.[4] In patients with right heart dysfunction, hepatic vein pulsatility increases and the retrograde pulses are exaggerated. With tricuspid regurgitation, right ventricular contraction during systole produces retrograde flow from the ventricle into the right atrium, and from the atrium into the hepatic veins. This causes an inverted systolic peak in the hepatic vein waveform (Figure 30-2).

PORTAL VEIN

The normal portal vein demonstrates continuous antegrade flow and provides approximately 75% of blood supply to the liver.[5] Although minor degrees of respiratory phasicity are reported,

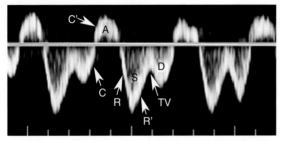

FIGURE 30-1 Normal hepatic waveform. As the right atrium contracts (C), flow out of the liver and toward the heart begins to slow and approach the baseline. It then reverses for a short phase and travels back into the liver (C'). As the right atrium starts to relax (R), flow in the hepatic vein converts from a retrograde direction to an antegrade direction and gradually increases in velocity, producing a rapid downslope in the hepatic vein waveform. As the right atrium progressively fills, flow out of the liver and into the right atrium begins to slow, and the Doppler signal starts to approach the baseline (R'). When the tricuspid valve opens (TV), the right atrium passively decompresses into the right ventricle, producing a second short phase of accelerating flow out of the liver. At this point, the right atrium starts to contract again, and the whole cycle is repeated. This process produces what is known as a triphasic pattern with retrograde pulses during atrial contraction (A) and two antegrade pulses during ventricular systole (S) and ventricular diastole (D).

these are difficult to appreciate with Doppler techniques since sampling is performed during suspended respiration.

Because the hepatic sinusoids separate the portal veins from the heart, the degree of portal vein pulsatility related to cardiac activity is considerably less than for the hepatic veins. However, some degree of portal vein pulsatility is normal and is well displayed on portal vein waveforms (Figure 30-3). Pulsatility can be quantified by using an index called the venous pulsatility index (VPI). The VPI is analogous to the arterial resistivity index and is calculated as the difference between the maximum velocity and the minimum divided by the maximum velocity. A very pulsatile waveform where the minimum velocity reached the baseline (i.e., 0 cm/sec) would have a VPI of 1. A completely nonpulsatile portal vein waveform would have a VPI of 0. Gallix and associates[6] showed that the mean VPI for the portal vein was 0.48 (± 0.31) in a group of normal individuals. A VPI of 0.48 means the minimum velocity is approximately half the maximum velocity.

Another way to quantify portal flow pulsatility is a simple ratio between the minimum and peak flow.[7] Using this approach, a flat waveform would have a portal vein pulsatility (PVP) of 1

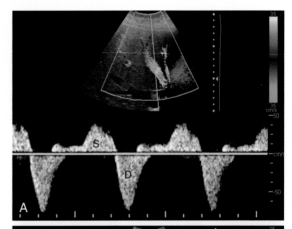

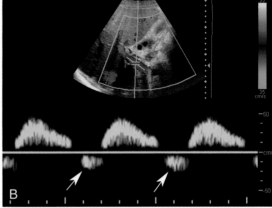

FIGURE 30-2 Right heart failure with tricuspid regurgitation and hepatic congestion. **A,** Hepatic vein waveform shows inversion of the systolic peak (S). Diastolic flow remains normal and below baseline (D). **B,** Portal vein waveform shows abnormal portal vein pulsatility with transient reversal of flow *(arrows)*.

and a very pulsatile waveform where the minimum velocity dropped to the baseline would have a PVP of 0. Wachsberg and colleagues[7] showed that 64% of normal patients had a PVP less than 0.54. That means that in a majority of patients the minimum velocity was less than half the peak velocity. Increased pulsatility in the portal vein is more prominent in thin individuals. As with the hepatic vein pulsatility, portal flow pulsatility can be blunted by a deep inspiration.

Right heart failure and tricuspid regurgitation may produce exaggerated portal vein pulsatility.[8] Given the degree of pulsatility that can be seen in normal patients, however, cardiac dysfunction should probably not be considered unless the portal pulsatility is so great that the minimum velocity reaches 0 or reverses (i.e., the VPI is at least 1; see Figure 30-2, *B.*).[9] It is also important to correlate the portal vein waveform with other

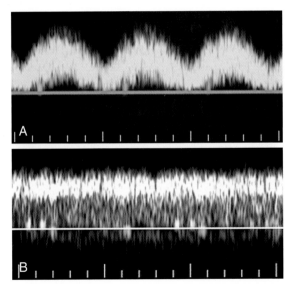

FIGURE 30-3 Normal portal vein waveforms. **A,** Portal vein waveform from a thin individual shows moderate pulsatility. Note: The flow velocity does not reach zero and does not reverse. **B,** Normal portal vein waveform from a different individual shows flat monophasic flow.

sonographic signs of heart dysfunction, including enlargement of the hepatic veins and IVC and alterations in the hepatic vein waveform.

There is considerable variation in the reported value for normal portal vein velocity. This variation is at least partially dependent on whether the maximum velocity or the time average mean velocity is being reported. Patriquin and co-workers[10] found that the maximum portal vein velocity ranged from 8 to 18 cm/sec in normal fasting adults and increased from 50% to 100% after eating. Haag and associates[11] found that the normal maximum portal vein velocity was 26.5 ± 5.5 cm/sec. Abu-Yousef and colleagues[9] and Kok and co-workers[12] found the maximum portal vein velocity to range from 16 to 31 cm/sec (mean 22 cm/sec) and from 11 to 39 cm/sec (mean 23 cm/sec), respectively. Zironi and associates[13] found that the normal mean portal velocity was 19.6 ± 2.6 cm/sec. Cioni and colleagues[14] found that the maximum velocity was 26.7 ± 3.2 cm/sec and the mean velocity was 22.9 ± 2.8 cm/sec. They considered the normal range for maximum portal vein velocity to be from 20 to 33 cm/sec. This variation in the reported range of normal makes it difficult to rely on portal velocities as a sign of portal hypertension. Very low velocities are a good indicator of portal hypertension, however; velocities in the normal range do not exclude the diagnosis.

One variation of portal vein flow is helical flow near the bifurcation. This can produce areas of localized flow reversal or apparent flow reversal and give the mistaken impression of portal vein flow reversal despite overall antegrade portal vein flow. Rosenthal and associates showed that this can be seen in 20% of patients with severe chronic liver disease. However, helical flow is also seen in approximately 2% of normal patients.[15] It is also seen following transjugular intrahepatic portosystemic shunts (TIPS), in patients following liver transplant, and in the setting of portal vein stenosis.

HEPATIC ARTERY

The hepatic artery waveform has a low resistance profile with broad systolic peaks, gradual deceleration from systole to diastole, and well-maintained diastolic flow throughout the cardiac cycle. This is similar to that of other solid parenchymal abdominal organs. The normal hepatic artery resistivity index ranges from 0.5 to 0.7. Evaluation of the hepatic artery is very important in liver transplant patients and will be considered in Chapter 34.

PORTAL HYPERTENSION

As mentioned earlier, chronic liver disease is the tenth most common cause of death in the United States, and alcoholism is the most common reason that Americans die of cirrhosis. Cirrhosis is the most common cause of portal hypertension with 60% of patients with cirrhosis having clinically significant portal hypertension.[1]

The precise pathophysiology of cirrhosis is unknown, but hepatic inflammation with regeneration is central to the process. Patients may be completely asymptomatic or experience complete hepatic decompensation. Mortality is largely related to complications of portal hypertension such as ascites (50%), variceal bleeding (25%), renal failure (10%), bacterial peritonitis (5%), and complications of ascites therapy (10%).[2]

Portal hypertension is defined as an increase in the gradient between the portal vein and IVC or hepatic veins of 10 to 12 mm Hg or greater. The easiest way to classify portal hypertension is to divide it into intrahepatic, extrahepatic, and hyperdynamic. Extrahepatic portal hypertension is subdivided into prehepatic (portal vein thrombosis [PVT], compression, and stenosis) and posthepatic (hepatic vein or IVC thrombosis, compression, or stenosis). Hyperdynamic refers to arteriovenous malformations or conditions that cause arterial portal fistulas. Extrahepatic and hyperdynamic portal hypertension are much less common than the intrahepatic category.

Intrahepatic portal hypertension includes presinusoidal and postsinusoidal causes. Presinusoidal causes are less common in Western countries and include hepatic fibrosis, sarcoidosis, schistosomiasis, and lymphoma. Postsinusoidal causes are much more common and include cirrhosis and venoocclusive disease. Since cirrhosis is so common, it is worth focusing on the sequence of events that occurs with cirrhosis.

Cirrhosis causes hepatocellular death, parenchymal degeneration, and regeneration. This leads to bridging fibrosis that causes increased resistance to blood flow in the sinusoids and the central venules that drain the sinusoids. Initially, increased portal pressures maintain portal vein flow volume. But as resistance to hepatic inflow progresses, it eventually equalizes with resistance to flow in portosystemic collaterals and portal flow starts to be diverted into the collaterals.

Ultimately, the resistance to flow through the sinusoids starts to affect arterial inflow so that arterial flow is shunted away from the sinusoids and into the portal vein system. This shunting occurs at a microscopic level in the sinusoids, peribiliary plexus, and the vasa vasorum of the portal vein. Initially, this produces portal vein flow reversal in isolated peripheral intrahepatic portal vein branches. As more and more peripheral branches reverse, flow in the major branches and the main portal vein also eventually reverse.[16]

VENOUS DIAMETER

There are a number of gray-scale signs of portal hypertension. Engorgement of the portal vein and its tributaries is an indicator of elevated pressures (Figure 30-4). Goyal and colleagues[17] prospectively compared portal vein diameter in 100 healthy subjects and 50 patients with portal hypertension. Keeping physiologic variables known to affect portal vein flow (such as fasting state, supine position, and deep inspiration) similar in both groups, they found that the upper limit of normal for portal vein diameter was 16 mm. Using this cutoff value, they achieved an overall sensitivity of 72%, accuracy of 91%, and specificity of 100% in diagnosing patients with suspected portal hypertension. Others, however,

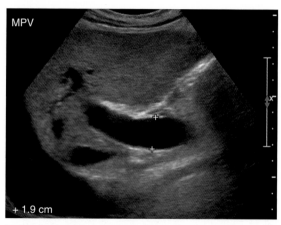

FIGURE 30-4 Portal vein enlargement in a patient with portal hypertension. Oblique view of the liver hilum shows a portal vein that measures 1.9 cm *(cursors)*. The upper limit of normal for portal vein diameter is between 1.3 and 1.6 cm.

have proposed 13 mm as the cutoff for upper limits of normal portal vein diameter.[18] The uncertainty about the normal value of portal vein diameter is one of the reasons that this parameter is not relied on to diagnose portal hypertension. While it is true that an unusually large portal vein is a reliable sign of portal hypertension, it is also unfortunately true that a normal-sized portal vein in no way excludes the diagnosis.

If one assumes that elevated portal pressure maximizes venous distention, it follows that little or no additional distention will occur when the portal vein outflow is indirectly restricted by sustained inspiration. Lack of caliber variation of the splenic and mesenteric vein during respiration is thus another parameter that has been investigated. In one study, this approach had a sensitivity of 80% and specificity of 100% in diagnosing portal hypertension.[19] As with portal vein diameter measurements, this method has not gained widespread utility, likely due to a combination of interobserver variability and difficulties in measurement accuracy.

PORTAL VEIN FLOW VELOCITY

Simple measurements of portal vein velocity are one of many Doppler techniques used to evaluate patients with suspected portal hypertension. A sensitivity of 88% and a specificity of 96% were achieved by Zironi and co-workers[13] using a mean portal vein velocity cutoff below 15 cm/sec. Haag and associates used a maximum portal vein velocity of 21 cm/sec as their cutoff for diagnosis of portal hypertension. Along with a portal vein diameter cutoff of 12.5 mm, they reported a sensitivity and specificity of 80%.[11] The differences in these two studies illustrate that the expected portal velocity values in normal subjects and cirrhotic patients vary considerably. Although portal velocities tend to decrease as portal pressures increase, the correlation is weak and is not statistically significant.[11,20] Sources of variability include interobserver variability, intermachine variability, presence of variable collateral pathways (especially recanalized umbilical veins), and variations caused by differences in patient positioning, different phases of respiration, different states of fasting, different exercise status, and different cardiac output.

Knowing that portal vein cross-sectional area typically increases and portal velocity typically decreases in the setting of portal hypertension has led some investigators to study the ratio of these parameters, assuming that it will increase dramatically with portal hypertension. The ratio of portal vein cross-sectional area and portal velocity is known as the congestion index. Moriyasu and colleagues[21] showed that the congestion index was 2.5 times higher in patients with cirrhosis and portal hypertension than in normal subjects. Sensitivities ranging from 67% to 95% have been achieved using congestion index measurements.[11,21] Unfortunately, the interobserver variability in area and velocity measurements is relatively high, and this variability is compounded when the parameters are combined in a ratio. Therefore, despite the theoretical value in this approach, optimistic results obtained in highly dedicated institutions may be difficult to reproduce in other centers.

HEPATIC ARTERY AND HEPATIC VEIN FLOW

When portal hypertension is caused by cirrhosis, hepatic artery flow may increase substantially as compensation for diminished portal vein flow. Ultimately, the bulk of liver blood flow is provided by the hepatic artery, which may become subjectively enlarged and tortuous on color flow examination (Figure 30-5) and show substantially increased blood flow on Doppler interrogation. Enlarged intrahepatic arteries can in fact simulate dilated bile ducts and produce a parallel channel sign (Figure 30-6). Unfortunately, the hepatic artery does not have the capacity to make up for the loss of portal vein flow, and persistent hepatic ischemia is a significant cause of ongoing hepatocyte damage and progression of fibrotic scarring.

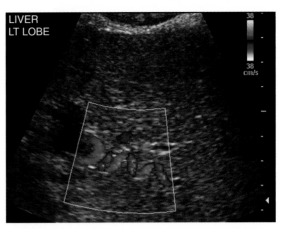

FIGURE 30-5 Tortuous hepatic artery in cirrhosis. Magnified transverse view of the left lobe of the liver shows a very tortuous intrahepatic branch of the left hepatic artery.

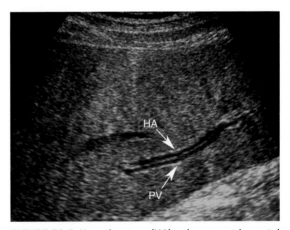

FIGURE 30-6 Hepatic artery (HA) enlargement in portal hypertension. Oblique view of the right lobe of the liver shows a parallel channel sign. This is traditionally considered a sign of intrahepatic bile duct dilatation. However, an enlarged hepatic artery can also produce the parallel channel sign. PV, portal vein.

Normal hepatic vein pulsatility is either blunted or completely eliminated in patients with cirrhosis. In fact, a higher Child-Pugh score and decreased survival rate have been shown to correlate with complete loss of hepatic vein pulsatility.[22] Although the mechanism for this loss of hepatic vein pulsatility is unclear, impression on the hepatic veins by regenerating nodules with resulting stenosis is a likely contributing factor.[23]

PORTOSYSTEMIC COLLATERALS

Although measurement of vessel diameters and velocities and calculation of various indices are helpful in some patients and used extensively

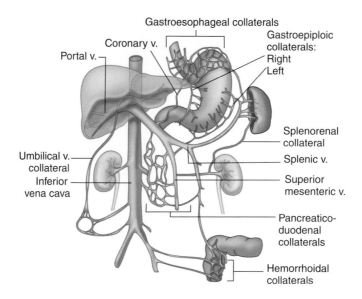

FIGURE 30-7 Diagram illustrating commonly encountered portal systemic collaterals in patients with portal hypertension. v., Vein.

in some institutions, the most widely used and reliable approach for the diagnosis of portal hypertension is the evaluation of portal systemic collaterals. Portal systemic collaterals can be divided into tributary and developed collaterals. Tributary collaterals are preexisting vessels that normally drain into the portal, splenic, and mesenteric venous systems. Blood flow in all tributaries should be directed toward the mesenteric, splenic, and portal veins.

The coronary vein, also known as the left gastric vein, is the most prevalent portal systemic collateral. It is identified angiographically in 80% to 90% of patients with portal hypertension.[24,25] Because its presence implies an increased risk for variceal hemorrhage, it is the most clinically important of the portal systemic collaterals. The coronary vein runs parallel to the left gastric artery between the two layers of the lesser omentum. It arises along the gastric pylorus and lesser curvature of the stomach and proceeds toward the esophageal hiatus, where it forms a U-shaped loop that returns inferiorly to drain into the portal system near the portal splenic confluence (Figure 30-7).

Using the left lobe of the liver as an acoustic window, the coronary vein can be identified sonographically as a vessel communicating with the superior aspect of the portal or splenic vein in the region of the confluence. It is located directly anterior to the bifurcation of the celiac axis or posterior to the common hepatic artery or the splenic artery (Figure 30-8, A and B). It is oriented in a slightly oblique plane, traveling superiorly and to the left of the portosplenic confluence and toward the gastroesophageal junction. Normal coronary vein blood flow, like all portal tributaries, should be directed toward the portal vein (Figure 30-8, C).

The normal coronary vein diameter should not exceed 5 to 6 mm.[10, 26-30] In approximately 25% of patients with portal hypertension, the coronary vein will become dilated. Unfortunately, variceal hemorrhage often occurs without coronary vein enlargement.[30] Demonstration of reversed flow in the coronary vein is a much earlier sign of portal hypertension than coronary vein enlargement. Wachsberg and co-workers[30] showed that Doppler demonstration of hepatofugal flow in the coronary vein occurs in 78% of patients with portal hypertension (Figure 30-9). Evaluation of the coronary vein is very important in patients with suspected portal hypertension since it may be the only portal systemic collateral visualized in up to 75% of patients. Preservation of hepatopetal coronary vein flow in patients with portal hypertension also has prognostic implications since it is associated with a low risk for variceal hemorrhage.

Short gastric veins and branches of the superior and inferior mesenteric veins are other tributaries of the portal system that can function as

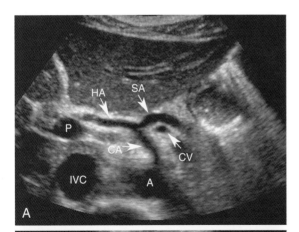

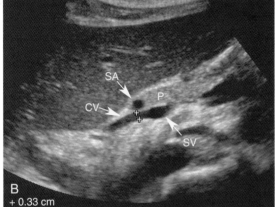

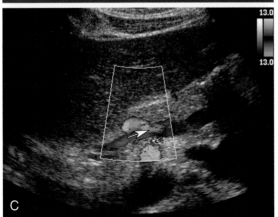

FIGURE 30-8 Normal coronary vein. **A,** Transverse gray-scale view of the epigastrium at the level of the celiac axis (CA) shows the coronary vein (CV) in cross section located posterior to the splenic artery (SA). Also seen on this image are the common hepatic artery (HA), the portal vein (P), the inferior vena cava (IVC), and the aorta (A). **B,** Sagittal view of the epigastrium through the body of the pancreas (P) shows the splenic vein (SV) posterior to the pancreas and the coronary vein (CV) extending superiorly from the splenic vein. In this individual the coronary vein measures 3.3 mm *(cursors)*. Also seen on this image is the splenic artery (SA). **C,** Sagittal color Doppler view similar to the gray-scale image shown in **B.** Note that flow direction in the normal coronary vein *(arrow)* is toward the splenic vein.

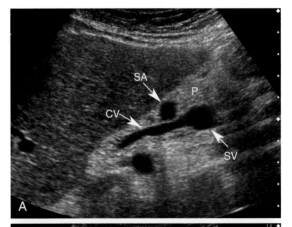

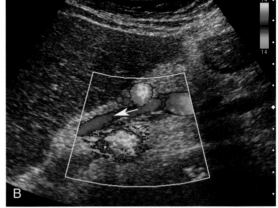

FIGURE 30-9 Coronary vein collateral in portal hypertension. **A,** Sagittal view of the epigastrium shows the coronary vein (CV) extending from the splenic vein (SV). The splenic artery (SA) and pancreas (P) are also seen on this image. **B,** Color Doppler view similar to the gray-scale view shown in **A** shows reversed flow *(arrow)* in the coronary vein directed away from the splenic vein.

portal systemic collaterals (Figure 30-10). The diagnosis of portal hypertension can be made whenever hepatofugal flow is identified in any of these vessels.

Vessels that are not normal portal tributaries but instead develop or recanalize in the setting of portal hypertension are referred to as developed collaterals. The umbilical vein is the easiest of these to identify (Figure 30-11). The remnant of the umbilical vein is located in the ligamentum teres. In some patients it can be identified in the liver as a hypoechoic band running within the fat of the ligamentum teres. It extends from the umbilicus to the anteriormost aspect of the umbilical segment of the left portal vein. In normal individuals the remnant measures less than 3 mm and contains no blood flow.

The umbilical vein is best seen by first identifying the umbilical segment of the left portal vein.

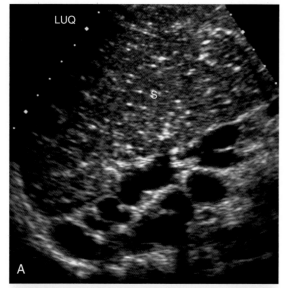

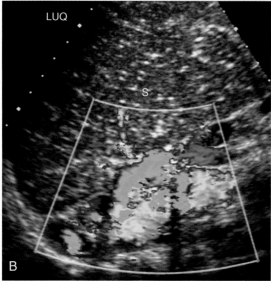

FIGURE 30-10 Short gastric collaterals in portal hypertension. **A,** Coronal view of the left upper quadrant through the spleen (S) shows multiple tortuous vessels medial to the spleen consistent with enlarged short gastric collaterals. Scattered small bright reflectors in the spleen are granulomas. **B,** Color Doppler view similar to gray-scale image in **A** shows flow throughout the short gastric collaterals.

The umbilical vein travels inferiorly from the umbilical segment of the left portal vein. After it exits the liver it extends inferiorly along the abdominal wall to the umbilical area and then extends further inferiorly to communicate with the inferior epigastric veins (see Figure 30-7). Ultimately, it communicates with the iliofemoral system and in this way diverts blood back to the systemic circulation. In most patients, a

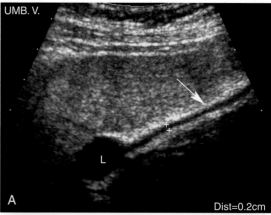

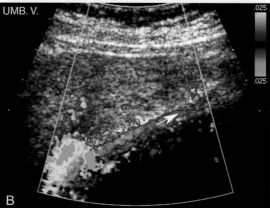

FIGURE 30-11 Small umbilical vein collateral in portal hypertension. **A,** Sagittal gray-scale view of the left lobe of the liver shows an umbilical vein collateral *(arrow)* communicating with the umbilical segment of the left portal vein (L). In this individual, the umbilical vein measures 2 mm in diameter *(cursors).* **B,** Sagittal color Doppler view shows hepatofugal flow *(arrow)* as the umbilical vein exits the liver.

recanalized umbilical vein appears as a variably sized, straight, single collateral within the central aspect of the ligamentum teres (Figure 30-12; see Figure 30-11). As it extends inferior to the liver, however, it begins to ramify into multiple periumbilical collaterals. In some patients with unusually large collaterals, particularly numerous and tortuous collaterals can be visualized around the umbilicus (Figure 30-13). When these periumbilical collaterals become so prominent that they are visible on physical examination, they are referred to as the caput medusae.

Gibson and associates[31] have shown that the normal remnant of the umbilical vein should not exceed 3 mm. Using this cutoff value, they were able to diagnose portal hypertension, without relying on Doppler, with a sensitivity of approximately 50%. By using Doppler and

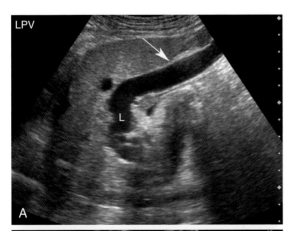

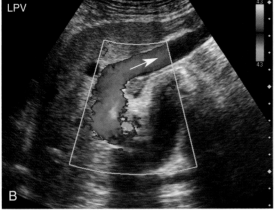

FIGURE 30-12 Large umbilical vein collateral in portal hypertension. **A,** Sagittal gray-scale view of the liver shows a large umbilical vein collateral *(arrow)* connecting to the umbilical segment of the left portal vein (L). **B,** Sagittal color Doppler view shows hepatofugal flow *(arrow)* as the umbilical vein exits the liver.

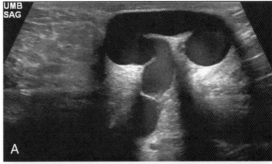

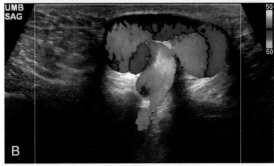

FIGURE 30-13 Sonographic caput medusae sign in portal hypertension. **A,** Sagittal magnified gray-scale view of the umbilicus shows enlarged tortuous vessels in the periumbilical region. **B,** Sagittal color Doppler view shows abundant blood flow within these periumbilical collaterals.

demonstrating hepatofugal flow in the umbilical vein, sensitivity increased to 80%. In fact, for diagnosing portal hypertension, sensitivity of Doppler evaluation of the umbilical vein was similar to endoscopic evaluation of varices in their population of patients.[31]

Based on the description above, it is clear that evaluation of either the umbilical vein or the coronary vein can lead to good sensitivity in diagnosing portal hypertension. Routinely scanning both potential collaterals will only increase sensitivity. Although these two collaterals are the easiest and most productive to analyze, there are other collaterals that can be detected sonographically, albeit with more difficulty in some cases. These include short gastric, splenoretroperitoneal, splenorenal, superior mesenteric, and inferior mesenteric collaterals. Large spontaneous portal systemic collaterals from the splenic hilum

or capsule to the left renal vein are known as splenorenal shunts. It is often difficult to trace these collaterals in continuity from the splenic vein to the renal vein. Fortunately, the detection of an enlarged left renal vein and multiple collaterals around the splenic hilum is generally enough to make the presumptive diagnosis of a splenorenal collateral. Splenoretroperitoneal collaterals communicate with lumbar veins, perivertebral vessels, or gonadal vessels. Superior mesenteric collaterals communicate with pancreaticoduodenal veins and retroperitoneal/perivertebral veins. Inferior mesenteric collaterals communicate with retroperitoneal veins and hemorrhoidal veins.

PORTAL VEIN FLOW REVERSAL

As mentioned earlier, flow reversal occurs in the portal veins as portal hypertension develops and progresses. This initially occurs in isolated peripheral portal vein branches.[16,32] This is easily detected with color Doppler since portal vein flow will be in the opposite direction as hepatic arterial flow, producing adjacent parallel vessels that are color coded in red and blue (Figure 30-14, *A*). It can be confirmed with pulsed Doppler by documenting venous and arterial flow

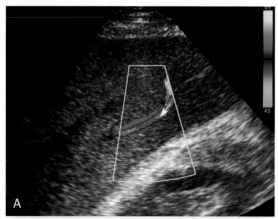

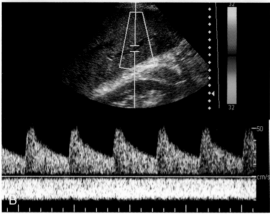

FIGURE 30-14 Intrahepatic portal vein flow reversal in portal hypertension. **A,** Color Doppler view of the right lobe of the liver shows two adjacent parallel vessels. The vessel color coded in red is the hepatic artery with hepatopetal blood flow directed toward the periphery of the liver *(black arrow)*. The vessel color coded in blue is the portal vein with reversed hepatofugal flow directed out of the liver *(white arrow)*. **B,** Pulsed Doppler waveform from the same two vessels shows hepatic arterial flow above the baseline and portal venous flow below the baseline. Normally, flow in the intrahepatic arteries and veins should be in the same direction, thus on the same side of the baseline.

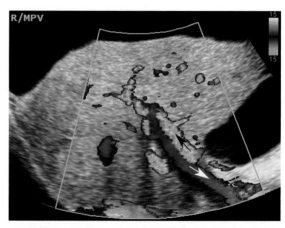

FIGURE 30-15 Flow reversal in the major portal veins in portal hypertension. Oblique view of the liver hilum shows reversed, hepatofugal flow in the right portal vein and main portal vein *(white arrow)*. There is antegrade flow in a prominent artery *(black arrow)*.

on opposite sides of the baseline (Figure 30-14, *B*). Eventually, as flow reverses in more portal vein branches, the main portal vein also reverses (Figure 30-15). Reversal of flow in the main portal vein typically indicates that portal hypertension is severe. It is not seen in early stages, and it is very important to realize that most patients with portal hypertension maintain antegrade flow in the main portal vein.

In addition to reversed flow, flow that alternates between antegrade and retrograde indicates sluggish flow and is another sign of portal hypertension. The alterations in flow direction may occur with the respiratory cycle or may be seen with varying the amount of pressure exerted on the liver by the transducer.[33]

In summary, the combination of gray-scale sonography and Doppler are valuable means for investigating suspected portal hypertension. Familiarity with the diagnostic implications and limitations of a variety of morphologic and hemodynamic alterations seen on gray-scale and Doppler findings is important in optimizing the sonographic analysis of these patients.

PORTAL VEIN THROMBOSIS

Evaluation of suspected PVT is probably the most common indication for a hepatic Doppler examination. PVT is most frequently a consequence of cirrhosis and portal hypertension, occurring in between 1% of early cirrhotic patients to up to 30% in advanced cirrhotic patients evaluated before liver transplantation.[34] Approximately 20% of all cases of PVT are due to cirrhosis. This is believed to be related to the sluggish portal vein flow in portal hypertension.[35] Malignancies (especially hepatic and pancreatic) are also responsible for approximately 20% of PVT due to direct invasion, extrinsic compression, or a hypercoagulable state.[34] Other causes include intra-abdominal inflammatory/infectious processes (i.e., diverticulitis, appendicitis, cholecystitis, inflammatory bowel disease), portal vein injury (splenectomy, intestinal resection, liver transplantation, TIPS, abdominal trauma), myeloproliferative diseases, and hypercoagulable

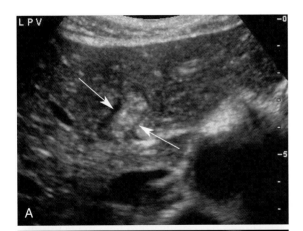

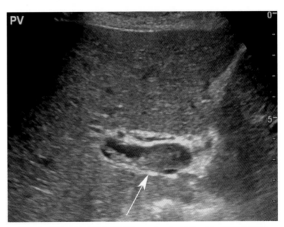

FIGURE 30-17 Isoechoic portal vein thrombosis. Oblique view of the liver hilum shows thrombus similar in echogenicity to the adjacent liver parenchyma partially occluding the portal vein *(arrow).*

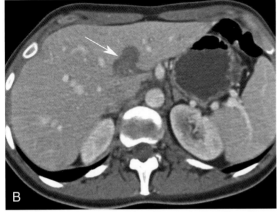

FIGURE 30-16 Hyperechoic portal vein thrombosis. **A,** Transverse view of the left lobe of the liver shows a segment of the left portal vein containing hyperechoic thrombus *(arrows).* **B,** Corresponding contrast-enhanced computed tomographic scan showing thrombus in the same segment of the left portal vein *(arrow).*

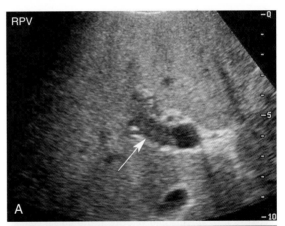

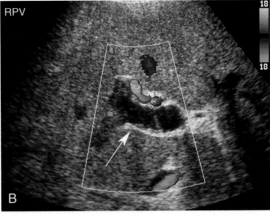

FIGURE 30-18 Hypoechoic portal vein thrombosis. **A,** Transverse gray-scale view of the right lobe of the liver shows thrombus filling the right portal vein *(arrow)* that is hypoechoic to the liver parenchyma. **B,** Transverse color Doppler view of the right lobe of the liver shows no detectable blood flow within the right portal vein *(arrow).*

states including pregnancy and oral contraceptives.[34,35] Clinical manifestations in acute PVT, when present, are typically related to intestinal congestion and ischemia and include pain, distension, diarrhea, gastrointestinal bleeding, and lactic acidosis. Chronic PVT may be completely asymptomatic or may present with varices or hypersplenism[34,35]

Sonographically, PVT may appear hyperechoic (Figure 30-16), isoechoic (Figure 30-17), hypoechoic (Figure 30-18), or anechoic. When the thrombus is clearly seen on gray-scale sonography, the diagnosis is straightforward. However, hypoechoic or anechoic thrombus can be difficult to distinguish from low-level artifactual echoes that are often seen in the portal vein. In such cases, color Doppler is important in establishing the diagnosis. With occlusive thrombus, no flow is detectable in the affected segment of the portal

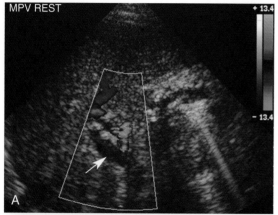

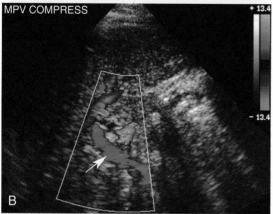

FIGURE 30-19 Slow portal vein flow simulating thrombosis. **A,** Oblique color Doppler view of the porta hepatis shows no detectable flow in the portal vein *(arrow)*. Low-level echoes in the portal vein may be due to thrombus or may be artifactual. **B,** Similar view of the porta hepatis obtained during compression of the lower abdomen. This augments mesenteric venous flow and increases flow volume and velocity in the portal vein so that it becomes detectable. *(Reproduced with permission from Robinson KA, Middleton WD, Al-Sukaiti R, et al: Doppler sonography of portal hypertension,* Ultrasound Q *25:3–13, 2009.)*

imaging, the possibility of very slow flow should also be considered. Careful attention should be paid to technical parameters that affect Doppler sensitivity so that detection of slow flow is maximized. Because portal vein flow increases after eating, postprandial scans can also help in detecting slow portal venous flow. Compression of the lower abdomen may also augment portal flow in a manner analogous to compression of the calf used to augment flow in the femoral veins (Figure 30-19). If flow remains undetectable despite these maneuvers, PVT is probably present. However, slow flow remains a possibility, and other tests should be considered to help make this distinction. Contrast-enhanced sonography is one such test that is extremely useful in making this distinction.[38] Contrast-enhanced magnetic resonance imaging is also very helpful.[39]

As mentioned above, the negative predictive value of Doppler is 98%.[36,37] This means that it is very unusual for portal thrombosis to be present when the Doppler examination is normal. One situation where that can happen is when color Doppler blooming artifact obscures focal nonobstructive thrombus (Figure 30-20). In such cases, the thrombus is usually easy to see on gray-scale images. This is another reason why it is critical to include both a careful gray-scale examination and Doppler examination whenever PVT is a possibility.

In addition to bland thrombus, tumor thrombus can occur, particularly as a complication of hepatocellular carcinoma. Macroscopic portal vein invasion is present in approximately 16% of patients undergoing hepatic resection for hepatocellular cancer. When present, this negatively affects both morbidity and mortality.

Certain gray-scale findings can be helpful in distinguishing bland thrombus and tumor thrombus. Tumor thrombus often expands the lumen of the portal vein, whereas bland thrombus rarely does. In addition, tumor thrombus may contain small cystic spaces, and this is uncommon in bland thrombus. Tumor invasion of the portal vein starts in the peripheral veins and then grows, along with its arterial supply, into the more central portal veins. Accordingly, arterial flow in tumor thrombus is usually hepatofugal (opposite the direction of the portal venous flow).[40] Visualization of internal vascularity in tumor thrombus on color Doppler and detection of an arterial signal on pulsed Doppler is relatively easy in some patients (Figure 30-21).

vein. With partially occlusive thrombus, a flow void is present in the affected segment.

Doppler sonography is generally recognized as the modality of choice for evaluation of suspected PVT. Sensitivity is 93%, specificity is 99%, positive predictive value is 97%, and negative predictive value is 98%.[36] As mentioned earlier, one limitation of color Doppler is that a patent portal vein may have very slow flow that cannot be detected with color Doppler.[37] Fortunately, this is becoming increasingly less common. Nevertheless, whenever the diagnosis of PVT is being entertained based on lack of detectable flow, but thrombus is not confirmed on gray-scale

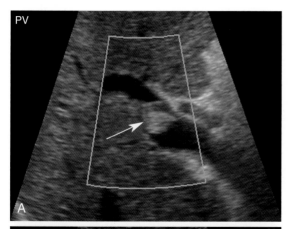

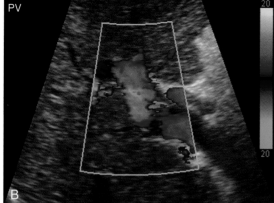

FIGURE 30-20 Color Doppler blooming artifact obscuring nonobstructive portal vein thrombosis. **A,** Oblique magnified view of the porta hepatis shows a hyperechoic focal thrombus in the portal vein lumen *(arrow).* **B,** Color Doppler view of the identical area shows blooming artifact obscuring the majority of the portal vein thrombus, making detection difficult.

In other patients however, tumor thrombus may be avascular on Doppler analysis[41] (Figure 30-22). Thus, detection of hepatofugal arterial flow in portal vein thrombus is diagnostic of tumor, but inability to detect internal Doppler signals does not necessarily mean that the thrombus is bland.

When it is necessary to obtain a tissue diagnosis in a patient with suspected hepatocellular carcinoma and tumor thrombus, it is safe to biopsy the thrombus in the portal vein.[42] This can be done as a fine-needle aspiration with a 22- to 25-gauge needle (Figure 30-22, *D*). Contrast-enhanced sonography has also been reported to be very sensitive in the diagnosis of tumor thrombus.[38] It is superior to spiral CT (computed tomography)[43] and actually exceeds fine-needle aspiration in some reports.[41]

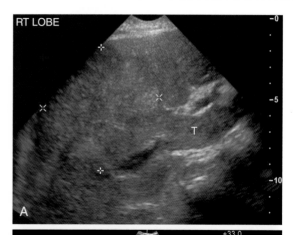

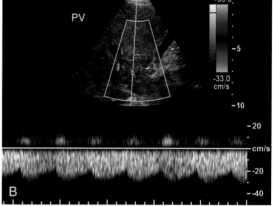

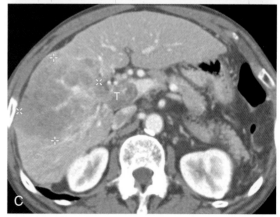

FIGURE 30-21 Portal vein tumor thrombus in a patient with hepatocellular carcinoma. **A,** Transverse gray-scale view of the right lobe of the liver shows a poorly marginated solid heterogeneous mass *(cursors)* in the right lobe of the liver. Tumor thrombus (T) extends directly from the mass into the portal vein. **B,** Oblique color Doppler image shows a small tumor vessel within the thrombus with a hepatofugal arterial signal on pulsed Doppler analysis. **C,** Contrast-enhanced computed tomographic scan shows the tumor in the right lobe *(cursors)* and the tumor thrombus in the portal vein (T).

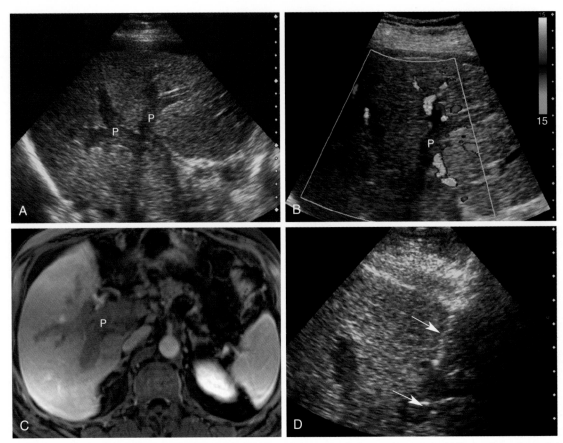

FIGURE 30-22 Portal vein tumor thrombus in a patient with hepatocellular carcinoma. **A,** Oblique view of the right lobe of the liver shows solid hypoechoic thrombus expanding the lumen of intrahepatic branches of the portal vein (P). **B,** Color Doppler view of one of these thrombosed portal vein branches shows flow in periportal arteries but no detectable flow within the portal vein thrombus. **C,** Transverse contrast-enhanced magnetic resonance scan of the liver shows a nonenhancing thrombus within the portal vein (P). **D,** Portal vein fine-needle aspiration. Magnified view of the liver periphery shows needle shaft and tip within the portal vein thrombus *(arrows)*. Cytologic analysis confirmed hepatocellular carcinoma.

One consequence of PVT is development of periportal venous collaterals in the hepatoduodenal ligament, referred to as cavernous transformation.[44,45] These collaterals can form relatively rapidly and have been documented to form as soon as 6 to 20 days after PVT.[46] Collateral venous flow, in addition to augmented hepatic arterial flow, may maintain relatively normal perfusion to the liver.[44] Although it is unusual, cavernous transformation may also develop when the portal vein is compromised but not completely thrombosed. When these collaterals are large enough and contain substantial blood flow, they can be seen in the porta hepatis as multiple tortuous vessels on grayscale and on color or power Doppler images (Figure 30-23).[46-48]

Although the thrombosed portal vein is usually apparent in the setting of cavernous transformation, it may be hard to identify and/or recognize if the thrombosed portal vein is thin and fibrosed or if the thrombus is isoechoic to the adjacent liver. In such cases, a single dominant periportal collateral may be mistaken for a patent main portal vein. Realizing that the normal portal vein travels deep to the right hepatic artery and periportal collaterals travel anterior to the right hepatic artery allows for proper interpretation in most instances. Enlarged, tortuous hepatic arteries can be another potential pitfall in the proper interpretation of cavernous transformation. Arterial enlargement usually occurs in the setting of cirrhosis and portal hypertension and can be distinguished from venous collaterals by Doppler waveform analysis.

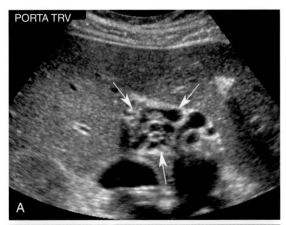

PORTA TRV

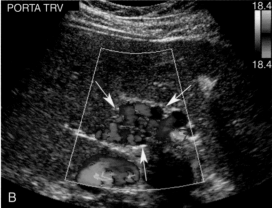

PORTA TRV   18.4

18.4

B

FIGURE 30-23 Cavernous transformation in a patient with portal vein thrombosis. **A,** Transverse view of the porta hepatis shows multiple tortuous vascular channels replacing the porta hepatis *(arrows)*. No defined portal vein is identified. **B,** Color Doppler view in the same area confirms flow within these periportal collaterals.

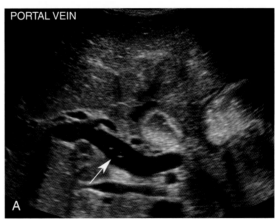

PORTAL VEIN

A

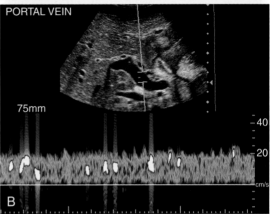

PORTAL VEIN

75mm

−40

−20

cm/s

B

FIGURE 30-24 Portal vein gas. **A,** Oblique view through the liver hilum shows two small bright reflectors within the lumen of the portal vein *(arrow)*. On real-time imaging, multiple similar reflectors were seen flowing throughout the portal venous system. **B,** Pulsed Doppler waveform (displayed with a reverse rainbow color map) from the portal vein shows multiple bright signals embedded within the portal vein signal. These represent the strong reflections from gas bubbles. Artifactual signal spikes are seen associated with many of these bubbles.

PORTAL VEIN GAS

Portal vein gas (PVG) can be due to a number of processes. Clearly the most important is bowel ischemia. When PVG is associated with ischemic bowel, the prognosis is poor. Other etiologies include diverticulitis, appendicitis, bowel distension, bowel obstruction, ulcer disease, inflammatory bowel disease, intestinal pneumotosis, abdominal abscess, sepsis, hypertrophic pyloric stenosis, gastrointestinal cancers, chronic obstructive pulmonary disease, corticosteroids, and following endoscopy and barium enemas. In these latter situations, the prognosis is good. Portal vein gas can also be idiopathic.[49]

PVG can be readily detected both on gray-scale and Doppler images.[50,51] As one would expect, small, mobile, bright reflectors are seen in the lumen of the portal vein and its branches on

gray scale (Figure 30-24, *A*). PVG can accumulate in the peripheral intrahepatic branches or liver parenchyma and cause bright linear reflectors or poorly defined areas of increased echogenicity. In the latter situation, PVG can potentially be confused with pneumobilia or parenchymal calcifications. The portal vein Doppler waveform typically shows periodic short, bright signals arising directly from the gas bubbles. Since these bubbles travel in the same direction and at the same velocity as the red blood cells in the portal vein, the bright signals arising from the gas are superimposed on the normal portal vein Doppler waveform (Figure 30-24, *B*). Because the gas signals are substantially stronger than the signals from red blood cells, they overload the Doppler receiver and frequently produce narrow artifactual spikes that extend on both sides of the baseline.

Because gas is such a strong reflector, sonography and Doppler analysis are extremely sensitive to PVG. In fact, the small quantities of gas that can be detected by sonography and Doppler generally has a much less ominous prognosis compared to the massive amounts of gas that are generally seen by radiography or the moderate amounts seen by CT.[49] It is also important to realize that detection of PVT by sonography and Doppler should not be questioned if subsequent radiographs or CTs are negative.[51-53]

Management of PVG depends on the etiology. In most situations, Doppler detection of PVG should be followed by careful sonographic inspection of the rest of the abdomen for possible etiologies. Close clinical assessment for possible bowel ischemia is critical. Contrast-enhanced CT also has an important role in evaluation of possible bowel-related pathology and ischemia.

HEPATIC VEIN OBSTRUCTION

Hepatic vein obstruction, also known as Budd-Chiari syndrome, can be due to thrombosis, compression, tumor infiltration, stenosis, or webs, and it can occur in the major hepatic veins, the IVC, or at a microscopic level. The most common cause is thrombosis, and most patients have one or more thrombotic risk factors, with oral contraceptives and myeloproliferative processes being most common.[54] In Asian populations, membranous obstruction of the IVC is common.[55] Although it is a rare disease with an estimated incidence of 1 in 2.5 million persons per year,[54] it is often included in the clinical differential diagnosis for patients with abdominal pain and acute onset of ascites. Although the majority of patients can be treated with anticoagulation, other options include TIPS, surgical shunting, and liver transplantation.[55]

The two most common findings on gray-scale sonography are overall hepatomegaly and selective hypertrophy of the caudate lobe.[56] Unfortunately, these are both very nonspecific. Hepatic vein thrombosis (HVT) itself appears like thrombus elsewhere in the body. It can range from hyperechoic to anechoic and can be occlusive or nonocclusive. In the acute setting, extensive HVT can manifest as hepatic failure, liver

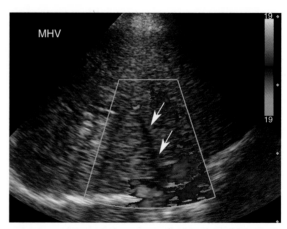

FIGURE 30-25 Hepatic vein thrombosis. Transverse view of the liver shows a poorly defined middle hepatic vein *(arrows)* with no detectable flow.

enlargement, and massive ascites. In such cases, gray-scale visualization of the hepatic veins may be very difficult. The hepatic veins may also be difficult to visualize in chronic cases, due to fibrosis and decreased size. Fortunately, there are a variety of hemodynamic consequences of HVT that can usually be detected with Doppler when the thrombosed vein itself cannot be detected.

The most obvious Doppler finding is lack of flow in the hepatic veins despite visualization of the veins on gray-scale images[57] (Figure 30-25). Because hepatic venous flow from obstructed segments cannot flow to the IVC in the normal way, collateral pathways develop[58] (Figure 30-26). The collaterals that are most frequently seen drain to unobstructed hepatic veins (such as accessory hepatic veins or caudate lobe veins), subcapsular veins, or portal veins. The caudate lobe is particularly important to evaluate because enlarged caudate veins (>3 mm) are present in approximately 50% of cases and in the absence of heart failure are a specific sign of Budd-Chiari syndrome.[55]

When collaterals develop, the hepatic vein that supplies the collateral will have reversed flow. This produces the typical appearance where one hepatic vein branch is flowing in a hepatofugal direction toward the IVC and a communicating vein is flowing away from the IVC in a hepatopetal direction (Figure 30-27). Because HVT isolates the hepatic vein from the right atrium, the pressure fluctuations in the right atrium do not get transferred to the patent portions of the hepatic vein. Therefore, the hepatic vein waveform loses its pulsatility and becomes

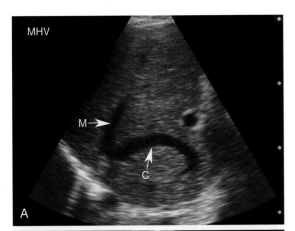

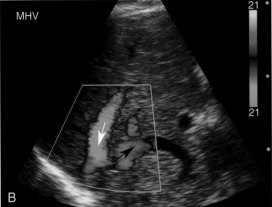

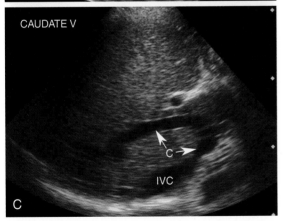

FIGURE 30-26 Hepatic vein thrombosis. **A,** Oblique view of the right lobe of the liver shows the middle hepatic vein (M) communicating with a collateral vessel (C) that is directed toward the caudate lobe. **B,** Color Doppler view similar to gray-scale view shown in **A** shows antegrade flow in the middle hepatic vein *(white arrow)* and reversed flow in the collateral vein *(black arrow).* **C,** Gray-scale view shows the collateral vein (C) communicating with veins in the caudate lobe and ultimately draining into the inferior vena cava (IVC).

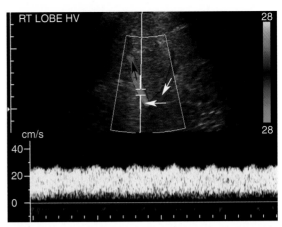

FIGURE 30-27 Hepatic vein thrombosis. Magnified color Doppler view of connecting hepatic veins shows antegrade flow in one vessel *(white arrow)* and reversed flow directed back into the liver *(black arrow)* in the other vessel. In this case the branch with reversed flow is supplying a collateral. Pulsed Doppler waveform analysis shows loss of the normal triphasic hepatic vein pulsatility.

monophasic (Figure 30-27). Other causes of blunted hepatic vein pulsatility include cirrhosis, diffuse metastatic disease, extrinsic compression of the vein, liver transplant rejection, other diffuse parenchymal diseases, and a deep inspiration. Finally, venous stenosis or webs can be seen as flow abnormalities and velocity elevations on color and pulsed Doppler.

Early investigations of Doppler ultrasound in making the diagnosis of HVT showed that the sensitivity was quite high.[59] Millener and colleagues[57] primarily relied on two criteria: (1) hepatic vein(s) seen on gray-scale imaging with no detectable flow or reversed flow on color Doppler and (2) hepatic vein(s) not seen on either gray-scale or color Doppler ultrasound, and they achieved a sensitivity of 100%. Unfortunately approximately 15% of patients with advanced cirrhosis but no HVT will have one or more hepatic veins that cannot be identified on either gray-scale or color Doppler. Therefore, the specificity of ultrasound was limited.[57] A more contemporary study has shown that Doppler ultrasound detected direct alterations of the hepatic veins and/or IVC in 98% of patients with Budd-Chiari syndrome.[56] Combining direct alterations of the veins and or IVC with a hypertrophied caudate lobe allowed for a specificity of 100%, and their absence excluded Budd-Chiari syndrome even if other suggestive signs were present. Sensitivity of Doppler is similar to magnetic resonance angiography.[59]

TRANSJUGULAR INTRAHEPATIC PORTOSYSTEMIC SHUNTS

TIPS has evolved into a common and well-accepted treatment for portal hypertension. The vast majority of shunts are placed in patients with variceal hemorrhage refractory to endoscopic and medical treatment and patients with refractory ascites. Other indications include Budd-Chiari syndrome, hepatorenal and hepatopulmonary syndromes, and hepatic hydrothorax. One-year mortality ranges from approximately 50% to 90% depending on the severity of liver disease and whether the procedure is performed emergently or electively. When covered stent-grafts are used, the technical success approaches 100%, and the one-year primary and secondary patency rates are approximately 80% and 99%.[60]

Doppler surveillance of patients following TIPS placement is somewhat controversial due to a lack of consensus on protocols to follow, parameters to measure, and criteria to use. Nevertheless, many centers rely heavily on Doppler sonography for follow-up of their TIPS patients.[61] The normal TIPS should have readily detectable flow throughout its lumen (Figure 30-28). Because the stent decompresses the high-pressure portal system directly into the low-pressure hepatic venous system, flow velocities in the stent are higher than typical for portal venous structures (Figure 30-29).[62] Although the normal range of TIPS velocities varies somewhat in different studies, a relatively widely accepted normal range is between approximately 90 and 190 cm/sec, and the normal post-TIPS portal vein velocity should be 30 cm/sec or greater.[63-65] An additional hemodynamic consequence seen in the majority of post-TIPS patients is that portal flow in the right and left portal vein reverses and is directed into the stent instead of into the liver[62] (Figure 30-28).

The major complications with TIPS are stenosis of the stent or the hepatic vein and complete thrombosis. The goal in monitoring these stents is to detect developing stenoses so they can be treated before development of clinical symptoms or complete thrombosis. Elevated velocities across the stenotic segment is a sign of intrastent stenosis. This is seen on color Doppler as focal areas of disturbed flow, color aliasing, and occasionally localized perivascular tissue vibration (Figure 30-30, *A*). When an abnormality is seen on color Doppler, pulsed

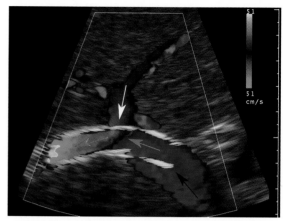

FIGURE 30-28 Normal transjugular intrahepatic portosystemic shunt (TIPS). Magnified view of the liver hilum shows a stent entering the portal vein at the junction of the right and main portal vein. Flow in the main portal vein *(black arrow)* and flow in the stent *(gray arrows)* are hepatopetal and directed into the liver. Flow in the right portal vein *(white arrow)* is directed in a retrograde manor toward the stent. *(Reproduced with permission from Middleton WD, Teefey SA, Darcy MD: Doppler evaluation of transjugular intrahepatic portosystemic shunts,* Ultrasound Q *19:56–70, 2003.)*

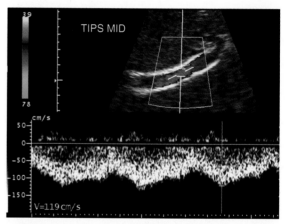

FIGURE 30-29 Normal transjugular intrahepatic portosystemic shunt (TIPS). Magnified color Doppler view of the stent shows flow throughout the stent lumen. Pulsed Doppler waveform shows normal slightly pulsatile flow with a velocity of 119 cm/sec.

Doppler waveforms can be obtained through the stenotic segments and velocities can be compared to nonstenotic segments (Figure 30-30, *B* and *C*). Velocities greater than 190 cm/sec in the stenotic segment and velocities less than 90 cm/sec in the nonstenotic segments are considered significant.[63] Low velocity (less than 30 cm/sec) in the main portal vein is another clue to TIPS dysfunction. When the stenosis occurs

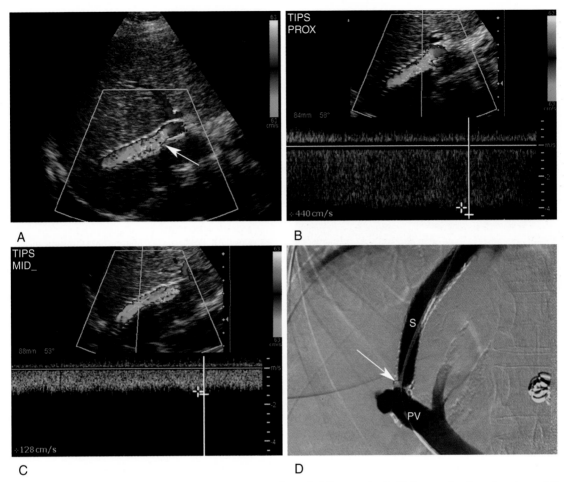

FIGURE 30-30 Transjugular intrahepatic portosystemic shunt (TIPS) stenosis. **A,** Oblique color Doppler view of the stent shows a focal area of aliasing and flow disturbance in the proximal segment *(arrow).* **B,** Pulsed Doppler waveform from the proximal stent confirms elevated velocity in this segment, reaching a maximum of 440 cm/sec. **C,** Pulsed Doppler waveform from the midstent shows a normal velocity of 128 cm/sec. **D,** Transjugular venogram of the stent (S) and portal vein (PV) shows a tight stricture at the junction of the stent and portal vein *(arrow).*

in the hepatic vein distal to the stent, flow in the hepatic vein that drains into the stent may reverse. Finally, conversion of left and/or right portal flow from the normal pattern of flow toward the stent to a pattern of flow away from the stent on follow-up scans indicates decreased flow going through the shunt. This type of flow conversion is usually a late manifestation of shunt dysfunction. Minor deviations from normal in single Doppler parameters typically do not indicate a significant stenosis. For instance, a portal vein velocity of 28 cm/sec would not be an indication for venography unless other abnormalities were present. Likewise, a slightly elevated maximum stent velocity or a slightly depressed minimum stent velocity would not

be indications for venography if they were isolated abnormalities. Stenosis is likely and intervention should be considered when multiple parameters are abnormal.[61] In addition, if sequential examinations have been performed, temporal trends in the various Doppler parameters are usually present and provide further evidence that a stenosis has developed.[65] In some patients, neointimal hyperplasia and hepatic vein or portal vein stenosis can be imaged directly as a narrowing in the flow lumen on color or power Doppler. When stent stenosis goes undetected, it can progress to complete thrombosis. This is usually easy to diagnose with Doppler since normal stent flow is relatively easy to detect (Figure 30-31).

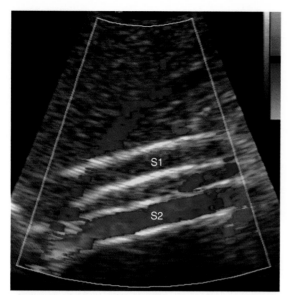

FIGURE 30-31 Transjugular intrahepatic portosystemic shunt (TIPS) thrombosis. Oblique view of the liver in a patient with dual parallel stents shows a thrombosed TIPS stent (S1) with no detectable flow adjacent to a patent stent (S2) with readily detectable blood flow. *(Reproduced with permission from Middleton WD, Teefey SA, Darcy MD: Doppler evaluation of transjugular intrahepatic portosystemic shunts,* Ultrasound Q *19:56–70, 2003.)*

REFERENCES

1. Fauci AS, et al: *Harrison's principles of internal medicine,* ed 17, USA, McGraw-Hill, 2008: 1972–1976.
2. Federle MP, et al: *Diagnostic imaging abdomen,* Salt Lake City, 2008, Amirsys. 1-40.
3. Abu-Yousef MM: Normal and respiratory variations of the hepatic and portal venous duplex Doppler waveforms with simultaneous electrocardiographic correlation, *J Ultrasound Med* 11:263–268, 1992.
4. Abu-Yousef MM: Duplex Doppler sonography of the hepatic vein in tricuspid regurgitation, *AJR Am J Roentgenol* 156:79–83, 1991.
5. Bombelli L, et al: Liver hemodynamic flow balance by image-directed Doppler ultrasound evaluation in normal subjects, *J Clin Ultrasound* 19:257–262, 1991.
6. Gallix BP, et al: Flow pulsatility in the portal venous system: A study of Doppler sonography in healthy adults, *AJR Am J Roentgenol* 169:141–144, 1997.
7. Wachsberg RH, Needleman L, Wilson DJ: Portal vein pulsatility in normal cirrhotic adults without cardiac disease, *J Clin Ultrasound* 23:3–15, 1995.
8. Duerinckx AJ, et al: The pulsatile portal vein in cases of congestive heart failure: Correlation of duplex Doppler findings with right atrial pressures, *Radiology* 176: 655–658, 1990.
9. Abu-Yousef MM, Milam SG, Farner RM: Pulsatile portal vein flow: A sign of tricuspid regurgitation on duplex Doppler, *AJR Am J Roentgenol* 155:785–788, 1990.
10. Patriquin H, et al: Duplex Doppler examination in portal hypertension: Technique and anatomy, *AJR Am J Roentgenol* 149:71–76, 1987.
11. Haag K, et al: Correlation of duplex sonography findings and portal pressure in 375 patients with portal hypertension, *AJR Am J Roentgenol* 172:631–635, 1999.
12. Kok T, et al: The value of Doppler ultrasound in cirrhosis and portal hypertension, *Scand J Gastroenterol Suppl* 230:82–88, 1999.
13. Zironi G, et al: Value of measurement of mean portal flow velocity by Doppler flowmetry in the diagnosis of portal hypertension, *J Hepatol* 16:298–303, 1992.
14. Cioni G, et al: Duplex-Doppler assessment of cirrhosis in patients with chronic compensated liver disease, *J Gastroenterol Hepatol* 7:382–384, 1992.
15. Rosenthal SJ, et al: Doppler ultrasound of helical flow in the portal vein, *Radiographics* 15:1103–1111, 1995.
16. Ralls PW: Color Doppler sonography of the hepatic artery and portal venous system, *AJR Am J Roentgenol* 155:517–525, 1990.
17. Goyal AK, Pokharna DS, Sharma SK: Ultrasonic measurements of portal vasculature in diagnosis of portal hypertension—a controversial subject reviewed, *J Ultrasound Med* 9:45–48, 1990.
18. Weinreb J, et al: Portal vein measurements by real time sonography, *AJR Am J Roentgenol* 139:497–499, 1982.
19. Bolondi L, et al: Ultrasonography in the diagnosis of portal hypertension: diminished response of portal vessels to respiration, *Radiology* 142:167–172, 1982.
20. Choi YJ, et al: Comparison of Doppler ultrasonography and the hepatic venous pressure gradient in assessing portal hypertension in liver cirrhosis, *J Gastroenterol Hepatol* 18:424–429, 2003.
21. Moriyasu F, et al: Congestion index of the portal vein, *AJR Am J Roentgenol* 146:735–739, 1986.
22. Ohta M, et al: Prognostic significance of hepatic vein waveform by Doppler ultrasonography in cirrhotic patients with portal hypertension, *Am J Gastroenterol* 90:1853–1857, 1995.
23. Lorenz J, Winsberg F: Focal hepatic vein stenosis in diffuse liver disease, *J Ultrasound Med* 15:313–316, 1996.
24. Burcharth F: Percutaneous transhepatic portography. Technique and application, *AJR Am J Roentgenol* 132: 177–182, 1979.
25. Nunez D Jr, et al: Portosystemic communications studied by transhepatic portography, *Radiology* 127:75–79, 1978.
26. Subramanyam BR, et al: Sonography of portosystemic venous collaterals in portal hypertension, *Radiology* 146:161–166, 1983.
27. Schmassman A, et al: Recurrent bleeding after variceal hemorrhage: predictive value of portal venous duplex sonography, *AJR Am J Roentgenol* 160:41–47, 1993.
28. Lafortune M, et al: The portal venous system measurements in portal hypertension, *Radiology* 151:27–30, 1984.
29. Dach JL, et al: Sonography of hypertensive portal venous system: Correlation with arterial portography, *AJR Am J Roentgenol* 137:511–517, 1981.
30. Wachsberg RH, Simmons MZ: Coronary vein diameter and flow direction in patients with portal hypertension: Evaluation with duplex sonography and correlation with variceal bleeding, *AJR Am J Roentgenol* 162:637–641, 1994.
31. Gibson RN, et al: Identification of a patent paraumbilical vein by using Doppler sonography: Importance in diagnosis of portal hypertension, *AJR Am J Roentgenol* 153:513–516, 1989.

32. Wachsberg RH, et al: Hepatofugal flow in the portal venous system: Pathophysiology, imaging findings, and diagnostic pitfalls, *Radiographics* 22:123–140, 2002.

33. Robinson KA, et al: Doppler sonography of portal hypertension, *Ultrasound Q* 25:3–13, 2009.

34. Ponziani FR, et al: Portal vein thrombosis: Insight into physiopathology, diagnosis, and treatment, *World J Gastroenterol* 16:143–155, 2009.

35. Fimognari FL, Violi F: Portal vein thrombosis in liver cirrhosis, *Intern Emerg Med* 3:213–218, 2008.

36. Bach AM, et al: Portal vein evaluation with US: Comparison to angiography combined with CT arterial portography, *Radiology* 201(1):149–154, 1996 Oct.

37. Tessler FN, et al: Diagnosis of portal vein thrombosis: Value of color Doppler imaging, *AJR Am J Roentgenol* 157:293–296, 1991.

38. Rossi S, et al: Contrast-Enhanced Versus Conventional and Color Doppler Sonography for the Detection of Thrombosis of the Portal and Hepatic Venous Systems, *AJR Am J Roentgenol* 186:763–773, 2006.

39. Cakmak O, et al: Role of contrast-enhanced 3D magnetic resonance portography in evaluating portal venous system compared with color Doppler ultrasonography, *Abdom Imaging* 33:65–71, 2008.

40. Dodd GD III, et al: Portal vein thrombosis in patients with cirrhosis: Does sonographic detection of intrathrombus flow allow differentiation of benign and malignant thrombus? *AJR Am J Roentgenol* 165:573, 1995.

41. Tarantino L, et al: Diagnosis of benign and malignant portal vein thrombosis in cirrhotic patients with hepatocellular carcinoma: Color Doppler US, contrast-enhanced US, and fine-needle biopsy, *Abdom Imaging* 31:537–544, 2006.

42. Dusenbery D, Dodd GD III, Carr BI: Percutaneous fine-needle aspiration of portal vein thrombi as a staging technique for hepatocellular carcinoma. Cytologic findings of 46 patients, *Cancer* 75:2057–2062, 1995.

43. Rossi S, et al: Contrast-enhanced ultrasonography and spiral computed tomography in the detection and characterization of portal vein thrombosis complicating hepatocellular carcinoma, *Eur Radiol* 18:1749–1756, 2008.

44. Sobhonslidsuk A, Reddy KR: Portal vein thrombosis: a concise review, *Am J Gastroenterol* 97:535–541, 2002.

45. Valla DC, Condat B: Portal vein thrombosis in adults: pathophysiology, pathogenesis and management, *J Hepatol* 32(5):865–871, 2000 May.

46. De Gaetano AM, et al: Cavernous transformation of the portal vein: Patterns of intrahepatic and splanchnic collateral circulation detected with Doppler sonography, *AJR Am J Roentgenol* 165:1151–1155, 1995.

47. Weltin G, et al: Duplex Doppler: Identification of cavernous transformation of the portal vein, *AJR Am J Roentgenol* 144:999–1001, 1985.

48. Kauzlaric D, Petrovic M, Barmeir E: Sonography of cavernous transformation of the portal vein, *AJR Am J Roentgenol* 142:383–384, 1984.

49. Sebastià C, et al: Portomesenteric vein gas: Pathologic mechanisms, CT findings, and prognosis, *Radiographics* 20:1213–1224, 2000.

50. Lafortune M, et al: Air in the portal vein: Sonographic and Doppler manifestations, *Radiology* 180:667–670, 1991.

51. Oktar SO, et al: Portomesenteric venous gas: Imaging findings with an emphasis on sonography, *J Ultrasound Med* 25:1051–1105, 2006.

52. Maher MM, et al: Portal venous gas: Detection by gray-scale and Doppler sonography in the absence of correlative findings on computed tomography, *Abdom Imaging* 26:390–394, 2001.

53. San Millan Ruiz D, de Perrot T, Majno PE: A case of portal venous gas secondary to acute appendicitis detected on gray scale sonography but not computed tomography, *J Ultrasound Med* 24:383–386, 2005.

54. Darwish Murad S, et al: EN-Vie (European Network for Vascular Disorders of the Liver). Etiology, management, and outcome of the Budd-Chiari syndrome, *Ann Intern Med* 151(3):167–175, 2009 Aug 4.

55. Bargallo X, et al: Sonography of Budd-Chiari syndrome, *AJR Am J Roentgenol* 187:33–41, 2006.

56. Boozari B, et al: Ultrasonography in patients with Budd-Chiari syndrome: Diagnostic signs and prognostic implications, *J Hepatol* 49(4):572–580, 2008 Oct.

57. Millener P, et al: Color Doppler imaging findings in patients with Budd-Chiari syndrome: Correlation with venographic findings, *AJR Am J Roentgenol* 161(2):307–312, 1993 Aug.

58. Ralls PW, et al: Budd-Chiari syndrome: Detection with color Doppler sonography, *AJR* 159:113–116, 1992.

59. Kane R, Eustace S: Diagnosis of Budd-Chiari syndrome: Comparison between sonography and MR angiography, *Radiology* 195:117–121, 1995.

60. Owen AR, et al: The transjugular intrahepatic portosystemic shunt (TIPS), *Clin Radiol* 64(7):664–674, 2009.

61. Middleton WD, Teefey SA, Darcy MD: Doppler evaluation of transjugular intrahepatic portosystemic shunts, *Ultrasound Q* 19:56–70, 2003.

62. Surratt RS, et al: Morphologic and hemodynamic findings at sonography before and after placement of a transjugular intrahepatic portosystemic shunt, *AJR Am J Roentgenol* 160:627–630, 1993.

63. Kanterman RY, et al: Doppler sonographic findings associated with transjugular intrahepatic portosystemic shunt (TIPS) malfunction, *AJR Am J Roentgenol* 168:467–472, 1997.

64. Feldstein VA, Patel MD, LaBerge JM: TIPS shunts: Accuracy of Doppler US in determination of patency and detection of stenoses, *Radiology* 201:141–147, 1996.

65. Dodd GD III, et al: Detection of transjugular intrahepatic portosystemic shunt dysfunction: Value of duplex Doppler sonography, *AJR Am J Roentgenol* 164(5):1119–1124, 1995 May.

ULTRASOUND ASSESSMENT OF NATIVE RENAL VESSELS

31

JOHN S. PELLERITO, MD, FACR, FSRU, FAIUM, and MARGARITA V. REVZIN, MS, MD

This chapter focuses on the duplex ultrasound assessment of the renal arteries and veins. The anatomy and principles of examination of the native renal vessels are considered first, followed by a discussion of renal vascular disorders, including renal artery stenosis and occlusion, aneurysms, arteriovenous fistulas (AVF) and arteriovenous malformations (AVMs), renal vein thrombosis, and tumor invasion of the renal veins. We finish with a discussion of renal artery stent evaluation with new diagnostic criteria for in-stent restenosis.

ANATOMY

Each kidney receives its arterial supply from one or more renal arteries. The renal arteries arise from the proximal abdominal aorta just below the origin of the superior mesenteric artery, which serves as a reference point (Figure 31-1). The right renal artery arises at an anterolateral location and passes posterior to the inferior vena cava (IVC). It is the only major vessel posterior to the IVC. The left renal artery generally arises from the lateral or posterolateral aspect of the aorta. Anterior to each renal artery runs a corresponding renal vein. Both vessels course anterior to the renal pelvis before entering the medial aspect of the renal hilum. The left renal vein lies *between* the superior mesenteric artery and the aorta (as opposed to the splenic vein, which lies *anterior* to the superior mesenteric artery). One of the most common anatomic variants of the renal venous system is a circumaortic left renal vein, in which one of the limbs of the left renal vein courses anterior to the aorta and another one runs posterior to it.

The right kidney is relatively inferior in its position, which explains a long downward course of the right renal artery, traversing behind the IVC and right renal vein. The left renal artery, on the other hand, arises below the right renal artery from the aorta and is more horizontally oriented. It has a direct upward course to the more superiorly positioned left kidney. Duplicate main renal arteries and polar accessory renal arteries occur in approximately 12% to 22% of patients.[1-8] Small accessory renal arteries may arise from the aorta or the iliac arteries and usually go unrecognized with ultrasound. Even duplicated main renal arteries may be overlooked sonographically.[1-5,9-15]

The main renal artery usually divides into five segmental arteries at the level of the renal hilum: the posterior, apical, upper, middle, and lower segmental renal arteries. The segmental arteries then course through the renal sinus and divide into the interlobar arteries, which are within the renal parenchyma. The interlobar arteries are in close proximity to the collecting system. The interlobar arteries divide into the arcuate arteries, which course around the medullary pyramids and lead to the interlobular arteries. The interlobular arteries give rise to the afferent arterioles, which feed each glomerulus. Blood flows from the glomerulus to the efferent arteries, which lead to the vasarecta, which, in turn, provides the network for venous drainage of the kidney.

The venous drainage follows the same branching pattern as the arteries. However, unlike the arterial system, multiple communications exist between the renal segments within the venous system.

PRINCIPLES OF EXAMINATION

Doppler ultrasound evaluation of the renal arteries is one of the most challenging tests to perform given the small size of the renal vessels, their depth, and variation in anatomy. It requires knowledge of the local anatomy, normal waveform physiology, and image optimization. With a little patience and experience, however, a sonographer can become adept at this study and perform the examination in a reasonable period

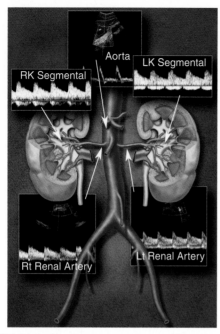

FIGURE 31-1 Renal artery anatomy with montage of normal Doppler waveforms. LK, left kidney; Lt, left; RK, right kidney; Rt, right.

of time. Literature reports indicate that as many as 95% of main renal arteries can be adequately examined in adult patients.[9-11,14,16] The key to the renal Doppler examination is accurate demonstration of the vascular anatomy. This requires an understanding of renal vascular anatomy, as well as the ability to recognize normal and abnormal Doppler waveforms.

Several imaging modalities are available to evaluate the renal vessels. Catheter angiography remains the gold standard examination but is limited by its invasive nature as well as the fact that it exposes patients to iodinated contrast material and radiation. Multidetector computed tomographic angiography (CTA) and contrast-enhanced magnetic resonance angiography (MRA) are less invasive alternatives to angiography. Both techniques have proven valuable in the demonstration of renal vascular disease. CTA offers higher resolution than MRA but also requires iodinated contrast material and is contraindicated in patients with renal failure. CTA also exposes patients to ionizing radiation. MRA usually requires intravenous contrast material (gadolinium-based agents), which may be contraindicated in patients with renal failure, and, in addition, is expensive and time consuming. MRA cannot be performed on claustrophobic patients or patients with metallic implants. Pressure measurements may be obtained only with catheter arteriography. CTA and MRA provide only anatomic information. Compared to these modalities, Doppler sonography is inexpensive and noninvasive and does not require contrast material. The Doppler examination also provides physiologic as well as anatomic information. Thus, Doppler can determine the hemodynamic significance of a lesion and can assess the need for intervention. Doppler examination also clarifies uncertain or indeterminate computed tomographic or magnetic resonance imaging diagnoses.

There are several key elements to a successful abdominal Doppler examination. Adequate patient preparation is important to reduce the amount of bowel gas, which produces scatter and attenuates the ultrasound beam. We recommend a 12-hour fast before examination. We prefer to schedule our renal Doppler studies in the morning, before patients have breakfast, to improve visualization of the vascular structures. We do not give any medication before the study. The examination is performed on a modern ultrasound unit, offering adequate gray-scale imaging as well as sensitive color, power, and pulsed Doppler modalities. We routinely utilize harmonic imaging during our investigations to improve resolution and decrease artifacts. The technical success of each study is also influenced by the degree of operator experience. We have had tremendous success by training dedicated sonographers and sonologists in the techniques required to perform complete renal Doppler studies in a timely manner. The best examiners share several characteristics: motivation, patience, and commitment to succeed. The learning curve is variable, requiring months to a year of experience, depending on the volume of cases performed.

TECHNIQUE

The study is performed using 2.5- to 5-MHz curved array transducers for adequate depth of penetration to visualize the abdominal aorta and its major branches: celiac, mesenteric, and renal arteries. Color flow imaging is an integral component of renal artery ultrasound examination. Color flow imaging is used to demonstrate patent renal arteries and detect flow disturbances that indicate stenosis. However, when used alone, this modality may give a false impression of renal artery stenosis, because atherosclerotic plaques can cause flow disturbances in vessels that are not significantly stenotic. A low pulse repetition frequency (PRF) setting may also produce an aliased signal in an area of normal velocity. Pulsed Doppler spectral analysis must be used in conjunction with color flow imaging, as it provides quantitative information through the measurement of blood flow velocity in the renal vessels.

There are a number of technical shortcuts that increase the likelihood of identifying the renal arteries in their entirety and decreasing the time of the examination. The first step is to optimize the gray-scale and color Doppler parameters so as to improve renal artery visualization as well as the conspicuity of flow-reducing lesions. Adjustment of the color Doppler parameters, including color gain, PRF (color velocity scale), and wall filter, is performed in areas of laminar flow, in either the aorta or a normal segment of a renal artery. Proper color Doppler adjustment allows the examiner to "screen" the vessel quickly for stenosis, because elevated velocities in stenotic regions then produce a color aliasing artifact that is readily apparent. The examiner can then place the Doppler sample volume at the site of flow disturbance to determine the highest peak systolic velocity (PSV).

In addition to optimization of the color Doppler parameters, the experienced sonographer utilizes all available acoustic windows to obtain velocity information from the renal arteries. The renal arteries can be visualized from an anterior abdominal approach through the abdominal wall, decubitus position through the liver and kidneys, and prone position with a posterior (translumbar) approach through the patient's back. In some patients, the anterior abdominal approach may not be feasible due to artifacts and attenuation from bowel gas or obesity. In addition to the anterior abdominal approach, we utilize the decubitus and prone windows to visualize the deep abdominal vessels. Our sonographers prefer the decubitus or oblique positions because they can use the liver and kidneys as acoustic windows to visualize the renal arteries. These windows allow the sonographers to obtain all the necessary color flow views and spectral Doppler samples from the renal arteries in a timely manner.

The spectral Doppler examination is performed with a small sample volume so as to obtain flow information from only the vessel of interest. Pulsed Doppler sampling is performed with angles of 60 degrees or less. We never use angles of greater than 60 degrees, because this artifactually increases the PSV measurement. The PRF is adjusted so that the waveforms are large and easy to read but without causing aliasing.

PROTOCOL

The protocol for our renal artery Doppler examination includes complete evaluation of the kidneys. Left and right decubitus patient positions are preferred for the kidney examination (left decubitus for the right kidney and vice versa). We note the echogenicity and thickness of the renal parenchyma and measure the kidney length. We also assess the kidneys for atrophy, scarring, hydronephrosis, calculi, or masses. We identify occult renal cell carcinomas each year during renal Doppler examinations.

We next perform a longitudinal survey of the abdominal aorta from the celiac artery to the iliac bifurcation and evaluate the amount of atherosclerotic plaque. This is done with both gray-scale and color flow Doppler. Gray-scale evaluation is important to assess for irregular plaque and ostial lesions (i.e., at the origin of the aortic branches), which may be obscured by color flow blooming. (*Blooming* refers to the tendency of the color flow Doppler image to extend beyond the vascular lumen, obscuring adjacent structures, including atherosclerotic plaque and the vessel wall.)

The presence of significant atherosclerotic plaque should increase the suspicion for possible ostial renal artery disease, particularly in older adult or diabetic patients. Conversely, the absence of plaque in the aorta decreases the likelihood of atherosclerotic renal artery stenosis. We also look for flow abnormalities at the origin of the celiac and superior mesenteric arteries that indicate significant stenosis. The size and location of abdominal aortic aneurysms are noted. Finally, angle-corrected PSV measurements are obtained from the abdominal aorta at the level of the renal arteries. These aortic velocity measurements are used to determine the renal artery–aorta velocity ratio, as discussed later.

Our protocol for the evaluation of renal arterial disease includes the direct examination of both renal arteries as well as sampling of the segmental branches in both renal hila. When possible, we locate the origin of the renal arteries on transverse images of the aorta using an anterior transducer approach.[17] We begin at the celiac axis or the superior mesenteric artery, because these are easily located, and move slightly caudad along the aorta until the origin of each renal artery is seen. The right renal artery is often easier to identify than the left with this approach and is relatively easy to follow to the renal hilum (Figure 31-2). The left renal artery is harder to follow all the way to the kidney from an anterior approach. The left renal artery may be better seen by positioning the patient in a *right* lateral decubitus position and scanning from a *left* posterolateral transducer approach,[18] using the left kidney as an acoustic window (Figure 31-3). An analogous approach can be used to visualize the distal right renal artery and its branches, with the patient in a *left* lateral decubitus position. In children, both renal arteries can sometimes be viewed simultaneously from a coronal approach through the left kidney. Transverse and sagittal sweeps of the abdominal aorta and kidneys are performed to identify duplicate renal arteries.

These arteries may arise from the inferior aorta or iliac arteries and can be followed to the renal hilum or either pole of the kidney (Figure 31-4).

Each renal artery should be examined with color flow imaging from its origin to the hilum of the kidney, including the main hilar branches. Look for areas of high-velocity flow, indicated by color shifts or aliasing, as well as turbulence-related flow disturbances, as these may be related to stenosis (Figure 31-5). Interrogate these areas with spectral Doppler analysis. We routinely obtain PSV measurements from the origin, proximal, mid, and distal segments of each renal artery. A small sample volume (1.5-2.0 mm), and an

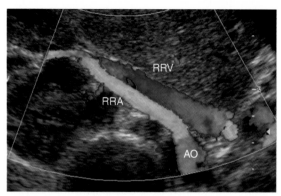

FIGURE 31-2 Color Doppler image displays the entire right renal artery (RRA) from the aorta (AO) to the renal hilum. Note that the anterior liver parenchyma serves as an acoustic window. RRV, right renal vein.

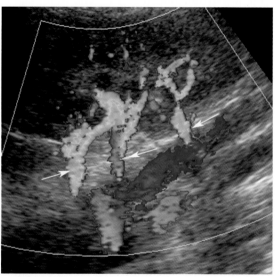

FIGURE 31-4 Multiple duplicate renal arteries *(arrows)* are identified on this longitudinal color Doppler image obtained through the left kidney.

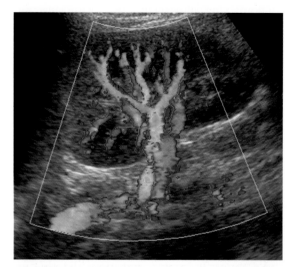

FIGURE 31-3 Color Doppler scan through the left kidney, obtained in the right lateral decubitus position, allows complete visualization of the left renal artery.

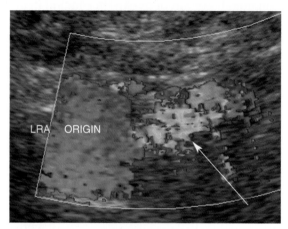

FIGURE 31-5 Focal color aliasing *(arrow)* represents high-velocity flow at the site of stenosis at the origin of the left renal artery (LRA).

angle of insonation of 60 degrees or less are used. Finally, waveforms are also obtained from the segmental arteries in the upper, mid, and lower poles of each kidney. Thus, at least seven waveforms are captured from each side. It is important to obtain clean, crisp waveforms with well-defined borders for analysis. This is accomplished by adjusting the spectral display so that the waveforms are large and easily measured.[19] This allows the examiner to readily determine the PSV, acceleration time or index, and the resistivity index (RI). The RI is the PSV minus the end-diastolic velocity, divided by the PSV. (The RI may be elevated in numerous conditions, including parenchymal renal disease, acute tubular necrosis, renal vein thrombosis, and urinary tract obstruction.)

The normal PSV range in adult renal arteries is 60 to 100 cm/sec. Normal renal artery waveforms demonstrate a rapid systolic upstroke with persistent forward flow in diastole (low-resistance bed) (Figure 31-6). An early systolic compliance peak (ESP) or notch may be seen in some patients.

Our philosophy on renal artery duplex ultrasound examination is quite pragmatic. We limit the amount of time allotted for our renal Doppler studies. In our experience, a complete renal artery Doppler examination can be performed in as little as 20 minutes. We never exceed 60 minutes. Experienced examiners can assess a patient quickly and determine if the study can be completed in a timely manner. Studies on difficult patients who cannot cooperate or are not "sonogenic" are aborted promptly, and an alternative study is recommended for further evaluation. It is also important to recognize that atherosclerotic renal artery disease is far and away the most common etiology of significant renal artery stenosis, and these lesions occur at the origin and proximal segments of the renal artery. We pay close attention to these segments in our older adult patients who are apt to have atherosclerotic obstructive lesions.[10,14] In younger adults, it is more important to see the entire renal artery, as these patients are more likely to have fibromuscular hyperplasia, which can affect the distal renal artery or the segmental branches.[13,20]

Improved visualization of renal arterial flow may be obtained with the use of ultrasound contrast (echo-enhancing) agents, which greatly increases the visibility of blood vessels. Ultrasound contrast may be particularly helpful in larger patients to visualize the renal arteries. In addition to reducing examination time, the use of these agents may enhance ultrasound visualization of multiple renal arteries and hilar branches. Ultrasound contrast agents are currently approved in the United States for echocardiography but may be used "off-label" for renal Doppler studies. Approval by the Food and Drug Administration for abdominal Doppler studies has not occurred as of this writing but is expected shortly.

VASCULAR DISORDERS

There are a variety of renal vascular disorders that affect the arteries and veins of the kidneys. These conditions may cause damage to the kidneys, renal failure, and/or hypertension. The most common vascular conditions affecting the

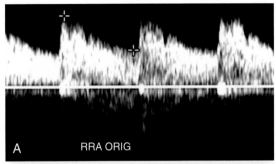

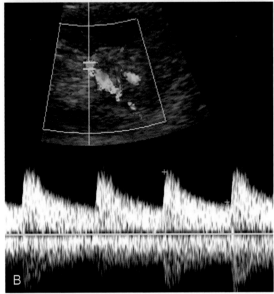

FIGURE 31-6 A, Normal Doppler waveform obtained at the origin of the right renal artery (RRA ORIG) demonstrates a low-resistance flow pattern with a rapid systolic upstroke and early systolic compliance peak. **B,** Waveforms obtained from a segmental artery branch, at the renal hilum, demonstrate normal waveform shape and acceleration.

renal arteries are renal artery stenosis (due to atherosclerosis or fibromuscular dysplasia [FMD]), renal artery occlusion, and renal artery aneurysm. Renal vein thrombosis can be seen with hypercoagulable states, malignancy (tumor thrombus), or propagation of clot from the IVC. Other renal vascular pathologies include arteriovenous fistula (AVF), vasculitis, and pseudoaneurysm.

RENAL ARTERY STENOSIS

Stenosis, or occlusion of a main renal artery or a duplicated renal artery, may cause renal ischemia, which in turn triggers the renin-angiotensin mechanism and causes hypertension. Renal artery stenosis can also cause or contribute to renal insufficiency by inducing renal parenchymal damage. The threshold level of renal artery stenosis that produces hypertension or ischemic damage is uncertain and probably varies from one patient to another. Studies suggest that ischemic nephropathy may be responsible for 5% to 22% of advanced renal disease in all patients older than 50 years.[21] From a hemodynamic perspective, renal artery obstruction is considered hemodynamically significant (or flow reducing) when the lumen diameter is narrowed by 50% to 60%.

It is estimated that 10% of the U.S. population has hypertension, and 3% to 5% of this group has renal arterial disease.[1,22] Although the latter percentages are small, renal artery disease represents the most common *correctable* cause of hypertension.[22] More recently, clinical interest has focused on the potential role of renal ischemia in the etiology of chronic renal insufficiency.[23,24] Once again, the potential correctability of renal artery stenosis has been stressed. Few kidney diseases can be cured, and it is understandable that clinicians should be keenly interested in a potentially curable disorder such as renal artery stenosis. Does this mean, however, that we should seek to diagnose renal artery disease in every patient with hypertension or renal insufficiency? To do so could be expensive and not cost-effective.[25] Furthermore, intervention for renal artery disease may be risky (e.g., arterial occlusion or rupture) and is not always successful. Considering these points, we believe that renal artery stenosis should be sought in the following groups of patients: (1) young patients with severe hypertension; (2) patients with rapidly accelerating hypertension or malignant hypertension; (3) patients with hypertension that is difficult to control despite a suitable treatment program; (4) patients with concomitant hypertension and deteriorating renal function; and (5) patients with renal insufficiency and discrepant kidney size (implying renal artery stenosis).[1,22-25]

Doppler Renal Artery Evaluation

As noted previously, color flow imaging is used to identify flow abnormalities that *may* be stenosis related, but spectral Doppler measurements provide quantitative data that are essential for determining the severity of stenosis. The following general comments about Doppler diagnosis of renal artery stenosis are noteworthy:

1. The principal ultrasound criterion for renal artery stenosis is Doppler-detected flow velocity elevation in the stenotic portion of the vessel.* Flow velocity is increased in proportion to the severity of luminal narrowing; therefore, spectral Doppler measurements can be used to approximate stenosis severity. Narrowed areas detected with color flow imaging must be carefully surveyed with the Doppler sample volume to ensure that the maximum flow velocity is identified.

2. Accurate assignment of the Doppler angle is essential for reliable measurement of stenosis-related velocity elevation, and a Doppler-to-vessel angle of 60 degrees or less is mandatory to ensure that velocity information is accurate.

3. Major stenoses are accompanied by post-stenotic flow disturbance (turbulence). Although disturbed flow is a useful beacon for the presence of stenosis, it is neither quantitative nor specific. Disturbed flow may occur without significant stenosis. Color bruit artifacts, however, usually indicate a significant flow abnormality.

4. Arterial waveforms within the kidney (segmental or interlobar arteries) may be scrutinized for evidence of damping, which is a downstream manifestation of renal artery stenosis. The most important downstream findings are the absence of an early systolic peak, a prolonged systolic acceleration time, and a reduced acceleration index (tardus-parvus waveform).[6,19,26,28-32]

Diagnostic Criteria

Normal blood flow in the renal artery and its branches has a low-resistance pattern with a rapid peak to systole and forward flow throughout

---

*References 1,13,14,16,20,26,27.

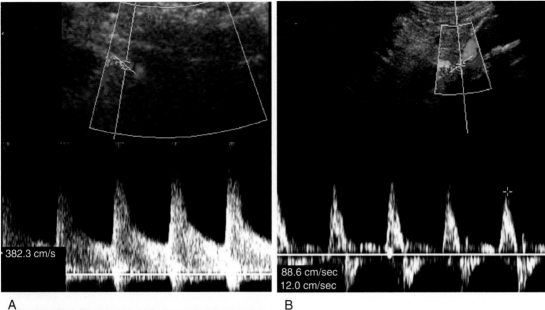

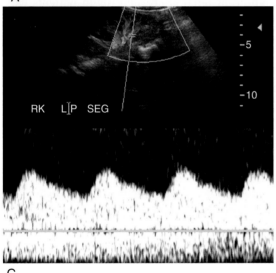

FIGURE 31-7 **A,** Renal artery stenosis. Pulsed Doppler interrogation of the right renal artery, at the site of color aliasing, reveals elevated peak systolic velocities (PSVs; 382.3 cm/sec.) **B,** Pulsed Doppler sampling of the aorta, at the level of the renal arteries, reveals a PSV of 88.6 cm/sec. The renal-aortic ratio is 4.3, consistent with significant renal artery stenosis. **C,** Renal hilar sampling reveals characteristic damping (tardus-parvus) of the segmental artery waveform. Note the absence of the early systolic peak, rounded contour, and prolonged systolic acceleration time. LP, lower pole; RK, right kidney; SEG, segmental artery.

diastole. The PSV in normal renal arteries ranges from 74 to 127 cm/sec in both adults and children.[17,20,33,34] Children tend to have slightly higher velocities than adults.

Numerous Doppler velocity criteria have been used to diagnose hemodynamically significant renal artery stenosis (defined generally as 50% to 60% diameter reduction).[†] The most universally accepted Doppler criteria are (1) PSV in the stenosis of 180 to 200 cm/sec or greater and (2) a renal artery to aortic ratio (RAR) exceeding 3.3 or 3.5.[1-3,10-12,16,20] The latter is

the ratio of peak systole in the stenotic portion of the renal artery divided by peak systole in the aorta at the renal artery level (Figure 31-7). Some authors have found PSV measurements, used alone, to be more accurate than the RAR.[3] In theory, the RAR compensates for hemodynamic variability between patients. Younger patients tend to have higher normal PSV flow in the aorta and branch vessels that can exceed 180 cm/sec without stenosis. Older adult patients, particularly patients with severe cardiac disease and poor cardiac output, may demonstrate lower PSVs, even in regions of stenosis.

[†]References 1-5,13,15,17,19,22,29,31,32,35-40.

Damping of *intrarenal* arterial signals is also a valuable criterion for diagnosis of renal artery stenosis. Damping is defined numerically with the acceleration index or the acceleration time. Both of these measures reflect the rate of systolic acceleration, which is slower than normal downstream from a hemodynamically significant stenosis. An acceleration index less than 300 cm/sec^2 or an acceleration time exceeding 0.07 second is considered abnormal and suggests a 60% or greater renal artery stenosis.[‡] Some authors use an acceleration time of 0.10 or 0.12 second as the cutoff for significant stenosis, which increases specificity.[1,2,35]

Intrarenal Waveform Assessment

An ideal survey method for renal artery stenosis would be accurate, quick, and easy. This is the appeal of *indirect* diagnosis of renal artery stenosis through the detection of damped Doppler waveforms in segmental or interlobar arteries within the kidney. For an experienced sonographer, the acquisition of intrarenal arterial Doppler signals is relatively easy, and, therefore, the examination is brief and successful in most individuals.

It has long been recognized that renal artery stenosis can cause pulsus tardus and parvus ("tardus parvus") changes in intrarenal arterial flow signals (see Figure 31-7).[36,37] It would be very convenient to simply look for these flow changes in the kidneys and thereby diagnose renal artery stenosis without the arduous task of finding and directly evaluating the renal arteries. Unfortunately, the accuracy of this diagnostic method is questionable. Several literature reports (based on acceleration time, acceleration index, and waveform shape changes) were promising, with sensitivity ranging from 89% to 95% and specificity ranging from 83% to 97% for main renal artery stenoses exceeding 60% or 70% diameter reduction.[2,19,28,31] But other literature reports, based on the same Doppler parameters, indicate poor results ranging from moderate accuracy to complete absence of correlation between Doppler and angiographic findings.[§] Because of these unfavorable results, this technique for diagnosis of renal artery stenosis has been largely abandoned as the sole diagnostic measure.

The question, then, is why doesn't intrarenal Doppler work? To begin with, it appears that intrarenal waveform findings are more accurate for high-grade renal artery stenoses exceeding 70% diameter reduction,[2,5,30] but even at high levels of stenosis, some patients do not have appreciable waveform damping. This is because the shape of intrarenal arterial waveforms is affected by multiple factors, including the stiffness (compliance) of the arteries, the resistance of the microcirculation, and inflow phenomena, such as renal artery stenosis.[39,40] In a patient with generalized arterial stiffness and/or high resistance in the microvasculature from parenchymal renal disease (e.g., diabetes-related nephropathy), the damping effects of a main renal artery stenosis may be obliterated (Figure 31-8). To make matters worse, damped intrarenal waveforms can occasionally be seen in the absence of significant renal artery stenosis in patients with aortic stenosis or aortic occlusion.

Because intrarenal Doppler waveform analysis has not been consistently accurate, we do not recommend the exclusive use of hilar waveform analysis for the diagnosis of renal artery stenosis. However, we do not ignore intra-arterial waveform findings either. We *always* evaluate acceleration and waveform shape in intrarenal arteries in conjunction with direct renal artery interrogation. The detection of abnormal waveforms, when present, confirms the hemodynamic significance of a main renal artery stenosis. Furthermore, damped intrarenal arterial signals may indicate occult stenosis or occlusion in the main renal artery, a duplicated renal artery, or a segmental artery. This is a particularly important finding when the direct examination is technically limited.

It has been suggested that the downstream effects of renal artery stenosis can be diagnosed merely by visual inspection of the shape of the segmental or interlobar Doppler waveforms.[19,26,35] Either the initial systolic peak is absent or the systolic peak is grossly rounded in patients with severe ipsilateral stenosis, as illustrated in Figures 31-7 and 31-9.

Loss of the ESP is associated with significant renal artery stenosis. The ESP is recognized as the initial acceleration phase in systole that is followed by a short acceleration phase then a second systolic peak. The ESP is not seen consistently in all patients. In our practice, some of the interpreting physicians choose visual inspection

---

[‡]References 1,2,6,14,19,28,31,35.
[§]References 5,6,13,26,27,38,39.

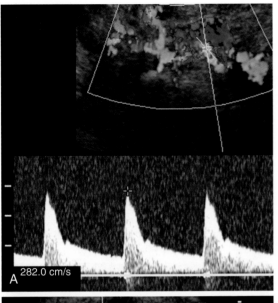

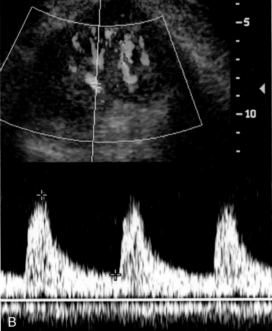

FIGURE 31-8 **A,** Elevated velocities (peak systolic velocity = 282 cm/sec) are identified in the left renal artery consistent with significant stenosis, confirmed with magnetic resonance angiography. **B,** Hilar waveforms obtained from the left kidney are normal in appearance. This is a false-negative finding obtained by indirect arterial sampling.

rather than acceleration index or acceleration time measurements for intrarenal waveform analysis.

Doppler assessment of the renal arteries is also valuable following revascularization with angioplasty, bypass, or stent placement.

Measurement of renal artery PSV is used to assess residual or recurrent stenosis after therapy. There is a reduction in PSV in the stenotic region following successful angioplasty and stent placement. Hilar waveforms will also return to normal appearance after successful treatment (see Figure 31-9).

Reported Results

Wide ranges of sensitivity (0%-98%) and specificity (37%-99%) have been reported for *direct* duplex detection of renal artery stenosis, based on either an elevated systolic velocity in the renal artery or an abnormal RAR.[∥] The disparate results of these studies are a reflection of selection bias, examiner experience, and statistical methods. For instance, several of the more successful studies were potentially biased because most or all of their patients were older adults, who, for the most part, have atherosclerotic stenoses at the renal artery origins. Because the origins of the renal arteries are the portions most easily visualized with ultrasound, greater accuracy may be expected in this population than in younger individuals, who may have more distal renal artery disease.[10-12,16] In addition, some studies included only successful Doppler examinations in statistical tabulation, whereas other studies included all examinations, regardless of the level of success or experience.

Despite the spread of reported results, it appears that *direct* duplex examination of the renal arteries is reasonably effective for diagnosis of clinically significant renal artery stenosis. With experience and good technique, the examiner is likely to attain sensitivity and specificity levels for adult patients in the vicinity of 90% for 60% or greater (diameter) stenosis in the proximal 4 cm (or so) of the main renal arteries.

Recently we performed a comparative analysis of the Doppler criteria for the diagnosis of renal artery stenosis. This included a retrospective review of greater than 3000 renal artery studies with correlations with conventional arteriography, CTA, and MRA. We assessed the performance of the PSV, RAR, RI, and presence of tardus-parvus waveforms for the detection of renal artery stenosis. The PSV greater than or equal to 200 cm/sec demonstrated the greatest accuracy (87%) compared to RAR greater than or equal to 3.5 (79%), RI greater than or equal to 0.8

[∥]References 1,11,12,14,19,27,29,36,37,41-44.

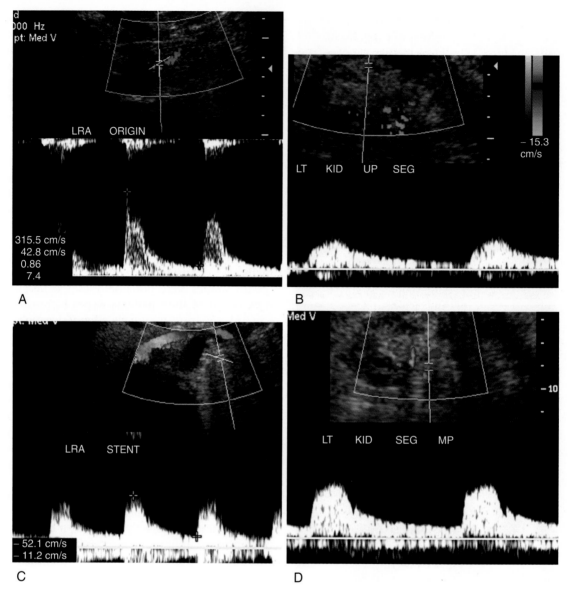

FIGURE 31-9 **A,** Elevated velocities (peak systolic velocity [PSV] = 315.5 cm/sec) are detected at the origin of the left renal artery (LRA ORIG) consistent with significant stenosis in this patient with hypertension. **B,** Typical tardus waveforms (delayed upstroke and rounded contour) are obtained from the left upper pole segmental artery in the left kidney (LT KID UP SEG). **C,** Following renal artery stent placement, PSVs in the left renal artery (LRA) return to the normal range (PSV = 52.1 cm/sec.). **D,** Pulsed Doppler waveforms obtained from the left midpole segmental artery demonstrate a return to normal appearance with normal upstroke (acceleration) and waveform shape. LT KID, left kidney; MP, midpole; SEG, segmental artery.

(50%), and tardus parvus waveforms (68%). The optimal threshold value for the PSV was 220 cm/sec with a sensitivity of 95%, specificity of 85%, and accuracy of 90%. The optimal threshold for RAR was 2.6 with a sensitivity of 87%, specificity of 85%, and accuracy of 86%. Tardus-parvus waveforms demonstrated high specificity (96%) and positive predictive value (92%) but overall low sensitivity (43%) in our study.

In our practice, we use a combination of the PSV and RAR in a similar fashion to the PSV and internal carotid artery/common carotid artery ratio for carotid examinations. The PSV greater than or equal to 200 cm/sec demonstrated the highest sensitivity (96%) and negative predictive value (95%), whereas the RAR greater than or equal to 3.5 demonstrated the highest specificity (93%) and positive predictive value (92%)

for significant renal artery stenosis. We always look for an elevated velocity at the site of stenosis and utilize the ratio to increase our confidence in the diagnosis. The RAR is particularly useful in cases where the renal PSV falls outside the normal range in patients with high- or low-flow states (i.e., cardiac or aortic disease). Cases with discordant findings are usually referred for additional imaging with CTA or MRA to clarify the diagnosis. Diagnostic accuracy for distal renal artery and segmental branch lesions may not be as good as that for more proximal stenoses, as discussed later.

Duplicate Artery Problems

In hypertensive patients, the documentation or exclusion of a renovascular etiology requires the assessment of the main renal artery, whether single or duplicate, and segmental arteries in the renal hilum. We use the term *duplicate main renal arteries* in reference to arteries that enter the renal hilum and supply segmental branches. Stenoses in duplicated main renal arteries can clearly cause hypertension and possibly renal insufficiency, in contrast to stenoses in small polar accessory arteries that are thought to rarely cause hypertension and are probably not a significant cause of renal insufficiency.[1,4,6-8,17] In medical literature reports, duplicate main renal arteries and polar accessory arteries are frequently called *accessory renal arteries*, which we feel is unfortunate, as they probably have considerably different importance from a clinical perspective.

Angiographic studies show that 12% to 22% of kidneys are supplied by more than one renal artery. Kliewer and associates[5] found that 15% of kidneys had double main renal arteries, and 13% had accessory arteries (usually at the poles of the kidney). Accessory arteries usually arise from the aorta but may also arise from the iliac arteries.

Unfortunately, the detection rate for multiple renal arteries with duplex ultrasound (including color flow imaging) seems to be quite poor. Hélénon and colleagues[13] reported detecting 30% of duplicate renal arteries with ultrasound, but they did not say whether these were double main renal arteries or polar arteries. They failed to detect 25% of main renal arteries, which apparently included some duplicated arteries. Melany and co-workers[15] visualized several duplicate main renal arteries with ultrasound contrast enhancement but failed to see three polar accessory arteries. In the literature reports of which we are aware, there is no clear indication of how reliably ultrasound visualizes duplicate main renal arteries, but there is some evidence that failure to detect these arteries adversely affects ultrasound accuracy.[2-5,9,11-13] In the study by Hansen and associates,[11] duplex ultrasound sensitivity for 60% (diameter) stenosis was 98% for single main renal arteries but only 67% for all renal arteries, including duplicate vessels.

It appears that polar accessory renal arteries rarely cause hypertension or significant ischemia; hence, one could argue that their visualization is unimportant. Gupta and colleagues[45] concluded from their study of 185 hypertensive patients that accessory renal arteries are not a direct cause of hypertension. Bude and co-workers,[46] in their study, found that accessory renal artery stenosis is an infrequent finding in hypertensive patients, occurring in 0.08% of the population, and concluded that examination should focus on detection of main renal artery stenosis. Duplicated main renal arteries, however, can be repaired, and their detection *is* clinically significant. The following scenario is easily envisioned: A normal renal artery is seen sonographically, but a second stenotic renal artery, the actual source of renal ischemia and hypertension, is overlooked. This limitation of sonography should be kept in mind, and a diligent search should be made for duplicate main renal arteries.

Segmental Branch Problems

As noted previously, atherosclerotic obstruction tends to occur at or near the origin of the main renal arteries and is detected quite easily with color flow sonography. Fibromuscular hyperplasia, however, can occur at any location from the origin of the vessel to the hilar segmental branches and may involve multiple branches. Statistical details are limited, but our experience and that of others suggest that duplex results are poorer for segmental branch stenoses than they are for the main renal artery.[5,13,20] For instance, Hélénon and colleagues[13] reported a sensitivity level of only 60% for hilar branch stenoses, and Kliewer and associates[5] reported missing three branch vessel stenoses with duplex examination. Stenoses in hilar branch vessels can be repaired with angioplasty,[47] so their detection in hypertensive patients is important. For this reason, we advise careful assessment of younger hypertensive patients who might have fibromuscular hyperplasia, and the use of angiographic procedures when hilar branch visualization is suboptimal.[2-8,13]

Although the RI, as measured in intrarenal arteries, is not reliable for diagnosing renal artery stenosis, it is proposed to have value in predicting the outcome of renal revascularization. Radermacher and colleagues[48] found that a renal RI greater than 0.8 reliably identifies patients with renal artery stenosis that are not likely to respond to revascularization. In their series of 5950 patients with hypertension, an RI greater than 0.8 before therapy was a strong predictor of worsening renal function and a lack of improvement in blood pressure, despite correction of renal artery stenosis. Elevation of the RI results from accentuated microvasculature resistance, which in turn indicates the presence of generalized renal parenchymal disease. There is much controversy concerning the role of RI in predicting response to revascularization. Cohn and co-workers[49] found no statistical difference in RIs before and after revascularization and concluded that intrarenal flow patterns alone are not sufficient to predict response to treatment. Garcia-Criado and associates[50] found that the RI and acceleration index were not useful parameters for predicting renal function outcome following renal artery revascularization.

DOPPLER WAVEFORM ABNORMALITIES IN NONVASCULAR RENAL DISEASE

Flow resistance within the renal parenchyma may be increased by a variety of pathologic processes, including urinary tract obstruction and a host of acute and chronic parenchymal disorders, including glomerulosclerosis, acute tubular necrosis, and pyelonephritis.[51,52] All of these conditions are associated with increased flow resistance in the microvasculature of the kidney, which causes the Doppler waveforms to exhibit *increased pulsatility.* This may be evident on visual inspection of waveforms or through pulsatility measures such as the pulsatility index or RI. The pulsatility index is the PSV minus the lowest diastolic velocity (including reversal flow) divided by the mean velocity. In normal kidneys, a large amount of diastolic blood flow is evident on visual inspection of the intrarenal Doppler signals, and the RI in segmental or intralobar arteries does not exceed 0.7.

An increase in vascular resistance (and pulsatility) in renal pathology is nonspecific with limited diagnostic value because it is multifactorial in origin. Increased pulsatility is of greatest diagnostic value when it is seen unilaterally, for in such cases, it implies an acute process such as urinary tract obstruction or renal vein obstruction

on the side with high pulsatility. High pulsatility may be apparent before significant urinary tract dilatation occurs.[51,52]

Another entity worth mentioning is tumor vascularity associated with solid renal masses. Solid masses such as renal cell carcinoma or oncocytomas may demonstrate significant neovascularity that is distinct from vascular disorders such as pseudoaneurysm or arteriovenous malformation. For example, patients with oncocytoma can reveal a characteristic spoke-wheel pattern of blood flow within the tumor, resembling a vascular pathology

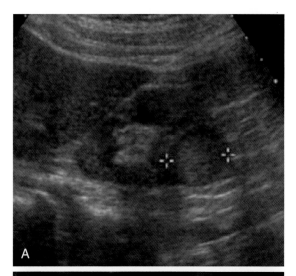

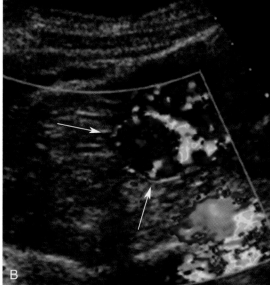

FIGURE 31-10 Renal oncocytoma. **A,** Gray-scale image demonstrates well-defined uniformly echogenic solid mass *(cursors)* eccentrically located in the right kidney. **B,** Color Doppler images reveal a spoke-wheel pattern of flow *(arrows)* within the mass highly suggestive of oncocytoma.

(Figure 31-10). Increased neovascularity is also commonly seen in renal cell carcinoma. Color and pulsed Doppler evaluation is helpful in characterization of indeterminate renal lesions identified on other modalities. Waveforms obtained from malignant tumors usually show a high-velocity, low-resistance pattern with velocities significantly higher than normally seen in renal arteries.

RENAL ARTERY OCCLUSION

Renal artery occlusion is diagnosed on the basis of the following findings: (1) absence of a visible main renal artery, (2) markedly reduced kidney size (smaller than 9 cm in length), and (3) either absence of detectable intrarenal blood flow or very low amplitude, damped intrarenal flow signals[1,3,10,16] (Figure 31-11).

Diagnostic accuracy for renal artery occlusion depends on reasonable color flow and spectral Doppler sensitivity at the level of the renal artery or kidney. That is, flow should be readily detected in other vessels at a similar depth or in the contralateral kidney before it is concluded that a renal artery is occluded. Although relatively few studies exist in the medical literature, it appears that duplex diagnosis of renal artery occlusion is reasonably accurate. Thirty-eight of 41 occluded arteries were correctly diagnosed in three published series, for an overall accuracy rate of 93%.[3,10,16]

False-positive diagnosis of renal artery occlusion can occur when visualization of the main renal artery is poor or the kidney is small for reasons other than arterial occlusion. False-negative results are caused by collateralization, which may occur via capsular or adrenal branches, and duplicate renal arteries. In the collateralized kidney, flow signals may well be present in the kidney parenchyma or in the renal hilum despite renal artery occlusion. Doppler waveforms may even be normal in the kidney in some cases, although tardus-parvus waveforms are typically seen.

RENAL VEIN THROMBOSIS

Renal vein thrombosis appears to be an underdiagnosed vascular disease because of the nonspecificity of clinical and radiographic findings.[53-55] Acute renal vein thrombosis usually presents with pain and hematuria, and it may occasionally cause thromboembolic complications, such as pulmonary embolism. Chronic renal vein thrombosis may be asymptomatic or may present with the nephrotic syndrome, hematuria, or renal failure.

The renal vein may be blocked by intraluminal tumor or thrombus formation or by extrinsic compression (possibly accompanied by secondary venous thrombosis). Associated or predisposing conditions include preexisting renal disease, renal cell carcinoma, hypercoagulable state, vena caval or ovarian vein thrombus (with extension to the renal veins), abdominal surgery, trauma, and dehydration. Primary renal disease is the most common predisposing factor, particularly the nephrotic syndrome and membranous glomerulonephritis.[55] Extrinsic retroperitoneal causes of renal vein thrombosis include acute pancreatitis, lymph node enlargement from a host of tumors, and retroperitoneal fibrosis. These conditions generally cause extrinsic compression of the vascular pedicle, predisposing to thrombosis.[53]

Renal vein thrombosis typically induces ischemic parenchymal damage in the kidney and acute renal failure.[53-55] The long-term effects of renal vein thrombosis are varied. The potential

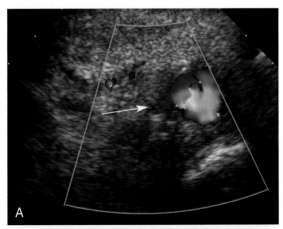
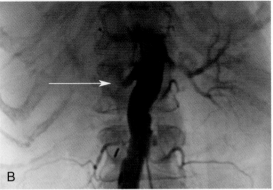

FIGURE 31-11 Occluded right renal artery. **A,** Transverse color flow image through the juxtarenal aorta demonstrates absence of flow in the expected location of the right renal artery with a small focal area of color at the level of the renal artery stump *(arrow)* as seen on the correlated conventional angiography **(B).**

exists for recanalization of the renal vein or the development of venous collaterals, and, in some cases, the kidney returns to a normal sonographic appearance. If the kidney is severely damaged, however, chronic changes become evident, including diminished kidney size and increased echogenicity (secondary to fibrosis).

The most easily detected ultrasound findings in *acute* renal vein occlusion[56-63] are kidney enlargement and altered parenchymal echogenicity, both of which are caused by parenchymal edema and in some cases by hemorrhage. Changes in echogenicity may include the following: (1) hypoechoic cortex with decreased corticomedullary differentiation, (2) hyperechoic cortex with preservation of corticomedullary differentiation, and (3) mottled heterogeneity accompanied by the loss of normal intrarenal architecture. In some cases, echogenic linear streaks of unknown origin course through the renal parenchyma. These streaks are thought to be pathognomonic for renal vein thrombosis.[58,59]

Kidney enlargement and altered parenchymal echogenicity are nonspecific findings, and the conclusive diagnosis of renal vein thrombosis depends on the direct identification of thrombus in the renal vein. With acute thrombosis, the renal vein is invariably enlarged, and Doppler signals are absent. A small trickle of flow may be present around the clot, and this may produce low-velocity, continuous Doppler signals (lacking respiratory phasicity). Recently formed thrombus is hypoechoic and in some cases appears anechoic. As a result, the thrombus may not be readily seen with gray-scale sonography and is detectable only with color flow imaging. Two additional pitfalls are noteworthy. First, venous flow may be present within the kidney itself, even though the renal vein is occluded, because large hilar collaterals may develop quickly. Second, very sluggish renal vein flow (as a result of more proximal obstruction or congestion) may mimic thrombosis, because the Doppler signal may be difficult to detect at very slow flow rates.

RENAL VEIN TUMOR EXTENSION

Tumor extension into the renal vein is most commonly associated with renal cell carcinoma, although renal lymphoma, transitional cell carcinoma, and Wilms' tumor can also propagate along the renal veins. Venous invasion is common in renal cell carcinoma, with gross involvement of the main renal vein occurring in 21% to 35% of patients with large tumors and IVC tumor extension in 5% to 10% of patients.[62,63] Vena cava invasion is approximately three times more common in right-sided tumors than in those on the left because of the shorter length of the right renal vein.[62,63] Preoperative diagnosis of venous tumor extension significantly influences surgical therapy. If no tumor is present, routine ligation of the renal vein may be performed through a flank incision, but if the renal vein is occluded by tumor and if the tumor extends into the IVC, a midline incision often is used, which may be extended cephalad to create a sternotomy if necessary.[63]

Contrast-enhanced computed tomography is the preferred method of investigation for intravenous tumor extension, supplemented when necessary with magnetic resonance imaging or sonography. The latter modality has cost and convenience advantages over magnetic resonance imaging and can often answer directed questions, such as the superior extent of the tumor within the IVC. Duplex sonography is not as accurate as computed tomography or magnetic resonance imaging for de novo detection of tumor extension into the renal vein, particularly on the left side, where the vein is frequently obscured by bowel gas.[64-70] If the renal vein and IVC are well visualized, sonographic accuracy is high (96% sensitivity, 100% specificity), but renal vein visualization is inadequate in 34% to 54% of patients, and the IVC is inadequately seen in 4% to 21% of cases.[65,68] Thus, the overall sensitivity of ultrasound for venous tumor extension may be as low as 18% for the renal veins and 33% for the IVC.[56]

As seen with ultrasound, renal vein tumor[51,52,66-70] is typically homogeneous and is low or intermediate in echogenicity. The tumor-containing renal vein is almost always distended to a distinctly abnormal size, and even the IVC may be distended when tumor infiltration is present (Figures 31-12 and 31-13). Differentiation between intravenous tumor and thrombus is accomplished through color flow detection of small blood vessels within the tumor thrombus.

RENAL ARTERY ANEURYSM

Normal renal artery size has a wide range with a mean of 4.5 to 5 mm at the ostium based on a person's gender.[71] Most renal artery aneurysms do not exceed 2 cm in diameter and are usually discovered incidentally during diagnostic

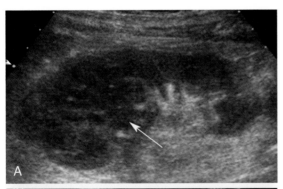

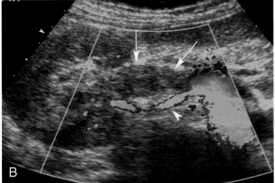

FIGURE 31-12 Renal vein thrombosis in a patient with renal cell carcinoma. **A,** Gray-scale image of the right kidney shows a loss of corticomedullary differentiation in the upper renal pole *(arrow).* **B,** Color Doppler image reveals an enlarged right renal vein filled with a heterogeneous material *(arrows)* compatible with a tumor thrombus. Note is made of a patent renal artery parallel to the enlarged renal vein *(arrowhead).*

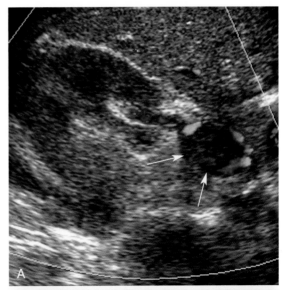

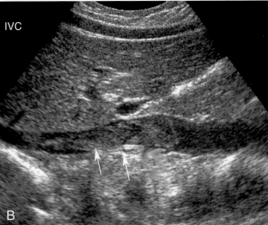

FIGURE 31-13 **A,** Hypoechoic thrombus *(arrows)* is identified in the main right renal vein. Color flow improves detection of the thrombus by demonstrating a filling defect in the vein lumen. **B,** Thrombus *(arrows)* extends into the inferior vena cava from the right renal vein.

procedures performed for other indications. Symptoms may develop from rupture, embolization of the peripheral vascular bed, or arterial thrombosis causing intrarenal ischemia or infarction.[72]

In the absence of trauma, renal artery aneurysms are rare (less than 0.1%). Most are saccular and noncalcified and tend to occur at the bifurcation of the main renal artery (Figure 31-14). Renal artery aneurysms are subdivided into two categories: extrarenal and intrarenal. Extrarenal aneurysms are caused by atherosclerosis and FMD. Depending on the type of FMD, the main renal artery may demonstrate a "string of beads" appearance on power Doppler or may show long segmental narrowing of the proximal, mid or distal aspects of the main renal artery (Figure 31-15). Intrarenal aneurysms are generally very small (microaneurysms) and multiple. Intrarenal aneurysms are seen in patients suffering from polyarteritis nodosa, a rare necrotizing vasculitis that affects the small and medium-sized

arteries of multiple organs, usually involving the renal (85%) and hepatic (65%) arteries. Microaneurysms range in size from 1 to 12 mm and classically are seen at branch points. Intrarenal microaneurysms can also be seen in patients with Wegener's granulomatosis, systemic lupus erythematosus, rheumatoid vasculitis, and drug abuse.[73-75] Angiomyolipoma are also associated with formation of berrylike aneurysms of intralobar and interlobular arteries.[76] Pseudoaneurysms are usually related to prior trauma (i.e., biopsy or arterial puncture) or infection that causes disruption of the arterial wall. The blood that escapes is confined by surrounding soft tissue and hematoma. A saccular outpouching or cavity

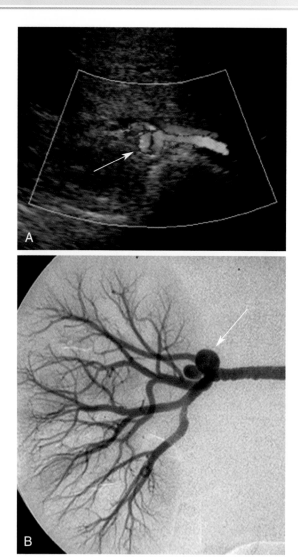

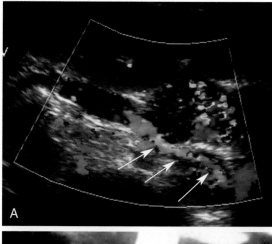

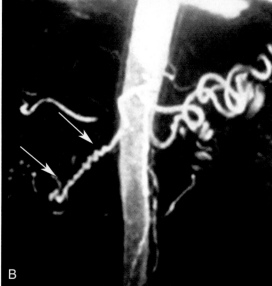

FIGURE 31-14 Renal artery aneurysm. **A,** Color Doppler image of the right renal artery reveals a focal saccular dilatation of the distal renal artery at the renal hilum that fills in with color *(arrow).* **B,** Conventional angiography of the same patient reveals contrast enhancement of the aneurysm *(arrow).*

FIGURE 31-15 Renal artery fibromuscular dysplasia (FMD). **A,** Color Doppler image of the right renal artery demonstrates a long segment of narrowing *(arrows)* of the proximal and mid portions of the renal artery. **B,.** Magnetic resonance angiography demonstrates a "string of beads" appearance *(arrows)* of the proximal and mid right renal artery characteristic of FMD.

is seen extending from the damaged vessel. Color Doppler demonstrates swirling blood flow in the cavity during real-time evaluation ("yin-yang" pattern) (Figure 31-16).

Management decisions are based on patient age and gender, severity of associated hypertension, anticipated pregnancy, and anatomic features of the aneurysm. Although aneurysm size greater than 2 cm is considered a threshold for surgical treatment, rupture of aneurysms less than 2 cm has been reported.[77] Young women, especially those with anticipated pregnancy, are considered to be at high risk for rupture. Treatment

of renal artery aneurysms is determined by the anatomic location of the aneurysm. Branch renal artery aneurysms are easily treated with embolization.[75] Aneurysms of the main renal artery may be treated with ligation and arterial bypass surgery, nephrectomy, or covered stent placement.[78]

ARTERIOVENOUS FISTULA AND ARTERIOVENOUS MALFORMATIONS

Renal arteriovenous malformations (AVMs) are abnormal communications between the intrarenal arterial and venous vessels. Renal AVMs are usually discovered during the evaluation for

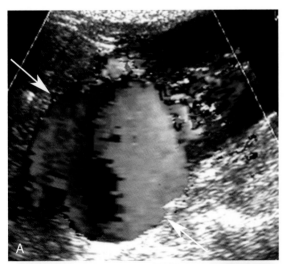

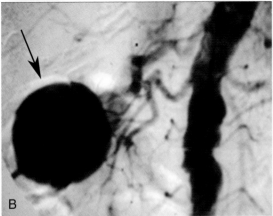

FIGURE 31-16 Renal artery pseudoaneurysm. **A,** Color flow examination shows a pseudoaneurysm sac *(arrows)* in the right kidney demonstrating characteristic yin-yang flow pattern. **B,** Conventional angiogram in the same patient reveals a large vascular mass *(arrow)* extending from the renal hilum that fills in with intravenous contrast.

gross hematuria. Renal AVMs are uncommon; the incidence range is 1 case per 1000 to 2500 patients.[79,80] There are two major types of AVMs: congenital (one-third) and acquired (two-thirds). The acquired type is predominately iatrogenic in origin. The term, *renal arteriovenous malformation,* usually refers to the congenital type of malformation. Two types of congenital renal AVMs are described: cirsoid (more common) and cavernous AVM. Congenital cirsoid AVMs have a dilated, corkscrew appearance, similar in appearance to a varicose vein. Cavernous AVMs have single dilated vessels.[81] Acquired renal AVMs are usually termed *renal arteriovenous fistulas* and represent as many as 75% to 80% of renal AVMs.[82] Idiopathic renal AVF represents less than 3% of renal AVMs.[83]

Percutaneous renal biopsy is the most common known cause of acquired renal AVF.[84] Trauma is a less common cause of acquired renal fistulas. In patients with hypertension following renal trauma, renal AVFs may occur in one-third of patients. In patients with penetrating trauma, AVFs may affect as many as 80% of patients with posttraumatic hypertension.[85] Trauma during ureteroscopy has recently been described as a cause of intrarenal AVF.[86] There is a theory that idiopathic AVFs arise from the spontaneous erosion or rupture of a renal artery into a nearby renal vein. AVMs are known to occur in the setting of malignancy. Hypervascular tumors, such as renal cell carcinoma, are characterized by extensive neovascularity and invasion into renal tissue and adjacent structures. Angiogenic tumor factors have been implicated and may explain the development of AVMs within renal tumors.

Turbulent flow within the renal parenchyma is a typical finding of AVF on renal ultrasound. The turbulence is very dramatic on color flow imaging, with a visible color bruit, caused by vibration of surrounding soft tissues (Figure 31-17). When the AVF is large, high-volume venous flow is observed and is indicated by elevated Doppler velocity measurements.[87]

The fistula itself is typically not visualized because the communication is small and the affected vessel is obscured by the surrounding bruit artifact. The diagnosis can be made by detection of high-velocity flow within the feeding artery and pulsatile flow within the affected vein. Hypertension and hematuria are typical clinical signs accompanying the fistula. High-output cardiac failure may occur with large fistulas.[88]

RENAL ARTERY STENTS AND THEIR EVALUATION

Renal artery stenosis that is caused by atherosclerotic disease is potentially curable with percutaneous transluminal angioplasty, endovascular stent placement, or surgical revascularization. These various therapies may improve or stabilize hypertension, preserve renal function, and prevent development of end-stage renal failure.[89-91]

Percutaneous stenting of the renal artery has become standard treatment for renal artery stenosis and is associated with a high technical success rate, with low periprocedural mortality (0.5%).[92,93] Although the technical success rate is high right after the procedure, the longer-term complication is the development of in-stent

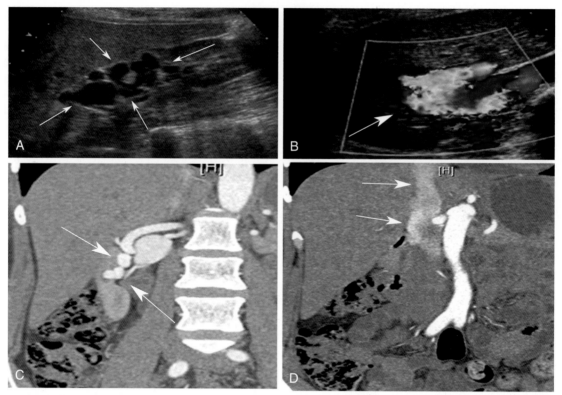

FIGURE 31-17 Renal arteriovenous malformation (AVM). **A,** Gray-scale image of the right kidney reveals multiple serpentine anechoic tubular structures *(arrows)*. **B,** Color Doppler image of the right kidney demonstrates color aliasing in the dilated feeding artery and draining vein of the AVM *(arrow)*. **C,** Computed tomographic (CT) angiography in this patient reveals multiple dilated enhancing vessels in the right renal cortex *(arrows)*. **D,** CT angiography reveals early fill-in of the suprarenal inferior vena cava *(arrows)*.

restenosis. Reported rates of 6% to 20 % for in-stent restenosis have been described.[94] Detection of in-stent renal artery restenosis is important to maintain renal artery patency and preserve renal function.[95,96] There are several modalities that are utilized for the assessment of renal artery stents, including conventional angiography, CTA, MRA, and Doppler ultrasound.

Conventional angiography, although accurate and reproducible, is limited for serial evaluation of renal artery stents because it is invasive with the potential for complications. It also requires exposure to ionizing radiation and iodinated contrast material. Iodinated contrast is associated with allergic reactions and is usually avoided in patients with renal insufficiency. This is important as many patients with renovascular disease have underlying renal dysfunction.

Noninvasive imaging techniques such as CTA, MRA, and Doppler ultrasound have also been used to detect renal artery in-stent restenosis.[97-104] CTA requires exposure to ionizing radiation and is also avoided in patients with renal insufficiency due to the nephrotoxic effects of iodinated contrast material. MRA is not suitable for renal artery stent evaluation due to the appearance of metallic artifacts that preclude adequate evaluation of the stent lumen. MRA also utilizes gadolinium as a contrast agent to opacify the renal arteries. Gadolinium agents carry the risk for nephrogenic systemic fibrosis, a potentially fatal disease, in patients with severely impaired renal function.[105-107]

Doppler ultrasound is gaining acceptance in the evaluation and long-term follow-up of patients after renal artery stent placement.[108-110] It is used to assess the success rate of the intervention itself, determine the baseline PSVs within the stent immediately after stent placement, and follow stent patency and identify long-term complications. There are few reports in the literature that describe the role of Doppler ultrasound for the diagnosis of in-stent renal artery restenosis. Bakker and associates[110] evaluated 33 renal artery stents in 24 patients for possible in-stent restenosis with digital subtraction angiography as a gold standard. They found that a threshold PSV greater than 226 cm/sec and RAR greater than 2.7 demonstrated sensitivities of 100% and 100% and specificities of 90% and 84%, respectively, in evaluation of significant (>50%) renal artery stenosis. The authors concluded that duplex ultrasound is sensitive for the detection of in-stent restenosis. In their series of 84 patients, Napoli and colleagues[109] evaluated 98 renal arteries treated with stent placement. They found that a PSV greater than 144 cm/sec and RAR greater than 2.5 were the threshold values for significant renal artery in-stent restenosis with sensitivities of 90% and 95% and specificities of 93% and 95%, respectively. The authors concluded that site-specific Doppler ultrasound criteria are valuable for the evaluation of renal artery in-stent restenosis. These authors did not evaluate the range of Doppler parameters for patent nonstenotic stents.

At our institution, we conducted a retrospective review of 98 Doppler renal stent evaluations to define Doppler parameters for patent renal artery stents immediately after stent placement, as well as appropriate duplex ultrasound criteria for identification of flow-reducing in-stent restenosis in the renal arteries. We found that the mean PSV in the patent nonstenotic stented renal arteries was 147.8 cm/sec with a median of 140.5 cm/sec (standard deviation [SD], 62.9). We also found that the mean stent/aortic ratio (SAR) in patent stents without stenosis was 1.88 with a median of 1.68 and SD of 1.2 (95% confidence interval [CI]). We also derived diagnostic criteria for the identification of in-stent renal artery restenosis using PSV and SAR values. The sensitivity and specificity for PSV greater than or equal to 240 cm/sec were shown to be 93% and 92%, respectively. For SAR greater than or equal to 3.2, the sensitivity and specificity for in-stent stenosis were shown to be 93% and 94%, respectively. The sensitivity and specificity for renal segmental artery tardus-parvus waveforms were shown to be 57% and 95%, respectively.

The protocol for evaluation of renal stents is similar to the native renal artery evaluation. The abdominal aorta is initially examined for evidence of significant atherosclerotic plaque, stenosis, or aneurysm. A PSV is obtained from the abdominal aorta to be used for the SAR. Following renal stent placement, the renal artery is evaluated in its entire length from the origin to the

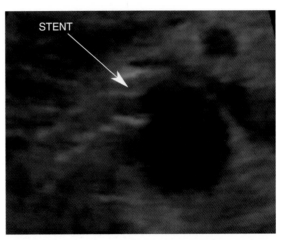

FIGURE 31-18 Renal artery stent. **A,** Gray-scale image of the juxtarenal abdominal aorta reveals a stent at the ostium of the right renal artery *(arrow).*

hilum. Gray-scale images provide optimal visualization of the stent as color flow may obscure the stent (Figure 31-18). Please note that most of the interventions are performed on patients with atherosclerotic disease, with a tendency for plaque to be near the origin of the renal arteries; therefore, the stents are typically placed near the origin of the renal artery. A small portion of the stent may protrude into the lumen of the aorta. Once gray-scale analysis is performed, color images are used to assess for flow disturbance (color aliasing). Color bruit artifacts are commonly seen at the site of significant renal artery in-stent restenosis. Subsequently, pulse Doppler is performed to record PSV measurements from within the stent as well as the origin, proximal, mid, and distal segments of the renal artery (Figure 31-19). Intrarenal waveforms are also obtained to assess for tardus parvus associated with significant in-stent restenosis.

The pitfalls and limitations of stent assessment are very similar to those encountered during the evaluation of native untreated renal arteries: overlying bowel gas, obesity, inability to breath-hold, and noncooperative patient. In addition, it has been postulated that patients with patent renal stents may have elevated PSVs throughout the stented renal artery when there is significant stenosis in the contralateral renal artery. This has also been identified in native arteries. Overestimation of stenosis in the presence of high PSV can be avoided by detection of additional signs of significant stenosis, including color and pulsed Doppler bruit artifacts,

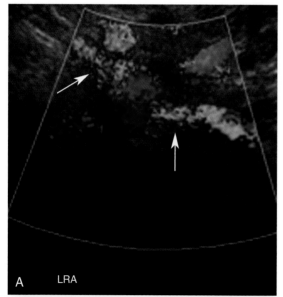

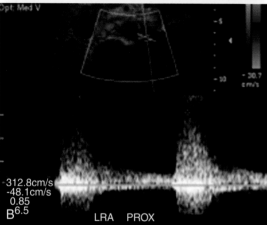

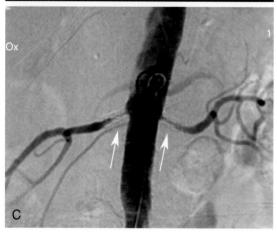

FIGURE 31-19 Renal in-stent restenosis. **A,** Color Doppler image through the transverse abdominal aorta demonstrates aliasing artifacts in both renal arteries treated with stents *(arrows)*. **B,** Spectral analysis of the left renal artery obtained at the level of the renal stent shows markedly elevated peak systolic velocity of 312 cm/sec, consistent with a hemodynamically significant in-stent restenosis. **C,** Angiography demonstrates severe in-stent stenoses within both renal arteries *(arrows)*.

poststenotic turbulence, and tardus-parvus waveforms. Analysis of Doppler parameters on the contralateral side is also helpful. In addition, patients with arrhythmia may present with fluctuating PSV complicating the determination of the actual PSV. Remember that baseline Doppler evaluation of renal artery stents is valuable for follow-up. Significant elevations in PSV on subsequent examinations may signify recurrent stenosis.

Acknowledgments. We would like to thank Saiedeh "Nanaz" Maghool for her expertise and enthusiasm and James Cooper, MD, for his wonderful illustrations. We also want to acknowledge Craig Greben, MD, James Naidich, MD, and Samuel Guzik for their assistance and guidance.

REFERENCES

1. Dawson DL: Noninvasive assessment of renal artery stenosis, *Semin Vasc Surg* 9:172–181, 1996.
2. Baxter GM, et al: Colour Doppler ultrasound in renal artery stenosis: Intrarenal waveform analysis, *Br J Radiol* 69:810–815, 1996.
3. Miralles M, et al: Value of Doppler parameters in the diagnosis of renal artery stenosis, *J Vasc Surg* 23:428–435, 1996.
4. Berland LL, et al: Renal artery stenosis: Prospective evaluation of diagnosis with color duplex US compared with angiography: Work in progress, *Radiology* 174:421–423, 1990.
5. Kliewer MA, et al: Doppler evaluation of renal artery stenosis: Interobserver agreement in the interpretation of waveform morphology, *Am J Roentgenol* 162:1371–1376, 1994.
6. Kliewer MA, et al: Early systole in the healthy kidney: Variability of Doppler US waveform parameters, *Radiology* 205:109–113, 1997.
7. Bakker J, et al: Renal artery stenosis and accessory renal arteries: Accuracy of detection and visualization with gadolinium-enhanced breath-hold MR angiography, *Radiology* 207:487–504, 1998.
8. De Cobelli F, et al: Renal artery stenosis: Evaluation with breath-hold, three-dimensional, dynamic, gadolinium-enhanced versus three-dimensional, phase-contrast MR angiography, *Radiology* 205:689–695, 1997.
9. Strotzer M, et al: Noninvasive assessment of renal artery stenosis: A comparison of MR angiography, color Doppler sonography, and intraarterial angiography, *Acta Radiol* 36:243–247, 1995.
10. Hoffmann U, et al: Role of duplex scanning for the detection of atherosclerotic renal artery disease, *Kidney Int* 39:1232–1239, 1991.
11. Hansen KJ, et al: Renal duplex sonography: Evaluation of clinical utility, *J Vasc Surg* 12:227–236, 1990.
12. Kohler TR, et al: Noninvasive diagnosis of renal artery stenosis by ultrasonic duplex scanning, *J Vasc Surg* 4:450–456, 1986.
13. Hélénon O, et al: Color Doppler US of renovascular disease in native kidneys, *Radiographics* 15:833–854, 1995.
14. Middleton WD: Doppler US evaluation of renal artery stenosis: Past, present, and future, *Radiology* 184:307–308, 1992.

15. Melany ML, et al: Ability of a phase shift US contrast agent to improve imaging of the main renal arteries, *Radiology* 205:147–152, 1997.

16. Olin JW, et al: The utility of duplex ultrasound scanning of the renal arteries for diagnosing significant renal artery stenosis, *Ann Intern Med* 122:833–838, 1995.

17. Strandness DE Jr: Duplex scanning in diagnosis of renovascular hypertension, *Surg Clin North Am* 70:109–117, 1990.

18. Isikoff MB, Hill MC: Sonography of the renal arteries: Left lateral decubitus position, *Am J Roentgenol* 134:1177–1179, 1980.

19. Stavros AT, et al: Segmental stenosis of the renal artery: Pattern recognition of tardus and parvus abnormalities with duplex sonography, *Radiology* 184:487–492, 1992.

20. Brun P, et al: Value of Doppler ultrasound for the diagnosis of renal artery stenosis in children, *Pediatr Nephrol* 11:27–30, 1997.

21. Van Ampting JM, et al: Prevalence of atherosclerotic renal artery stenosis in patients starting dialysis, *Nephrol Dial Transplant* 18:1147–1151, 2003.

22. Aristizabal D, Frohlich ED: Hypertension due to renal arterial disease, *Heart Dis Stroke* 1:227–234, 1992.

23. Wilcox CS: Ischemic nephropathy: Noninvasive testing, *Semin Nephrol* 16:43–52, 1996.

24. Meyrier A: Renal vascular lesions in the elderly: Nephrosclerosis or atheromatous renal disease? *Nephrol Dial Transplant* 11(Suppl 9):45–52, 1996.

25. Blaufox MD, et al: Cost efficacy of the diagnosis and therapy of renovascular hypertension, *J Nucl Med* 37:171–177, 1996.

26. Postma CT, et al: Pattern recognition of loss of early systolic peak by Doppler ultrasound has a low sensitivity for the detection of renal artery stenosis, *J Hum Hypertens* 10:181–184, 1996.

27. Pederson EB, et al: Diagnosing renal artery stenosis: A comparison between conventional renography, captopril renography and ultrasound Doppler in a large consecutive series of patients with arterial hypertension, *Blood Press* 5:342–348, 1996.

28. Nazzal MM, et al: Renal hilar Doppler analysis is of value in the management of patients with renovascular disease, *Am J Surg* 174:164–168, 1997.

29. Handa N, et al: A new accurate and non-invasive screening method for renovascular hypertension: The renal artery Doppler technique, *J Hypertens* 6(Suppl):458–460, 1988.

30. Kliewer MA, et al: Renal artery stenosis: Analysis of Doppler waveform parameters and tardus-parvus pattern, *Radiology* 189:779–787, 1993.

31. Patriquin HB, et al: Stenosis of the renal artery: Assessment of slowed systole in the downstream circulation with Doppler sonography, *Radiology* 184:470–485, 1992.

32. LaFortune M, et al: Renal arterial stenosis: Slowed systole in the downstream circulation—experimental study in dogs, *Radiology* 184:475–478, 1992.

33. Stanley JC: Renal vascular disease and renovascular hypertension in children, *Urol Clin North Am* 11:451–463, 1984.

34. Strandness DE Jr: *Duplex Scanning in Vascular Disorders*, New York, 1990, Lippincott-Raven. p 240.

35. Isaacson JA, Neumyer MM: Direct and indirect renal arterial duplex and Doppler color flow evaluations, *J Vasc Technol* 19:309–316, 1995.

36. Handa N, et al: Efficacy of echo-Doppler examination for the evaluation of renovascular disease, *Ultrasound Med Biol* 14:1–5, 1988.

37. Nichols BT, et al: Non-invasive detection of renal artery stenosis, *Bruit* 8:26–29, 1984.

38. Isaacson JA, et al: Noninvasive screening for renal artery stenosis: Comparison of renal artery and renal hilar duplex scanning, *J Vasc Technol* 19:105–110, 1995.

39. van der Hulst VPM, et al: Renal artery stenosis: Endovascular flow wire study for validation of Doppler US, *Radiology* 100:165–168, 1996.

40. Bude RO, et al: Pulsus tardus: Its cause and potential limitations in detection of arterial stenosis, *Radiology* 190:779–784, 1994.

41. Greene ER, et al: Noninvasive characterization of renal artery blood flow, *Kidney Int* 20:523–529, 1981.

42. Taylor DC, et al: Duplex ultrasound scanning in the diagnosis of renal artery stenosis: A prospective evaluation, *J Vasc Surg* 7:363–369, 1988.

43. Avasthi PS, Voyles WF, Greene ER: Noninvasive diagnosis of renal artery stenosis by echo-Doppler velocimetry, *Kidney Int* 25:824–829, 1984.

44. Dubbins PA: Renal artery stenosis: Duplex Doppler evaluation, *Br J Radiol* 59:225–229, 1986.

45. Gupta A, Tello R: Accessory renal arteries are not related to hypertension risk: a review of MR angiography data, *Am J Roentgenol* 182:1521–1524, 2004.

46. Bude RO, et al: Is it necessary to study accessory arteries when screening the renal arteries for renovascular hypertension? *Radiology* 226:411–416, 2003.

47. Fujitani RM, Murray SP: Surgical methods for renal revascularization, *Semin Vasc Surg* 9:198–217, 1996.

48. Radermacher J, et al: Use of Doppler ultrasonography to predict the outcome of therapy for renal artery stenosis, *N Engl J Med* 344:410–417, 2001.

49. Cohn EJ, et al: Can intrarenal duplex waveform analysis predict successful renal artery revascularization? *J Vasc Surg* 28:471–481, 1998.

50. García-Criado A, et al: Value of Doppler sonography for predicting clinical outcome after renal artery revascularization in atherosclerotic renal artery stenosis, *J Ultrasound Med* 24:1641–1647, 2005.

51. Platt JF, et al: Duplex Doppler US of the kidney: Differentiation of obstructive from nonobstructive dilatation, *Radiology* 171:515–517, 1989.

52. Platt JF, et al: Intrarenal arterial Doppler sonography in patients with nonobstructive renal disease: Correlation of resistive index with biopsy findings, *Am J Roentgenol* 154:1223–1227, 1990.

53. Keating MA, Althausen AF: The clinical spectrum of renal vein thrombosis, *J Urol* 133:938–945, 1985.

54. Clark RA, Wyatt GM, Colley D: Renal vein thrombosis: An underdiagnosed complication of multiple renal abnormalities, *Radiology* 132:43–50, 1979.

55. Llach F, Papper S, Massry SG: The clinical spectrum of renal vein thrombosis: Acute and chronic, *Am J Med* 69:819–827, 1980.

56. Rosenberg ER, et al: Ultrasonic diagnosis of renal vein thrombosis in neonates, *Am J Roentgenol* 134:35–38, 1980.

57. Paling MR, Wakefield JA, Watson LR: Sonography of experimental acute renal vein occlusion, *J Clin Ultrasound* 13:647–653, 1985.

58. Metreweli C, Pearson R: Echographic diagnosis of neonatal renal venous thrombosis, *Pediatr Radiol* 14:105–108, 1984.

59. Lalmand B, et al: Perinatal renal vein thrombosis, *J Ultrasound Med* 9:437–442, 1990.

60. Rosenfield AT, et al: Ultrasound in experimental and clinical renal vein thrombosis, *Radiology* 137:735–741, 1980.

61. Taylor KJW, Burns PN: Duplex Doppler scanning in the pelvis and abdomen, *Ultrasound Med Biol* 11:643–658, 1985.

62. Goncharenko V, et al: Incidence and distribution of venous extension in 70 hypernephromas, *Am J Roentgenol* 133:263–265, 1979.

63. Levine E: Malignant renal parenchymal tumors in adults. In Pollack HM, editor: *Clinical Urography: An Atlas and Textbook of Urological Imaging*, Philadelphia, 1990, WB Saunders, pp 1216–1291.

64. Goldstein HM, Green B, Weaver RM Jr: Ultrasonic detection of renal tumor extension into the inferior vena cava, *Am J Roentgenol* 130:1083–1085, 1978.

65. Schwerk WB, Schwerk WN, Rodeck G: Venous renal tumor extension: A prospective US evaluation, *Radiology* 156:491–495, 1985.

66. Didier D, et al: Tumor thrombus of the inferior vena cava secondary to malignant abdominal neoplasms: US and CT evaluation, *Radiology* 162:83–89, 1987.

67. Dubbins PA, Wells I: Renal carcinoma: Duplex Doppler evaluation, *Br J Radiol* 59:231–236, 1986.

68. London NJM, et al: A prospective study of the value of conventional CT, dynamic CT, ultrasonography and arteriography for staging renal carcinoma, *Br J Urol* 64:209–217, 1989.

69. Roubidoux MA, et al: Renal carcinoma: Detection of venous extension with gradient-echo MR imaging, *Radiology* 182:269–272, 1992.

70. Thomas JL, Bernardino ME: Neoplastic-induced renal vein enlargement: Sonographic detection, *Am J Roentgenol* 136:75–79, 1981.

71. Turba UC, et al: Normal renal arterial anatomy assessed by multidetector CT angiography: are there differences between men and women? *Clin Anat* 22(2):236–242, 2009.

72. Tham G, et al: Renal artery aneurysms: natural history and prognosis, *Ann Surg* 197:348–352, 1983.

73. Henke PK, et al: Renal artery aneurysms: a 35-year clinical experience with 252 aneurysms in 168 patients, *Ann Surg* 234:454–463, 2001.

74. Bulbul MA, Farrow GA: Renal artery aneurysms, *Urology* 40:124–126, 1992.

75. Klein GE, et al: Endovascular treatment of renal artery aneurysms with conventional non-detachable microcoils and Guglielmi detachable coils, *Br J Urol* 79:852–860, 1997.

76. Yamakado K, et al: Renal angiomyolipoma: Relationships between tumor size, aneurysm formation and rupture, *Radiology* 225:78–82, 2002.

77. English WP, et al: Surgical management of renal artery aneurysms, *J Vasc Surg* 40:53–60, 2004.

78. Chuansheng Z, et al: Visceral and renal artery aneurysms: a pictorial essay on endovascular therapy, *Radio-Graphics* 26:1687–1704, 2006.

79. Takaha M, Matsumoto A, Ochi K: Intrarenal arteriovenous malformation, *J Urol* 124:315–331, 1980.

80. Cho K, Stanley J: Non-neoplastic congenital and acquired renal arteriovenous malformations and fistulas, *Radiology* 129:333–343, 1978.

81. Kopchick JH, et al: Congenital renal arteriovenous malformations, *Urology* 17:13–17, 1981.

82. Messing E, Kessler R, Kavaney PB: Renal arteriovenous fistulas, *Urology* 8:101–107, 1976.

83. Shah SR, et al: Large arteriovenous malformation in kidney mimicking cyst, *Indian J Radiol Imaging* 10:35–36, 2000.

84. Bennet AR, Wiener SN: Intrarenal arteriovenous fistula and aneurysm: a complication of percutaneous renal biopsy, *Am J Roentgenol* 95:372–382, 1965.

85. McAlhany JC, et al: Renal arteriovenous fistula as a cause of hypertension, *Am J Surg* 122:117, 1971.

86. Tiplitsky SI, et al: *J Endourol* 21(5):530–532, May 2007.

87. Naganuma H, et al: Renal arteriovenous malformation: sonographic findings, *Abdom Imaging* 26:661–663, 2001.

88. Hirai S, et al: High-output heart failure caused by a huge renal arteriovenous fistula after nephrectomy: report of a case, *Surg Today* 31(5):468–470, 2001.

89. Leertouwer TC, et al: Stent placement for renal arterial stenosis: where do we stand? A meta-analysis, *Radiology* 216:78–85, 2000.

90. Dworkin LD: Controversial treatment of atherosclerotic renal vascular disease: the cardiovascular outcomes in renal atherosclerotic lesions trial, *Hypertension* 48:350–356, 2006.

91. Hirsch AT, et al: ACC/AHA 2005 Practice guidelines for the management of patients with peripheral arterial disease (lower extremity, renal, mesenteric, and abdominal aortic): a collaborative report from the American Association for Vascular Surgery/Society for Vascular Surgery, Society for Cardiovascular Angiography and Interventions, Society for Vascular Medicine and Biology, Society of Interventional Radiology, and the ACC/AHA Task Force on Practice Guidelines (Writing Committee to Develop Guidelines for the Management of Patients With Peripheral Arterial Disease): endorsed by the American Association of Cardiovascular and Pulmonary Rehabilitation; National Heart, Lung, and Blood Institute; Society for Vascular Nursing; TransAtlantic Inter-Society Consensus; and Vascular Disease Foundation, *Circulation* 113:e463–e654, 2006.

92. Jokhi PP, et al: Experience of stenting for atherosclerotic renal artery stenosis in a cardiac catheterization laboratory: technical considerations and complications, *Can J Cardiol* 25(8):e273–e278, 2009.

93. White CJ: Catheter-based therapy for atherosclerotic renal artery stenosis, *Circulation* 113:1464–1473, 2006.

94. Zeller T, et al: Restenosis after stenting of atherosclerotic renal artery stenosis: is there a rationale for the use of drug-eluting stents? *Catheter Cardiovasc Interv* 68(1):125–130, 2006.

95. Vignali C, et al: Predictive factors of in-stent restenosis in renal artery stenting: a retrospective analysis, *Cardiovasc Interv Radiol* 28:296–302, 2005.

96. Shammas NW, et al: Clinical and angiographic predictors of restenosis following renal artery stenting, *J Invas Cardiol* 16:10–13, 2004.

97. Goldman CK, Chi YW: Magnetic resonance, computed tomographic, and angiographic imaging of peripheral arterial disease. In Mohler E, Jaff M, editors: *Peripheral arterial disease*, 1st edition, 2008, American College of Physicians, pp 53–72.

98. Lookstein RA: Impact of CT angiography on endovascular therapy, *Mt Sinai J Med* 70:367–374, 2003.

99. Dong Q, et al: Diagnosis of renal vascular disease with MR angiography, *Radiographics* 19:1535–1554, 1999.

100. Lenhart M, et al: Stent appearance at contrast-enhanced MR angiography: in vitro examination with 14 stents, *Radiology* 217:173–178, 2000.

101. Maintz D, et al: Multislice CT angiography of the iliac arteries in the presence of various stents: in vitro evaluation of artifacts and lumen visibility, *Invest Radiol* 36:699–704, 2001.

102. Maintz D, et al: Revealing in-stent stenoses of the iliac arteries: comparison of multidetector CT with MR angiography and digital radiographic angiography in a Phantom model, *Am J Roentgenol* 179:1319–1322, 2002.

103. Bartels LW, et al: MR imaging of vascular stents: effects of susceptibility, flow, and radiofrequency eddy currents, *J Vasc Interv Radiol* 12:365–371, 2001.

104. Spuentrup E, et al: Artifact-free coronary magnetic resonance angiography and coronary vessel wall imaging in the presence of a new, metallic, coronary magnetic resonance imaging stent, *Circulation* 111:1019–1026, 2005.

105. Richmond H, et al: Nephrogenic systemic fibrosis: relationship to gadolinium and response to photopheresis, *Arch Dermatol* 143:1025–1030, 2007. *Erratum in: Arch Dermatol* 143:1565, 2007.

106. Marckmann P: Nephrogenic systemic fibrosis: epidemiology update, *Curr Opin Nephrol Hypertens* 17:315–319, 2008.

107. Wertman R, et al: Risk of nephrogenic systemic fibrosis: evaluation of gadolinium chelate contrast agents at four American universities, *Radiology* 248:799–806, 2008.

108. Radermacher J, et al: Use of Doppler ultrasonography to predict the outcome of therapy for renal-artery stenosis, *N Engl J Med* 344:410–417, 2001.

109. Napoli V, et al: Duplex ultrasonographic study of the renal arteries before and after renal artery stenting, *Eur Radiol* 12:796–803, 2002.

110. Bakker J, et al: Duplex ultrasonography in assessing restenosis of renal artery stents, *Cardiovasc Interv Radiol* 22:475–480, 1999.

DUPLEX ULTRASOUND EVALUATION OF THE UTERUS AND OVARIES

32

JOHN S. PELLERITO, MD, FACR, FSRU, FAIUM

Duplex and color Doppler imaging have become a routine part of the ultrasound evaluation of the female pelvis.[1] These techniques are utilized for both transabdominal and endovaginal examinations. The combination of Doppler ultrasound with endovaginal scanning is particularly valuable for gynecologic investigations because there is improved resolution and increased sensitivity to blood flow. The term *endovaginal color flow Doppler imaging* (EVCF) is used to describe this pairing of techniques.[2] We routinely utilize Doppler ultrasound in a number of different applications, including the following:

1. Identification of the dominant follicle or corpus luteal cyst in patients with pelvic pain or suspected ectopic pregnancy
2. Detection of placental tissue in abnormal intrauterine pregnancy, ectopic pregnancy, and retained products of conception
3. Diagnosis of ovarian torsion
4. Characterization of ovarian and adnexal masses
5. Detection of a number of uterine abnormalities, including fibroids, polyps, and tumors, as well as vascular abnormalities such as arteriovenous malformation and the pelvic congestion syndrome.

EVCF offers several advantages over endovaginal scans without Doppler. Integration of Doppler signal information into the sonographic analysis allows for specific tissue characterization and recognition of normal and abnormal flow patterns and may eliminate the need for computed tomographic or magnetic resonance imaging correlation in many cases. EVCF also improves the detection of blood flow compared with transabdominal scans with color Doppler. The endovaginal probe is closer to the areas of interest, so there is enhanced detection of vessel patency and tissue vascularity. This is extremely helpful in cases when the

demonstration of blood flow is critical to the diagnosis (i.e., ovarian torsion).

TECHNICAL ISSUES

Because the technical aspects of color flow imaging are covered in Chapter 3, this chapter emphasizes just the key points pertinent to pelvic sonography. Similar to other color and pulsed Doppler examinations, Doppler evaluation of the uterus and ovaries should be considered a dynamic process, requiring adjustment of the color flow parameters according to the type of examination. Using the manufacturer's settings (presets) is a good starting point for any examination. They serve as a general guide and can be adjusted to improve visualization of blood flow. Presets are helpful to novice or beginner sonographers and sonologists, particularly when the initial demonstration of color flow is suboptimal but critical for diagnosis.

It is important to remember that color, power, and pulsed Doppler images are based on the same physical principles but display different information.[3] Color Doppler images are based on the mean velocity display of reflected frequency shifts. In other words, the frequencies reflected from the moving red blood cells are averaged over time and presented on the image. Color Doppler displays a range of velocities on the image but does not provide absolute or peak systolic velocity information. Pulsed Doppler is used to determine the peak velocity at a particular location.

Power (amplitude) Doppler images are determined by the strength or amplitude of the returning Doppler shifts.[4] The frequency shifts are amplified and displayed along with the grayscale information. Power Doppler provides three to five times increased sensitivity to blood flow, compared with color flow imaging. There is less dependence on the angle of insonation, so flow can be demonstrated at angles close to 90 degrees. Thus, very weak Doppler shifts are presented on the power Doppler image. Advantages of power Doppler include improved vascular detail, faster localization of blood flow for pulsed Doppler sampling, and assessment of global tissue perfusion.

Power Doppler images do not demonstrate color aliasing or direction of flow. This is not a significant limitation, as determination of flow direction or aliasing is achieved with color flow or pulsed Doppler sampling. Power Doppler is also susceptible to the same pitfalls associated with incorrect color flow settings as with color Doppler imaging. In general, there are three parameters that should always be checked to ensure optimal color and power Doppler imaging:

1. Color velocity range or pulse repetition frequency (PRF)
2. Color gain
3. Wall filter

These settings should be adjusted to improve the detection of color flow for each study, as they are fundamental to the detection of low-flow states.[3] To detect low-velocity flow, we decrease the PRF, increase the color gain, and/or decrease the wall filter settings. When flow velocities are high and we want to reduce the degree of color noise or aliasing in the image, we increase the PRF or color velocity scale, decrease the color gain, and/or increase the wall filter. Experience and practice with different parameter settings will increase understanding of the interrelationships between these settings and lead to improved detection of flow. As always, the focal zone should be placed near the region of interest.

Most studies are performed with transducers in the 2.5- to 5-MHz range for transabdominal studies. Endovaginal scans utilize frequencies in the 5- to 10-MHz range. For pulsed Doppler evaluation, angle correction is performed when the direction of flow can be ascertained. We use no angle correction (0 degrees) for tiny or tortuous vessels in the pelvis when the direction of flow cannot be determined. A small sample volume is important for spectral analysis to avoid obtaining signals from multiple sources.

NORMAL ANATOMY AND HEMODYNAMICS

A thorough sonographic evaluation of the uterus and ovaries is usually performed in conjunction with Doppler assessment for blood flow.

We usually begin our evaluation with the uterus and then turn our attention to the adnexa and evaluation of the ovaries. The uterus is a pear-shaped, midline structure that is usually easy to identify (Figure 32-1). Measurements of the length, width, and anteroposterior diameter of the uterus should be obtained. We also evaluate the thickness of the endometrium as well as the cervix and the presence and location of any uterine masses. The ovaries are variable in shape and location. Although the ovaries can be identified with either transabdominal or endovaginal scanning, a combination of techniques may be necessary for complete evaluation. The ovaries are also measured in three dimensions. The presence of cysts or masses is noted and correlated with the menstrual cycle.

Color and pulsed Doppler examination requires knowledge of the vascular anatomy and hemodynamic changes of the female pelvis. The vessels most frequently examined in the pelvis include the iliac, uterine, and ovarian arteries and veins (see Figure 32-1).[5] These vessels may be identified with both transabdominal and endovaginal imaging. EVCF affords improved resolution and vascular detail compared with the transabdominal approach.

The uterine artery is a branch of the internal iliac artery and penetrates the uterus at the lower uterine segment (see Figure 32-1, *B*). Uterine artery branches course toward the uterine fundus and cervix as well as toward the ovaries in the broad ligament. Color and pulsed Doppler sampling of the uterine artery reveals high-impedance, low diastolic flow in the nongravid state.[5] A characteristic diastolic "notch" is usually noted (Figure 32-2). Identification of the notch is helpful in characterizing waveforms found in the uterus and adnexa as originating from the uterine artery. There is a gradual decrease in resistance to flow in the spectral samples obtained from the uterine arteries during the second trimester of pregnancy. The decrease in resistance and resistivity index is related to increased blood flow, particularly in diastole, necessary for normal placental and fetal growth. Continuous low-resistance blood flow should be detected in the placenta and umbilical arteries supplying the fetus.

Each ovary receives a dual blood supply, as shown in Figure 32-1, *A*. The ovarian artery originates from the abdominal aorta and descends to the pelvis. The ovary also receives branches from

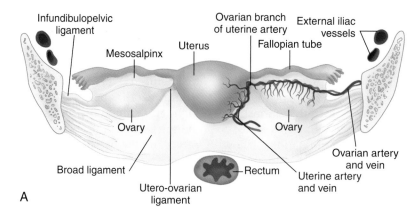

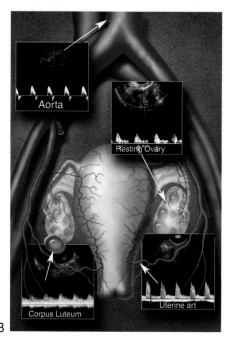

FIGURE 32-1 **A,** Normal pelvic anatomy. **B,** Montage of normal pelvic Doppler waveforms.

the uterine artery that course along the broad ligament. Blood flow patterns observed during color and pulsed Doppler sampling of the ovary vary depending on the phase of the ovulatory cycle. Low-velocity, high-impedance waveforms are usually noted early in menses into the follicular phase. (Figure 32-3). This is seen during the first menstrual week, when the ovaries are dormant and before the formation of the dominant follicle and corpus luteal cyst.[6]

The luteal phase coincides with the extrusion of the mature egg or oocyte and formation of the corpus luteal cyst. Thickening of the cyst walls is seen with gray-scale imaging. Color Doppler demonstrates a ring of vascularity ("ring of fire" pattern) around the luteal cyst, related to

formation of tiny vessels in the walls of the cyst.[7] Pulsed Doppler shows a marked increase in peak systolic and end-diastolic velocities (Figure 32-4). The increased velocities are related to neovascularization of the corpus luteum, required for oocyte maturation and hormonal activity.[8]

I originally described the "ring of fire" color flow pattern to represent the increased vascularity noted around the periphery of an extrauterine gestational sac.[9] Subsequently, it became very clear that a similar pattern of peripheral blood flow occurs with the formation of a corpus luteal cyst. In fact, we look for the ring of increased vascularity in the ovary to locate and characterize luteal cysts. It should be clear that the "ring of fire" color flow pattern alone cannot distinguish

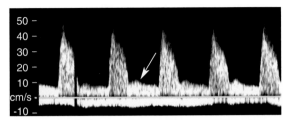

FIGURE 32-2 Normal uterine artery waveform. Pulsed Doppler evaluation reveals a high-resistance waveform with the early diastolic "notch" *(arrow)*.

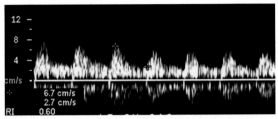

FIGURE 32-3 Normal follicular phase ovarian waveform. Pulsed Doppler evaluation of the ovary during the first week of the menstrual cycle reveals low-velocity systolic and diastolic flow.

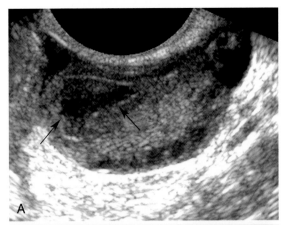

A

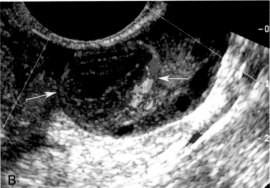

B

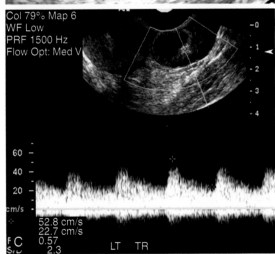

C

between ectopic pregnancies and luteal cysts. Investigators have tried to identify discriminating Doppler parameters to distinguish luteal from ectopic flow.[10,11] This is difficult due to overlap in peak systolic velocity and resistivity index measurements between luteal cysts and ectopic pregnancies. The origin of the Doppler signal, from within the ovary or from an adnexal mass, allows more accurate characterization of a corpus luteal cyst or ectopic pregnancy than velocity or resistivity index alone. Therefore, we do not use Doppler to distinguish luteal from ectopic flow but to localize the site of origin of the signals to determine their significance.

Color and pulsed Doppler signals obtained from a postmenopausal ovary have low peak systolic velocities similar to ovaries in the follicular phase[7] (Figure 32-5). This is typical of ovaries in the resting state. Because postmenopausal ovarian vessels carry low-velocity flow, this vascularity may be very difficult to visualize with conventional color Doppler flow settings. Low color velocity scale (PRF) and color wall filter adjustments may be necessary to detect postmenopausal ovarian blood flow. Power Doppler imaging improves the visualization of ovarian flow, particularly in postmenopausal women. Because postmenopausal ovaries no longer ovulate, they remain relatively quiescent and are associated with little or no diastolic flow.

FIGURE 32-4 A, Corpus luteal cyst. Gray-scale image demonstrates a hypoechoic lesion with echogenic borders *(arrows)*. **B,** Color Doppler shows a ring of increased color flow *(arrows)* around the periphery of the corpus luteal cyst. **C,** Pulsed Doppler demonstrates increased systolic and diastolic velocities associated with the vascular ring.

CURRENT APPLICATIONS

Current applications of transabdominal scanning and EVCF include identification of the corpus luteal cyst, detection of intrauterine placental

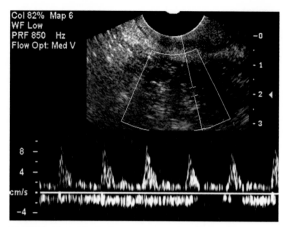

FIGURE 32-5 Normal postmenopausal ovarian wave-form. Pulsed Doppler demonstrates typical low-velocity, high-resistance flow.

flow, diagnosis of ectopic pregnancy and retained products of conception, evaluation for ovarian torsion, and characterization of adnexal masses and uterine abnormalities.

CORPUS LUTEAL CYST

Identification of the dominant follicle or corpus luteal cyst has proven extremely helpful in patients who present with pelvic pain, adnexal mass, or ectopic pregnancy. Ovarian cysts are the most common cause of acute pelvic pain in premenopausal patients.[12] The pain is usually associated with enlargement of the cyst during the midportion of the menstrual cycle and precedes cyst rupture and the release of fluid.

Simple ovarian cysts are easily characterized by their lack of internal echoes; smooth, thin walls; and posterior sound enhancement. Complex ovarian cysts can be much harder to characterize as benign ovarian cysts. Hemorrhagic cysts may be filled with low-level echoes and are not easily recognized, as they become isoechoic to the ovarian parenchyma. These cysts may also contain solid regions and septations and may resemble ovarian neoplasms.

Color and pulsed Doppler are important tools for the characterization of complex ovarian cysts. Color Doppler can demonstrate the ring of increased vascularity in the wall of the corpus luteal cyst (Figure 32-6). As mentioned earlier, the peripheral vascularity is related to neovascularization associated with the formation of the corpus luteal cyst.[8] The increased blood flow identified with color Doppler is associated with elevated peak systolic velocities and low-resistance flow.

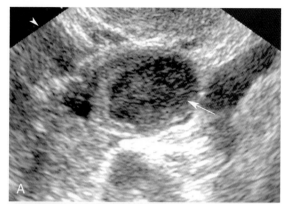

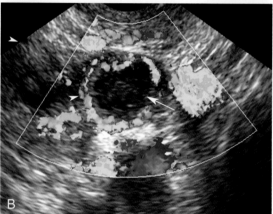

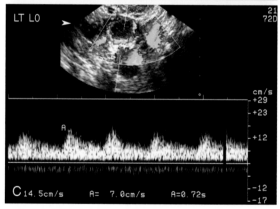

FIGURE 32-6 **A,** Hemorrhagic ovarian cyst. A hypoechoic lesion (arrow) is seen within the ovary, which contains low-level heterogeneous echoes consistent with hemorrhage. **B,** Color Doppler demonstrates a "ring of fire" (arrowhead) around the hemorrhagic cyst (arrow). Note that there is no color flow within the hemorrhagic component. **C,** Pulsed Doppler demonstrates low-resistance flow consistent with luteal flow.

Dillon and colleagues[13] demonstrated a peak systolic velocity of 27 ± 10 cm/sec and a resistivity index of 0.44 ± 0.09 for corpus luteal cysts. The demonstration of peripheral vascularity with color or power Doppler increases the conspicuity of the corpus luteal cyst, even when it is filled with blood and is isoechoic to ovarian tissue on gray-scale images. The lack of vascularity within the central part of the lesion suggests it is a hemorrhagic cyst.[12] This is particularly helpful when gray-scale evaluation demonstrates wall thickening, nodules, or septations within the cyst cavity. The absence of flow within the cyst cavity suggests that any solid material within the cyst is likely related to hematoma or retracting clot and not tumor (Figure 32-7). A follow-up ultrasound study 6 to 8 weeks later, during the first week of a subsequent menstrual cycle, is recommended to assess for complete resolution of the complex cyst and to exclude the possibility of tumor.

The recognition of the corpus luteal cyst also aids in the diagnosis of ectopic pregnancy. Approximately 85% to 90% of ectopic pregnancies occur on the same side as the corpus luteal cyst.[9] Identification of the corpus luteum determines the side of ovulation and directs the examiner to the expected site of the ectopic pregnancy (Figure 32-8). Color and pulsed Doppler also play a role in the identification and follow-up of ectopic pregnancy, which is our next topic of discussion.

ECTOPIC PREGNANCY

Ectopic pregnancy occurs in approximately 2% of pregnancies and is the leading cause of pregnancy-related deaths during the first trimester.[14] There is a rising incidence of ectopic pregnancy that is related to the following:

An increased number of patients at risk
New techniques that allow earlier diagnosis
Improved treatment for salpingitis and ectopic pregnancy
Increased utilization of ovulation induction and assisted reproduction techniques

The vast majority of ectopic pregnancies occur in the fallopian tube, usually in the ampullary region. Less commonly, ectopic pregnancies will be seen in the cornual region (interstitial portion of the fallopian tube), in the cervical canal, or within a cesarean defect. Abdominal and intraovarian pregnancies are rare.

It is important to understand and solicit risk factors from patients with suspected ectopic pregnancy.[15] Any process that produces scarring or obstruction of the fallopian tube predisposes to ectopic pregnancy. The obstruction may be related to prior pelvic surgery or tubal ligation, prior ectopic pregnancy, or history of pelvic inflammatory

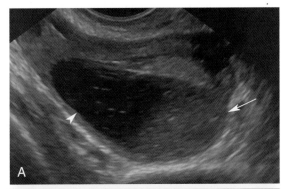
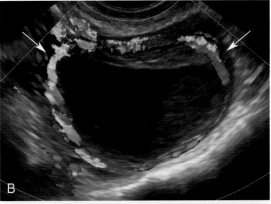
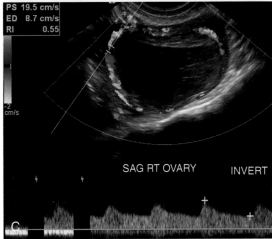

FIGURE 32-7 Hemorrhagic cyst. **A,** A heterogeneous complex lesion is identified in the ovary, with solid *(arrow)* and fluid *(arrowhead)* components. **B,** Color Doppler demonstrates flow around the periphery of the mass *(arrows)* but no central or internal flow. **C,** Pulsed Doppler evaluation reveals classic luteal flow signals. A follow-up examination after 8 weeks demonstrated resolution of the lesion.

disease or salpingitis. The use of an intrauterine contraceptive device or the "morning after" pill may also increase the risk for ectopic pregnancy. In vitro fertilization also increases the rate of ectopic pregnancy because of multiple risk factors,

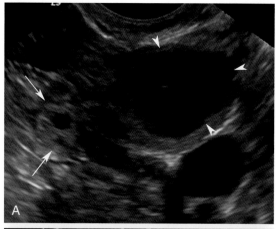

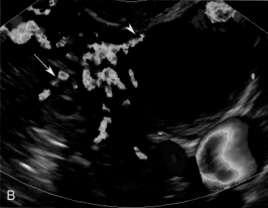

FIGURE 32-8 A, A well-defined extrauterine gestational sac *(arrows)* is identified on the same side as a hemorrhagic corpus luteal cyst *(arrowheads)* in the left ovary. **B,** Color Doppler reveals flow within the wall of the ectopic pregnancy *(arrow)* and in the wall of the corpus luteal cyst *(arrowhead).*

including infertility, ovulation induction, and embryo transfer with retrograde migration of the embryo into the fallopian tube. Infertility is associated with multiple anatomic and physiologic conditions that increase risk for ectopic pregnancy. Other risk factors include prior cesarean section, in utero exposure to diethylstilbestrol, and sterilization.

The clinical presentation of ectopic pregnancy is variable; however, a positive pregnancy test, pelvic pain, an adnexal mass, and/or vaginal bleeding raise clinical suspicion for this condition. The classic triad of pelvic pain, adnexal mass, and vaginal bleeding occurs only in approximately 45% of patients.[16] Patients may be asymptomatic or have focal or generalized pelvic or abdominal pain.

Earlier diagnosis of ectopic pregnancy is possible due to improved sonographic techniques and increased awareness of the disease. Early

detection reduces the risk for tubal rupture and significant hemorrhage. The evaluation for ectopic pregnancy usually includes a combination of endovaginal sonography and serum human chorionic gonadotropin (hCG) titers. Diagnostic laparoscopy is considered the gold standard and is usually reserved for difficult cases.

The sonographic findings associated with ectopic pregnancy include absence of a normal intrauterine pregnancy, a pseudogestational sac (described later), a live extrauterine embryo, pelvic fluid, and an adnexal mass. A common sonographic feature is the extrauterine gestational sac or "tubal ring." This appears as a ring-shaped adnexal mass with a thick wall, similar in appearance to a doughnut or life preserver. Occasionally, a complex or solid adnexal mass is identified, related to pelvic hematoma or hematosalpinx. The complex appearance of the mass is usually related to bleeding or rupture of the ectopic pregnancy. A live embryo is seen less commonly but provides the highest positive predictive value for the diagnosis of ectopic pregnancy.

PLACENTAL FLOW

In the absence of a normal intrauterine pregnancy, color and pulsed Doppler imaging can demonstrate features of placental flow in the uterus or adnexa.[10] The presence or absence of placental flow in the uterus is an extremely valuable finding in the evaluation for suspected ectopic pregnancy, for when it is present in the uterus, the focus of examination shifts toward an abnormal intrauterine pregnancy rather than an extrauterine gestation. Placental flow is related to invasion of the endometrium by growing trophoblastic (placental) tissue. As the trophoblast grows into the uterine tissue, the maternal spiral arteries will shunt arterial blood into the intervillous sinusoids. This results in relatively high-velocity, low-resistance blood flow that is readily detected with color Doppler imaging (Figure 32-9). Pulsed Doppler examination of intrauterine placental flow reveals a peak systolic velocity greater than 21 cm/sec, and the impedance decreases to a mean resistivity index of 0.44 ± 0.09.[17] The increased vascularity related to trophoblastic implantation is detected 36 to 50 days after the last menstrual period.

Detection of the flow characteristics related to placentation is invaluable in the identification of gestational tissue in the uterus or in the adnexa. A peak systolic velocity cutoff at 21 cm/sec or more is utilized to characterize placental flow in the

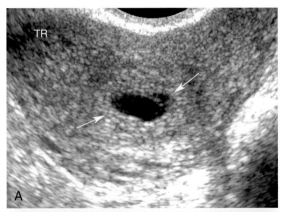

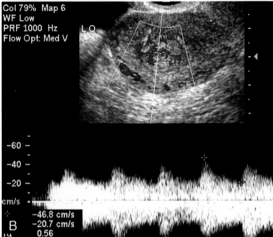

FIGURE 32-9 **A,** Endovaginal sonography reveals a gestational sac *(arrows)* within the endometrial canal. **B,** Color Doppler demonstrates increased flow around the gestational sac. Pulsed Doppler waveforms show characteristic high-velocity, low-resistance flow signals with a peak systolic velocity of 47 cm/sec.

uterus. We utilize no (0-degree) angle correction for the pulsed Doppler examination, as the vessels are too small to determine the direction of flow. Despite the 0-degree angle correction, Doppler is remarkably sensitive for the detection of placental flow when the peak systolic velocity is greater than 21 cm/sec. The detection of placental flow in the uterus confirms the presence of a normal or abnormal intrauterine pregnancy. In general, pulsed Doppler interrogation of a normal embryo is not performed due to potential bioeffects related to cavitation and heating.

PSEUDOGESTATION

Color and pulsed Doppler can also distinguish between an abnormal intrauterine pregnancy and a pseudogestational sac related to ectopic pregnancy. The sonographic appearance of "pseudosacs" ranges from endometrial thickening to a fluid collection in the endometrial canal. Unlike normal intrauterine gestational sacs, pseudosacs tend to be oval and located centrally in the endometrial cavity rather than eccentrically placed in the endometrium. They do not demonstrate a double decidual reaction, yolk sac, or embryo. They also do not exhibit placental flow, an important discriminatory factor (Figure 32-10). Doppler sampling of the area surrounding the pseudosac will demonstrate velocities less than 21 cm/sec. Dillon and colleagues[17] showed that Doppler findings were 100% specific in the identification of pseudogestational sacs.

VALUE OF DOPPLER FOR EVALUATION OF ECTOPIC PREGNANCY

The diagnosis of ectopic pregnancy is based on the finding of a cystic, complex, or solid mass, separate from the uterus and ovaries, in a pregnant patient. Color Doppler is helpful in cases of ectopic pregnancy when the gray-scale findings are not diagnostic and increased vascularity is identified in the adnexa (Figure 32-11). In a study of 155 patients with suspected ectopic pregnancy, my colleagues and I [9] found that placental flow was observed in 85% (55 of 65) of patients with ectopic pregnancy. Color and pulsed Doppler showed a sensitivity of 95% and specificity of 98% for the detection of ectopic pregnancy. We have been able to distinguish ectopic pregnancy from hematoma, bowel loops, and other adnexal masses on the basis of increased color flow (Figure 32-12). Color and pulsed Doppler have also proven useful in cases of interstitial (cornual) and cervical ectopic pregnancies when no significant mass is identified but there is increased flow on color and power Doppler examination (Figure 32-13).

Color and pulsed Doppler are also utilized to assess for persistent abnormal flow after treatment for ectopic pregnancy. There is a trend toward nonsurgical treatment of small, uncomplicated ectopic pregnancies with methotrexate or careful clinical follow-up. Doppler is used to assess for absence or persistence of placental flow after treatment or during follow-up. Ultrasound may show persistence or increase in size of the adnexal mass after methotrexate administration.[15] Serial sonograms may be required to

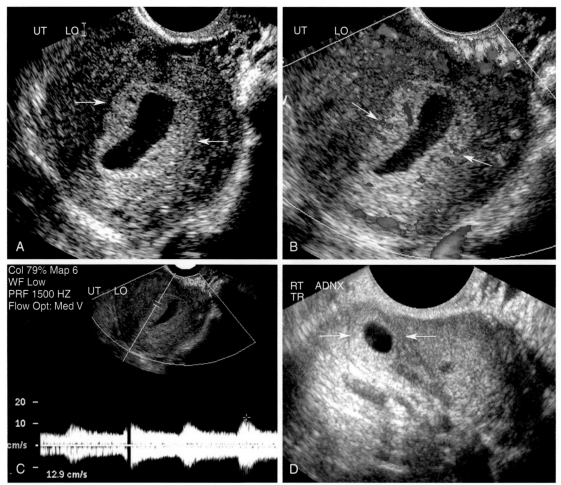

FIGURE 32-10 **A,** Endovaginal scan reveals a well-defined sac-like structure *(arrows)* within the endometrial canal in a patient with a positive human chorionic gonadotropin titer and vaginal bleeding. This finding may be related to an abnormal intrauterine pregnancy or pseudogestational sac associated with an ectopic pregnancy. **B,** Color Doppler demonstrates flow in the myometrium and vessels associated with the intrauterine sac *(arrows)*. **C,** Spectral analysis of the vessels around the sac demonstrates low-velocity signals (<21 cm/sec) consistent with a pseudogestational sac. **D,** Examination of the right adnexa demonstrates a ring-shaped mass *(arrows)* consistent with an ectopic sac.

demonstrate resolution of placental flow following methotrexate.

PITFALLS

As previously mentioned, one must use caution when interpreting color and pulsed Doppler images. There is significant overlap in the appearance of placental and luteal flow. Intrauterine and extrauterine gestational sacs, as well as corpus luteal cysts, exhibit the "ring of fire" appearance. Similarly, both placental and luteal waveforms demonstrate indistinguishable low-resistance arterial flow. The origin of the color Doppler signals must be considered for accurate diagnosis. Because intraovarian ectopic pregnancies are extremely rare (less

than 1% of all ectopics),[18] increased flow obtained from within the ovary likely represents luteal flow.

These techniques work very well in the appropriate clinical setting, but other pathologies may demonstrate high-velocity, low-resistance flow patterns that simulate placental flow. For example, fibroids or polyps can demonstrate similar low-resistance signals. The gray-scale features usually allow identification of the fibroid or polyp as the source of the signals. Other pathologies, such as endometritis, may demonstrate low-resistance signals similar to placental flow, but in the case of endometritis, the clinical situation prompts the correct diagnosis. Certain adnexal pathologies may also demonstrate signals that simulate placental flow. The keys to correct diagnosis relate to

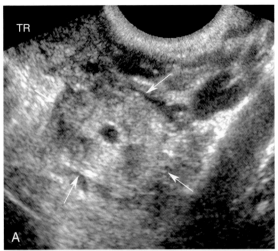

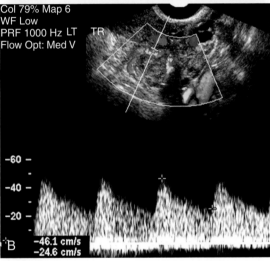

FIGURE 32-11 A, A poorly defined hypoechoic region *(arrows)* is identified in the left adnexa, separate from the ovary, in this patient with a positive human chorionic gonadotropin titer and pelvic pain. The finding is suspicious for an ectopic pregnancy. **B,** Color Doppler demonstrates increased flow within the mass. Pulsed Doppler shows high-velocity, low-impedance waveforms consistent with placental flow in this patient with proven ectopic pregnancy.

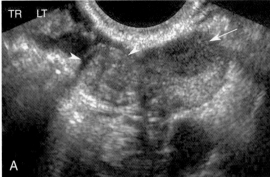

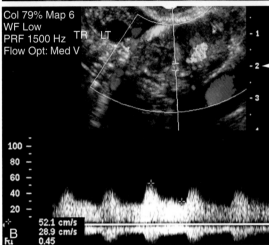

FIGURE 32-12 A, Endovaginal scan shows a round, solid region *(arrowheads)* adjacent to the left ovary in this pregnant patient with pain and vaginal bleeding. The differential diagnosis included hematoma, bowel, and ectopic pregnancy. Note that the left ovary contains a hemorrhagic luteal cyst *(arrow).* **B,** Color Doppler reveals increased flow within the tissue. Pulsed Doppler demonstrates high-velocity, low-resistance signals consistent with trophoblastic flow. Increased flow will not be seen in bowel or hematoma, and the findings are consistent with ectopic pregnancy.

relevant clinical information and recognition of the source of the Doppler waveforms.

Pitfalls can occur when the site of Doppler insonation is not clear. The most common pitfall is confusing a corpus luteal cyst with an ectopic pregnancy. Both the corpus luteal cyst and the ectopic pregnancy may present with a cystic, ring-shaped mass and low-resistance arterial signals. This situation is resolved by recognizing that the corpus luteal cyst is located within the ovary and is not a separate adnexal mass. A mass that cannot be separated from the ovary is unlikely to represent an ectopic pregnancy for reasons mentioned

previously. Another important diagnostic clue is that the ectopic sac is usually more echogenic than the corpus luteal cyst and ovarian tissue.[19-20] Other potential pitfalls include a tubo-ovarian abscess, endometrioma, pedunculated fibroid, ovarian malignancy, or other pelvic tumor or abscess. The location of Doppler flow and the clinical scenario should allow for correct diagnosis.

In summary, the value of color Doppler in the evaluation of ectopic pregnancy includes the following:

Diagnosis of an abnormal intrauterine pregnancy through identification of placental flow associated with a spontaneous miscarriage or incomplete abortion

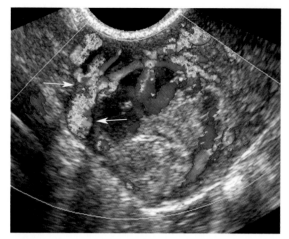

FIGURE 32-13 This cornual pregnancy was identified on the basis of increased color flow signals *(arrows)* in the absence of a sac or significant mass.

Absence of placental flow in a pseudogestational sac

Detection of placental flow in the adnexa when the gray-scale findings are not diagnostic or no mass is identified

Identification of retained products of conception following delivery or after therapeutic abortion

Assessment of therapeutic efficacy following methotrexate or laparoscopic surgery

RETAINED GESTATIONAL TISSUE

Identification of placental flow is also useful in the diagnosis of retained products of conception and gestational trophoblastic neoplasia. We use color and pulsed Doppler to assess for retained placental tissue after spontaneous miscarriage or therapeutic abortion and in patients following delivery (Figure 32-14). Retained products may be suspected clinically due to persistent vaginal bleeding or elevated hCG titer. Color Doppler is able to demonstrate foci of placental tissue, even in the absence of an appreciable soft tissue endometrial mass or fluid collection (Figure 32-15). Pulsed Doppler sampling in the region of increased color flow reveals peak systolic velocity measurements greater than 21 cm/sec, consistent with retained placental tissue. Conversely, the absence of placental flow in an endometrial mass suggests retained clot. Dillon and co-workers[13] reported that persistent high-velocity, low-resistance flow was noted in half of patients studied after therapeutic abortion. This increased vascularity spontaneously resolved over the next

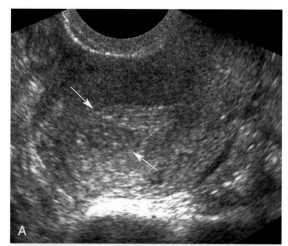

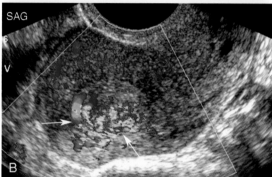

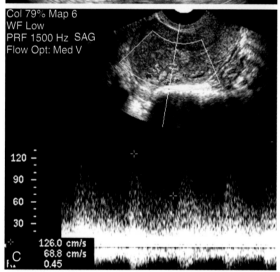

FIGURE 32-14 A, Endovaginal scan reveals a thickened, heterogeneous endometrium *(arrows)* in this patient following incomplete abortion. **B,** Color Doppler shows markedly increased vascularity *(arrows)* in the region of endometrial thickening suggestive of retained products of conception. **C,** Pulsed Doppler demonstrates high-velocity (126 cm/sec), low-resistance (resistivity index = 0.45) flow consistent with placental flow and retained products of conception.

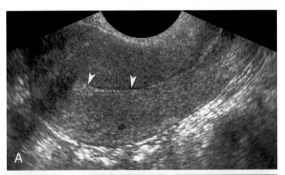

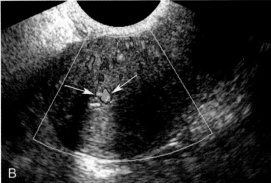

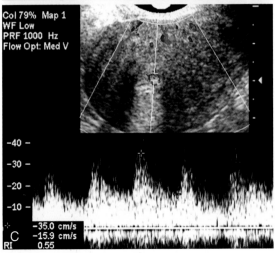

FIGURE 32-15 **A,** This patient presented with persistent vaginal bleeding after delivery. Endovaginal scan reveals no evidence of endometrial thickening or mass *(arrowheads).* **B,** Color Doppler demonstrates a focus of increased vascularity in the endometrium *(arrows)* consistent with retained products of conception. **C,** Pulsed Doppler confirms the presence of placental flow (peak systolic velocity = 35 cm/sec) within the area of abnormal vascularity. Subsequent dilatation and curettage revealed products of conception.

few days. This is a pitfall for retained placental tissue, and treatment decisions in the first week after therapeutic abortion or dilatation and curettage should be based on clinical factors and not Doppler findings.

GESTATIONAL TROPHOBLASTIC DISEASE

Gestational trophoblastic disease, or molar disease, is an uncommon complication of pregnancy. The clinical and sonographic presentations are variable. Typically, patients present in early pregnancy with symptoms and signs of threatened abortion, and with elevated serum hCG levels, usually greater than 100,000 mIU/mL.[21] Sonographic examination of the uterus demonstrates an echogenic mass, which may appear complex. The molar tissue is usually extremely vascular and easily seen with color and power Doppler. Moles demonstrate multiple arteriovenous shunts with high-velocity, low-resistance blood flow. The detection of increased color flow is helpful when small amounts of tissue are noted on the grayscale image. Myometrial invasion of molar tissue can also be identified by the presence of abnormal color flow extending into the myometrium.

OVARIAN TORSION

Ovarian torsion represents approximately 3% of gynecologic emergencies.[22] Thus, ovarian torsion occurs less commonly than other gynecologic problems. The differential diagnosis includes other etiologies of acute pelvic pain, including ruptured ovarian cyst, pelvic inflammatory disease, appendicitis, renal colic, or bowel obstruction.[23] Duplex and color Doppler evaluation is the best noninvasive modality for the evaluation of ovarian torsion. Immediate diagnosis and surgical intervention are required to avoid irreversible ovarian injury.

Torsion occurs more commonly in premenopausal patients and is related to partial or complete twisting of the vascular pedicle, usually due to ovarian or adnexal mass or swelling. The mass may be an ovarian or broad ligament cyst or neoplasm. The mass or broad ligament serves as the fulcrum for the torsion. Less commonly, torsion may be related to displacement or compression by a pelvic mass or enlarged uterus. Torsion occurs more commonly on the right side, which may be related to increased space and absence of the sigmoid colon. A hypermobile adnexa or abnormal attachment may also predispose to torsion. There is also increased incidence of torsion with pregnancy.[24-25] Unexplained pelvic pain in the setting of an abnormal ovary should put ovarian torsion near the top of the differential diagnosis.

Most patients with torsion present with ovarian enlargement or ovarian mass, which serves as the focal point for torsion. Typical sonographic findings include an enlarged ovary or adnexal mass, which may be cystic, complex, or solid.[24] The ovary may be edematous and associated with free fluid. An enlarged ovary in an unusual location, including the midline above the uterus, flank, or in the cul-de-sac, should raise suspicion for torsion.

The diagnosis of ovarian torsion relies on the failure to detect arterial and venous flow within the ovarian parenchyma (Figure 32-16).[23,24,26-28] The absence of flow within the torsed ovary during color flow, power, and pulsed Doppler is diagnostic.

Color Doppler may also demonstrate a coiling or twisting of the vascular pedicle (Figure 32-17).[29] The "whirlpool sign" was described as the definitive sign of ovarian torsion on Doppler imaging.[30] Absent or reversed diastolic flow in the ovarian vessels or within the ovarian parenchyma also suggests torsion. Other abnormal flow patterns are associated with ovarian torsion. Detection of arterial flow without venous flow was noted in 50% of cases of proven torsion in one study.[31] A nonpulsatile, low-velocity venous-like pattern may occur that likely represents subtotal vascular occlusion with blunted, monophasic arterial flow signals (Figure 32-18). Rarely, normal ovarian flow has also been detected in ovarian torsion.

There are important pitfalls to the diagnosis of ovarian torsion. Arterial signals may be detected from within the ovary when there is partial, or less than 360-degree, twisting of the vascular pedicle. This may be related in part to the dual arterial supply to the ovaries. Lack of intraovarian venous signals or damped arterial waveforms detected during pulsed Doppler interrogation should increase suspicion for partial or incomplete torsion. The patient with "missed" or chronic torsion may present with absent internal vascularity and flow around the periphery of the ovary. The peripheral vascularity is related to reactive inflammation and scarring, similar to the "halo sign" associated with testicular torsion. The patient with intermittent torsion may present with episodic pain. Doppler examination may reveal increased hyperemic flow during periods of detorsion. The patient's pain is typically relieved following detorsion. All color flow parameters must be optimized to ensure that the absence of flow is not related to technical factors, including high PRF, high wall filter, or low color gain settings. Power Doppler is very helpful to demonstrate low-velocity flow in

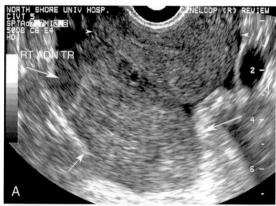

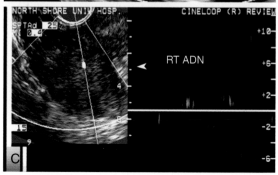

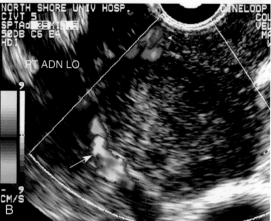

FIGURE 32-16 A, Endovaginal scan demonstrates a large right adnexal mass *(arrows)* behind the uterus *(arrowheads)* in this patient with acute pelvic pain. **B,** Color Doppler demonstrates flow in the adjacent right iliac artery *(arrow)* and parametrial vessels *(arrowhead)* but no flow in the right adnexal mass. **C,** Pulsed Doppler confirms the absence of flow in the right adnexal mass. Surgical exploration identified right ovarian torsion.

the ovary when flow is not appreciated with color Doppler imaging.

Ovarian torsion remains a challenging diagnosis, and close correlation between clinical examination and Doppler findings is usually required. Clinical signs and symptoms associated with ovarian torsion include the following, in order of frequency: abdominal pain, ovarian enlargement,

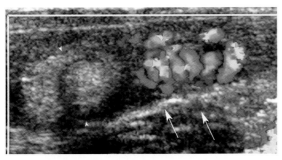

FIGURE 32-17 Color Doppler shows coiling or twisting of the vascular pedicle *(arrows)* in this patient with proven ovarian torsion. Note the absence of color flow in the ovary *(arrowheads)*.

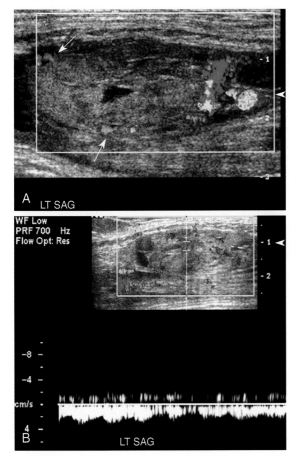

FIGURE 32-18 **A,** This patient presented with left adnexal pain. Endovaginal color flow Doppler imaging demonstrates an enlarged heterogeneous ovary with scattered internal blood vessels *(arrows)*. **B,** Spectral Doppler reveals nonpulsatile low-velocity waveforms suggestive of partial ovarian torsion, proven at laparoscopy.

vomiting, absence of ovarian venous flow, and leukocytosis.[31] An enlarged ovary with clinical signs should suggest ovarian torsion, even when flow is present. An ovary located in an unusual location, such as in the cul-de-sac or at the uterine fundus, should also raise suspicion for ovarian torsion.

CHARACTERIZATION OF ADNEXAL MASSES

Ultrasound is utilized to detect neovascularity associated with malignant tumors.[32] Color Doppler demonstrates clusters of small abnormal tumor vessels within malignant masses and assists in placement of the sample volume for pulsed Doppler examination. Pulsed Doppler typically demonstrates high-velocity, low-resistance flow within cancers. These flow patterns are related to increased flow through tumor vessels, arteriovenous shunting, and absence of muscular media in the walls of tumor vessels. Power Doppler appears to improve visualization of malignant vascularity compared with conventional color flow imaging. Doppler techniques have proven valuable in the evaluation of cancers of the breast, kidney, liver, and prostate gland.

Color and pulsed Doppler is also used to characterize adnexal masses (Figure 32-19).[33-38] Spectral tracings from ovarian cancer demonstrate high-velocity and/or low-impedance monophasic waveforms with no diastolic notch. Although color Doppler can demonstrate malignant neovascularity associated with ovarian cancers, there is considerable overlap between benign and malignant Doppler signals.[39,40] Apart from ovarian cancer, corpus luteal cysts, fibroids, endometriomas, abscesses, and other benign tumors can have similar low-impedance signals. The similarities in blood flow patterns between these entities limits the value of Doppler in their characterization.

Before Doppler evaluation, gray-scale morphologic findings were used to identify ovarian cancer. Thick cyst walls, complex masses, mural nodules, and septations more than 2 mm in thickness are associated with malignancy.[41] Like the Doppler findings, these features are nonspecific and overlap with benign lesions. Studies[42-45] have shown that a combination of morphologic and Doppler features increases specificity for the diagnosis of ovarian cancer. Scoring systems have been devised to assist in the recognition and characterization of ovarian cancer. In a study of 172 adnexal masses, my colleagues and I[44] showed that a scoring system consisting of elevated ovarian volume, abnormal morphologic features, and the detection of high-velocity, low-impedance flow in the abnormal solid components demonstrated a sensitivity of 95% and specificity of

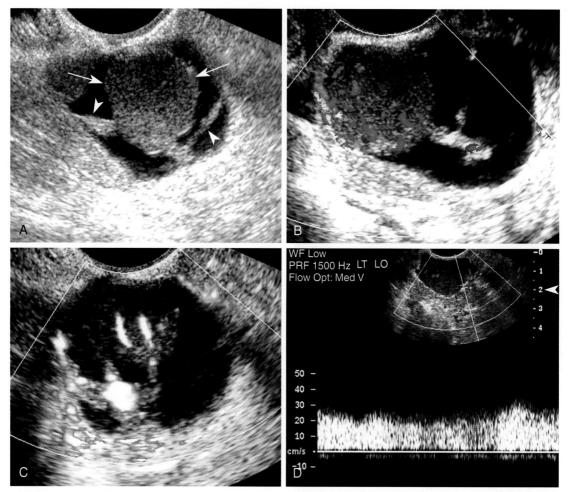

FIGURE 32-19 A, Endovaginal scan demonstrates a complex adnexal mass with a central solid component *(arrows)* and septations *(arrowheads)* in this postmenopausal patient. **B,** Color Doppler reveals flow in the central component and septation, suggestive of malignancy. **C,** Power Doppler demonstrates increased flow throughout all the solid components of the adnexal mass. **D,** Pulsed Doppler reveals high-velocity, low-resistance signals consistent with malignant vascularity in this ovarian cancer.

92% for the detection of ovarian cancer. Brown and associates[43] reviewed 211 pelvic masses and demonstrated a sensitivity and specificity of 93% for a combination of gray-scale and Doppler parameters. Their scoring system included the presence of nonhyperechoic solid components, free fluid, absent or thick septations, and central location of blood flow. Both studies concluded that the identification of abnormal tumor vascularity within the complex and solid components of ovarian tumors has proven useful in the diagnosis of malignancy.

These Doppler findings are particularly useful in postmenopausal patients with adnexal masses. Normal postmenopausal ovaries are typically quiescent and small, with low-velocity (<20 cm/sec), high-resistance (resistivity index

≥ 0.7) flow. Confusion with corpus luteal cysts, endometriosis, and pelvic inflammatory disease should not occur in this age-group. The presence of an adnexal mass with high-velocity, low-impedance signals raises considerable suspicion for carcinoma in an older adult patient.

Recent studies have shown that contrast-enhanced ultrasound examinations can distinguish ovarian cancers from benign lesions by their enhancement patterns.[46] Malignant masses have greater peak enhancement, longer washout time, and increased vascular volume than benign masses.

UTERINE ABNORMALITIES

Color Doppler also plays a role in the evaluation of uterine pathology. Through the demonstration of increased vascularity, color Doppler may improve the definition of fibroids and endometrial polyps. Fibroids may be highly vascular, and the vascularity is typically identified along the periphery of the mass. Spectral analysis may reveal high-velocity, low-resistance flow, similar to tumor signals seen in ovarian cancer. This is a significant pitfall for the misdiagnosis of ovarian cancer when there is an adnexal mass (subserosal fibroid) and the normal ispsilateral ovary is not identified with certainty.

Color Doppler is especially helpful for confirming that a solid adnexal mass is a subserosal fibroid. We look for the vascular pedicle attachment between the fibroid and the uterine body to confirm the nature of the mass (Figure 32-20). Correlation with magnetic resonance imaging is helpful for difficult cases, when the uterine attachment is not well visualized. Color Doppler may also play a role in the evaluation of fibroid vascularity following uterine artery embolization. We also utilize Doppler in the emergency setting to evaluate for fibroid degeneration in the setting of pelvic pain. The absence of flow in an uterine mass that is tender on examination can confirm fibroid degeneration.

Uterine polyps may present as focal endometrial thickening or a mass. Identification of a feeding vessel assists in the characterization of focal endometrial lesions as polyps (Figure 32-21). Sonohysterography improves the visualization of endometrial polyps and determines the size and number of endometrial lesions.

The value of color and pulsed Doppler in the evaluation of endometrial carcinoma is controversial.[47,48] Color Doppler imaging may be utilized to display abnormal vascularity associated with endometrial thickening. Low-impedance blood flow identified within a thickened endometrium during pulsed Doppler examination has been noted with endometrial carcinoma.[49] As is the case with adnexal masses, there is considerable overlap between the Doppler appearances of benign and malignant conditions. Low-resistance signals are also associated with endometrial hyperplasia, polyps, submucosal fibroids, adenomyosis, endometritis, molar disease, and placental tissue. Doppler studies may aid in the determination of the extent of tumor invasion and guide biopsy to regions of increased blood flow.[50]

We have had success with the identification of enlarged, tortuous parauterine vessels in patients with the pelvic congestion syndrome. Patients with this syndrome may present with complaints

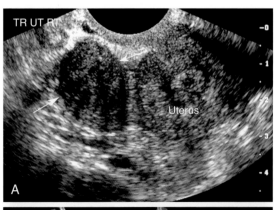

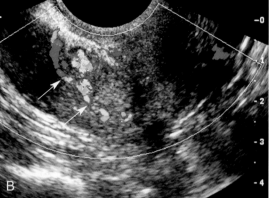

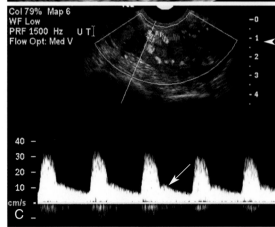

FIGURE 32-20 **A,** A solid hypoechoic mass *(arrows)* is identified adjacent to the uterus in this patient with pelvic pain. **B,** Color Doppler demonstrates the vascular pedicle *(arrows)* to this subserosal fibroid. **C,** Pulsed Doppler interrogation of the vascular pedicle reveals characteristic uterine artery waveforms with the diastolic notch *(arrow).*

of nonspecific, chronic pelvic pain. Patients are usually premenopausal and multiparous with a history of pelvic pain for at least 6 months. Findings associated with pelvic congestion syndrome include enlarged pelvic varices greater than 5 mm in diameter, dilated left ovarian vein greater than 5 mm in diameter, dilated uterine arcuate veins,

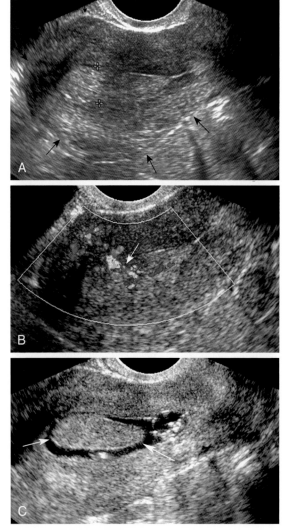

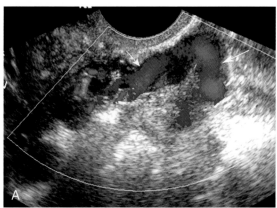

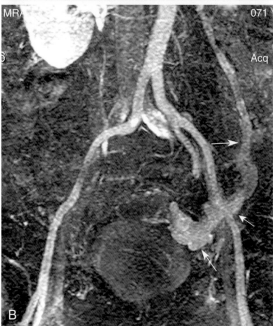

FIGURE 32-21 **A,** Endovaginal scan reveals endometrial thickening *(cursors)* within the uterus *(arrows)* in this patient with irregular vaginal bleeding. **B,** Color Doppler demonstrates a feeding vessel *(arrow)* to the region of endometrial thickening consistent with a polyp. **C,** Sonohysterography confirms the presence of an endometrial polyp *(arrows)*.

FIGURE 32-22 **A,** Color Doppler reveals large left parametrial venous varices *(arrows)* in this patient with chronic pelvic pain. **B,** Delayed three-dimensional magnetic resonance venography reveals large left venous varices *(arrows)* consistent with pelvic congestion syndrome.

polycystic changes in the ovaries, and reversal of flow in the dilated veins with the Valsalva maneuver.[51] Large venous varices are well visualized with endovaginal color Doppler imaging (Figure 32-22). Magnetic resonance imaging is also utilized to assess for evidence of enlarged vessels, abdominal or pelvic mass, or venous thrombosis.

Uncommon vascular lesions, including uterine vascular malformations, are also identified with color Doppler. Uterine arteriovenous malformations may appear as focal areas of uterine heterogeneity or a cystic, complex, or tubular mass, with or without prominent parametrial vessels on gray-scale imaging. Color Doppler will demonstrate increased vascularity in the region of the arteriovenous malformation.[52] Pulsed Doppler will reveal high-velocity, low-resistance arterial signals consistent with arteriovenous shunting (Figure 32-23).

CONCLUSIONS

Multiple useful applications of color and pulsed Doppler are described for the evaluation of female pelvic disorders, and Doppler is currently

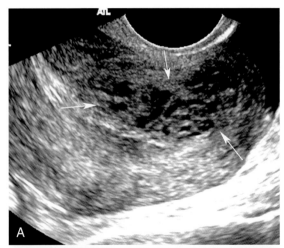

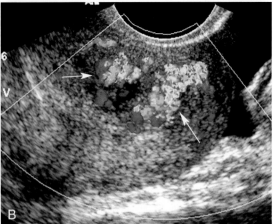

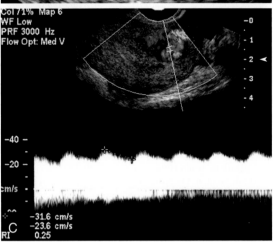

FIGURE 32-23 **A,** Endovaginal scan shows a complex region with cystic spaces *(arrows)* in the uterus in this postpartum patient with pelvic pain. **B,** Color Doppler demonstrates tremendous vascularity in this region with turbulent flow *(arrows).* **C,** Pulsed Doppler waveforms show marked low-resistance arterial flow consistent with an arteriovenous shunt pattern. This was confirmed at arteriography with subsequent embolization.

a routine component of obstetric and gynecologic sonography. Attention to technique and understanding of color flow parameters is key to maximum sensitivity. Integration of clinical and sonographic information, as well as recognition of diagnostic pitfalls, improves diagnostic accuracy and reduces misinterpretation.

Acknowledgments. I would like to recognize Kenneth J.W. Taylor, MD, for his dedication, innovations, and outstanding contributions to the field of pelvic Doppler.

REFERENCES

1. Taylor KJ, et al: Doppler color imaging. Obstetric and gynecologic applications, *Clin Diagn Ultrasound* 27:195–223, 1992.
2. Pellerito JS, Taylor KJW, Case CQ: Current applications of endovaginal color flow imaging, *Radiology* 193(P):395, 1994.
3. Pellerito JS, et al: Common pitfalls of endovaginal color flow imaging, *Radiographics* 15:37–47, 1995.
4. Rubin JM, et al: Power Doppler US: A potentially useful alternative to mean frequency-based color Doppler US, *Radiology* 190:853–856, 1994.
5. Taylor KJ, Burns PN, Wells PNT: Ultrasound Doppler flow studies of the ovarian and uterine arteries, *Br J Obstet Gynaecol* 92:240–246, 1985.
6. Hata K, et al: Change in ovarian arterial compliance during the human menstrual cycle assessed by Doppler ultrasound, *Br J Obstet Gynaecol* 97:163, 1990.
7. D'Agostino C, Pellerito JS: Color and pulsed Doppler imaging of the pelvic vasculature and pelvic organs, *J Vasc Tech* 19(5–6):331–335, 1995.
8. Parsons AK: Imaging the human corpus luteum, *J Ultrasound Med* 20:811–819, 2001.
9. Pellerito JS, et al: Ectopic pregnancy: evaluation with endovaginal color flow imaging, *Radiology* 183:407–411, 1992.
10. Taylor KJ, et al: Ectopic pregnancy: duplex Doppler evaluation, *Radiology* 173:93–97, 1989.
11. Atri M: Ectopic pregnancy versus corpus luteal cyst revisited: best Doppler predictors, *J Ultrasound Med* 22:1181–1184, 2003.
12. Pellerito JS: Acute pelvic pain. In Benson CB, Arger PH, Bluth EI, editors: *Ultrasonography in obstetrics and gynecology: a practical approach,* New York, 2000, Thieme Publishers, pp 10–19.
13. Dillon EH, et al: Endovaginal pulsed and color flow Doppler in first trimester pregnancy, *Ultrasound Med Biol* 19:517–525, 1993.
14. NCHS: *Advanced report of final mortality statistics, 1992* Report No. 43(Suppl), Hyattsville, MD, 1994, U.S. Department of Health and Human Services, Public Health Service, CDC.
15. Levine D: Ectopic pregnancy. In Callen PW, editor: *Ultrasonography in obstetrics and gynecology,* ed 4, Philadelphia, 2000, WB Saunders, pp 912–934.
16. Schwartz R, Di Pietro DL: B-hCG as a diagnostic aid for suspected ectopic pregnancy, *Obstet Gynecol* 56:197, 1980.

17. Dillon EH, Feyock AL, Taylor KJW: Pseudogestational sacs: Doppler US differentiation from normal or abnormal intrauterine pregnancies, *Radiology* 176:359–364, 1990.

18. Chow TT, Lindahl S: Ectopic pregnancy, *J Clin Ultrasound* 7:217–218, 1979.

19. Frates MC, Visweswaran A, Laing FC: Comparison of tubal ring and corpus luteum echogenicities: a useful differentiating characteristic, *J. Ultrasound Med* 20:27–31, 2001.

20. Stein MW, et al: Sonographic comparison of the tubal ring of ectopic pregnancy with the corpus luteum, *J Ultrasound Med* 23:57–62, 2004.

21. Taylor KJW, Schwartz PE, Kohorn EI: Gestational trophoblastic neoplasia: diagnosis with Doppler US, *Radiology* 165:445–448, 1987.

22. Hibbard LT: Adnexal torsion, *Am J Obstet Gynecol* 152:456–461, 1985.

23. Albayram F, Hamper UM: Ovarian and adnexal torsion. Spectrum of sonographic findings with pathologic correlation, *J Ultrasound Med* 20:1083–1089, 2001.

24. Pena JE, et al: Usefulness of Doppler sonography in the diagnosis of ovarian torsion, *Fertil Steril* 73:1047–1050, 2000.

25. Bider D, et al: Clinical, surgical and pathologic findings of adnexal torsion in pregnant and nonpregnant women [review], *Surg Gynecol Obstet* 173:363–366, 1991.

26. Halvie MA, Silver TM: Ovarian torsion: Sonographic evaluation, *J Clin Ultrasound* 17:327–332, 1989.

27. Rosado WM Jr, et al: Adnexal torsion: Diagnosis by using Doppler sonography, *AJR Am J Roentgenol* 159:1251–1253, 1992.

28. Fleischer AC, et al: Color Doppler sonography of adnexal torsion, *J Ultrasound Med* 14:523–528, 1995.

29. Lee EJ, et al: Diagnosis of ovarian torsion with color Doppler sonography: depiction of twisted vascular pedicle, *J Ultrasound Med* 17:83–89, 1998.

30. Boopathy Vijayaraghavan S: Sonographic whirlpool sign in ovarian torsion, *J Ultrasound Med* 23:1643–1649, 2004.

31. Shadinger LL, et al: Preoperative sonographic and clinical characteristics as predictors of ovarian torsion, *J Ultrasound Med* 27:7–13, 2008.

32. Taylor KJ, et al: Correlation of Doppler US tumor signals with neovascular morphologic features, *Radiology* 166:57–62, 1988.

33. Fleischer AC, et al: Assessment of ovarian tumor vascularity with transvaginal color Doppler sonography, *J Ultrasound Med* 10:295–297, 1991.

34. Weiner Z, et al: Differentiating malignant from benign ovarian tumors with transvaginal color flow imaging, *Obstet Gynecol* 79:159, 1992.

35. Fleischer AC, et al: Color Doppler sonography of ovarian masses: a multiparameter analysis, *J Ultrasound Med* 12:41, 1993.

36. Brown DL, et al: Ovarian masses: can benign and malignant lesions be differentiated with color Doppler US? *Radiology* 190:333, 1994.

37. Pellerito JS, et al: Endovaginal color flow imaging of palpable adnexal masses, *J Ultrasound Med* 12:559, 1993.

38. Jain KA: Prospective evaluation of adnexal masses with endovaginal gray-scale and duplex and color Doppler US: correlation with pathologic findings, *Radiology* 191:63, 1994.

39. Hamper UM, et al: Transvaginal color Doppler sonography of adnexal masses: differences in blood flow impedance in benign and malignant lesions, *AJR Am J Roentgenol* 160:1225–1228, 1993.

40. Levine D, et al: Sonography of ovarian masses: poor sensitivity of resistive index for identifying malignant lesions, *AJR Am J Roentgenol* 162:1355, 1994.

41. Lerner JP, et al: Transvaginal ultrasonographic characterization of ovarian masses with an improved, weighted scoring system, *Am J Obstet Gynecol* 170:81–85, 1994.

42. Kurjak A, Predanic M: New scoring system for prediction for ovarian malignancy based on transvaginal color Doppler sonography, *J Ultrasound Med* 11:631, 1992.

43. Brown DL, et al: Benign and malignant ovarian masses: Selection of the most discriminating gray-scale and Doppler sonographic features, *Radiology* 208:103–110, 1998.

44. Pellerito JS, et al: Endovaginal color flow scoring system: a sensitive indicator of pelvic malignancy, *Radiology* 193(P):276, 1994.

45. Taylor KJW, Schwartz PE: Screening for early ovarian cancer, *Radiology* 192:1–10, 1994.

46. Fleischer AC, et al: Advances in sonographic detection of ovarian cancer: depiction of tumor neovascularity with microbubbles, *AJR Am J Roentgenol* 194:343–348, 2010.

47. Bourne TH, et al: Detection of endometrial cancer in postmenopausal women by ultrasonography and color flow imaging, *BMJ* 301:369, 1990.

48. Nalaboff KM, Pellerito JS, Ben-Levi E: Imaging the endometrium: disease and normal variants, *Radiographics* 21:1409–1424, 2001.

49. Bourne TH, et al: Detection of endometrial cancer by transvaginal ultrasonography with color flow imaging and blood flow analysis: a preliminary report, *Gynecol Oncol* 40:253–259, 1991.

50. Fleischer AC: Sonographic assessment of endometrial disorders, *Semin Ultrasound CT MR* 20:259–266, 1999.

51. Park SJ, et al: Diagnosis of pelvic congestion syndrome using transabdominal and transvaginal sonography, *AJR Am J Roentgenol* 182(3):683–688, 2004.

52. Polat P, et al: Color Doppler US in the evaluation of uterine vascular abnormalities, *Radiographics* 22:47–53, 2002.

DUPLEX ULTRASOUND EVALUATION OF THE MALE GENITALIA

33

CAROL B. BENSON, MD

This chapter has two components; the first considers duplex ultrasound assessment of the scrotal contents, and the second describes the role that ultrasound and Doppler play in the diagnosis of erectile dysfunction. In both sections, emphasis is given to color Doppler imaging and Doppler waveform analysis, in keeping with the focus of the text.

THE SCROTUM

ANATOMY AND NORMAL SONOGRAPIC FEATURES

The anatomy of the scrotum, testis, and epididymis is illustrated in Figures 33-1 and 33-2. As seen with ultrasound, the normal testis is homogeneous and medium in echogenicity (Figure 33-3), with a smooth outer border but no visible capsule.[1-9] In adults, each testis measures 3 to 5 cm in long axis and 2 to 3 cm in short axis. The testes are relatively hypoechoic before the age of puberty and increase in echogenicity with adulthood . The mediastinum testis is seen regularly as a strongly echogenic band running along one side of the testis. The epididymis is similar to or slightly less echogenic than the testis. Its echotexture may be somewhat heterogeneous.

The arterial and venous anatomy of the testes is illustrated in Figures 33-4 and 33-5. In postpubertal boys and adults, blood vessels[4-7,10,11] are normally visible in and about the testis with color flow sonography (Figure 33-6). The capsular arteries, which course around the periphery, and the centripetal arteries, which penetrate the parenchyma, are commonly seen. Blood flow in the centripetal arteries is from the capsule inward. Testicular veins follow the same pattern as the arteries and generally are readily visualized. Differentiation between arteries and veins is possible only with spectral Doppler. In some normal individuals, one or more large artery/vein pair(s) may traverse the testis obliquely from the mediastinum to the opposite capsule.[4,5] These "transmediastinal" vessels may be visible on gray-scale imaging and should not be mistaken for pathology.

Arterial blood flow in the testis and epididymis characteristically exhibits a low-resistance pattern on Doppler spectral waveforms, including continuous flow during diastole (Figure 33-7). In contrast, a high-resistance flow pattern is seen in extragonadal arteries, which are part of the cremasteric system. These arteries are occasionally visualized along the course of the spermatic cord. It is important not to mistake extragonadal flow signals for testicular flow. Peak systolic velocity in testicular arteries ranges from 4 cm/sec to 19 cm/sec (mean, 9.7 cm/sec), and end-diastolic velocity, from 1.6 cm/sec to 6.9 cm/sec (mean, 3.6 cm/sec).[11] These values permit quantitative assessment of arterial flow when a sufficiently long arterial segment is visualized with color flow, allowing for angle correction of the Doppler signal. When angle correction is not possible, spectral Doppler features are evaluated qualitatively.

SONOGRAPHIC TECHNIQUE

A linear array transducer with a frequency output of 7 MHz or higher is used to examine the testes, unless the scrotum is severely swollen and lower frequencies are required to achieve sufficient penetration of the ultrasound beam. A towel is draped over the penis for the sake of modesty and to keep it against the abdomen and out of the way of the testicular scan. For best results, place a towel across the patient's legs to prop up and support the scrotum.

The first step in scanning the scrotal contents is to get oriented. Long- and short-axis images of each testis and epididymis, including long- and short-axis testis dimensions, should be recorded. A composite transverse view showing both testicles

559

simultaneously is also obtained, as this view is essential for comparing testicular echogenicity and testicular vascularity. If both testes cannot be viewed simultaneously on a transverse view, separate images should be recorded side by side, using identical ultrasound settings. When pathologic findings are present, they should be portrayed in whatever image plane best documents the abnormality, but long- and short-axis views should be used whenever possible as an aid to orientation.

The color flow examination may be conducted with color Doppler or power Doppler. In either case, the pulse repetition frequency must be set to detect very low velocity flow and the wall filter

must be low. Relatively high color gain settings typically are needed, as the testicular vessels are quite small and produce weak Doppler signals. One method to improve visualization of flow is to increase the color gain until color artifacts appear in the image and then slightly decrease the color gain setting to reduce these artifacts. It is important to make the Doppler spectral waveforms appear large on the images by using an appropriate spectral display scale. If the waveforms are small, it is difficult to assess pulsatility patterns and compare testicular flow from one side to the other.

SCROTAL MASSES

Masses and mass-like lesions of the scrotal contents may be caused by cysts, tumors, hematomas, inflammation, and abscesses. The location of the pathology, the gray-scale appearance, and the Doppler flow features are diagnostic in many cases.

Testicular Cysts

Cysts of the testis* are idiopathic and benign. They also are fairly common, seen with increasing frequency with increasing age and present in approximately 8% of adults at sonography. Most intratesticular cysts are located near the mediastinum testis and are not palpable. They are typically small, measuring less than 1 cm in diameter,

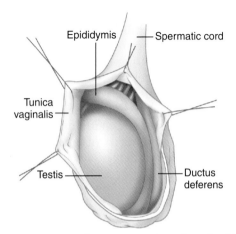

FIGURE 33-1 Scrotal anatomy. Each testis and epididymis is suspended in a sac lined by the tunica vaginalis.

_____

*References 1,2,6,7,9,12.

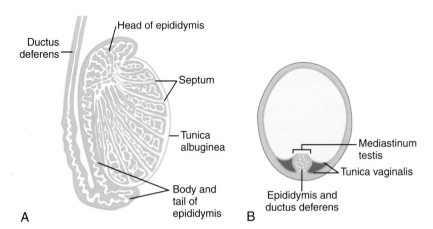

FIGURE 33-2 Testicular anatomy. **A,** The testis is encapsulated by a tough fibrous layer called the tunica albuginea and is divided into chambers by fibrous septa that are not visible with ultrasound. Myriad seminiferous tubules converge at the head of the epididymis, where they coalesce to form a single, but highly convoluted, tube that ultimately becomes the ductus deferens. For descriptive purposes, the epididymis is divided into the head (located superiorly), the body, and the tail (located inferiorly). **B,** The tunica vaginalis is a thin tissue layer that envelops the testis and epididymis and lines the scrotal sac, forming the mediastinum testis. The arrangement is analogous to the chest, where the pleura envelops the lungs, lines the chest cavity, and encloses the mediastinum of the thorax.

and are thought to arise from the rete testes, the convergence of intratesticular tubules at the mediastinum. These cysts may be single or multiple. Sometimes, in the presence or absence of discrete cysts, a region of dilated tubules is seen in the vicinity of the mediastinum, representing a

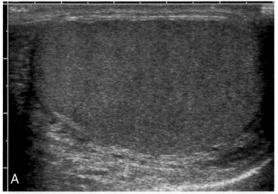

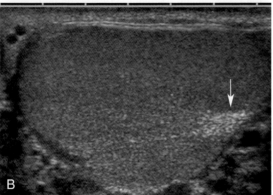

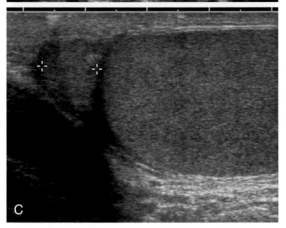

FIGURE 33-3 Normal sonography of the testes and epididymis. **A,** This longitudinal view of a normal testis demonstrates homogeneous texture and medium-level echogenicity. **B,** On this transverse image, the mediastinum testis is visible as a more echogenic region *(arrow)* on one side of the testis. **C,** Longitudinal views show the head of the epididymis *(cursors)* capping the superior pole of the testis.

dilated rete testis.[13] Cysts located on the testicular surface are almost always tunical cysts, arising in the tunica albuginea, the fibrous layer that encapsulates the testis. Tunical cysts may be palpable, prompting ultrasound investigation.

The most important point about testicular cysts and a dilated rete testis is distinguishing these benign lesions from other pathologies, including tumors and abscesses. Testicular cysts (Figure 33-8) have the following sonographic features: (1) anechoic contents, (2) sharply defined borders and invisible wall, (3) enhanced through-transmission of ultrasound, and (4) no blood flow within or surrounding the cyst (other than normal testicular vessels). Cysts meeting these criteria are benign and inconsequential and require no follow-up. A dilated rete testis appears as small serpiginous tubular structures clustered in the mediastinum (Figure 33-9).

Testicular Neoplasms

Testicular neoplasms are most often primary testicular tumors of germ cell origin (Table 33-1).[1,2,14] These neoplasms occur most frequently between the ages of 25 and 35 years and almost always are malignant. The prognosis generally is excellent, however, and 5-year survival is 95%, overall, assuming timely treatment with surgery, radiation therapy, and/or chemotherapy.[15] Less common testicular neoplasms arise from the stromal parenchyma and are either Sertoli or Leydig cell tumors. Rarely, nontesticular malignancies involve the testicle, including leukemia and lymphoma and metastatic disease. Testicular tumors usually present in one of two ways: as a palpable mass or with sudden pain and swelling due to hemorrhage. It is not uncommon for the latter presentation to

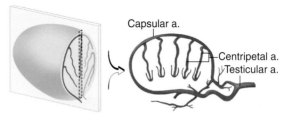

FIGURE 33-4 Vascular anatomy of the testis. The testicular (or spermatic) artery follows the course of the epididymal body through the mediastinum testis and gives off "capsular" branches that circle the periphery of the testis, beneath the tunica albuginea. The capsular arteries give off centripetal arteries that course through the testis toward the mediastinum and then loop back for a short distance as the recurrent rami. The venous drainage (not shown) parallels the arterial distribution. a., artery.

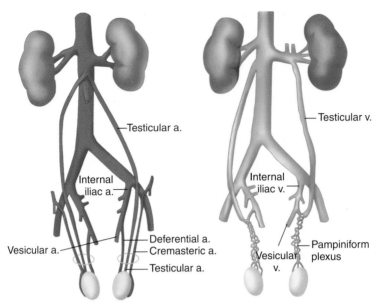

FIGURE 33-5 Arterial supply and venous drainage of the scrotal contents. Each testicular artery arises from the aorta and extends directly to the testicle and epididymis, following the course of the spermatic cord and the body of the epididymis. Structures other than the testis and epididymis receive arterial flow via the cremasteric and deferential branches, which originate from the internal iliac arteries, as shown. Although the testicular arteries provide the principal arterial supply to the testis and epididymis, anastomotic channels exist among all of the scrotal arteries, permitting collateral flow. The venous drainage of each testis and epididymis is via a network of tiny veins called the pampiniform plexus. This network gradually coalesces to form two or three veins that follow the spermatic cord and unite as the testicular (spermatic) vein. On the left, the spermatic vein drains into the ipsilateral renal vein, and on the right, the spermatic vein drains into the inferior vena cava. a., artery; v., vein.

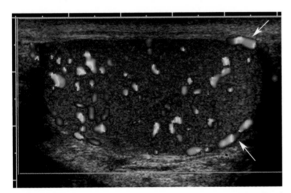

FIGURE 33-6 Normal testicular vessels. Longitudinal image shows the capsular artery *(arrows)* and intraparenchymal vessels with color Doppler.

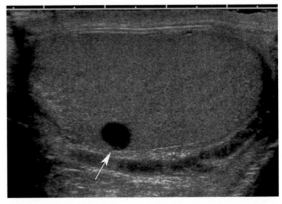

FIGURE 33-8 Testicular cyst. This long-axis image shows a testicular cyst *(arrow).*

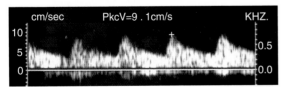

FIGURE 33-7 Low-resistance Doppler waveforms of normal testicular and epididymal flow. PkcV, peak systolic velocity.

follow minor trauma. Tumors may also present with symptoms of epididymitis. A small number of patients present with signs and symptoms resulting from metastatic testicular cancer, such as back pain from retroperitoneal disease.

Ultrasound can distinguish intratesticular from extratesticular pathology with extremely high accuracy.[1] Nevertheless, ultrasound generally cannot differentiate among histologic types of testicular

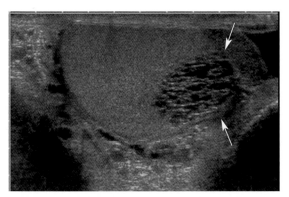

FIGURE 33-9 Dilated rete testis. In the mediastinum of the testis are dilated, serpiginous tubular structures *(arrows)* representing the dilated rete testis.

TABLE 33-1 **Classification of Testicular Malignant Neoplasms**
Testicular malignancies of germ cell origin (95%)
Seminoma
Embryonal cell carcinoma
Teratocarcinoma
Choriocarcinoma
Mixed germ cell carcinoma
Other primary testicular malignancies
Sertoli cell carcinoma
Leydig cell carcinoma
Metastases
Leukemia
Lymphoma
Genitourinary primaries
Other primaries (e.g., lung)

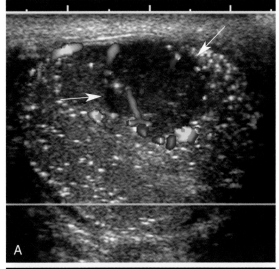

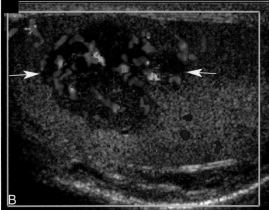

FIGURE 33-10 Seminoma. **A,** Color Doppler sonogram of small testicular seminoma *(arrows)* demonstrating a few blood vessels at the periphery and within the malignant testicular tumor. The punctate, strong reflections are caused by microlithiasis, which has been associated with increased risk for testicular neoplasia. **B,** Color Doppler sonogram of another seminoma demonstrating hypervascularity of the tumor *(arrows)* compared with the surrounding testicular parenchyma.

tumors, nor can it generally differentiate between malignant (common) and benign (uncommon) neoplasms. Most testicular tumors are well-defined hypoechoic intratesticular masses, but some may be poorly marginated or grossly infiltrating.[†] They may exhibit some degree of internal heterogeneity due to hemorrhage and/or necrosis, and calcification is occasionally present. Vascularity is evident within testicular neoplasms on color Doppler images and is a very important feature used to distinguish tumors from avascular structures such as cysts, hematomas, and abscesses. Testicular tumor vascularity (Figure 33-10) is variable; however, most malignant tumors are hypervascular compared to the surrounding normal testicular parenchyma.[4,9-11,14,17,18] The distribution of tumor blood vessels also is variable, with some lesions showing an orderly distribution of blood vessels and others, a chaotic distribution. Large avascular

areas may be present in a testicular tumor, when necrosis or hemorrhage is present. Spectral Doppler generally shows low-resistance flow within tumor vessels, which is typical of malignant neoplasms regardless of location. Flow velocities may be elevated substantially in markedly hypervascular tumors, but flow may be in the normal range in mildly hypervascular lesions or lesions with less flow. In general, the larger the testicular tumor, the more hypervascular it will be.[11]

Testicular microlithiasis, scattered small calcifications in the testicular parenchyma as shown in Figure 33-10, *A,* has been associated with increased

[†]References 1,7,9,11,14,16-18.

risk for testicular cancer in some series, but the level of risk and follow-up requirements remain controversial.[17,19-21]

Testicular Tumor Mimics

Lesions that can mimic the appearance of neoplasms include abscesses, inflamed areas or focal orchitis (without frank abscess formation), contusions, hematomas, and infarcts.[1,7,9,14,22-24] The sonographic appearance of these lesions is nonspecific, as discussed later. Color and spectral Doppler features are of considerable importance in differentiating among these etiologies. Although blood flow is absent within abscesses, infarcts, and hematomas, blood flow signals can be detected at the periphery of abscesses.

Epididymal Cysts

Epididymal cysts[1,2,7,9,14] are much more common than testicular cysts, being found in about 40% of adult males examined sonographically.[1] Most are located in the epididymal head, but cysts may occur anywhere in the epididymis. They may be single, multiple, unilateral, or bilateral. In some cases they are palpable, while in others they are found incidentally. Unlike testicular cysts, epididymal cysts may be septated or even multilocular. Most are 2 to 3 mm in diameter, but larger cysts are also common, and occasionally they may be several centimeters in size. The etiology of epididymal cysts is not entirely clear, although some are spermatoceles, which are encapsulated collections of sperm.

The great majority of epididymal cysts have the same sonographic features as those described previously for testicular cysts, but there are other variations. Some may be septated or multilocular, and others may contain diffuse or dependent low-level echoes (Figure 33-11). When evaluating epididymal cysts sonographically, it is most important to document that benign epididymal cysts have no solid components, have exquisitely thin walls, and show no internal blood flow on color Doppler examination.

Other Epididymal Masses

Other than cysts, the only common mass lesions of the epididymis are hematomas, abscesses, and inflammatory masses.[‡] Tumors of the epididymis are uncommon and usually benign. Their sonographic features are not well described in

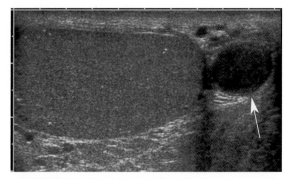

FIGURE 33-11   Complex epididymal tail cyst. Longitudinal image demonstrating a cyst *(arrow)* containing internal echoes within the tail of the epididymis.

the medical literature. An important characteristic, however, is the presence of blood flow within the tumor, which is not present in hematomas or abscesses. Hematomas of the epididymis or spermatic cord usually occur in the context of recognized trauma but may occur spontaneously and in association with vigorous exercise. An epididymal hematoma usually presents as a hard, palpable (and possibly tender) mass that may mimic a neoplastic mass on physical examination. On ultrasound, a hematoma usually has a nonspecific, hypoechoic, or heterogeneous appearance. Most importantly, blood flow is absent in and around the lesion (except for normal vessels) on color flow examination. Abscesses and inflammatory masses are differential considerations and are discussed later.

EPIDIDYMITIS AND ORCHITIS

Infection is the most common cause of acute scrotal pain and tenderness.[14] In the great majority of cases, the infection[§] is caused by sexually transmitted organisms (principally *Neisseria gonorrhoeae* and *Chlamydia trachomatis*) that "ascend" through the genital tract. The tail of the epididymis is infected first, and then the infection spreads throughout the epididymis (epididymitis). The infection may then extend to the testis (orchitis) and finally to the scrotal cavity, generating an infected hydrocele.[9]

Ultrasound is a very useful method for confirming the diagnosis of epididymitis or orchitis and for excluding other pathologies that may cause acute scrotal pain or swelling. The key findings are enlargement and decreased echogenicity of the affected structures, accompanied by

‡References 1,2,8,14,23,24.

§References 2,6,7,9,11,12,18,22,25-27.

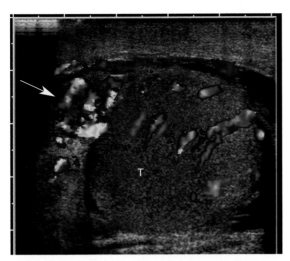

FIGURE 33-12 Epididymo-orchitis. Longitudinal image of testis and epididymis demonstrating hypervascularity of the epididymis *(arrow)* and mildly decreased echogenicity in the upper pole of the testis (T) adjacent to the epididymis.

increased blood flow (hyperemia) on color and spectral Doppler examination[I] (Figure 33-12). Because orchitis may be present by the time the patient seeks care, involvement of both the testis and epididymis may be evident sonographically; however, in some patients, epididymal involvement may predominate. A hydrocele (excess scrotal fluid) often is present, and the scrotal wall may become edematous and/or inflamed. In some cases of epididymitis/orchitis, the ultrasound findings may be dramatic. In other instances, findings are less obvious and are based solely on side-by-side comparison of epididymal size, echogenicity, and blood flow. Obviously, side-by-side comparison is not helpful in cases of symmetrical, bilateral infection; nevertheless, hyperemia of the scrotal contents may still be evident in such cases. It is noteworthy that a focal, hypoechoic area of inflammation may be seen in the periphery of the testis, adjacent to an infected epididymal head.[28] This should not be mistaken for a testicular tumor but should be followed to resolution with antibiotic treatment.

The sonographic diagnosis of epididymo-orchitis generally is straightforward, but mimics occasionally may cause misdiagnoses; namely, hyperemia following detorsion of a testis (considered later) and diffusely infiltrating lymphoma or leukemia.[29,30] The epididymis and testis usually return to a normal sonographic appearance following an episode of infection, but in severe cases, testicular atrophy or infarction may occur. Atrophy is a noteworthy complication of mumps orchitis.

Abscesses may occur in the epididymis or testis in severe cases of scrotal infection. These appear as heterogeneous masses or as fluid collections with irregular walls, sometimes containing diffuse or dependent debris. Increased blood flow due to hyperemia may be apparent in the surrounding tissues, either focally or diffusely. In our experience, testicular abscesses are seen acutely rather than as chronic processes. Epididymal abscesses, however, may be chronic, and, as a result, hyperemia may not be evident, causing a chronic abscess to be indistinguishable from other extratesticular masses.

In unusual cases of acute epididymo-orchitis, infection may spread to the scrotal sac, producing an infected hydrocele. The sonographic manifestation is echogenic debris within the hydrocele fluid, either diffusely or dependently, and possible loculation of the hydrocele. These findings are nonspecific, however, and may also be seen with chronic hydroceles in the absence of active infection. Therefore, infected hydrocele should be suggested only when there are concomitant findings of acute infection in the epididymis and/or testis.

Most cases of epididymo-orchitis are treated successfully and resolve, but untreated or incompletely treated cases may present with findings of chronic epididymitis, which may be manifested as diffuse thickening and heterogeneity of the epididymis or as a focal, heterogeneous epididymal mass. As noted previously, increased blood flow may not be a feature of chronic epididymitis. Hydrocele may also be present and may be loculated or may contain echogenic material.

VARICOCELE

Varicocele, or dilatation of the pampiniform venous plexus, is a common cause of a palpable epididymal mass and scrotal discomfort.[¶] In some individuals, a varicocele contributes to low sperm count, decreased sperm motility, and infertility. These problems have been attributed to persistent, hyperemia-induced elevation of testicular temperature, but the real cause may be more complex and is not known with certainty.

The veins of the pampiniform plexus drain the testis and epididymis and are normally quite

[I]References 2,6,7,9,11,22,25-27.

[¶]References 1,2,7,9,12,31,32.

small, but may dilate because of valvular incompetence and/or elevated pressure, forming a tangle of enlarged veins along the course of the spermatic cord and epididymis. In unusual cases, dilated veins may even extend into the substance of the testis.[33] Varicoceles are more common on the left side of the scrotum than the right, possibly due to elevated pressure in the left testicular vein. The left testicular vein inserts into the left renal vein, which drapes across the aorta and may be compressed between the aorta and superior mesenteric artery, raising venous pressure. The right testicular vein drains into the inferior vena cava directly and is not subject to compressive effects. Because of the left-side predominance of varicocele, the possibility of neoplastic testicular vein obstruction or compression (due to intra-abdominal lymphadenopathy) should be considered when a varicocele is isolated to the right cord/epididymis.

Varicocele usually is a clinical diagnosis, as the tangle of veins is easily palpated and feels like a "bunch of worms." Ultrasound is required when the nature of the palpable mass is unclear or when pain or tenderness is present, as well as in men who experience infertility. Varicocele is diagnosed with color flow ultrasound when numerous veins of unusually large size are seen along the spermatic cord or epididymis, as shown in Figure 33-13. In all cases, the extent of the varicosities should be documented, and the largest veins should be measured, as discussed later. The presence of reflux within the veins can be investigated by having the patient perform the Valsalva maneuver during color flow observation. Normal pampiniform veins are barely detectable, so from one perspective, a varicocele can be diagnosed whenever veins of unusual size and number are readily seen. More specific diagnosis may be important, however, in men with pain or infertility, in whom a decision must be made concerning the potential benefit of therapy. In this respect, veins 2 mm in diameter or less are generally regarded as not substantially dilated, while larger veins are considered varicose, especially those with a diameter of 3 mm or larger.[2,12,31,32] This definition includes veins reaching this size with the patient in positions not typically used during ultrasound examination (e.g., standing, squatting) and in any state of respiration, including straining or performing a Valsalva maneuver. The demonstration of reflux in the veins is further evidence of potential clinical significance.

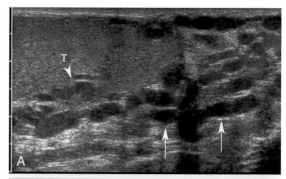
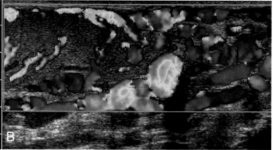

FIGURE 33-13 Varicocele. **A** and **B,** Gray-scale and color Doppler imaging shows serpiginous veins *(arrows)* posterior and inferior to the testis representing the varicocele, as well as extension of the varicocele into the testis (T, *arrowhead*).

Although these sonographic criteria are used in an attempt to define the clinical significance of a varicocele, decisions concerning the need for venoocclusive therapy are multifactorial and are more a matter of clinical judgment than of specific ultrasound criteria.

TESTICULAR TORSION

Torsion refers to twisting of the testis within the scrotal sac, such that the arteries and veins are compressed and blood flow is compromised.[#] Torsion usually occurs in children or young adults, and two peaks of incidence have been noted: the neonatal period and puberty. Torsion in neonates is typically extravaginal. That is, the entire contents of the scrotum twist on the spermatic cord, including the parietal and visceral layers of the tunical vaginalis. The torsion often occurs prenatally and is seen in neonates of high birth weights.[41]

In children and young adults, torsion is typically intravaginal, in which the parietal tunica vaginalis remains intact, while the scrotal contents inside the parietal tunica twist. The torsion results from abnormal mobility of the testis, due

#References 2,9,11,12,18,22,25,26,34-40.

to narrow attachment of the testis to the scrotal wall by the reflection of the tunica vaginalis (see Figure 33-2). Normally, the parietal layer of the tunica vaginalis lines the inner wall of the scrotal sac until it reaches the edge of the testicle, where it reflects over the testicle, forming the visceral layer of the tunica vaginalis. The portion of the testicle that is not covered by the visceral layer of the tunica vaginalis is closely held against the scrotal wall and called the "bare area." Vessels and tubules from the spermatic cord enter and leave the testicle across the bare area. When the bare area is abnormally small (an abnormality called the "bell clapper deformity"), the attachment of the testicle to the scrotal wall is narrow and the testicle is at risk for torsion due to twisting at this attachment. The pathologic sequence of events begins when the spermatic cord twists, with a rotation of at least 360 degrees, at the bare area. This causes venous obstruction, leading to swelling and increased pressure inside the testicle and within the spermatic cord. Subsequently, arterial flow becomes occluded and testicular ischemia results, progressing to infarction if detorsion does not occur surgically or spontaneously.

The pathologic process of torsion can be divided into acute torsion, during which the testicle suffers ischemia but can be saved if detorsion occurs, and missed torsion, the stage after which testicular infarction has occurred to the point that the testicle cannot be saved even if detorsed. The testicle is almost always salvageable during the first 6 to 10 hours of torsion and is progressively less likely to be salvageable thereafter. In virtually all cases of torsion lasting more than 24 hours, the testicle cannot be saved.**

Color Doppler ultrasound has become the predominant imaging method for diagnosing testicular torsion, although occasionally scintigraphy is still used. Ultrasound imaging with Doppler is reported to be 86% to 100% sensitive and virtually 100% specific for diagnosing testicular torsion.[34-38,42-45]

Early on after torsion occurs, the testicle may appear normal in echotexture. During this time, the only abnormal gray-scale sonographic findings may be in the spermatic cord and epididymis, which may appear as a thick echogenic structure with acoustic shadowing due to twisting.[39,40] On Doppler, blood flow

will be diminished or absent in the testicle and the knotted cord and epididymis. As the torsion persists and blood flow remains occluded, the testicle becomes enlarged and mildly hypoechoic, due to swelling and edema. At this time, a small hydrocele is sometimes seen. With color Doppler, flow remains diminished or absent in the testicle and epididymis. If there is further progression to the development of testicular necrosis, the testicle becomes mottled and heterogeneous with hypoechoic areas, and the scrotal wall becomes thickened. Once the testicle becomes heterogeneous, the likelihood of successful salvage is extremely low.[46]

Gray-scale and Doppler findings are key to the diagnosis of testicular torsion. The examination should begin with gray-scale, including side-by-side comparison of testicular size and echogenicity and assessment of the epididymis to look for the knotted cord (Figure 33-14). Color Doppler should then be performed for side-by-side assessment of blood flow. With testicular torsion, differences in perfusion, including absence or marked diminution of blood flow on the affected side, will be found. If blood flow is still present on the affected side, spectral waveforms typically demonstrate high-resistance flow, as compared with the low-resistance flow in the normal testicle.

Rarely, detorsion of the testicle occurs before the sonographic and Doppler assessment.[6,18,25,26] In such cases, the affected testicle may be hyperemic as compared with the normal testicle. In these cases, the knot of the twisted cord and epididymis will not be present.

With neonatal or extravaginal torsion, the key findings are swelling of the testis with generalized decreased echogenicity and absence of blood flow in the affected testis (Figure 33-15). Sometimes, fluid is seen in two spaces surrounding the testis, an inner collection within the parietal tunica vaginalis and a rim of fluid outside the parietal tunica. A rim of peripheral vascularity may be seen in the tissues surrounding an avascular testis with a missed or chronic torsion. This is likely due to inflammation or hyperemia of the adjacent tissues. This may correlate to the "halo sign" on a nuclear medicine image that is considered pathognomonic for missed testicular torsion. It is important to recognize that this flow is outside the testicle.

There are several pitfalls with respect to testicular torsion diagnosis.[2,18,22,25,26] First, blood

---

**References 2,11,18,22,25,26.

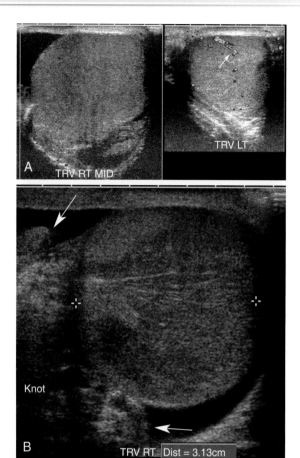

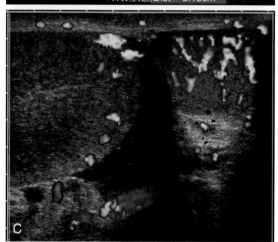

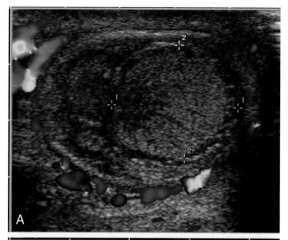

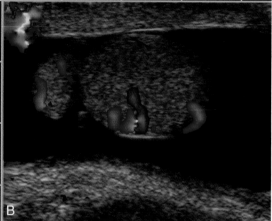

FIGURE 33-15 Neonatal testicular torsion. **A,** Longitudinal sonogram of neonatal scrotum demonstrating extravaginal torsion. The swollen testis *(cursors)* and epididymis maintain their anatomic relationship because both the parietal and visceral layers of the tunical vaginalis have torsed with the testicle. Note absent blood flow within the scrotal contents, with a peripheral rim of color flow in the scrotal wall. **B,** The contralateral testis and epididymis are normal in appearance with normal vascularity and are surrounded by a small hydrocele.

FIGURE 33-14 Testicular torsion. **A,** Transverse (TRV) views of right (RT) and left (LT) testicles demonstrate flow in several vessels on the left *(arrow)* and no flow in the right testicle due to acute torsion. The right testicle is markedly swollen and hypoechoic compared with the left. **B,** Transverse view of right torsed testis *(cursors)* in a different patient demonstrates swelling of the testis with geographic areas of decreased echogenicity. A small hydrocele is present. Part of the knot of the twisted cord and epididymis (Knot, *arrows*) is seen adjacent to the testicle. **C,** Color Doppler images show marked swelling of the right testicle with decreased color Doppler signals as compared to the smaller, well-perfused left testicle.

flow is cut off completely only with fairly marked levels of torsion (360 degrees or greater). With lesser degrees of torsion, Doppler may be subtly abnormal or even normal. Second, appreciating side-by-side differences in blood flow may be problematic in young children and neonates, because the testicles may be small and blood flow may be difficult to detect even in a normal testicle.[47,48] Third, a torsed testis may undergo spontaneous detorsion, followed by a period of hyperemia. If the testis is examined during the hyperemic period, increased blood flow may be mistaken for orchitis.

SCROTAL TRAUMA

Penetrating scrotal trauma usually requires surgical exploration and is not generally the subject of ultrasound examination. Ultrasound is useful, however, in concussion or crush injuries of the scrotum, which are difficult to evaluate clinically because of pain and scrotal swelling.[9,11,22,26,49-54] The primary role of ultrasound is to determine whether the testes are intact and to assess perfusion. Improved salvage of traumatized testes can be achieved if testicular rupture is recognized early and treated surgically. When testicular rupture is likely, based on the nature of the crush/contusion injury, then surgery is required, and ultrasound may not have a role in patient management. Sonography is most useful when conservative (nonsurgical) management is anticipated. If the testes appear intact, conservative management is supported, but if there is evidence of rupture or if there are large nonperfused areas or a complete lack of perfusion (due to torsion), surgery is necessary.

A large hematocele (blood-filled scrotum) typically is present in trauma patients due to hemorrhage from the testis or other scrotal contents. The injured testis may be heterogeneous due to hematoma formation or infarction. Focal hematomas vary in echogenicity according to their age. Acute hematomas tend to be moderately echogenic, and older hematomas, hypoechoic. Infarcted areas are isoechoic or hypoechoic. Color Doppler shows absent perfusion in both hematomas and infarcted areas; therefore, this does not differentiate one from the other. Fractures of the testicular tissue may be visualized as hypoechoic clefts that may or may not be associated with disruption of the tunica albuginea (testicular surface). If the testicular surface is clearly disrupted or tissue is extruded from the testis, the term *testicular rupture* is used, and this finding implies disruption of the tunica albuginea. This distinction is important, as fractures may not be surgical lesions, whereas rupture is generally treated surgically. The most useful signs of testicular rupture are contour irregularity of the testicle, the detection of a frank cleft in the testicular surface, or the detection of extruded testicular tissue.[9,48,50,53,54] Heterogeneity is also associated with rupture due to intratesticular hemorrhage and contusion, but this finding may also be present without rupture.

The epididymis also may be injured, with or without associated testicular injury. Epididymal trauma is manifested by swelling and heterogeneity due to hemorrhage. Focal hematoma formation may also occur.

Color Doppler is used in blunt testicular injury to detect avascular areas representing infarction of testicular parenchyma or hematoma formation. Color Doppler may also detect the absence of venous or arterial flow due to posttraumatic torsion of the testis. Finally, large scrotal hematoceles may cause sufficient pressure to obstruct venous drainage, which is diagnosed through the absence of venous flow signals on Doppler examination.

The value of ultrasound in nonpenetrating scrotal trauma is well recognized, yet it appears that sonography is a less-than-perfect diagnostic method.[49-54] Statistics are limited because published series are small; however, it is clear that ultrasound cannot detect fractures reliably and even misses testicular rupture in some cases; furthermore, some testes that appear ruptured (even with apparent extrusion of testicular tissue) are found at surgery to be intact. In the latter cases, it appears that thrombus adherent to the testis may mimic tunica rupture and tissue extrusion. Epididymal injuries also may be difficult to detect due to absence of sonographic findings or obscuration by adherent thrombus.

ERECTILE DYSFUNCTION

PENILE ANATOMY

The normal penis comprises three columns of spongy tissue, each encased by a dense fibrous sheath. Two of the columns, the paired corpora cavernosa, lie in parallel on the dorsal side of the penis. Each corpus cavernosum contain multiple sinusoidal spaces with smooth muscle in their walls, and it is this spongy tissue that expands and fills with blood during an erection. The tunica albuginea is the dense fibrous sheath that encapsulates the sinusoidal tissue, providing structure and support when the penis is erect.

Along the ventral side of the penis runs the corpus spongiosum. This column of spongiosal tissue surrounds the urethra, which remains in a collapsed state except during active urination. The corpus spongiosum is usually smaller than the corpora cavernosa, except at its distal end, where it broadens to form the glans penis. The spongiosal tissue of the corpus spongiosum expands somewhat with erection but not to the extent that the cavernosal tissues expand. The

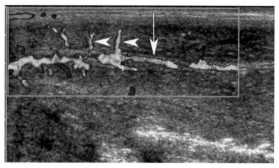

FIGURE 33-16 Cavernosal artery and helicine branches. Longitudinal color Doppler sonogram of corpus cavernosum demonstrating flow in the cavernosal artery *(arrow)* that courses through the middle of the corpus cavernosum. Small helicine branches *(arrowheads)* extend radially from the cavernosal artery.

three columns of tissue are surrounded by a layer of subcutaneous tissue and skin.

Arterial blood supply to the penis is via bilateral penile arteries, each a branch of the internal pudendal artery. The penile artery has two main branches, the dorsal artery and the cavernosal artery. The dorsal artery travels along the dorsal side of the penis lateral to the midline dorsal vein and supplies blood to the glans penis and the corpus spongiosum. It has few or no branches before it reaches the glans penis. The cavernosal artery travels centrally within the corpus cavernosum and supplies blood to the cavernosal sinusoids via multiple branches called helicine arteries that extend radially from the cavernosal artery (Figure 33-16). Most men have a single cavernosal artery on each side; however, anatomic variants of cavernosal blood supply are common. In some cases, the cavernosal artery arises from the dorsal artery. In other cases, more than one cavernosal artery is present. During the generation of an erection, flow in the cavernosal arteries and helicine branches is markedly increased.

The venous drainage from the corpora cavernosa is via small veins that perforate the tunica albuginea to drain into the deep dorsal vein. Toward the base of the penis are small crural veins that drain into the deep pelvic veins to the internal pudendal vein. When the penis is erect and the corpora cavernosa are expanded, the small draining veins are occluded by stretching of the tunica albuginea.

ERECTILE FUNCTION

The physiologic process of a normal erection begins with increased parasympathetic motor nervous activity to the penis, involving sacral nerves two, three, and four. The parasympathetic motor activity causes the smooth muscle in the walls of the cavernosal sinusoids to relax, allowing the sinusoids to expand and decreasing the resistance to incoming blood flow. At the same time, the cavernosal arteries dilate and carry increased blood flow into the penis. The sinusoids fill with blood, and the corpora cavernosa expand and stretch to become rigid. With expansion of the corpora cavernosa, the draining veins are occluded, preventing blood from leaving the dilated sinusoids. Once the cavernosal sinusoids are filled, the cavernosal arterial blood flow decreases because of increased resistance within the corpora cavernosa. Continued parasympathetic nervous activity maintains the erection.[55]

Normal erectile function requires normal psychologic health, normal endocrine balance, intact innervation to the penis, normal cavernosal sinusoids, adequate arterial blood supply, and normal venous occlusion with erection. Abnormalities of any of these systems may lead to erectile dysfunction. Impotence can be classified as organic, in which a physiologic abnormality is present, or psychogenic, in which impotence is due to psychologic factors. Among men with previously normal erectile function who seek medical attention for impotence, an organic cause is found in 50% to 90%.[56-58]

The vast majority of patients with organic impotence have hemodynamic abnormalities: arterial insufficiency, venous incompetence, or both. Arteriogenic impotence occurs as a result of stenoses or occlusions that limit blood flow to the penis even in the presence of parasympathetic stimulation. If maximum flow is inadequate to fill the cavernosal sinusoids, tumescence and rigidity cannot occur. Without adequate filling of the corpora cavernosa, draining veins are not occluded but rather continue to carry blood away from the corpora cavernosa.[55,59] Arteriogenic impotence occurs most commonly in men with risk factors for atherosclerosis, including diabetes mellitus, hypertension, hypercholesterolemia, and smoking.[60-63]

Patients with mild to moderate arterial insufficiency in the absence of venous incompetence can often be successfully treated with oral pharmacologic therapy, such as sildenafil citrate (Viagra), vardenafil (Levitra), and tadalafil (Cialis).[64] Patients with severe arterial insufficiency usually require a penile implant to restore sexual function.[55]

Venous incompetence results from failure of occlusion of the draining veins, despite adequate filling of the cavernosal sinusoids. Patients may experience partial erections, but rigidity cannot be fully achieved or maintained.

Other penile abnormalities, including scarring within the corpora cavernosa or involving the tunica albuginea, may also cause impotence. Scarring or fibrosis of sinusoidal tissue prevents that area of the corpora from expanding when an erection is developing. The sinusoidal tissue around the scar fills with blood and pulls on the abnormal area, causing penile curvature. If the scarring is severe, expansion of the surrounding sinusoids may also cause pain, leading to detumescence.

When scarring affects the tunica albuginea that surrounds the corpora cavernosa, the tunica becomes thickened and may even calcify. Calcified plaques of the tunica are called *Peyronie's disease*. Plaques involving the tunica albuginea most often cause painless curvature with erection. Sometimes, as with cavernosal plaques, there may be enough pain from the plaque with an erection that detumescence results.

SONOGRAPHY

Sonographic evaluation of the penis is performed with high-frequency (7 MHz or higher) linear transducers. The transducer is placed directly on the penis, and longitudinal and transverse images are obtained. The corpora of the normal penis have homogeneous echotexture. The two corpora cavernosa should be symmetric in size (Figure 33-17). The tunica albuginea surrounding the cavernosal tissue appears as a thin echogenic line encasing the corpora. Within the corpora cavernosa, the bright walls of the cavernosal arteries may be seen in some areas (Figure 33-18). The corpus spongiosum is usually smaller than the corpora cavernosa but has similar echogenicity to the flaccid corpora. The urethra cannot be seen when it is collapsed.

When the penis is erect, the corpora cavernosa are larger, and the spongiosal tissue has a speckled appearance with small anechoic areas representing dilated sinusoids, separated by the brightly echogenic sinusoidal septa (Figure 33-19). The cavernosal arteries are dilated, and their walls are brightly echogenic (Figure 33-20) because they are surrounded by blood-filled sinusoids.

Scarring of the corpora cavernosa or tunica albuginea can be diagnosed by ultrasound. Scars of the corpora cavernosa appear as irregular echogenic areas within the corpora (Figure 33-21). With an erection and dilatation of the surrounding sinusoids, the scars become more prominent

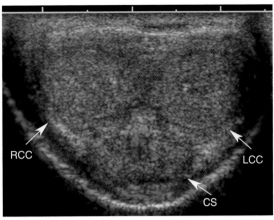

FIGURE 33-17 Normal nonerect penis. Transverse sonogram demonstrating two symmetric corpora cavernosa—right corpus cavernosum (RCC; *arrow*) and left corpus cavernosum (LCC; *arrow*)—dorsally and the corpus spongiosum (CS; *arrow*) ventrally. The tunica albuginea encapsulates the corpora cavernosa.

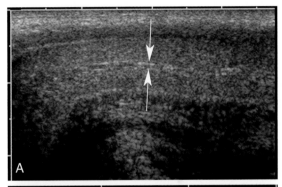

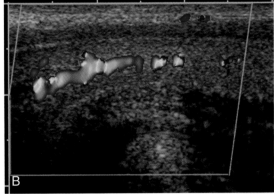

FIGURE 33-18 Cavernosal artery in nonerect penis. **A,** Longitudinal sonogram of a corpus cavernosum demonstrating cavernosal artery *(arrows)* within sinusoidal tissue. The walls of the cavernosal artery are echogenic. **B,** Color Doppler demonstrating flow within the cavernosal artery.

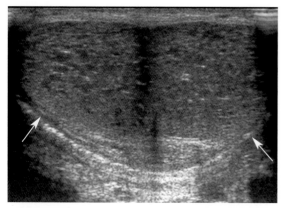

FIGURE 33-19 Erect penis. Transverse sonogram demonstrating the enlarged corpora cavernosa *(arrows)* with a speckled appearance because of blood-filled sinusoids.

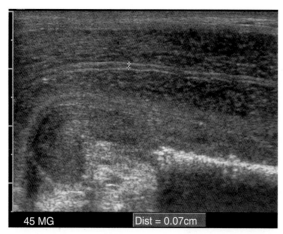

FIGURE 33-20 Cavernosal artery in erect penis. Longitudinal sonogram of the right corpus cavernosum demonstrating the cavernosal artery *(cursors)* with brightly echogenic walls running through blood-filled sinusoids.

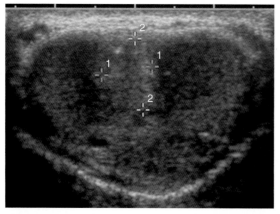

FIGURE 33-21 Sinusoidal scarring. Transverse sonogram demonstrating echogenic plaque *(cursors)* in the midline extending into both corpora cavernosa.

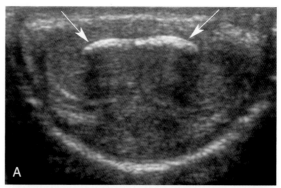

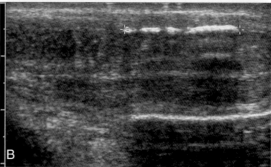

FIGURE 33-22 Peyronie's disease. **A,** Transverse sonogram demonstrating brightly echogenic calcified plaque *(arrows)* across the dorsal surface of the corpora cavernosa. **B,** Longitudinal sonogram of calcified plaque *(cursors).*

and easier to delineate. Tunical plaques appear sonographically as focal areas of thickening of the tunica albuginea. Calcification in the plaque is brightly echogenic and casts an acoustic shadow (Figure 33-22).

DOPPLER EVALUATION

Color Doppler and pulsed Doppler assessments are used to evaluate the hemodynamic function of the penis in patients who do not respond to a trial of oral pharmacologic agents.[64] Doppler assessment is performed before and after intracavernosal injection of a vasoactive pharmacologic agent to induce and maintain an erection. Either papaverine or prostaglandin E_1, both of which induce an erection by causing sinusoidal smooth muscle relaxation and dilatation of the cavernosal arteries, can be used. The dose for papaverine is usually 30 to 60 mg, and that for prostaglandin E_1, 10 to 15 μg. The pharmacologic substance is injected directly into one corpus cavernosum using a small-gauge needle. A single injection acts on both corpora via multiple communications across the intercavernosal septum. Before injection, some examiners place a tourniquet at the base of the

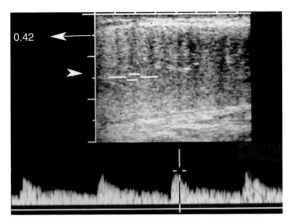

FIGURE 33-23 Normal cavernosal arterial waveform. Longitudinal sonogram with the Doppler waveform below, taken after injection of papaverine, demonstrating normal high velocities and low-resistance flow. Peak velocity is 42 cm/sec (0.42 m/sec; *arrow*).

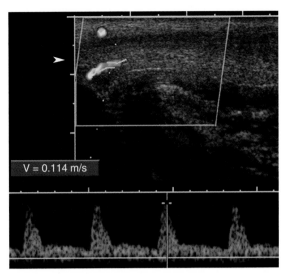

FIGURE 33-24 Color Doppler assessment of cavernosal artery. Longitudinal sonogram with the color Doppler image taken before the development of an erection, demonstrating low-velocity flow in the cavernosal artery.

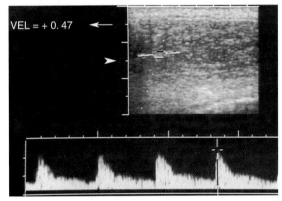

FIGURE 33-25 Cavernosal arterial waveform during the generation of erection. Longitudinal sonogram with a Doppler waveform below demonstrating low-resistance flow with normal peak systolic velocity of 47 cm/sec (0.47 m/sec; *arrow*).

penis to prolong the local effect of the agent, leaving the tourniquet in place for 2 to 3 minutes until Doppler assessment is begun. Immediately after injection, some examiners use vibratory stimulation or ask the patient to manually stimulate the penis to promote the action of the drug.

Initial Doppler assessment before injection entails obtaining Doppler waveforms from both cavernosal arteries and measuring the peak systolic velocity in each. Once the injection has been given, Doppler assessment should begin 2 to 3 minutes later by again obtaining cavernosal arterial waveforms and measuring the peak systolic velocity in each (Figure 33-23). The waveforms are most easily obtained by scanning from the dorsal side of the penis, using color Doppler assessment to help localize the cavernosal artery. Angle correction of 60 degrees or less must be maintained during pulsed Doppler interrogation. Arterial waveforms should be obtained at 2- to 3-minute intervals until the peak systolic velocity is above 35 cm/sec or has reached a plateau. Once the penis has reached maximal tumescence or a maximal peak systolic velocity, usually 8 to 10 minutes after injection or as long as 15 to 20 minutes in anxious patients,[65-68] the end-diastolic velocities are measured from both cavernosal arterial waveforms. At this time, blood flow is also assessed in the deep dorsal vein by scanning the vein from the ventral side of the penis using color Doppler or pulsed Doppler assessments.[58,65-67,69-71]

The blood flow in men with normal hemodynamic function follows a predictable pattern during generation of an erection. Initially, in the flaccid state, Doppler waveforms of the cavernosal arteries demonstrate a high-resistance pattern, with relatively low peak systolic velocity, but usually greater than 13 cm/sec,[72] and absent or reverse diastolic flow (Figure 33-24), and no flow is demonstrated in the deep dorsal vein. Two to three minutes after intracorporal injection of papaverine or prostaglandin E_1, the smooth muscles in the cavernosal sinusoids relax, leading to increased arterial inflow and a low-resistance arterial waveform, typified by high diastolic flow (Figure 33-25). As the high flow continues in the cavernosal arteries and the sinusoids fill, the waveform changes to a higher-resistance

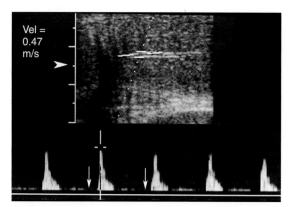

FIGURE 33-26 Cavernosal arterial waveform after full erection is achieved. Longitudinal sonogram with a Doppler waveform below demonstrating sharp systolic peaks with normal peak systolic velocity of 47 cm/sec and absent end-diastolic flow *(arrows)*.

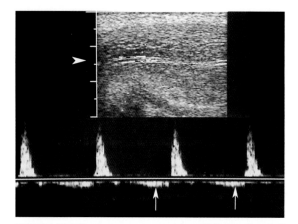

FIGURE 33-27 Cavernosal arterial waveform after full erection is achieved. Longitudinal sonogram with the Doppler waveform below demonstrating sharp systolic peaks and reverse end-diastolic flow *(arrows)*.

pattern with sharp systolic peaks and diminished or absent diastolic flow (Figure 33-26). The peak systolic velocity increases over the first several minutes after injection, up to a maximum that exceeds 35 cm/sec in most normal men.[69,73-75] Because some men who achieve normal erections have peak systolic velocities between 30 and 35 cm/sec, these patients with peak flows of 30 cm/sec or greater may be classified as normal.[61,66,71] With full tumescence, peak systolic velocities decline and there is absent or even reversed end-diastolic flow (Figures 33-26 and 33-27). At this point, no flow should be seen in the deep dorsal vein with color Doppler examination.

Deviation from this normal pattern may be diagnostic of arterial or venous disease. Arterial insufficiency is best diagnosed using the maximum

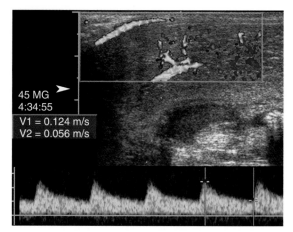

FIGURE 33-28 Arterial insufficiency. Cavernosal arterial waveform with arterial insufficiency. Longitudinal sonogram with color and spectral Doppler of cavernosal artery demonstrating an abnormally low peak systolic velocity of 12.4 cm/sec (V1 = 0.124 m/s) and persistent forward diastolic flow.

cavernosal arterial systolic velocity, as good correlation has been demonstrated between this measurement and findings at angiography.[59,76] The lower the peak systolic velocity, the greater the degree of severity of arterial disease. Patients with maximum systolic velocities below normal, in the range of 25 to 30 cm/sec, usually have mild to moderate arterial insufficiency. Patients with maximum velocities less than 25 cm/sec usually have severe arterial insufficiency[††] (Figure 33-28). A discrepancy in maximum velocities of greater than 10 cm/sec between right and left sides is also usually indicative of some degree of arterial insufficiency. In the flaccid state, a peak systolic velocity less than 13 cm/sec also suggests arterial insufficiency, but this parameter has lower sensitivity than Doppler measurements obtained during pharmacologically induced erection.[72]

Although the maximum systolic velocity correlates fairly well with arterial function of the penis, there are limitations to this diagnostic method. Patient anxiety can diminish the arterial response to the vasoactive pharmacologic agents to the point that maximum velocities fall below the normal range despite normal arterial function. A similar decrease may be found in some patients with psychogenic impotence.[78] In general, the maximum systolic velocity is lower in patients with psychogenic impotence and normal arterial function than in patients without this condition.[75] Patients with variants of

[††]References 56,61,69,71,74,77.

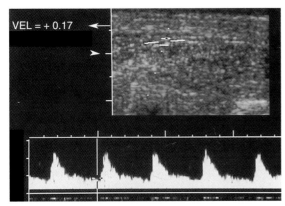

FIGURE 33-29 Venous incompetence. Longitudinal sonogram with the Doppler waveform below demonstrating persistent diastolic flow at 17 cm/sec (0.17 m/sec; *arrow*).

cavernosal arterial anatomy, such as duplicated cavernosal arteries on one side, may have peak systolic velocities less than 30 cm/sec despite normal arterial flow. For this reason, when more than one artery is seen, conclusions about arterial function cannot be drawn if the maximum systolic velocity is less than 30 cm/sec.[79]

Doppler sonography can also be helpful for diagnosing venous incompetence, as a number of findings suggest this diagnosis when arterial function is normal. This diagnosis should be suspected in any patient who fails to generate an adequate erection despite normal cavernosal arterial Doppler waveforms.[58,69] The Doppler findings most suggestive of venous incompetence are flow in the dorsal vein or persistent cavernosal arterial diastolic flow above 5 cm/sec (Figure 33-29). Demonstration of dorsal vein flow, via either color Doppler or pulsed Doppler assessment (Figure 33-30), is consistent with dorsal venous incompetence.[61,71,80] Persistently high diastolic flow without evident dorsal venous flow suggests venous leakage through the crural veins, as flow in these veins cannot be detected by Doppler sonography.

Although Doppler sonography can suggest the diagnosis of venous insufficiency, it is not the modality of choice for evaluating this disorder. Cavernosometry and cavernosography are preferable. Cavernosometry, performed with vasoactive pharmacologic agents, is the most accurate method for making the diagnosis. When venous incompetence is found, cavernosography provides anatomic delineation of the abnormal venous pathways.[80-83]

Venous competence can be assessed by Doppler only if arterial function is normal. Patients

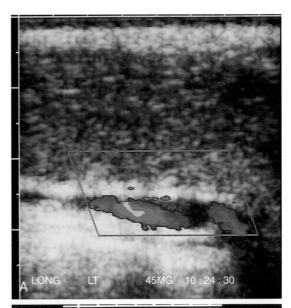

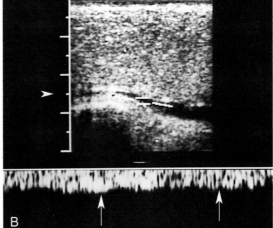

FIGURE 33-30 Venous incompetence. **A,** Longitudinal color Doppler sonogram demonstrating flow in the dorsal vein. **B,** Longitudinal sonogram with the Doppler waveform below demonstrating flow in the dorsal vein *(arrows)*. Note that imaging is done from the ventral aspect of the penis.

with arterial insufficiency may have too little arterial inflow to expand the sinusoids enough to occlude the draining veins, and hence, these patients can have persistent venous flow regardless of whether the veins are intrinsically competent. For this reason, the results of the Doppler assessment of the cavernosal arteries should be kept in mind when evaluating for venous leakage. If the maximum systolic velocities in the cavernosal arteries are within the normal range, then further assessment for venous competence can be performed. If a diagnosis of arterial insufficiency is made based on abnormally low peak systolic velocities, conclusions about venous competence cannot be drawn from the arterial waveform or Doppler assessment of the dorsal vein.[58]

PRIAPISM

Priapism is a persistently erect or engorged penis without sexual stimulation. The type of priapism can be classified based on the amount of flow to the penis while it is engorged as low-flow or high-flow priapism. Low-flow priapism results from occlusion of the draining veins from the penis, trapping blood in the sinusoids and leading to thrombosis. This form of priapism can lead to ischemia of the corpora cavernosa and, if left untreated, cavernosal scarring. Low-flow priapism may be seen in association with diseases complicated by a hypercoagulable state, such as sickle cell anemia or leukemia. High-flow priapism can result from trauma with arterial rupture leading to intracavernosal arteriovenous shunting. It can also result from misuse of medication that causes prolonged sinusoidal smooth muscle relaxation.[84]

Color Doppler sonography is key to the diagnosis of priapism.[85-89] With low-flow priapism, minimal flow is seen in the cavernosal arteries, which demonstrate high-resistance flow. The sinusoidal spaces may be hypoechoic rather than anechoic if thrombosis has occurred. With high-flow priapism, color and spectral Doppler will demonstrate high flow in the cavernosal arteries and flow in the helicine branches. The dilated cavernosal sinusoids will be anechoic.

REFERENCES

1. Doherty FJ: Ultrasound of the nonacute scrotum, *Semin Ultrasound CT MRI* 12:113–156, 1991.
2. Gerscovich EO: High-resolution ultrasonography in the diagnosis of scrotal pathology: I. Normal scrotum and benign disease, *J Clin Ultrasound* 21:355–373, 1993.
3. Hamm B, Fobbe F: Maturation of the testis: Ultrasound evaluation, *Ultrasound Med Biol* 21:143–147, 1995.
4. Middleton WD, Bell MW: Analysis of intratesticular arterial anatomy with emphasis on transmediastinal arteries, *Radiology* 189:157–160, 1993.
5. Fakhry J, Khoury A, Barakat K: The hypoechoic band: A normal finding on testicular sonography, *AJR Am J Roentgenol* 153:321–323, 1989.
6. Luker GD, Siegel MJ: Color Doppler sonography of the scrotum in children, *AJR Am J Roentgenol* 163:649–655, 1994.
7. Ragheb D, Higgins JL: Ultrasonography of the scrotum, technique, anatomy and pathologic entities, *J Ultrasound Med* 21:171–185, 2002.
8. Black JAR, Patel A: Sonography of the normal extratesticular spaces, *AJR Am J Roentgenol* 167:503–506, 1996.
9. Winter T: Ultrasonography of the scrotum, *Appl Radiol* 31:9–18, 2002.
10. Middleton WD, Thorne DA, Melson GL: Color Doppler ultrasound of the normal testis, *AJR Am J Roentgenol* 152:293–297, 1989.
11. Horstman WJ, et al: Color Doppler US of the scrotum, *Radiographics* 11:941–957, 1991.
12. Watson LR, et al: Applied scrotal sonography, *Appl Radiol* 20:27–35, 1991.
13. Brown DL, et al: Cystic testicular mass caused by dilated rete testis: sonographic findings in 31 cases, *AJR Am J Roentgenol* 158:1257–1259, 1992.
14. Gerscovich EO: High-resolution ultrasonography in the diagnosis of scrotal pathology: II. Tumors, *J Clin Ultrasound* 21:375–386, 1993.
15. Horner MJ, Ries LAG, Krapcho M, et al, editors: SEER Cancer Statistics Review, 1975-2006, National Cancer Institute. Bethesda, MD, http://seer.cancer.gov/csr/1975_2006.
16. Lerner DM, et al: Color Doppler US in the evaluation of acute scrotal disease, *Radiology* 176:355–358, 1990.
17. Middleton WD, Teefey SA, Santillan CS: Testicular microlithiasis: Prospective analysis of prevalence and associated tumor, *Radiology* 224:425–428, 2002.
18. Luker GD, Siegel MJ: Pediatric testicular tumors: Evaluation with gray-scale and color Doppler US, *Radiology* 191:561–564, 1994.
19. Cast JE, et al: Testicular microlithiasis: Prevalence and tumor risk in a population referred for scrotal sonography, *AJR Am J Roentgenol* 175:1703–1706, 2000.
20. Ahmad I, et al: Testicular microlithiasis: prevalence and risk of concurrent and interval development of testicular tumor in a referred population, *Int Urol Nephrol* 39:1177–1181, 2007.
21. Miller FN, et al: Testicular calcification and microlithiasis: association with primary intra-testicular malignancy in 3,477 patients, *Eur Radiol* 17:363–369, 2007.
22. Tumeh SS, Benson CB, Richie JP: Acute diseases of the scrotum, *Semin Ultrasound CT MRI* 12:115–130, 1991.
23. Oh C, et al: Sonographic demonstration, including color Doppler imaging, of recurrent sperm granuloma, *J Ultrasound Med* 19:333–335, 2000.
24. Frates MC, et al: Solid extratesticular masses evaluated with sonography: Pathologic correlation, *Radiology* 204:43–46, 1997.
25. Paltiel HJ, et al: Acute scrotal symptoms in boys with an indeterminate clinical presentation: Comparison of color Doppler sonography and scintigraphy, *Radiology* 207:223–231, 1998.
26. Paltiel HJ: Sonography of pediatric scrotal emergencies, *Ultrasound Q* 16:53–71, 2000.
27. Gordon LM, Stein SM, Ralls PW: Traumatic epididymitis: Evaluation with color Doppler sonography, *AJR Am J Roentgenol* 166:1323–1325, 1996.
28. Lentini JF, Benson CB, Richie JP: Sonographic features of focal orchitis, *J Ultrasound Med* 8:61–365, 1989.
29. Mazzu D, Greffrey RB, Ralls PW: Lymphoma and leukemia involving the testicles: Findings on gray-scale and color Doppler sonography, *AJR Am J Roentgenol* 164:645–647, 1995.
30. Yang DM, et al: Lymphoma of the testis and epididymis mimics chronic inflammation upon sonography, *J Clin Ultrasound* 37:242–244, 2009.

31. Winkelbauer FW, et al: Doppler sonography of varicocele: Long-term follow-up after venography and transcatheter sclerotherapy, *J Ultrasound Med* 13:953–958, 1994.

32. Graif M, et al: Varicocele and the testicular-renal venous route: Hemodynamic Doppler sonographic investigation, *J Ultrasound Med* 19:627–631, 2000.

33. Kessler A, et al: Intratesticular varicocele: gray scale and color Doppler sonographic appearance, *J Ultrasound Med* 24:1711–1716, 2005.

34. Weber DM, Rosslein R, Fliegel C: Color Doppler sonography in the diagnosis of acute scrotum in boys, *Eur J Pediatr Surg* 10:2241, 2000.

35. Baker LA, et al: An analysis of clinical outcomes using color Doppler testicular ultrasound for testicular torsion, *Pediatrics* 105:604–607, 2000.

36. Nussbaum-Blask AR, et al: Color Doppler sonography and scintigraphy of the testis: A prospective, comparative analysis in children with acute scrotal pain, *Pediatr Emerg Care* 18:67–71, 2002.

37. Burks DD, et al: Suspected testicular torsion and ischemia: Evaluation with color Doppler sonography, *Radiology* 175:815–821, 1990.

38. Kravchick S, et al: Color Doppler sonography: Its real role in the evaluation of children with highly suspected testicular torsion, *Eur Radiol* 11:1000–1005, 2001.

39. Baud C, et al: Spiral twist of the spermatic cord: A reliable sign of testicular torsion, *Pediatr Radiol* 28:950–954, 1998.

40. Arce JD, Cortes M, Vargas JC: Sonographic diagnosis of acute spermatic cord torsion. Rotation of the cord: A key to the diagnosis, *Pediatr Radiol* 32:485–491, 2002.

41. Traubici J, et al: Testicular torsion in neonates and infants: sonographic features in 30 patients, *AJR Am J Roentgenol* 180:1143–1145, 2003.

42. Waldert M, et al: Color Doppler Sonography Reliably Identifies Testicular Torsion in Boys, *Urology* 75:1170–1174, 2010.

43. Rattansingh A, Adamson B, Cosgrove D: Bidirectional flow within the intratesticular arteries caused by microvenous thrombosis secondary to testicular torsion, *J Ultrasound Med* 28:817–821, 2009.

44. Baldisserotto M: Scrotal emergencies, *Pediatr Radiol* 39:516–521, 2009.

45. Pepe P, et al: Does color Doppler sonography improve the clinical assessment of patients with acute scrotum? *Eur J Radiol* 60:120–124, 2006.

46. Kaye JD, et al: Parenchymal echo texture predicts testicular salvage after torsion: potential impact on the need for emergent exploration, *J Urol* 180(4S):1733–1736, 2008.

47. Luker GD, Siegel MJ: Scrotal US in pediatric patients: Comparison of power and standard color Doppler US, *Radiology* 198:381–385, 1996.

48. Albrecht T, et al: Power Doppler US of the normal prepubertal testis: Does it live up to its promises? *Radiology* 203:227–231, 1997.

49. Lupetin AR, et al: The traumatized scrotum, *Radiology* 148:203–207, 1983.

50. Micallef M, et al: Ultrasound features of blunt testicular injury, *Injury* 32:23–26, 2001.

51. Corrales JG, et al: Accuracy of ultrasound diagnosis after blunt testicular trauma, *J Urol* 150:1834–1836, 1993.

52. Martinez-Pineiro L Jr, et al: Value of testicular ultrasound in the evaluation of blunt scrotal trauma without haematocele, *Br J Urol* 69:286–290, 1992.

53. Learch TJ, Hansch LP, Ralls PW: Sonography in patients with gunshot wounds of the scrotum: Imaging findings and their value, *AJR Am J Roentgenol* 165:879–883, 1995.

54. Kim SH, et al: Significant predictors for determination of testicular rupture on sonography: a prospective study, *J Ultrasound Med* 26:1649–1655, 2007.

55. Krane RJ, Goldstein I, Tejada IS: Impotence, *N Engl J Med* 321:1648–1659, 1989.

56. Krysiewicz S, Mellinger BC: The role of imaging in the diagnostic evaluation of impotence, *AJR Am J Roentgenol* 153:1133–1139, 1989.

57. Paushter DM: Role of duplex sonography in the evaluation of sexual impotence, *AJR Am J Roentgenol* 153:1161–1163, 1989.

58. Benson CB, Vickers MA Jr, Aruny J: Evaluation of impotence, *Semin Ultrasound CT MR* 12:176–190, 1991.

59. Benson CB, Aruny JE, Vickers MA Jr: Correlation of duplex sonography with arteriography in patients with erectile dysfunction, *AJR Am J Roentgenol* 160:71–73, 1993.

60. Kaufman JM, et al: Evaluation of erectile dysfunction by dynamic infusion cavernosometry and cavernosography (DICC), *Urology* 41:445–451, 1993.

61. Kadioglu A, Erdogru T, Tellaloglu S: Evaluation of penile arteries in papaverine-induced erection with color Doppler ultrasonography, *Arch Esp Urol* 48:654–658, 1995.

62. Corona G, et al: Cardiovascular risk engines can help in selecting patients to be evaluated by dynamic penile color Doppler ultrasound, *J Endocrinol Invest* 31:1058–1062, 2008.

63. Kendirci M, et al: The effect of vascular risk factors on penile vascular status in men with erectile dysfunction, *J Urol* 178:2516–2520, 2007.

64. Aversa A, Sarteschi LM: The role of penile color-duplex ultrasound for the evaluation of erectile dysfunction, *J Sex Med* 4:1437–1447, 2007.

65. Govier FE, et al: Timing of penile color flow duplex ultrasonography using a triple drug mixture, *J Urol* 153:1472–1475, 1995.

66. Schwartz AN, et al: Evaluation of normal erectile function with color flow Doppler sonography, *AJR Am J Roentgenol* 153:1155–1160, 1989.

67. Meuleman EJH, et al: Penile pharmacological duplex ultrasonography: A dose-effect study comparing papaverine, papaverine/phentolamine and prostaglandin E_1, *J Urol* 148:63–66, 1992.

68. Shabsigh R, et al: Evaluation of vasculogenic erectile impotence using penile duplex ultrasonography, *J Urol* 142:1469–1474, 1989.

69. Benson CB, Vickers MA: Sexual impotence caused by vascular disease: Diagnosis with duplex sonography, *AJR Am J Roentgenol* 153:1149–1153, 1989.

70. Broderick GA, Arger P: Duplex Doppler ultrasonography: Noninvasive assessment of penile anatomy and function, *Semin Roentgenol* 28:43–56, 1993.

71. Quam JP, et al: Duplex and color Doppler sonographic evaluation of vasculogenic impotence, *AJR Am J Roentgenol* 153:1141–1147, 1989.

72. Corona G, et al: Penile Doppler ultrasound in patients with erectile dysfunction (ED): role of peak systolic velocity measured in the flaccid state in predicting arteriogenic ED and silent coronary artery disease, *J Sex Med* 5:2623–2634, 2008.

73. Hampson SJ, et al: Independent evaluation of impotence by colour Doppler imaging and cavernosometry, *Eur Urol* 21:27–31, 1992.

74. Herbener TE, et al: Penile ultrasound, *Semin Urol* 12: 320–332, 1994.

75. Iacovo F, Barra S, Lotti T: Evaluation of penile deep arteries in psychogenic impotence by means of duplex ultrasonography, *J Urol* 149:1262–1264, 1993.

76. Mueller SC, et al: Comparison of selective internal iliac pharmacoangiography, penile brachial index and duplex sonography with pulsed Doppler analysis for the evaluation of vasculogenic (arteriogenic) impotence, *J Urol* 143:928–932, 1990.

77. Mueller SC, Lue TF: Evaluation of vasculogenic impotence, *Urol Clin North Am* 15:65–76, 1988.

78. Allen RP, et al: Comparison of duplex ultrasonography and nocturnal penile tumescence in evaluation of impotence, *J Urol* 151:1525–1529, 1994.

79. Mancini M, et al: The presence of arterial anatomical variations can affect the results of duplex sonographic evaluation of penile vessels in impotent patients, *J Urol* 155:1919–1923, 1996.

80. Vickers MA, Benson CB, Richie JR: High-resolution ultrasonography and pulsed-wave Doppler for detection of corporo-venous incompetence in erectile dysfunction, *J Urol* 43:1125–1127, 1990.

81. Gall H, et al: Diagnosis of venous incompetence in erectile dysfunction, *Urology* 35:2238, 1990.

82. Rudnick J, Bodecker R, Weidner W: Significance of intracavernosal pharmacological injection test, pharmacocavernosography, artificial erection and cavernosometry in the diagnosis of venous leakage, *Urol Int* 46:338–343, 1991.

83. Vickers MA, et al: The current cavernosometric criteria for corporo-venous dysfunction are too strict, *J Urol* 147: 614–617, 1991.

84. Cherian J, et al: Medical and surgical management of priapism, *Postgrad Med J* 82:89–94, 2006.

85. Bertolotto M, et al: Color Doppler appearance of penile cavernosal-spongiosal communications in patients with high-flow priapism, *Acta Radiol* 49:710–714, 2008.

86. Volgger H, Pfefferkorn S, Hobisch A: Posttraumatic high-flow priapism in children: noninvasive treatment by color Doppler ultrasound-guided perineal compression, *Urology* 70:590.e3–590.e5, 2007.

87. Bartsch G Jr, et al: High-flow priapism: colour-Doppler ultrasound-guided supraselective embolization therapy, *World J Urol* 22:368–370, 2004.

88. Mentzel HJ, et al: High-flow priapism in acute lymphatic leukaemia, *Pediatr Radiol* 34:560–563, 2004.

89. Parascani R, et al: Arteriovenous intracavernous post-traumatic fistula: clinical management and treatment by superselective embolization, *Urology* 63:380–382, 2004.

EVALUATION OF ORGAN TRANSPLANTS

34

MAHAN MATHUR, MD; DANIEL T. GINAT, MD, MS;
DEBORAH RUBENS, MD; and LESLIE M. SCOUTT, MD

Organ transplantation has become the treatment of choice for end-stage renal and liver disease (with the exception of diffuse metastatic liver disease or hepatocellular carcinoma that has extended beyond the liver). Advances in organ procurement, human leukocyte antigens (HLA) matching, surgical technique, and immunosuppression regimens have substantially improved mortality and morbidity and also significantly improved quality of life following organ transplantation. This chapter reviews the role of ultrasound (US) in the workup of graft dysfunction in the patient following renal and hepatic transplantation.

RENAL TRANSPLANTATION

Renal transplantation has become the gold standard treatment for patients with end-stage renal disease.[1] Improvements in surgical technique, coupled with advances in immunosuppressant therapy, careful imaging, and clinical graft surveillance have resulted in improved patient and graft survival as well as improved quality of life when compared to dialysis alone.[1,2] It is currently estimated that deceased donor (DD) renal transplantation extends the average life expectancy of the recipient by 7 to 10 years and living related donor transplantation by 15 to 20 years.[3] These benefits are reflected in a 31% increase in the number of renal transplants performed in the United States from 1998 through 2007 as well as an 86% rise in the number of candidates on the renal transplant waiting list.[4] The United Organ Procurement and Transplant Network reported that 17,357 renal transplants were performed in the United States in 2008 and that 108,000 patients remain on the waiting list in 2010.[5] Despite utilization of living related, living nonrelated, and deceased donors (DDs), organ shortage remains the major rate-limiting factor for renal transplantation in the United States.

Causes of allograft failure are numerous, ranging from rejection to drug toxicity, urinary tract obstruction, and vascular thrombosis or stenosis. However, the clinical presentations of these conditions overlap, and findings such as renal failure, low-grade fever, elevated white blood cell count, and pain are nonspecific. Hence, time course since transplantation, imaging, and ultimately renal biopsy play key roles in determining patient management by differentiating between underlying pathology that requires surgical or percutaneous intervention from conditions that can be managed medically. US has become the imaging modality of choice for the evaluation of both the immediate and long-term complications of renal transplants because US is noninvasive, radiation-free, and relatively inexpensive.[6] In addition, US may be helpful in guiding interventional diagnostic and therapeutic procedures. Other imaging modalities that may be used to evaluate patients following renal transplantation include radionuclide scintigraphy, magnetic resonance angiography, and computed tomography (CT). These modalities are typically used to further delineate an abnormality first identified on US or to investigate a particular clinical question following a negative or equivocal sonogram.

PRETRANSPLANT WORKUP

Renal transplantation may be performed with HLA-matched DDs or HLA-matched living donors (LDs) that are either related or unrelated. Survival outcomes are best for LD renal transplants.[5] In addition to the history, physical examination, and regular laboratory workup, pretransplant evaluation of the living renal transplant donor generally includes cross-sectional imaging to evaluate the renal anatomy for congenital anomalies and to exclude underlying pathology.[1] The vascular anatomy of the donor kidney is particularly important, as preoperative knowledge of the number, length, location, and branching patterns of the renal arteries aid the surgeon in his/her surgical approach.[7] In the past, conventional angiography was the procedure of choice, but technical advances have made CT angiography and magnetic resonance angiography viable alternatives, both showing good correlation with surgical findings.[7,8] In general, the left kidney is preferred for harvesting as the renal vein is longer.

SURGICAL TECHNIQUE

The renal transplant is preferentially placed in the extraperitoneal space in the right iliac fossa because the sigmoid colon limits space on the left. Intraperitoneal placement may occasionally be performed in children. For DD renal transplants, a small oval portion of the aortic wall surrounding the renal ostium, known as a Carrel patch, is often harvested along with the intact main renal artery and anastomosed in an end-to-side fashion with the external iliac artery (EIA; Figure 34-1). With LD renal transplants, the

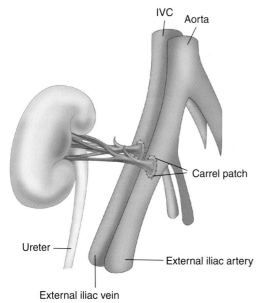

FIGURE 34-1 Schematic diagram demonstrating the most common surgical anastomoses performed in a deceased donor (DD) renal transplant. The Carrel patch is a small circumferential rim of the aortic wall surrounding the ostium of the donor main renal artery. This allows for a larger arterial anastomosis as well as less potential for injury and manipulation of the main renal artery in comparison to the direct end-to-side approach necessary for a living donor (LD) renal transplant because the surrounding aortic wall cannot be harvested. Hence, renal artery stenosis is less common in DD than in LD renal transplants. IVC, inferior vena cava.

main renal artery is directly anastomosed either end to side with the EIA or less commonly end to end with the internal iliac artery. However, end-to-end anastomoses are more likely to stenose or thrombose.[9] The main renal artery is implanted into a region of the recipient EIA without significant atherosclerotic burden as determined by palpation. In the case of multiple renal arteries, a variety of surgical approaches can be used, including multiple individual end-to-side anastomoses, harvest of a larger Carrel patch including the origins of all the main and accessory renal arteries, or the creation of a "Y-graft" of the smaller to the dominant renal artery. The main renal vein (MRV) is anastomosed end to side to the external iliac vein (Figure 34-2, *E*). Urinary drainage is created via a ureteroneocystostomy, whereby the ureter is tunneled into the dome of the bladder, resulting in an orifice superior to the native ureterovesicular junction (UVJ), although variations such as implantation of the ureter into an interposed bowel segment are also sometimes performed.[2] A stent is commonly placed in the ureter (Figure 34-2, *F*) to reduce the incidence of ureteral stricture and extravasation of urine. Stents are usually removed after 2 weeks to 3 months. The placement of perinephric drains has been reported to decrease the incidence of lymphocele formation (personal communication, Yale Transplant Service).

NORMAL ULTRASOUND FINDINGS

The renal transplant is evaluated with gray-scale and color and pulse Doppler imaging. Relatively high frequency transducers (5 MHz) can often be used owing to the more superficial location of the renal allograft in the pelvis in comparison to the native kidney. The renal length is measured in maximal sagittal dimension and may increase following transplantation because of compensatory hypertrophy. However, changes in size from one examination to the next may indicate underlying pathology. Corticomedullary differentiation is typically more pronounced with the renal cortex relatively echogenic and the medullary pyramids more hypoechoic in comparison to the native kidney.[10,11] The renal pelvis is usually slightly dilated, which is thought to be secondary to multiple factors, including increased volume of urine production (one kidney doing the work of two), denervation of the autonomic nervous system, and perhaps minor dysfunction at the surgical UVJ.[11] However, dilatation of the infundibulum and/or calyces should raise the suspicion for a distal ureteral obstruction.[11]

Color and spectral Doppler evaluation of the renal parenchyma, the main renal artery and vein, including their anastomoses, and the recipient iliac vessels are routinely obtained (Figure 34-2, A to E). On color or power Doppler interrogation, a normal transplant should demonstrate parenchymal blood flow arborizing out to the renal capsule without focal areas of decreased vascularity. Peak systolic velocity (PSV) in both the main renal artery and EIA is measured. PSV in the transplanted main renal artery may be elevated in comparison to the native main renal artery, with an upper limit of normal of approximately 200 to 250 cm/sec, likely due to acute angle of takeoff from the EIA and/or tortuosity of the main renal artery. The spectral tracing of the normal renal artery (Figure 34-2, B to D) in the transplanted kidney has a sharp systolic upstroke and continuous forward diastolic flow, reflecting the presence of a low-resistance peripheral vascular bed, and is similar in appearance to the spectral tracing of a normal native renal artery. The resistivity index (RI) of the intraparenchymal renal arteries is measured at the upper, mid, and lower poles in the segmental and interlobar vessels. The normal RI should be less than 0.7 (see Figure 34-2, D). An RI greater than 0.8 is considered abnormal. On the other hand, the recipient EIA should demonstrate a high-resistance waveform pattern with absent or reversed diastolic flow. The MRV is interrogated to demonstrate patency and exclude renal vein thrombosis. Flow may be slightly pulsatile due to close proximity to the adjacent main renal artery. At our institutions, a baseline examination is performed immediately following surgery and subsequently as clinically indicated.

COMMON PARENCHYMAL CAUSES OF GRAFT DYSFUNCTION

The most common causes of renal transplant failure include acute tubular necrosis (ATN), rejection (hyperacute, acute, and chronic), and drug toxicity. Clinical presentation is typically nonspecific except in regard to time of onset. Hyperacute rejection, for example, typically presents in the recovery room, and ATN most commonly is noted 2 to 3 days after transplantation, whereas acute or chronic rejection and drug toxicity present later. Similarly, sonographic findings are also nonspecific and unpredictable. Both increased as

well as decreased echogenicity of the renal parenchyma, indistinct but also increased or decreased corticomedullary differentiation, decreased visibility of the renal sinus, and allograft swelling with or without increased cortical thickness have all been described.[6] Spectral Doppler findings may include an elevated RI greater than 0.80, which is a nonspecific finding of renal dysfunction likely reflecting increased peripheral vascular resistance from a myriad of factors, including anything that can cause interstitial edema.[6] Conversely, a normal RI does not exclude underlying pathology. While serial measurements of RI may be helpful to determine progression or therapeutic efficacy of intervention, biopsy with serologic correlation remains the gold standard for diagnosis of the underlying cause of graft failure in most cases.[11-20]

ATN is the most common cause of graft dysfunction in the immediate postoperative period, occurring in up to 34% of DD renal transplants.[14,15] Ischemic insult to the renal transplant parenchyma before revascularization is typically the primary cause of ATN. Risk factors include prolonged ischemic time (>24 hours), hypotension or excessive blood loss during surgery, prolonged illness or intensive care unit stay of the donor, a donor without spontaneous cardiac activity, and reperfusion injury. ATN is unusual in LD renal transplants unless problems, such as hypotension, occur during surgery. ATN typically begins 2 to 3 days postoperatively, but can be severe and develop immediately following the transplant procedure. While some degree of ATN may persist for up to 3 months, most cases resolve within 2 to 3 weeks, although 10% to 30% of patients may require temporary dialysis.[16] Of note, it is believed that the process of tubular repair increases the risk for later development of acute rejection.[13] While the surgeon knows preoperatively which donor kidneys are at risk and can recognize a lack of "pinking up" of the kidney once it is revascularized, the clinical presentation of renal failure and decreased urine output in patients with ATN is nonspecific. Nor are gray-scale US findings helpful in making the diagnosis. On Doppler US interrogation, decreased diastolic flow or increase in RI is typical of ATN (Figure 34-3) but is also a nonspecific finding seen in many causes of graft dysfunction. In general, the higher the RI, the worse the ATN, and actual reversal of diastolic flow may be observed in extreme cases.[21] An RI greater

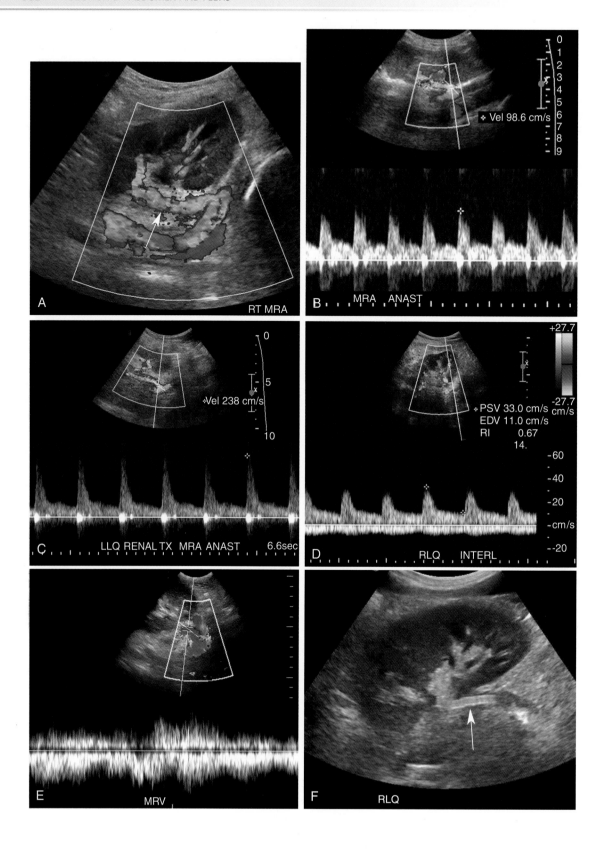

FIGURE 34-2 Doppler ultrasound findings in a normal renal transplant. **A,** End-to-side anastomosis of the main renal artery (MRA) *(arrow)* with the recipient external iliac artery. The transplant is located in the right (RT) lower quadrant. **B,** In another patient, pulsed Doppler waveform at the arterial anastomosis (ANAST) has a sharp systolic upstroke, continuous forward diastolic flow, and a peak systolic velocity (PSV) of 99 cm/sec. **C,** In a third patient, PSV is higher, 238 cm/sec, at the MRA anesthesia, but there was no narrowing on the gray-scale image, no distal turbulence or tardus-parvus waveform changes, and the patient did not have hypertension. In the normal patient, PSV may be elevated close to 200-250 cm/sec at the MRA anastomosis, particularly immediately postoperatively. Increased PSV may be due to slight torquing of the vessel, postsurgical edema, increased flow through the single artery, or secondary to acute angle of takeoff from the iliac vessel. **D,** Pulsed Doppler tracing from an interlobar artery (INTERL) demonstrates a sharp systolic upstroke and continuous forward diastolic flow with a resistivity index (RI) of 0.67. Note intraparenchymal venous flow below the baseline. **E,** Duplex Doppler image of the end-to-side venous anastomosis of the main renal vein (MRV) with the recipient external iliac vein reveals no narrowing and no color aliasing. Note transmission of respiratory variation. The spectral tracing may be flat, however, in some cases due to compression from the transplanted kidney. **F,** Note tubular structure with two echogenic parallel lines *(arrow)* in the renal hilum. A stent *(arrow)* is often left for up to 3 months in the ureter to promote healing without stricture or extravasation of urine. Stent placement decreases the likelihood that a patient will develop a urinoma.

than 0.73 30 minutes postoperatively has been described as strongly predictive of the development of ATN.[22]

Hyperacute rejection occurs in the immediate (<24 hours) postsurgical period, usually in the recovery room, and is extremely rare in today's practice due to preoperative HLA matching. Doppler interrogation may not be able to detect parenchymal blood flow because of intense vasospasm and interstitial edema. Hence, findings may mimic renal artery thrombosis (RAT). If blood flow is seen, diastolic flow is typically absent or even reversed and the RI is markedly elevated.[21]

Acute rejection is estimated to occur in up to 20% to 40% of all renal transplants and usually develops within 1 to 3 weeks to months after transplantation.[19] However, new immunosuppressant regimens have decreased the incidence of acute rejection in recent years.[19] Most patients are asymptomatic, but flu-like symptoms, graft tenderness, and low-grade fever along with deteriorating renal function are occasionally reported. Patients may present with a rapid rise (>25%) of serum creatinine level over a 1- to 2-day period.[17,18,20] Swelling of the graft, pruning of parenchymal blood flow, and increased RI are nonspecific findings in moderate to severe cases on Doppler US examination. However, these are nonspecific findings, and diagnosis requires biopsy. In most cases, acute rejection can be treated with steroids or by increasing immunosuppression. However, an episode of acute rejection is an indicator of future transplant failure.[23]

Chronic rejection manifests as a progressive decline in renal function beginning at least 3 months after surgery and may ultimately lead to renal failure.[6] A prior episode of acute rejection is the most common predisposing risk factor. Gray-scale imaging may demonstrate a decrease in kidney length with a thinned and echogenic cortex. The RI may be increased on spectral Doppler interrogation.[6]

Cyclosporine and tacrolimus (calcineurin inhibitors) are extremely effective immunosuppressive agents. However, both are nephrotoxic, causing renovascular constriction and interstitial fibrosis. Reactivation of polyomavirus is associated with these drugs and is also reported to cause nephropathy. Since the clinical presentation, time course, and Doppler US findings of drug toxicity and chronic rejection are indistinguishable, differentiation between these two causes of renal failure requires biopsy and careful correlation with serum drug levels.[11,19,20]

Pyelonephritis may cause diffuse or focal areas of either increased or decreased echogenicity. A segmental infarct may cause a similar focal appearance, although an infarct is often more sharply marginated and wedge shaped. A segmental infarct will also be avascular on color or power Doppler interrogation (Figure 34-4).

VASCULAR COMPLICATIONS

Doppler US is considered the primary screening modality for the diagnosis of vascular complications. Vascular complications occur in less than 10% of renal allograft recipients[24] but are

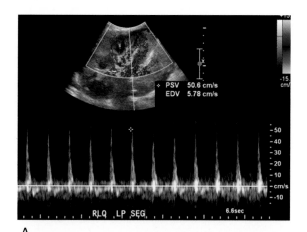
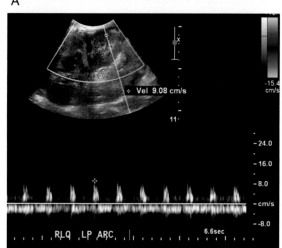
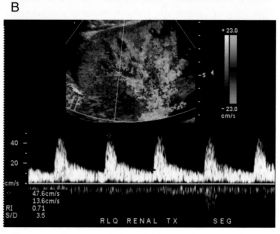

FIGURE 34-3 Acute tubular necrosis (ATN). Two days after deceased donor renal transplantation the patient developed decreased urine output and increasing serum creatinine levels. Duplex Doppler ultrasound (US) examination reveals no evidence of hydronephrosis, but tracings from the segmental (SEG; **A**) and arcuate (ARC; **B**) arteries reveal no evidence of diastolic flow with a resistivity index (RI) of 1.0. In this time frame, increase in RI is most often due to ATN. Repeat US in 3 weeks **(C)** demonstrates improvement in diastolic flow and a normal RI of 0.71. Renal function was now normal. Note the normal venous flow below the baseline. TX, transplant.

often treatable causes of graft dysfunction. Renal artery and renal vein thrombosis tend to occur in the immediate postoperative course, whereas stenoses of these vessels typically develop more than 5 to 6 months following transplantation. Postbiopsy complications include arteriovenous fistulas (AVFs) and pseudoaneurysms (PSAs).

RAT typically occurs very early in the postoperative period. Immediate diagnosis is critical so that thrombectomy or thrombolysis can be performed to prevent graft loss. RAT has a reported incidence of less than 1% and is more common in LD transplant recipients, in patients with complex arterial anastomoses, and in pediatric transplants due to the small size of the main renal artery.[2,12,24] Acute and hyperacute rejection, underlying hypercoagulable states, arterial kinks, arterial dissections, vessel size mismatch, ATN, prolonged ischemic time, or faulty surgical technique have all been reported as underlying causes of RAT.[2,12,19,20] Clinically, patients with RAT present with acute anuria and tenderness over the graft.[2] On color, power, or spectral Doppler US, neither arterial nor venous flow will be seen distal to the site of occlusion[2,10,12,19,24-26] (Figures 34-5 and 34-6). The kidney may appear relatively hypoechoic and enlarged on gray-scale imaging. Focal or segmental infarcts occur most commonly in the setting of embolus, acute rejection, cytomegalovirus (CMV) infection, vasculitis, separate anastomosis of a small polar artery, or scarring due to injury from the perfusion catheter. On US, focal infarcts typically manifest as well-defined wedge-shaped to round avascular masses or regions. Echogenicity is variable depending upon the time course and whether or not hemorrhage into the infarct has occurred (see Figure 34-4). Focal pyelonephritis may have a similar appearance.

Renal vein thrombosis (RVT) has a reported incidence of approximately 5%.[2] It usually occurs within the first postoperative week, and patients also present with abrupt onset of oliguria, graft swelling, and tenderness.[12] If detected

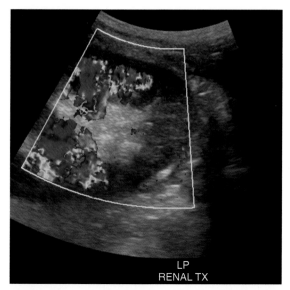

FIGURE 34-4 Focal renal infarct. Note complete absence of color flow to the lower pole (LP) of the renal transplant (TX). Focal infarcts may be due to embolus, infection, or progression of distal or branch stenosis in the main renal artery due to periprocedural injury of the arterial wall from the perfusion catheter or cellular infiltration of the vessel wall due to rejection. Occasionally an accessory main renal artery with a separate, small anastomosis may thrombose, causing a polar infarct.

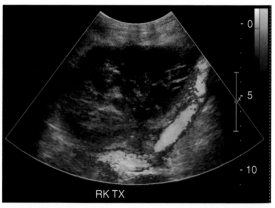

FIGURE 34-5 Renal artery thrombosis. Note complete absence of blood flow signals to the entire transplanted kidney on this sagittal power Doppler image. This patient presented with acute pain as well as anuria 1 day postoperatively. The patient was returned to the operating room immediately following the ultrasound examination, and an arterial thrombectomy was performed. Although blood flow was restored, the patient developed severe acute tubular necrosis requiring dialysis. Eventually renal function recovered.

early, thrombectomy may prevent graft loss. However, nephrectomy and retransplantation are required if infarction has already occurred by the time of diagnosis.[2] Predisposing risk factors include hypotension, hypercoagulable states, acute rejection, anastomotic stenosis, venous compression from perinephric fluid collections, and propagation of an underlying clot in the iliac vein[2,12,19,20,24-26] (Figure 34-7). RVT occurs slightly more commonly in transplants placed in the left iliac fossa, possibly due to compression of the left iliac vein by the overlying artery and aorta. Gray-scale findings are nonspecific and include enlargement of the renal graft with decreased parenchymal echogenicity.[12] The MRV may be enlarged and filled with hypoechoic thrombus, although acute thrombus can be anechoic. Doppler interrogation will demonstrate absence of venous flow associated with increased resistance in the renal arteries to the point of reversed diastolic flow (Figure 34-8).[2,12,19,20,24-26] However, reversal of diastolic arterial flow alone (i.e., without demonstration of concomitant absence of venous flow) is a nonspecific finding and can be seen in patients with hyperacute rejection, severe ATN, and compression of the renal parenchyma

by surrounding fluid collections, resulting in the Page kidney phenomenon (Figure 34-9).[15,21]

Renal artery stenosis (RAS) is the most common vascular complication in renal transplants, with an incidence ranging from 1% to 12%.[12,19,20,24] RAS is more common in LD than DD transplants because harvesting of the main renal artery with a Carrel patch likely protects the renal ostium in a DD transplant. End-to-end anastomoses have the highest risk for developing RAS.[9] As with RAT, the incidence of RAS is higher in patients with complex arterial anastomoses and in pediatric transplants. Stenosis generally occurs after 3 months and within the first 3 years after transplantation. Patients present with new onset or worsening of severe, refractory hypertension.[2,12,24,25] On physical examination, a bruit may be audible over the transplanted kidney.[2] Causes of RAS are postulated to include intimal fibrosis/scarring, faulty surgical technique, vessel injury from the perfusion catheter, allergic reaction to the suture material, and rejection.[2,12,19,20,24-26] Stenoses occur most commonly at the main renal artery anastomosis. Distal stenoses are infrequent and may be a sign of allograft rejection or prior dissection and/or endothelial damage from the perfusion catheter.[2] In the early postoperative period, compression, kinking, or torquing of the renal artery may cause a functional RAS, particularly in patients with an

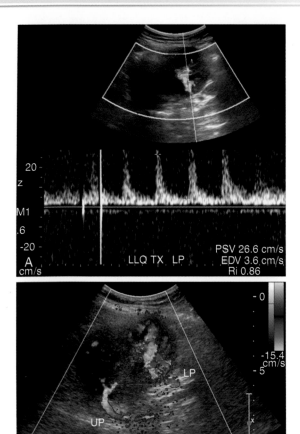

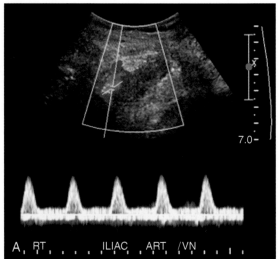

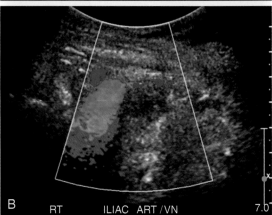

FIGURE 34-6 Renal artery thrombosis. This living related donor transplant had two main renal arteries (MRAs) with separate end-to-side anastomoses with the recipient external iliac artery. **A,** Postoperative baseline duplex Doppler examination in the recovery room demonstrates no evidence of flow in the parenchyma of the upper pole, and the more superior MRA could not be identified. Relatively poor diastolic flow with a resistivity index (RI) of 0.96 is noted in a segmental artery to the lower pole (LP). The transplant is located in the left lower quadrant (LLQTX). Findings are consistent with acute thrombosis of the MRA to the upper pole. It was thought that swelling of the upper pole caused compression of the LP, resulting in increased peripheral vascular resistance and decreased diastolic flow with resulting increase in RI. **B,** Following surgical thrombectomy, flow is restored to the upper pole and the superior MRA is now well seen. Note increased flow to the LP as well.

FIGURE 34-7 Deep venous thrombosis. This patient presented with leg pain and swelling following transplantation. Duplex Doppler image **(A)** and color Doppler image **(B)** demonstrate flow in the right (RT) external iliac artery (ART) (red) but no flow in the adjacent external iliac vein (VN). Note echoes within the external iliac vein (EIV)—tubular in **A** and round in **B**—inferior to the external iliac artery consistent with acute deep venous thrombosis. External compression of the pelvic veins from the transplanted kidney may result in slow flow in the EIV, increasing the risk for developing deep venous thrombosis. Extension of thrombus from the EIV is an uncommon cause of renal vein thrombosis in the transplanted kidney.

excessively long or redundant vascular pedicle (see later). In such cases, stenosis of the MRV with or without elevated Doppler velocities is usually observed. Stenosis in the native EIA near the arterial anastomosis due to atherosclerosis or clamp injury can mimic RAS clinically as well as on Doppler US examination.[2]

On color Doppler imaging, focal color aliasing indicates high-velocity flow and localizes the site of the stenosis.[6,12] Pulsed Doppler criteria include (1) PSV greater than 200 to 250 cm/sec, (2) PSV velocity ratio of at least 2:1 between the PSV at the stenosis and the arterial segment proximal to the stenosis, (3) spectral broadening of the arterial waveform immediately distal to the stenosis, and (4) a tardus-parvus waveform in the distal intraparenchymal vessels[2,12,19,20,25-32]

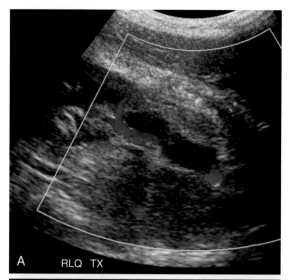

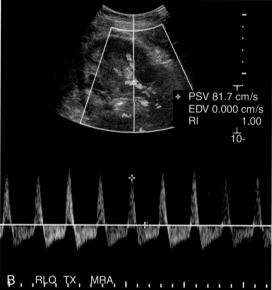

FIGURE 34-8 Renal vein thrombosis (RVT). **A,** Color Doppler image demonstrates no flow in the main renal vein anterior to the main renal artery (red) in a transplant (TX) in the right lower quadrant (RLQ). **B,** Duplex Doppler waveform demonstrates a high-resistance pattern in the main renal artery (MRA) with reversed diastolic flow. While RVT is the most common cause of such a waveform pattern in the immediate postoperative period, it is a nonspecific finding and may be seen in hyperacute rejection, severe acute tubular necrosis, and compression of the renal parenchyma by surrounding fluid collections (Page kidney; see Figure 34-9).

(Figure 34-10). However, PSV at the main renal artery anastomosis is often much higher than the PSV at the origin of the native main renal artery due to tortuosity of a redundant artery, acute angle of takeoff from the EIA, or increased flow volume.[26] Therefore, some authors advocate

using a PSV of 300 cm/sec as a diagnostic threshold.[27] Still, increased PSV is not as specific a finding of RAS in the transplanted kidney as it is in the native renal artery. Tardus-parvus waveforms, either identified subjectively or by measuring acceleration time greater than 70 to 100 msec, add specificity to the diagnosis,[26,28] although the presence of this waveform pattern merely indicates a proximal stenosis somewhere—which also could be at the level of the EIA, aorta, or even aortic valve. The sensitivity of Doppler US for the detection of RAS has been reported to range from 87% to 94% with specificities of 86% to 100%, but these vary depending upon the specific Doppler criteria. Higher thresholds increase specificity at the expense of sensitivity.[27-31] Therefore, due to the lack of specificity of Doppler US findings and the fact that most hypertensive renal transplant recipients do not have RAS, confirmatory imaging with non–contrast-enhanced magnetic resonance angiography is often suggested. Administration of gadolinium is generally avoided in renal transplant recipients, especially those with reduced renal function, due to the risk for nephrogenic systemic fibrosis. Similarly, iodinated intravenous contrast is also avoided due to the risk for renal failure. RAS may be treated via percutaneous transluminal angioplasty, arterial stenting, or less commonly, surgical revascularization.[2]

Renal vein stenosis (RVS) is an uncommon vascular complication and is usually caused by extrinsic compression from an adjacent perinephric fluid collection or perivascular fibrosis.[6] Duplex Doppler US findings include narrowing of the vessel with focal color aliasing and high velocities in the region of stenosis (Figure 34-11).[25] No specific Doppler or gray-scale criteria have been established to grade RVS, and the clinical significance of RVS is debatable, although a threefold to fourfold increase in velocity at the stenosis has been reported as possibly clinically significant in a patient with renal dysfunction.[26,32] Stenting is the treatment of choice.

Biopsy of the renal cortex is frequently performed to establish the etiology of allograft dysfunction.[2] Complications of this procedure include hematomas, AVFs, and PSAs. Most postbiopsy perinephric hematomas are small and do not require treatment unless they are expanding and/or compressing the renal parenchyma or vascular pedicle.[33] Most AVFs and PSAs are also small, clinically insignificant, and will resolve spontaneously. PSAs greater than 2 cm in

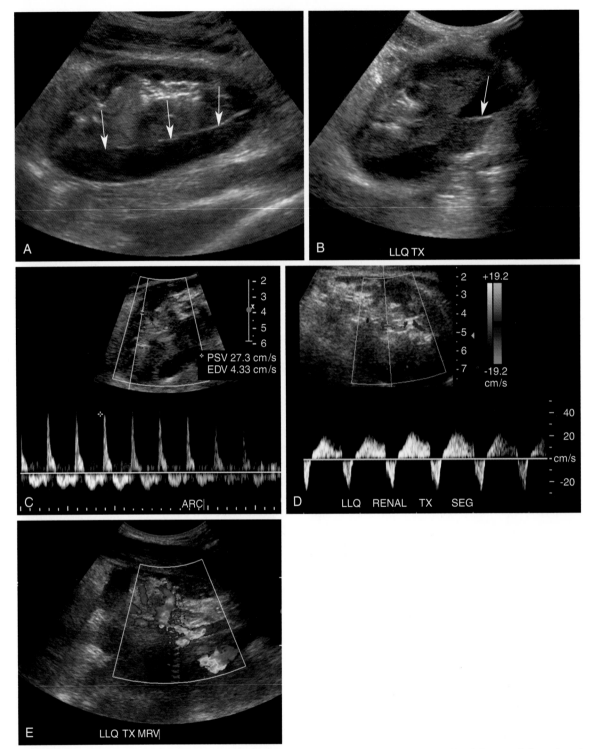

FIGURE 34-9 Page kidney. This patient presented with pain and decreased urine output 1 day following living related donor transplantation. Sagittal **(A)** and oblique transverse **(B)** gray-scale images demonstrate a complex fluid collection surrounding the kidney and distorting the renal parenchyma (*arrows* in **A**). A fluid/fluid level is noted (*arrow* in **B**). LLQ, left lower quadrant. Findings are consistent with a large subcapsular hematoma with hematocrit level compressing the renal parenchyma. Spectral Doppler tracings demonstrate reversed diastolic flow, similar to Figure 34-8, *B,* in the arcuate (ARC; **C**) and segmental (SEG; **D**) arteries. However, color Doppler image of the renal hilum **(E)** demonstrates venous flow (blue) in the main as well as parenchymal renal veins. In this case the reversed diastolic flow was caused by the Page kidney phenomenon (i.e., increased peripheral vascular resistance due to compression of the renal parenchyma from the surrounding hematoma). Unfortunately, despite surgical decompression, severe acute tubular necrosis developed, and the kidney never regained function and had to be removed.

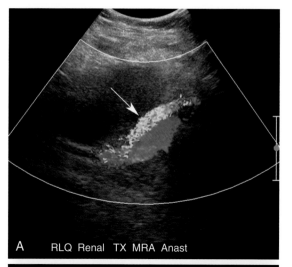

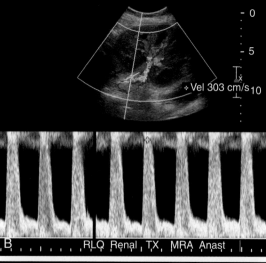

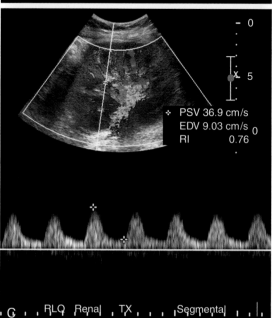

FIGURE 34-10 Renal artery stenosis (RAS). This patient presented with severe hypertension 6 months following living donor renal transplantation. **A,** Color Doppler image demonstrates focal color aliasing *(arrow)* in the main renal artery (MRA) above the main renal vein (blue). TX, transplant; RLQ, right lower quadrant. Spectral Doppler tracings reveal marked increase in peak systolic velocity (PSV) of 303 cm/sec at the main renal artery anastomosis (Anast; **B**) and mild horizontal sloping of systolic upstroke (tardus-parvus waveform) in a segmental artery **(C)**. These findings are consistent with the diagnosis of RAS. The presence of the tardus-parvus waveform increases the specificity of the Doppler finding of increased PSV at the MRA anastomosis since an elevated PSV can be seen in some patients without RAS. The focal color aliasing and increased PSV in the MRA help to locate the site of the stenosis.

diameter and large AVFs resulting in renal ischemia, hematuria, or congestive heart failure will require percutaneous embolization.[2,12,19,20,25] The incidence of clinically important AVFs and PSAs is significantly reduced if US guidance is used to ensure that the renal sinus containing the larger segmental arteries and veins is avoided. A tangential approach through the cortex is safest. Extrarenal AVFs and PSAs are usually due to faulty surgical technique, breakdown of the anastomosis, or infection and generally require intervention due to their large size and risk for rupture (Figure 34-12).

Damage to both the artery and vein may result in a fistulous connection (AVF) between these two structures.[2,12,19,20,24-26] Color Doppler imaging may demonstrate disorganized color signals outside the normal borders of the vessels, termed a soft tissue bruit, a finding attributed to perifistula soft tissue vibration. Focal color aliasing will also be observed due to high-velocity flow within the feeding artery.[2,12,32] Spectral Doppler interrogation demonstrates a characteristic high-velocity, low-resistance waveform within the feeding artery and pulsatile high-velocity flow in the draining vein (Figure 34-13).* Dilatation of the draining vein may mimic a cystic structure on gray-scale imaging.

Escape of blood through a puncture in the arterial wall may lead to the formation of a PSA. Extra-arterial flow is contained by a pseudocapsule formed by compression of the surrounding

*References 2,12,19,20,24-26,32.

FIGURE 34-11 Renal vein stenosis (RVS). **A,** Color Doppler image reveals focal color aliasing *(long arrow)* at the site of the anastomosis of the main renal vein (MRV) with the external iliac vein (EIV) in this renal transplant (TX) placed in the right lower quadrant (RLQ). The main renal vein to the upper pole is indicated by the short arrow. The external iliac artery is indicated in red. **B,** Spectral Doppler tracing from the EIV demonstrates a velocity of 15 cm/sec in comparison to a velocity of over 200 cm/sec in the MRV at the anastomosis **(C)**. Velocity ratio is over 13:1, consistent with a tight stenosis of the MRV. In the setting of renal failure, stent placement would be advised. Without evidence of graft dysfunction, however, the clinical significance of this finding is uncertain, and ultrasound follow-up would be recommended.

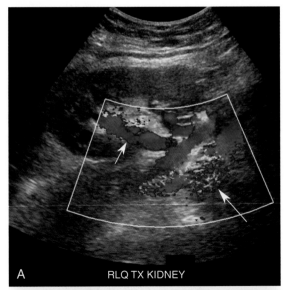

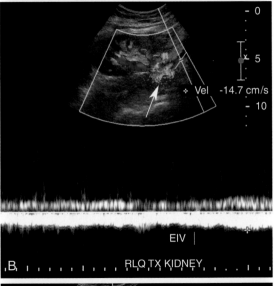

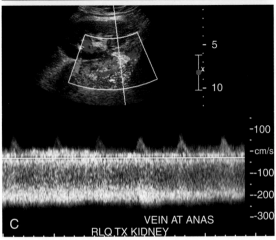

soft tissues.[12] Gray-scale imaging will demonstrate an anechoic cyst-like structure that may contain intraluminal thrombus.[†] On color imaging, a "yin-yang" pattern (red on one side and blue on the other) of swirling blood flow will be seen in the PSA, and a characteristic "to-and-fro" pattern with flow above the baseline heading toward the PSA in systole and reversed flow or flow below the baseline heading away from the PSA in diastole will be observed in the neck of the PSA (Figure 34-14).[‡]

Torsion of the vascular pedicle is a rare complication occurring when the transplant is placed within the peritoneal cavity or when the main renal artery and MRV are excessively long and redundant.[34] Torsion presents early in the post-operative period and may be complete or partial.[34] Clinical signs are nonspecific, with patients complaining of abdominal tenderness and swelling.[25,34] Early recognition of this complication is of paramount importance as surgical revision or detorquing is necessary to improve blood flow to the transplanted kidney and to prevent the development of RAT, RVT, or ATN—although long-term outcomes remain poor.[34] Minimal degrees of torsion may resolve spontaneously as the kidney settles in the iliac fossa and surrounding swelling/hemorrhage is reabsorbed. Gray-scale imaging may demonstrate malrotation of the kidney, with the hilum pointing anteriorly rather than posteriorly.[34] Twisting of the ureter may result in hydronephrosis and thickening of the uroepithelium. Color Doppler findings are variable, ranging from

†References 2,12,19,20,24-26,32.
‡References 2,12,19,20,24-26,32.

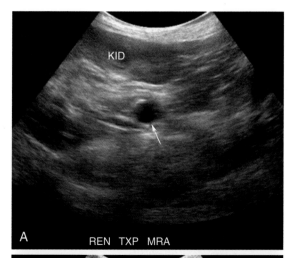

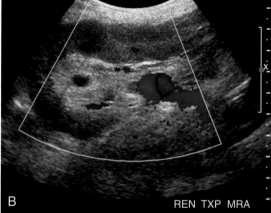

FIGURE 34-12 Extrarenal pseudoaneurysm (PSA). **A,** Oblique sagittal gray-scale image of the renal hilum demonstrates an anechoic round structure *(arrow)* above the main renal artery (MRA) in a renal transplant (REN TX). KID, kidney. **B,** Color Doppler image demonstrates a yin-yang pattern of swirling blood flow diagnostic of a PSA. Due to the size and extrarenal location, bleeding would likely be extensive if rupture were to occur.

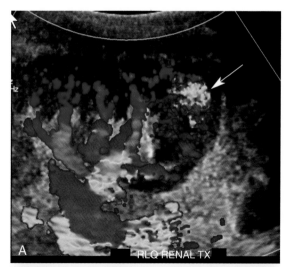

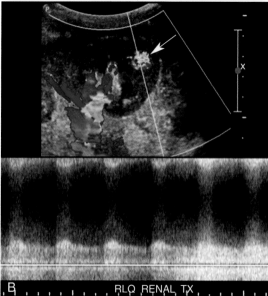

FIGURE 34-13 Arteriovenous fistula (AVF). This patient with a renal transplant (TX) in the right lower quadrant (RLQ) underwent renal biopsy to assess the cause of renal failure 2 days previously. **A,** Color Doppler image of the lower pole demonstrates a focal area of color aliasing *(arrow)* indicative of high-velocity flow. **B,** spectral Doppler tracing from this area demonstrates an arterial waveform with high peak systolic as well as high end-diastolic velocity consistent with an arteriovenous shunt. These findings are diagnostic of an AVF *(arrow).* The draining vein demonstrated a pulsatile high-velocity waveform (not shown). The amount of blood shunted through the fistula cannot be determined by Doppler ultrasound. Since most AVFs will close spontaneously, follow-up is generally recommended unless there are signs of graft ischemia, hematuria, or congestive heart failure, in which case percutaneous embolization is the treatment of choice.

normal to reversal of arterial diastolic flow. Torsion should be suspected in the immediate postoperative period if increased blood flow velocity is noted in adjacent portions of the main renal artery and vein at a location distal to the anastomoses. If torsion is complete, Doppler findings may be indistinguishable from RAT and RVT and no parenchymal blood flow will be detected.[34]

PERINEPHRIC FLUID COLLECTIONS

Perinephric fluid collections include hematomas, seromas, lymphoceles, urinomas, and abscesses and are extremely common. While US is useful in delineating the size and presence of a fluid collection as well as the significance of any mass

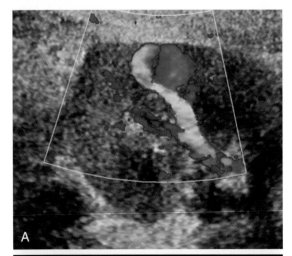

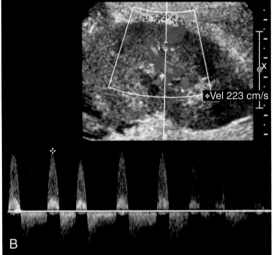

FIGURE 34-14 Intrarenal pseudoaneurysm (PSA). **A,** Transverse color Doppler image of the transplanted kidney demonstrates a round area with a yin-yang pattern (red/blue) of color flow consistent with a PSA. Note color aliasing with turquoise and yellow speckled color pattern in the feeding vessel (neck), indicating high-velocity flow. **B,** Pulsed Doppler tracing in the neck of the PSA reveals a classic to-and-fro blood flow pattern with flow heading toward the PSA in systole and away from the PSA in diastole.

effect upon the renal allograft, the gray-scale and color Doppler appearances are nonspecific.[9] Differentiating between these entities is typically based on the time course of the findings and symptoms, although definitive diagnosis may require percutaneous aspiration.[2] Any of these fluid collections may become superinfected and form an abscess. Hence, correlation with white blood cell count, fever, and tenderness is critical, although signs and symptoms of infection may be masked by immunosuppression.

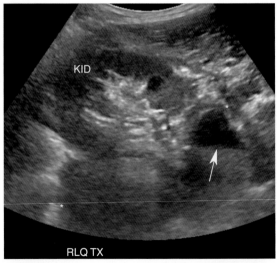

FIGURE 34-15 Perinephric hematoma. Baseline study performed in the recovery room. Note large, complex lobular echogenic fluid collection (*) medial and inferior to the transplanted kidney (KID). Most perinephric collections identified immediately postoperatively will be hematomas. In addition, there is a fluid/fluid or "hematocrit" level *(arrow),* suggesting that this is a hematoma. Most postoperative hematomas are small and clinically insignificant. However, because this large hematoma adjacent to the vascular pedicle was observed to grow during the course of the ultrasound examination, the patient was returned to the operating room to evacuate the hematoma and to tie off the bleeding vessel.

Small postoperative perinephric hematomas are extremely common, perhaps ubiquitous, and most resolve spontaneously. Hematomas may also occur following biopsy or pelvic trauma. Large or expanding hematomas that displace the kidney, compressing the vascular pedicle or ureter, can respectively cause vascular compromise or hydronephrosis and may require surgical decompression (Figure 34-15).[2] A subcapsular hematoma may compress the renal parenchyma (Figure 34-16), resulting in renal dysfunction or ischemia, and require aspiration or surgical debridement. Rarely, the entire kidney may be compressed by a surrounding hematoma resulting in a Page kidney that results in renal ischemia and/or hypertension. In this setting, the increased peripheral vascular resistance caused by extrinsic compression of the kidney can diminish or even reverse diastolic flow (RI > 0.80) (see Figure 34-9).[33] On gray-scale imaging, acute hematomas are usually echogenic, becoming more anechoic and complex over time (see Figures 34-9, 34-15, and 34-16).

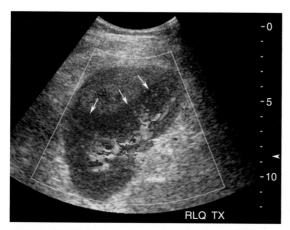

FIGURE 34-16 Subcapsular hematoma. Note echogenic avascular area conforming to the contour of the kidney but compressing and scalloping the renal cortex *(arrows)* in a patient presenting with pain following renal biopsy.

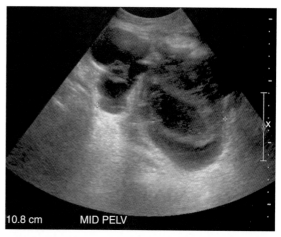

FIGURE 34-17 Lymphocele. Note large complex, septated fluid collection *(cursors)* medial to the kidney (not shown). This was an incidental finding in a patient evaluated 8 weeks after transplantation.

Layering of blood or a hematocrit level (see Figures 34-9 and 34-15) may rarely be seen.[2] A subcapsular collection will distort, compress, or scallop the renal parenchyma (see Figure 34-16). The subcapsular collection will not have any internal vascularity on Doppler interrogation.

Urinomas are relatively uncommon post-transplant fluid collections with an incidence of approximately 1%.[35] They typically occur within the first 2 weeks after surgery and may be due to extravasation of urine from the calyces, renal pelvis, ureter, or ureteroneocystostomy.[2] Leakage from the ureteroneocystostomy anastomosis may be due to surgical technique or ureteral necrosis from ischemia and/or rejection. The blood supply to the ureter is more tenuous than to the rest of the transplant, and ischemia due to poor blood supply and/or cellular infiltration from rejection may cause either necrosis, breakdown of the anastomosis, or ureteral stricture. Proximal or perihilar extravasation is more likely due to underlying obstruction (clot, calculi, debris, fungal balls) or ureteral stricture from instrumentation.[6] Patients with urinomas can present with abdominal tenderness, decreased urine output, and discharge from the wound.[6] On US, urinomas are well-defined anechoic fluid collections typically found between the renal graft and bladder.[2] Internal septations are uncommon in urinomas, thereby helping to distinguish them from hematomas or lymphoceles.[6] Interval increase in size of an anechoic fluid collection is also suggestive of a urinoma. Complications include superinfection

with abscess formation or rupture resulting in urinary ascites.[2]

Lymphoceles typically develop 4 to 8 weeks after surgery with a prevalence ranging from 0.5% to 20%.[2] Often an incidental finding, lymphoceles can compress the ureter and vascular pedicle, resulting in hydronephrosis and/or increased velocity in the main renal vein or artery. Rarely, lymphoceles may result in swelling of the scrotum, labia, or lower extremities.[6] Internal septations are often seen on US, but lymphoceles are typically anechoic. Lymphoceles are found most often medial to the renal transplant[2] but may occur anywhere surrounding the kidney (Figure 34-17). Large lymphoceles causing hydronephrosis or mass effect require surgical marsupialization or percutaneous drainage.[2] Recurrence rates are diminished with prolonged catheter drainage and sclerotherapy.[36,37]

On US, a perinephric abscess typically appears as a complex fluid collection containing low-level echoes. Increased peripheral vascularity may be present. However, the diagnosis of abscess must be strongly considered in any transplant recipient with signs and symptoms of infection and a perinephric fluid collection independent of the US appearance. Diagnosis is confirmed with aspiration, Gram stain, and culture.

Urinary tract obstruction occurs in less than 5% of renal transplants, usually occurring within the first 6 months.[2,6,35] Obstruction may be secondary to a variety of causes, including extrinsic compression from adjacent fluid collections, strictures from ischemia or rejection, or intraluminal obstruction of the collecting system from blood clot (Figure 34-18), calculi (Figure 34-19), fungus balls, or papillary necrosis.[2] The vast majority of strictures occur within the distal third of the ureter, most frequently at the UVJ, and are due to ischemia or poor surgical technique.[2] Renal transplant patients are at increased risk for calculi formation (see Figure 34-19) with a reported incidence of 1% to 2%, likely due to hypercalcemia from persistent secondary hyperparathyroidism.[38] Even patients

with obstructive renal calculi are usually asymptomatic secondary to denervation of the transplanted kidney.[2] Hematuria and/or intraluminal blood clot can be seen in the setting of renal biopsy,[39] necrosis/ischemia of the collection system, or tumor (see later), and, if observed, a careful search for underlying AVF, PSA, or mass should be made. Reliable sonographic diagnosis of urinary tract obstruction may be challenging, as some degree of mild to moderate pelvicaliectasis may be seen in nonobstructed transplant

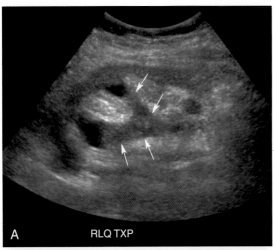

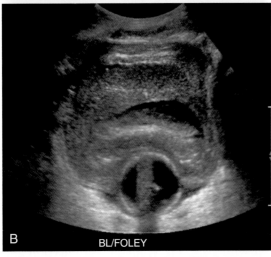

FIGURE 34-18 Hemorrhage in the collecting system. This patient presented with hematuria following renal biopsy. Other images (not shown) demonstrated an arteriovenous fistula. **A,** Gray-scale image demonstrates distention of the intrarenal collecting system with echogenic material (clot; *arrows*). Pyonephrosis could have a similar ultrasound appearance but different clinical presentation consistent with infection and pyuria. **B,** Transverse gray-scale image demonstrates that the bladder (BL) is also filled with echogenic layering clot/hemorrhage. A Foley catheter is present in the bladder lumen.

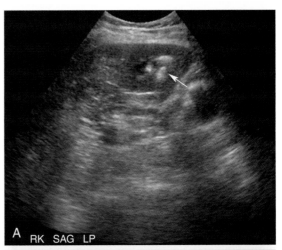

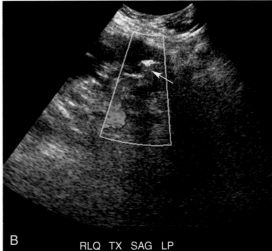

FIGURE 34-19 Renal calculi. **A,** Gray-scale sagittal (SAG) image demonstrates three echogenic foci at the lower pole (LP) of the transplanted kidney *(arrow)*. Although these do not shadow, a color Doppler image **(B)** demonstrates twinkle artifact *(arrow)*, confirming that at least one of these echogenic foci is a renal calculus. These stones are nonobstructing, and the patient is asymptomatic. However, patients may be asymptomatic even during passage of stones as the transplanted kidney is denervated.

patients.[2] However, dilatation of the minor calyces suggests underlying obstruction, and evaluation of the allograft after voiding may be helpful to exclude reflux. In a patient with pelvicaliectasis, an otherwise unexplained increase in RI (>0.70) suggests underlying obstruction (Figure 34-20).

NEOPLASM

Renal transplant recipients have a substantially increased risk for developing cancers, most commonly lymphoma and skin cancers, due to prolonged immunosuppression.[40] However, rectal and cervical carcinomas and renal cell carcinoma in either the native or transplanted kidney (Figure 34-21) occur at an increased frequency.[2,6,41] Posttransplant lymphoproliferative disorder (PTLPD) is reported in approximately 0.9% to 2.5% of renal transplant recipients.[42-44]

Reactivation of the Epstein-Barr virus and possibly CMV infection in the setting of immunosuppression is thought to result in a monoclonal proliferation of B cells.[6,12,42-44] The disease spectrum ranges from a mild mononucleosis flu-like syndrome to a high-grade solid lymphoma.[42] Early PTLPD tends to affect younger patients within the first year after transplantation. These patients often do well with antiviral therapy and decrease in the level of immunosuppression. Late-onset PTLPD is a more aggressive disorder with poor prognosis and tends to present more than 2.5 years after transplant.[21] Although any solid organ may be affected, common presentations include solid parenchymal renal masses (Figure 34-22, A), diffuse parenchymal infiltration (Figure 34-22, B), or perihilar lymphadenopathy that can compress or encase the ureter and vascular pedicle.[6,42-44]

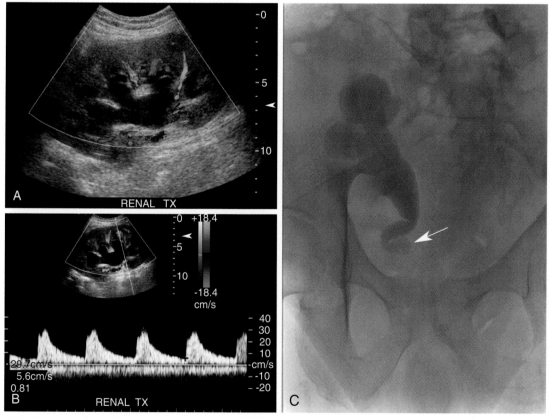

FIGURE 34-20 Hydronephrosis. **A,** Sagittal color Doppler image of a renal transplant (TX) demonstrates dilatation of the collecting system. While mild dilatation of the collecting system in the transplanted kidney is common due to increased urine output and loss of the autonomic nervous system, the dilatation of the calyces and of the infundibulum suggests obstruction. In addition, pulsed Doppler waveforms **(B)** show decreased diastolic flow and increased resistive index of 0.81. These findings imply that the collecting system is obstructed and that the obstruction is physiologically significant since it causes increased vascular resistance. **C,** Percutaneous nephrostogram reveals a stricture of the distal ureter *(arrow)* and hydronephrosis.

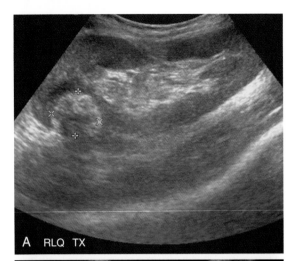

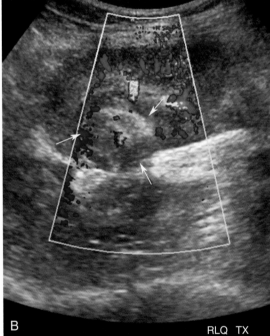

FIGURE 34-21 Renal cell carcinoma in a transplanted kidney. **A,** Sagittal gray-scale image of a renal transplant (TX) in the right lower quadrant (RLQ) reveals a heterogeneous echogenic mass *(cursors)* at the upper pole. **B,** Color Doppler image demonstrates vascularity within the mass *(arrows)*, confirming its solid nature. Although an angiomyolipoma (AML) could be echogenic, AMLs are usually not so heterogeneous or vascular and are unlikely to develop de novo in a renal transplant. This mass was proven on biopsy to be a renal cell carcinoma and was treated with nephron-sparing surgery.

FUTURE DIRECTIONS

Contrast-enhanced ultrasound (CE-US) with intravenous injection of microbubbles is a developing methodology for the evaluation of organ perfusion and cortical enhancement patterns.

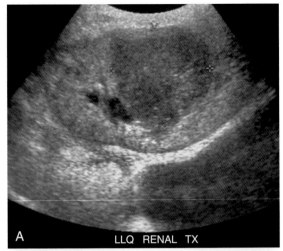

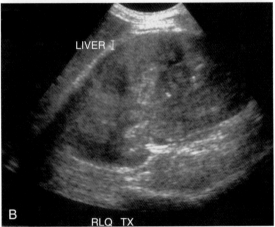

FIGURE 34-22 Posttransplant lymphoproliferative disorder (PTLPD). **A,** Sagittal gray-scale image of a renal transplant (TX) in the left lower quadrant (LLQ) demonstrates a large focal hypoechoic area *(calipers)* involving the renal cortex and sinus. On biopsy, this proved to be PTLPD. **B,** Sagittal gray-scale image from another patient with PTLPD demonstrates that the transplanted kidney is markedly enlarged, extending up to the lower surface of the liver. The kidney is also markedly hypoechoic with loss of the normal renal ultrasound architecture. This is an example of the diffuse infiltrative form of PTLPD.

Although not approved by the Food and Drug Administration in the United States, intravenous US contrast agents are used extensively elsewhere and provide superior visualization of the transplant vascularity, including the anastomoses of the renal artery and vein as well as cortical perfusion. CE-US has the potential to improve sonographic visualization of vessels and tissue perfusion in otherwise nondiagnostic examinations, to detect subtle cortical perfusion defects, to characterize focal masses, and to distinguish high-grade renal artery stenosis from vessel kinking and RAT.[45,46]

Elastography is another evolving sonographic technique that can be used to measure tissue stiffness. Initial reports have suggested that an increase in parenchymal cortical stiffness is a sensitive indicator of subclinical chronic rejection.[47]

CONCLUSIONS

Renal transplantation remains the best treatment option in patients with end-stage renal disease. US is a noninvasive modality that is the first-line imaging tool of choice in evaluating renal transplants presenting with symptoms or renal failure. While US findings are frequently nonspecific, duplex Doppler imaging, when combined with clinical parameters, is excellent at depicting the early abnormalities that may be seen with ATN, rejection, vascular complications, or perinephric collections. The presence of an elevated RI, while a nonspecific indicator of transplant dysfunction, may provide important corroborative evidence of the clinical significance of gray-scale or other Doppler findings. Although further research is needed, new developments with CE-US and elastography hold promise for further improvement of both the sensitivity and specificity of US diagnosis in the renal transplant recipient with the aim of earlier intervention when the graft is still salvageable.

HEPATIC TRANSPLANTATION

The first liver transplant was performed in 1963 at the University of Colorado Health Sciences Center by Starzl and colleagues.[48] Currently, liver transplantation is increasingly considered the optimal treatment for patients with many causes of acute or chronic liver failure. Common indications for liver transplantation are listed in Table 34-1.[49,50] In patients with hepatocellular carcinoma (HCC) the Milan criteria, namely the presence of a single HCC less than 5 cm or fewer than three HCCs less than 3 cm each in diameter, is the most commonly accepted guideline for transplantation.[51] Contraindications for hepatic transplantation are listed in Table 34-2.[49] In 2008, a total of 6318 deceased donor and living donor hepatic transplants were performed, and 16,865 patients remain on the waiting list as of March 2011.[4] Priority for transplantation is assigned on the basis of the highest estimated short-term mortality. With improvement in immunosuppression regimens and surgical technique, the 1-year, 5-year, and 10-year unadjusted

TABLE 34-1 Indications for Liver Transplantation[49,50]

Cirrhosis: complications, including liver failure
Hepatocellular carcinoma (Milan criteria apply)
Hepatitis (chronic hepatitis B, chronic hepatitis C, autoimmune)
Acetaminophen (Tylenol) overdose
Primary biliary cirrhosis
Primary sclerosing cholangitis
Hemachromatosis
Wilson's disease

TABLE 34-2 Contraindications for Liver Transplantation

Absolute
  Extrahepatic malignancy (not in remission)
  Hepatocellular carcinoma >5 cm or more than three tumors >3 cm in diameter
  Diffuse infiltration of the liver by malignancy
  Complete thrombosis of the portal and superior mesenteric veins
  Active or uncontrolled systemic infection
  Active substance or alcohol abuse
  Severe cardiopulmonary disease (significant surgical comorbidity)
  Noncompliance
Relative
  Age
  Cholangiocarcinoma
  Portal vein thrombosis
  Refractory infection, including human immunodeficiency virus (HIV)
  Previous malignancy
  Psychiatric disorder
  Poor social support

survival rates for patients following deceased donor orthotopic transplantation is 88.4%, 73.8%, and 60.0%, respectively, and 91%, 79%, and 69.9%, for recipients of living donor hepatic transplants.[4] Primary nonfunction of the graft is the primary cause of graft failure and loss. However, vascular and biliary complications as well as perioperative bleeding and infection also contribute to mortality and morbidity. Prompt identification of postoperative complications is imperative for preempting graft failure and optimizing patient outcomes. Doppler US is considered the first-line imaging modality of choice for evaluating the transplanted liver, particularly if vascular complications are suspected. US also has an important role in evaluating peritransplant fluid collections. However, the diagnosis of rejection in the liver transplant requires biopsy because imaging is nondiagnostic. This section describes the role of US in evaluating common postoperative complications of hepatic transplantation.

SURGICAL TECHNIQUE

Most liver transplants are performed with orthotopic implantation of deceased donor whole liver grafts. Other options include living donor segmental liver transplantation and reduced-size or split deceased donor allografts that are most commonly used for pediatric patients. Three basic vascular anastomoses in addition to the biliary anastomosis are performed during liver transplantation: hepatic artery (HA), portal vein (PV), and inferior vena cava (IVC; Figures 34-23 and 34-24). The exact type of anastomotic technique depends upon whether the liver is from a living vs deceased donor, whole vs partial liver, and whether there are congenital anomalies in the donor or recipient and disease in the recipient vessels or common bile duct (CBD).[52]

The HA anastomosis is most commonly performed by harvesting the deceased donor celiac axis via a Carrel patch (surrounding rim of deceased donor aortic wall) or common hepatic-splenic artery branch point and creating a "fish-mouth" end-to-end anastomosis with the recipient HA at the left/right HA bifurcation or at the origin of the gastroduodenal artery. A short, diseased recipient HA or celiac axis may require the use of a donor external iliac artery interposition graft anastomosed directly to the recipient aorta. The PV anastomosis is most commonly an end-to-end anastomosis between the donor and recipient main PVs. In the setting of preexisting PV/superior mesenteric vein thrombosis in the recipient, a jump graft derived from the donor external iliac vein may be required to connect the unaffected portion of the recipient superior mesenteric vein (or more rarely recipient renal vein) with the donor PV. Traditionally, the donor IVC was placed as an interposition graft requiring both a suprahepatic and infrahepatic IVC end-to-end anastomosis with the recipient IVC (see Figure 34-23). However, currently a "piggyback" approach (see Figure 34-24) is preferred. With this technique, the suprahepatic donor IVC is anastomosed end-to-side with the recipient hepatic venous confluence, and the donor infrahepatic IVC is tied off distally. Caudate veins draining directly into the infrahepatic donor IVC generally keep this part of the vessel patent. The advantages of the piggyback technique include decreased operating room time, creation of only one anastomosis, maintenance of recipient caval flow during surgery (no need for venous bypass), and decreased retroperitoneal dissection, which decreases the likelihood of hemorrhage and blood loss. In modified right lobe liver transplants, interposition grafts (external iliac artery or saphenous vein) are used for middle hepatic vein (HV) reconstruction.

Biliary drainage is usually accomplished via an end-to-end anastomosis between the donor

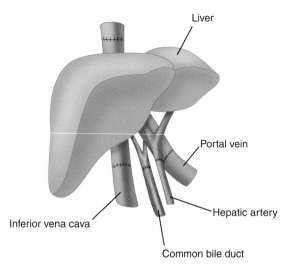

FIGURE 34-23 Schematic diagram demonstrating common anastomoses in a whole liver deceased donor transplant with an interposition inferior vena cava graft.

Liver

Portal vein

Hepatic artery

Inferior vena cava

Common bile duct

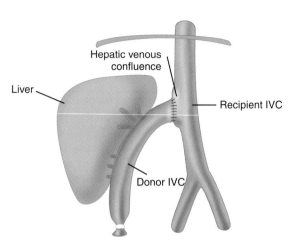

FIGURE 34-24 Schematic diagram demonstrating a "piggyback" anastomosis of the inferior vena cava (IVC) in a liver transplant.

Hepatic venous confluence

Liver

Recipient IVC

Donor IVC

CBD and the recipient common hepatic duct. Cholecystectomy is routinely performed. Disease in the recipient CBD or common hepatic duct mandates creation of a choledochojejunostomy. Currently, placement of a temporary T-tube is avoided due to the perceived increased risk for bile leaks.

NORMAL POSTOPERATIVE ULTRASOUND FINDINGS

At our institutions, Doppler US screening is performed on a daily basis for at least the first 3 days postoperatively and subsequently at 1, 6, and 12 months following liver transplantation. US examination is usually performed using 2- to 5-MHz curved array transducers depending upon body habitus. Multiple acoustic windows, including transabdominal, intercostal, and subcostal, may be required, particularly in the immediate postoperative period due to the presence of overlying bandages.[53] The intercostal approach is well suited for visualizing the posterior right hepatic lobe vessels, whereas the subcostal approach is helpful for scanning the junction of the HVs and IVC. Gray-scale evaluation of the liver parenchyma, biliary tree, and perihepatic space is performed. Color and pulsed Doppler interrogation of the main and intrahepatic HAs and PVs; the right, middle, and left HVs; and the IVC, as well as their anastomoses, is included in the examination. RI, PSV, and acceleration time (determined as the time interval between end diastole and the first systolic peak), should be measured in the main and intraparenchymal HAs.

The normal HA waveform has a sharp systolic upstroke with an acceleration time of less than 0.08 seconds and an RI in the range of 0.5 to 0.8 (Figure 34-25. A). The normal PSV at the HA anastomosis should be less than 200 cm/sec, although PSV may be falsely elevated in a tortuous, redundant vessel due to inappropriate Doppler angle correction.[50,54,55] However, in the early postoperative period, the RI may exceed 0.8 in normal grafts. This increase in RI is most likely due to increased hepatic vascular resistance and decreased compliance caused by reperfusion edema. Since the RI will usually normalize between 3 and 7 days following transplantation, a patient with an elevated RI should be followed with serial US examinations. Imaging with other more invasive modalities is generally not warranted. Increases in RI during the immediate postoperative period have not been associated

with increased risk for biliary complications, graft failure, or death.[56-61] If there is clinical concern or if a Doppler signal cannot be obtained from the HA in the immediate postoperative period, the patient can be rescanned 20 to 30 minutes after a trial of nifedipine, a potent vasodilator. If the HA is normal, arterial flow with an RI of 0.5 to 0.8 should be seen following the administration of nifedipine (Figure 34-26). An increased postoperative RI is often present in grafts from older donors (>50 years), grafts experiencing extended preoperative and intraoperative ischemic times, and cholestatic disease in the recipient.[56-61] On the other hand, progression from an initial waveform demonstrating a normal amount of diastolic flow to one with absent diastolic flow and a dampened systolic peak should raise concern for impending HA thrombosis and further imaging with CT angiography, magnetic resonance angiography, or angiography should be considered.[62] In addition, early increased diastolic flow in the HA, with the RI less than 0.6, has been reported to have 100% sensitivity and near-80% specificity as a predictor of impending vascular complications, although a decreased RI is not associated with the increased likelihood of developing biliary complications.[56,62]

The normal PV waveform is monophasic with continuous flow toward the liver and can have slight respiratory phasicity (see Figure 34-25, B). Mismatch between the donor and recipient PV may be seen and is particularly common in pediatric transplants and should not be mistaken for a stenosis of the PV. The normal HVs and IVC should demonstrate a triphasic waveform pattern reflecting right heart pressure (see Figure 34-25, C to F). A monophasic waveform in the HVs or IVC is considered a nonspecific indicator of abnormality such as proximal obstruction, thrombosis, or stenosis and, therefore, should be followed closely. However, a monophasic waveform in the HVs can occasionally be seen due to compression (ascites or large transplanted liver in a small space) or during a deep breath hold. Loss of phasicity in the HVs is not believed to be associated with transplant rejection. Accentuated cardiac pulsatility transmitted to the PVs and HVs (Figure 34-27) in the immediate postoperative period may be due to tricuspid regurgitation, right heart failure, or volume overload. This is a relatively common but transient postoperative finding.

In addition to Doppler US, intravenous CE-US may be useful for further delineating the

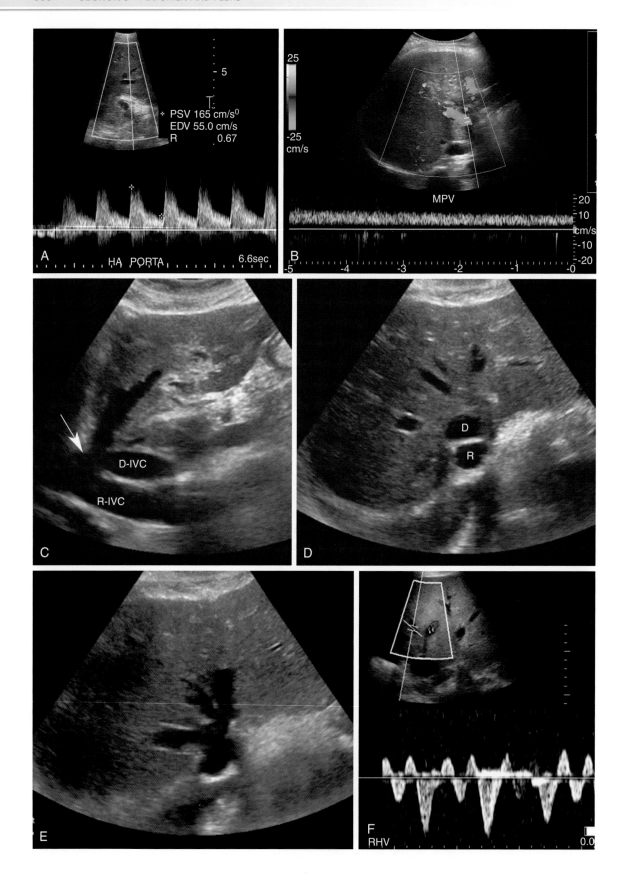

FIGURE 34-25 Spectral Doppler waveforms in a normal liver transplant. **A,** Duplex Doppler tracing from the main hepatic artery (HA) in the porta hepatis. Note sharp systolic upstroke with continuous forward diastolic flow. The resistive index (RI) is 0.67. The intrahepatic arteries from each transplanted lobe should also be sampled and have a similar waveform. **B,** Duplex Doppler tracing from the main portal vein (MPV). Note continuous hepatopetal flow toward the transplanted liver. Slight respiratory variation is a normal finding but is not seen in this case. The intrahepatic portal veins from each transplanted lobe should also be sampled and are expected to have a similar waveform. **C,** Sagittal gray-scale image of a piggyback inferior vena cava (IVC) anastomosis. The superior aspect of the donor inferior vena cava (D-IVC) is sutured to the recipient hepatic confluence *(arrow)*, and the distal end is tied off. Blood flow from small hepatic veins draining the caudate lobe directly into the D-IVC generally keep it patent. recipient inferior vena cava, R-IVC. **D,** Transverse gray-scale image demonstrates the donor (D) and recipient (R) IVC in cross section. **E,** More superior transverse gray-scale image at the level of the donor hepatic confluence in the same patient as in **C** and **D**. **F,** Spectral Doppler tracing from the right hepatic vein (RHV). Note pulsatile triphasic waveform reflecting changes in right atrial pressure. Waveforms in the IVC and all hepatic veins should appear similar.

transplant vasculature as it is more sensitive to low-velocity blood flow signals.[63-66]

VASCULAR COMPLICATIONS

Doppler US is an accurate modality for evaluating vascular complications and should be considered the first-line imaging modality of choice. Sensitivities and specificities are listed in Table 34-3.[67] Representative diagnostic color and spectral Doppler US parameters are listed in Table 34-4. CT angiography, magnetic resonance angiography, and angiography serve as adjunctive modalities in indeterminate cases.

Hepatic artery thrombosis (HAT) is the most common vascular complication following hepatic transplantation with an estimated incidence of 4% to 12% in adult recipients and up to 40% in pediatric recipients.[50,68,69] HAT most often occurs within 6 weeks after transplantation but can develop several years later. HAT has a very high mortality rate if retransplantation or thrombectomy/thrombolysis, often followed by vascular reconstruction, is not immediately performed. Most patients ultimately require retransplantation.[62,70] Since the HA provides the sole vascular supply to the biliary system in liver transplant patients, HAT may result in biliary necrosis leading to bile leaks, bilomas, biliary strictures, and superinfection with abscess formation, cholangitis, and hepatic infarcts. Therefore, clinical presentation includes fulminant liver failure due to hepatic necrosis, biliary necrosis, bile leak, bacteremia, and sepsis. Risk factors include size mismatch in the donor and recipient arteries, small vessels (especially common in pediatric transplants), underlying HA or celiac artery stenosis, complex arterial reconstruction (especially with

an interposition graft), prolonged ischemic time for the donor liver, ABO blood type incompatibility, acute rejection, surgical technique, prior liver transplantation, and possible CMV infection.[70-73] On Doppler US, HAT manifests as absence of flow in the main and intrahepatic arteries (Figure 34-28). HA waveforms that evolve from a normal flow pattern to decreasing diastolic flow and dampening of the PSV have been described as predictors of impending HAT.[62] Doppler US has a reported accuracy of approximately 92% for the diagnosis of HAT.[72] Poor technique, low-velocity blood flow due to poor cardiac output or hypotension, high-grade HA stenosis, and severe vasospasm can also result in poor or non-visualization of Doppler flow signals in the hepatic arteries and therefore mimic HAT. Repeat US following administration of nifedipine (see earlier) or CE-US may improve visualization of blood flow signals in the normal HA and diminish the need for angiographic confirmation.[63-66] Collateral arterial flow to the transplanted liver may develop in patients with HAT, especially in children. A tardus-parvus waveform suggestive of HA stenosis (see later) may be observed in the intraparenchymal HAs and thus lead to a false-negative interpretation in patients with arterial flow to the liver from collateral vessels. Hepatic infarcts (see Figures 34-28, *B* to *D*, 34-36, and 34-37), abscesses, and biliary necrosis with bile leaks and biliary ductal dilatation are common findings in patients with HAT, and if noted should prompt careful evaluation of the hepatic arteries for thrombosis or stenosis.

Hepatic artery stenosis (HAS) is the second most common vascular complication following hepatic transplantation with an estimated

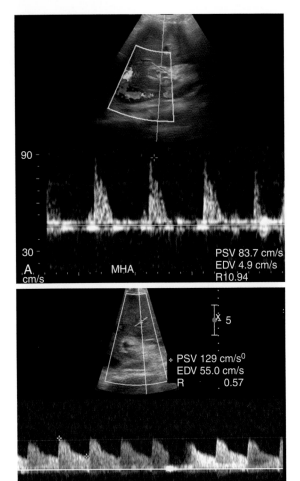

FIGURE 34-26 High-resistance arterial waveform. **A,** Spectral Doppler tracing from the main hepatic artery (MHA) within 24 hours postoperatively demonstrates nearly complete absence of diastolic flow. While this was initially thought to be a harbinger of hepatic artery thrombosis, it is actually a quite common finding postoperatively, likely due to increased vascular hepatic resistance secondary to swelling and/or interstitial edema of the graft and typically resolves within 3 days. If there is clinical concern, repeat imaging 20 to 30 minutes following the administration of nifedipine (a vasodilator) can be performed as was done in **B.** Note that diastolic flow is now normal in the left hepatic artery (LT HA). The resistive index (RI) is 0.57.

incidence of 2% to 11%.[70,74] HAS can be either an early or late finding.[70,74] Predisposing risk factors include injury from surgical clamps and intra-arterial catheters, poor surgical technique, and rejection.[53] Stenosis most commonly occurs at the anastomosis. HAS can also lead to biliary ischemia and necrosis, resulting in hepatic dysfunction and even graft loss. The characteristic

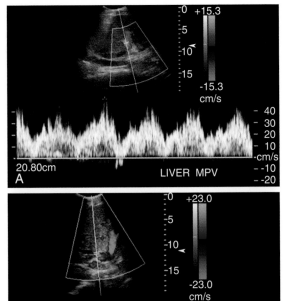

FIGURE 34-27 Congestive heart failure. Spectral tracings from the main portal vein (MPV; **A**) and middle hepatic vein (MHV; **B**) demonstrate markedly pulsatile flow patterns with dramatic increase in the size of the "a-wave" in **B** consistent with right heart failure.

TABLE 34-3 Sensitivities and Specificities of Doppler Ultrasound for Liver Transplantation Vascular Complications

Site of Complication	Sensitivity (%)	Specificity (%)
Hepatic artery	60-92*	86-97
Portal vein	73-100	95-100
Outflow veins	70-99	Up to 100

*The sensitivity for extrahepatic segments of the hepatic artery is lower than for intrahepatic segments.

Doppler US features of HAS include focal narrowing of the artery and increased PSV with poststenotic dilatation and turbulent flow. PSVs exceeding 200 cm/sec have been reported to have a 96% positive predictive value for HAS.[75] Distal tardus-parvus waveforms with an acceleration time greater than 80 msec and an RI less than 0.5 are also suggestive of HAS (Figure 34-29) and may be the only finding if the HAS is too

TABLE 34-4 Doppler Ultrasound Parameter Abnormalities for Liver Transplant Vascular Complications

Complication	Acceleration Time(s)	Resistive Index	Pulsatility Index	Waveform	Peak Anastomotic Velocity (cm/sec)	Anastomotic-Preanastomotic Velocity (ratio)	Peak Systolic Velocity (cm/sec)
Hepatic artery stenosis	>0.08	<0.5		Tardus-parvus			>200
Pseudoaneurysm				To-and-fro			
Hepatic artery-to-portal vein fistula				Focal low-resistance flow in the feeding artery and arterialization of flow in the affected portal vein branch			
Portal vein stenosis				Monophasic or reversed	>125	>2.5-3:1	
Outflow vein stenosis			<0.45	Monophasic or reversed		>3-4:1	

central to be visualized on US due to shadowing from overlying bowel gas or surgical scarring.[56,75,76] The sensitivity and specificity of this tardus-parvus waveform is reportedly approximately 73%.[75] Another study reports that this waveform along with an RI less than 0.5 is the most sensitive indicator of HAS or impending HAT.[77] A similar Doppler waveform may be seen in the first 24 to 48 hours following transplantation due to peripheral hepatic vasodilatation in response to reperfusion injury. Hence, the tardus-parvus waveform is a much more specific finding for the presence of HAS 48 hours after transplantation. In addition, a very low grade HAS may not show these Doppler US findings. Therefore, if unexplained biliary problems exist, CT angiography or angiography should be considered even if the US examination is normal.[50,68] Another pitfall resulting in a false-positive diagnosis of HAS is the presence of collateral arterial flow with a tardus-parvus waveform in the setting of HAT. Treatment options for HAS include stent placement, angioplasty, surgical revision, and retransplantation.

Hepatic artery PSAs are uncommon, occurring in only about 1% of liver transplants. Although asymptomatic in most patients and an incidental finding, PSAs are an extremely serious vascular complication due to the risk for hemorrhage from rupture.[78] Most posttransplant PSAs are extrahepatic, arising at the anastomosis as a consequence of surgical breakdown or HA angioplasty. However, intrahepatic PSAs may be mycotic in origin or develop secondary to iatrogenic injury following percutaneous biopsy or biliary intervention.[79] PSAs appear as cystic lesions in continuity with the HA on gray-scale US. Color Doppler interrogation will depict the classic yin-yang blood flow pattern due to swirling blood within the PSA, confirming that the structure is not a simple fluid collection (Figure 34-30). A to-and-fro pattern with flow above the baseline heading toward the PSA in systole and below the baseline heading away from the PSA in diastole will be observed on spectral waveforms obtained from the neck of the PSA when the communicating neck is narrow. A more disorganized flow pattern will be noted with a wide neck. CT angiography, magnetic resonance angiography, and angiography can confirm the diagnosis. Treatment options include percutaneous embolization, exclusion with covered stent placement, or surgical revision.[80]

Hepatic artery to portal vein fistulas (AVFs) are extremely uncommon and most often arise following liver biopsy. Indeed, the incidence of HA

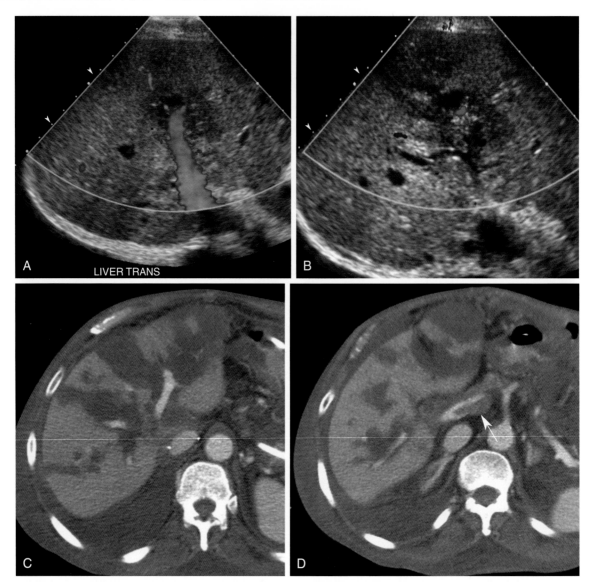

FIGURE 34-28 Hepatic artery thrombosis. **A,** Transverse (TRANS) color Doppler image demonstrates flow in the main portal vein (red) but no evidence of flow in the adjacent main hepatic artery, which is not visualized. **B,** Color Doppler image 2 days later again reveals intrahepatic portal venous flow, but no arterial tracings could be obtained. Note wedge-shaped area of decreased echogenicity centrally around the portal triads extending toward the liver capsule consistent with infarction. **C** and **D,** Contrast-enhanced computed tomographic scans demonstrating multiple wedge-shaped nonperfused areas of low density consistent with multiple infarctions and areas of liver necrosis. No contrast enhancement of the hepatic arteries is identified, confirming hepatic artery thrombosis. A filling defect in the main portal vein *(arrow)* in **D** is indicative of coexistent nonocclusive portal vein thrombosis.

to PV fistulas is estimated to be as high as 50% following liver biopsy performed in the first week following transplantation.[54] However, most are small and resolve spontaneously. The characteristic Doppler US findings for HA to PV fistulas include color aliasing and a soft tissue bruit at the site of the fistula, arterialization of flow in the draining branch of the PV, and isolated low-resistance, high-velocity flow in the feeding HA

(Figure 34-31). Reversal of blood flow in the affected PV may also occur, but this is a very uncommon finding.[53]

Portal vein thrombosis (PVT) is diagnosed in about 1% to 3% of liver transplant recipients.[53,56,64,69,70] Risk factors for PVT include previous PV surgery (including transjugular intrahepatic portosystemic shunt [TIPS]), history of PVT in the recipient, hypercoagulable

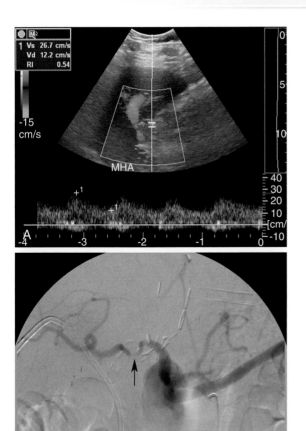

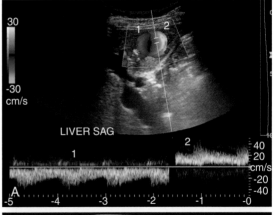

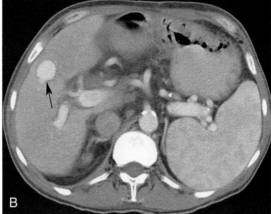

FIGURE 34-30 Intrahepatic pseudoaneurysm (PSA). **A,** Sagittal (SAG) duplex Doppler image of the liver demonstrates a round area of color flow demonstrating the classic yin-yang (blue/red) flow pattern of a patent PSA in this transplant following liver biopsy. Bidirectional flow in the lumen of the PSA is confirmed on the spectral tracing. **B,** Contrast-enhanced computed tomographic scan demonstrates the intraparenchymal-enhancing PSA (arrow).

FIGURE 34-29 Hepatic artery stenosis. **A,** Spectral Doppler tracing of the distal main hepatic artery (MHA) demonstrates a tardus-parvus waveform indicative of a proximal stenosis. Increased velocity at the site of the stenosis in the MHA may not be observed on Doppler ultrasound examination when the MHA anastomosis is central and/or obscured by overlying bowel gas. Doppler interrogation of the distal MHA and intraparenchymal hepatic arteries is performed in patients presenting with evidence of dilated bile ducts, bilomas, or abnormal liver function tests consistent with biliary tract abnormalities in order to look for the tardus-parvus waveform indicative of a more central stenosis. **B,** Angiogram documents the stenosis of the main hepatic artery (arrow).

conditions, vessel redundancy, donor vs recipient vessel diameter mismatch, and injury during surgery.[53,56,64,69,70] Clinical manifestations range from portal hypertension with gastrointestinal bleeding and ascites to liver dysfunction/failure and peripheral edema.[81] Doppler US examination reveals lack of blood flow most commonly

in the extrahepatic portal venous segment. Non-occlusive thrombus appears as a hypoechoic filling defect on gray-scale or color Doppler imaging (Figure 34-32), although acute thrombus may be anechoic. Over time, the thrombus progressively becomes more echogenic and the PV becomes narrowed. Cavernous transformation may also develop. US is believed to be extremely sensitive and specific for the diagnosis of PVT.[53,56,64,69,70] Management can range from thrombolysis or thrombectomy, stent placement or angioplasty to surgical revision with a jump graft.

Portal vein stenosis (PVS) is diagnosed on US by focal narrowing of the main PV (<2.5 mm) and usually occurs at the anastomosis. On Doppler US, the reported diagnostic criteria include peak PV velocities >125 cm/sec or peak velocity ratio of

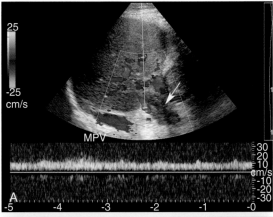

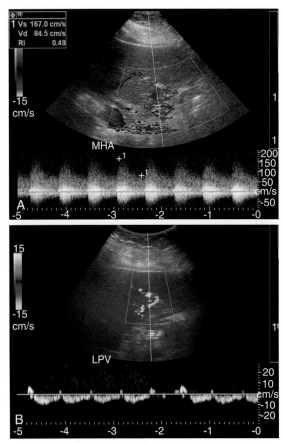

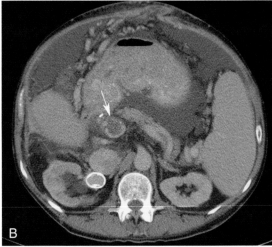

FIGURE 34-31 Arteriovenous fistula (AVF). **A,** Duplex Doppler tracing reveals a color bruit in the soft tissues surrounding the main hepatic artery (MHA), indicative of high-velocity flow. Spectral tracing confirms increased peak systolic velocity and end-diastolic velocity. **B,** Duplex Doppler image of the left lobe of the liver reveals a pulsatile waveform in the left portal vein (LPV) as well as an adjacent tangle of small vessels. This constellation of findings is consistent with a small AVF. This patient was asymptomatic 3 days following percutaneous liver biopsy.

FIGURE 34-32 Portal vein thrombosis (PVT). **A,** Duplex Doppler image of the main portal vein (MPV) demonstrates internal echoes within the lumen *(arrow)* and peripheral flow (red) with a normal waveform consistent with partially occlusive PVT. **B,** Contrast-enhanced computed tomographic scan demonstrates a filling defect in the MPV *(arrow)*, confirming the ultrasound findings in **A.**

the main PV at the stenosis to prestenosis velocity greater than 2.5 to 3:1 (Figure 34-33).[80,81] Care must be taken not to confuse vessel size mismatch with a true PVS, particularly in the pediatric transplant population. Comparison to baseline examinations is, therefore, critical.

HV or IVC thrombosis and/or stenosis are uncommon findings in liver transplants with an incidence of under 2%.[54,68,70] Factors that predispose to IVC or HV thrombosis include hypercoagulable states, underlying stenosis, and injury during surgical manipulation of the vessels. Stenosis may be due to vessel kinking or size mismatch, compression by large hematomas or other

fluid collections, and severe graft edema.[54,68,70] Patients may present with hepatomegaly, lower extremity edema, pleural effusions, and ascites, although some patients with mild degrees of stenosis may be completely asymptomatic. Thus, the clinical significance of a mild stenosis is uncertain. Intraluminal echoes will be noted on gray-scale US in patients with IVC or HV thrombosis. No blood flow signals are detected if the thrombosis is occlusive. In nonocclusive thrombosis, blood flow signals will be documented in the peripheral venous branches (Figure 34-34). In patients with hepatic or IVC stenosis, Doppler interrogation will reveal increased blood flow velocity at the site of narrowing and focal color aliasing. A threefold to fourfold increase

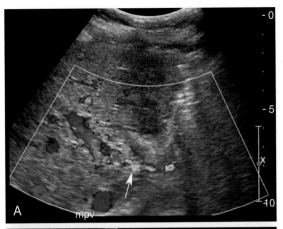

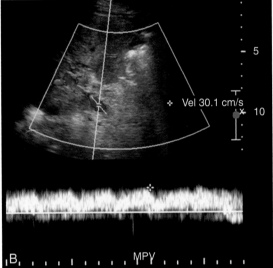

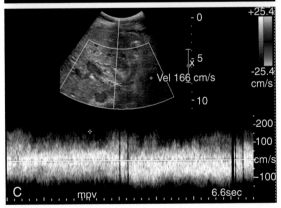

FIGURE 34-33 Portal vein stenosis (PVS). **A,** Color Doppler image demonstrating narrowing and focal color aliasing of the main portal vein (MPV). Spectral tracing from the MPV proximal to the stenosis **(B)** demonstrates a velocity of 30 cm/sec in comparison to 166 cm/sec obtained at the site of the stenosis **(C)**. Ratio is 5.5. While the clinical significance of PVS is uncertain, stenting could be considered in the setting of abnormal liver function tests and no other explanation.

in blood flow velocity has been suggested as being indicative of a significant stenosis.[50,54] A suprahepatic IVC stenosis or central HV thrombosis may cause a monophasic waveform in the peripheral HVs.[68,82,83] Dampening of the hepatic venous waveforms with a pulsatility index of less than 0.45 is suggestive of outflow stenosis.[81,83] As with PVS, care must be taken not to confuse mismatch in vessel size with a true IVC or HV stenosis. Angioplasty or stent placement is the treatment of choice.

PERIHEPATIC FLUID COLLECTIONS

Perihepatic hematomas and right-sided pleural effusions are extremely common postoperatively. Most are small and resolve spontaneously. However, intervention may be required if the hematoma or pleural effusion significantly increases in size or causes symptoms such as falling hematocrit or respiratory distress. Hematomas are often found inferior to the left lobe of the liver, in Morison's pouch, in the gallbladder fossa, or in the falciform ligament. Echogenicity is variable and often complex. Most acute hematomas are echogenic, becoming more hypoechoic to anechoic over time (Figure 34-35). Hematomas are avascular. Anechoic fluid collections may be difficult to differentiate from bilomas without aspiration. Superinfection is suggested by the presence of gas (although postoperative air and Surgicel may mimic this appearance) and clinical presentation. Whether internal echoes are due to blood or infection cannot be differentiated by US. Diagnosis requires aspiration. The role of US in evaluating fluid collections, therefore, is to localize fluid, to assess for change in size or echogenicity of the collection, and to guide intervention.

INTRAHEPATIC COLLECTIONS OR MASSES

Intrahepatic abscess formation most often occurs in the setting of liver infarction or biliary necrosis in a patient with HAT or HAS.[50] On US, a complex fluid collection of variable echogenicity will be observed (Figure 34-36). The outer margins may be irregular and thickened surrounding a more hypoechoic to anechoic center. The presence of echogenic speckles with ring-down artifact is indicative of air and is a highly specific finding for abscess in an intrahepatic fluid collection. An abscess will be centrally avascular but may demonstrate increased peripheral vascularity.

A geographic hypoechoic area in the liver parenchyma near the portal triads of either increased

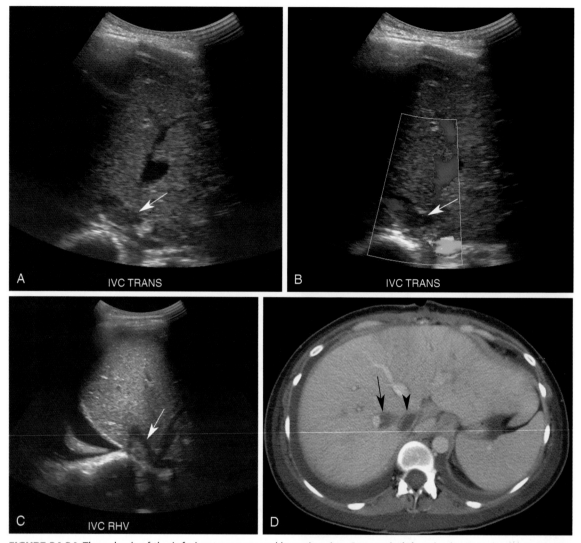

FIGURE 34-34 Thrombosis of the inferior vena cava and hepatic veins. Gray-scale **(A)** and color Doppler **(B)** transverse (TRANS) images of the liver demonstrate intraluminal echoes indicative of thrombus in the inferior vena cava (IVC; *arrows*). The thrombus extends into the right hepatic vein (RHV; *arrow* in **C**). Note the right pleural effusion and collapsed lung, both common findings after liver transplantation. **D,** Thrombus in the RHV *(arrow)* and IVC *(arrowhead)* is confirmed on contrast-enhanced computed tomographic scan demonstrating filling defects in the vessels.

or decreased echogenicity is a worrisome finding for biliary necrosis (Figure 34-37) or hepatic ischemia (see Figures 34-28 and 34-37). Hepatic infarcts are typically well defined and round or peripheral and wedge shaped, but may be more geographic in configuration. Echogenicity is variable. Central necrosis and liquefaction may occur.

The presence of a new solid intraparenchymal mass should raise concern for malignancy, either recurrent tumor or PTLPD. The overall incidence of PTLPD seems to be slightly higher in liver than in renal transplants, particularly in children.[84] PTLPD may present as single or multiple liver

masses, diffuse infiltration of the liver, or a portal mass encasing the portal vessels and CBD. Extrahepatic disease, including lymphadenopathy and involvement of other organs, is slightly more common than intrahepatic involvement.[68] Liver transplant recipients are also at increased risk for developing malignancies, especially squamous cell or basal cell skin cancers, Kaposi's sarcoma (see earlier discussion of neoplasms in renal transplants), and non-Hodgkin's lymphoma.[50,68] Most cancers develop 2 to 6 years after transplantation. Risk is likely related to degree of immunosuppression, previous viral infection (hepatitis B,

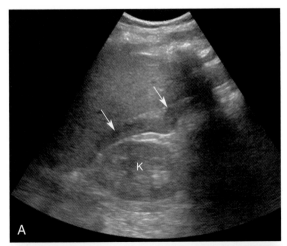

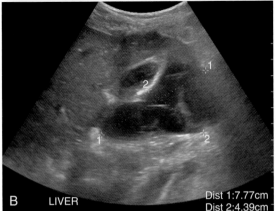

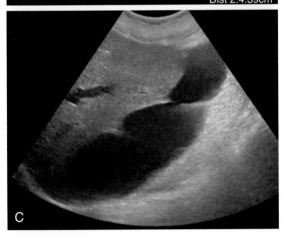

FIGURE 34-35 Perihepatic fluid collections. **A,** Gray-scale image of the right upper quadrant demonstrates an elongated complex, echogenic collection between the inferior surface of the liver and the right kidney (K) consistent with hematoma. Small perihepatic hematomas are seen in most liver transplant recipients immediately postoperatively and usually resolve spontaneously. **B,** Larger, more complex hematoma *(cursors)* in a different patient. In an asymptomatic patient a hematoma of this size would still likely be followed closely for interval increase in size or drop in hematocrit. Surgical exploration/evacuation or angiography to embolize a "bleeder" is recommended in a patient with an enlarging perihepatic hematoma or evidence of significant blood loss. Aspiration would be performed in patients with fever or elevated white blood cell count to exclude superinfection. **C,** Large anechoic perihepatic collection in a different patient. The findings are nonspecific. While resolving hematomas may become anechoic, a biloma or loculated ascites could have a similar appearance.

hepatitis C, Epstein-Barr, herpes, and CMV), and possibly history of alcohol abuse.[50,68]

BILIARY COMPLICATIONS

Biliary complications are estimated to occur in 5% to 15% of liver transplant recipients[76,85-87] and are more common in patients following right lobe living donor transplantation. Patients may present with symptoms ranging from abdominal discomfort to sepsis. Leakage of bile at the CBD anastomosis may form bilomas or leak freely into the peritoneal cavity and tends to occur in the first month after transplantation. Bile leakage is best detected via cholangiography, endoscopic retrograde cholangiopancreatography (ERCP), or cholescintigraphy as the US appearance of bile leakage may mimic ascites, hematoma, or even abscess. Bile leakage from biliary necrosis of the intrahepatic ducts or distal CBD is usually indicative of HAT or HAS[68,76,85-87] and on US may mimic hypoechoic periportal edema (see Figure 34-37). Most biliary strictures occur at the anastomotic site secondary to scarring or fibrosis. More peripheral strictures are usually due to biliary ischemia from HAT or HAS, infectious cholangitis, or recurrent primary sclerosing cholangitis and have a much worse prognosis.[68] Sloughing of the biliary mucosa may cause intraluminal echoes in the bile ducts.[50] Biliary strictures do not always cause biliary ductal dilatation in the transplant patient. Therefore, if there is high clinical suspicion of biliary pathology, further imaging with magnetic resonance cholangiopancreatography (MRCP), ERCP, or percutaneous transhepatic cholangiography is warranted even if there is no evidence of biliary ductal dilatation on US or CT.[68] As mentioned previously, the presence of biliary complications, particularly intrahepatic pathology, should prompt evaluation of the hepatic artery for HAT or HAS.

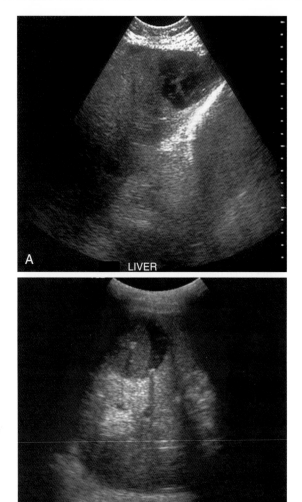

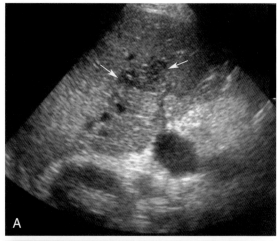

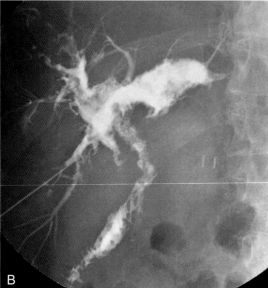

FIGURE 34-36 Hepatic abscess. **A,** Note complex hypoechoic rounded area at the tip of the left lobe of the liver in a febrile patient. This patient had a distal segmental hepatic artery thrombosis (not shown), resulting in a focal hepatic infarct, which became superinfected. **B,** Note complex round and sharply marginated collection in another patient with a hepatic abscess and hepatic artery thrombosis. Note heterogeneity of surrounding liver parenchyma due to diffuse ischemia.

FIGURE 34-37 Biliary necrosis. **A,** Gray-scale image of the liver demonstrates a periportal geographic area of decreased echogenicity *(arrows)* as well as an inferior ill-defined area of increased echogenicity. These findings are worrisome for bile leakage and hepatic ischemia. Patients with such findings should be carefully evaluated for biliary and hepatic artery abnormalities. It can be difficult to document dilatation of the bile ducts in transplant patients, however. **B,** Cholangiogram demonstrates irregularity and dilatation of the biliary tree as well as a focal collection of contrast or biloma. Findings are consistent with extensive biliary necrosis.

CONCLUSIONS

Doppler US is the primary screening modality of choice for the evaluation of vascular complications related to liver transplantation, including HA, PV, and HV/IVC thrombosis or stenosis as well as less common vascular complications such as hepatic artery PSA and arterioportal fistula. Familiarity with the different types of hepatic transplants and surgical anastomoses as well as the appearance of Doppler US waveforms in normal hepatic vessels following transplantation is critical for interpretation. Careful attention to the status of the HA should be paid in the setting of biliary tract pathology since the HA provides the sole blood supply to the transplanted biliary tree. US also plays an important role in evaluating peritransplant fluid collections and parenchymal abnormalities in the symptomatic patient but is not helpful in the evaluation of hepatic transplant rejection.

REFERENCES

1. Neipp M, et al: Renal transplantation today, *Arch Surg* 394:1–16, 2009.
2. Akbar SA, et al: Complications of renal transplantation, *Radiographics* 25:1335–1356, 2005.
3. Brown ED, et al: Complications of renal transplantation: evaluation with US and radionuclide imaging, *Radiographics* 20:607–622, 2000.
4. *2009 Annual report of the U.S. Organ Procurement and Transplantation Network and the Scientific Registry of Transplant Recipients: transplant data 1998-2008*: U.S. Department of Health and Human Services, Health Resources and Services Administration, Division of Transplantation, Rockville, MD; United Network for Organ Sharing, Richmond, VA. http://www.ustransplant.org/annual_reports/current/chapter_index.htm.
5. United Network for Organ Sharing and Scientific Registry data: *Data from the Organ Procurement and Transplantation Network*. Available online: http://www.unos.org.
6. Brown ED, et al: Complications of renal transplantation: evaluation with US and radionuclide imaging, *Radiographics* 20:607–622, 2000.
7. Sahani DV, et al: Multi-detector row CT in evaluation of 94 living renal donors by readers with varied experience, *Radiology* 235:905–910, 2005.
8. Israel GM, et al: Comprehensive MR imaging in the preoperative evaluation of living donor candidates for laparoscopic nephrectomy: initial experience, *Radiology* 225:427–432, 2002.
9. Irshad A, et al: A review of sonographic evaluation of renal transplant complications, *Curr Probl Diagn Radiol* 37:67–79, 2008.
10. Baxter GM: Ultrasound of renal transplantation, *Clin Radiol* 56:802–818, 2001.
11. Cosgrove DO, Chan KE: Renal transplants: what ultrasound can and cannot do, *Ultrasound Q* 24:77–87, 2008.
12. Friedewald SM, et al: Vascular and nonvascular complications of renal transplants: sonographic evaluation and correlation with other imaging modalities, surgery, and pathology, *J Clin Ultrasound* 33:127–139, 2005.
13. Daly PJ, et al: Delayed graft function: a dilemma in renal transplantation, *BJU Int* 96:498–501, 2005.
14. Shoskes DA, Shahed AR, Kim S: Delayed graft function. Influence on outcome and strategies for prevention, *Urol Clin North Am* 28:721–732, 2001.
15. Rao KV, Kjellstrand CM: Post transplant acute renal failure: A review, *Clin Exp Dial Apheresis* 7:127–143, 1983.
16. Perico N, et al: Delayed graft function in kidney transplantation, *Lancet* 364:1814–1827, 2004.
17. Chudek J, et al: The intrarenal resistance parameters measured by duplex Doppler ultrasound shortly after kidney transplantation in patients with immediate, slow and delayed graft function, *Transplant Proc* 49:15–20, 2005.
18. Datta R, et al: Role of duplex Doppler and power Doppler sonography in transplanted kidneys with acute renal parenchyma dysfunction, *Australas Radiol* 49:15–20, 2005.
19. Parthipun A, Pilcher J: Renal transplant assessment: sonographic imaging, *Ultrasound Clin* 5:379–399, 2010.
20. Langer JE, Jones LP: Sonographic evaluation of the renal transplant, *Ultrasound Clin* 2:73–88, 2007.
21. Lockhart ME, et al: Reversed diastolic flow in the renal transplants: perioperative implications versus transplants older than 1 month, *AJR Am J Roentgenol* 190:650–655, 2008.
22. Tranquart F, et al: The use of perioperative Doppler ultrasound as a screening test for acute tubular necrosis, *Transpl Int* 6:14–17, 1993.
23. Pirsch JD, et al: Determinants of graft survival after renal transplantation, *Transplantation* 61:1581–1585, 1996.
24. Hohnke C, et al: Vascular complications in 1200 kidney transplantations, *Transplantation Proc* 19:3691–3692, 1987.
25. O'Neill WC, Baumgarten DA: Ultrasonography in renal transplantation, *Am J Kidney Dis* 39:663–678, 2002.
26. Dodd G, et al: Imaging of vascular complications associated with renal transplantation, *AJR Am J Roentgenol* 157:449–459, 1991.
27. Patel U, Khaw KK, Highes NC: Doppler ultrasound for the detection of renal transplant artery stenosis—threshold peak systolic velocity needs to be higher in low-risk or surveillance population, *Clin Radiol* 58:772–777, 2003.
28. Gottlieb RH, et al: Diagnosis of renal artery stenosis in transplanted kidneys: value of Doppler waveform analysis of intrarenal arteries, *AJR Am J Roentgenol* 65:1441–1446, 1995.
29. Li J, et al: Evaluation of severe transplant renal artery stenosis with Doppler sonography, *J Clin Ultrasound* 31:135–141, 2003.
30. de Morais RH, et al: Duplex Doppler sonography of transplant renal artery stenosis, *J Clin Ultrasound* 31:135–141, 2003.
31. Loubeyre P, et al: Transplanted renal artery: detection of stenosis with color Doppler US, *Radiology* 203:661–665, 1997.
32. Tublin ME, Dodd GD III: Sonography of renal transplantation, *Radiol Clin North Am* 33:447–459, 1995.
33. Heffernan E, et al: Page kidney after renal allograft biopsy: sonographic findings, *J Clin Ultrasound* 37:226–229, 2009.
34. Wong-You-Cheong JJ, et al: Torsion of intraperitoneal renal transplants: imaging appearances, *AJR Am J Roentgenol* 171:1355, 1998.
35. Makisalo H, et al: Urological complications after 2084 consecutive kidney transplantations, *Transplant Proc* 29:152–153, 1997.
36. Montalvo BM, et al: Percutaneous sclerotherapy of lymphoceles related to renal transplantation, *J Vasc Interv Radiol* 7:117–123, 1996.
37. Kuzuhara K, et al: Ethanol ablation of lymphocele after renal transplantation: a minimally invasive approach, *Transplantation Proc* 29:147–150, 1997.
38. Cho DK, et al: Urinary calculi in renal transplant recipients, *Transplantation* 45:899–902, 1988.
39. Boschiero LB, et al: Renal needle biopsy of the transplant kidney: vascular and urologic complications, *Urol Int* 48:130–133, 1992.
40. Vajdic CM, et al: Cancer incidence before and after kidney transplantation, *JAMA* 296:2823–2831, 2006.
41. Bretan PN Jr, et al: Chronic renal failure: a significant risk factor in the development of acquired renal cysts and renal cell carcinoma, *Cancer* 57:1871–1879, 1986.
42. Jain M, et al: Post-transplant lymphoproliferative disorder after live donor renal transplantation, *Clin Transpl* 19:668–673, 2005.
43. Kew CE, et al: Posttransplant lymphoproliferative disorder localized near the allograft in renal transplantation, *Transplantation* 69:809–814, 2000.

44. Lopez-Ben R, et al: Focal posttransplantation lympho-proliferative disorder at the allograft hilum, *AJR Am J Roentgenol* 175:14–17, 2000.

45. Kay DH, et al: Ultrasonic microbubble contrast agents and the transplant kidney, *Clin Radiol* 64:1081–1087, 2009.

46. Jimenez C, et al: Ultrasonography in kidney transplantation: Values and new developments, *Transplant Rev* 23:209–213, 2009.

47. Arndt R, et al: Noninvasive evaluation of renal allograft fibrosis by transient elastography – a pilot study, *Transpl Int* 3:871–877, 2010.

48. Starzl TE, et al: Homotransplantation of the liver in humans, *Surg Gynecol Obstet* 117:659–676, 1963.

49. O'Leary JG, Lepe R, Davis GL: Indications for Liver Transplantation, *Gastroenterology* 134:1764–1776, 2008.

50. Crossin JD, Muradali D, Wilson SR: US of liver transplants: Normal and abnormal, *Radiographics* 23:1093–1114, 2003.

51. Mazzaferro V, et al: Liver transplantation for the treatment of small hepatocellular carcinomas in patients with cirrhosis, *N Engl J Med* 334:693–699, 1996.

52. Catalano OA, et al: Vascular and biliary variants in the liver: Implications for liver surgery, *Radiographics* 28:359–378, 2008.

53. Saad WE, et al: Noninvasive imaging of liver transplant complications, *Tech Vasc Interv Radiol* 10:191–206, 2007.

54. Singh AK, et al: Postoperative imaging in liver transplantation: What radiologists should know, *Radiographics* 30:339–351, 2010.

55. Brody MB, Rodgers SK, Horrow MM: Spectrum of normal or near-normal sonographic findings after orthotopic liver transplantation, *Ultrasound Q* 24:257–265, 2008.

56. Uzochukwu LN, Bluth EI, Smetherman DH: Early postoperative hepatic sonography as a predictor of vascular and biliary complications in adult orthotopic liver transplant patients, *AJR Am J Roentgenol* 185:1558–1570, 2005.

57. García-Criado A, et al: Doppler ultrasound findings in the hepatic artery shortly after liver transplantation, *AJR Am J Roentgenol* 193:128–135, 2009.

58. García-Criado A, et al: Significance of and contributing factors for a high resistive index of Doppler sonography of the hepatic artery immediately after surgery: prognostic implications for liver transplant recipients, *AJR Am J Roentgenol* 181:831–838, 2003.

59. Kok T, et al: Doppler ultrasound of the hepatic artery and vein performed daily in the first two weeks after orthotopic liver transplantation. Useful for the diagnosis of acute rejection? *Invest Radiol* 31:173–179, 1996.

60. Propeck PA, Scanlan KA: Reversed or absent hepatic arterial diastolic flow in the liver transplants shown by duplex sonography: a poor predictor of subsequent hepatic artery thrombosis, *AJR Am J Roentgenol* 152:1199–1201, 1992.

61. Hedegard WC, et al: Hepatic arterial waveforms on early posttransplant Doppler ultrasound, *Ultrasound Q* 27:49–54, 2011.

62. Nolten A, Sproat IA: Hepatic artery thrombosis after liver transplantation: temporal accuracy of diagnosis with duplex US and the syndrome of impending thrombosis, *Radiology* 198:553–559, 1996.

63. Vaidya S, et al: Liver transplantation: vascular complications, *Ultrasound Q* 23:239–253, 2007.

64. Berry JD, Sidhu PS: Microbubble contrast-enhanced ultrasound in liver transplantation, *Eur Radiol* 14(Suppl 8):P96–P103, 2004.

65. Hom BK, et al: Prospective evaluation of vascular complications after liver transplantation: comparison of conventional and microbubble contrast-enhanced US, *Radiology* 241:267–274, 2006.

66. Sidhu PS, et al: Microbubble ultrasound contrast in the assessment of hepatic artery patency following liver transplantation: Role in reducing frequency of hepatic artery angiography, *Eur Radiol* 14: 21–20, 2004.

67. Tamsel S, et al: Vascular complications after liver transplantation: evaluation with Doppler US, *Abdom Imaging* 32:339–347, 2007.

68. Caiado AH, et al: Complications of liver transplantation: Multimodality imaging approach, *Radiographics* 27:1401–1417, 2007.

69. Quiroga S, et al: Complications of orthotopic liver transplantation: Spectrum of findings with helical CT, *Radiographics* 21:1085–1110, 2001.

70. Wozney P, et al: Vascular complications after liver transplantation: A 5 year experience, *AJR Am J Roentgenol* 147:657–663, 1986.

71. Langnas AN, et al: Vascular complications after orthotopic liver transplantation, *Am J Surg* 161:76–82, 1991.

72. Flint EW, et al: Duplex sonography of hepatic artery thrombosis after liver transplantation, *AJR Am J Roentgenol* 151:481–483, 1998.

73. Errocal T, et al: Pediatric liver transplantation: A pictorial essay of early and late complications, *Radiographics* 26:1187–1209, 2006.

74. Sanchez-Bueno F, et al: Hepatic artery complications after liver transplantation, *Clin Transplant* 8:399–404, 1994.

75. Dodd GD, et al: Hepatic artery stenosis and thrombosis in transplant recipients: Doppler diagnosis with resistive index and systolic acceleration time, *Radiology* 192:657–661, 1994.

76. Friedewald SM, et al: Vascular and nonvascular complications of liver transplants: Sonographic evaluation and correlation with other imaging modalities and findings at surgery and pathology, *Ultrasound Q* 19:71–85, 2003.

77. Vit A, et al: Doppler evaluation of arterial complications of adult orthotopic liver transplantation, *J Clin Ultrasound* 31:339–345, 2003.

78. Fistouris J, et al: Pseudoaneurysm of the hepatic artery following liver transplantation, *Transplant Proc* 38:2679–2682, 2006.

79. Ginat DT, et al: Stent-graft placement for management of iatrogenic hepatic artery branch pseudoaneurysm after liver transplantation, *Vasc Endovascular Surg* 43:513–517, 2009.

80. Marshall MM, et al: Hepatic pseudoaneurysms following liver transplantation: incidence, presenting figures and management, *Clin Radiol* 56:579–587, 2001.

81. Chong WK, Beland JC, Weeks SM: Sonographic evaluation of venous obstruction in liver transplants, *AJR Am J Roentgenol* 188:515–521, 2007.

82. Kim KW, et al: Doppler sonographic abnormalities suggestive of venous congestion in the right lobe graft of living donor liver transplant recipients, *AJR Am J Roentgenol* 188:239–245, 2007.

83. Ko EY, et al: Hepatic vein stenosis after living donor liver transplantation: evaluation with Doppler US, *Radiology* 229:806–810, 2003.

84. Jain A, et al: Posttransplant lymphoproliferative disorders in liver transplantation: A 20 year experience, *Ann Surg* 236:429–437, 2002.

85. Letourneau JG, Castaneda-Zunega WR: The role of radiology in the diagnosis and treatment of biliary complications after liver transplantation, *Cardiovasc Intervent Radiol* 13:278–283, 1990.

86. Stratta RJ, et al: Diagnosis and treatment of biliary tract complications after orthotopic liver transplantation, *Surgery* 106:675–683, 1989.

87. Lerut J, et al: Biliary tract complications in human orthotopic liver transplantation, *Transplantation* 43:47–51, 1987.

SCREENING FOR VASCULAR DISEASE

35

JOSEPH F. POLAK, MD, MPH

Medical screening is the process of using a diagnostic algorithm to detect a disease or the susceptibility to develop a disease. A screening process can consist of a medical history, a blood sample for measuring a marker such as cholesterol, or a medical image targeting a certain morphologic or functional trait. The screening process is normally applied to a patient population with predefined characteristics. The ultimate applicability of the screening process requires weighing of the benefits to the population or "average" individual against the costs of the process. This form of public health screening has to be distinguished from the benefits and disadvantages of performing "individual" screening with the costs borne not by society but by the individual being screened. The latter scenario will not be discussed in this chapter.

This chapter focuses on application of B-mode and Doppler ultrasound imaging to individuals without any clinical signs or manifestations of arterial disease. The goal is to identify from a large group of individuals a smaller subset with the disease so that an intervention can be performed. This approach is one of primary prevention. This means that the patient being screened is *asymptomatic and without any clinical signs.*

Certain clinical scenarios will not be discussed in this chapter. For example, a patient with prior lower extremity bypass surgery who has an ankle-arm index measurement or a Doppler ultrasound study of the graft is not considered as being screened since the patient obviously has peripheral vascular disease. The patient is undergoing surveillance, a form of secondary prevention (i.e., a diagnostic test is used to identify a subset of the patient population that might have an abrupt occlusion of a bypass graft). In another scenario, a patient who recently had a stroke then undergoes a carotid ultrasound examination. This is not considered to be screening. This patient is being managed as part of a clinical workup. The goal

is to detect the presence of a significant carotid artery stenosis and potentially correct it. This can also be considered as being secondary prevention since the patient already has the clinical outcome and the goal is to prevent recurrent strokes.

This chapter, after reviewing some generic aspects of screening, will address three different aspects of screening: use of color Doppler ultrasound to detect significant carotid artery stenoses in asymptomatic individuals, the use of ultrasound to detect abdominal aortic aneurysms, and the use of ultrasound to detect high-risk individuals for the presence of subclinical atherosclerosis.

DEFINITION AND TYPES OF SCREENING

What is screening? The different elements of a screening process were clearly presented in a World Health Organization (WHO) bulletin published in 1968.[1] These basic principles are listed in Table 35-1. It is obvious that certain criteria have to be met in order to make the screening process a success. Each of these criteria will be discussed when we review the three screening protocols described in this chapter.

In addition to these basic principles, it is important to remember that the word *screening* has multiple meanings. Three specific types of screening are described in the WHO bulletin: selective screening, mass public health screening, and surveillance (Table 35-2).

SELECTIVE SCREENING

The selective screening approach is the application of a diagnostic test to a predetermined asymptomatic population that has certain risk factors. These risk factors are identified by other means than the screening tool. For example, a clinical history of cigarette smoking is a risk factor for aneurysm formation. The yield of an abdominal ultrasound will therefore be greater in smokers than in nonsmokers. The problem with this approach is that the individual who has never smoked can still have an aneurysm, although the odds are much lower than for the smoker. He/she will unfortunately not meet the criteria for screening.

MASS PUBLIC SCREENING

The second type of screening is a mass public screening. This approach is to apply the same test to the whole population. Mass screening does not necessarily mean that everybody is screened. Often, a specific demographic criterion such as age, sex, or geographic location is used to focus the process. Testing young children for thyroid hormone levels is such an example. The basic limitation with this approach is cost.

SURVEILLANCE SCREENING

The third type of screening is surveillance screening, and its implications are often ignored. One of the WHO criteria indicates that the disease being screened for has a well-defined natural history and that an intervention is available to treat it. The finding of an ectatic aorta, while not quite an aneurysm, in a patient is such an example. Although the diagnosis of an aneurysm has not been made, the patient is at increased risk for developing an aneurysm. The patient will need monitoring since the risk for aneurysm formation is increased. The appropriate time interval for the surveillance examinations needs to be determined and justified.

SCREENING FOR ASYMPTOMATIC CAROTID STENOSIS

The goal of this type of screening is the detection of individuals who are asymptomatic, at risk for stroke, and would benefit from an operative intervention, currently carotid endarterectomy. The Doppler screening test has to be compared to the results of carotid angiography since the benefits of carotid endarterectomy are measured based on the arteriogram and not the Doppler ultrasound examination. This assumes that there is a cut-point above which, by arteriography, a carotid stenosis is considered significant and

---

TABLE 35-1 Principles of Screening Presented by Wilson and Jungner*

1. The condition sought should be an important health problem.
2. There should be an accepted treatment for patients with recognized disease.
3. Facilities for diagnosis and treatment should be available.
4. There should be a recognizable latent or early symptomatic stage.
5. There should be a suitable test or examination.
6. The test should be acceptable to the population.
7. The natural history of the condition, including development from latent to declared disease, should be adequately understood.
8. There should be an agreed policy on whom to treat as patients.
9. The cost of case-finding (including diagnosis and treatment of patients diagnosed) should be economically balanced in relation to possible expenditure on medical care as a whole.
10. Case-finding should be a continuing process and not a "once and for all" project.

*From Wilson JMG, Jungner G: *Principles and practice of screening for disease,* Geneva, 1968, World Health Organization.

TABLE 35-2 Differences Between Types of Screening

	Selective Screening	Mass Screening	Surveillance Screening
Advantages	Appropriate for individuals	Applied to whole population	Applied to subset with precursor lesion and at highest risk for developing a clinical outcome
	Decrease in costs as compared to mass screening	Unlikely to miss individuals at risk	Permits timing of intervention
Disadvantages	Expensive: high cost per individual	Expensive: low cost but for many individuals	Expensive: repeat examinations over time
	Even low-risk individuals might have the lesion	False positives are very likely	Requires motivation to have repeat examinations
	Requires individual motivation	Large infrastructure needed to perform reliable test	Psychologic effect of having a biological "time bomb"

an intervention is justified. The question then becomes how accurate is a Doppler ultrasound in detecting the stenosis and grading it as compared to arteriography?

DEFINING ACCURACY OF DOPPLER ULTRASOUND

Accuracy of Doppler ultrasound is measured as the sensitivity and specificity of the Doppler ultrasound examination and shown in Table 35-3. A derived value, the negative predictive value is also very important. One would believe that the positive predictive value of a test would be more important than the negative predictive value; however, this is not the case. A screening Doppler examination has to be as sensitive as possible when compared to the gold standard measurement made by arteriography. While we would like to make sure that the individuals that we classify as negative are without significant stenosis, we need to set a Doppler velocity threshold low enough so that individuals with disease are not being missed. However, by setting a low screening threshold, we detect not only individuals with significant stenosis but also individuals without disease, and the false-positive rate is very high. This leads to a low positive predictive value and a high negative predictive value (Table 35-4).

This is the basic dilemma of any screening test: the sensitivity has to be set very high. Therefore, in order to screen a population for asymptomatic carotid artery stenosis, the Doppler velocity threshold for a given degree of stenosis is set lower than normal, and many individuals are misclassified as having a significant stenosis. The overall performance of the process is also affected by disease prevalence.

DOPPLER ULTRASOUND IN LARGE TRIALS OF ASYMPTOMATIC PATIENTS

Diagnostic Performance

Two multicenter trials have used Doppler velocity measurements to identify individuals with significant carotid artery stenosis (≥60% diameter narrowing)[2,3] who would then undergo carotid endarterectomy. The Asymptomatic Carotid Atherosclerosis Study (ACAS)[2] investigators used carotid Doppler ultrasound as a screening test but with the intent of ensuring that almost all individuals who went on to carotid arteriography and surgery would have a lesion of at least 60% in their carotid artery. For this reason, the selected Doppler velocity threshold was set to a high enough value so that 95% of selected individuals would have a lesion causing a diameter narrowing of 60% or more.[2] This approach yielded a high positive predictive value and also resulted in a low negative predictive value. In essence, many individuals who likely had carotid artery stenoses above 60% were missed.

The ACAS trial[2] gives insights into the use of carotid Doppler ultrasound as a screening tool. On the technical side, lessons to be learned from this study are the need for strict adherence to a quality control process, adherence to strict protocols, and selection of an appropriate ultrasound imaging device. On the practical side, ACAS

TABLE 35-3 Key Parameters for a Screening Test

	Disease Present	Disease Absent
Test positive for disease	a	b
Test negative for disease	c	d
Total	a + c	b + d

Sensitivity: a/(a + c)
Specificity: d/(b + d)
Disease prevalence: (a + c)/(a + c + b + d)
Positive predictive value: a/(a + b)
Negative predictive value: d/(c + d)

TABLE 35-4 Estimated Rates of Detection of Disease and False Positives for a High-Accuracy Diagnostic Test* †

Prevalence	Sensitivity/ Specificity	True Positive	False Positives	Positive Predictive Value	Negative Predictive Value
10%	90%/90%	180	162	52.6%	98.8%
	95%/85%	190	270	41.3%	99.4%
5%	90%/90%	90	171	34.5%	99.4%
	95%/85%	95	285	25%	99.7%

*Calculations are based on 2000 individuals being screened with disease prevalence of 10% and 5%.
†Calculations are based on equations shown in Table 35-3. Estimates of the true positives and false positives can be extrapolated for larger populations by multiplying the numbers in these columns by (number in population /2000).

showed the relatively low cost-effectiveness of screening asymptomatic individuals suitable for carotid endarterectomy.

Although the overall sensitivity of carotid Doppler in all ACAS centers was not measured, the overall specificity of carotid ultrasound was above 97%.[4] Carotid ultrasound was, however, used according to a very strict protocol. Qualifying centers needed to show a strong correlation between Doppler measurements and the results of carotid arteriography. Marked variations between centers and outlier centers with poor accuracy of carotid Doppler[4] improved with new instrumentation selection and a standardized imaging protocol.[5] The success of carotid ultrasound in ACAS was based on the use of a standard imaging protocol, a certification program for both sonographers and vascular laboratories, and the implementation of a quality assurance program supervised by a central coordinating center.

Effect of Ultrasound Devices

Differences in imaging devices or imaging protocols likely affected the diagnostic performance of Doppler ultrasound in ACAS[6-8] and are therefore likely to affect any screening process that looks at detecting significant carotid artery stenosis in the population. The variability of carotid Doppler ultrasound is measurable at the level of individual laboratories and for different imaging devices,[7,9] confirming the observations made in ACAS.[5] Despite this variability, carotid Doppler ultrasound is likely to perform well as a screening tool. The European Asymptomatic Carotid Surgery Trial (ACST) used locally derived parameters to define percent stenosis by carotid ultrasound and achieved outcome results very similar to those of the ACAS study.[3]

Defining Thresholds

The effectiveness of carotid artery screening is dependent on the reliability of Doppler velocities to estimate the degree of percent stenosis in the carotid artery. Results are compared to those of arteriography, the gold standard. Since carotid Doppler ultrasound has a sensitivity and specificity of less than 100%, there will always be false positives and false negatives. Falsely elevated Doppler velocity measurement leads to extra costs, as a risk to the patient, when individuals without disease go on to the intervention (false positives). Conversely, individuals with disease

can be missed because of falsely low Doppler velocity readings and excluded from the benefits of an intervention (false negative).

The use of carotid Doppler ultrasound to detect the presence of "significant" disease requires the selection of a velocity parameter and of a threshold value for this parameter. Based on ACAS[5] and on a consensus recommendation,[10] the internal carotid artery peak systolic velocity is the most reliable of the Doppler velocity parameters and should be used. A strategy that relies on the power Doppler image[11] can help triage patients, but this adds an intermediate step and is therefore not likely to be cost-effective. A peak systolic velocity value of 125 cm/sec should suffice for detecting a 50% diameter carotid artery stenosis.[10,12] Detection of a 70% carotid artery stenosis can be done using a value of 230 cm/sec,[7,10,13] although this value may show greater interlaboratory variability.[7] A value of 260 cm/sec has been reported for stenosis greater than or equal to 60%,[14] but is higher than that reported for lesions causing 70% or greater stenosis (230 cm/sec).[13] Of the two, the lower threshold of 230 cm/sec seems more suitable since it has high sensitivity and therefore fewer individuals with disease are likely to be missed (Figure 35-1).

AN OVERVIEW OF OVERALL EFFECTIVENESS

The value of the screening process also depends on the degree of stenosis used to determine the need for a surgical intervention. ACAS results show a benefit of carotid endarterectomy for

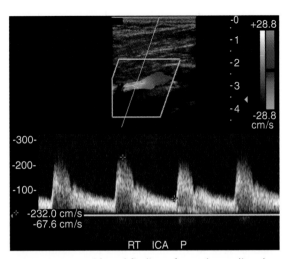

FIGURE 35-1 Incidental finding of a peak systolic velocity of slightly greater than 230 cm/sec in a patient without symptoms who participated in a screening program.

stenosis of 60% or greater as a relative risk reduction of 55%. This, however, translates to an absolute risk reduction, at 5 years, of 5.9%, or slightly more than 1 morbidity event for slightly less than 100 operated patients each year. Data from a European study also shows an absolute risk reduction of 5.3% over 5 years.[3] Based on the data from these studies, 94 to 98 asymptomatic patients with significant (>60% diameter stenosis) need to have carotid endartertectomy performed in order to prevent one stroke. This shows that the yield of the screening process is very low since a large number of patients need to be screened and of the small proportion of identified patients, a large number need to undergo surgery in order to prevent one stroke.

It is the combination of the yield of positive examinations and the yield of the intervention that needs to be factored into an evaluation of the efficacy of the screening process.

Some of the answers to some of these issues can be derived from epidemiologic studies in which carotid ultrasound has been used to estimate the degree of stenosis. In the Cardiovascular Health Study (CHS), a multicenter study of 5888 individuals age 65 years or more, carotid Doppler velocity measurements were used to measure the severity of carotid disease. The prevalence of lesions causing velocities above 250 cm/sec was 1.03%[15] and a still-low 5.5 % for lesions causing Doppler velocities above 150 cm/sec.[15] Figure 35-2 shows on the y-axis the proportion of individuals who are likely to have a Doppler velocity below the value listed on the x-axis. Only a small proportion of the population being screened has values above a selected

threshold. Using data from CHS[15] and assuming that individuals with Doppler velocities above 250 cm/sec warrant an intervention, 1030 out of 100,000 individuals age 65 years or more presenting for screening each year would be candidates for endarterectomy. Based on ACAS/ACST, approximately 10.8 strokes would be prevented if the 1030 underwent the intervention. The cost of 100,000 carotid ultrasounds has to be added to the cost of 1030 endarterectomies to give a rough appreciation of the efficacy of using Doppler ultrasound to screen for asymptomatic individuals. Even if we account $100 for the Doppler examination and $2000 for the surgery, the saved "strokes" cost $ 12,060,000. The net cost for saving one stroke each year is $1,117,000. This does not take into account the cost of investigating false-positive Doppler ultrasound studies.

This simple cost-effectiveness evaluation shows the high cost and relatively low yield of screening for significant asymptomatic carotid artery stenosis.[16]

SURVEILLANCE

There are few observational data on which to base recommendations for monitoring patients with less than 60% carotid artery stenosis.[17] A Doppler value between 175 cm/sec and 260 cm/sec seems to identify a subset of patients with higher risk for progression.[17] There are few data useful to help identify individuals with lesser degrees of stenosis that might be at risk for progression. An interesting clinical question is whether or not a clinical protocol should grade the extent of plaque as either present or absent or into finer subjective groupings. If all plaques that are not

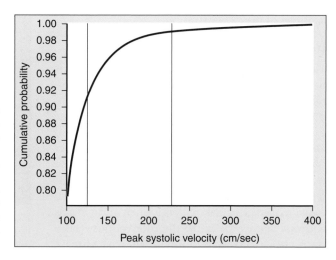

FIGURE 35-2 Based on prevalence data in the general population, this graph summarizes the probability of a patient having a Doppler velocity below the value on the intercept. For example, the intercept for 125 cm/sec corresponds to a likelihood of less than 92%. The likelihood of having a Doppler velocity above 125 cm/sec, which corresponds to a 50% stenosis, is therefore slightly more than 8%. The prevalence of a Doppler velocity above 230 cm/sec, corresponding to a 70% stenosis, is less than 1% in the general population.

hemodynamically significant, say with velocities less than 125 cm/sec, are lumped together, then surveillance is hard to justify given the large number of individuals with small plaques. If plaques are graded in categories such as 1% to 24% and 25% to 49% or 1% to 15% and 16% to 49%, then the subset of larger plaques could be submitted to selective surveillance. This assumes that larger plaques are more likely to make the transition to significant stenosis than smaller plaques, an early hypothesis[18] that has been poorly studied.[19]

EXTENT OF THE EXAMINATION

Performance of the carotid ultrasound examination as a screening test should mimic as closely as possible a diagnostic ultrasound examination of the carotid arteries. Based on epidemiologic studies, the minimum would include a peak systolic velocity at the point of aliasing on a color Doppler image of the internal carotid artery and good gray-scale images confirming the presence of a plaque.

SUMMARY

In itself, screening for asymptomatic carotid artery stenosis might have some benefit to the individual, but it is not a cost-effective process (Table 35-5).

ABDOMINAL ANEURYSM SCREENING

OVERVIEW

Ultrasound screening for the presence of abdominal aortic aneurysm has been a justified expenditure in the United States since 2007. The original proposal of Screening Abdominal Aortic Aneurysm Very Efficiently (SAAAVE) and recommendations by the U.S. Preventive Health Task Force[20] led to the adoption by the Centers for Medicare and Medicaid Services (CMS) of a policy that permits the use of one abdominal screening ultrasound examination in men of 65 years or more. This is a selective screening since this specifically applies to men, individuals who have smoked 100 cigarettes or more during their life, and also individuals with a family history of aneurysm formation.

VALIDITY OF B-MODE (GRAY-SCALE) ULTRASOUND

In contrast to carotid artery stenosis screening with Doppler ultrasound, the gray-scale abdominal ultrasound examination is considered a gold standard for the detection of aortic aneurysms.

The discussion regarding sensitivity and specificity is therefore not a consideration when evaluating the value of this imaging approach (Figure 35-3). Implicitly, this pushes aortic abdominal screening toward being cost-effective since consideration does not have to be given to the engendered false-positive cases. Validation has been documented by comparing associations between ultrasound-measured abdominal aortic diameters and risk factors.[21] The technique is therefore assumed to be its own gold standard, although the reproducibility of the ultrasound

TABLE 35-5 Screening for Asymptomatic "Significant" Carotid Artery Stenosis

WHO Principles of Screening	Applicability
The condition sought should be an important health problem.	Risk for stroke estimated at greater than 5% per year.
There should be an accepted treatment for patients with recognized disease.	Carotid endarterectomy / carotid stent.
Facilities for diagnosis and treatment should be available.	Part of routine clinical care.
There should be a recognizable latent or early symptomatic stage.	Precursor significant stenoses can become symptomatic.
There should be a suitable test or examination.	Carotid ultrasound.
The test should be acceptable to the population.	Noninvasive.
The natural history of the condition, including development from latent to declared disease, should be adequately understood.	Presence of plaque and plaque size linked to likelihood of developing significant stenotic lesions.
There should be an agreed policy on whom to treat as patients.	Debatable as to overall number of strokes prevented.
The cost of case-finding (including diagnosis and treatment of patients diagnosed) should be economically balanced in relation to possible expenditure on medical care as a whole.	Relatively expensive.
Case-finding should be a continuing process and not a "once and for all" project.	Implementable if costs are not factored in.

WHO, World Health Organization.

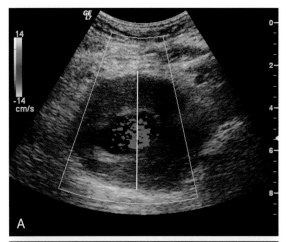

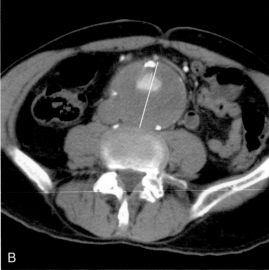

FIGURE 35-3 A, Incidental finding of a 6-cm aneurysm in a patient who presented with syncope. Note the small lumen *(in red)* as compared to the total size of the aneurysm *(white line)*. **B,** Corresponding computed tomogram confirming the presence of a 6-cm aneurysm. The yellow line is the lumen diameter, and the white line is the full diameter of the aneurysm.

examination might be slightly worse than that of computed tomography.[22,23]

The effect of the ultrasound device has not been addressed in any of the large published studies on aortic screening. Unlike Doppler ultrasound measurements of internal carotid artery stenosis, the reproducibility and accuracy of B-mode ultrasound does not seem to be an issue in large multicenter studies.

SURVEILLANCE

The natural history of abdominal aortic aneurysms is that of progressive growth ultimately leading to rupture. The association between aneurysm size and the risk for rupture has been well documented in observational studies made with ultrasound examinations or in historical series relying on measurements made by arteriography.[24-26]

The threshold for determining the level of significance of an abdominal aneurysm has been set at 5.5 cm since the risk for rupture increases dramatically at this point and above. However, it can be argued that the size range between 5 and 5.5 cm in aortic diameters marks a transition zone where the risk for rupture starts to increase significantly. The screening exercise is therefore not limited to detecting the presence of only large aneurysms. The presence of any aneurysm is considered to be the starting point of a surveillance protocol. The presence of an aneurysm, assuming a 3.0 cm threshold, indicates that the patient is at continued risk over time since aneurysms tend to grow. The growth rates, although roughly proportional to aneurysm size,[27] are considered to be in the range of 1 to 2 mm/yr for most small aneurysms.[28] Unfortunately, some individuals can show more rapid growth rates. Appropriate selection of a surveillance interval is controversial. For example, as soon as an aneurysm is detected, a second examination should likely be performed within 6 months to confirm that the aneurysm is not showing rapid expansion. The time interval between examinations then will depend on the size of the aneurysm, typically yearly for aneurysms 3 to 4 cm in size and possibly increasing to every 6 months when the aneurysm transitions from 4 to 5 cm. By 5 cm, the relative risk and benefits of an intervention should be carefully weighed. The time interval between visits will vary from 3 to 6 months. The timing is chosen to detect possible rapid expansion and help schedule an elective intervention, either using an open surgical technique with bypass graft or tube graft placement or by means of an endovascular approach and endograft insertion.

While a relative increase in aortic diameter of 50% is used as a definition of an aneurysm, there are many instances in which smaller areas of aortic dilatation can be detected. These areas where the increase in relative diameter is 20% or more correspond to areas of ectasia (Figure 35-4). Typically these bulges measure 3.0 cm or less.[29] Despite their small size, these lesions should be considered precursors of aortic aneurysm. Although their expansion rates tend to be low,[30] rapid expansion to values above 4.0 cm can occur

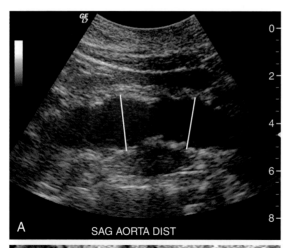

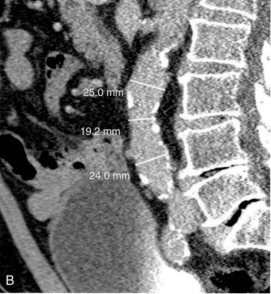

FIGURE 35-4 **A,** Small bulge in the abdominal aorta identified by the white lines. The diameters are less than 3.0 cm. **B,** The corresponding computed tomogram confirms the areas of ectasia, greater than the baseline diameter of 1.9 cm yet below the 3.0-cm cut-point. The clinical significance of this finding is controversial.

in a small percentage of cases. Surveillance intervals of 2 years seem reasonable based on what data there are in the literature.[29,30]

Ultrasound surveillance of aortic aneurysm size is more easily justified than surveillance for asymptomatic carotid artery stenosis. From an outcome point of view, an abdominal aortic aneurysm of 5.5 cm or larger carries with it a well-documented risk for death through rupture above 5% per year. Carotid ultrasound detection of a significant stenosis (≥60%) carries an excess risk of 1% to 2% for stroke and not necessarily

death. Serial measurements of abdominal aortic aneurysm size are very consistent, and progression can be readily measured. Progression of clinically significant carotid artery stenosis has been less well documented, and measurement variability of Doppler velocities is greater than that of gray-scale images used for aortic imaging.

EXTENT OF THE EXAMINATION

The examination will typically include an evaluation of the full length of the aorta from the diaphragm to the iliac artery bifurcation. The proximal common iliac arteries should be evaluated to detect the extension of an abdominal aortic aneurysm, the primary formation of an aneurysm, or the presence of iliac artery involvement.[31]

A gray-scale frequency of 3 to 3.5 MHz or greater is normally used, and a curved array transducer offers the most flexibility. The basic images stored are transverse images of the proximal, mid, and distal abdominal aorta with the associated diameter measurements. Measurements are made outer wall to outer wall. Although anteroposterior and transverse diameter measurements are made, the anteroposterior measurements are more reliable since they are based on the reflection of the ultrasound beam from the aortic wall interfaces. The major caveat is the need for the sonographer to reorient the imaging plane perpendicular to the axis of the aorta. Transverse measurements of the common iliac artery diameters are also made.

Sagittal images can be used to confirm the anteroposterior measurements. The sagittal images also offer the ability to detect the presence of early aortic ectasia, a relative enlargement of the aortic diameter of 20% or more but less than 50% (see Figure 35-4).

The reported 95% confidence intervals for replicate measurements of the abdominal aorta are 4.0 mm based on transverse images, although these are likely lower if sagittal images are also used. Serial changes of less than 4.0 mm should be considered to be within the measurement error of the technique.[22]

SUMMARY

Ultrasound screening for abdominal aortic aneurysms is recognized as being cost-effective and is now implemented for men in the United States (Table 35-6). The differences between men and women when it comes to disease prevalence and

TABLE 35-6 Screening for Abdominal Aortic Aneurysm

WHO Principles of Screening	Applicability
The condition sought should be an important health problem.	Risk for rupture linked to death is well documented.
There should be an accepted treatment for patients with recognized disease.	Aortic grafting or endograft.
Facilities for diagnosis and treatment should be available.	Part of routine clinical care.
There should be a recognizable latent or early symptomatic stage.	Ectatic aorta and small aneurysms.
There should be a suitable test or examination.	Abdominal ultrasound.
The test should be acceptable to the population.	Noninvasive and accepted as gold standard.
The natural history of the condition, including development from latent to declared disease, should be adequately understood.	Well documented.
There should be an agreed policy on whom to treat as patients.	Mild debate on waiting until 5.5 cm vs 5.0 cm.
The cost of case-finding (including diagnosis and treatment of patients diagnosed) should be economically balanced in relation to possible expenditure on medical care as a whole.	Relatively expensive but cost-effective for men.
Case-finding should be a continuing process and not a "once and for all" project.	Normal aorta at 65 years of age makes it unlikely a large aneurysm will develop before death from other causes.

WHO, World Health Organization.

possibly disease outcome suggest this should also be considered for women.

SCREENING FOR CARDIOVASCULAR DISEASE: RISK AND SUBCLINICAL CARDIOVASCULAR DISEASE

Until now, the discussion has focused on the use of ultrasound to detect instances where there is a clear-cut morbidity, stroke or aortic aneurysm rupture, and accepted surgical or endovascular interventions. However, these are late manifestations of cardiovascular disease. In this section, the use of ultrasound as a means of screening and detecting young individuals that might have very early evidence of cardiovascular disease and are therefore at high risk for future cardiovascular events in the next few decades of life are discussed.

CARDIOVASCULAR RISK FACTORS

Studies like the Framingham Heart Study[32] helped define specific parameters associated with the likelihood of developing myocardial infarctions. These parameters are the Framingham Risk Score variables and include age, history of diabetes, history of smoking, systolic blood pressure, and cholesterol levels (low-density-lipoprotein cholesterol as a positive risk and high-density-lipoprotein cholesterol as protective).[33] These

measures became recognized as risk factors for cardiovascular events and, therefore, risk factors for cardiovascular disease.

SUBCLINICAL CARDIOVASCULAR DISEASE

Cardiovascular disease develops early and progresses over time. Autopsy studies on young individuals suffering sudden traumatic death show progressive involvement of different arterial beds with atherosclerotic lesions with age even in the 20s and 30s.[34] The presence of these atherosclerotic lesions and plaques is also associated with the basic cardiovascular risk factors mentioned in the preceding paragraph.[35]

However, it is increasingly understood that cardiovascular events occur in the background of a certain level of atherosclerosis and that atherosclerosis is a system-wide disease. Clinical cardiovascular events mark the transition from asymptomatic subclinical disease to clinical disease. The odds of the patient having a clinical event increase with the extent of atherosclerotic burden and can be compared to the progressive increase of an undersea volcano that, with time, reaches the surface (Figure 35-5). Although patients have myocardial infarctions because of coronary thrombosis at the site of a culprit lesion,[36] autopsy studies have shown that there is global involvement of the coronary arteries by plaques causing significant stenoses.[37,38] Atherosclerosis is a systemic disease. Plaque in the carotid artery is more likely present if

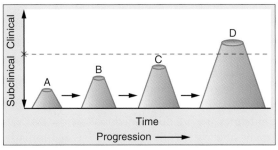

FIGURE 35-5 Representation of the progression of subclinical cardiovascular disease. Here the extent of atherosclerotic burden is represented as an undersea volcano. The likelihood of a transition between subclinical disease (*A, B,* and *C*) and clinical disease (stroke, myocardial infarction; *D*) increases with the extent of subclinical disease. The bigger the volcano (subclinical disease), the more likely it is to reach the surface (transit to a clinical event). This does not preclude a rapid evolution from a lower level of subclinical disease to a symptomatic event. The likelihood of this occurring decreases with lower burdens of subclinical disease.

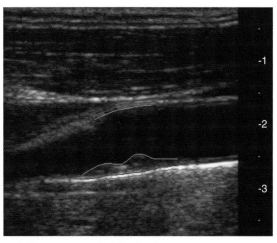

FIGURE 35-6 Examination conducted as part of an epidemiologic study. A plaque is present in the proximal internal carotid artery of a 40-year-old man (between the green line and the blue line). This is a finding suggestive of a larger atherosclerotic burden than expected for a man of that age.

there is plaque in the coronary artery.[39] Presence of carotid artery plaque is therefore a surrogate measure of coronary artery disease. In the Framingham study, a value of 25% or greater diameter stenosis in the internal carotid artery has served to identify individuals with atherosclerotic disease.[40,41] Two consensus meetings on using carotid artery ultrasound for screening individuals for the presence of early atherosclerosis have proposed that a carotid artery wall thickness of 1.5 mm or more is also a measure of atherosclerotic plaque.[42,43] The presence of relatively small focal carotid lesions in the carotid system can therefore serve as a surrogate for the determination of atherosclerotic burden in young individuals (Figure 35-6). These measurements are semiquantitative and subjective yet can serve as a powerful noninvasive tool for determining the effects of risk factor exposure on the arterial system. The absence of a plaque in the carotid arteries is also a good index of a low risk for coronary disease.[44]

These measures have not been routinely applied in the clinic, but observational studies suggest that they are good markers of early atherosclerosis.

QUANTITATIVE MEASURES OF CAROTID ARTERY WALL THICKNESS

In 1986, a group of investigators described a strong association between the presence of atherosclerosis and ultrasound measurement of the wall thickness of the aortic wall. The wall

thickness is measured as the intima-media thickness (IMT) and defined as the distance between the leading edge of the lumen-to-wall interface to the interface between the media and adventitia in the artery wall. This measurement, also performed at the carotid artery wall, correlates with the presence of cardiovascular risk factors (hypercholesterolemia and smoking).[45,46] Carotid ultrasound studies performed in large populations (Atherosclerosis Risk in Communities [ARIC] [47] and Kuopio heart studies[48]) showed early a clear association between focal lesions in the internal carotid artery and common carotid artery IMT.

Whereas the common carotid artery wall thickening is a more diffuse process, the internal carotid artery wall thickness is a measure of carotid plaque. As such, increased internal carotid IMT corresponds to increased degrees of carotid artery stenosis, with measurements of internal carotid artery wall thickness correlating to the extent of subjectively graded percentage stenosis.[15]

IMT AND PREDICTION OF INCIDENT EVENTS

IMT measurements performed in different population groups have shown predictive power for incident events: IMT is a marker for future myocardial infarction as well as for stroke.[49-51]

EFFECT OF EQUIPMENT

Selection of the ultrasound device and the expertise of the sonographer are likely important factors for obtaining precise wall thickness measurements. Differences in ultrasound device selection might explain differences in the ability to evaluate internal carotid artery IMT measurements when comparing the high rate of internal carotid IMT measurements in the CHS[52] and Coronary Artery Risk Development in Young Adults (CARDIA) [53] studies to the lower rates in the ARIC[54] and the Rotterdam[55] studies. High-resolution transducer of at least 5 MHz and typically 7 MHz or above are used. The ideal imaging device has not been formally identified. Different investigators have used imaging devices made by different ultrasound companies, but no systematic comparisons have been made. Modern digital ultrasound devices give more reproducible measurements than the older generation analog devices.[56]

IMAGE ANALYSIS AND IMT AS A MEASURE OF ATHEROSCLEROTIC BURDEN

The simplest methodology for measuring wall thickness is to use calipers to measure IMT directly on the image screen, a hard copy image, or a digital image. IMT measurements made with digital calipers on the ultrasound image screen show a relation to cardiovascular risk factors,[57] but these are not as strong as those made on imaging workstations.[53] A series of crosshairs separated by approximately 1 mm can also be placed along the artery wall and used to measure IMT[58]; however, continuous measurements are more precise[59] and can be used to calculate the mean and maximal IMT values. The mean of the maximal IMT values in the common and internal carotid arteries shows the strongest association with cardiovascular outcomes.

Edge detection algorithms can also be applied to the processing of digitally stored carotid images. The performance of these edge detectors has been well evaluated for the far wall of the common carotid artery. Phantom studies have shown some increase in the precision of IMT measurement as compared to data from human readers.[60]

CRITERIA FOR "POSITIVE" IMT VALUES

There are two approaches proposed for IMT as a screening test. The first is to use IMT as a supplemental measurement added to the traditional cardiovascular risk factors. This is, in fact, a form of selective screening. It is not clear if this approach adds predictive value in identifying individuals at risk for cardiovascular events.[55] A major limitation of this approach is the lack of a standardized range of normal IMT values. Although some authors have proposed various values such as 0.8 mm, 0.7 mm, or 1.0 mm, the fact that IMT increases with age[61] needs to be factored into these calculations.

The second, as proposed by the Screening for Heart Attack Prevention and Education (SHAPE) guidelines, is to identify individuals whose IMT values lie above the 75th percentile.[62] This approach, although rational, has not been tested as an effective screening strategy. It also requires a range of normal values.

IMT MEASUREMENT PROTOCOL

IMT measurements are made at the level of the common carotid artery, as well as in the proximal internal carotid artery. After a survey of the carotid arteries in the transverse plane, imaging is done in a longitudinal plane. The ultrasound beam is perpendicular to the artery wall being interrogated (wall parallel to the surface of the transducer). Two key landmarks are used in an IMT protocol. The carotid artery bulb is the dilatation of the distal common carotid artery that corresponds to the proximal internal carotid artery sinus. The flow divider identifies where the internal and external carotid artery walls are joined. Typically, a 1-cm-long segment of the IMT is measured in the distal common carotid artery before the carotid artery bulb. In some of the IMT literature, the bulb is defined as ending at the flow divider (Figure 35-7) so that the IMT measurement made there includes only a portion of the internal carotid artery sinus.[54] The internal carotid artery IMT is measured over a distance of 1 cm starting from the flow divider and moving to the left. In other IMT imaging protocols, the common carotid artery IMT is measured 0.5 to 1 cm below the bulb (Figure 35-8) in an area free of plaque.[43] The bulb measurement is extended to include the internal carotid artery sinus in yet other protocols.[63]

Significant differences exist in the measurement protocols. A simple approach has been proposed: measure the common carotid artery mean IMT and the maximal IMT in the internal carotid arteries. Again, the lack of normal ranges of values limits the application of this protocol.

APPLICABILITY

The use of IMT as a screening tool assumes the detection of early manifestations of atherosclerosis in relatively young patients but still above

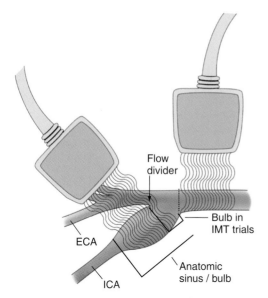

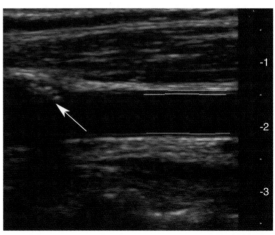

FIGURE 35-7 This diagram shows the difference between the standard approach to intima-media thickness (IMT) measurements in the common carotid artery (CCA) bulb and the corresponding level of the internal carotid artery (ICA) sinus. Plaque formation preferentially occurs in the ICA sinus, beyond the narrow limits defined by the region between the flow divider and the beginning of the carotid bulb. ECA, external carotid artery.

FIGURE 35-8 Variant of an intima-media thickness (IMT) protocol in which the IMT is measured in the common carotid artery 1 cm below the bulb. Note the presence of plaque in the internal carotid artery sinus *(arrow)* despite the relatively thin far-wall common carotid artery IMT (distance between the green and blue lines).

TABLE 35-7 Screening for Subclinical Disease with IMT

WHO Principles of Screening	Applicability
The condition sought should be an important health problem.	Atherosclerotic lesions are the number one cause of death.
There should be an accepted treatment for patients with recognized disease.	Early lifestyle intervention and lipid and blood pressure–lowering therapies.
Facilities for diagnosis and treatment should be available.	Not yet part of routine clinical care; poorly standardized.
There should be a recognizable latent or early symptomatic stage.	Measurement based on thicker than expected IMT for age.
There should be a suitable test or examination.	Carotid ultrasound.
The test should be acceptable to the population.	Noninvasive and accepted as gold standard.
The natural history of the condition, including development from latent to declared disease, should be adequately understood.	Well documented in older adults; inferred from studies of middle-age individuals.
There should be an agreed policy on whom to treat as patients.	Consensus not yet reached.
The cost of case-finding (including diagnosis and treatment of patients diagnosed) should be economically balanced in relation to possible expenditure on medical care as a whole.	Relatively expensive and requires quality assurance and standardization.
Case-finding should be a continuing process and not a "once and for all" project.	Measurement can be repeated; time interval to be determined but likely between 2 and 5 years.

IMT, intima-media thickness; WHO, World Health Organization.

45 years of age. The possible justification of this approach is the availability of various pharmacologic therapies and lifestyle changes that can act on the development of atherosclerosis over time. This preventive strategy makes sense at the level of the individual but is difficult to justify financially (Table 35-7).

CONCLUSIONS

Ultrasound imaging can be used as a screening test. Applicability is very successful and recognized for the detection and monitoring of abdominal aortic aneurysms. The approach is likely not cost-effective for imaging the carotid arteries in order to detect asymptomatic carotid stenoses in need of surgical or endovascular interventions.

The applicability of a more general screening of atherosclerosis and subclinical disease with IMT measurements coupled with internal carotid artery plaque measurements is being investigated. It is part of screening guidelines, but the overall efficacy has not yet been proven.

REFERENCES

1. Wilson JMG, Jungner G: *Principles and practice of screening for disease*, Geneva, 1968, World Health Organization.
2. Executive Committee for the Asymptomatic Carotid Atherosclerosis Study: Endarterectomy for asymptomatic carotid artery stenosis, *JAMA* 273:1421–1428, 1995.
3. Halliday A, et al: Prevention of disabling and fatal strokes by successful carotid endarterectomy in patients without recent neurological symptoms: Randomised controlled trial.[erratum appears in Lancet. 2004 Jul 31; 364(9432):416], *Lancet* 363:1491–1502, 2004.
4. Howard G, et al: An approach for the use of Doppler ultrasound as a screening tool for hemodynamically significant stenosis (despite heterogeneity of Doppler performance). A multicenter experience. Asymptomatic Carotid Atherosclerosis Study investigators, *Stroke* 27:1951–1957, 1996.
5. Schwartz SW, et al: Consistency of Doppler parameters in predicting arteriographically confirmed carotid stenosis. Asymptomatic Carotid Atherosclerosis Study investigators, *Stroke* 28:343–347, 1997.
6. Criswell BK, et al: Evaluating institutional variability of duplex scanning in the detection of carotid artery stenosis, *Am J Surg* 176:591–597, 1998.
7. Kuntz KM, et al: Duplex ultrasound criteria for the identification of carotid stenosis should be laboratory specific, *Stroke* 28:597–602, 1997.
8. Ranke C, et al: Standardization of carotid ultrasound: A hemodynamic method to normalize for interindividual and interequipment variability, *Stroke* 30:402–406, 1999.
9. Fillinger MF, et al: Carotid duplex criteria for a 60% or greater angiographic stenosis: Variation according to equipment, *J Vasc Surg* 24:856–864, 1996.
10. Grant EG, et al: Carotid artery stenosis: Gray-scale and Doppler US diagnosis–Society of Radiologists in Ultrasound consensus conference, *Radiology* 229:340–346, 2003.
11. Bluth EI: Power Doppler imaging to evaluate flow-limiting stenoses, *Radiology* 221:557–558, 2001.
12. Polak JF, et al: Internal carotid artery stenosis: Accuracy and reproducibility of color-Doppler-assisted duplex imaging, *Radiology* 173:793–798, 1989.
13. Hunink MG, et al: Detection and quantification of carotid artery stenosis: Efficacy of various Doppler velocity parameters, *AJR Am J Roentgenol* 160:619–625, 1993.
14. Moneta GL, et al: Screening for asymptomatic internal carotid artery stenosis: Duplex criteria for discriminating 60% to 99% stenosis, *J Vasc Surg* 21:989–994, 1995.
15. Polak JF, et al: Sonographic evaluation of carotid artery atherosclerosis in the elderly: Relationship of disease severity to stroke and transient ischemic attack, *Radiology* 188:363–370, 1993.
16. U.S. Preventive Services Task Force: Screening for carotid artery stenosis: U.S. Preventive Services Task Force recommendation statement.[erratum appears in Ann Intern Med. 2008 Feb 5;148(3):248], *Ann Intern Med* 147:854–859, 2007.
17. Lovelace TD, et al: Optimizing duplex follow-up in patients with an asymptomatic internal carotid artery stenosis of less than 60%, *J Vasc Surg* 33:56–61, 2001.
18. Roederer GO, et al: The natural history of carotid arterial disease in asymptomatic patients with cervical bruits, *Stroke* 15:605–613, 1984.
19. Johnson BF, et al: Clinical outcome in patients with mild and moderate carotid artery stenosis, *J Vasc Surg* 21:120–126, 1995.
20. Fleming C, et al: Screening for abdominal aortic aneurysm: A best-evidence systematic review for the U.S. Preventive Services Task Force, *Ann Intern Med* 142:203–211, 2005.
21. Lederle FA, et al: The aneurysm detection and management study screening program: Validation cohort and final results. Aneurysm Detection and Management Veterans Affairs Cooperative Study Investigators, *Arch Intern Med* 160:1425–1430, 2000.
22. Singh K, et al: Intra- and interobserver variability in ultrasound measurements of abdominal aortic diameter. The tromsø study, *Eur J Vasc Endovasc Surg* 15:497–504, 1998.
23. Singh K, et al: Intra- and interobserver variability in the measurements of abdominal aortic and common iliac artery diameter with computed tomography. The tromsø study, *Eur J Vasc Endovasc Surg* 25:399–407, 2003.
24. Mortality results for randomised controlled trial of early elective surgery or ultrasonographic surveillance for small abdominal aortic aneurysms. The UK small aneurysm trial participants, *Lancet* 352:1649–1655, 1998.
25. Lederle FA, et al: Rupture rate of large abdominal aortic aneurysms in patients refusing or unfit for elective repair, *JAMA* 287:2968–2972, 2002.
26. Vardulaki KA, et al: Growth rates and risk of rupture of abdominal aortic aneurysms.[erratum appears in Br J Surg 1999 Feb;86(2):280], *Br J Surg* 85:1674–1680, 1998.
27. McCarthy RJ, et al: Recommendations for screening intervals for small aortic aneurysms, *Br J Surg* 90:821–826, 2003.

28. Santilli SM, et al: Expansion rates and outcomes for the 3.0-cm to the 3.9-cm infrarenal abdominal aortic aneurysm, *J Vasc Surg* 35:666–671, 2002.

29. d'Audiffret A, et al: Fate of the ectatic infrarenal aorta: Expansion rates and outcomes, *Ann Vasc Surg* 16: 534–536, 2002.

30. Basnyat PS, et al: Natural history of the ectatic aorta, *Cardiovasc Surg* 11:273–276, 2003.

31. Lee ES, et al: Implementation of an aortic screening program in clinical practice: Implications for the Screen for Abdominal Aortic Aneurysms Very Efficiently (SAAAVE) act, *J Vasc Surg* 49:1107–1111, 2009.

32. Dawber TR: *The Framingham study. The epidemiology of atherosclerotic disease. A Commonwealth Fund Book,* Cambridge, MA, and London, England, 1980, Harvard University Press.

33. Wilson PW, et al: Prediction of coronary heart disease using risk factor categories, *Circulation* 97:1837–1847, 1998.

34. Strong JP, et al: Prevalence and extent of atherosclerosis in adolescents and young adults: Implications for prevention from the Pathobiological Determinants of Atherosclerosis in Youth Study, *JAMA* 281:727–735, 1999.

35. McGill HC Jr, et al: Effects of serum lipoproteins and smoking on atherosclerosis in young men and women. The PDAY Research Group. Pathobiological Determinants of Atherosclerosis in Youth, *Arterioscler Thromb Vasc Biol* 17:95–106, 1997.

36. Mann JM, Davies MJ: Vulnerable plaque. Relation of characteristics to degree of stenosis in human coronary arteries, *Circulation* 94:928–931, 1996.

37. Haft JI, et al: Development of significant coronary artery lesions in areas of minimal disease. A common mechanism for coronary disease progression, *Chest* 94:731–736, 1988.

38. Kragel AH, et al: Morphometric analysis of the composition of atherosclerotic plaques in the four major epicardial coronary arteries in acute myocardial infarction and in sudden coronary death, *Circulation* 80:1747–1756, 1989.

39. Wyman RA, et al: Ultrasound-detected carotid plaque as a predictor of cardiovascular events, *Vasc Med* 11: 123–130, 2006.

40. Selhub J, et al: Association between plasma homocysteine concentrations and extracranial carotid-artery stenosis, *N Engl J Med* 332:286–291, 1995.

41. Wilson PW, et al: Cumulative effects of high cholesterol levels, high blood pressure, and cigarette smoking on carotid stenosis, *N Engl J Med* 337:516–522, 1997.

42. Stein JH, et al: Use of carotid ultrasound to identify subclinical vascular disease and evaluate cardiovascular disease risk: A consensus statement from the American Society of Echocardiography Carotid Intima-Media Thickness Task Force. Endorsed by the society for vascular medicine, *J Am Soc Echocardiogr* 21:93–111, 2008. quiz 189–190.

43. Touboul PJ, et al: Mannheim carotid intima-media thickness consensus (2004-2006). An update on behalf of the advisory board of the 3rd and 4th watching the risk symposium, 13th and 15th European stroke conferences, Mannheim, Germany, 2004, and Brussels, Belgium, *Cerebrovasc Dis* 23:75–80, 2007.

44. Brook RD, et al: A negative carotid plaque area test is superior to other noninvasive atherosclerosis studies for reducing the likelihood of having underlying significant coronary artery disease, *Arterioscler Thromb Vasc Biol* 26:656–662, 2006.

45. Pignoli P, et al: Intimal plus medial thickness of the arterial wall: A direct measurement with ultrasound imaging, *Circulation* 74:1399–1406, 1986.

46. Poli A, et al: Ultrasonographic measurement of the common carotid artery wall thickness in hypercholesterolemic patients. A new model for the quantitation and follow-up of preclinical atherosclerosis in living human subjects, *Atherosclerosis* 70:253–261, 1988.

47. Heiss G, et al: Carotid atherosclerosis measured by B-mode ultrasound in populations: Associations with cardiovascular risk factors in the ARIC study, *Am J Epidemiol* 134:250–256, 1991.

48. Salonen R, Salonen J: Determinants of carotid intima-media thickness: A population-based ultrasonography study, *J Intern Med* 229:225–231, 1991.

49. Chambless LE, et al: Association of coronary heart disease incidence with carotid arterial wall thickness and major risk factors: The atherosclerosis risk in communities (ARIC) study, 1987-1993, *Am J Epidemiol* 146: 483–494, 1997.

50. Hodis HN, et al: The role of carotid arterial intima-media thickness in predicting clinical coronary events, *Ann Intern Med* 128:262–269, 1998.

51. O' Leary DH, et al: Carotid-artery intima and media thickness as a risk factor for myocardial infarction and stroke in older adults. Cardiovascular Health Study Collaborative Research Group, *N Engl J Med* 340:14–22, 1999.

52. O'Leary DH, et al: Distribution and correlates of sonographically detected carotid artery disease in the cardiovascular health study. The CHS Collaborative Research Group, *Stroke* 23:1752–1760, 1992.

53. Polak JF, et al: Segment-specific associations of carotid intima-media thickness with cardiovascular risk factors: The Coronary Artery Risk Development in Young Adults (CARDIA) study, *Stroke* 41:9–15, 2010.

54. Howard G, et al: Carotid artery intimal-medial thickness distribution in general populations as evaluated by B-mode ultrasound. ARIC Investigators, *Stroke* 24: 1297–1304, 1993.

55. del Sol AI, et al: Is carotid intima-media thickness useful in cardiovascular disease risk assessment? The rotterdam study, *Stroke* 32:1532–1538, 2001.

56. Baldassarre D, et al: Reproducibility validation study comparing analog and digital imaging technologies for the measurement of intima-media thickness, *Stroke* 31:1104–1110, 2000.

57. Baldassarre D, et al: Carotid artery intima-media thickness measured by ultrasonography in normal clinical practice correlates well with atherosclerotic risk factors, *Stroke* 31:2426–2430, 2000.

58. Atherosclerosis Risk in Communities Study protocol manual 6: *ultrasound assessment, part B:* Chapel Hill, NC, 1989, Ultrasound reading ARIC Coordinating Center. Version 1:68–70.

59. Wendelhag I, et al: Ultrasound measurement of wall thickness in the carotid artery: Fundamental principles and description of a computerized analysing system, *Clin Physiol* 11:565–577, 1991.

60. Selzer RH, et al: Evaluation of computerized edge tracking for quantifying intima-media thickness of the common carotid artery from B-mode ultrasound images, *Atherosclerosis* 111:1–11, 1994.

61. Howard G, et al: Does the association of risk factors and atherosclerosis change with age? An analysis of the combined ARIC and CHS cohorts. The Atherosclerosis Risk in Communities (ARIC) and Cardiovascular Health Study (CHS) investigators, *Stroke* 28:1693–1701, 1997.

62. Naghavi M, et al: From vulnerable plaque to vulnerable patient–part III: Executive summary of the Screening for Heart Attack Prevention and Education (SHAPE) task force report, *Am J Cardiol* 98:2H–15H, 2006.

63. O' Leary DH, et al: Use of sonography to evaluate carotid atherosclerosis in the elderly. The Cardiovascular Health Study. CHS Collaborative Research Group, *Stroke* 22:1155–1163, 1991.

CORRELATIVE IMAGING

36

JOSEPH F. POLAK, MD, MPH, and JOHN S. PELLERITO, MD, FACR, FSRU, FAIUM

OVERVIEW

The current trend in cardiovascular imaging is to increase reliance on noninvasive approaches, to minimize complications linked to invasive imaging, and to reserve invasive techniques for therapeutic interventions.

Arteriography, still the gold standard, is now being performed with greater speed and lower complication rates than in previous decades. This has been achieved with the use of smaller catheters and decreased procedure times linked to digital technologies.

A new facet to the use of traditional x-rays has been the development of computed tomographic angiographic methods. This partly noninvasive approach relies on the intravenous administration of iodinated contrast material. In addition to rapidly obtaining traditional cross-sectional images, the image sets can be reprojected and rendered as three-dimensional (3D) data sets.

Magnetic resonance imaging displays soft tissue images similar to those made with computed tomography (CT) but without the need for ionizing radiation. In addition, specially designed magnetic pulse sequences can be used to create magnetic resonance angiograms. Magnetic resonance angiography (MRA) can be performed with or without the administration of intravenous contrast material containing gadolinium.

Doppler ultrasound imaging has strengths and weaknesses when compared to these other imaging modalities. This chapter reviews different aspects of each of these imaging approaches and compares their diagnostic efficacy.

ARTERIOGRAPHY

Arteriography remains the gold standard examination for the evaluation of patients before any vascular intervention. Current techniques allow for outpatient diagnostic studies to be performed with extremely low morbidity and mortality. The rapid film changers of the 1970s and 1980s have been replaced by completely digital imaging technologies. The iodinated contrast media have lower associated complications with the adoption of nonionic and low-osmolar compounds.

Imaging of vascular structures is dependent on producing x-rays, filling the vessels of interest with iodinated contrast, and recording the images generated (Figure 36-1).

EQUIPMENT AND PRINCIPLES

The basic physical principle behind diagnostic angiography is the production of x-rays that are attenuated in the body to different degrees, related roughly to the electron density in the soft tissues. Vascular structures must first be filled with an electron-dense substance, iodinated contrast material, before they can be clearly visualized. The amount injected and electron density of the material itself must be sufficient to permit preferential visualization by the x-ray imaging device.

The penetrability of x-rays in soft tissues relates directly to the energy of the x-ray photons and is described by the kilovoltage. For angiography, it is usually set between 70 and 80 kV but can be adjusted based on the amount of contrast seen on the final films. Lowering the kilovoltage will improve the contrast between objects on the film, but it will deliver more radiation to the patient. Increasing the kilovoltage increases penetration of the x-ray beam but reduces image contrast.

The x-ray tube defines the area from which x-rays are produced, and the x-ray beam is further focused by collimators (lead screens that reduce the size of the beam to fit the body part being imaged as closely as possible).

A large space is required to comfortably hold the equipment and personnel needed for patient care during the procedure. The room is usually based around the x-ray tube, a patient table, and an x-ray detector. Most digital imaging systems have a C-arm configuration with the x-ray tube coupled to the x-ray detector by a C-shaped bracket. The patient lies on a table situated between the tube and the detector (Figure 36-2). Imaging device configuration varies considerably in sophistication, from small portable systems to table-mounted systems equipped with

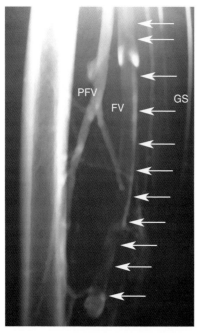

FIGURE 36-1 Venogram of the upper thigh using traditional cut-film venography. Cut-film technique has been replaced by digital imaging techniques. Note the filling defect *(arrowheads)* in the femoral vein (FV) due to acute thrombus. PFV, profunda femoral vein; GS, great saphenous vein.

moving tables for the performance of runoff arteriography.

DIGITAL IMAGING

The resolution of digital images is dependent on the size of the imaging detector, either a phosphor tube intensifier or increasingly, a solid state detector, and the matrix size of the digital image. Large image fields that cover up to 16 inches need a large matrix size such as 1024 by 1024 pixels to give 1.3 line pairs per millimeter of spatial resolution.

Most units allow for "single-station" imaging at a fixed location over an arterial segment or venous segment. More expensive configurations with a moving table can provide multiple station "bolus-chasing" images for imaging of the lower extremity runoff arteries.

Digital subtraction builds on digital imaging by obtaining one or several "mask" images before radiographic contrast injection. The mask image is then subtracted digitally from the images with contrast to display the areas containing contrast only (Figure 36-3). Patient movement during injection causes an imaging "mismatch,", as does respiratory excursion. Full patient cooperation remains necessary for high-quality imaging. Digital subtraction techniques can result in reduction of the amount of contrast agent needed by twofold to threefold.

GENERAL PRINCIPLES: ARTERIAL

Vascular access sites are determined by the pattern of disease. Standard arterial access is the common femoral artery because it is a large vessel

FIGURE 36-2 Diagram showing the differences between traditional x-ray detectors and digital imaging technologies. Not only has the x-ray detector been replaced by solid state detectors, but the signals are fed directly to a computer for processing.

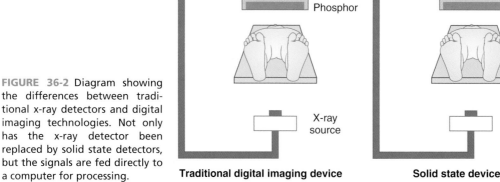

Traditional digital imaging device **Solid state device**

and has low complication rates historically. The axillary artery has a smaller caliber than the common femoral artery, but with the brachial plexus intimately wrapped around it in the brachial fascia, nerve-related complications are possible (0.4%-9.5%). Because of the risk for nerve injury, low brachial artery punctures, at midarm and performed under ultrasound guidance, are preferred. Direct popliteal artery punctures can also be performed but are limited by the increased rate of complications and are reserved for highly specific indications by experienced angiographers and not commonly used.

Puncture of vascular prosthetic grafts is commonly seen in the patient population coming to angiography. Graft puncture can be more difficult because of the fibrosis that surrounds the graft.

GENERAL PRINCIPLES: VENOUS

Lower extremity venography is performed during continued fluoroscopic monitoring of contrast being injected into a pedal vein. Normally the patient is placed on a tilt table so that gravity can help distend the veins. Full opacification of the veins is needed to exclude deep vein thrombosis.

Common femoral vein punctures are performed when the iliac veins or the inferior vena cava has to be studied. Large volumes of contrast, typically 30 to 40 mL, are then rapidly injected while digital venography is performed.

Direct ultrasound-guided punctures into the popliteal or tibial veins are occasionally done during venous interventions.

Upper extremity venography is occasionally performed to map the anatomy of the upper extremity veins. Most often, upper extremity venography is done during an intervention, typically venous thrombolysis to treat an acute deep venous thrombosis of the upper extremity veins.

CONTRAST AGENT ADMINISTRATION

The amount and rate of contrast agent injection depends on the size of the vessel segment being studied and the amount of blood flow. The highest injection rates are used when injecting into the proximal ascending and descending aorta (70-80 mL injected at a rate of 30-40 mL/sec). Selective studies of the mesenteric vasculature can require large volumes of contrast (up to 50-60 mL at rates of 3-5 mL/sec) in order to opacify both the artery branches and mesenteric veins. Lower extremity runoff studies are conducted by sequentially shifting the imaging field of view over the leg arteries during the injection of a bolus of 60 to 90 mL at a rate of 6 to 10 mL/sec. Unilateral arterial studies of the arms and legs require 20 to 30 mL.

The general trend toward the use of nonionic contrast agents has been driven by the decrease in pain, discomfort, and contrast reactions seen when these agents are used. Low-osmolar ionic contrast agents are also available.

Administration of iodinated contrast material is not indicated when renal function is depressed. Below an estimated glomerular filtration rate (GFR) of 30 mL/min per 1.73 m^2, contrast is relatively contraindicated unless the patient is on dialysis. Contrast is administered cautiously and with a hydration protocol when the estimated GFR is between 30 and 60 mL/min per 1.73 m^2. There are no contraindications, except for possible allergic reactions, for estimated GFR above 60 mL/min per 1.73 m^2.

ACCURACY AND REPRODUCIBILITY

The diagnostic accuracy of angiography has been verified by direct surgical correlations. It has been accepted as the gold standard. There are possible limitations in the carotid artery and peripheral arterial systems. In cases of near-occluded carotid arteries, the small amount of contrast that enters the distal internal carotid artery does not permit adequate evaluation of the diameter and quality of the artery. Direct surgical verification is needed to confirm suitability for endarterectomy.

In the lower extremity arteries, opacification of the peripheral runoff vessels in the leg and foot is sometimes not possible. The use of "on-table"

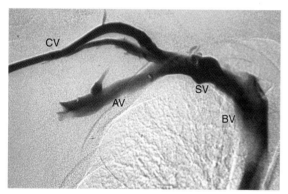

FIGURE 36-3 Right upper extremity venogram using digital technique. Note the absence of the bones. A faint outline of the ribs can be seen as a result of mild respiratory motion. AV, axillary vein; BV, brachiocephalic vein; CV, cephalic vein; SV, subclavian vein.

arteriograms in the operative suite while the patient is under anesthesia has been suggested as a possible way of circumventing this problem in some patients.

Multiple projections are often needed to improve visualization of arterial lesions, related to the fact that arterial lesions tend to be eccentric. Rotational arteriography is another approach to more precisely estimating the degree of stenotic narrowing in an artery.

COMPLICATIONS

Complications are mostly linked to local access sites. Formation of pseudoaneurysms and hematomas increases with catheter size and procedure time as well as the duration of postprocedural groin compression of common femoral arteries. Arteriovenous fistulas are more likely with punctures made lower down the thigh.

Contrast allergy rates are much lower than rates seen for intravenous injections.

Local complications such as dissections and subintimal injuries are linked to poor catheter placement and can be caused by rapid contrast injection. Due to these potential complications, arteriography is not recommended for serial examinations. Recent concerns regarding radiation exposure, particularly in young and pregnant patients, also drive the tendency toward other less-invasive modalities.

CONTRAINDICATIONS

Contrast allergy is a relative contraindication. In general, premedication with steroids and the selection of a different contrast material significantly decrease the risk for severe allergic reaction. Poor renal function is also a relative contraindication.

COMPUTED TOMOGRAPHY ANGIOGRAPHY

Computed tomographic angiography (CTA) has multiple vascular applications. Essentially any arterial bed that can be studied with arteriography, including the pulmonary arteries, can be examined with CTA. Advances in multidetector technologies and imaging processing have made these examinations very cost-effective.

EQUIPMENT

CT scanners have evolved continuously since their introduction in 1979. The first multidetector (four-slice) scanner was used in 1998. Currently,

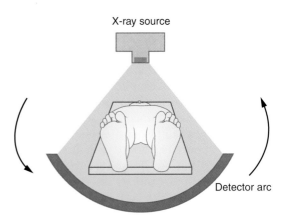

FIGURE 36-4 Diagram showing a typical computed tomographic detector setup. An x-ray source projects x-rays through the body as it rotates. The x-ray beam creates a "fan beam," thereby increasing the efficiency for capturing imaging information.

state-of-the-art scanners use a fan-shaped x-ray beam and an arc of x-ray detectors opposite the beam, both mounted on a ring surrounding the patient (Figure 36-4). This rotates to encompass a 360-degree circle around the patient. Rotation times are now shorter than half a second. Fast table speeds and thin slice width allow submillimeter (isotropic) resolution.

CT was originally performed as a "step-and-shoot" approach: one image was obtained during a 360-degree rotation of the detector, and then the patient table moved to the next position for the next image acquisition. The current approach is to use helical or spiral imaging (Figure 36-5). Rather than sequentially acquiring data at fixed distances, these devices continuously acquire data as the patient is moved at a constant rate through the scanner. The addition of multiple detectors, currently 16 and often 64 or more, permits coverage of larger distances with each rotation of the detector (Figure 36-6). For example, if a 64-detector array scans over a 40-mm-long segment, each rotation of the gantry can cover a slice thickness of 40 mm with an effective slice thickness less than 1 mm.

PHYSICAL PRINCIPLES

The x-ray detectors are used to measure the attenuated x-ray beam after it has passed through the patient. These data are digitally manipulated to calculate a cross-sectional image. Images are displayed with a gray scale of -1000 Hounsfield units (air) to over 1000 Hounsfield units (bone),

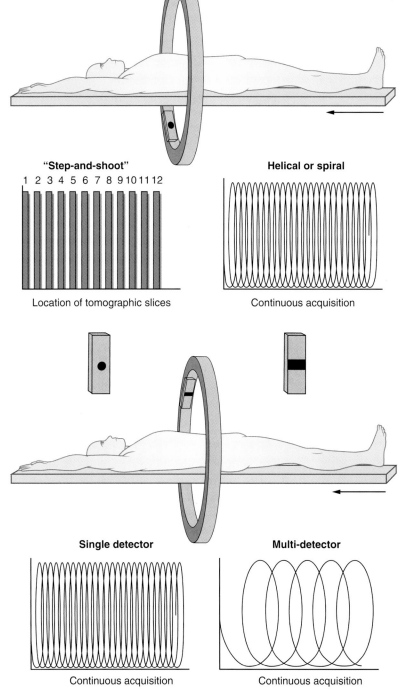

"Step-and-shoot"
1 2 3 4 5 6 7 8 9 10 11 12

Location of tomographic slices

Helical or spiral

Continuous acquisition

FIGURE 36-5 Diagram showing the difference between "step-and-shoot" computed tomographic imaging *(left)* and spiral imaging *(right).* With step and shoot, the table with the patient on it is moved by a given increment, a picture is taken, and the table is moved again by the same increment before another picture is taken. This is repeated as often as needed to cover the region of interest. With spiral imaging, the table is fed in a continuous fashion during the rotation of the x-ray tube and detectors. This covers the region of interest more rapidly than the step-and-shoot approach.

Single detector

Continuous acquisition

Multi-detector

Continuous acquisition

FIGURE 36-6 Diagram showing the difference between single-detector *(left)* and multiple-detector *(right)* computed tomographic scanners. Since the detector array is wider on the right, it takes a lower number of rotations to cover the region of interest. Acquisition times are dramatically shortened.

on a television monitor, normally with a format of 512 × 512 pixels.

TECHNIQUE

In CTA, the x-ray data are continuously acquired during a single breath hold while the patient is moved through the x-ray beam of the gantry. Iodinated contrast is simultaneously injected intravenously to enhance vessels at a rate of 3 to 5 mL/sec depending on the application. The acquired data are reconstructed to produce multiple slices of preselected thicknesses. The data are then reconstructed and displayed as axial slices or rendered in a 3D format. A display of vascular structures can be achieved when a maximum intensity projection (MIP) algorithm is applied. This projects only the brightest pixel along each ray path. The image data set can also be manipulated and displayed in a format resembling the multiple projections used in conventional angiography or in selected coronal and sagittal planes.

CTA can be used to carefully evaluate the soft tissues. In this, it is superior to angiography. A simple example is the evaluation of abdominal aortic aneurysm. The CT angiogram can depict the extent of thrombus deposition in the aorta, an evaluation that is not possible by arteriography. CT spiral angiograms can record abdominal vessels to the third-order branches from the aorta (Figure 36-7). The limited spatial resolution restricts visualizing smaller arterial branches. Constraints in the amount of contrast that can be injected make it difficult to follow long vessels such as those found in the extremities.

Timing of the arrival of contrast in the target arterial segment is critical. Optimal performance of the 3D formatting programs requires a maximal amount of contrast agent in the artery segment while minimizing venous opacification. Selecting the appropriate timing interval is key

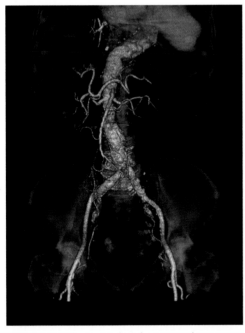

FIGURE 36-7 Volume-rendered computed tomographic angiogram with partial visualization of the bones. This type of display is useful since it can be reoriented in three-dimensional space in order to visualize vessels of interest on different projections.

to optimizing image quality. A simple strategy follows: a small bolus of contrast is administered first. Images are taken and used to time the appearance of contrast material in the vessels of interest. The time from injection to visualization of contrast on the CT image is used to protocol the study for optimal data acquisition. For imaging of the pulmonary arteries, the quality is limited by patient motion, and acquisition must take place during a breath hold, typically 15 to 20 seconds. Bolus-tracking algorithms are also available on modern CT scanners that automatically detect the arrival of contrast material in the target vessel and initiate scanning through the area of interest.

With spiral CTA, the operator selects the speed of acquisition or the effective rate at which the patient is moved through the gantry. Final slice thickness and the distance between slices depend on these parameters but can be further modified by the operator at the time of image reconstruction.

ACCURACY AND REPRODUCIBILITY

CT pulmonary angiography has essentially replaced pulmonary arteriography. The validation studies have mostly been done on the basis of outcomes study. The basic outcome used in pulmonary embolism is the absence of recurrent thromboembolic disease over a 3-month period if the study is called negative.

The overall accuracy of the technique for the detection and grading of arterial stenoses is competitive with arteriography in all arterial beds. The basic limitations for CTA are characterizing lesions in arterial segments with diameters smaller than 1 mm, difficulty visualizing the smaller visceral branches, and heavy arterial calcification that can hinder visualization of luminal patency.

COMPLICATIONS

Complications of CT angiography include contrast allergy. Serious contrast reactions requiring treatment occur in approximately 1 to 2 per 1000 examinations with high-osmolar contrast materials and 1 to 2 per 10,000 with low-osmolar contrast materials. The actual mortality rate is very low, by some estimates 1 per 40,000 and by others less than 1 per 170,000 contrast administrations.[1]

Additional complications include local problems due to incorrect placement of intravenous catheters and the possibility of contrast extravasation. Since large volumes of intravenous contrast may be administered, infiltration of the soft tissues may occur at the site of injection. This may result in significant pain, swelling, and loss of local soft tissues.[2]

CONTRAINDICATIONS

Poor renal function and a history of contrast allergy are relative contraindications as discussed in the section on arteriography. The rate of contrast reactions is slightly greater than those experienced during intra-arterial injections. In addition, imaging is complicated by the fact that the patient can occasionally experience claustrophobia.

As with conventional angiography, there is considerable concern regarding potential radiation-related cancer risk. Risk projection models estimate approximately 29,000 future cancers related to CT scans performed in the United States in 2007.[3,4] In general, CTA is associated with greater radiation dose than conventional nonangiographic CT studies.

MAGNETIC RESONANCE ANGIOGRAPHY

The truly noninvasive modality of MRA operates on a completely different physical principle than radiography. It competes with CTA for evaluating the aorta and its major branches. In the carotid arteries and the runoff arteries of the legs, it has shown similar and sometimes superior accuracy to other noninvasive tests such as Doppler sonography. In certain circumstances it might even be superior to arteriography for evaluating the runoff arteries of the foot.

There are three forms of MRA. The first type is unenhanced, that is, no contrast material is administered, and flowing blood itself proves an intrinsic contrast medium when specific pulse sequences are applied. The second type is enhanced. Contrast media consisting of gadolinium complexes is injected, and studies resembling those possible with CTA are obtained. Cost and availability are current major limitations that limit the widespread application of MRA. Limitations in the current technology limit its use for evaluating moving structures (pulmonary vessels) and for looking at fine detail (vessels <1 mm in diameter).

A third type of MRA is referred to as the phase-sensitive imaging. The phase-sensitive methods rely on the acquisition of paired images, each with a different sensitivity to flowing blood. These images are acquired in either two or three directions and amalgamated into a final 3D image. It is limited to relatively small volumes and often used for imaging the intracerebral arteries.

EQUIPMENT AND PRINCIPLES

For imaging, the patient is placed into a large-bore magnet operating at magnetic field strengths typically at or above 1.5 tesla. This causes the majority of tissue protons to align with the magnetic field. Additional coils generate radio frequency (RF) signals and magnetic field gradients. RF pulses are applied to the volume of tissue to be imaged and can select portions of the body through a combination of RF pulse shape and synchronous application of a magnetic field gradient. These pulses disturb the alignment of the protons as they are oriented in the static magnetic field. As the protons realign to their resting state in the magnet, they emit characteristic RF energy themselves, forming the basis of the MR image.

Signal intensity of various tissues on an MR image can be manipulated by the various pulse sequences used. It is first dependent on the proton density of the tissue interrogated. The relaxation and release of energy as protons in the tissues return to their original orientation is referred to as spin-lattice relaxation, or T1. Spin-spin relaxation, or T2 effects, cause loss of signal by dephasing of protons. Different tissues, including blood, have different combinations of T1 and T2 characteristics accounting for their different appearance on MR images.

Imaging of flowing blood with unenhanced MRA is performed mostly with rapid gradient echo sequences. It is called time-of-flight imaging when the signal of blood flowing in one direction is displayed. Gradient echo sequences use RF pulses of very short duration that are applied very rapidly to the same slice location. Static protons in the selected slice quickly become saturated. As flowing blood enters the imaging slice, these fresh protons give off a strong signal (Figure 36-8). Since blood is continually replaced by the inflow of unsaturated protons, it appears bright (Figure 36-9). This effect is known as flow-related enhancement and is the basis of time-of-flight MRA (TOF MRA). Areas of signal loss occur when slow-moving blood becomes saturated or when blood flow is no longer perpendicular to

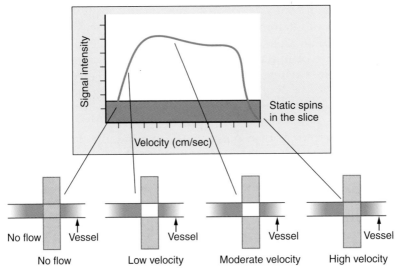

FIGURE 36-8 Time-of-flight principle. Static or slowly moving blood loses signal because of the repeated application of radiofrequency energy in the magnet *(bottom)*. Blood moving at mild to moderate velocities transits through the imaging slice before it can absorb too much energy and is able to generate magnetic resonance (MR) signals *(top left and center)*. Finally, blood moving very quickly through the imaging plane is not exposed to sufficient radiofrequency energy to generate an MR signal, or the blood has moved outside of the slice when it generates an MR signal *(top right)*.

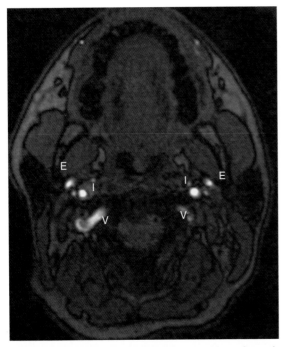

FIGURE 36-9 This time-of-flight acquisition through the neck emphasizes white structures representing the internal carotid *(I)*, external carotid *(E)*, and vertebral *(V)* arteries. The right vertebral artery is dominant (left of image) and has stronger flow signals than the left vertebral artery. Note that a special pulse sequence is used to apply radiofrequency energy to venous blood that is about to flow into the imaging plane. This saturates the blood in the vein so that it cannot generate a magnetic resonance signal.

the plane of the slice and can mimic a stenotic lesion or occlusion.

Gradient-refocused sequences, when applied to large volumes, saturate the signal from tissues within these large volumes. When a contrast material with paramagnetic characteristics enters this volume, it will cause a local increase in signal intensity. This is the basic principle of contrast-enhanced MRA (CE-MRA). The basic limitation of this approach is the time and duration when the contrast material is present in sufficient concentration to cause this peak in signal. Typically, as with CTA, the transit of contrast in the artery lasts approximately 10 to 20 seconds. The imaging sequence must therefore be tailored to image the whole volume in this time interval. This requires use of techniques that decrease the spatial resolution of the image. Ultimately, the technique can incorporate short repeated acquisition times and create the appearance of a contrast arteriogram. Newer contrast agents allow for increased circulation time and the ability to scan for longer periods due to prolonged vascular enhancement.

TECHNIQUE

There is no specific preparation required. The acquisition of the selected MR angiogram normally requires the delineation of the specific vascular bed that is to be studied. This is normally achieved by an initial series of images referred

2-D TOF MRA

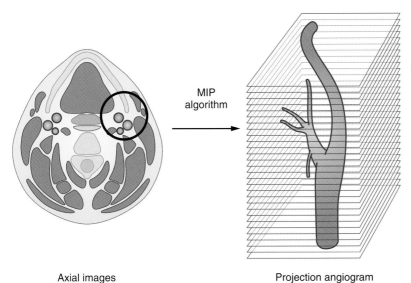

MIP
algorithm

Axial images   Projection angiogram

FIGURE 36-10 This figure demonstrates the process for creating a time-of-flight image. Multiple small slices are acquired (typically 1 mm in thickness or slightly more) and are projected so that the maximal-intensity pixel is represented in one selected projection. This is called a maximum intensity projection (MIP) algorithm.

to as the localizer sequence. The MR angiogram sequence of choice is then applied in the selected anatomic region.

Image display can be in any of the selected imaging planes (i.e., transverse, coronal, sagittal, or any combined oblique orientation). The algorithm most often used is the MIP algorithm, applicable to both time-of-flight (Figure 36-10) and Gadolinium contrast imaging. The target region must be located near the center of the magnet, thereby requiring the near-complete introduction of the patient into the bore of the magnet (Figure 36-11, *A*). The addition of a moving table makes it possible to image the lower extremity arteries during the injection of a bolus of gadolinium contrast (Figure 36-11, *B*).

ACCURACY AND REPRODUCIBILITY

Accuracy is dependent on the technique in use. TOF MRA is well recognized as being reliable in the carotid arteries and in selective portions of the lower extremities. As a gradient-refocused technique, it can be used to evaluate the major veins in the abdomen and pelvis.

CE-MRA has high accuracies in the thorax for evaluating dissections and is a very competitive modality for the evaluation of most arterial beds. A major limitation with CE-MRA is the time needed to cover large volumes and the associated decrease in spatial resolution. For example, MRA offers limited resolution of the visceral branches of the superior mesenteric arteries.

CONTRAINDICATIONS

Claustrophobia and the presence of biomaterials likely to be affected by magnetic fields are the two major contraindications. Most patients with pacemakers and defibrillators cannot be imaged since the magnetic field will disable the device. Patients that need close monitoring of their vital signs can only be placed in the magnet with great care.

Poor renal function is another contraindication. Patients with an estimated GFR of less than 30 mL/min per 1.73 m^2 are at high risk for developing nephrogenic systemic fibrosis (NSF), a diffuse multisystem disease with high mortality rates.[5] The risk for NSF for patients with estimated GFRs of 30 to 60 mL/min per 1.73 m^2 is much lower but still needs to be considered.

COMPLICATIONS

Possible complications of MR imaging are associated with the large magnetic fields in use. The sound generated by the rapidly switching field gradients can cause auditory discomfort and may require earplugs or headphones. Surgical devices, such as intracerebral aneurysm clips, can move and cause local vessel injury. Small radiopaque metallic bodies, especially if lodged close to the eyes, can cause local heating and possibly move and disrupt the surrounding soft tissues. Indwelling vascular stents and metallic implants produce imaging artifacts that render the study nondiagnostic. Overestimation of arterial stenosis, a common pitfall, occurs due

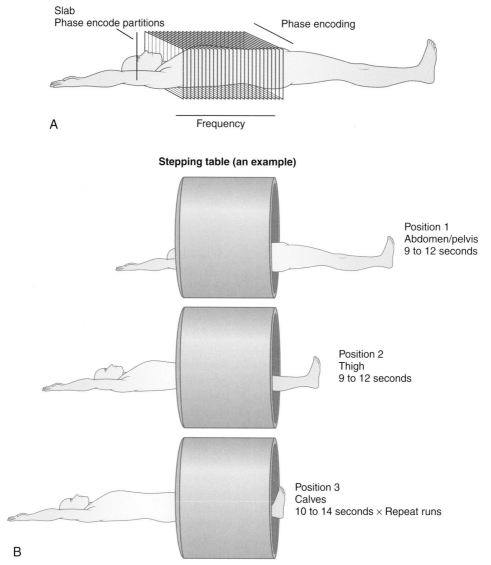

FIGURE 36-11 A, Example of the encoding scheme used for image acquisition. The size of the region and its thickness determine the acquisition time. **B,** During bolus chasing, the patient is moved into the magnet so that imaging takes place when the concentration of gadolinium is highest in the region being imaged.

to intravoxel dephasing or turbulent flow with disruption of the flow stream. Vascular calcifications are not visualized on conventional MR sequences.

OVERVIEW AND CORRELATIVE FINDINGS

CEREBROVASCULAR DISEASE[6-11]

Conventional arteriography is the gold standard for the evaluation of the carotid bifurcation and the intracerebral arteries. It is occasionally done before carotid endarterectomy and is part of the procedure for carotid stent placement.

Spiral CT has a diagnostic accuracy sufficiently high to be considered an effective screening test for the evaluation of carotid bifurcation disease and the detection of intracerebral aneurysms. Imaging reformats, including 3D renditions of the carotid bifurcation, permit consistent grading of stenosis severity (Figure 36-12). As compared to arteriography, there is a loss in spatial resolution that might affect the characterization of band-like lesions

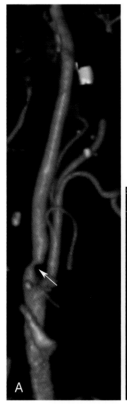

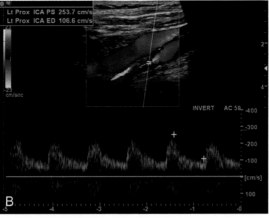

Lt Prox ICA PS 253.7 cm/s
Lt Prox ICA ED 106.6 cm/s

INVERT   AC 59

FIGURE 36-12 A, Volume rendering of a carotid computed tomographic angiogram. The stenotic lesion in the right internal carotid artery is easily visualized *(arrow).* **B,** Corresponding Doppler ultrasound shows a significant stenosis with a peak systolic velocity of 254 cm/sec.

of fibromuscular dysplasia. The aortic arch is easily accessible to this technique, and the origin of the great arteries can be readily evaluated. The source images as well as the projection angiogram are reviewed in all cases before making a diagnosis. This examination can be completed in 5 minutes.

MRA has high diagnostic accuracy and is considered an effective screening test for detecting the presence of significant carotid lesions. This applies mostly to time-of-flight techniques, with the observation that CE-MRA is even more accurate. The spatial resolution is lower than for CTA. A stenotic lesion seen on 2-D time-of-flight images can either cause luminal narrowing (Figure 36-13) or the appearance of a zone of signal loss, or flow gap, that can used to infer the presence of a significant (>50%) stenosis. The 3D time-of-flight sequences are less sensitive to the artifacts generated by flowing blood and can depict a high-grade stenosis as an area of focal narrowing. These images are, however, more susceptible to artifacts generated by patient motion. The source images as well as the projection angiogram are reviewed in all cases before making a diagnosis.

CE-MRA can be used to evaluate the aortic arch and include the carotid arteries. The intracerebral branches can be evaluated by either time-of-flight or contrast-enhanced techniques, but the phase-contrast approach is typically used, especially if contrast cannot be given. An examination of the carotid arteries by itself takes 10 to 15 minutes for one full set of sequences. It is, however, done in most instances as part of a more complete evaluation of the brain, thereby accounting for a longer examination time.

The accuracy of color Doppler imaging in combination with pulsed Doppler sonography is approximately 90%. There are some limitations to the use of sonography in the carotid arteries. The first is the presence of calcifications of 1 cm or more in length that affect the accuracy of sonography and the measurement of accurate Doppler velocities. Visualization of left common carotid or right brachiocephalic origin stenoses is not always possible. This pitfall may be circumvented when the stenosis is severe enough to cause a pressure drop that affects the waveform in the downstream carotid artery. The combination of a delayed upstroke—tardus—and low-amplitude—parvus—signal can detect the more

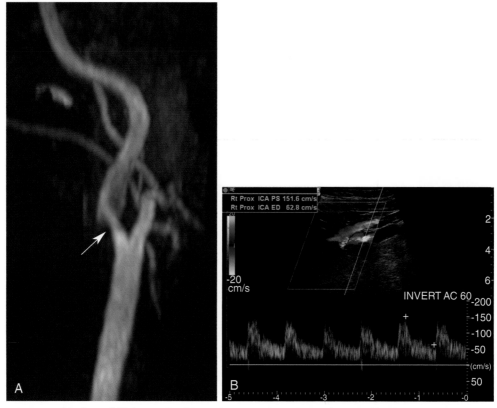

FIGURE 36-13 **A,** This time-of-flight maximal intensity projection image of a carotid bifurcation shows an apparent luminal narrowing in the proximal internal carotid artery *(arrow)*. **B,** The corresponding Doppler ultrasound confirms the presence of a lesion with peak systolic velocity of 152 cm/sec, close to the 50% cut-point of 125 cm/sec.

severe stenoses. Luckily, such a scenario is not common. Tandem lesions in the intracerebral portion of the carotid artery can easily be missed with sonography. The importance of these lesions in patients undergoing carotid endarterectomy is, fortunately, not critical when patient outcome is evaluated following surgery. Neartotal occlusions may be difficult to detect and to differentiate from total occlusions. All imaging techniques perform surprisingly well at this task.

PERIPHERAL ARTERIAL DISEASE[12]

Arteriography is principally used as a road map to guide surgical or endovascular interventions. Short focal lesions that are few in number are suitable for angioplasty and possible stent placement. More complex multilevel disease will likely benefit from bypass surgery that requires an accurate depiction of the extent of arterial disease and a clear-cut identification of the level below which arterial lesions are no longer significant. In diabetics, for example, the pedal arch must often be visualized since the tibioperoneal branches are almost always involved by disease. Arteriography is also used to identify stenotic lesions developing in native arteries, bypass grafts, and stents after endovascular interventions.

CTA has yet to replace arteriography. Spiral CTA can serve as a surgical road map, but the spatial resolution is much less than that of arteriography. A normal or near-normal examination can be used to exclude significant disease. CTA is limited when multilevel and complex lesions cause nonvisualization of segments because of the differences in the timing and arrival of contrast material. However, CTA is especially valuable for evaluating the pelvic arteries. Visualization of the soft tissues surrounding the major arteries to the leg can also help identify infections, fluid collections, and various perivascular masses that may arise following surgery. It is very useful for evaluating aneurysm disease, determining the degree of luminal thrombus, and evaluating perianeurysmal fluid. CTA is also commonly used in the setting of trauma, allowing rapid identification of significant vascular injury in addition to relevant

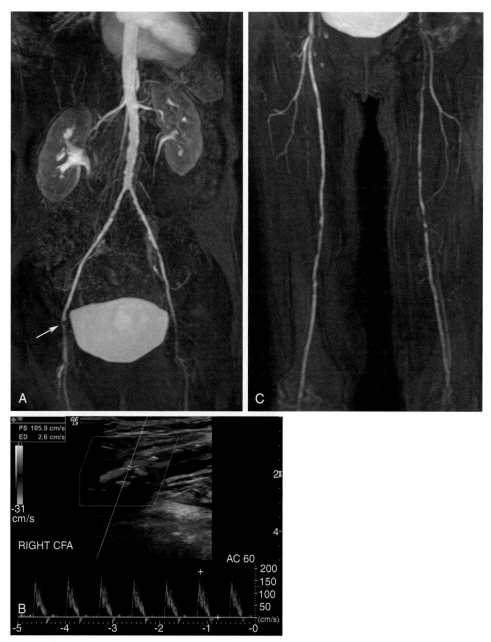

FIGURE 36-14 A, This gadolinium magnetic resonance angiographic (MRA) image is the first station of a bolus chase runoff. The iliac arteries are well visualized. A moderate stenosis is seen at the origin of the common femoral artery *(arrow).* **B,** The Doppler sampling of the common femoral artery confirms the presence of a lesion with a moderate elevation in velocity (186 cm/sec). **C,** The second station of the bolus chase MRA is shown. This station is focused on the thigh level. Diffuse arterial occlusive changes are observed in both superficial femoral arteries. The third station would demonstrate the calf arteries (not shown).

soft tissue findings of visceral organ injuries and fractures.

MRA has shown superiority to arteriography for evaluating the distal runoff arteries of the calf and foot. This observation was made for time-of-flight MRA of the calf, where it is often difficult for contrast material to reach the distal arteries when

there is multilevel disease. Imaging of the proximal arteries in the thigh and pelvis is very reliable when the injection of gadolinium compounds is coupled to the use of moving tables (Figure 36-14). Separate imaging of the calf arteries using rapid imaging sequences can create image sets that resemble lower extremity arteriograms

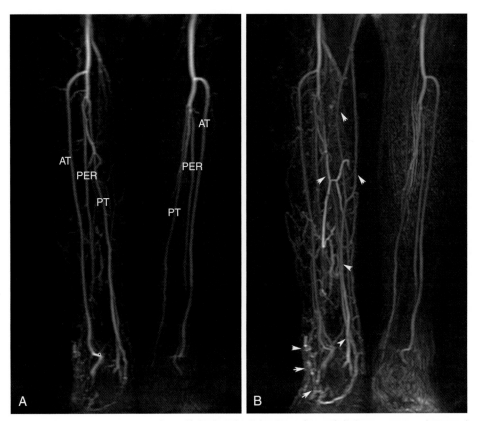

FIGURE 36-15 **A,** Dynamic acquisition at the calf during the injection of a gadolinium compound. Note the detail of the anterior tibial (AT), posterior tibial (PT), and peroneal (PER) arteries. **B,** Early filling of the superficial veins *(arrowheads)* is seen in this patient with reactive cellulitis in the distal calf and foot.

(Figure 36-15). Evaluation of bypass grafts is limited since surgical clips create artifacts that mimic graft stenoses.

Color Doppler imaging is the gold standard examination for graft surveillance. A severely compromised graft will typically have a peak systolic velocity of 45 cm/sec or below. This simple velocity criterion is not sensitive for detecting early graft dysfunction since one-half to two-thirds of all grafts with stenoses will be missed. Typical examinations need to include full-length scans of the bypass graft with Doppler waveform analysis at all sites of suspected stenoses. Elevations in velocities causing more than a doubling of the peak systolic velocity indicate stenoses of greater than 50% diameter narrowing. Interventions are likely when velocity ratios reach 4 or more.

Evaluation of native peripheral arterial lesions is most reliable in the femoropopliteal segments. The accuracy of Doppler sonography is close to 90%. The technique is especially well suited for the detection of occluded arterial segments, where the accuracy is closer to 95%. Doppler

sonography can help triage patients for endovascular interventions when lesions are solitary and focal and for bypass surgery for long occlusions and multilevel disease. Sonographic evaluation of the iliac arteries is slightly less reliable. The careful interrogation of the runoff vessel, although feasible, is less accurate, especially for the peroneal artery, although improved color sensitivity on newer Doppler units and the addition of ultrasound contrast agents can improve the quality of this application.

RENOVASCULAR DISEASE[13-15]

Arteriography has been used as a screening test for renal artery stenoses since it has the highest accuracy for estimating stenosis severity and has high reliability for identifying multiple renal arteries. It is best suited for identifying peripherally located lesions in the intrarenal arterial branches and involvement by fibromuscular disease.

CTA is highly reliable for the evaluation of proximal renal artery disease. It can image the proximal renal branches in an efficient fashion and also identify, in most cases, the presence of fibromuscular dysplasia. It has high accuracy in evaluating accessory renal arteries. It can also image the surrounding soft tissues and potentially detect the rare case of adrenal pheochromocytoma that can cause hypertension.

MRA is highly accurate for the detection of renal artery stenoses (Figure 36-16). Accuracies of higher than 90% may apply to very proximal stenoses and cases where solitary renal arteries are present. The accuracy is highest with the use of gadolinium contrast agents. The technique is limited in the evaluation of renal arteries after stent placement.[16] An important pitfall of MRA is overestimation of stenosis.

Doppler sonography for the detection and grading of renal artery stenoses requires a dedicated sonographer and a high level of expertise. The most reliable and technically demanding approach is direct interrogation of the proximal renal arteries as they originate from the aorta. The accuracy of the technique is likely near 90% in experienced laboratories. Detection of accessory renal branches remains a limitation of the study, although some authors argue that stenoses in these small branches are not clinically important. The primary velocity criteria are a peak systolic velocity greater than 200 cm/sec in the stenotic segment and a renal-aortic ratio (RAR) of 3.5 or greater. (The RAR is the peak systolic velocity measured in the stenotic segment of the renal artery divided by the peak systolic velocity in the aorta.). The second type of renal artery evaluation looks at the waveforms obtained from the segmental arteries in the renal hilum. A delayed systolic upstroke or low-amplitude/low-resistance waveform is thought to indicate severe proximal renal artery lesions. The technique is very useful for following the results of percutaneous angioplasty and stent placement.

MESENTERIC ARTERIES[17-20]

Arteriography offers the best overall performance for evaluating the mesenteric branches. The evaluation of the mesenteric arteries includes a full visualization of the celiac trunk and its major branches as well as opacification of both the superior and inferior mesenteric arteries. Patients typically have chronic mesenteric ischemia if two of these three arteries are occluded or involved by high-grade stenoses. Patients presenting with acute symptoms of abdominal pain rarely have an acute occlusion of the proximal artery but will likely have an acute embolus lodged in the more peripheral branches of the superior mesenteric artery. The presence of nonocclusive mesenteric ischemia is a diagnosis based on the angiographic appearance of diffuse narrowing of the arterial branches with focal areas of dilatation, causing a beaded appearance. This entity is associated with low cardiac output states and may occur in association with an embolic event and is treated by aggressive catheter-directed pharmacoangiography.

CTA displays the proximal 3 to 6 cm of the mesenteric arteries and the hepatic branches out to the periphery of the liver with great detail. It loses diagnostic accuracy in the subbranches of the mesenteric arteries because of motion and the relatively low contrast volume reaching these distal branches. For this reason, CTA cannot be used to exclude the presence of an embolus or to detect evidence of nonocclusive mesenteric ischemia, although the newer generation of scanners permit visualization of the tertiary branches in most cases. CTA can demonstrate bowel wall thickening, fluid, and pneumatosis, indirect signs of ischemic injury.

MRA is well suited for evaluating the main trunks of the mesenteric branches and the more proximal hepatic and splenic arteries. MRA is subject to long acquisition times, motion artifacts, and artifacts from metallic implants and requires contrast material for optimal visualization of the abdominal branch vessels.

The role of sonography in the mesenteric arteries is mainly for the detection of proximal or origin stenoses and occlusions. Ultrasound is not useful for cases of acute embolization or nonocclusive mesenteric ischemia. Peak systolic velocity cutoff values for defining significant (>60% diameter reduction) stenoses of the mesenteric arteries are 200 cm/sec for the celiac artery and inferior mesenteric artery and 275 cm/sec for the superior mesenteric artery.

PULMONARY ARTERIES

CT pulmonary angiography has essentially replaced catheter angiography for the evaluation of patients with suspected pulmonary embolism (Figure 36-17).

MRA plays a minor role at this time, although it may be used to visualize the proximal pulmonary artery branches.

FIGURE 36-16 **A,** Abdominal magnetic resonance angiogram showing a high-grade stenosis of the right renal artery *(arrow).* The proximal portion of the splenic artery (SA) is not seen because the image plane did not include the abdomen anterior to the aorta. The origins of the superior mesenteric artery and the celiac axis are therefore not visualized. **B,** The intrarenal Doppler tracings show a tardus-parvus appearance consistent with a high-grade proximal renal artery stenosis. **C,** Poststenotic turbulence is identified in the proximal right renal artery with evidence of higher Doppler velocity signals greater than 200 cm/sec *(arrowheads)* on the same tracing.

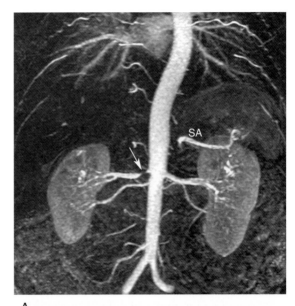

A

AORTIC DISEASE

Angiography has traditionally been used as a road map before aortic aneurysm surgery. The major role of arteriography is to plot the relative location of the aneurysm with respect to the renal arteries and other arterial branches. This affects the surgical approach as well as the extent of the surgery. Angiography is, however, less reliable when it comes to documenting the size and extent of the aneurysm and especially involvement by thrombus. The aortogram is considered the gold standard examination for aortic dissection. It is used to confirm the site of entry of the dissection and the exit point. Proximal tears involving the ascending aorta are treated surgically. Dissections originating below the origin of the left subclavian artery are treated medically, barring complicating circumstances such as retrograde extension of the dissection or involvement of major visceral branches into the false lumen of the dissection.

CTA plays a major role before aortic aneurysm repair. The technique is routinely used to define the presence of aortic aneurysms and to determine their size (Figure 36-18). It is also used to evaluate the relative position of the major arterial branches. The appropriate sizing of aortic endografts is dependent on obtaining accurate measurements of the aortic lumen and measurements of the branch points. CTA is also a gold standard for monitoring the results of endograft placement. CTA can document the presence of acute and chronic aortic dissections. The thrombosed false lumen is easily seen even when conventional aortography fails.

MRA is an acceptable approach to define the presence of aortic aneurysms. It can also visualize dissections and the relative location and involvement of the major visceral branches.

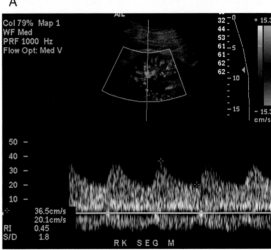

B

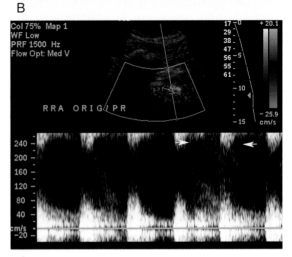

C

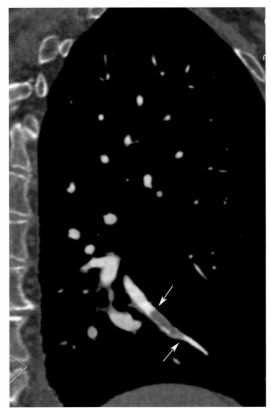

FIGURE 36-17 Filling defect in the anterolateral branch of the lower lobe pulmonary artery *(arrows)* is consistent with an acute pulmonary embolism.

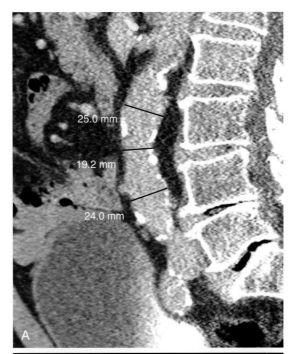

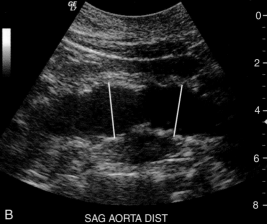

SAG AORTA DIST

FIGURE 36-18 A, Computed tomographic scan reformatted in a sagittal plane shows an ectatic aorta measuring less than the 3.0-cm cut-point for an aneurysm. **B,** Corresponding ultrasound showing the same regions of ectasia.

Sonography is considered to be a gold standard for the evaluation of abdominal aortic aneurysms. The technique shows great reproducibility and can be used to monitor aneurysm growth and plan possible surgical interventions. It is less reliable when it comes to identifying the level of the aneurysm with respect to the main renal artery branches or accessory branches and the actual course of the artery. It can also be reliably used to assess for endograft function, principally by serial estimates of a stabilized or decreasing size of the aneurysm sac. Ultrasound has also been used to evaluate for direct and indirect signs of graft endoleak, although CTA is considered the primary modality for this application.

TRAUMA

Arteriography can detect arterial disruptions, dissections, and even vasospastic changes associated with arterial trauma.

CTA is mostly used to confirm the presence of contrast extravasation following traumatic injuries. A common complication of trauma is arterial pseudoaneurysm. Direct visualization of the feeding arterial branch is occasionally possible.

MRA is ill suited for evaluating this type of patient due to its susceptibility to image degradation by motion and difficulties in patient monitoring.

The use of sonography following trauma is principally directed at determining the presence of arterial occlusion, dissection, and pseudoaneurysms and distinguishing them from hematoma.

If a pseudoaneurysm is identified in the context of an iatrogenic femoral artery injury following catheterization, then transcutaneous injection of thrombin may be therapeutic. If the lesion arose following surgery or following knife or bullet wounds, then surgery should be considered.

VASOSPASTIC DISEASE

Increased vascular reactivity is more likely to affect the smaller muscular arterial branches. Raynaud's phenomenon, typically considered a vasospastic disease, may be mimicked clinically by other pathologic states such as a vasculitis or peripheral embolic phenomena. Arteriography can help differentiate these pathologic entities.

CTA is of limited value in patients with vasospastic diseases. It can help exclude the presence of proximal subclavian or axillary artery aneurysms that can coexist with peripheral embolization.

MRA can be used to exclude more proximal arterial lesions that might mimic vasospastic diseases.

Doppler sonography can be used to map flow velocities and arterial responses to stimuli known to induce vasospasm. This application is very useful for determining the therapeutic efficacy of specific vasodilator therapies.

CONGENITAL DISEASE

Arteriography plays a significant diagnostic and therapeutic role in the management of various congenital arteriovenous malformations (AVMs). Selective arteriography can be used to embolize feeding arteries and minimize blood loss before surgical interventions.

CTA has limited application in making the diagnosis of AVMs. The appearance is nonspecific and can mimic any other hypervascular mass.

CE- MRA can be used to detect AVMs that are not clinically suspected. Time-resolved imaging sequences demonstrate early venous filling with AVMs and arteriovenous fistulas.

Sonography can be used to delineate AVMs and arteriovenous fistulas. Ultrasound can be used to guide percutaneous ablation of superficial AVMs.

VASCULITIS

The diagnosis of vasculitis is normally made by the presence of diffuse arterial narrowing rather than focal lesions. In younger patients with more central lesions, the diagnosis of Takayasu's arteritis should be considered. Specific signs of polyarteritis nodosa, small aneurysms in the kidneys, are seen in 50% of patients with this form of vasculitis. In older patients, Buerger's disease preferentially affects the more peripheral arteries and is related to a long history of smoking.

The diagnosis of vasculitis can be made by combining diffuse luminal narrowing with diffuse arterial wall thickening on CTA. In younger patients, the diagnosis of Takayasu's aortitis should be considered when the wall thickness is greater then a few millimeters. Small vessel vasculitides are more difficult to image.

MRA can also show diffuse wall thickening on pulse sequences that are used to image soft tissues rather than vessels. The wall of the artery can also show contrast enhancement because of the active inflammation.

The presence of vasculitis is normally indicated by the observation of thickening in the artery wall. Such a finding has been mostly described in patients with Takayasu's arteritis. Ultrasound may play a role in identifying wall thickening, luminal narrowing, and associated inflammation in selected vessels, such as the temporal or peripheral arteries.

NEOPLASTIC DISEASES

Arteriography is now rarely used for the diagnosis of either primary or metastatic neoplasms. Its role has migrated to a therapeutic adjunct in cases in which therapeutic embolization might be needed.

CTA is the modality of choice for detecting neoplastic lesions and evaluating their size and relationship to feeding vessels.

MRA is useful for characterizing neoplastic lesions but limited compared to CTA for evaluating the feeding vessels.

Doppler sonography is helpful in the diagnosis and characterization of neoplastic lesions. The observation of tumor vascularity increases suspicion for malignancy. Tumor vascularity is identified as relatively high velocity (>25 cm/sec) flow with a low-impedance flow pattern. Ultrasound is also used to confirm that a structure is a lymph node based on the appearance and typical arterial blood flow into the hilum. Malignant infiltration may replace the normal fatty hilum and alter the normal architecture of lymph nodes.

CONCLUSIONS

Noninvasive imaging approaches such as CTA and MRA complement duplex ultrasound and, when combined in different permutations, can offer diagnostic information equivalent if not superior to what is available with contrast arteriography.

REFERENCES

1. Incidence of adverse effects: *Manual on contrast media version 7*, 2010, American College of Radiology. 17–18. http://www.acr.org/secondarymainmenucategories/quality_safety/contrast_manual.

2. Adverse effects of iodinated contrast media: *Manual on contrast media version 7*, 2010, American College of Radiology. 19–23. http://www.acr.org/secondarymainmenu categories/quality_safety/contrast_manual.

3. Berrington de Gonzalez A, et al: Projected cancer risks from computed tomographic scans performed in the United States in 2007, *Arch Intern Med* 169:2071–2077, 2009.

4. Smith-Bindman R, et al: Radiation dose associated with common computed tomography examinations and the associated lifetime attributable risk of cancer, *Arch Intern Med* 169:2078–2086, 2009.

5. Nephrogenic systemic fibrosis: *Manual on contrast media version 7*, 2010, American College of Radiology. 49–55. http://www.acr.org/secondarymainmenucategories/quality_safety/contrast_manual.

6. Chappell FM, et al: Carotid artery stenosis: Accuracy of noninvasive tests—individual patient data meta-analysis, *Radiology* 251:493–502, 2009.

7. Debrey SM, et al: Diagnostic accuracy of magnetic resonance angiography for internal carotid artery disease: A systematic review and meta-analysis, *Stroke* 39:2237–2248, 2008.

8. Jahromi AS, et al: Sensitivity and specificity of color duplex ultrasound measurement in the estimation of internal carotid artery stenosis: A systematic review and meta-analysis, *J Vasc Surg* 41:962–972, 2005.

9. Koelemay MJW, et al: Systematic review of computed tomographic angiography for assessment of carotid artery disease, *Stroke* 35:2306–2312, 2004.

10. Nederkoorn PJ, van der Graaf Y, Hunink MGM: Duplex ultrasound and magnetic resonance angiography compared with digital subtraction angiography in carotid artery stenosis: A systematic review, *Stroke* 34:1324–1332, 2003.

11. Provenzale JM, Sarikaya B: Comparison of test performance characteristics of MRI, MR angiography, and CT angiography in the diagnosis of carotid and vertebral artery dissection: A review of the medical literature, *AJR Am J Roentgenol* 193:1167–1174, 2009.

12. Collins R, et al: A systematic review of duplex ultrasound, magnetic resonance angiography and computed tomography angiography for the diagnosis and assessment of symptomatic, lower limb peripheral arterial disease, *Health Technol Assess* 11:iii-iv, xi-xiii, 1–184, 2007.

13. Schoenberg SO, et al: Renal MR angiography: Current debates and developments in imaging of renal artery stenosis, *Semin Ultrasound CT MR* 24:255–267, 2003.

14. Tan KT, et al: Magnetic resonance angiography for the diagnosis of renal artery stenosis: A meta-analysis, *Clin Radiol* 57:617–624, 2002.

15. Vasbinder GB, et al: Diagnostic tests for renal artery stenosis in patients suspected of having renovascular hypertension: A meta-analysis, *Ann Intern Med* 135:401–411, 2001.

16. Spuentrup E, et al: Metallic renal artery MR imaging stent: Artifact-free lumen visualization with projection and standard renal MR angiography, *Radiology* 227:897–902, 2003.

17. Armstrong PA: Visceral duplex scanning: Evaluation before and after artery intervention for chronic mesenteric ischemia, *Perspect Vasc Surg Endovasc Ther* 19:386–392, 2007.

18. Aschoff AJ, et al: Evaluation of acute mesenteric ischemia: Accuracy of biphasic mesenteric multi-detector CT angiography, *Abdom Imaging* 34:345–357, 2009.

19. Meaney JF, et al: Gadolinium-enhanced MR angiography of visceral arteries in patients with suspected chronic mesenteric ischemia, *J Magn Reson Imaging* 7:171–176, 1997.

20. Moriwaki Y, et al: Usefulness of color Doppler ultrasonography (CDUS) and three-dimensional spiral computed tomographic angiography (3D-CT) for diagnosis of unruptured abdominal visceral aneurysm, *Hepatogastroenterology* 49:1728–1730, 2002.

ACCREDITATION AND THE VASCULAR LABORATORY

37

SANDRA KATANICK, RN, RVT, FSVU, CAE

The Intersocietal Commission for the Accreditation of Vascular Laboratories (ICAVL) has been providing voluntary accreditation for noninvasive vascular laboratories since 1991. The ICAVL was conceived during the 1989 American Institute of Ultrasound in Medicine annual conference by several visionaries in the field, including Christopher Merritt, MD; Brian Thiele, MD; D. Eugene Strandness, MD; and Anne Jones, RN, BSN, RDMS, RVT, FSVU. They realized that a multispecialty effort to standardize the field was needed because of the rapid growth of noninvasive vascular imaging and the fact that it was being performed by multiple specialties with no defined standards for training and experience, examination performance, or interpretation. This chapter will address the ICAVL history and current process for laboratory accreditation.

HISTORY AND ORGANIZATIONAL STRUCTURE

The mission of ICAVL in 1989 was to develop a program that would ensure high-quality patient care by providing a mechanism of peer review that would encourage and recognize the provision of quality noninvasive vascular diagnostic testing regardless of setting (i.e., hospital, office, clinic) or specialty. In order to do this, it was necessary to develop and maintain a process of accreditation. This consisted of the establishment of requirements for accreditation and a mechanism for the peer-review evaluation of applicant laboratories to verify that they were compliant with these accreditation requirements. The program was designed to be educational in nature, as well as to provide a mechanism for recognition of those laboratories providing quality diagnostic testing.

Following the initial meeting in 1989 with two representatives each from the American Institute of Ultrasound in Medicine, the Society for Vascular Surgery, and the Society for Vascular Ultrasound, all other professional societies with an interest in noninvasive vascular testing were invited to appoint two representatives to this new organization and share in the initial funding and commitment necessary to develop a comprehensive accreditation program for vascular laboratories. The other founding sponsoring organizations included the American Academy of Neurology / the American Society of Neuroimaging, the American College of Radiology, the International Society for Cardiovascular Surgery (North American chapter), the Society of Vascular Medicine and Biology, and the Society of Diagnostic Medical Sonographers. The initial work proposed standards for noninvasive vascular testing that encompassed the following: (1) requirements for medical and technical personnel experience, including training and a definition of their duties; (2) appropriate indications for physiologic testing and ultrasound imaging; (3) well-defined testing protocols such as acquisition techniques, including views and measurements; (4) requirements for reporting and record keeping; and (5) processes for ongoing quality assurance. Once the standards were composed, the board of directors developed an application process that could adequately assess a laboratory's compliance with all of these standards.

In 1991, 10 laboratories were selected to pilot the application for accreditation and assist the ICAVL in assessing the adequacy of the application designed to evaluate the actual quality of the laboratory. After several edits, the final ICAVL *Essentials and Standards* and application package were released in late 1991.

In 1993 and 1995, several sponsoring organizations were added to provide additional expertise and perspective to the accreditation program. These organizations were the American College of Cardiology, the Joint Section on Cerebrovascular Surgery/American Association of Neurological Surgeons and Congress of Neurological Surgeons, the Society of Interventional Radiology, and the Society of Radiologists in Ultrasound.

ICAVL ACCREDITATION AS A MODEL

In 1996, the American Society of Echocardiography explored options for echocardiography accreditation and solicited the ICAVL to develop a program specifically for echocardiography using the ICAVL model as a template. In late 1996, the Intersocietal Commission for the Accreditation of Echocardiography Laboratories (ICAEL) was incorporated as a not-for-profit organization. The American College of Cardiology, the Society of Pediatric Echocardiography, and the Society of Diagnostic Medical Sonography were invited to participate in this program. The ICAEL piloted their application process in mid-1997 and accepted their first applications for accreditation in late 1997. It was then that the IAC (Intersocietal Accreditation Commission) was formed to provide management and oversight for these two intersocietal accreditation programs.

Following the success of the ICAVL and ICAEL, the nuclear medicine community approached the IAC to develop an accreditation program for nuclear cardiology, nuclear medicine, and positron emission tomography (PET). Following the incorporation of nuclear cardiology, the Intersocietal Commission for the Accreditation of Magnetic Resonance Laboratories (ICAMRL) was formed in 2000 for magnetic resonance imaging (MRI) and the Intersocietal Commission for the Accreditation of Computed Tomography Laboratories (ICACTL) was formed in 2006 for computed tomography (CT) examinations. At that time, the various IAC organizations decided that it would be prudent to consider a reorganization so that all accrediting bodies would fall under one umbrella that would continue to support the IAC mission of accreditation: "dedicated to promoting high quality health care by providing a peer review process of laboratory accreditation."

IAC MERGER

On April 1, 2008, following nearly 18 months of reorganization planning, the IAC filed Articles of Merger in the State of Maryland. All IAC members (ICAVL, ICAEL, Intersocietal Commission for the Accreditation of Nuclear Medicine Laboratories [ICANL], ICAMRL, and ICACTL) were officially made divisions of IAC and ceased operations as independently incorporated organizations. The merger provided greater efficiency through unified accounting practices and streamlining of accreditation policies with the organization now functioning under the IAC bylaws and an IAC board of directors. These streamlined business practices enabled the individual accrediting divisions to focus on the important tasks related to recognizing and improving the provision of quality patient care through quality diagnostic imaging, thus allowing the IAC to provide increased value and services to participating laboratories.

Each of the five divisions (ICAVL, ICAEL, ICANL, ICAMRL, and ICACTL) continues to be guided by an individual division board, functions under self-approved policies and procedures, and has a significant degree of autonomy over the ongoing development of its standards, respective to the division's accreditation programs. The sponsoring organizations of each division continue to nominate board members.

Increased participation in the accreditation program has resulted in dramatic growth, as reflected by the IAC combined staff of 40 individuals, along with a volunteer network of 98 board members and hundreds of application reviewers and site visitors.

Benefits of the merger include the creation of a single IAC online accreditation application for all five divisions and the granting of discounts for applications made in multiple modalities. This single application portal streamlines the process for laboratories seeking IAC accreditation in more than one imaging modality.

ICAVL STANDARDS

Currently all IAC division standards are reviewed and revised every 2 years at a minimum, or more frequently if indicated. Over time, the ICAVL has modified its standards and the application process in an effort to better assess the quality of the laboratory and to improve the quality of vascular testing. Laboratories are required to review the standards when revisions are published and are expected to maintain compliance with the most current revisions. In 2010, the ICAVL underwent a significant review and restructuring of the standards document. The current ICAVL *Standards* is now published on the ICAVL website as a single document with seven major parts: part I—organization, and parts II through VII—vascular laboratory testing. There are six specific areas of vascular laboratory testing: extracranial cerebrovascular, intracranial cerebrovascular, peripheral arterial, peripheral venous, visceral vascular, and screening. Each part is divided into nine specific subsections, and laboratories can apply for accreditation for any area(s) of testing that they provide. The *Standards* can be reviewed and downloaded at any time at www.icavl.org.

PART I—ORGANIZATION

The organization standard has six sections: supervision and personnel; support services; physical facilities; examination interpretation, reports, and records; patient safety and confidentiality; and multiple sites and mobile services. Following is a brief summary of each section.

Supervision and Personnel

The section on supervision and personnel includes specific requirements for qualifications, training, and experience for all medical and technical personnel; responsibilities for each staff person; and requirements for ongoing continuing medical education. For physicians, there are four pathways to document training and experience: formal training, informal training, established practice, and physician credential for vascular interpretation. For technologists, all technical directors must have a vascular credential—registered vascular technologist (RVT), registered vascular specialist (RVS), or registered technologist (vascular specialist) (RT[VS])—and each technologist must perform a minimum number of examinations. All staff technologists will require a vascular credential by 2017. If the technical director is not on site full-time, an appropriately credentialed sonographer who is a member of the technical staff must be present in the laboratory in the absence of the technical director and assume the duties of the technical director.

Support Services

Ancillary personnel (e.g., clerical, nursing, transport) necessary for safe and efficient patient care must be provided.

Physical Facilities

Examinations must be performed in a setting that provides for patient and technical staff safety, comfort, and privacy. There must also be

adequate space for interpretation and storage of supplies and records.

Examination Interpretation, Reports, and Records

All studies must be interpreted and reported by the medical director or a member of the medical staff. Requirements for standardized reporting and the timeliness of final reports are outlined. The section also includes a list of specific components that must be included in every report, as well as guidelines for the generation and retention of examination records for all studies performed.

Patient Safety and Confidentiality

Guidelines for patient safety and confidentiality are provided.

Multiple Sites and Mobile Services

Specific requirements for multiple sites and mobile testing, including supervision and staffing, are outlined.

PARTS II TO VII

Parts II to VII represent all of the various vascular testing areas for which laboratories can apply for accreditation: extracranial cerebrovascular, intracranial cerebrovascular, peripheral arterial, peripheral venous, visceral vascular, and screening. Each testing section includes the following: indications, equipment, protocols, techniques, documentation, diagnostic criteria, interpretation, quality assurance, and procedure volumes.

Indications

All testing must be performed for appropriate clinical indications.

Equipment

All equipment used for testing must provide accurate data. Each testing area describes the specific minimum testing equipment required for imaging and nonimaging procedures and specific standards for equipment quality control.

For duplex testing, an ultrasound system with color Doppler capabilities is required. In addition, that system must have transducers operating at the appropriate imaging and Doppler frequency ranges for the type of study performed. The system must also have hard copy recording capabilities and have routine maintenance performed.

Protocols

Each examination performed in the laboratory must have a written protocol that includes the equipment, techniques, anatomic extent, and documentation required.

Techniques

Appropriate techniques must be used for each evaluation to assess for the presence of any abnormalities and to document their severity, location, extent, and, whenever possible, etiology.

Documentation

Each examination performed in the laboratory must provide documentation as required by the protocol that is sufficient to allow proper interpretation.

Diagnostic Criteria

Each examination performed in the laboratory must have a single set of written, validated diagnostic criteria to interpret the presence of disease and to document its severity, location, extent, and, whenever possible, etiology.

Interpretation

Study interpretation must be performed by the medical director or a member of the medical staff using the documented findings and the diagnostic criteria and must indicate the absence or presence of abnormalities in the sites and vessels that were examined.

Quality Assurance

Quality assurance must be performed according to a written policy. The policy must include correlations with other imaging modalities and/or surgical findings. For venous testing, since venography is virtually obsolete, repeat scanning or overreading is an acceptable alternative. In general, each testing section requires a minimum number of correlations in a 3-year period (generally at least 30) with a greater than 70% accuracy. Documentation of the correlations must be maintained, and a minimum of two vascular laboratory quality assurance meetings must be held annually to discuss the results and address any discrepancies or difficult cases. Minutes of these meetings must be maintained.

Procedure Volumes

Volumes must be sufficient to maintain proficiency in examination techniques and interpretation. There are recommendations for minimum volumes for each type of testing. However, these minimum numbers are not absolute requirements, and accreditation can be granted even when the volume is low provided the cases submitted with the application adhere to the standards.

PAYMENT POLICIES

In July 2008, Congress passed and overrode a presidential veto of the Medicare Improvements for Patients and Providers Act (MIPPA). This law now mandates accreditation of facilities that provide advanced diagnostic imaging services by 2012. The Department of Health and Human Services designated three acceptable accreditation bodies in January 2010. Per the language in the legislation, advanced diagnostic imaging services are defined as "diagnostic magnetic resonance imaging, computed tomography, and nuclear medicine (including positron emission tomography)." Other diagnostic imaging services, including x-ray examination, **ultrasound**, and fluoroscopy were excluded from the law. Although many organizations involved in vascular ultrasound provided comments that ultrasound should be included, the bill was passed with the exclusion of ultrasound. Therefore, for the outpatient, Part B Medicare provider, accreditation requirements for cardiovascular and general ultrasound remain voluntary.

There are more than 30 states and jurisdictions that have published local coverage determinations (LCDs) for Medicare Part B; however, their enforcement remains weak or nonexistent and generally only occurs on postpayment audit. In 2003, the Medicare contracting payment system was mandated to undergo reform. Since the inception of Medicare, the Centers for Medicare and Medicaid Services (CMS) has contracted out vital program operational functions (e.g., claims processing, provider and beneficiary services, appeals) to a set of contractors known as Medicare fiscal intermediaries (FIs) and carriers. Under the new Medicare administrative contractor (MAC) contracting authority, CMS has 6 years, between 2005 and 2011, to complete the transition of Medicare fee-for-service (FFS) claims-processing activities from the FIs and carriers to the MACs. With their change to MACs and as consolidation of policies occur, the least restrictive policy can be adopted without the need for public comment. Therefore, some of the existing policies may be removed as the MAC consolidation continues, and others may be edited. A list of payment policies relative to vascular ultrasound can be found at http://www.intersocietal.org/icavl/main/payment_policies.htm. Although efforts are made to keep this list up-to-date, the ICAVL relies on the medical community to keep it informed.

UNITED HEALTHCARE

In 2007, United Healthcare, a major health care insurer, announced a nationwide imaging accreditation program that would require providers of outpatient/private practice MRI, CT, nuclear medicine, and echocardiography services to become accredited by either the IAC or the American College of Radiology by the third quarter of 2008. The date was subsequently extended to 2012. Although general and vascular ultrasound were excluded from this policy, United Healthcare continues to state that those procedures will be considered for future reimbursement policies.

It is clear from the many quality initiatives in imaging, on both the federal and private payer sides, that ultrasound will and should be included in future policies.

CURRENT ICAVL STATISTICS

For the past 9 out of 10 years, the number of ICAVL-accredited vascular laboratories has remained fairly consistent (Figure 37-1). In 2009 and 2010, the number increased, possibly because of the perception that vascular ultrasound was included with the imaging accreditation initiatives introduced by the federal government and United Healthcare. It has also been noted that with the increase in applications received by all IAC divisions, including ICAVL, the quality of the applications and the imaging in general has deteriorated (Figure 37-2). Currently there are 1293 ICAVL-accredited laboratories at 1933 sites, and 46% of those are in hospitals.

BENEFITS OF ACCREDITATION

Although the absolute number of imaging facilities in the United States is unknown, it is evident that only a small percentage apply for accreditation on a voluntary basis. Because the goal of

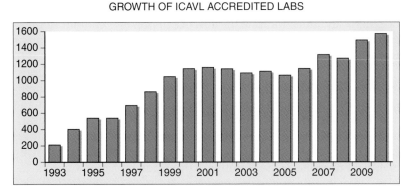

FIGURE 37-1 Number of accredited vascular laboratories enrolled in the Intersocietal Commission for the Accreditation of Vascular Laboratories (ICAVL) program. The number was relatively stable after 2000-2001 and shows recent growth after 2006.

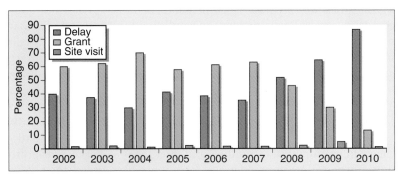

FIGURE 37-2 This graph summarizes the results of the review process for laboratories applying for accreditation. The relative number of candidate laboratories showing deficiencies and therefore a source of deferment (delay) has increased since 2007. ICAVL, Intersocietal Commission for the Accreditation of Vascular Laboratories.

accreditation is to actually improve the quality of imaging through a peer-review process, the benefits remain unknown to those that choose not to apply. For those that have applied, the improvement in the quality of the imaging is particularly evident at reaccreditation.[1] Several studies have been published demonstrating the reduced number of repeat examinations,[2] as well as the benefits of an ongoing quality assurance and correlation program.[3] Accreditation also demonstrates to patients and referring physicians the commitment that the laboratory has demonstrated to provide quality imaging.

REFERENCES

1. Abuhamad AZ, et al: The accreditation of ultrasound practices: impact on compliance with minimum performance guidelines, *J Ultrasound Med* 23:1023–1029, 2004.
2. Brown WO, et al: Reliability of extracranial carotid artery duplex ultrasound scanning: value of vascular laboratory accreditation, *J Vasc Surg* 39(2):366–371, 2004.
3. Stanley DG: The importance of the Intersocietal Commission for the Accreditation of Vascular Laboratories (ICAVL) certification of noninvasive peripheral vascular tests: the Tennessee experience, *J Vasc Ultrasound* 28(2):65–69, 2004.

INDEX

Page numbers followed by "*f*" indicate figures; "*b*" boxes; "*t*" tables.